THIRD EDITION

Traumatic Brain Injury

Rehabilitation, Treatment, and Case Management

EDITED BY MARK J. ASHLEY, Sc.D.

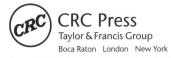

CRC Press
Taylor & Francis Group
Boca Raton   London   New York

CRC Press is an imprint of the
Taylor & Francis Group, an **informa** business

CRC Press
Taylor & Francis Group
6000 Broken Sound Parkway NW, Suite 300
Boca Raton, FL 33487-2742

© 2010 by Taylor and Francis Group, LLC
CRC Press is an imprint of Taylor & Francis Group, an Informa business

No claim to original U.S. Government works

Printed in the United States of America on acid-free paper
10 9 8 7 6 5 4 3 2 1

International Standard Book Number: 978-1-4200-7194-8 (Hardback)

Library of Congress Cataloging-in-Publication Data

Traumatic brain injury : rehabilitation, treatment, and case management / edited by Mark J. Ashley.
-- 3rd ed.
    p. ; cm.
Includes bibliographical references and index.
ISBN 978-1-4200-7194-8 (hardcover : alk. paper)
1. Brain damage--Patients--Rehabilitation. I. Ashley, Mark J. II. Title.
[DNLM: 1. Brain Injuries--rehabilitation. 2. Case Management. WL 354 T77795 2010]

RC387.5T74 2010
617.4'81044--dc22   2009042540

Visit the Taylor & Francis Web site at
http://www.taylorandfrancis.com

and the CRC Press Web site at
http://www.crcpress.com

Contents

Part I Medical Themes

Part II   Allied Health Themes

Part III   Case Management Themes

Preface

The third edition of this text marks a longevity extending over 14 years—a remarkable life for such a text. Many of the chapters in this book have been present since the first edition and have been continuously updated. The second edition saw a number of new chapters added, and the third edition is no different. Since the publication of the first edition, a great deal of change has come to the field that largely affects access to treatment. As the health care marketplace has evolved, however, the needs of people who sustain brain injury have not.

A major question that has arisen during the past several years concerns disease processes initiated by brain injury. Chronic disease processes require continued medical interventions and management. In some diseases, we arrest the disease processes, mitigate the disease progression, or manage the consequences of disease progression. The key point is that we remain medically active, to varying degrees, in the management of the disease. This is less the case following brain injury, yet there is ample evidence of disease progression. Brain injury has been historically viewed as an event in time, resulting in an injury that heals. In actuality, the brain does not heal in the traditional sense. In fact, as the brain attempts to accommodate for structural damage, a combination of residual and new structures must react to the functional demands defined by the environment to determine which skills are to be reacquired and, to the extent possible, must provide the neural capacity to support that function.

Another question rests in whether allied health professionals adequately understand the fundamentals of plasticity in neurorehabilitation and whether these principles are represented in interventions undertaken following brain injury. A central issue is the degree to which rehabilitative medicine understands and respects aspects of neurophysiologic function. Together, these questions address how structures in the brain develop, function, respond to, and ultimately manipulate the organism and environment.

We have yet to define the terminal rehabilitative potential for various injuries to the brain. At the same time that access to treatment following brain injury has been extremely attenuated, calls for evidence-based medicine approaches are increasing. A consistent theme in a number of the chapters herein relates to truncations in treatment duration during the past three decades. The literature shows that decrements in length of stay (LOS) witnessed from the 1970s to 1990 were probably advantageous and related to improved understanding of brain injury rehabilitation, its potential, and its limitations. More recent decrements in LOS, however, have been driven by benefits restrictions that view rehabilitation as something other than medicine. Consequently, at the very time that calls for evidence-based medicine have increased, the population to be studied has become heavily biased by diminished access to treatment, severely restricted treatment intensity, and treatment standards derived by averaging surveys of clinical practice patterns that are significantly influenced by financially motivated payer-based utilization review practices that universally truncate LOS and artificially restrict ultimate recovery of function.

The literature provides strong support for several important variables in the practice of rehabilitative medicine following brain injury. These include intensity, timing, duration, and expertise of treatment. Neural plasticity occurs in response to environmentally induced experiential demand. Treatment intensity and duration speak to the intentional provision of hierarchically designed and delivered experiential demand to guide nearly pluripotent, trophic factor-enriched, residual neural structure plasticity. Of course, plasticity is not solely responsible for recovered function. Metabolic stabilization, unmasking, genetic alteration, and genesis of vascular, glial, and neural structures combine to provide additional substrate by which recovered function is subserved. Traditional rehabilitation therapies provide an essential component to recovered function when they are expertly executed and thus provide the proper experiential demand for neurophysiologic genesis, neural plasticity, cortical reorganization, and network remodeling. The brain responds to all environmental stimuli following injury, and either adaptive or maladaptive plasticity occurs. Thus, rehabilitation should provide greater assurance for adaptive plasticity although, certainly, improper or inexpert execution of rehabilitative interventions can result in maladaptive plasticity.

The push for function, although commendable, can result in maladaptive plasticity. Take rehabilitation following stroke, for example. Functional orientation causes therapists to encourage the compensatory use of an unaffected upper extremity in the presence of a hemiparesis following injury. At this precise time, upregulation of trophic factors is occurring as the brain also identifies available pathways for motor function in the unaffected, contralateral hemisphere. Neurons are chemically primed to take on function, and the environmentally induced experiential demand created by well-intentioned, although poorly informed, therapists is to facilitate functional recovery by encouraging the person to learn to do all things with the single unaffected extremity, with a goal of using the affected extremity ultimately as "an assist." So now, the brain increases cortical representation for the exercised, unaffected, and already well-represented unaffected extremity. Instead, interventions that assist the brain in identification of unmasked, ipsilateral motor pathways in an unaffected hemisphere is more logical and more closely mirrors the cortical reorganization associated with constraint-induced treatment. However, this approach requires substantially greater intensity and duration of treatment and may be slower in achieving functional recovery. Greater intensity and longer treatment duration equate to more money, however. Hence, the dilemma in neurologic rehabilitation in today's health care climate.

New frontiers are emerging as brain injury becomes better recognized as disease causative or accelerative. Although molecular approaches to injury mitigation within the first 48 hours of injury have proved elusive, the search for such strategies in the weeks, months, and years following injury may hold great promise. Combination therapies that consider endocrine, metabolic, mitochondrial, myelin, lipid metabolism, and neurotransmitter systems along with controlled, hierarchically designed and delivered environmentally induced experiential demand (properly instituted traditional rehabilitative therapies) now constitute fresh horizons in medical rehabilitation and disease management following brain injury. Given the opportunity, we are on the verge of new treatment paradigms that view brain injury as causative of disease and rehabilitation as the medicine.

Rehabilitation following brain injury maybe more properly viewed as facilitated adaptive plasticity, cortical reorganization, and network remodeling. By their very nature, accomplishing these requires time and effort, and each is heavily dependent upon both time and effort. Research investment in identification of those interventions that can further either the rate or extent of recovery may result in accelerated rates of recovery and/or further the overall extent of recovery.

Acquisition of function within the central nervous system occurs at a surprisingly rapid rate; however, it is, nonetheless, rate restricted. Clearly, differences exist across injuries with regard to injury severity and resultant disease processes that affect rate and extent of recovery of function. Some injuries are so extensive as to seemingly prevent recovery

of function altogether. Overall, rate restriction is influenced by a large number of metabolic, neurophysiologic, genetic, and exogenous environmental factors, not to mention that
neural structures respond to environmental stimuli and cannot distinguish well between
those stimuli that promote adaptive versus maladaptive plasticity. The challenge is to
understand how to affect positively the rate and extent of angiogenesis, gliogenesis, synaptogenesis, and neurogenesis, as well as to improve overall metabolic function across the
central nervous system after injury. Residual structures that take on extraordinary function following injury experience additional metabolic demands, and the attendant consequences of heightened metabolic activity may be problematic for an already compromised
metabolic milieu. Some of the newer chapters and many of the revised chapters in this
book provide insight into these mechanisms and potential avenues to address beneficial
alteration of these facets of neurophysiologic recovery of function.

Finally, we must consider the extent to which different disease processes exist following
brain injury. Differences in disease processes can be expected for individuals with varying
neuroendocrine disorders, lipid metabolism disorders, injury locations, injury size, serum
extravasation, axonal injury, myelin formation and repair disruption, metabolic stress and
recovery, mitochondriopathy, neurotransmitter production and transport deficiencies,
immune system activation, and disruptions of primary sensory information processing
systems. Development of biomarkers that enable objective of measurement dysfunction may enable more exacted disease treatment and management along the postinjury
time continuum. Targeted interventions across these dimensions may prove beneficial in
achieving heightened function for the person with brain injury.

Editor

Mark J. Ashley, ScD, CCC-SLP, CCM, CBIS, is founder and president/CEO of Centre for Neuro Skills, which has operated postacute brain injury rehabilitation programs since 1980 at facilities in Bakersfield, California; Encino, California; and Irving, Texas. Dr. Ashley serves on the board of directors of the Brain Injury Association of America, is the immediate past chair, and serves on the Chairman's Circle. He also serves on the board of directors of the California Brain Injury Association and is the current Chair. Dr. Ashley founded the Centre for Neuro Skills Clinical Research and Education Foundation, a nonprofit research organization.

Dr. Ashley received his master's degree in speech pathology and a doctorate of science from Southern Illinois University in Carbondale, Illinois. He is an adjunct professor for the University's Department of Communication Disorders and Sciences in the College of Education, specializing in brain injury and cognitive deficits. Dr. Ashley is a licensed speech–language pathologist in California and Texas and is a certified case manager.

Contributors

Sam S. Andrews
Craig Hospital
Englewood, Colorado

Jessica G. Ashley
Centre for Neuro Skills
Bakersfield, California

Mark J. Ashley, ScD, CCC-SLP, CCM, CBIS
Centre for Neuro Skills
Bakersfield, California

Matthew J. Ashley
University of California, Irvine
Irvine, California

Susan M. Ashley, MS, CCC-SLP, CCM, CBIS
Centre for Neuro Skills
Bakersfield, California

Sorin G. Beca, MD
Stark Diabetes Center
University of Texas Medical Branch, Galveston
Galveston, Texas

Juan J. Bermejo, PhD, FAAA
Bakersfield, California

Amy Berryman, OTR, MSHSA
Craig Hospital
Englewood, Colorado

Patti Blau, PhD
Department of Physical Therapy
The University of Texas Southwestern Medical Center
Dallas, Texas

Ronald A. Browning, PhD
Departments of Physiology and Pharmacology
Southern Illinois University School of Medicine
Southern Illinois University
Carbondale, Illinois

Velda L. Bryan, PT, CBIS
Centre for Neuro Skills
Bakersfield, California

Kimberley Buytaert-Hoefen, PhD
Food and Drug Administration
Department of Health and Human Services
Denver, Colorado

Charles D. Callahan, PhD
Memorial Health Systems
Springfield, Illinois

Steven J. Cloud, PhD
University of Southern Mississippi
Hattiesburg, Mississippi

Fofi Constantinidou, PhD, CCC-SLP
Department of Psychology
University of Cyprus
Nicosia, Cyprus

Roberta DePompei, PhD
School of Speech–Language Pathology and Audiology
The University of Akron
Akron, Ohio

Deborah Lynne Doherty
Kentfield, California

William L. E. Dussault, AAL
Dussault Law Group
Seattle, Washington

Michael G. Elliott, MPT, PT, CBIS
Centre for Neuro Skills, Los Angeles
Encino, California

David A. Gelber, MD
Springfield Clinic Neuroscience Institute
Springfield, Illinois

Kenneth A. Gerhart, PT, MS
Craig Hospital
Englewood, Colorado

Fernando Gomez-Pinilla, PhD
University of California, Los Angeles
Los Angeles, California

Wayne A. Gordon, PhD
Department of Rehabilitation Medicine
Mount Sinai School of Medicine
New York, New York

Stephanie L. Hanson, PhD, ABPP(Rp)
College of Public Health and Health
    Professions
University of Florida
Gainesville, Florida

**David W. Harrington, MBA, OTR/L,
CBIST**
Centre for Neuro Skills
Bakersfield, California

Richard E. Helvie, MD
Centre for Neuro Skills
Bakersfield, California

Theresa D. Hernández, PhD
Department of Psychology and
    Neuroscience
University of Colorado
Boulder, Colorado

Kenneth R. Hosack, MS
Craig Hospital
Englewood, Colorado

Brett E. Kemker, PhD
University of Southern Mississippi
Hattiesburg, Mississippi

Thomas R. Kerkhoff, PhD, ABPP(Rp)
College of Public Health and Health
    Professions
University of Florida
Gainesville, Florida

Rose Leal
Centre for Neuro Skills
Bakersfield, California

Robert P. Lehr, Jr., PhD
Emeritus, Department of Anatomy
School of Medicine
Southern Illinois University
Carbondale, Illinois

Paul M. Levisohn, MD
School of Medicine Neuroscience
    Program
and
The Children's Hospital
University of Colorado Denver
Aurora, Colorado

Brent Masel, MD
Transitional Learning Center at Galveston
Galveston, Texas

Zenobia Mehta
Centre for Neuro Skills
Bakersfield, California

Ronald L. Morton, MD, FACS
Bakersfield, California

John R. Muma, PhD
University of Southern Mississippi
Hattiesburg, Mississippi

Dean K. Naritoku, MD
Departments of Neurology and
    Pharmacology
Southern Illinois University School of
    Medicine
Springfield, Illinois

Joe Ninomiya, Jr.
Centre for Neuro Skills
Bakersfield, California

Chris H. Persel
Centre for Neuro Skills
Bakersfield, California

Craig S. Persel, BA
Centre for Neuro Skills
Montreal, Quebec, Canada

Leigh Anne Randa
Seattle Pacific University
Seattle, Washington

Karen Rasavage, OTR
Craig Hospital
Englewood, Colorado

David L. Ripley, MD, MS, CRC
Craig Hospital
and
School of Medicine
University of Colorado

Peter S. Roland, MD
Department of Otolaryngology
University of Texas Southwestern Medical
    Center
Dallas, Texas

Sandeep Sharma, PhD
University of California, Los Angeles
Los Angeles, California

**Penelope S. Suter, OD, FCOVD, FABDA,
FNORA**
Bakersfield, California

Zoë N. Swaine, MS
College of Public Health and Health
    Professions
University of Florida
Gainesville, Florida

Robin D. Thomas, PhD
Department of Psychology
Miami University
Oxford, Ohio

Theodore Tsaousides, PhD
Department of Rehabilitation
    Medicine
Mount Sinai School of Medicine
New York, New York

Janet Siantz Tyler, PhD
Neurologic Disabilities Support
    Project
University of Kansas Medical
    Center
Kansas City, Kansas

Jay M. Uomoto, PhD
Defense Centers of Excellence
    for Psychological Health and
    Traumatic Brain Injury
Silver Spring, Maryland

Randall J. Urban, MD
Department of Internal Medicine
University of Texas Medical
    Branch, Galveston
Galveston, Texas

Jill Stelley Virden, MS, CTRS
Craig Hospital
Englewood, Colorado

Alan Weintraub, MD
Rocky Mountain Regional Brain
    Injury System
Craig Hospital
Englewood, Colorado

Rhonda M. Williams, PhD
School of Medicine
University of Washington
and
VA Puget Sound Health Care
    System
Seattle, Washington

**Jan Wood, CRC, CCM, CDMS, CLCP,
MSCC, RTC**
JMW Associates Life Care Plans
Santa Clarita, California

Part I

Medical Themes

1

Neurologic Examination of the Patient with Traumatic Brain Injury

David A. Gelber and Charles D. Callahan

CONTENTS

1.1 Introduction

The neurologist often has a key role in the evaluation and management of patients with traumatic brain injury (TBI), especially during the emergent and acute phases of care delivery. As rehabilitation commences, the neurologist may be involved as a consultant or may play a more active role overseeing the rehabilitation process, depending on the nature of his or her practice and the degree to which physiatric services are available. The role of the neurologist in the rehabilitation of the patient with TBI includes defining the extent of neurologic damage, reviewing pharmacologic issues as they affect central nervous function, identifying and managing neurologic complications such as posttraumatic seizures, and presenting information in a manner that is of maximal use to allied health professionals, family members, and the patient. This chapter provides a review of the neurologic examination, which will foster effective interaction between the neurologist and other rehabilitation professionals.

The brain and supporting structures are extremely vulnerable to traumatic injury. Patients with TBI are often left with significant physical, cognitive, and behavioral sequelae requiring prolonged hospitalization and the need for postacute rehabilitation programs. In the postacute setting, it is the physician's role to perform an adequate patient evaluation, including conducting a detailed history, and physical and neurologic examination, and, in conjunction with the rest of the rehabilitation team, developing a comprehensive rehabilitation program to address each patient's particular needs.

The extent of brain injury and residual deficits varies from patient to patient, depending upon the nature of the insult and localization of brain injury. Penetrating or open head wounds resulting from skull fracture or gunshot wound, for example, most often cause focal brain injury at the site of impact as a result of contusion, laceration, hemorrhage, or necrosis of underlying brain tissue.[1] Closed head acceleration/deceleration injuries typically cause coup or contrecoup insults to the brain, resulting in polar injuries to the frontal, temporal, and, occasionally, the occipital lobes. Diffuse axonal injury also commonly occurs as a result of shearing of axons within myelin sheaths, leading to injury to the subcortical white matter.[2] Brain structures most vulnerable to this type of injury include the corpus callosum, superior cerebellar peduncles, basal ganglia, and periventricular white matter.[3] In addition to direct traumatic injury, the brain may also be damaged as a result of complications of head injury, including edema, hypoxia, posttraumatic infarction, and hydrocephalus.[4] Apoptosis of neurons and glia can occur at the site or distant from the injury because trauma may affect expression of certain survival promoter and death-inducing proteins.[5,6]

Generally speaking, the severity of brain injury is predictive of functional outcome. Poorer functional outcomes are associated with increased patient age, presence of intracranial hemorrhage, abnormal motor responses, impaired eye movements or pupillary responses, hypotension, hypoxemia, hypercarbia, and increased intracranial pressure.[7,8] With the most severe injuries, patients may have prolonged coma, severe cognitive and behavioral sequelae, and marked motor and sensory deficits, leading to profound functional impairments. At the other end of the spectrum, mild brain injuries may result in the *persistent postconcussion syndrome*, marked by concentration, memory, and behavioral manifestations, as well as headache and vertigo, but without sensory or motor deficits.[9,10]

The neurologic examination is a key element in the evaluation of the patient with traumatic brain injury. The focus of the examination, however, differs depending on the stage of patient recovery. In the acute patient, the neurologic examination serves to localize the site and extent of brain injury, allowing the physician to develop a plan of acute medical and surgical management. In addition, serial neurologic examinations performed during the first few days or weeks following injury provide useful information regarding prognosis for recovery.

The purpose of the neurologic examination in the postacute rehabilitation setting is different from that performed during the acute stages following TBI. The most important aspect of the examination in the postacute setting is to identify the specific physical, neurologic, cognitive, and behavioral deficits that will potentially limit the patient from a functional standpoint. Hemiparesis, for example, may affect a patient's ability to perform independent transfers, ambulate safely, or dress without help. Spasticity may impede nursing care, limit bed mobility, and cause difficulty with wheelchair seating and ambulation. Identifying these deficits and related functional impairments allows the rehabilitation team to set appropriate functional goals and to develop a comprehensive rehabilitation program to address the patient's needs. It is also important for the "rehab" team to be able to identify specific deficits and potential limitations to patients' family members and caregivers, to allow them to adjust to these changes and to make adequate plans for the patient's return to home and reentry into the community.

In the postacute setting, the physician must also be able to distinguish deficits that are a direct consequence of the TBI from those that are the result of medical complications. These potential complications include heterotopic ossification, posttraumatic hydrocephalus, posttraumatic epilepsy, intracranial and systemic infections, and medication side effects. Failure to identify medical complications will delay appropriate treatment and could place the patient at risk of permanent impairment.

This chapter details the neurologic examination of the patient with TBI during the postacute recovery period. Emphasis is placed on identifying neurologic deficits that are commonly associated with TBI. Functional impairments, particularly as they relate to rehabilitation, are reviewed. Last, medical complications that are commonly encountered in TBI rehabilitation are briefly discussed.

1.2 Evaluation of the Traumatic Brain Injury Patient in the Postacute Setting

The initial evaluation of the patient with TBI should include a detailed history. Because most of these patients have some cognitive impairment, the history may need to be obtained from medical records and from family members. Important details of the injury include the nature of the head injury (open or closed); whether the brain injury was focal or diffuse; the presence and duration of coma and posttraumatic amnesia; complicating conditions (hemorrhage, hypoxia, hypertension, posttraumatic seizures); associated systemic injuries (including spinal cord or peripheral nerve injury); the presence of intoxicants (drugs or alcohol);[11] and prior history of brain illness or injury.

One of the most important factors in assessing patients with TBI is the patient's premorbid cognitive and behavioral status. Assessment should include a history of substance abuse or psychiatric illness. Level of education and employment status should also be obtained. Younger patients will have school records, often including results of previous formal cognitive testing, that can provide some objective picture of premorbid cognitive skills. Additional information can be sought from family members or employers.

A physical examination should be performed on all patients. General observation should include assessment of the patient's level of consciousness; posture in bed; and presence of any external catheters or tubes (tracheostomy, gastrostomy tube, Foley catheter). The skin should be carefully examined for signs of breakdown (decubitus ulcers) or rash. Because concomitant skeletal injuries are common, a thorough musculoskeletal examination should be performed, with careful attention to any abnormal posturing of limbs, skeletal deformities, or limited range of motion at joints. Careful examination of the lungs, heart, and abdomen should also be performed to rule out infection or other pathologic processes.

Last, a detailed neurologic examination should be performed. This should include a detailed assessment of mental status, cranial nerves, motor system, sensory system, reflexes, coordination, and posture and gait (Table 1.1).

TABLE 1.1

Components of the Neurologic Examination in the Patient with TBI

Mental status
Level of consciousness
Orientation
Attention and concentration
Memory
Calculations
Speech and language
Spatial orientation/perception
Affect, mood, and behavior
Cranial nerves
Motor
Muscle bulk
Muscle tone
Muscle strength
Abnormal movements
Sensation
Primary sensory modalities
Cortical sensory function
Coordination
Reflexes
Posture and gait

1.3　The Neurologic Examination

1.3.1　Examination of Mental Status

Cognition and behavioral deficits are typical of TBI and often are the features most related to chronic functional disability. Manifestations include disorders of attention, learning and memory, language, perception, and executive functions. Although a formal detailed cognitive assessment is usually performed by the neuropsychologist and speech pathologist, useful information may be obtained from simple testing at bedside. Areas that should be assessed include level of consciousness, orientation, attention and concentration, memory, calculations, speech and language, spatial orientation and perceptual skills, affect, mood, and behavior.

1.3.1.1　Level of Consciousness

An altered level of consciousness may occur during the acute stage following TBI as a result of diffuse injury to the cerebral hemispheres or damage to the brainstem reticular formation. Other contributing factors include hypoxia, cerebral edema with increased intracranial pressure, and infection. Altered consciousness is often accompanied by confusion, disorientation, and anterograde amnesia, particularly if the limbic structures are affected.

Impairment in the level of consciousness may also be evident in the postacute rehabilitation setting, either because of residual brain injury or secondary factors such as metabolic abnormalities (hypernatremia, hypoglycemia, uremia, and so forth), posttraumatic seizures, posttraumatic hydrocephalus, or medication side effects. Deterioration in level of consciousness should always alert the physician to the possibility of one of these complications. From a functional standpoint, an altered or deteriorating level of consciousness will obviously interfere with a patient's ability to participate actively in rehab therapies and will shift the focus of therapy to more passive activities, such as muscle stretching and range-of-motion exercises.

Level of consciousness is easily assessed at bedside by observation and is best described by noting the patient's response to various levels of stimulation. Terms often used to describe altered levels of consciousness include *lethargy* (arousal to voice), *stupor* (arousal to vigorous physical stimulation), or *coma* (unresponsiveness to pain or other external stimuli).[12]

1.3.1.2　Orientation

Confusion and disorientation are common sequelae of TBI and are often associated with an altered level of consciousness. Disorientation most often results from diffuse cerebral injury, particularly that involving limbic structures, but can also be caused by factors such as metabolic abnormalities or even emotional factors. It is generally accepted that the duration of posttraumatic disorientation is related to brain injury severity and outcome, with shorter periods of orientation impairment offering the more favorable prognosis. Beyond this, the methods and meanings of acute orientation deficits, often referred to as *posttraumatic amnesia* (or PTA), continue to spark debate.[13]

During the bedside examination, orientation is assessed by asking the patient his name; the date (day of week, month, year); and location (name of hospital, floor number, room number, and so on).

1.3.1.3 Attention and Concentration

Attention and concentration are often impaired in patients with diffuse head injuries, particularly with insults to the frontal lobes.[14] Slowing of cognitive functioning and distractibility are also common findings.[15] These impairments can significantly affect a patient's progress in therapies because of inattention, slowness in performing cognitive tasks, and diminished ability to carry over information from day to day.

Attention and concentration may be informally evaluated during the course of the neurologic examination. Patients may have difficulty attending to the interview and may be easily distracted by external stimuli, such as hallway activity or roommates. Speed of cognitive processing may also be grossly assessed by noting the patient's response time to questions or commands. Serial sevens subtraction or backward spelling tasks are also commonly used in mental status screening exams.

1.3.1.4 Memory

Both long- and short-term memory may be affected in the head-injured patient as a result of direct injury to the mesial temporal lobes and thalamus.[3] In addition, areas that subserve memory, such as the hippocampus, are extremely sensitive to anoxic and hypotensive injury, which often occurs in patients with TBI.[16] There are a number of small series that suggest a possible benefit of hyperbaric oxygen in these individuals.[17–19]

Although old (retrograde) memory may be involved, new learning deficits (anterograde memory impairment) are a hallmark feature of moderate to severe TBI. Noting the diffuse nature of TBI (vs. focal stroke or neoplasm), deficits in verbal and visual–spatial memory are common, although the degree varies for each patient. Other cognitive impairments, such as poor concentration and apathy, may also interfere with encoding of new memories such that "forgetting" may actually be secondary to a primary attentional disorder.

The duration of posttraumatic amnesia is an important prognostic factor with regard to recovery.[20] Patients with prolonged posttraumatic amnesia tend to have more residual cognitive impairment and overall poorer functional outcome. Memory impairment may seriously limit patients' progress in the rehabilitation program, especially if the ability to learn new information is affected and the carryover of information learned in therapies is limited.

At bedside, immediate, recent, and remote memory can be evaluated. Immediate memory is primarily a function of information registration and is most dependent on attention and concentration. It is usually spared following TBI, except during the early recovery period or when other factors, such as medication side effects or metabolic encephalopathy, affect patients' ability to attend to task.[14] Immediate memory can be assessed by asking the patient to repeat immediately three objects named. Alternatively, one can use digit span testing. The examiner gives a series of digits at a rate of one per second and asks the patient to repeat these, both forward and backward. A normal individual can repeat seven digits forward and six in reverse order. In testing recent memory, the patient can be asked to recall three objects in 3 or 5 minutes. Recent memory can also be assessed by asking the patient simple historical questions, such as: What did you have for breakfast this morning? Remote memory may be assessed by asking the patient about events in the past, his address or telephone number, names of children, anniversary dates, and so forth. Again, remote memory is typically preserved, although it may be impaired during the acute confusional period.

1.3.1.5 Calculations

Acutely, problems with calculations reflect attentional deficits. However, focal injury to the dominant parietal lobe may result in more chronic impairment of mathematic skills. Deficits may limit the patient functionally in terms of his ability to manage finances or to participate in basic community activities such as shopping.

Calculation skills can easily be assessed at bedside by having patients perform serial subtraction of sevens from 100. Other tasks, such as counting change, or more complex multiplication or division problems can be administered. One must take premorbid educational history into account when interpreting the results of these tests.

1.3.1.6 Speech and Language

Language skills are commonly impaired in TBIs that involve the dominant hemisphere. Difficulty with spoken and written languages or problems with language processing may result. Language deficits are usually accompanied by other cognitive impairments.[21] The most common feature of traumatic aphasia is anomia, characterized by difficulty naming, word-finding deficits, and paraphasic errors.[22] Wernicke's (fluent or receptive) aphasia occurs less commonly following TBI. It is caused by focal injury to the dominant temporal lobe and is characterized by fluent paraphasic speech, with impaired comprehension and repetition.[23] Broca's (nonfluent or expressive) aphasia is more common in penetrating-type head injuries resulting from a lesion of the dominant frontal lobe. Broca's aphasia is characterized by nonfluent speech with disturbed prosody and perseveration. Other language disorders associated with TBI include echolalia (repetition of others) and palilalia (repetition of self).[4] Injuries to the medial frontal cortex, caudate nucleus, and globus pallidus, especially those that disrupt dopaminergic pathways connecting frontal lobe and basal ganglia structures, can result in apathy, abulia, and akinetic mutism. This is commonly seen following head injuries in children and in recovery from coma. A number of small series have reported improvement in these conditions with dopaminergic agonists such as bromocriptine, carbidopa/levodopa, and amantadine, or psychostimulants including methylphenidate and amphetamine.[24–26] Stuttering has also been reported following injuries to the right or left internal capsules, frontal white matter, and striatum.[27] Higher level language skills may also be affected, often becoming apparent as the aphasia resolves. Problems include difficulty with complex auditory processing, spelling, sentence construction, synonyms, and antonyms, and with abstract language skills such as picture description.[28]

Dysarthria, or impairment in articulation, is also a common sequela of TBI caused by weakness and incoordination of the tongue and pharyngeal muscles. Deficits range from mild inarticulation to unintelligible speech, with the pattern depending on the location of brain injury.[23] Lesions of the hypoglossal nerve cause unilateral tongue weakness and difficulty articulating lingual consonants (t, d, l, r, n). Weakness of the soft palate results in nasal speech characterized by an abnormal resonance to sounds.[29] Patients with pronounced facial weakness often have difficulty with labial and dentilabial consonants (p, b, m, w, f, v). Bilateral involvement of corticobulbar pathways results in "pseudobulbar" speech, characterized by slow, labored speech with imprecise articulation and a harsh, "strained" quality. Cerebellar lesions are associated with dysrhythmic speech, with irregularity of pitch and loudness. Injury to the basal ganglia may result in jerky, dysrhythmic speech with associated choreoathetosis, or slowed, slurred speech lacking inflection and modulation, associated with parkinsonian features.

Speech and language deficits clearly cause functional impairments, limiting a patient's ability to communicate effectively and to interact verbally with those around him. This not only affects the rehabilitation program but also has serious implications in terms of a patient's interaction with others and in eventually being able to live independently in the community.

Although a comprehensive evaluation is typically performed by the speech pathologist or neuropsychologist, basic aspects of speech and language can be assessed at bedside during the neurologic examination. The physician should observe the patient's spontaneous speech for fluency and syntax. Receptive language skills can be evaluated by having the patient follow one-, two-, and three-step verbal and written commands. Often, patients with receptive language impairments can "hide" their deficits through reliance upon subtle nonverbal cues of the examiner. Families may argue that an aphasic patient is understanding more than is true as a result of this effect. The keen examiner may test for this by using subtle misdirection. An example would be to ask the patient to "point to the floor" while simultaneously pointing their hand to the ceiling. The receptively impaired patient will mimic the examiner's movement, having misunderstood the verbal instruction. Similarly, counterintuitive commands such as "touch your right hand to your right elbow" can be used. Finally, asking questions without offering voice inflection or head nods/gestures will often result in a confused nonresponse by such patients with receptive language deficits.

Patients should be asked to name various common objects. Repetition can be assessed by asking the patient to repeat "no ifs, ands, or buts." Patients can be asked to read the newspaper or daily menu aloud and to write from dictation. Articulation can be grossly assessed by listening to the patient's speech during the interview by having the patient repeat certain test phrases such as "Methodist Episcopal."

1.3.1.7 Spatial Orientation/Perception

Patients with focal injuries to the nondominant parietal lobe will often have difficulty with spatial orientation and perceptual tasks. This may manifest as constructional apraxia, characterized by difficulty drawing or copying geometric designs. Disorders of body image may also be evident, manifested by a dressing apraxia, or neglect of the contralateral side of the body. The most serious form of neglect is anosognosia, or the inability of one to recognize one's own deficits.

Perceptual impairments and neglect are a serious hindrance to progress in the rehabilitation program. Patients with poor spatial orientation often wander or get lost. Patients with neglect are a safety risk because they often do not appreciate or pay attention to their deficits. Inattention to the affected side may cause a patient to roll over accidentally on a paretic arm or dangle it in the spokes of a wheelchair. Patients may be unable to negotiate their wheelchairs safely down a hallway or to turn into an open doorway without striking a wall.

Constructional praxis may be assessed at bedside by having the patient draw simple geometric figures, such as a square or triangle, or more complex forms, such as two intersecting pentagons. Patients should be able to bisect a line at the midline and draw an accurate clock face. Neglect can often be identified at bedside by observation. The patient may not attend to his affected side or may ignore his motor or sensory deficits, or miss food or other desired items positioned in the impaired hemispace.

1.3.1.8 Affect, Mood, and Behavior

Affect is an external facial expression (smile, frown, tear, laugh), whereas mood refers to an internal emotional state (happiness, sadness, fear, anger). Although affect can be observed, mood can only be revealed by the patient. Inferring the internal mood state of the patient with neurologic injury through observation only (in other words, relying upon affect in isolation) should be avoided. Neurologic emotional lability (pseudobulbar) syndromes may remove the correlation of an affective display (tearfulness) with its typically associated mood (sadness). It is recommended that both mood and affect be evaluated independently—affect through direct observation and mood by asking the patient.

Disturbances of affect and mood are common during the early recovery period following TBI, especially upon recovery from coma,[3,30] but may be seen years after injury.[31] Acute patients may experience delirium with disorientation and confusion, distractibility, restlessness, irritability, hallucinations, and delusions. These manifestations are most common in patients who have evidence of frontal or temporal lobe damage.[32] Delirium may also be caused by medication side effects, metabolic abnormalities, or infection.

Later during the recovery period, a change in personality, affect, and mood may be evident as a result of damage to the frontal lobes and limbic structures. Patients may be irritable and aggressive, demonstrate childish behavior, and show exaggeration of their premorbid personality. Other common features of frontal lobe injury include emotional disinhibition, emotional blunting, diminished drive and initiative, egocentricity, perseveration, mental rigidity, affective lability, loss of temper control, and impatience.[3,14] Patients with lesions of the basomedial frontal cortices demonstrate impairment in social judgment and in sexual control.[3] Patients with injury to the dorsolateral frontal cortices also demonstrate difficulty with "executive skills," or the inability to plan and execute a complex task.[14]

Both behavioral absences and excesses may be difficult to manage and, left unaddressed, can complicate or even sabotage the rehab process. Patients who are apathetic and lack initiative often do not put forth the maximum effort in therapies. Patients who demonstrate lack of impulse control, aggressiveness, and sexual inappropriateness are often disruptive not only to staff but also to other patients participating in the program. Furthermore, family members may have difficulty adjusting to a change in the patient's behavior. It is important for the physician and rehab team to identify these behavioral abnormalities, to develop an optimal behavior modification program to minimize disruptive behavior, and to design the most effective overall rehabilitation strategies to address these problems.

Although not usually assessed formally during the neurologic examination, behavior and affect can be observed during the patient interview. Further information regarding patient behavior can be obtained from nursing staff, and from more detailed testing can be performed by the rehabilitation neuropsychologist. Premorbid behavioral status should be ascertained from family members. Typically, post-TBI behavior is a complex product of premorbid personality, the brain injury itself, and emotional reactions to that injury.

1.3.2 Cranial Nerve Examination

1.3.2.1 Cranial Nerve I

Modern research has indicated that olfactory dysfunction (anosmia) is a common, although commonly undetected, sequela of TBI. Recent studies using standardized assessments reveal an incidence of 13% to 50% following TBI.[33,34] Notably, approximately 40%

of anosmic patients are unaware of their sensory loss. For this reason, reliance upon self-and/or family report of anosmia is ill-advised.[35]

Impairment in detection and/or recognition of smell occurs as a result of shearing injury to olfactory pathways that extend from the olfactory epithelium through the cribriform plate to the entorhinal cortex.[36,37] Notably, occipital blows are five times more likely to lead to such shearing injury than are frontal blows.[38] It has long been recognized that anosmia can lead to functional impairments, including diminished life satisfaction, interference with certain occupations, and potential safety problems resulting from the inability to detect signs of danger, such as smoke or the smell of spoiled food. Beyond this, anosmia may serve as a unique marker for impairment of orbital frontal lobe "executive" systems.[39,40] Evidence now suggests that post-TBI patients with anosmia have a greater incidence of frontal lobe-mediated executive skill deficits, which places them at risk for poor vocational and community integration outcomes.[34,35,41]

Smell may be assessed at bedside by having the patient identify various common odors such as tobacco or cloves. Noxious stimuli, such as ammonia, should be avoided because these stimulate the trigeminal nerve rather than the olfactory nerve. Standardized "scratch-and-sniff" measures are now commercially available and offer the advantages of ease of administration and demonstrated validity.[42]

1.3.2.2 Cranial Nerve II

The optic nerve and anterior visual pathways are affected in approximately 5% of TBI patients,[43] with 3% experiencing persistent visual field defects, impaired visual acuity, or blindness.[44] Loss of vision occurs most commonly following frontal injuries, particularly if there are fractures of the orbital bones. The optic nerve and pathways may be injured as a result of shear forces, mechanical stretching, contusion, or vascular insufficiency.[45,46] Deficits include monocular blindness resulting from retinal or optic nerve injury, bitemporal hemianopsia resulting from ischemia of the optic chiasm, homonymous hemianopia resulting from injury to the optic radiations, and cortical blindness resulting from lesions of the calcarine cortex. The latter is particularly common after head injury in children and is usually transient.[34]

Functionally, visual impairment results in diminished personal pleasure and may limit the patient's mobility resulting from impaired visual acuity and altered depth perception. In the rehab setting, visual impairments may lead to difficulty with wheelchair propulsion and ambulation, and may cause safety concerns. Patients may have difficulty performing daily care, ultimately leading to a loss of independence. Community reentry skills, such as returning to work or resumption of driving, may also be affected.

Optic nerve function is assessed by pupillary response, funduscopic examination, visual field testing, and measurement of visual acuity. In comatose patients, optic nerve function is best assessed by the pupillary response. In the case of unilateral optic nerve injury, neither the ipsilateral nor the contralateral pupil constricts when light is shone in the affected eye. Both pupils constrict, however, when light is shone in the unaffected eye. An afferent pupillary defect may also be demonstrated by the swinging flashlight test. When the light is swung back and forth from eye to eye, the pupil on the affected side will dilate as the light is swung to that eye (Marcus Gunn phenomenon). In long-standing optic nerve atrophy, the optic disc may appear pale on funduscopic examination. The presence of papilledema suggests the possibility of posttraumatic hydrocephalus or increased intracranial pressure of other cause and warrants further investigation.

Visual acuity may be impaired as a result of traumatic injury to the orbit and optic nerve or because of diffuse injuries to the occipital lobe. Acuity may be assessed at bedside by having the patient read a handheld Snellen acuity chart or Rosenbaum near-vision card,[47] or by bedside reading materials such as a newspaper or menu. Visual fields are assessed at bedside by confrontation testing. Each eye should be tested separately with comparison of the patient's visual fields with the examiner's.

1.3.2.3 Cranial Nerves III, IV, and VI

Injury to the oculomotor, trochlear, or abducens nerves occurs in 2% to 8% of patients following head injury. These nerves may be injured in the orbit as a result of orbital wall fractures, or in the cavernous sinus as a result of basilar skull fractures.[48–50] Delayed injury to these nerves can occur years after TBI because of the development of carotid–cavernous sinus fistulas.[51,52] The cranial nerve nuclei or intranuclear pathways may also be injured as a result of brainstem contusion or hematoma.[53] Injury may result in eye deviation, dysconjugate gaze, or abnormal head postures, with subjective complaints of diplopia. Supranuclear or conjugate gaze paresis may result from injury to the gaze centers in the frontal or parietal lobes, horizontal gaze center in the pons, or vertical gaze centers in the midbrain. Diplopia, or gaze paresis, may cause functional impairment by interfering with patients' visual–motor tasks, whereas accommodation difficulty may interfere with one's ability to read or perform close-up tasks.[54]

Eye movements are evaluated by having the patient track an object in the six cardinal positions of gaze. The inability to move the eye upward, inward, or downward, with preserved lateral movement suggests injury to the oculomotor nerve. This is often accompanied by ptosis and pupillary dilatation. Injury to the trochlear nerve is manifested by the inability to intort the eye or move it downward, often accompanied by head tilt to the nonaffected side.[55] The inability to move the eye laterally, with preservation of other ocular movements, suggests injury to the abducens nerve. In the comatose individual, eye movements can be assessed by oculocephalic or oculovestibular testing (see Section 1.3.2.6, Cranial Nerve VIII).

1.3.2.4 Cranial Nerve V

A trigeminal nerve lesion occurs in 3.6% of head-injured patients.[56] The injury is most commonly extracranial as a result of facial fracture and can involve any or all of the branches of the trigeminal nerve. Rarely, the trigeminal nerve may be injured as a result of trauma to the brainstem or as a result of basilar skull fracture involving the petrous bone.[57] In the latter instance, associated hearing loss and ipsilateral facial weakness are common.

Complete injury to the sensory branches of the trigeminal nerve results in hemianesthesia of the face, whereas partial injuries often result in facial pain.[58] Involvement of the ophthalmic branch leads to corneal anesthesia and potential corneal abrasion. Motor branch involvement results in weakness of the muscles of mastication and impairment of chewing. Loss of sensation in the mouth may cause pocketing of food and increases the risk of aspiration.

In the comatose patient, trigeminal nerve sensory function can be assessed by testing the corneal reflex (sensory limb). In alert, attentive patients, facial sensation can be evaluated with pinprick or cotton swab in the three nerve divisions. Trigeminal motor function can be tested by assessing masseter and pterygoid muscle strength. With trigeminal nerve injury, the jaw will deviate toward the affected side.

1.3.2.5 Cranial Nerve VII

The facial nerve is injured in approximately 3% of head-injured patients, most commonly as a result of temporal bone fractures.[59] Associated hearing loss is common. Brainstem trauma may also result in injury to the facial nerve nucleus. Facial nerve injury results in ipsilateral weakness in muscles of the upper and lower face. Injury to the corticobulbar pathways, resulting from lesion of the frontal lobe, internal capsule, or upper brainstem, also results in facial weakness, but spares the upper facial musculature.

Facial nerve injury can cause significant functional impairments. The inability to close the eye fully and an impairment in lacrimation can lead to corneal dryness, abrasion, and pain. Facial weakness may impair swallowing or cause a flaccid dysarthria. Hemifacial spasm can develop early after traumatic injury.[60]

Facial nerve function can be assessed in the comatose patient by the corneal reflex (motor limb). In the attentive patient, facial muscle strength can be assessed by asking the patient to smile, purse the lips, whistle, raise the eyebrows or forehead, and close the eyes.

1.3.2.6 Cranial Nerve VIII

Both the cochlear and vestibular nerves may be injured as a result of head trauma. Hearing loss occurs in 18% to 56% of head-injured patients[61] as a result of injury to the inner ear and related structures. Longitudinal fractures of the temporal bone, most commonly caused by a blow to the temporoparietal area, result in conductive hearing loss resulting from dislocation and disruption of the ossicles.[62] Transverse fractures of the temporal bone, caused by occipital or frontal blows, cause sensorineural hearing loss, vertigo, and disequilibrium resulting from direct injury to the acoustic nerve, trauma to the cochlea, or injury to the labyrinths.[63,64] Lesions of the auditory or vestibular nuclei occur rarely as a consequence of brainstem contusions. There is not much functional impairment resulting from hearing loss, because the deficit is usually unilateral. Vestibular insults are usually more problematic, leading to dizziness and difficulties with balance and coordination.

Hearing may be evaluated at bedside by whisper or finger rub. Air and bone conduction are assessed by the Rinne and Weber tests. Patients with suspected hearing loss should be referred for more detailed audiometric evaluation. In comatose patients, brainstem auditory evoked potential testing can provide useful information regarding the integrity of the auditory pathways.[65]

The presence of direction-fixed horizontal nystagmus usually suggests unilateral vestibular injury. Vertical nystagmus usually results from direct brainstem injury. Nystagmus may also occur as a consequence of medications, particularly anticonvulsants. In the comatose individual, vestibular function may be assessed by testing the oculocephalic reflexes (doll's eyes) and oculovestibular reflexes (ice-water calorics). In testing the oculocephalic reflex, rapid turning of the head results in conjugate eye deviation to the opposite side. Injury to the vestibular apparatus or vestibular pathways results in absence of eye deviation. Dysconjugate eye movements suggest injury to the internuclear pathways in the brainstem. In performing oculovestibular testing, the patient's head is tilted to 30°, and the external auditory canal is irrigated with ice water. A normal response is characterized by tonic conjugate deviation of the eyes toward the side of irrigation. In an awake individual, there may be nystagmus, with the fast component directed away from the site of irrigation. Injury to the vestibular pathways results in failure of eye deviation, whereas injury to the internuclear brainstem pathways results in dysconjugate eye movements.

Patients with suspected injury to the vestibular pathways may be more formally assessed with electronystagmography.

1.3.2.7 Cranial Nerves IX and X

The glossopharyngeal and vagus nerves are only rarely affected in TBI, usually the result of basilar skull fracture with extension into the foramen magnum.[66] These nerves are responsible for laryngeal and pharyngeal sensory and motor function, respectively, with injury resulting in impaired phonation and swallowing.

Glossopharyngeal and vagus nerve function are assessed at bedside by the gag reflex. The reflex is diminished or absent on the side of nerve injury. In addition, the palate and uvula may be deviated to the opposite side. The gag reflex may be pathologically brisk when there are lesions of the corticobulbar pathways bilaterally, usually a consequence of extensive injury to the frontal lobes or deep white matter. There is usually an associated pseudobulbar affect, characterized by emotional lability and spastic tetraparesis.

1.3.2.8 Cranial Nerve XI

The spinal accessory nerve supplies motor function to the ipsilateral sternocleidomastoid and trapezius muscles. This nerve is affected only rarely in head injury, occasionally seen following basilar skull fractures.

Spinal accessory nerve function is assessed by testing sternocleidomastoid muscle (lateral neck rotation to the opposite side) and trapezius muscle (ipsilateral shoulder shrug) strength. Impairment results in weakness of these muscles.

1.3.2.9 Cranial Nerve XII

The hypoglossal nerve provides motor function to the ipsilateral tongue. This nerve is also only rarely affected in head-injured patients as a result of basilar skull fractures or injury to the atlantooccipital region.[66] Injury results in swallowing difficulties resulting from the inability to manipulate the food bolus in the mouth.

The hypoglossal nerve is tested by having the patient stick out the tongue. Injury results in deviation of the tongue to the ipsilateral side.

1.3.3 Motor Examination

1.3.3.1 Muscle Bulk

In the traumatic brain-injured patient, generalized muscle atrophy may occur as a result of disuse following prolonged coma or immobility. Focal muscle atrophy always suggests lower motor neuron injury and should alert the physician to possible peripheral nerve, plexus, or nerve root injury. A peroneal neuropathy, for example, may arise secondary to a dislocated knee or as a consequence of an excessively tight lower extremity cast, resulting in foot drop and atrophy of the anterior compartment of the lower leg. The median, ulnar, radial, and sciatic nerves may also be injured as a result of skeletal injury or impingement by heterotopic bone. Brachial plexus or cervical root injuries are common in motorcycle accidents, particularly when the patient lands on his neck and shoulder.

Muscle bulk is generally assessed by observation. Focal atrophy can be discerned by comparing the circumference of the limb in question to the opposite side.

1.3.3.2 Muscle Tone

Various abnormalities of muscle tone may develop in the head-injured patient. Spasticity is the most common type of tone abnormality seen in brain-injured patients. Spasticity is defined as a velocity-dependent increase in resistance to passive movement, predominantly affecting the flexor groups in the upper extremities and extensor groups in the lower extremities. Tone may also be increased in the truncal muscles. Spasticity results from injury to the corticospinal tracts and is usually associated with muscle weakness, hyperreflexia, and an extensor plantar reflex response (Babinski's sign).[67] Rigidity is defined as an increase in resistance to passive movement, independent of velocity, and is most prominent in the flexor muscle groups of the upper and lower limbs. Cogwheel rigidity may result from direct injury to the basal ganglia; however, this is more common as a consequence of anoxia or a side effect of neuroleptic medications. Paratonia, or the inability of a patient to relax his muscles voluntarily during passive movement, is seen as a consequence of bilateral frontal lobe injury. Hypotonia, or diminished muscle tone, is occasionally seen as a consequence of cerebellar injury.

Increased tone may cause pain in the affected limb and may impede rehabilitation by limiting mobility and transfer skills, performance of nursing care, and activities of daily living. Spasticity in the upper extremity may hamper fine dexterity and may limit the ability to perform daily care. Neck and head control may be impaired, leading to difficulties with grooming and feeding skills. Spasticity of the pharyngeal and laryngeal muscles may impair articulation, phonation, swallowing, and breathing. Increased tone in the trunk musculature leads to problems in positioning in bed, wheelchair seating, standing, and ambulation.[67] Treatment of TBI patients with an increase in muscle tone should include daily range-of-motion exercises. Bracing and splinting can be utilized. Medications such as baclofen, tizanidine, diazepam, and dantrolene have been shown to be effective in reducing spasticity.[68] For patients who do not respond to or who are unable to tolerate oral medications, placement of an intrathecal baclofen pump may be considered. This has been formally approved for management of spasticity secondary to TBI.[69,70] Botulinum toxin injections are often of benefit in patients with more focal spasticity—in other words, an increase in muscle tone isolated to a few muscle groups.[71,72]

If a routine program of passive stretching is not performed, fixed-joint contractures may develop; these occur most commonly at the wrist, elbow, knee, and ankle. Patients with ankle plantar flexion contractures may not have an adequate base of support to transfer safely. Contractures of the hip and knee may limit a patient's ability to stand and ambulate. Contractures of the hip adductors may limit access to the perineal area, causing problems with catheter care and skin breakdown. Patients may have difficulty turning in bed or positioning themselves properly in the wheelchair, ultimately leading to pressure ulcerations on contact points (greater trochanters, sacrum, and heels).

Muscle tone is evaluated by passively moving the upper and lower extremities with the patient fully relaxed. Movements that are commonly tested include flexion/extension of the wrist, pronation/supination of the forearm, flexion/extension of the elbow, and flexion/extension of the knee or hip.

Range of motion of all joints should also be carefully assessed. Limited range of motion is suggestive either of contracture of that joint or heterotopic ossification, particularly if there is evidence of bony overgrowth in the joint region.[73] Heterotopic ossification will be discussed in more detail later in this text.

1.3.3.3 Muscle Strength

The two most common patterns of muscle weakness following TBI are hemiparesis and tetraparesis resulting from injury to the corticospinal tracts in the cerebral hemispheres or brainstem. Weakness is usually accompanied by spasticity and hyperreflexia. Focal muscle weakness should raise the suspicion of a superimposed nerve root, plexus, or peripheral nerve injury.

Muscle weakness causes obvious functional limitations, depending on its distribution and severity. Patients with severe tetraparesis often are unable even to roll in bed without assistance and may need help with simple daily care such as feeding and grooming. Although patients with hemiparesis usually require less physical assistance, they are often unable to transfer or ambulate independently and usually require help with daily care.

Primary movers of the fingers, wrists, elbows, shoulders, neck, ankles, knees, and hips should be assessed. It is important to position the patient properly while conducting muscle strength testing to ensure that the muscle being tested is appropriately isolated from other muscles with similar function. Strength is most commonly graded on the following scale[29]:

0   No muscle contraction noted

1   Flicker of movement (0%–10% of normal movement)

2   Movement through partial range of motion with gravity eliminated (11%–25% of normal movement)

3   Movement through full range of motion against gravity (26%–50% of normal movement)

4   Movement through full range of motion, against gravity, with minimal resistance from the examiner (51%–75% of normal movement)

5   Normal muscle power (76%–100% of normal movement)

1.3.3.4 Abnormal Movements

Abnormal postures or motor movements may result directly from TBI or as a consequence of medication side effects (Table 1.2). Dystonia, defined as inappropriate and prolonged contraction of muscles resulting in distortion of the limb,[74] can occur secondary to injury to the basal ganglia or as a side effect of neuroleptic medications.[74–76] Similarly, dyskinesias, characterized by insuppressible, stereotyped automatic movements of the limbs or orofacial musculature, may also result from basal ganglia injury or from medication side effects.[77] Choreoathetosis, or slow, writhing, spasmodic involuntary movements of the limbs or facial musculature, is most commonly seen as a side effect of anticonvulsants,

TABLE 1.2

Movement Disorders Associated with TBI

Dystonia
Dyskinesia
Choreoathetosis
Ballismus
Tremor
Myoclonus
Asterixis
Parkinsonism

dopaminergic medications, adrenergic medications, oral contraceptives, or antipsychotic medications, but may also result from traumatic injury to the basal ganglia.[78] Ballismus, characterized by violent flinging of the proximal upper extremity, may occur from direct injury or hemorrhage in the subthalamic region.[76] Tremor has also been reported as a consequence of head injury. Most frequent is a postural or kinetic tremor that may involve the head or upper or lower extremities.[79]

Myoclonus is defined as sudden, brief, shocklike involuntary muscle contractions. These can be focal, segmental, or generalized, and may be stimulus induced.[80] Myoclonus has also been reported as a direct consequence of head injury, often associated with cerebellar, basal ganglia, or pyramidal signs.[81]

Myoclonus may also result from complications including metabolic abnormalities (renal or hepatic failure, hyponatremia, or hypoglycemia); medication side effects (L-dopa); or hypoxic brain injury.[80] Asterixis is defined as an involuntary lapse of posture occurring at a joint during tonic muscle contraction. This is usually detected as a wrist flap while holding the arms outstretched with the wrists extended. Asterixis has been reported as a consequence of injury to the thalamus, internal capsule, midbrain, or parietal cortex, but is more commonly associated with toxic/metabolic encephalopathy (hepatic or renal failure) or the use of anticonvulsant medications.[82] Posttraumatic parkinsonism has also been described as a result of blunt head injury.[83]

Abnormal movements interfere with both gross and fine motor function by inhibiting normal coordinated movements. These hamper the ability to perform activities of daily living such as feeding or grooming, and interfere with fine motor activities such as buttoning or pulling zippers. Abnormal postures may interfere with wheelchair positioning, sitting balance, standing, and ambulation.

1.3.4 Sensory Examination

Sensory perception is often affected in patients with TBIs, although the sensory deficits are usually overshadowed by motor and cognitive impairments. Injury to the thalamus results in impairment of all sensory modalities on the contralateral face and body. With parietal lobe injuries, there is preservation of pain and temperature sensation, although patients are unable to localize the site of sensory stimulation. In addition, joint position sense, stereognosis (the ability to identify shapes and objects by touch), and graphesthesia (the ability to recognize figures written on the skin) are also impaired. Sensory neglect is often apparent, particularly if the nondominant parietal lobe is involved.

Sensory deficits may lead to serious functional impairments. A patient's inability to detect or localize pain may result in body injury as the result of the patient's lack of awareness and inability to protect the affected extremity. This is even a greater problem in patients who demonstrate neglect. Impaired upper extremity joint position sense may significantly affect a patient's ability to perform daily care, such as feeding or grooming, because of the inability to detect and control accurately limb position in space. Lack of feeling in the hands may also impair fine motor movements, making buttoning or fastening snaps difficult. Lower extremity sensory deficits may lead to difficulties with transfer and ambulation because of difficulties with accurate foot placement and balance. Patients with impaired sensation are at increased risk of developing pressure ulcerations, particularly if there is associated spasticity and impaired mobility.[84]

Patients' responses to sensory testing are highly subjective and dependent on factors that include level of consciousness, attention, and concentration. In a patient with a depressed level of consciousness, only gross sensory testing can be performed. In this case, sensory testing involves evaluation of the patient's grimace or motor response (e.g., withdrawal of limb) to a painful stimulus.

In an alert, cooperative patient, bedside sensory testing should include assessment of the primary sensory modalities, which include pain, light touch, vibration, and joint position sense. Responses should be compared from side to side and between upper and lower extremities. If the primary sensory modalities are intact, higher cortical sensory functions can be assessed. Graphesthesia can be evaluated by asking the patient to identify a letter or number traced in the palm of the hand. Stereognosis is tested by having the patient identify an object or shape placed in the hand. Localization of a sensory stimulus can be evaluated by touching a body part with either a pin or cotton swab and asking the patient to identify specifically the area of stimulation. Sensory neglect can be assessed by double simultaneous stimulation. Patients with neglect will be able to detect a stimulus on either limb when tested individually but will neglect the affected side when the limbs are stimulated at the same time.

1.3.5 Coordination

Coordination is modulated by various central and peripheral nervous system structures, including the corticospinal tracts, basal ganglia, cerebellum, and sensory pathways. Most severe TBIs cause diffuse structural injury and can affect any of these systems. Injury to the corticospinal tracts results in muscle weakness and slowing of gross and fine motor tasks. Basal ganglial lesions cause slowed initiation of movement and bradykinesia. Cerebellar injury may result in limb and truncal ataxia; dysmetria (inability to gauge distance, speed, and power of movement, resulting in an overshoot or undershoot of the target); dysdiadochokinesia (impairment in performance of rapid alternating movements); dyssynergia (decomposition of movement, resulting in lack of speed and skill in performing complex motor movements); and intention tremor.[26] Sensory pathway insults, particularly those involving the posterior columns, cause ataxia resulting from impaired proprioception.

Incoordination can affect a patient's ability to perform either gross or fine hand movements necessary to perform daily care. Patients may have difficulty bringing food to the mouth and may need assistance with dressing, particularly with buttons, snaps, and shoelaces. Writing may be illegible. Truncal ataxia may impair sitting and standing balance, causing problems with wheelchair seating, standing, and ambulation.

Upper extremity coordination can be assessed by various bedside tests. During finger-to-nose testing, the patient alternates between touching his nose and touching the examiner's finger held at arm's length from the patient. The smoothness and accuracy of the movement are noted, looking for evidence of dysmetria, dyssynergia, or intention tremor. Rapid alternating movements can be evaluated in several ways. Patients can be asked to flex and extend the fingers quickly, rapidly oppose the tips of the index finger and thumb, alternate hand patting between the palmar and dorsal surface (pronation/supination), or alternate touching the tip of the thumb to the tips of each finger in succession. The speed of movement, rhythm, smoothness of movement, and accuracy should be assessed.

Lower extremity coordination can be evaluated by the heel-to-knee-to-toe test. The patient is asked to touch his heel to his knee and slide his heel up and down his lower leg. Again, the smoothness and accuracy of movement are assessed. Alternatively, the patient can be asked to draw a figure eight or circle in the air with his great toe. Rapid alternating movements can be evaluated by asking the patient to tap his foot rapidly or repeat a pattern of tapping.

1.3.6 Reflexes

Evaluation of muscle stretch reflexes helps localize the sites of brain injury. Hyperactive reflexes suggest injury to the corticospinal tracts and are associated with muscle weakness, spasticity, and an extensor plantar response (Babinski's sign). Hypoactive reflexes occur most commonly with diseases or injuries of the lower motor neuron. Focal hyporeflexia, particularly if involving one reflex or reflexes in a single limb, should always raise the suspicion of a spinal root, plexus, or peripheral nerve injury. Diffuse hyporeflexia is most often associated with peripheral neuropathy (e.g., secondary to diabetes, chronic alcohol abuse, or renal disease), but also occurs with cerebellar injury.

The presence or exaggeration of other reflexes also helps localize brain injury. A hyperactive jaw jerk (masseter reflex) suggests bilateral corticospinal tract injury above the level of the mid pons. The presence of primitive reflexes, also called *frontal release signs* (i.e., sucking, grasp, and snout reflexes), suggests bifrontal or diffuse cerebral injury. The biceps, triceps, brachioradialis, patellar, and Achilles muscle stretch reflexes are most commonly tested. Responses are graded on a 0- to 4-point scale[29]:

0 Absent reflex

1 Diminished reflex

2 Normal reflex

3 Hyperactive reflex, although not necessarily pathologic

4 Pathologically hyperactive reflex, with clonus or spread to other muscles in the ipsi- or contralateral limb

The plantar response can be elicited in a number of ways. The most common maneuvers are the Babinski technique (performed by stimulating the sole of the foot with a blunt object) and the Chaddock maneuver (performed by stimulating the lateral aspect of the foot). A normal response is plantar flexion of the toes, whereas an abnormal response is characterized by dorsiflexion of the great toe with fanning of the other toes.

1.3.7 Posture and Gait

TBI, because of injury to the motor and sensory systems, commonly results in abnormalities in posture and stance, and difficulty walking. Patients with spastic hemiparesis may have difficulty standing because of trunk instability and may be unable to weight shift adequately to ambulate safely. If ambulation is possible, there may be significant gait deviation. Weak hip flexors and ankle dorsiflexors result in impaired swing-through of the limb and inadequate toe clearance during the swing phase of gait. Spasticity and contractures may limit range of motion at the hip, knee, and ankle. Decreased arm swing and circumduction of the lower extremity may be noted. Assistive devices (walker, cane) and lower extremity orthoses may be necessary. Patients with basal ganglial injury often demonstrate a stooped posture and shuffling gait. Patients with marked proprioceptive deficits may have difficulty with foot placement and balance.

The patient should be observed in a sitting and, if possible, standing position for assessment of posture and static balance. Patients can be asked to stand with their feet together and arms outstretched, or to stand on one leg to maintain their balance. Dynamic balance reactions can be tested by pushing the patient off balance, noting whether he is able to maintain his position, and whether he demonstrates protective reflex reactions. If the patient is able to ambulate, gait should be assessed. Attention should be given to position of the patient's head and trunk, and whether arm swing is normal and symmetric. The movement of the patient's pelvis and hip, knee, ankle, and foot should also be observed. Balance and coordination can be further assessed by having the patient attempt to walk heel-to-toe in a straight line (tandem gait).

1.4 Change in Status

One of the difficulties in patient assessment is distinguishing deficits that are directly the result of the TBI from those that are secondary to systemic disease or complications of the head injury. At any point during the patient's recovery, deterioration in neurologic status should always alert the physician to the possibility of such a complication. These include development of posttraumatic epilepsy, hydrocephalus, central nervous system or systemic infections, and toxic/metabolic encephalopathies.

1.4.1 Posttraumatic Epilepsy

Epileptic seizures occur in 2.5% to 5% of patients with TBI. These are most commonly secondarily generalized tonic–clonic seizures, although approximately 20% are of complex partial type, manifested by staring, interruption of speech, and automatisms.[85–87] Early epilepsy (i.e., seizures occurring within the first week following injury) is most common in children younger than 5 years and in adults with depressed skull fracture or intracranial hemorrhage. Late epilepsy begins months to years following injury and is felt to be secondary to an epileptogenic scar.

Any alteration in level of consciousness, particularly if intermittent and associated with abnormal motor movements, should raise the suspicion of an epileptic seizure. An electroencephalogram is necessary to document seizure activity electrically and to localize the seizure focus. Urgent neuroimaging is warranted to rule out the possibility of an acute structural brain lesion such as hemorrhage or abscess. The possibility of metabolic abnormalities such as hypoglycemia, hyponatremia, hypomagnesemia, or underlying infection (systemic or central nervous system) can lower seizure threshold and should also be considered.

1.4.2 Hydrocephalus

Ventricular dilatation is seen in 29% to 72% of patients following TBI.[88] This is most often a consequence of diffuse brain injury with compensatory ventricular enlargement (hydrocephalus ex vacuo). Hydrocephalus may also develop as a result of impairment in the flow or absorption of cerebrospinal fluid.[89] The true incidence of posttraumatic extraventricular obstructive hydrocephalus, characterized by ventricular enlargement without concomitant enlargement of the sulci, is probably approximately 8%,[90] with the incidence of symptomatic hydrocephalus less than 1%.[91]

Symptoms of hydrocephalus range from loss or alteration of consciousness to the classic triad of normal pressure hydrocephalus, which includes urinary incontinence, gait apraxia, and memory deficits. Any patient with a deteriorating level of consciousness or the clinical features of normal pressure hydrocephalus should be evaluated with head computed tomography or magnetic resonance imaging. Additional studies (lumbar puncture, radionuclide cisternography) may also be necessary for diagnosis.

1.4.3 Infection

Intracranial infections, including meningitis, brain abscess, or encephalitis, can occur in patients following TBI. Most susceptible are patients with a basilar skull fracture with extension into the paranasal sinuses or middle ear, or those who have had intracranial surgery.[92] Signs and symptoms of intracranial infection include fever, nuchal rigidity, depressed level of consciousness, and focal neurologic signs, including seizures. Workup should include a neuroimaging procedure of the brain. If there is no evidence of a mass lesion, a lumbar puncture should be performed.

Systemic infections (e.g., urinary tract infection or pneumonia) can also cause fever and depressed level of consciousness, especially in patients with underlying brain injury. Seizure threshold is also lowered in these individuals. Any change in patient behavior, deterioration in level of consciousness, or development of breakthrough seizures should raise the possibility of infection. Workup should be guided toward locating the source of infection so that appropriate treatment can be instituted as quickly as possible.

1.4.4 Toxic/Metabolic Encephalopathy

Toxic encephalopathy resulting from medication side effects is common in the head-injured population. Any change in the patient's behavior, depressed level of consciousness, or sudden appearance of a movement disorder should raise the suspicion of a medication side effect. The most common offenders include sedatives/hypnotics, neuroleptics, and anticonvulsants. Fortunately, these side effects are usually reversible upon cessation of the medication. Other causes for encephalopathy, such as infection or metabolic abnormalities (hyponatremia, hypernatremia, hypocalcemia, hypoglycemia, hyperglycemia, and so on), should be ruled out.

1.4.5 Endocrinologic Dysfunction

Pituitary hormonal insufficiency can occur after TBI. Those at greatest risk include patients with low Glasgow Coma Scale scores, diffuse brain swelling, associated hypoxic or hypotensive events, or concurrent subarachnoid hemorrhage.[93] Laboratory screening of pituitary function, including thyroid, gonadotrophin, cortisol, and growth hormone levels, should be considered in these high-risk individuals.

1.4.6 Depression

The onset of severe mood disorders following TBI can mimic other neurologic complications and can impede the rehabilitation process. Persons recovering from severe TBI are at a two to five times higher risk of developing depressive illness compared with the general population.[94] Therefore, distinguishing transitory sadness from depression (the former responds to subsequent good news whereas the latter does not) and knowing when and how to intervene is critical.[95] The involvement of a rehabilitation neuropsychologist within the interdisciplinary treatment team affords tremendous benefits in this regard, because the careful analysis of premorbid, injury-related, and adjustment-to-injury variables is needed. Should the presence of a clinical mood disorder be established, the availability of modern serotonin agonist antidepressants (selective serotonin reuptake inhibitors [SSRIs]), which are often "activating," offer significant advantages over first-generation agents. This is because the older drugs, especially the tricyclic compounds, are often sedating and require extended titration to reach clinically effective dosages. In the TBI population with the near-universal goals of increased attentional clarity and safe mobility, excessive sedation is clearly contraindicated. In addition, the rapid action and relatively benign side-effect profile of the SSRIs generally make them a much better choice for use with patients with TBI. Often, it is a combination of medication and psychotherapy that is most effective in assisting the patient to adapt to the chronic psychosocial changes resulting from TBI.

1.5 Summary

The neurologist has a key role to play in the medical and therapeutic management of the TBI patient in the postacute rehabilitation environment. The role extends beyond cursory neurologic examination, encompassing occasionally complex neurologic diagnosis and management. The neurologist should be comfortable in interfacing with physiatry, otolaryngology, psychiatry, neuropsychology, and all allied health professionals to formulate an optimum approach to comprehensive postacute rehabilitation of the TBI patient.

References

1. Adams, J. H., Graham, D., Scoff, G., Parker, L. S., and Doyle D., Brain damage in fatal non-missile head injury, *Journal of Clinical Pathology*, 33(12), 1132–1145, 1980.
2. Adams, J. H., Graham, D. I., and Jennett, B., The structural basis of moderate disability after traumatic brain damage, *Journal of Neurology, Neurosurgery and Psychiatry*, 71(4), 521–524, 2001.
3. McAlllster, T. W., Neuropsychiatric sequelae of head injuries, *Psychiatric Clinics of North America*, 15(2), 395–413, 1992.
4. Levin, H. S., Aphasia after head injury, in M. T. Sarno (Ed.), *Acquired Aphasia*, Academic Press, San Diego, CA, 455–498, 1991.
5. Raghupathi, R., Graham, D. I., and McIntosh, T. K., Apoptosis after traumatic brain injury, *Journal of Neurotrauma*, 17(10), 927–938, 2000.
6. Werner, C. and Engelhard, K., Pathophysiology of traumatic brain injury, *British Journal of Anaesthesia*, 99(1), 4–9, 2007.
7. Prasad, M. R., Ewing-Cobbs, L., Swank, P. R., and Kraner, L., Predictors of outcome following traumatic brain injury in young children, *Pediatric Neurosurgery*, 36(2), 64–74, 2002.
8. MRC Crash Trial Collaborators, Predicting outcome after traumatic brain injury: Practical prognostic models based on large cohort of international patients, *British Journal of Medicine*, 336(764), 425–429, 2008.
9. Yang, C. C., Tuy, K., Hua, M. S., and Huang, S. J., The association between the postconcussive symptoms and clinical outcomes for patients with mild traumatic brain injury, *Journal of Trauma*, 62(3), 657–663, 2007.
10. Bigler, E. D., Neuropsychology and clinical neuroscience of persistent post-concussion syndrome, *Journal of the International Neuropsychologic Society*, 14(1) 1–22, 2008.

11. Tate, P. S., Freed, D. M., and Bombardier, S., Traumatic brain injury: Influence of blood alcohol level on post-acute cognitive function, *Brain Injury*, 13(10), 767–784, 1999.

12. Plum, F. and Posner, J. B., *The Diagnosis of Stupor and Coma*, F.A. Davis, Philadelphia, PA, 1985.

13. Parker, R. S., *Concussive Brain Trauma: Neurobehavioral Impairment and Maladaption*, CRC Press, Boca Raton, FL, 2001.

14. Brooks, N., Behavioral abnormalities in head injured patients, *Scandinavian Journal of Rehabilitational Medicine*, 17 (Suppl.), 41–46, 1988.

15. Bennett-Levy, J. M., Long-term effects of severe closed head injury on memory: Evidence from a consecutive series of young adults, *Acta Neurologica Scandinavica*, 70(4), 285–298, 1984.

16. Bigler, E. D. and Alfano, M., Anoxic encephalopathy: Neuroradiological and neuropsychological findings, *Archives of Clinical Neuropsychology*, 3(4), 383–396, 1988.

17. Ren, H., Wang, W., and Ge, Z., Glasgow Coma Scale, brain electric activity mapping and Glasgow Outcome Scale after hyperbaric oxygen treatment of severe brain injury, *Chinese Journal of Traumatology*, 4(4), 239–241, 2001.

18. Neubauer, R. A., Gottlieb, S. F., and Pevsner, N. H., Hyperbaric oxygen for treatment of closed head injury, *Southern Medical Journal*, 87(9), 933–936, 1994.

19. Tinianow, C. L., Tinianow, T. K., and Wilcox, M., Effects of hyperbaric oxygen on focal brain contusions, *Biomedical Sciences Instrumentation*, 36, 275–281, 2000.

20. McFarland, K., Jackson, L., and Gelle, G., Post-traumatic amnesia: Consistency-of-recovery and duration-to-recovery following traumatic brain impairment, *Clinical Neuropsychologist*, 15(1), 59–68, 2001.

21. Groher, M. E., Communication disorders in adults, in M. Rosenthal, E. R. Griffith, M. R. Bond, and J. D. Miller (Eds.), *Rehabilitation of the Adult and Child with Traumatic Brain Injury*, F. A. Davis, Philadelphia, PA, 148–162, 1990.

22. Lambon, R., Sage, K., and Roberts, J., Classical anomia: A neuropsychological perspective on speech production, *Neuropsychologia*, 38(2), 186–202, 2000.

23. Sarno, M. T., Buonaguro, A., and Levita, E., Characteristics of verbal impairment in closed head injured patients, *Archives of Physical Medicine and Rehabilitation*, 67(6), 400–405, 1986.

24. Robinson, R. G., Boldue, P. L., and Price, J. R., Two-year longitudinal study of post-stroke mood disorders: Diagnosis and outcome at one and two years, *Stroke*, 18(5), 837–843, 1987.

25. Muller, U. and Von Cannon, Y., The therapeutic potential of bromocriptine in neuropsychological rehabilitation of patients with acquired brain damage, *Progress in Neurophychopharmacology and Biological Psychiatry*, 18(7), 1103–1120, 1994.

26. Mann, R. S., Fogel, B. S., and Hawkins, J., et al., Apathy: A treatable syndrome, *Journal of Neuropsychiatry and Clinical Neurosciences*, 7, 23–30, 1995.

27. Ludlow, C. L., Rosenberg, J., Salazar, A., Graftnan, J., and Smutok, M., Site of penetrating brain lesions causing chronic acquired stuttering, *Annals of Neurology*, 2(1), 60–66, 1987.

28. Thomsen, I. V., The patient with severe head injury and his family, *Scandinavian Journal of Rehabilitational Medicine*, 6(4), 180–183, 1974.

29. Haerer, A. F., *DeJong's The Neurologic Examination*, 5th ed., Lippincott, Philadelphia, PA, 1992.

30. Lishman, W. A., Brain damage in relation to psychiatric disability after head injury, *British Journal of Psychiatry*, 114(509), 373–410, 1968.

31. Lezak, M. D., Relationships between personality disorders, social disturbances, and physical disability following traumatic brain injury, *Journal of Head Trauma Rehabilitation*, 2(1), 57–69, 1987.

32. Thomsen, I. V., Late outcome of very severe blunt head trauma: A 10–15 year second follow-up, *Journal of Neurology, Neurosurgery and Psychiatry*, 47(3), 260–268, 1984.

33. Costanzo, R., DiNardo, L., and Reiter, E., Head injury and olfaction, in R. Doty (Ed.), *Handbook of Olfaction and Gustation*, Marcel Dekker, New York, 1038–1053, 2003.

34. Callahan C. D. and Hinkebein, J., Neuropsychological significance of anosmia following traumatic brain injury, *Journal of Head Trauma Rehabilitation*, 14(6), 581–587, 1999.

35. Callahan C. D. and Hinkebein, J. H., Assessment of anosmia after traumatic brain injury: Performance characteristics of the University of Pennsylvania Smell Identification Test, *Journal of Head Trauma Rehabilitation*, 17(3), 251–256, 2002.

36. Varney, N. R., Pinkston, J. B., and Wu, J. C., Quantitative PET findings in patients with post-traumatic anosmia, *Journal of Head Trauma Rehabilitation*, 16(3), 253–259, 2001.
37. Hendriks, A. P. J., Olfactory dysfunction, *Rhinology*, 26(4), 229–251, 1988.
38. Costanzo, R. M. and Zasler, N. D., Epidemiology and pathophysiology of olfactory and gustatory dysfunction in head trauma, *Journal of Head Trauma Rehabilitation*, 7(1), 15–24, 1992.
39. Malloy, P. F. and Richardson, E. D., The frontal lobes and content-specific delusions, *Journal of Neuropsychiatry and Clinical Neurosciences*, 6, 455–465, 1994.
40. Varney, N. R. and Bushnell, D., NeuroSPECT findings in patients with posttraumatic anosmia: A quantitative analysis, *Journal of Head Trauma Rehabilitation*, 13(3), 63–72, 1998.
41. Varney, N. R. and Menefee, I., Psychosocial and executive deficits following closed head injury: Implications for orbital frontal cortex, *Journal of Head Trauma Rehabilitation*, 8(1), 32–44, 1993.
42. Doty, R. L., Yousem, D. M., Pham, L. T., Kreshak, A. A., Geckle, R., and Lee, W. W., Olfactory dysfunction in patients with head trauma, *Archives of Neurology*, 54(9), 1131–1140, 1997.
43. Gjerris, F., Traumatic lesions of the visual pathways, in P. J. Vinken and C. W. Bruyn (Eds.), *Handbook of Clinical Neurology*, Vol. 24, North Holland Publishing, Amsterdam, 27–57, 1976.
44. Roberts, A. H., *Severe Accidental Head Injury: An Assessment of Long-Term Prognosis*, Macmillan Press, London, 1979.
45. Hoyt, C. S., Brain injury and the eye, *Eye*, 21(10), 1285–1289, 2007.
46. Granaraj, L., Gilliland, M. G., Yahya, R. R., Rutka, J. T., Drake, J., Dirks, P., and Levin, A. V., Ocular manifestations of crush head injury in children, *Eye*, 21(1), 5–10, 2007.
47. Kline, L. B., Morawetz, R. B., and Swaid, S. N., Indirect injury of the optic nerve, *Neurosurgery*, 14(6), 756–764, 1984.
48. Takeuchi, S., Takasoto, Y., Masaoka, H., Hayakawa, T., Otani, N., Yoshino, Y., and Yatsushiga, H., Isolated traumatic oculomotor nerve palsy caused by minor head trauma, *Brain and Nerve*, 60(5), 555–558, 2008.
49. Dhaliwal, A., West, A. C., Trobe, J. D., and Musch, D. S., Third, fourth, and sixth cranial nerve palsies following closed head injury, *Journal of Neuro-Ophthalmalogy*, 26(1), 4–10, 2006.
50. Suchoff, I. B., Kapoor, N., Waxman, R., and Ference, W., The occurrence of ocular and visual dysfunctions in an acquired brain-injury patient sample, *Journal of the American Optometric Association*, 70(5), 301–308, 1999.
51. Dubov, W. E. and Bach J. R., Delayed presentation of a carotid–cavernous sinus fistula in a patient with traumatic brain injury, *American Journal of Physical Medicine and Rehabilitation*, 70(5), 178–180, 1991.
52. Miller, N. R., Diagnosis and management of dural carotid–cavernous sinus fistulas, *Neurosurgical Focus*, 23(5), E13, 2007.
53. Schmeck, M. J., Smith, R., and Moster, M., Isolated bilateral abducens nerve palsy associated with traumatic prepontine hematoma, *Seminars in Ophthamology*, 22(1), 21–24, 2007.
54. Ciuffreda, K. J., Kapoor, N., Rutner, D., Suchoff, I. B., Han, M. E., and Craig, S., Occurrence of oculomotor dysfunctions in acquired brain injury: A retrospective analysis, *Optometry*, 78 (4), 155–167, 2007.
55. Keane, J. R., Fourth nerve palsy: Historical review and study of 215 inpatients, *Neurology*, 43(12), 2439–2443, 1993.
56. Yadav, Y. R. and Khosia, V. K., Isolated 5th to 10th cranial nerve palsy in closed head trauma, *Clinical Neurology and Neurosurgery*, 93(1), 61–63, 1991.
57. Schecter, A. D. and Anziska, B., Isolated complete post-traumatic trigeminal neuropathy, *Neurology*, 40(10), 1634, 1990.
58. Dubner, R. and Ron, K., Brainstem mechanism of persistent pain after injury, *Journal of Orofacial Pain*, 18(4), 299–305, 2004.
59. Rafferty, M. A., McConn Welsh, R., and Walsh, M. A., A comparison of temporal bone fracture classification systems, *Clinical Otolaryngology*, 31(4), 287–291, 2006.
60. Wang, H. C., Lu, C. H., Lee, R. J., Yang, T. M., and Hung K. S., Post-traumatic hemifacial spasm, *Journal of Clinical Neuroscience*, 13(6), 681–683, 2006.

61. Kochhar, L. K., Deka, R. C., Kacker, S. K., and Raman, E. V., Hearing loss after head injury, *Ear, Nose, and Throat Journal*, 69(8), 537–542, 1990.

62. Sakai, C. S. and Mateer, C. A., Otological and audiological sequelae of closed head trauma, *Seminars in Hearing*, 5(2), 157–174, 1984.

63. Nelson, J. R., Neuro-otologic aspects of head injury, in R. A. Thompson and J. R. Green (Eds.), *Advances in Neurology: Complications of Nervous System Trauma*, Vol. 22, Raven Press, New York, 107–123, 1979.

64. Fitzgerald, D. C., Persistent dizziness following head trauma and perilymphatic fistula, *Archives of Physical Medicine and Rehabilitation*, 76(11), 1017–1020, 1995.

65. Fitzgerald, D. C., Head trauma: Hearing loss and dizziness, *Journal of Trauma*, 40(3), 488–496, 1996.

66. Delamont, R. S. and Boyle, R. S., Traumatic hypoglossal nerve palsy, *Clinical and Experimental Neurology*, 26, 239–241, 1989.

67. Gelber, D. A. and Jozefczyk, P. B., Therapeutics in the management of spasticity, *Neurorehabilitation and Neural Repair*, 13(1), 5–14, 1999.

68. Gelber, D. A. and Jeffery, D. R. (Eds.), *Clinical Evaluation and Management of Spasticity*, Humana Press, Totowa, NJ, 2002.

69. Meythaler, J. M., Pharmacology update: Intrathecal baclofen for spastic hypertonia in brain injury, *Journal of Head Trauma Rehabilitation*, 12(1), 87–90, 1997.

70. Francisco, G. E., Latorie, J. M., and Ivanhoe, C. B., Intrathecal baclofen therapy for spastic hypertonia in chronic traumatic brain injury, *Brain Injury*, 21(3), 335–338, 2007.

71. Yablon, S. A., Agana, B. T., Ivanhoe, C. B., and Boake, C., Botulinum toxin in severe upper extremity spasticity among patients with traumatic brain injury: An open-labeled trial, *Neurology*, 47(4), 939–944, 1996.

72. Van Rhijn, J., Molenaers, G., and Ceulemans, B., Botulinum toxin type A in the treatment of children and adolescents with an acquired brain injury, *Brain Injury*, 19(5), 331–335, 2005.

73. Garland, D. E. and Rhoades, M. E., Orthopedic management of brain-injured adults: Part II, *Clinical Orthopaedics and Related Research*, 131, 111–122, 1978.

74. Marsden, C. D., Obeso, J. A., Zarranz, J. J., and Lang, A. E., The anatomical basis of symptomatic hemidystonia, *Brain*, 108(2), 463–483, 1985.

75. Flanagan, S. R., Kwasnica, C., Brown, A. W., Elovic, E. P., and Kothari, S., Congenital and acquired brain injury. 2. Medical rehabilitation in acute and subacute settings, *Archives of Physical Medicine and Rehabilitation*, 89(3), S9–S14, 2008.

76. King, R. B., Fuller, C., and Collins, G. H., Delayed onset of hemidystonia and hemiballismus following head injury: A clinicopathological correlation, case report, *Journal of Neurosurgery*, 94(2), 309–314, 2001.

77. Alves, R., Barbosa, E., and Scaff, M., Hemiparkinsonism and levodopa-induced dyskinesias following focal nigral lesion, *Movement Disorders*, 21(12), 2267–2268, 2006.

78. Robin, J. J., Paroxysmal choreoathetosis following head injury, *Annuals of Neurology*, 2, 447–448, 1977.

79. Umemura, A., Samadani, U., Jaggi, J. L., Hurtig, H. I., and Baltuch, G. H., Thalamic deep brain stimulation for post traumatic action tremor, *Clinical Neurology and Neurosurgery*, 106(4), 280–283, 2004.

80. Fahn, S., Marsden, C. D., and Van Woert, M. H., Definition and classification of myoclonus, in S. Fahn, C. D. Marsden, and M. H. Van Woert (Eds.), *Advances in Neurology: Myoclonus*, Vol. 43, Raven Press, New York, 1–5, 1986.

81. Jacob, P. C. and Chand, R. P., A posttraumatic thalamic lesion associated with contralateral action myoclonus, *Movement Disorders*, 14(3), 512–514, 1999.

82. Young, R. R. and Shahani, B. T., Asterixis: One type of negative myoclonus, in S. Fahn, C. D. Marsden, and M. H. Van Woert (Eds.), *Advances in Neurology: Myoclonus*, Vol. 43, Raven Press, New York, 137–156, 1986.

83. Bhatt, M., Desai, J., Mankodi, A., Elias, M., and Wadia, N., Posttraumatic akinetic–rigid syndrome resembling Parkinson's disease: A report in three patients, *Movement Disorders*, 15(2), 313–317, 2000.

84. Donovan, W. H., Garber, S. L., Hamilton, S. M., Krouskop, T. A., Rodriguez, G. P., and Stal, S., Pressure ulcers, in J. A. DeLisa (Ed.), *Rehabilitation Medicine*, Lippincott, Philadelphia, PA, 476–491, 1988.

85. Jennett, B., Post-traumatic epilepsy, in M. Rosenthal, E. R. Griffith, M. R. Bond, and J. D. Miller (Eds.), *Rehabilitation of the Adult and Child with Traumatic Brain Injury*, F.A. Davis, Philadelphia, PA, 89–93, 1990.

86. Skandsen, T., IvarLund T., Fredrilksli, O., and Vik, A., Global outcome, productivity and epilepsy 3–8 years after severe head injury: The impact of injury severity, *Clinical Rehabilitation*, 22(7), 653–662, 2008.

87. Wang, H. C., Chang, W. N., Chang, H. W., Ho, J. T., Yang, T. M., Lin, W. C., Chuang, Y. C., and Lu, C. H., Factors predictive of outcome in post-traumatic seizures, *Journal of Trauma*, 64(4), 883–888, 2008.

88. Beyeri, B. and Black, P., Posttraumatic hydrocephalus, *Neurosurgery*, 15(2), 257–261, 1984.

89. Kishore, P. R. S., Lipper, M. H., Girevendulis, A. K., Becker, D. P., and Vines, F. S., Post-traumatic hydrocephalus in patients with severe head injury, *Neuroradiology*, 16(1), 261–265, 1978.

90. Gudeman, S. K., Kishore, P. R. S., Becker, U. P., Lipper, M. H., Girevendulis, A. K., Jeffries, B. F., and Butterworth, J. F., Computed tomography in the evaluation of incidence and significance of post-traumatic hydrocephalus, *Neuroradiology*, 141(2), 397–402, 1981.

91. Narayan, R. K., Gokaslan, Z. L., Bontke, C. F., and Berrol, S., Neurologic sequelae of head injury, in M. Rosenthal, E. R. Griffith, M. R. Bond, and J. D. Miller (Eds.), *Rehabilitation of the Adult and Child with Traumatic Brain Injury*, F.A. Davis, Philadelphia, PA, 94–106, 1990.

92. Miller, J. D., Pentland, B., and Berrol, S., Early evaluation and management, in M. Rosenthal, E. R. Griffith, and J. D. Miller (Eds.), *Rehabilitation of the Adult and Child with Traumatic Brain Injury*, F.A. Davis, Philadelphia, PA, 21–33, 1990.

93. Kelly, D. F., Gonzalo, I. T., Cohan, P., Berman, N., Swerdolff, R., and Wang C., Hypopituitarism following traumatic brain injury and aneurysmal subarachnoid hemorrhage: A preliminary report, *Journal of Neurosurgery*, 93(5), 743–752, 2000.

94. Eames, P. G., Distinguishing the neuropsychiatric, psychiatric, and psychological consequences of acquired brain injury, in R. L. Wood and T. M. McMillan (Eds.), *Neurobehavioral Disability and Handicap Following Traumatic Brain Injury*, Psychology Press, East Sussex, UK, 29–45, 2001.

95. Prigatano, G. P., *Principles of Neuropsychological Rehabilitation*. Oxford University Press, New York, 1991.

2

Posttraumatic Epilepsy and Neurorehabilitation

Theresa D. Hernández, Paul M. Levisohn,
Kimberley Buytaert-Hoefen, and Dean K. Naritoku

CONTENTS

2.1 Introduction

Two percent of patients with traumatic brain injury (TBI) experience early seizures, defined as occurring while the patient is still experiencing the direct effects of the head injury, usually within the first 24 hours of injury, although up to 2 weeks later in those with severe head trauma.[1] There is a 3.6-fold increase in late seizures (after the acute effects of head trauma have resolved). The majority of these late-occurring seizures take place during the first year following TBI, although some increased risk continues for 4 years after the trauma. By definition, the occurrence of multiple seizures (two or more) is defined as epilepsy. Although epilepsy (i.e., late-occurring seizures) has long been recognized as a common sequel to brain injury, progress in understanding the pathophysiology and treatment of posttraumatic epilepsy has been limited. Therefore, clinicians have little information regarding appropriate therapy of posttraumatic epilepsy, and as a result, therapy of posttraumatic epilepsy has remained empirical and arbitrary. The decision to initiate or withhold antiepileptic drug (AED) therapy has far-reaching implications for rehabilitation of the traumatic brain-injured patient. Inappropriate use of anticonvulsants may cause unnecessary cognitive impairment in those persons not requiring medication. At the same time, experimental data suggest that certain types of seizures may retard functional improvement during recovery from brain injury, whereas other types have no deleterious consequences. Thus, it is crucial to differentiate patients who will require and benefit from AED therapy from those who will not.

2.2 Evaluation of Episodic Behavioral Changes

Episodes of abnormal behavior occur commonly after severe head injuries and present a diagnostic challenge for the treating physician. There are many potential etiologies for these episodes; therefore, it is crucial to determine the correct diagnosis to select the most appropriate and efficacious therapies to avoid iatrogenic complications. Several disease entities result in fluctuations of mental status in the posttraumatic brain-injured state. These include posttraumatic encephalopathy, seizures, postictal state, and numerous encephalopathies of toxic and metabolic etiologies. Episodic dyscontrol and disinhibition from frontal injury may occur. The encephalopathy caused by the posttraumatic state is discussed in detail by Gelber elsewhere in this volume. Mentation and attention tend to fluctuate in the patient with TBI and may be mistaken for seizures, especially when there is a superimposed encephalopathy of another etiology. Simple staring spells are rarely the result of seizures in the setting of TBI. Nonepileptic spells (psychogenic seizures) and misinterpretation of behaviors by caregivers may be difficult to differentiate from epileptic seizures. Metabolic encephalopathies are characterized by fluctuating mentation and may also be mistaken for seizures. Inappropriate use of AEDs in these situations will not only be ineffective but may also result in worsening of confusion or agitation.

There are many common etiologies for acute encephalopathies. Medication-induced encephalopathies rank among the most common and easily remedied causes of confusional states. As a result of the brain injury, patients with TBI possess a lower tolerance to the central nervous system (CNS) side effects of psychotropic drugs and other medications. Medications with anticholinergic properties are tolerated especially poorly and should be avoided because of their tendency to cause confusion, hallucinations, and memory loss, especially in older patients.[2,3] Antihistamines and many over-the-counter preparations fall into this category and are often overlooked as causes of transient or prolonged confusion. Several centrally acting sedatives, especially benzodiazepines and barbiturates, have extremely long half-lives. From a pharmacokinetic standpoint, long half-lives result in a greater interval before steady state is achieved; thus, adverse effects on the CNS may not be apparent until several days after the start of medications, and cause and effect may not be apparent. As a general rule, sedative agents (including benzodiazepines, opioids, and barbiturates) exacerbate encephalopathies; therefore, they frequently aggravate confusion or agitation in patients with TBI and should be avoided. Other drugs commonly used in the patient with TBI may have profound effects on the CNS. The medication list should always be reviewed for histamine antagonists (e.g., cimetidine) and narcotics for the possibility that they are inducing the confusional state.

Several systemic derangements are commonly associated with the posttraumatic state. Head injury may cause the syndrome of inappropriate antidiuretic hormone and result in hyponatremia, which, in turn, may cause confusion. Systemic infections are common in the patients with TBI because of reduced mobility and presence of indwelling catheters. Any infection may manifest as an abrupt decline in mental status or agitation. An acute decline or fluctuation in mental status may herald a pulmonary, urinary tract, or wound infection. In patients with open head injuries and skull fractures, the possibility of a CNS infection should always be considered when there is an abrupt decline in mental status. When in doubt, a lumbar puncture must be performed, after careful assessment for potential causes of increased intracranial pressure (ICP). Hypoxia may also cause agitation and confusion and is commonly caused by pulmonary emboli from deep venous thrombosis or fat emboli. Stroke is usually not a cause of global cognitive dysfunction except in cases of multifocal, brainstem, or diencephalic strokes.

Syncope (fainting) may be confused with seizures, especially if there is associated tonic posturing. As the patient loses consciousness, there is dimming of vision, and the patient appears pale and clammy. The patient generally falls limply to the ground or slumps over, if sitting. Occasionally, a brief tonic or tonic–clonic seizure occurs, adding to the confusion regarding the diagnosis. In contrast to epileptic seizures, the patient with a syncopal episode generally regains consciousness and orientation rather quickly. Medications such as tricyclic antidepressants, beta blockers, and neuroleptics may result in systemic hypotension and lead to syncope.

Panic disorder may mimic epilepsy and is frequently seen in patients after trauma. Panic episodes may be mistaken for complex partial seizures because of altered consciousness that may occur. Panic episodes and other spells of psychogenic etiology are often misdiagnosed as medically intractable seizures, and these diagnoses should be considered in patients who are not responsive to antiepileptic medications. A careful history will help sort out this differential diagnosis. Typically, in the case of a panic attack, the patient complains of feeling dissociated, smothered, and in need of fresh air. The patient may have perioral numbness, tingling of digits, and a feeling of impending doom. Generally, full awareness of surroundings is retained and the patient is able to maintain conversation. Episodes of syncope may occur in patients with panic disorder. They are usually brief and vasovagal in nature. As opposed to patients with complex partial seizures, those with syncope resulting from panic attacks generally retain full awareness and can maintain a conversation until there is loss of consciousness. AEDs are ineffective for panic disorder, whereas alprazolam and imipramine are very effective.[4]

2.3 Clinical Evaluation of Seizures

Seizures should be considered when episodes of discrete and stereotypic behaviors occur with altered or lost consciousness. Although an electroencephalogram (EEG) is often supportive, the diagnosis of epilepsy must be made on clinical grounds. The patient may provide only a vague or incomplete history and the diagnosis often depends on a careful history taken from observers. Seizures are distinct, stereotyped episodes, with a definite start and end. With the exception of status epilepticus, seizure usually lasts only a few minutes. Afterward, mentation will often clear within a few minutes with return to baseline, although postictal somnolence may persist. Prolonged confusion of hours to days is rarely caused by seizures and should alert the clinician to the possibility of other causes mentioned earlier. Directed aggression is not seen during seizures or the postictal state, although confusion and undirected aggressive behaviors may be seen.

Under the International Classification of Seizures,[5] seizures are classified by whether they appear to start from a localized cortical region (partial or localization-related seizures) or from the entire brain at once (primary generalized seizures). Partial seizures are further divided by whether they impair consciousness (complex partial seizures) or not (simple partial seizures). Partial seizures are caused by localized cortical abnormalities and tend to be acquired in nature, whereas primary generalized seizures are often caused by genetic factors. The partial-onset seizure category encompasses seizure types that previously went under several terminologies, including Jacksonian, psychomotor, and temporal lobe seizures. Tonic–clonic ("grand mal") seizures that result from spread of the ictus from a focal onset are described as partial seizures with secondary generalization.

The distinction in seizure onset has important implications for the pathophysiology and therapy of the seizure. AEDs tend to be selective for the seizure type and are analogous to cardiac antiarrhythmic drugs, which are fairly selective for arrhythmia type. Because posttraumatic seizures occur as a result of localized injury to the cerebral cortex, the resulting seizures are usually of partial onset, with or without secondary generalization. The behavioral manifestations of posttraumatic seizures relate to area of onset, usually in the penumbra of injury. Thus, injuries to the convexity of the brain often result in sensory or primary motor manifestations at seizure onset, such as a migrating paresthesias or twitching and jerking of an extremity. Seizures of the temporal lobe may result in psychic phenomena such as a sensation of fear or déjà vu, followed by automatisms, whereas frontal seizure foci often result in aversive motor or more complex behaviors, described as *hypermotor.*

During typical complex partial seizures, the patient will often stare and become nonresponsive or poorly responsive to commands. Automatisms frequently occur and take the form of lip smacking and swallowing or chewing (oral–alimentary automatisms), and fidgeting with objects. Although the patient may spontaneously speak or seem to respond to commands, the language is inappropriate to the situation. The patient may affirm or disagree when questioned but usually gives little more than simple responses and does not follow complex commands. Generally, combativeness occurs only when the person is restrained. Thus, when directed aggression occurs, such as seeking out and striking a staff member, the episode most likely is a conscious act and not the result of a seizure. After a complex partial seizure, there is often a several-minute period of confusion and disorientation, which represents the postictal state. The patient will often feel tired or exhausted and will frequently go to sleep. When present, a history of postictal confusion and lethargy often helps to identify episodes as seizures because they generally do not occur or are brief with spells of other etiologies. Amnesia for the event is often noted in patients with complex partial seizures. Seizures emanating from the frontal lobes may be confused with nonepileptic events resulting from the bizarre nature of the seizures (hypermotor) reported, occasionally without impaired consciousness and without a period of postictal mental change.

In patients with TBI, tonic–clonic (convulsive) seizures result from secondary generalization—in other words, spread of the seizure from the seizure focus at the site of trauma to other parts of the brain, especially the brainstem, which appears to moderate the initial tonic phase of the convulsion.[6] Thus, the tonic–clonic seizure episode often begins as a brief simple or complex partial seizure. The warning, or "aura," that patients often describe is actually the beginning of a seizure that is perceived while the person is conscious and is actually a simple partial seizure.

Tonic–clonic seizures consist of two phases: the tonic phase and the clonic phase. These phases are easily identified with a careful history. During the tonic phase, there is a sudden stiffening of all extremities. The epileptic cry may occur during this phase as a result of sudden diaphragmatic contraction. After a brief period, the extremities become tremulous. As the tremor slows in frequency, it evolves into a rhythmic jerking motion—the clonic phase. As the seizure ends, the jerking slows and ceases. After a tonic–clonic seizure, the person is invariably groggy and disoriented for several minutes. Absence of the tonic phase or postictal confusion and somnolence in a person with convulsive behavior should raise the question of nonepileptic episodes, including psychogenic seizures. However, the postictal state may be fleeting or indiscernible after brief complex partial seizures, and absent following simple partial seizures. Thus, a minimal or absent postictal state does not exclude seizures when convulsive activity does not occur. A recent monograph by Lüders and Noachtar[7] is a useful reference for defining the clinical semiology of seizures.

Acute medical management is similar for both partial and tonic–clonic seizures. If semiconscious, the patient should be gently directed away from harm. During a convulsion, the patient should be rolled to one side to avoid aspiration if vomiting occurs. Contrary to common belief, the tongue cannot be swallowed or bitten off, and objects should never be forced into the patient's mouth. Insertion of hard objects, such as spoons or "bite sticks," may break teeth and cause serious complications of fragment aspiration and pneumonia. A soft oral airway may be used, if it is easily inserted. If available, oxygen via face mask may be provided, as well as suction, if needed.

Epilepsy, by definition, consists of recurrent seizures. As with seizures, epilepsies have been classified. In the instance of epilepsy, the classification is into epilepsy syndromes, defined by seizure type, EEG features, etiology, and natural history.

Primary generalized epilepsies, including absence ("petit mal"), myoclonic, and generalized convulsive epilepsy, commonly begin during childhood or adolescence and are usually idiopathic or genetic in etiology. These epilepsies are diagnosed by their distinctive patterns on the EEG, which consist of bilateral synchronous epileptiform patterns. Their onset in patients following TBI is highly unusual and should be considered coincidental. It is important to identify these epilepsy syndromes because primary generalized seizures, especially absence and myoclonic seizures, do not respond to, or may be worsened by, medications used for partial-onset seizures, such as phenytoin, carbamazepine, and oxecarbazepine.[8,9] It is important to note that epilepsy itself may result in trauma and TBI, and preexisting epilepsy should be considered in patients with TBI and primary generalized epilepsy.[10]

2.4 Etiologic Considerations

Risk factors for posttraumatic epilepsy have been examined in several population studies. However, it is difficult to resolve the relative risk of specific characteristics of injury, such as presence of intracranial bleeding and depth of injury, because these markers tend not to be independent variables. For example, although concussion (with loss of consciousness) has been considered a risk factor for posttraumatic epilepsy, patients with mild concussive injury alone have only a 0.6% risk of seizures within 5 years, which is not significantly increased over the incidence of new seizures in the general population.[1]

Data from World War II, the Korean War, and the Vietnam War have provided information on risk factors for posttraumatic epilepsy. Overall, the risk for epilepsy following nonmissile head injury was 24% in World War II[11] and 12% during the Korean War.[12] Interestingly, the risk of epilepsy following penetrating missile injury was about 35% for both World War II and the Korean War, but was much higher (53%) in the Vietnam War.[13] The differences between studies on Vietnam War veterans and previous war veterans may relate both to improved care of head injury and differences in the nature of injuries. In particular, high-velocity rifles were used in combat during the Vietnam War and, when combined with improved surgical care, may have resulted in a greater percentage of survivors with epileptogenic lesions. TBI is an important source of morbidity in survivors of war-induced injury in the Iraq and Afghanistan wars. Explosion or blast injury is the most common cause of war injuries in the current conflicts in Iraq and Afganistan.[14,15] The effect of blast-induced TBI on subsequent development of posttraumatic encephalopathy is unknown.[16] There are no data on the risk of posttraumatic epilepsy resulting from blast-induced TBI.

Risk factors have also been studied in nonmilitary injuries. As mentioned earlier, mild head injuries do not present an increased risk of posttraumatic epilepsy. The incidence of posttraumatic epilepsy after moderate head injuries is 1.6%, and 11.6% after severe injuries.[1] On review of military and nonmilitary injuries, similar risk factors appear. Early seizures (onset less than 1 week after TBI) also appear to be a risk factor for subsequent seizures in several series,[17] but the increased risk appears to be dependent on the severity of head injury.[1] In civilian head injuries, early seizures are not predictive of seizure recurrence when the head injury is mild, yet do appear to increase risk in moderate to severe injuries.[1] In children, seizures occurring immediately after minor head trauma are more common, although not necessarily predictive of subsequent epilepsy.[1] The time of seizure onset also appears to be predictive of seizure recurrence. In wartime injuries, early seizures are associated with seizure recurrence, and the risk of seizure recurrence increases if the onset is greater than 1 week.[18] More recently, Angeleri et al.[19] reported that the risk of posttraumatic epilepsy was 8.58% higher for those individuals with early seizures, and 3.43% greater for individuals with frontal or temporal lesions on computed tomographic (CT) scanning. The degree of hypoperfusion in the temporal lobes as detected by single photon emission computed tomography has also been correlated with posttraumatic epilepsy.[20] Also associated with the increased risk of posttraumatic epilepsy (+3.49%) was the presence of an EEG focus at 1 month.

The risk of posttraumatic epilepsy in the presence of an intracerebral hematoma was estimated at 21% in nonmilitary injuries.[1] However, Guidice and Berchou[21] found intracerebral hematomas *not* to be predictive of posttraumatic epilepsy. This may be a result of the fact that CT scans were used routinely in all head-injured patients at their center. Earlier studies, which did not utilize CT scanning, would not have detected intracerebral hemorrhage in milder cases that did not require surgery or cerebral angiography. Alternatively, other studies have argued that the most predictive factor for posttraumatic seizures is focal CT abnormalities.[17,22] Brain contusion with subdural hematoma was predictive of posttraumatic epilepsy in a population-based study.[23] In one small series, the development of posttraumatic epilepsy was correlated with the presence of bone fragments on CT scan studies[24]; however, the scope of this study could not establish whether the risk of bone fragments was independent of injury severity. The type of skull fracture also tends to predict the likelihood of posttraumatic epilepsy. Greater risk occurs in patients with depressed skull fractures,[1,17] whereas linear convexity or basilar fractures carry an intermediate risk. The value of acute magnetic resonance imaging (MRI) studies in predicting posttraumatic epilepsy is unclear, although a relationship between abnormalities on magnetic transfer MRI and posttraumatic epilepsy has been reported.[25] Final risk factors for posttraumatic epilepsy include duration of coma,[1,21,23] genetic susceptibility to epilepsy,[26,27] and age older than 65 years.[23]

When the epidemiologic studies are viewed as a group, it appears that the severity of brain injury best predicts whether posttraumatic epilepsy will occur. Although there is debate on the relative risk of any single factor, it is likely that most identified risk factors are indicators of a high degree of brain injury, rather than being specific etiologies. Furthermore, posttraumatic epileptogenesis is probably dependent on several pathophysiologic mechanisms (discussed later in this chapter), which may explain in part the large number of identified risk factors.

2.5 Diagnostic Investigations of Posttraumatic Seizures

The evaluation of the first seizures in adults is focused on determining the presence of a possibly treatable CNS lesion and on defining the risk for recurrence with an EEG. There is evidence that supports the use of EEG brain imaging with CT or MRI as part of the routine neurodiagnostic evaluation of adults presenting with an apparent unprovoked first seizure. Laboratory tests, such as blood counts, blood glucose, and electrolyte panels (particularly sodium), lumbar puncture, and toxicology screening may be helpful as determined by the specific clinical circumstances based on the history, and physical and neurologic examinations, but there are insufficient data to support or refute recommending any of these tests for the routine evaluation of adults presenting with an apparent first unprovoked seizure.[28]

The EEG is a useful tool for evaluating patients with episodic behavioral changes. Interictal abnormalities, such as epileptiform spikes or sharp waves, are often present in patients with epilepsy. A difficulty arises in that interictal abnormalities are transient, much like the seizures they attempt to detect. Thus, a normal EEG does not exclude the possibility of epilepsy. Conversely, an abnormal EEG alone does not diagnose epilepsy. As discussed in later sections, there are important consequences of AED therapy; thus, it is crucial that patients with TBI not be treated solely on the basis of EEG findings. The EEG does provide supportive evidence of a seizure disorder when it is clinically suspected, and its greatest utility lies in its ability to help identify whether the seizure onset is partial or generalized. Despite its limitations, the EEG is one of the most important tests in evaluating epilepsy because it provides electrophysiologic information that cannot be obtained from any other laboratory investigation.

For example, a retrospective study of EEG findings in patients with head injury revealed no predictive value of focal or generalized EEG abnormalities.[29] However, this study included all abnormalities and did not specifically assess the risk of epileptiform patterns. The EEG is valuable as a prognostic factor in persons who have already experienced a seizure. The interictal hallmark of epilepsy is the epileptiform spike or sharp wave. When well formed and definite, focal spikes are predictive of seizure recurrence in both brain-injured patients[30] and in patients with seizures of unidentified causes.[31] Focal EEG findings 1 month following TBI was associated with an increased risk of subsequent epilepsy in a prospective study of risk factors following an early seizure.[19]

The value of *prolonged* EEG monitoring after TBI has been promoted as a means of detecting subclinical seizures and even predicting posttraumatic epilepsy.[32] Postinjury EEG assessment revealed that subclinical seizures occur frequently despite anticonvulsant drug administration.[32] As many as 22% of TBI individuals have postinjury seizures within the first 2 weeks,[32] many of which are subclinical. Postinjury EEG monitoring may help define the affect of seizure activity on patient outcomes, especially with regard to the risk for subsequent epilepsy.

The EEG study should follow the technical guidelines of the American EEG Society.[33] To summarize briefly, all studies should utilize at least 16 channels of EEG recording to allow for adequate spatial resolution and localization of EEG abnormalities. Gold disk electrodes should be used and attached to the scalp with either collodion or electrode paste to ensure low electrical impedance. Needle electrodes should not be used because of their high impedance and the potential risk of blood-borne pathogens. Standard EEG montages should be used, per recommendations of the American EEG Society. Digital EEG recordings are now routinely obtained, which allows for reformatting the montages, if necessary. Drowsiness and sleep-enhanced expression of epileptiform abnormalities and recording during these stages of consciousness must be performed. The patient should be partially sleep deprived during the night prior to the EEG study because this will increase the probability of recording epileptiform abnormalities and avoid the need for sedation.

There has been much debate regarding the advantages of special EEG electrodes used to improve the detection of interictal abnormalities. Nasopharyngeal electrodes are now rarely used. Standard scalp electrodes with high-distance electrode montages are as effective as nasopharyngeal electrodes at detecting epileptiform abnormalities and are considerably more comfortable.[34,35] Other scalp electrodes (such as T1 and T2 electrodes) increase sensitivity to temporal spikes.[36]

Prolonged EEG recording may be extremely useful in cases when the cause of altered mental status episodes cannot be ascertained by conventional means and the spells occur with enough frequency to be detected within the designated recording period. Twenty-four-hour ambulatory EEG monitoring is usually available at larger medical centers. These devices continually record EEG and electrocardiographic activity for 1 to 2 days and may be performed on an outpatient basis. Newer digital equipment allows for higher quality recordings than was possible in the past, with analogue recordings that were often limited to eight channels. Nevertheless, there are several limitations to ambulatory recording. Artifact makes interpretation of ambulatory EEGs difficult, and technologists must review large amounts of data. Because EEG technicians or other health care staff are not present to observe the recording, it may be difficult later to sort artifact from true abnormalities during playback. Moreover, if a diary is not carefully maintained during the recording period or the patient is unable to trigger the alarm on the recording unit reliably, it may not be possible to correlate the episodes in question with the EEG or electrocardiogram, or the episode may even be missed entirely.

Video EEG monitoring involves continuous recording of EEG, electrocardiographic, and other electrophysiologic data with simultaneous video recording of behavior. These studies allow precise correlation of behavioral changes with electrophysiologic data to determine the exact etiologies of the behavioral episodes. Such monitoring is costly and requires hospital admission; however, it may provide the only means to obtain definitive and conclusive information.

2.6 Potential Epileptogenesis Associated with Psychotropic Medications

Behavioral and affective disorders are common after TBI, and it is often necessary to treat the brain-injured patient with psychotropic medications. Of concern is whether these agents lower seizure threshold. In high doses, tricyclic antidepressants induce seizures, but it is less clear to what extent they are proconvulsant at clinically effective doses. Many reports of tricyclic-induced seizures are retrospective and do not take into account the normal incidence of new-onset seizures. When drug monitoring has been instituted to avoid high levels, the risk has been estimated at only 0.4%.[37] Although a 0.2% risk of seizures has been estimated for fluoxetine therapy on the basis of preclinical trials, fluoxetine is anticonvulsant in experiments using epileptic rodents with convulsive seizures.[38] In a retrospective study of persons with depression and established epilepsy, antidepressant therapy actually improved seizure frequency in the majority (56%) of patients.[39] This raises the question of whether this positive effect on seizure control occurs indirectly (i.e., through improvement of depression) or, instead, by directly raising seizure threshold. Interestingly, a double-blind placebo study has demonstrated imipramine to be effective adjunctive antiepileptic therapy in intractable atonic, myoclonic–astatic epilepsy and absence epilepsy in subjects without affective problems.[40,41] Thus, at nontoxic levels, tricyclic antidepressants may have anticonvulsant properties for certain seizure types, despite being proconvulsant at toxic levels. This bimodal response is frequently seen in other drugs with anticonvulsant properties, such as phenytoin and lidocaine.

The ability of tricyclic antidepressants to increase seizure frequency may be selective for seizure type. For example, a selective increase of tonic–clonic seizures may occur with the use of imipramine or maprotiline in patients with mixed seizure types.[41] Neuroleptics are frequently utilized during the posttraumatic state for agitated behavior and there are several reports of their proconvulsant effect. Unfortunately, little data exist on the actual risks of antidepressants and neuroleptics in the setting of TBI. However, from existing information on these agents, it appears that the actual clinical risk of seizure exacerbation by psychotropic medications is small and is usually far outweighed by the need to manage effectively a severe affective or disruptive state in patients with TBI.[42] Thus, these medications should be used when necessary for psychiatric and behavioral problems. As a caveat, although neuroleptics may not pose a risk for seizures after TBI, there are data showing that the administration of these drugs is detrimental to neurobehavioral recovery in this population.[43]

2.7 Therapy for Posttraumatic Epilepsy

It is common practice to initiate AEDs following acute TBI as prophylaxis against seizures. In acute treatment of severe brain injury, acute prophylactic treatment with AEDs, especially phenytoin and fosphenytoin, is common. Jones et al.[44] have recently demonstrated that levetiracetam is equal in efficacy to phenytoin in acute treatment in patients with severe TBI. With fewer drug–drug interactions, levetiracetam may become the preferred AED for acute TBI. Such treatment decreases the risk of early seizures but does not appear to prevent late-occurring seizures—that is, posttraumatic epilepsy. Studies on acute prophylaxis regarding the use of newer AEDs, other than levetiracetam, are lacking.[45,46]

Long-term prophylactic treatment with AEDs has not been shown to prevent subsequent development of posttraumatic epilepsy. As described in later sections, and based on a meta-analysis of anticonvulsant prophylaxis trials,[47] as well as a practice parameter published by the American Academy of Neurology, there are clearly no firm data to justify long-term prophylactic AED therapy in patients with TBI who have not experienced a late-occurring seizure.[46] Although some advocate prophylactic use of Mg^{++}, a clinical trial failed to demonstrate efficacy of magnesium sulfate used acutely for protection from posttraumatic epilepsy.[48]

It is appropriate to treat those who experience late-occurring seizures—that is, post-traumatic epilepsy. Initiation of AED therapy should begin only after careful evaluation of the patient, and after seizures have been clearly identified. Almost all clinicians will begin therapy after two seizures have occurred, but there is debate regarding whether therapy should be initiated after the first seizure. Many clinicians will not treat a single seizure without recurrence; others *will* treat, depending on the situation. Selection of AED therapy must be based on several factors, including efficacy for seizure type and side effects. A specific AED may be quite selective for seizure type, thus necessitating seizure classification. Posttraumatic epilepsy is caused by focal or multifocal injury and consists of partial-onset seizures and secondarily generalized tonic–clonic seizures. Accordingly, appropriate AEDs for posttraumatic epilepsy are those used for partial-onset seizures. The most commonly used AEDs are listed in Table 2.1.

The effectiveness of AED in the treatment of epilepsy of all etiologies has been extensively examined. A multicenter, double-blind, randomized study compared the efficacy of phenytoin, carbamazepine, primidone, and phenobarbital against partial-onset seizures. All the drugs were equally efficacious in terms of seizure control.[49] However, barbiturates were tolerated poorly, resulting in a high dropout rate in these treatment groups.

Similar results were obtained in a British study involving patients with newly diagnosed partial-onset epilepsy that compared the efficacy of carbamazepine, phenytoin, and valproic acid.[50] Valproic acid exhibited the same efficacy as phenytoin and carbamazepine against partial-onset seizures and convulsion, suggesting its usefulness for these seizure types. A Veterans' Administration study compared the efficacy of carbamazepine to valproic acid for partial-onset seizures and indicated a modest but significantly lower efficacy of valproic acid against complex partial seizures.[51] Nevertheless, valproic acid appeared to be equally effective to carbamazepine against secondarily generalized tonic–clonic seizures. Because valproic acid is generally well tolerated, it should be considered for patients who are unresponsive or intolerant to carbamazepine. Kwan and Brodie[52] likewise have found that carbamazepine, valproate, and lamotrigine all had equal efficacy in newly diagnosed patients with epilepsy, although tolerability differed. More patients on carbamazepine changed medication as a result of adverse events than those on the other two drugs.[52]

All AEDs may cause significant problems with adverse effects, especially neurotoxicity, and may pose problems for patients with TBI. Indeed, several AEDs commonly cause ataxia at high levels and may also exacerbate gait abnormalities at lower levels, in some patients. This may present a problem to the patient who is returning to ambulation. There is a significant incidence of hyponatremia in carbamazepine-treated patients older than 25 years of age,[53] as well as in those taking oxcarbazepine.[54] Postural tremor is a common side effect of valproic acid that may pose a problem to patients with TBI and can be particularly troublesome in patients who are prone to postural tremor. The tremor is reversible, dose dependent, and responds to a dose reduction or other medications that block essential tremor (propranolol, primidone). Because the barbiturates, including phenobarbital and primidone, are poorly tolerated and result in a high incidence of cognitive impairment, they should not be used as first-line drugs, but rather should be used in patients refractory to other antiepileptic medications. All AEDs carry the potential for cognitive impairment, and attention to their potential effects on CNS function is necessary.[55]

Ten new AEDs (felbamate, gabapentin, lamotrigine, levetiracetam, oxcarbazepine, pregabalin, rufinamide, tiagabine, topiramate, and zonisamide) have been approved by the Food and Drug Administration (FDA) since 1993, predominantly for use as adjunctive therapy in partial-onset seizures. In general, they appear to have high therapeutic indices (i.e., a wide window between efficacy and toxicity) and have been demonstrated

TABLE 2.1

Guide to AED Dosing and Adverse Effects

Medication, Target Dose (pediatric dose), mg/kg/day	Target Serum Levels, µg/mL	Type of Idiosyncratic Effect	Type of Dose-Related Effect	Type of Age-Specific/ Other Effect
Carbamazepine, 1000–2000 (10–30)	4–12	Dermatologic rash, including Stevens-Johnson, rare hematologic, hepatic	Vertigo, visual disturbance (diplopia), leukopenia	Hyponatremia in adults, leukopenia, liver induction, myoclonus in patients with generalized spike wave on electroencephalogram
Ethosuximide, 1000 (15–40)	40–100	Leukopenia, systemic lupus erythematosus, nephrotic syndrome, rash	Sedation, GI upset	Behavioral
Felbamate, 2400–3600 (45–60)	30–100	Aplastic anemia, hepatic failure, rash (rare)	Anorexia, insomnia, headache, irritability	Aplastic anemia, drug interactions
Gabapentin, 1800–3600 (30–100)	4–20	Rash (rare)	Somnolence, irritability, weight gain	Renal excretion, no drug interactions
Lamotrigine, 300–500 (1–15); dose depends on concomitant medication	3–20	Rash, hypersensitive reaction	Ataxia, diplopia, GI upset, headache	Rash (1%–5% in children), Stevens-Johnson
Levetiracetam, 1200–3000 (20–100)	5–50	None reported to date	Somnolence, ataxia	Agitation, aggression, depression
Oxcarbazepine, 1200–2400 (15–45)	Monohydroxy derivative: 10–55	Rash (25% cross-reactivity with carbamazepine)	CNS, diplopia	Hyponatremia (3% of adults)
Phenobarbital, 60–120 (2–6)	15–40	Rash, Stevens-Johnson, systemic lupus erythematosus	Somnolence, irritability	Possible irreversible cognitive effects, liver induction
Phenytoin, 200–600 (4–8)	10–20	Rash (5%–10%), hematologic, hepatic, lymphadenopathy, others	Cosmetic, CNS, ataxia, nystagmus	Elevated LFTs, induction, reduced vitamin D, cerebellar degeneration?
Pregabalin, 150–600 mg/ day (no established pediatric dose)	None established	Edema, weight gain	Dizziness, sleepiness, ataxia, headache	Avoid abrupt discontinuation, also approved for pain (SCHEDULE V substance)
Primidone, 750–2000 (5–20)	4–12	Rash	Sedation, irritability, GI upset	Similar to phenobarbital
Rufinamide, 400–3200 (10–45)	None established	Multiorgan hypersensitivity syndrome	Somnolence, ataxia	Indicated for Lennox–Gastaut syndrome

(continued)

TABLE 2.1 (continued)

Guide to AED Dosing and Adverse Effects

Medication, Target Dose (pediatric dose), mg/kg/day	Target Serum Levels, μg/mL	Type of Idiosyncratic Effect	Type of Dose-Related Effect	Type of Age-Specific/ Other Effect
Tiagabine, 32–56 (0.25–1.25)	5–70	Psychiatric	CNS, tremor, weakness, gastroesophageal reflux, gait difficulty	
Topiramate, 200–400 (5–25)	3–25	Rash (rare), acute glaucoma (rare)	Somnolence, memory disturbance, renal stones, paraesthesia	Language and cognitive disturbance (especially with polypharmacy), oligohidrosis
Valproic acid, 750–1500 (20–60)	50–150	Hepatic failure, pancreatitis	Tremor, weight gain, alopecia, sedation and cognitive changes, thrombocytopenia, prolonged bleeding time	Hepatic failure (1 in 500 younger than age 2 on polypharmacy), elevated LFTs; GI upset with syrup; incidence of polycystic ovary syndrome unknown; liver enzyme inhibition; teratogenicity
Vigabatrin, maximum of 3000 (49–100)	—	Visual field constriction, sedation, CNS	Psychiatric symptoms (rare), visual field constriction	Especially effective for infantile spasms and tuberous sclerosis
Zonisamide, 200–600 (4–10)	10–30	Rash, hematologic, hepatic	Renal stones, anorexia, somnolence	Oligohidrosis in children, cross-sensitivity with sulfa drugs

For newer drugs, doses, levels, and adverse effects are based on reported clinical experience and not on adequate scientific information from clinical trials in most cases. Some medications do not have Food and Drug Administration approval for children. The package insert for each medication lists potential adverse effects, warnings, and so forth. CNS, central nervous system; GI, gastrointestinal; LFT, liver function test.

to be effective and safe in controlled studies.[56–59] Improved pharmacokinetics provide an additional advantage of some of these newer AEDs, including renal clearance, the lack of significant protein binding, and the absence of CyP450 induction.[59] However, serious idiosyncratic adverse effects can occur. The use of felbamate has been restricted by the FDA for use in severe, intractable epilepsy because of a significant risk of aplastic anemia estimated by the FDA to be 1 in 2000. Lamotrigine is associated with a risk of serious rash in approximately 1 in 1000 patients, usually at onset of therapy. Vigabatrin has not been approved for use in the United States, in part because of potential retinal toxicity. In addition, treatment-emergent side effects can be troublesome. For example, topiramate is associated with word-finding difficulties in some patients, particularly at higher doses or when the drug is used in polypharmacy. Gabapentin may cause weight gain and somnolence. Levetiracetam may cause behavioral side effects. Although monitoring serum drug levels, complete blood counts, and liver function tests are not required with most of the new AEDs (with the notable exception of felbamate), the difficulty in assessing the clinical status of patients with significant traumatic encephalopathy may make such monitoring advisable. Practitioners should take advantage of published reviews of these drugs in textbooks and journals to familiarize themselves with their use.

In a systematic review of efficacy and tolerability of the newer AEDs, Marson and Chadwick[60] found no statistical differences between gabapentin, lamotrigine, tiagabine, topiramate, vigabatrin, and zonisamide. Nevertheless, the addition of these new drugs will provide alternatives for patients who do not tolerate or respond to current AEDs. Undoubtedly, they will be tested in posttraumatic epilepsy and may provide a better armamentarium for this problem.

In general, all AEDs should be introduced slowly to avoid problems with neurotoxicity, including somnolence and altered mental status. If introduced too quickly, carbamazepine may cause severe dizziness; lamotrigine may precipitate a serious rash. However, when multiple seizures or status epilepticus occurs, loading with phenytoin is often effective in controlling seizures. For intravenous use, fosphenytoin is better tolerated than phenytoin. Valproic acid is also available for intravenous use and can be used in relatively high doses, acutely, if necessary. Levetiracetam is also available for intravenous administration and appears to be well tolerated at therapeutic starting doses. The intravenous preparations of these drugs may be useful for patients who are unable to take oral medications (e.g., after surgical procedures). With all AEDs, clinical efficacy and tolerability determine appropriate dosing. Most of the newer AEDs do not have well-established therapeutic plasma levels, but, nevertheless, the presence of significant traumatic encephalopathy may make determination of AED plasma levels appropriate. Drug plasma levels may be utilized to provide a rough guideline for therapy but should not be used as the sole indicator of therapy or toxicity.[61] It should be noted that plasma steady state is not achieved for up to seven half-lives of a medication, so that levels are rarely useful acutely after dosing changes.

Phenytoin is unique among the commonly used AEDs in that it saturates binding sites at therapeutic levels, which results in zero-order kinetics. As a result of nonlinear kinetics, there is a proportionate increase of serum level at low doses of phenytoin, but at therapeutic levels, small increments result in marked elevations of levels.[62] In addition, phenytoin and valproic acid compete for protein binding, increasing the potential for dose-related toxicity and making routine measurements of phenytoin levels inappropriate when used in combination with valproate. Rather, unbound phenytoin levels should be obtained through reference laboratories because they are not routinely available in most hospital laboratories. Also of note are the kinetics of Dilantin Kapseals, which allow once-a-day dosing, not true for phenytoin suspension or chewable 50-mg tablets. Extended release formulations of several AEDs are now available, including levetiracetam and valproate, allowing for once-a-day dosing, which may aid in adherence to dosing regimens.

The use of phenytoin, carbamazepine, and oxcarbazepine suspensions may be useful in patients who cannot swallow tablets or capsules. However, care must be taken to shake the bottle adequately before administering a dose to allow for even distribution of drug in the solution. Levetiracetam and phenobarbital are available as solutions. Lamotrigine, levetiracetam, and zonisamide can be dissolved and given as a solution. Both valproic acid and topiramate are available as sprinkle capsules, but they cannot be given through gastric tubes because of the tendency of the sprinkles to adhere to the tubing.

Several AEDs have been evaluated for their potential neuroprotective effects, including antiepileptogenicity, in both experimental and clinical studies. Temkin[47] performed a meta-analysis of 47 studies of the effectiveness of anticonvulsant drug administration for seizure prevention and antiepileptogenicity. Of these, 13 were conducted after TBI. There was no good evidence to support that anticonvulsant drug administration after TBI is antiepileptogenic in the long term, although acutely (within the first week), there was seizure reduction associated with phenytoin,[63] carbamazepine,[64] and levetiracetam.[44] Temkin[47] emphasizes the need for "rigorous clinical trials" (p. 522) to determine the drug's antiepileptogenic effects as well as any neurobehavioral costs. She goes further to state that "[c]linical use of any drug to prevent epileptogenesis should be avoided until clinical trials have proven the drug to be effective for that purpose."[47, p. 522] More recently, after the completion of additional clinical trials, this same sentiment is echoed: "None of the drugs studied (phenytoin, phenobarbital, their combination, carbamazepine, valproate, or magnesium) has shown reliable evidence that they prevent, or even suppress, epileptic seizures after TBI."[65, p. 10]

It is likely that there are individual differences in response to, and tolerance of, any given AED. Therefore, additional medications should be tried in patients who have failed to respond to, or who are unable to tolerate, initial treatment. In all cases, the therapeutic plan should strive for a single AED regimen. Monotherapy has been shown to be more efficacious than polytherapy and minimizes toxicity, drug interactions, and cost.[66] Patients who fail to respond to two or more AEDs used in appropriate doses are likely to remain resistant to pharmacotherapy. Other options, such as epilepsy surgery, should be considered in patients who are resistant to medication treatment.

2.8 Mechanisms and Models of Posttraumatic Epilepsy

When considering the appropriate treatment of posttraumatic epilepsy, it is worthwhile to understand the mechanisms whereby trauma leads to the epileptogenic state. Studies of posttraumatic epileptogenesis implicate several potential pathologic etiologies that may result in a seizure focus. These etiologies can be broadly separated into those related to the acute or primary insult (i.e., penetration of parenchyma, shearing forces, and disruption of the blood–brain barrier) and those caused by late or secondary sequelae (i.e., vascular disruption, cicatricial pulling, and synaptic reorganization). Given the wide variations of brain injury and complications, it is unlikely that any single mechanism is responsible for posttraumatic epileptogenesis. Thus, posttraumatic epileptogenesis probably utilizes combinations of several mechanisms, many of which are supported by scientific studies and concur with clinical aspects of this type of epilepsy.

In 1930, Foerster and Penfield[67] induced seizure activity by electrical stimulation of areas surrounding a gunshot lesion of cerebral cortex. These findings suggested the presence of an epileptic zone, or penumbra, surrounding the site of injury. Furthermore, retraction of dura that had become adherent to the damaged cortex also triggered seizures. They concluded that posttraumatic seizures are most likely to occur after dural penetration, which induces formation of scar tissue between brain and dura, and subsequent pulling of the ipsilateral and, sometimes, contralateral hemispheres toward the lesion, as a result of contraction brought about by normal maturation of the scar (cicatricial contraction).[67] This hypothesis is supported by clinical findings that head injuries associated with dural penetration are associated with the highest incidence of posttraumatic epilepsy (27%–43%).[27]

Additional putative mechanisms include glial cell proliferation and damage to blood vessels, axon collaterals, and the blood–brain barrier, each of which is known to precipitate brain injury.[68] Jasper[68] hypothesized that the toxicity of extravasated blood increases neuronal activity abnormally in some brain regions and disrupts blood flow in others. These pathophysiologic changes could result in the alternating periods of seizure activity and functional neuronal depression that characterize acute status epilepticus induced by brain contusion.[68] Alternatively, damage to inhibitory axon collaterals by shearing forces may result in reduction of inhibitory tone and excessive depolarization that ultimately produce seizure discharges.[68] Overt penetration of dura and disruption of brain parenchyma may not be absolute requisites for posttraumatic epilepsy.

Lowenstein et al.[69] reported that extradural fluid percussion induces profound decreases in hippocampal hilar neurons and hyperexcitability of dentate granule cells in rodents. Postinjury hyperexcitability in the granule cell and molecular layer of the dentate gyrus has been shown to be persistent (observable at 15 weeks) and pervasive (e.g., bilateral).[70] Measures taken at earlier time points throughout the hippocampus revealed dramatic physiologic and receptor-mediated disruptions in excitatory–inhibitory balance, with the changes being time dependent and only observable ipsilateral to the site of TBI.[71,72] Thus, even nonpenetrating brain injury can cause pathologic changes in distal structures, possibly tipping the balance in favor of posttraumatic seizures. These findings could help explain the emergence of posttraumatic epilepsy in persons with milder, low-velocity head injuries who do not appear to have frank penetration of dura or intracerebral bleeding.

Because penetrating brain injuries carry the greatest risk for posttraumatic epilepsy, disruption in the blood–brain barrier[73] and/or alterations in blood flow may play a role. Not only does brain injury disrupt vascularization at the site of damage, but areas "downstream" from the insult are also affected. Disruption in blood flow could bring about both ischemic and hypoxic conditions that produce significant increases in synaptic glutamate release and decreased inactivation of glutamate. Overactivation of glutamate receptors, including N-methyl-D-aspartate (NMDA) receptor activation, results in excessive Ca^{++} influx,[74] which promotes phosphorylation of the γ-aminobutyric acid A ($GABA_A$) receptor to its nonfunctional, desensitized state.[75] Trauma has also been associated with GABA-mediated Ca^{++} influx,[76,77] which would not only lead to depolarization, but also would potentially lead to cell death. Loss of inhibitory neurons, coupled with other trauma-induced disruptions in normal brain function, could result in a state that both primes the brain for acute seizures and provides the foundation for long-term epileptogenic changes.

A related hypothesis implicates blood breakdown products, particularly hemosiderin, in the cellular events that lead to epileptogenesis. An important role for iron deposition has been supported by experimental studies in animals. Subpial iontophoresis of ferrous or ferric chloride into the sensorimotor cortex of cat or rat induces a chronic epileptic focus with many striking similarities to lesions in human posttraumatic epilepsy.[78,79] Electrocorticographic seizure activity is observed within 48 hours after injection, and behavioral convulsions occur between 48 hours and 5 days. These abnormalities recur spontaneously and persist for more than 12 weeks after injection.[79] Examination of the iron-induced focus reveals many histopathologic changes found in posttraumatic epileptic foci from humans.[78,79] A meningocerebral cicatrix, consisting of fibroblasts and iron-laden macrophages, surrounds the iron injection cavity with neuronal loss and gliosis occurring next to the injection site. Hypertrophied astrocytes encompass the entire iron focus. It has been hypothesized that a cascade of events is initiated by the iron focus, resulting in the genesis of a posttraumatic epileptic focus. Breakdown of blood from brain injury-induced extravasation creates iron deposits that may induce free radical oxidant formation and subsequent lipid peroxidation.[80] In support of this hypothesis is the finding that antioxidant administration reduces the incidence of iron-induced seizure activity.[80]

The possibility of hemosiderin deposition leading to posttraumatic epilepsy has also been studied in humans.[19] After TBI, magnetic resonance images were utilized to detect the presence of hemosiderin, gliosis, or both. Eighty-one percent of patients showed evidence of hemosiderin deposits. Although there was no correlation between the presence of hemosiderin, alone, and posttraumatic epilepsy, the presence of cortical hemosiderin surrounded by a "gliotic wall" was significantly correlated with the development of post-traumatic epilepsy.

The mechanisms discussed so far largely address seizure activity that occurs acutely following brain injury. However, the onset of posttraumatic seizures is bimodal; the highest incidence occurs during the first week (early-onset seizures; Figure 2.1) with a secondary peak occurring at about 6 months.[81] This latency suggests there is a maturation process resulting in the genesis of an epileptic focus. Because the latent period can last months to years after the insult in humans,[81] most of what we know about the mechanisms underlying posttraumatic epileptogenesis comes from animal models.

Modeling posttraumatic epilepsy in animals poses quite a challenge. First, not only is it difficult to evoke spontaneous seizures secondary to TBI, chronically monitoring animals to determine when (and if) subconvulsive versus convulsive seizures occur is an enormous task. Second, because the goals of animal models vary, it may not be possible to test all aspects of interest in every model. For example, a model of posttraumatic epilepsy that attempts to mimic the postinsult latent period may not allow for neurobehavioral assessment of acute postinsult seizures or anticonvulsant drug administration. In addition, such a model may not use trauma as the precipitating event. Alternatively, a model designed to assess postinjury neurobehavioral change may not allow for the assessment of the spontaneous epileptogenic process. With these limitations in mind, discussion of some of the animal models is worthwhile.

Status epilepticus, induced by excitotoxins (e.g., kainic acid or pilocarpine)[83,84] or electrical stimulation,[85–87] has been proposed to share commonalities with posttraumatic epileptogenesis.[88] The initial precipitating insult of prolonged seizures is followed by a latent period, after which spontaneous seizures occur. Like experimentally induced TBI, status epilepticus results in dramatic and significant morphologic, physiologic, and neurochemical alterations. Indeed, the insult-associated plasticity and neuronal reorganization seen after experimentally induced insult via seizures or frank trauma appears to share similarities.[88,89] Likewise, another useful model involves the cortical "undercut method" in which the initial brain insult is followed by a dormant period after which cortical epilepsy is evident.[90] More recently, a model of posttraumatic epilepsy[91,92] has been developed that shows spontaneous seizures following severe lateral fluid percussion injury. Seizure activity and convulsive behavior were captured via ongoing video and EEG monitoring after lateral injury. Much like human posttraumatic epilepsy, the rodent posttraumatic epilepsy model also exhibits a latent period between injury and seizure onset, and once initiated, seizure activity progressively increases over time. Indeed, this transition from TBI to posttraumatic epilepsy has been proposed as an excellent model in rodents[93] and humans[94] within which to study potential antiepileptogenic drug efficacy. Despite this promising advance, this model has not been utilized to characterize fully the degree to which seizure activity and postinjury drug administration affect the process of *recovery from the brain injury itself*. For this reason, it is worth discussing the kindling model of epileptogenesis, which has been combined with a focal cortical lesion to model posttraumatic seizures, posttraumatic epilepsy, and the neurobehavioral consequences of these, as well as their treatment.[95,96]

The kindling model of epileptogenesis is a highly reliable phenomenon whereby a brain region can be rendered permanently epileptic when subjected to brief, repeated electrical stimulations that, alone, would not induce behavioral seizures.[97] Clinical evidence that "seizures beget seizures" is supported by a prospective study of unselected patients with new onset of seizures that demonstrated that the probability of seizure control

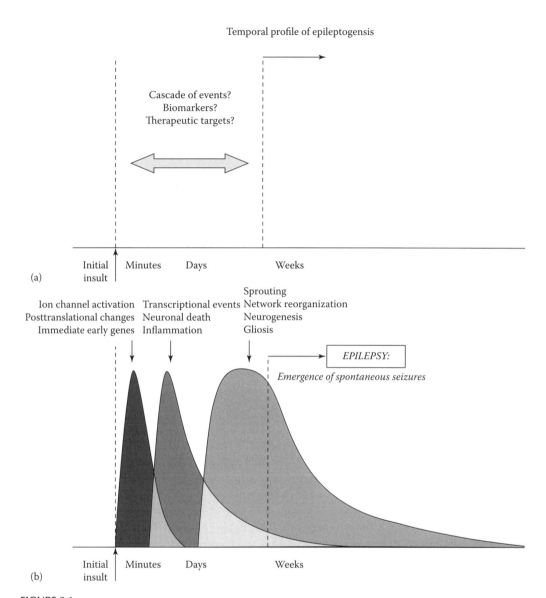

FIGURE 2.1

Time course of epileptogenesis. (a) An initial insult, such as TBI and/or status epilepticus occurs, followed by a "latent period" that lasts weeks to months or even years prior to the onset of spontaneous seizures. This latent period represents a period during which a cascade of molecular and cellular events alters network excitability to result in spontaneous epileptiform activity. This latent period is also an opportunity for biomarker development and therapeutic intervention. (b) The cascade of events that is currently suggested by experimental evidence can be classified temporally following the initial insult. Early changes occur within seconds to minutes, including induction of immediate early genes and posttranslational modification of receptor and ion channel-related proteins. Within hours to days, there can be neuronal death, inflammation, and altered transcriptional regulation of genes such as growth factors. A later phase that lasts weeks to months includes morphologic alterations such as mossy fiber sprouting, gliosis, and neurogenesis. (From Jensen, F. E., *Epilepsia*, 50(Suppl. 2), 1–3, 2009. With permission.)

was inversely related to the number of seizures experienced prior to initiation of AED therapy.[98,99] Furthermore, the time interval between seizures appears to decrease with subsequent episodes in untreated patients.[100]

The kindling paradigm in which the brain "learns" to seize has been used to study epileptogenesis and neuronal plasticity. Typically, electrical stimulation is administered by an implanted depth electrode and, initially, results only in a brief, localized epileptiform discharge on EEG, without a behavioral response. With continued daily stimulation, there are progressive increases in duration of both EEG epileptiform discharges and motor seizure activity.

The resulting convulsive behavior evolves through stages that are highly reproducible from animal to animal and may be graded by levels of behavioral severity.[101] Stage 0 is no behavioral response, stage 1 consists of chewing motion, and stage 2 consists of head nodding. At stage 3, the animal displays clonus jerking of forelimbs, and at stage 4 there is forelimb clonus with rearing onto hind limbs. The fifth and most severe stage consists of forelimb clonus with rearing and falling.

Electrical kindling of seizure activity induces neuronal changes within the brain that result in more severe generalized seizures from a stimulus that initially produced only focal seizure activity. Numerous transient and long-term changes occur during, and as a result of, electrical kindling, with the most dramatic being seen within the excitatory and inhibitory amino acid transmitter systems.[102–107] For example, kindling significantly reduces neuronal sensitivity to GABA; the changes are long lasting and may be seen at 4 and 12 weeks after the last fully kindled (stage 5) seizure.[108–111] Loss of sensitivity to GABA evolves during the course of kindling and correlates with seizure severity.[108] These changes are believed to result from a compensatory desensitization of the receptor in response to increased GABA release during the electrical kindling process.[112,113] Thus, the very mechanisms utilized by the brain to suppress kindling appear to be counterproductive and ultimately facilitate the kindling process.

Because sequelae of brain injury also elicit aberrations in the excitatory and inhibitory tone,[71] using the kindling model to produce postinjury epileptogenesis is a useful tool, particularly in combination with focal cortical damage. In this model,[95,96] injury severity is controlled using a reproducible focal cortical lesion[114,115] that induces behavioral deficits in animals similar to those seen in humans with brain injury.[116] This focal cortical lesion in animals does not routinely produce spontaneous convulsions, yet it does lower the seizure threshold in the amygdala. In our laboratory, we observed a 37% decrease in stage 5 seizure threshold following cortical lesion in comparison with fully kindled animals without lesions. Electrical kindling of the amygdala after focal cortical lesion is a useful and unique model because it allows for the study of the neurobehavioral affect of epileptogenesis (with and without anticonvulsant drug administration), while still controlling seizure severity, timing, and number.

2.9 Posttraumatic Seizures, Epilepsy, and Anticonvulsant Prophylaxis: Implications for Neurobehavioral Recovery

Brain damage resulting from TBI can significantly impair physical, cognitive, and social function. Recovery from such deficits can be variable, and permanent neurologic disability occurs in as many as 90,000 survivors of brain injury in the United States each year.[117]

These disabilities are further compounded by posttraumatic epilepsy, which results not only in spontaneous and unpredictable seizure recurrence, but also in toxicities associated with AED therapies. Individuals with posttraumatic epilepsy pose a special case, in that they are neither patients with only a brain injury, nor patients having only epilepsy. Thus, the treatment requirements for posttraumatic epilepsy extend well beyond those available for either the epilepsy or brain injury alone. This makes it difficult to generalize from the anticonvulsant drug toxicity and efficacy profiles obtained from epileptic subjects without brain injury, and few anticonvulsant drugs have been systematically investigated in patients with TBI alone.[43,46,118–120] Treatment strategies that acknowledge these complexities will improve patient quality of life.

The controversy surrounding whether anticonvulsants should be administered prophylactically requires assessing the potential neurobehavioral affect of seizures versus the risk of AED administration.[118,121,122] Anticonvulsants are often administered after brain injury even though they have not been found to be effective in preventing later development of posttraumatic epilepsy.[46,47] Several early studies suggested a beneficial effect of prophylactic anticonvulsant therapy,[123,124] but later controlled studies failed to support these findings.[65] For example, when studied in a double-blind, placebo-controlled, randomized manner, phenytoin administered following TBI had no affect on the later development of epilepsy, although it did reduce the incidence of early seizures (i.e., those occurring within the first week after injury).[45,63]

The lack of effectiveness of anticonvulsant drugs in preventing posttraumatic epilepsy is also paralleled in experimental kindling studies. Although many AEDs may block fully kindled convulsions in animals, they do not prevent the kindling process and do not prevent the increases in seizure severity. Specifically, phenytoin and carbamazepine may block seizures, but do not consistently prevent epileptogenesis from occurring.[125,126] In contrast, phenobarbital and benzodiazepines do appear to be antiepileptogenic in that they are effective in slowing the progression of amygdala-kindled seizures.[127–129] Valproic acid has also been found to retard the rate of amygdala kindling, but only when used at high doses with significant toxicities.[130,131] Antagonists that directly compete for the NMDA receptor inhibit the progression of electrically kindled seizures but have relatively less effect on seizures after kindling has been achieved.[132] This suggests a potential antiepileptogenic role of NMDA receptor antagonists that is independent of their ability to block acute seizures. A full-scale trial in which magnesium, which blocks the NMDA channel, was administered after TBI failed to show neurobehavioral benefits or antiepileptogenic effects.[64] Other transmitters have been targeted to determine their antiepileptogenicity in the kindling model as well. Administration of the alpha adrenergic receptor agonist clonidine can significantly retard the rate of evolution of kindled seizure stage; but, by itself, it does not block the fully established kindled seizure.[133,134] Thus, a key role of noradrenergic neurotransmission in the regulation of epileptogenesis has been proposed.[135,136]

The search for effective *antiepileptogenic* drugs may necessitate a change in current experimental drug development paradigms so that potential prophylactic drugs may be screened. Use of models of epilepsy, rather than acute seizures, holds great promise for the future development of antiepileptogenic drugs. These models include the electrical kindling paradigm, studies in genetically seizure-prone animals, and models in which the focal insult (e.g., status epilepticus, cortical "undercut," fluid percussion injury) is followed by a latent period and epilepsy.[88,90–92] Ultimately, however, the effectiveness of a drug as an antiepileptogenic agent will require prospective, placebo-controlled trials in TBI and other high-risk patients, with simultaneous assessment of neurobehavioral recovery.

Currently available AEDs do not appear to affect the pathophysiologic processes resulting in spontaneous seizure recurrence, and may be merely masking the outward manifestations of seizure activity. The question is: Does this come at a cost to the patient with TBI? The neurobehavioral effects of anticonvulsant drug therapy are known. Indeed, it has been argued that, because brain injury carries only an approximate 5% risk for posttraumatic epilepsy, the remaining 95% needlessly receive anticonvulsant medication[137] without evidence of the desired benefit. None of the drugs tested most rigorously to date display any antiepileptogenic effects, and some do not effectively suppress early seizure activity after TBI.[65] Patients with TBI may be unnecessarily exposed to the toxicities of anticonvulsant administration at a time when the brain is highly vulnerable to adverse drug effects. Even in normal volunteers, AEDs cause significant cognitive impairment, albeit minor in many cases.[138] Barbiturates commonly cause cognitive impairment, even at low doses.[139] For many drugs, however, toxic levels can account for some of their untoward effects. For example, it was initially suggested that carbamazepine induced less cognitive impairment than phenytoin.[140] When the data were reexamined so that patients with toxic phenytoin levels were removed from the study, no significant differences in cognitive impairment could be found between treatments.[141] A subsequent study, which maintained levels in therapeutic ranges, verified these findings.[139] Although valproic acid is thought to cause minimal problems with cognition, withdrawal of this medication improved psychometric scores.[142] In a study that included completely randomized assignment of drug versus placebo, phenytoin administration after TBI was associated with impaired function on several neuropsychological measures of cognition, which are among the most common and disabling problems faced by individuals with brain injury.[118] Phenytoin and carbamazepine have each been shown to affect psychomotor function adversely following brain injury, although this is reversible upon drug discontinuation.[120] The newer AEDs have not been studied for their effects on cognitive function in patients with TBI, although in individuals with epilepsy, many of these drugs exhibit a better neuropsychological profile than the older drugs[55,143] These negative consequences of treatment with AEDs on cognitive functioning are not surprising when one considers anticonvulsant drugs can adversely affect cognitive function in *nonbrain-injured individuals*[138,144,145] and that drug sensitivity is greater after brain injury. To address these issues, it has been recommended that anticonvulsant prophylaxis be utilized in high-risk patients (e.g., those with severe TBI) and only for the first week after injury.[46,146]

Animal studies addressing these issues paint a similarly negative picture. For example, if diazepam is administered during the first 3 weeks after unilateral anteromedial cortex damage, recovery from somatosensory deficits is delayed indefinitely.[115] Even if diazepam is administered only for the first 7 days after brain damage, recovery is significantly delayed.[147,148] Phenobarbital also appears to interfere with somatosensory and motor recovery following brain damage in rats and nonhuman primates,[149,150] as does phenytoin.[151] Not all anticonvulsant drugs have been found to be detrimental after brain damage in animals. Carbamazepine[152] and vigabatrin[153] had no affect on recovery from somatosensory deficits. As a caveat, however, when an anticonvulsant dose of vigabatrin was coadministered against subconvulsive kindled seizures, recovery was impeded.[154] Similarly detrimental to functional recovery was phenobarbital administration prior to evoked subconvulsive seizures.[155] These data suggest that the interaction between anticonvulsant drugs and subclinical seizures after brain insult are detrimental to functional recovery, and the net effect is greater than either factor alone. There may be some value in EEG monitoring after TBI,[19,32] not only as a means of detecting subclinical seizures, but also of influencing treatment strategies that optimize neurobehavioral outcome.

There are several potential mechanisms by which anticonvulsants may adversely affect the recovering brain. First, these drugs suppress repetitive firing, which is important for long-term potentiation, a phenomenon associated with learning. Long-term potentiation is discussed in Chapter 13 in this volume. Second, barbiturates and benzodiazepines directly modulate the $GABA_A$ receptor and increase neuronal inhibition. That there is a link between enhanced postsynaptic GABA-mediated inhibition and impaired functional recovery is well established.[115,147–150,156–158] Likely mechanisms include toxicity of excessive intracellular Cl^-[159,160] and Ca^{++}[76,77] associated with GABA postinjury, GABA receptor-dependent excitotoxicity,[161] and decreases in growth factor production attributed to GABA augmentation.[162] Finally, suppression of repetitive firing or general CNS depression could be counterproductive following brain injury, especially because neuronal depression already occurs as a consequence of brain injury. This condition of postinjury neuronal depression has been referred to as *diaschisis*,[163] which is the temporary disruption of neuronal activity in undamaged areas functionally related to injured areas.

Evidence that diaschisis occurs after brain injury has been well established with measures of blood flow, metabolism, electrical activity, and neurotransmitter levels.[164–167] Moreover, this depression of neuronal activity after brain injury has been correlated with behavioral deficits, and restoration of normal neuronal activity correlates with behavioral recovery.[168–170] The use of positron emission tomography has made it possible to measure posttraumatic neural depression after brain injury in humans. Measures of cerebral glucose metabolism clearly show a state of metabolic depression postinjury, and the relationship between this and functional level depends on outcome measures utilized, although persistent metabolic disturbances after TBI, especially within critical periods, has been linked to poorer outcome.[171] In general, the level of posttraumatic neural depression is commensurate with the precipitating insult and correlates with outcome. The more severe the insult, the greater the posttraumatic neural depression; the greater the posttraumatic neural depression, the greater the behavioral deficit.[172]

Based on the brain's functionally depressed state after trauma, it has been hypothesized that posttraumatic seizures may be the result of adaptive mechanisms initiated by the injured brain in its attempt to restore normal neuronal activity. For this to be the case, the neurobehavioral consequences of seizures would need to be associated with improved recovery or no deleterious effect (e.g., neutral). Experimental data in animal studies suggest the effects of seizures are not uniform, and greatly depend on seizure type, severity, and frequency. For example, mild or infrequent seizures have been found to improve recovery.[173–175]

At first blush, these data may seem counterintuitive. However, when the entire array of neural and functional consequences of seizures are considered, a complex, yet fairly clear, picture emerges that is dependent on the timing, type, and severity of postinjury seizures. For example, using an animal model of posttraumatic epilepsy (described earlier in this chapter), it appears that the affect of seizures is bimodal. Convulsive seizures (stage 1) during the 6-day postlesion critical period are detrimental to the recovery process, whereas subconvulsive seizures (stage 0) have no functional affect.[95,176] This effect is time dependent and hemisphere specific, in that stage 1 kindled seizures occurring on postlesion day 7 or later have no affect on the recovery process. Moreover, contralaterally kindled seizures exert no affect on recovery, regardless of when they occur. We propose that the occurrence of early stage 0 kindled seizures after cortical lesion models early posttraumatic seizures, whereas the occurrence of early stage 1 kindled seizures after lesion models posttraumatic epilepsy. As such, our results suggest that the occurrence of early posttraumatic seizures does not adversely affect recovery from the brain injury, but early posttraumatic epilepsy blocks recovery completely. Potential mechanisms for the behavioral effects of early posttraumatic seizures (stage 0) versus early posttraumatic epilepsy (stage 1) include fibroblast growth factor 2 (FGF-2). Specifically, stage 0 seizures exert no affect on the time course of peak FGF-2 expression, whereas stage 1 seizures block this important neurotrophic contributor to functional recovery.[177] Moreover, early posttraumatic seizures followed by the later development of posttraumatic epilepsy had no affect on functional recovery and no affect on FGF-2 expression. In contrast, even a single epileptic seizure (stage 1) within the 6-day postlesion critical period in our model blocked recovery for the duration of testing, in addition to blocking FGF-2 expression. Interestingly, kindled seizures in nonbrain-injured animals have been associated with neurogenesis,[178,179] which may contribute in a positive or negative way to the recovery process, depending upon whether these new cells replace lost ones, make functionally relevant connections, or contribute to aberrant plasticity (e.g., excitability that might contribute to epileptogenesis).

There is other evidence that seizure effects vary. Clinical studies have shown that simple abnormal EEG activity is associated with impaired cognition[180] and that response time is impaired even during single focal interictal spikes in humans.[181] Learning is also impaired in young rodents undergoing repetitive and frequent audiogenic seizures.[132] In contrast, repetitive kindled seizures do not appear to affect most aspects of learning,[182,183] although some components of learning (e.g., acquisition) are affected by the transition from partial to generalized seizures.[182] There are some data suggesting that the seizure activity and convulsive behavior, in and of itself, may not be responsible for adverse cognitive effects. Instead, opioid receptor activation may be responsible. Pentylenetetrazol (PTZ)-kindled animals failed to exhibit impairments on the Morris Water Maze when the opioid antagonist naloxone was administered prior to PTZ kindling,[184] even though both groups of PTZ-kindled animals exhibited the same degree of seizure activity. Taken together, these data suggest that, although in some situations seizures may inhibit learning, the seizure activity in and of itself may not be sufficient to impair learning. Instead, it is the underlying physiologic processes (e.g., opioid activation) that seizures trigger that leads to deficits. Finally, brief seizures do not necessarily cause brain damage,[107] yet prolonged seizures cause neuronal death via excitotoxicity.[88,185] This latter type of seizure activity following trauma would likely contribute to further cell death or interfere with the plasticity underlying recovery processes.

Although seizures, per se, may not be detrimental to functional outcome, there is significant evidence suggesting that *posttraumatic epilepsy* poses significant problems for rehabilitation of the patients with TBI.[186] The uncertainty caused by randomly occurring loss of consciousness places yet an additional barrier to independence. At worst, uncontrolled epilepsy may necessitate placement in specialized care facilities and, at the least, may prohibit driving privileges. Uncontrolled seizures are also associated with a significant risk of trauma and unexpected death ("SUDEP").[187] Some data suggest the affect of posttraumatic epilepsy on neurorehabilitation may extend beyond these social aspects and could actually impede brain recovery. World War II veterans with head injury who developed posttraumatic epilepsy had a lower survival rate than veterans without epilepsy.[188] The incidence and severity of cognitive deficit in hemiplegic children is highly correlated with the presence of seizure activity, independent of the amount of cerebral damage.[189] A retrospective study of head-injured patients demonstrated that functional measures were lower in patients who developed posttraumatic epilepsy upon entry into rehabilitation than those who did not. Although both groups improved significantly, functional outcome remained lower in the epileptic group.[190] More important, these studies could not address the question of whether the results were the result of seizures, injury severity, or anticonvulsant drug administration. Haltiner et al.[191] were able to tease apart some of these issues. When injury severity is controlled, neither late posttraumatic seizures nor posttraumatic epilepsy had an influence on neuropsychological outcome measures.

To delineate effectively the neurobehavioral affect of seizures versus epilepsy following TBI in humans, it is necessary to know when and if the patient is having seizures. To this end, Vespa et al.[32] continuously monitored patients after TBI for up to 14 days. Twenty-two percent of these individuals had clinically evident or nonclinically evident seizures. When comparing outcome between these individuals and those in the nonseizure group, it appears that seizures are not necessarily detrimental. For example, both groups exhibited increased ICP after brain injury, but the overall ICP was actually greatest in the nonseizure group. Cerebral perfusion pressure was slightly, although significantly, lower in the nonseizure group. There was no difference between the groups in terms of length of stay nor in outcome (Glasgow outcome score); both good and poor outcomes were equally likely regardless of whether there had been seizures. Even though there was a greater mortality rate within the seizure group, this could be fully accounted for by those individuals with status epilepticus. If these individuals were removed from the analysis, it appeared that the seizure group had a lower mortality rate than the nonseizure group. It is also worth noting that Vespa et al.[192] have shown postinjury seizures can be correlated with elevated glutamate levels as assessed by intracerebral microdialysis. Elevated glycerol, a marker of membrane damage, was reported in one patient with posttraumatic status and in another with posttraumatic electrographic events without status.[193] It remains unclear whether these results are only specific to instances of postinjury status epilepticus or are generalizable to other types of recurrent seizure events. Moreover, what any of these findings mean for functional outcome has yet to be determined.

In summary, experimental data suggest the effect of seizures on functional recovery of the injured brain is not uniform and depends on seizure type, timing, and severity. Specifically, recurrent and/or severe seizures may have a negative affect on recovery, whereas mild, infrequent seizures may be associated with improved behavioral recovery or may be without neurobehavioral consequence. Thus, it is only when the seizures are severe enough to cause further brain damage, or frequent enough to develop into epilepsy, that they appear to be detrimental to behavioral recovery and quality of life.

2.10 Conclusions

The accurate diagnosis of episodic behaviors is crucial to providing the most appropriate therapy for patients with TBI. Although posttraumatic epilepsy is a common entity, it may be difficult to recognize. Posttraumatic epilepsy must be carefully distinguished from other types of behavioral spells because either unnecessary AED therapy or uncontrolled seizures may potentially impair neurologic recovery. Currently, there is little evidence to support prophylactic use of anticonvulsants in patients with TBI. Their use in this way does not prevent epileptogenesis clinically, and much data implicate negative effects on cognition and recovery of brain function. Thus, AED therapy should be withheld until there is a bona fide diagnosis of epilepsy (i.e., at least two separate seizure events that are not the result of transient metabolic derangements). After the diagnosis of epilepsy is secure, effective therapy should be initiated promptly to prevent the deleterious effects of uncontrolled seizures on brain recovery. Future research will need to address whether control of posttraumatic epilepsy improves functional outcome and whether these gains outweigh the adverse effects of AED drug therapy. In addition, the mechanisms of posttraumatic seizures will need to be better understood so that therapies that prevent epileptogenesis may be achieved.

References

1. Annegers, J. F., Grabow, J. D., Groover, R. V., Laws, E. R., Elveback, L. R., and Kurland, L. T., Seizures after head trauma: A population study, *Neurology*, 30(7 pt. 1), 683–689, 1980.
2. McEvoy, J. P., McCue, M., Spring, B., Mohs, R. C., Lavori, P. W., and Farr, R. M., Effects of amantadine and trihexyphenidyl on memory in elderly normal volunteers, *American Journal of Psychiatry*, 144(5), 573–577, 1987.
3. Potamianos, G. and Kellett, J. M., Anti-cholinergic drugs ad memory: The effects of benzhexol on memory in a group of geriatric patients, *British Journal of Psychiatry*, 140(4), 470–472, 1982.
4. Cross-National Collaborative Panic Study, Second Phase Investigators, Drug treatment of panic disorder: Comparative efficacy of alprazolam, imipramine, and placebo, *British Journal of Psychiatry*, 160(2), 191–202, 1992.
5. Commission on Classification and Terminology of the International League Against Epilepsy, Proposal for revised clinical and electroencephalographic classification of epileptic seizures, *Epilepsia*, 22(4), 268–278, 1981.
6. Browning, R. A. and Nelson, D. K., Modification of electroshock and pentylenetetrazol seizure patterns in rats after precollicular transections, *Experimental Neurology*, 93(3), 546–556, 1986.
7. Lüders, H. O. and Noachtar, S. (Eds.), *Epileptic Seizures, Pathophysiology and Clinical Semiology,* Churchill Livingston, Philadelphia, 2000.
8. Snead, O. C., III and Hosey, L. C., Exacerbation of seizures in children by carbamazepine, *New England Journal of Medicine*, 313(15), 916–921, 1985.
9. Gelisse, P., Worsening of seizures by oxcarbazepine in juvenile idiopathic generalized epilepsies, *Epilepsia*, 45, 1282–1286, 2004.
10. Buck, D., Baker, G. A., Jacoby, A., Smith, D. F., and Chadwick, D. W., Patients' experiences of injury as a result of epilepsy, *Epilepsia*, 38(4), 439–444, 1997.
11. Walker, A. E. and Jablon, S., A follow up study of head-wounds in World War II, *Veterans' Administration Monograph*, Veterans Administration, Washington, DC, 1961.
12. Caveness, W. F., Walker, A. E., and Ascroft, P. B., Incidence of posttraumatic epilepsy in Korean veterans as compared with those from World War I and World War II, *Journal of Neurosurgery*, 19(2), 122, 1962.
13. Salazar, A. M., Jabbari, B., Vance, S. C., Grafman, J., Amin, D., and Dillon, J. D., Epilepsy after penetrating head injury, I. Clinical correlates: A report of the Vietnam Head Injury Study, *Neurology*, 35(10), 1406–1414, 1985.
14. Warden, D., Military TBI during the Iraq and Afghanistan wars, *Journal of Head Trauma Rehabilitation*, 21(5), 398–402, 2006.
15. Okie, S., Traumatic brain injury in the war zone, *New England Journal of Medicine*, 352(20), 2043–2047, 2005.
16. Taber, K. H., Warden, D. L., and Hurley, R. A., Blast-related traumatic brain injury: What is known?, *Journal of Neuropsychiatry and Clinical Neurosciences*, 18(2), 141–145, 2006.
17. Pagni, C.A., Posttraumatic epilepsy: Incidence and prophylaxis, *Acta Neurochirurgica*, 50 (Suppl.), 38–47, 1990.
18. Weiss, G. H. and Caveness, W. F., Prognostic factors in the persistence of posttraumatic epilepsy, *Journal of Neurosurgery*, 37(2), 164–169, 1972.

19. Angeleri, F., Majkowski, J., Cacchio, G., Sobieszek, A., D'Acunto, S., Gesuita, R., Bachleda, A., Polonara, G., Krolicki, L., Signorino, M., and Salvolini, U., Posttraumatic epilepsy risk factors: One-year prospective study after head injury, *Epilepsia*, 40(9), 1222–1230, 1999.

20. Mazzini, L., Cossa, F. M., Angelino, E., Campini, R., Pasote, I., and Monaco, F., Posttraumatic epilepsy: Neuroradiologic and neuropsychological assessment of long-term outcomes, *Epilepsia*, 44(4), 569–574, 2003.

21. Guidice, M. A. and Berchou, R. C., Post-traumatic epilepsy following head injury, *Brain Injury*, 1(1), 61–64, 1987.

22. D'Alessandro, R., Tinuper, P., Ferrara, R., Cortelli, P., Pazzaglia, P., Sabattini, L., Frank, G., and Lugaresi, E., CT scan prediction of late post-traumatic epilepsy, *Journal of Neurology, Neurosurgery and Psychiatry*, 45(12), 1153–1155, 1982.

23. Annegers, J. F. and Coan, S. P., The risks of epilepsy after traumatic brain injury, *Seizure*, 9(7), 453–457, 2000.

24. Askenasy J. J. M., Association of intracerebral bone fragments and epilepsy in missile head injuries, *Acta Neurologica Scandiviavica*, 79(1), 47–52, 1989.

25. Kumar, R., Gupta, R. K., Husain, M., Vatsal, D. K., Chawla, S., Rathore, R. K., and Pradhan, S., Magnetization transfer MR imaging in patients with posttraumatic epilepsy, *AJNR American Journal of Neuroradiology*, 24(2), 218–224, 2003.

26. Hughes, J. R., Post-traumatic epilepsy in the military, *Military Medicine*, 151(8), 416–419, 1986.

27. Caveness, W. F., Meirowsky, A. M., Rish, B. L., Mohr, J. P., Kistler, J. P., Dillon, J. D., and Weiss, G. H., The nature of posttraumatic epilepsy, *Journal of Neurosurgery*, 50(5), 545–553, 1979.

28. Krumholz, A. Wiebe, S. Gronseth, G. Shinnar, S., Levisohn, P., Ting, T., Hopp, J., et al., Quality Standards Subcommittee of the American Academy of Neurology, American Epilepsy Society, practice parameter: Evaluating an apparent unprovoked first seizure in adults (an evidence-based review): Report of the Quality Standards Subcommittee of the American Academy of Neurology and the American Epilepsy Society, *Neurology*, 69(21), 1996–2007, 2007.

29. Jennett, B. and van de Sande, J., EEG prediction of post-traumatic epilepsy, *Epilepsia*, 16(2), 251–256, 1975.

30. Courjon, J., A longitudinal electro-clinical study of 80 cases of post-traumatic epilepsy observed from the time of the original trauma, *Epilepsia*, 11(1), 29–36, 1970.

31. van Donselaar, C.A., Schimsheimer, R.- J., Geerts, A. T., and Declerck, A. C., Value of the electro-encephalogram in adult patients with untreated idiopathic first seizures, *Archives of Neurology*, 49(3), 231–237, 1992.

32. Vespa, P. M., Nuwer, M. R., Nenov, V., Ronne-Engstrom, E., Hovda, D. A., Bergsneider, M., Kelly, D. F., Martin, N. A., and Becker, D. P., Increased incidence and impact of non-convulsive and convulsive seizures after traumatic brain injury as detected by continuous electroencephalographic monitoring, *Journal of Neurosurgery*, 91(5), 750–760, 1999.

33. American EEG Society, Guidelines in EEG, *Journal of Clinical Neurophysiology*, 3(2), 131–168, 1986.

34. Starkey, R. R., Sharbrough, F. W., and Drury I., A comparison of nasopharyngeal with ear and scalp electrodes using referential and bipolar technique, *Electroencephalography and Clinical Neurophysiology*, 58(2), 117–118, 1984.

35. Sperling, M. R. and Engel, J., Jr., Electroencephalographic recording from the temporal lobes: A comparison of ear, anterior temporal, and nasopharyngeal electrodes, *Annals of Neurology*, 17, 510–513, 1985.

36. Sharbrough, F. W., Commentary: Extracranial EEG evaluation, in J. Engel, Jr. (Ed.), *Surgical Treatment of the Epilepsies*, Raven Press, New York, 167–171, 1987.

37. Preskorn, S. H. and Fast, G. A., Tricyclic antidepressant induced seizures and plasma drug concentration, *Journal of Clinical Psychiatry*, 53(5), 160–162, 1992.

38. Dailey, J. W., Yan, Q. S., Mishra, P. K., Burger, R. L., and Jobe, P. C., Effects of fluoxetine on convulsions and on brain serotonin as detected by microdialysis in genetically epilepsy-prone rats, *Journal of Pharmacology and Experiment Therapeutics*, 260(6), 533–540, 1992.

39. Ojemann, L. M., Baugh-Bookman, C., and Dudley, D. L., Effect of psychotropic medications on seizure control in patients with epilepsy, *Neurology*, 37(9), 1525–1527, 1987.

40. Fromm, G. H., Amores, C. Y., and Thies, W., Imipramine in epilepsy, *Archives of Neurology*, 27(3), 198–204, 1972.

41. Fromm, G. H., Wessel, H. B., Glass, J. D., Alvin, J. D., and Van Horn, G., Imipramine in absence and myoclonic–astatic seizures, *Neurology*, 28(9 pt. 1), 953–957, 1978.

42. Kanner, A. M., The use of psychotropic drugs in epilepsy: What every neurologist should know, *Seminars in Neurology*, 28, 379–388, 2008.

43. Goldstein, L. B., Prescribing of potentially harmful drugs to patients admitted to hospital after head injury, *Journal of Neurology, Neurosurgery and Psychiatry*, 58(6), 753–755, 1995.

44. Jones, K. E., Puccio, A. M., Harshman, K, J., Falcione, B., Benedict, N., Jankowitz, B. T., Stippler, M., et al., Levetiracetam versus phenytoin for seizure prophylaxis in severe traumatic brain injury, *Neurosurgical Focus*, 25(4), E3, 2008.

45. Schierhout, G. and Roberts, I., Anti-epileptic drugs for preventing seizures following acute traumatic brain injury (update of Cochrane Database of Systematic Reviews, CD000173, 920, 2000), *Cochrane Database of Systematic Reviews*, 4, CD000173, 2001.

46. Chang, B. S. and Lowenstein, D. H., Practice parameter: Antiepileptic drug prophylaxis in severe traumatic brain injury. Report of the Quality Standards Subcommittee of the American Academy of Neurology, *Neurology*, 60(1), 10–16, 2003.

47. Temkin, N. R., Antiepileptogenesis and seizure prevention trials with antiepileptic drugs: Meta-analysis of controlled trials, *Epilepsia*, 42(4), 515–524, 2001.

48. Temkin, N. R., Anderson, G. D., Winn, H. R., Ellenbogen, R. G., Britz, G. W., Schuster, J., Lucas, T., et al., Magnesium sulfate for neuroprotection after traumatic brain injury: A randomised controlled trial, *Lancet Neurology*, 6(1), 29–38, 2007.

49. Mattson, R. H., Cramer, J. A., Collins, J. F., Smith, D. B., Delgado-Escueta, A. V., Browne, T. R., Williamson, P. D., et al., Comparison of carbamazepine, phenobarbital, phenytoin, and primidone in partial and secondarily generalized tonic–clonic seizures, *New England Journal of Medicine*, 313(3), 145–151, 1985.

50. Callahan, N., Kenney, R. A., O'Neill, B., Crowley, M., and Goggin, T., A prospective study between carbamazepine, phenytoin and sodium valproate as monotherapy in previously untreated and recently diagnosed patients with epilepsy, *Journal of Neurology, Neurosurgery and Psychiatry*, 48(7), 639–644, 1985.

51. Mattson, R. H., Cramer, J. A., and Collins, J. F., A comparison of valproate with carbamazepine for the treatment of complex partial seizures and secondarily generalized tonic–clonic seizures in adults. The Department of Veterans Affairs Epilepsy Cooperative Study No. 264 Group, *New England Journal of Medicine*, 327(11), 765–771, 1992.

52. Kwan, P. and Brodie, M. J., Effectiveness of first antiepileptic drug, *Epilepsia*, 42(10), 1255–1260, 2001.

53. Kalff, R., Houtkooper, M. A., Meyer, J. W., Goedhart, D. M., Augusteijn, R., and Meinardi, H., Carbamazepine and serum sodium levels, *Epilepsia*, 25(3), 390–397, 1984.

54. Sachdeo, R. D, Wasserstein, A., Mesenbrink, P. J., and D'Souza, J., Effects of oxcarbazepine on sodium concentration and water handling, *Annals of Neurology*, 51, 613–620, 2002.

55. Arif, H., Bushsbaum, R., Weintraub, D., Pierro, J., Resor, Jr., S. R., and Hirsch, L. J., Patient-reported cognitive side effects of antiepileptic drugs: Predictors and comparison of all commonly used antiepileptic drugs, *Epilepsy and Behavior*, 14(1), 202–209, 2009.

56. Anonymous, Gabapentin in partial epilepsy, UK Gabapentin Study Group, *Lancet*, 335(8698), 1114–1117, 1990.

57. Leppik, I. E., Deifuss, F. E., Pledger, G. W., Graves, N. M., Santilli, N., Drury, I., Tsay, J. Y., et al., Felbamate for partial seizures: Results of a controlled clinical trial, *Neurology*, 41(11), 1785–1789, 1991.

58. Loiseau, P., Yuen, A. W. C., Duche, B., Menager, T., and Arne-Bes, M. C., A randomized double-blind placebo-controlled crossover add-on trial of lamotrigine in patients with treatment-resistant partial seizures, *Epilepsy Research*, 7(2), 136–145, 1990.

59. Holland, K. D., Efficacy, pharmacology, and adverse effects of antiepileptic drugs, *Neurologic Clinics*, 19(2), 313–345, 2001.

60. Marson, A. G. and Chadwick, D., Comparing antiepileptic drugs, *Current Opinion in Neurology*, 9(2), 103–106, 1996.

61. Pellock, J. M. and Willmore, L. J., A rational guide to routine blood monitoring in patients receiving antiepileptic drugs, *Neurology*, 41(7), 961–964, 1991.

62. Browne, T. R. and Chang, T., Phenytoin biotransformation, in R. Levy, R. Mattson, B. Meldrum, J. K. Penry, and F. E. Dreifuss (Eds.), *Antiepileptic Drugs*, 3rd ed., Raven Press, New York, 197–213, 1989.

63. Temkin, N. R., Dikmen, S. S., Wilensky, A. J., Keihm, J., Chabal, S. and Winn, H. R., A randomized, double blind study of phenytoin for the prevention of posttraumatic seizures, *New England Journal of Medicine*, 323(8), 497–502, 1990.

64. Glötzner, F. L., Haubitz, I., Miltner, F., Kapp, G., and Pflughaupt, K. W., Anfallsprophylxe mit Carbamazepin nach schweren Schadelhirnverletzungen, *Neurochirurgia (Stuttg)*, 26(3), 66–79, 1983 [abstract in English].

65. Temkin, N. R., Preventing and treating posttraumatic seizures: The human experience, *Epilepsia*, 50(Suppl. 2), 10–13, 2009.

66. Schmidt, D., Reduction of two-drug therapy in intractable epilepsy, *Epilepsia*, 24(3), 368–376, 1983.

67. Foerster, O. and Penfield, W., The structural basis of traumatic epilepsy and results of radical operation, *Brain*, 53(pt. 2), 99–119, 1930.

68. Jasper, H. H., Pathophysiological mechanisms of post-traumatic epilepsy, *Epilepsia*, 11(1), 73–80, 1970.

69. Lowenstein, D. H., Thomas, M. J., Smith, D. H., and McIntosh, T. K., Selective vulnerability of dentate hilar neurons following traumatic brain injury: A potential mechanistic link between head trauma and disorders of the hippocampus, *Journal of Neuroscience*, 12(12), 4846–4853, 1992.

70. Golarai, G., Greenwood, A. C., Feeney, D. M., and Connor, J. A., Physiological and structural evidence for hippocampal involvement in persistent seizure susceptibility after traumatic brain injury, *Journal of Neuroscience*, 21(21), 8523–8537, 2001.

71. Reeves, T. M., Lyeth, G. G., Phillips, L. L., Hamm, R. J., and Povlishock, J. T., The effects of traumatic brain injury on inhibition in the hippocampus and dentate gyrus, *Brain Reserach*, 757(1), 119–132, 1997.

72. Reeves, T. M., Zhu, J., Povlishock, J. T., and Phillips, L. L., The effect of combined fluid percussion and entorhinal cortical lesions on long-term potentiation, *Neuroscience*, 77(2), 431–444, 1997.

73. Seiffert, E., Dreier, J. P., Ivens, S., Bechmann, I., Tomkins, O., Heinemann, U., and Friedman, A., Lasting blood–brain barrier disruption induces epileptic focus in the rat somatosensory cortex, *Journal of Neuroscience*, 24(36), 7829–7836, 2002.

74. Choi, D. W., Calcium-mediated neurotoxicity: Relationship to specific channel types and role in ischemic damage, *Trends in Neurosciences*, 11(10), 465–469, 1988.

75. Chen, Q. X., Steltzer, A., Kay, A. R., and Wong, R. K. S., GABA-A receptor function is regulated by phosphorylation in acutely dissociated guinea-pig hippocampal neurons, *Journal of Physiology*, 420(1), 207–221, 1990.

76. Van den Pol, A.N., Obrietan, K., and Chen, G., Excitatory actions of GABA after neuronal trauma, *Journal of Neuroscience*, 16(13), 4283–4292, 1996.

77. Van den Pol, A. N., Reversal of GABA actions by neuronal trauma, *Neuroscientist*, 3(5), 281–286, 1997.

78. Willmore, L. J., Sypert, G. W., and Munson, J. B., Recurrent seizures induced by cortical iron injection: A model of posttraumatic epilepsy, *Annals of Neurology*, 4, 329–336, 1978.

79. Willmore, L. J., Sypert, G. W., Munson, J. B., and Hurd, R. W., Chronic focal epileptiform discharges induced by injection of iron into rat and cat cortex, *Science*, 200(4349), 1501–1503, 1978.

80. Rubin, J. J. and Willmore, L. J., Prevention of iron-induced epileptiform discharges in rats by treatment of antiperoxidants, *Experimental Neurology*, 67(3), 472–480, 1980.

81. Paillas, J. E., Paillas, N., and Bureau, M., Post-traumatic epilepsy: Introduction and clinical observations, *Epilepsia*, 11(1), 5–15, 1970.

82. Jensen, F. E., Introduction: Posttraumatic epilepsy: Treatable epileptogenesis, *Epilepsia*, 50(Suppl. 2), 1–3, 2009.

83. Coulter, D. A., Epilepsy-associated plasticity in gamma-amino butyric acid receptor expression, function, and inhibitory synaptic properties, *International Review of Neurobiology*, 45, 237–252, 2001.

84. Heillier, J. L., Patrylo, P. R., Buckmaster, P. S., and Dudek, F. E., Recurrent spontaneous motor seizures after repeated low-dose systemic treatment with kainate: Assessment of a rat model of temporal lobe epilepsy, *Epilepsy Research*, 31(1), 267–282, 1998.

85. Halonen, T., Nissinen, J., and Pitkanen, A., Chronic elevation of brain GABA levels beginning two days after status epilepticus does not prevent epileptogenesis in rats, *Neuropharmacology*, 40(4), 536–550, 2001.

86. Pitkanen, A. and Halonen, T., Prevention of neuronal cell damage in the temporal lobe by vigabatrin and carbamazepine in experimental status epilepticus, *Epilepsia*, 35(Suppl. 8), 64, 1994.

87. Sloviter, R. S., Decreased hippocampal inhibition and a selective loss of interneurons in experimental epilepsy, *Science*, 235(4784), 73–76, 1987.

88. Pitkanen, A. and Halonen, T., Prevention of epilepsy, *Trends in Pharmacological Sciences*, 19(7), 253–254, 1998.

89. Wuarin, J.- P. and Dudek, F. E., Excitatory synaptic input to granule cells increases with time after kainate treatment, *Journal of Neurophysiology*, 85(3), 1067–1077, 2001.

90. Li, H. and Prince, D.A., Synaptic activity in chronically injured, epileptogenic sensory–motor cortex, *Journal of Neurophysiology*, 88(1), 2–12, 2002.

91. D'Ambrosio, R., Fairbanks, J. P., Fender, J. S., Born, D. E., Doyle, D. L., and Miller, J. W., Post-traumatic epilepsy following fluid percussion injury in the rat, *Brain*, 127(2), 1–11, 2004.

92. Kharatishvili, I., Nissinen, J. P., McIntosh, T. K., and Pitkänen, A., A model of posttraumatic epilepsy induced by lateral fluid percussion brain injury in rats, *Neuroscience*, 140(2), 685–697, 2006.

93. Pitkänen, A., Immonen, R. J., Gröhn, O. H. J., and Kharaishvili, I., From traumatic brain injury to posttraumatic epilepsy: What animal models tell us about the process and treatment options, *Epilepsia*, 50(Suppl. 2), 21–29, 2009.

94. Diaz-Arrastia, R., Agostini, M. A., Madden, C. J., and Van Ness, P. C., Posttraumatic epilepsy: The endophenotypes of a human model of epileptogenesis, *Epilepsia*, 50(Suppl. 2), 14–20, 2009.

95. Hernandez, T. D. and Warner, L. A., Kindled seizures during a critical post-lesion period exert a lasting impact on behavioral recovery, *Brain Research*, 673, 208–216, 1995.

96. Hernandez, T. D., Warner, L. A., and Montanez, S., The neurobehavioral consequences of kindling, in M. Corcoran and S. Moshe (Eds.), *Kindling 5*, Plenum Press, New York, 361–376, 1998.

97. Goddard, G. V., McIntyre, D. C., and Leech, C. K., A permanent change in brain function resulting from daily electrical stimulation, *Experimental Neurology*, 25(3), 295–330, 1969.

98. Reynolds, E. H., Early treatment and prognosis of epilepsy, *Epilepsia*, 28(2), 97–106, 1987.

99. Anonymous, Randomized clinical trial on the treatment of the first epileptic seizure. Scientific background, rationale, study design and protocol: First seizure trial group, *Italian Journal of Neurological Sciences*, 14(4), 295–301, 1993.

100. Elwes, R. D., Johnson A. L., and Reynolds E. H., The course of untreated epilepsy, *British Medical Journal*, 297(6654), 948–950, 1988.

101. Racine, R. J., Modification of seizure activity by electrical stimulation: II. Motor seizure, *Electroencephalography and Clinical Neurophysiology*, 32(3), 281–294, 1972.

102. Martin, D., McNamara, J. O., and Nadler, J. V., Kindling enhances sensitivity of CA3 hippocampal pyramidal cells to NMDA, *Journal of Neuroscience*, 12(5), 1928–1935, 1992.

103. McNamara, J. O., Bonhaus, D. W., Shin, C., Crain, B. J., Gellman, R. L., and Giacchino, J. L., The kindling model of epilepsy: A critical review, *Critical Reviews in Clinical Neurobiology*, 1(4), 341–391, 1985.

104. McNamara, J. O., Bonhaus, D. W., and Nadler, J. V., Novel approach to studying N-methyl-D-aspartate receptor function in the kindling model of epilepsy, *Drug Development Research*, 17(4), 321–330, 1989.

105. Represa, A. and Ben-Ari, Y., Kindling is associated with the formation of novel mossy fibre synapses in the CA3 region, *Experimental Brain Research*, 92(1), 69–78, 1992.

106. Sutula, T., Xiao-Xian, H., Cavazos, J., and Scott, G., Synaptic reorganization in the hippocampus induced by abnormal functional activity, *Science*, 239(4844), 1147–1150, 1988.

107. Tuunanen, J. and Pitkanen, A., Do seizures cause neuronal damage in rat amygdala kindling?, *Epilepsy Research*, 39(2), 171–176, 2000.

108. Hernandez, T. D. and Gallager, D. W., Development of long-term subsensitivity to GABA in dorsal raphe neurons of amygdala-kindled rats, *Brain Research*, 582, 221–225, 1992.

109. Hernandez, T. D., Rosen, J. B., and Gallager, D. W., Long-term changes in sensitivity to GABA in dorsal raphe neurons following amygdala kindling, *Brain Research*, 517, 294–300, 1990.

110. Kamphuis, W., Gorter, J. A., and Lopes da Silva, F. H., A long-lasting decrease in the inhibitory effect of GABA on glutamate responses of hippocampal pyramidal neurons induced by kindling epileptogenesis, *Neuroscience*, 41(2–3), 425–431, 1991.

111. Kapur, J., Michelson, H. B., Buterbaugh, G. G., and Lothman, E. W., Evidence for chronic loss of inhibition in the hippocampus after kindling: Electrophysiological studies, *Epilepsy Research*, 4(2), 90–99, 1989.

112. During, M. J., Craig, J. S., Hernandez, T. D., Anderson, G. M., and Gallager, D. W., Effect of amygdala kindling on the in vivo release of GABA and 5-HT in the dorsal raphe nucleus of freely moving rats, *Brain Research*, 584, 36–44, 1992.

113. Kamphuis, W., Huisman, H., Dreijer, A. M. C., Ghijsen, W. E. J. M., Verhage, M., and Lopes da Silva, F. H., Kindling increases the K$^+$-evoked Ca^{2+}-dependent release of endogenous GABA in area CA1 of rat hippocampus, *Brain Research*, 511, 63–70, 1990.

114. Barth, T. M., Jones, T. A., and Schallert, T., Functional subdivisions of the rat somatic sensorimotor cortex, *Behavioural Brain Research*, 39(1), 73–95, 1990.

115. Schallert, T., Hernandez, T. D., and Barth, T.M., Recovery of function after brain damage: Severe and chronic disruption by diazepam, *Brain Research*, 379, 104–111, 1986.

116. Schwartz, A. S., Marchak, P. L., Kreinick, C. J., and Flynn, R. E., The asymmetric lateralization of the tactile extinction in patients with unilateral cerebral dysfunction, *Brain*, 102(4), 669–684, 1979.

117. Goldstein, M., Traumatic brain injury: A silent epidemic, *Annals of Neurology*, 27, 327, 1990.

118. Dikmen, S. S., Temkin, N. R., Miller, B. M., Machamer, J., and Winn, R., Neurobehavioral effects of phenytoin prophylaxis of posttraumatic seizures, *Journal of the American Medical Association*, 265(10), 1271–1277, 1991.

119. Dikmen, S. S., Machamer, J. E., Winn, H. R., Anderson, G. D., and Temkin, N. R., Neuropsychological effects of valproate in traumatic brain injury: A randomized trial, *Neurology*, 54(4), 895–902, 2000.

120. Smith, K. R., Goulding, P. M., Wilderman, D., Goldfader, P. R., Holterman-Hommes, P., and Wei, F., Neurobehavioral effects of phenytoin and carbamazepine in patients recovering from brain trauma: A comparative study, *Archives of Neurology*, 51(7), 753–755, 1994.

121. Hernandez, T. D., Preventing post-traumatic epilepsy after brain injury: Weighing the costs and benefits of anticonvulsant prophylaxis, *Trends in Pharmacological Sciences*, 18(2), 59–62, 1997.

122. Hernandez, T. D. and Naritoku, D. K., Seizures, epilepsy and functional recovery following traumatic brain injury: A reappraisal, *Neurology*, 48(4), 803–806, 1997.

123. Wohns, R. N. and Wyler, A. R., Prophylactic phenytoin in severe head injuries, *Journal of Neurosurgery*, 51(4), 507–509, 1979.

124. Servit, Z. and Musil, F., Prophylactic treatment of posttraumatic epilepsy: Results of a long-term follow-up in Czechoslovakia, *Epilepsia*, 22(3), 315–320, 1981.

125. McNamara, J. O., Rigsbee, L. C., Butler, L. S., and Shin, C., Intravenous phenytoin is an effective anticonvulsant in the kindling model, *Annals of Neurology*, 26, 675–678, 1989.

126. Weiss, S. R. B. and Post, R. M., Carbamazepine and carbamazepine-10, 11-epoxide inhibit amygdala-kindled seizures in the rat but do not block their development, *Clinical Neuropharmacology*, 10(3), 272–279, 1987.

127. Schmutz, M., Klebs, K., and Baltzer, V., Inhibition or enhancement of kindling evolution by antiepileptics, *Journal of Neural Transmission*, 72(3), 245–257, 1988.
128. Löscher, W. and Hönack, D., Comparison of the anticonvulsant efficacy of primidone and phenobarbital during chronic treatment of amygdala-kindled rats, *European Journal of Pharmacology*, 162(2), 309–322, 1989.
129. Silver, J. M., Shin, C., and McNamara, J. O., Antiepileptogenic effects of conventional anticonvulsants in the kindling model of epilepsy, *Annals of Neurology*, 29, 356–363, 1991.
130. Löscher, W., Fisher, J. E., Nau, H., and Honack, D., Valproic acid in amygdala-kindled rats: Alterations in anticonvulsant efficacy, adverse effects, and drug and metabolite levels in various brain regions during chronic treatment, *Journal of Pharmacology and Experimental Therapeutics*, 250(3), 1067–1078, 1989.
131. Young, N. A., Lewis, S. J., Harris, Q. L. G., Jarrot, H. B., and Vajda, F. J. E., The development of tolerance to the anticonvulsant effects of clonazepam, but not sodium valproate, in the amygdaloid kindled rat, *Neuropharmacology*, 26(11), 1611–1614, 1987.
132. Holmes, G. L., Thompson, J. L., Marchi, T. A., Gabriel, P. S., Hogan, M. A., Carl, F. G., and Feldman, D. S., Effects of seizures on learning, memory, and behavior in the genetically epilepsy-prone rat, *Annals of Neurology*, 27, 24–32, 1990.
133. Gellman, R. L., Kallianos, J. A., and McNamara, J. O., Alpha-2 receptors mediate an endogenous noradrenergic suppression of kindling development, *Journal of Pharmacology and Experimental Therapeutics*, 241(3), 891–898, 1987.
134. Pelletier, M. R. and Corcoran, M. E., Intra-amygdaloid infusions of clonidine retard kindling, *Brain Research*, 598, 51–58, 1992.
135. Burchfiel, J. and Applegate, C. D., Stepwise progression of kindling: Perspectives from the kindling antagonism model, *Neuroscience and Behavioral Reviews*, 13(4), 289–299, 1989.
136. Dailey, J. W., Mishra, P. K., Ko, K. H., Penny, J. E., and Jobe, P. C., Noradrenergic abnormalities in the central nervous system of seizure-naive genetically epilepsy-prone rats, *Epilepsia*, 32(2), 168–173, 1991.
137. Pellock, J. M., Who should receive prophylactic antiepileptic drug following head injury?, *Brain Injury*, 3(2), 107–108, 1989.
138. Meador, K. J., Loring, D. W., Allen, M. E., Zamrini, M. D., Moore, B. A., Abney, O. L., and King, D. W., Comparative cognitive effects of carbamazepine and phenytoin in healthy adults, *Neurology*, 41(10), 1537–1540, 1991.
139. Meador, K. J., Loring, D. W., Huh, K., Gallagher, B. B., and King, D. W., Comparative cognitive effects of anticonvulsants, *Neurology*, 40(3 pt. 1), 391–394, 1990.
140. Dodrill, C. B. and Troupin, A. S., Psychotropic effects of carbamazepine in epilepsy: A double-blind comparison with phenytoin, *Neurology*, 27(6), 1023–1028, 1977.
141. Dodrill, C. B. and Troupin, A. S. Neuropsychological effects of carbamazepine and phenytoin: A reanalysis, *Neurology*, 41(1), 141–143, 1991.
142. Gallassi, R., Morrreale, A., Lorusso, S., Procacciaanti, G., Lugaresi, E., and Baruzzi, A., Cognitive effects of valproate, *Epilepsy Research*, 5(2), 160–164, 1990.
143. Loring, D. W., Marino, S., and Meador, K. J., Neuropsychological and behavioral effects of antiepilepsy drugs, *Neuropsychology Review*, 17(4), 413–425, 2007.
144. Lee, S., Sziklas, V., Andermann, F., Farnham, S., Risse, G., Gusafson, M., Gates, J., Penovich, P., Al-Asmi, A., Dubeau, F., and Jones-Gotman, M., The effects of adjunctive topiramate on cognitive function in patients with epilepsy, *Epilepsia*, 44(3), 339–347, 2003.
145. Massagli, T. L., Neurobehavioral effects of phenytoin, carbamazepine, and valproic acid: Implications for use in traumatic brain injury, *Archives of Physical Medicine and Rehabilitation*, 72(3), 219–226, 1991.
146. American Academy of Physical Medicine and Rehabilitation, Practice parameter: Antiepileptic drug treatment of posttraumatic seizures. Brain Injury Special Interest Group of the American Academy of Physical Medicine and Rehabilitation, *Archives of Physical Medicine and Rehabilitation*, 79(4), 594–597, 1998.

147. Hernandez, T. D., Jones, G. H., and Schallert, T., Co-administration of the benzodiazepine antagonist Ro15-1788 prevents diazepam-induced retardation of recovery, *Brain Research*, 487, 89–95, 1989.

148. Hernandez, T. D., Kiefel, J., Barth, T. M., Grant, M. L., and Schallert, T., Disruption and facilitation of recovery of function: Implication of the gamma-aminobutyric acid/benzodiazepine receptor complex, in M. Ginsbergand and W. D. Dietrich (Eds.), *Cerebro-Vascular Diseases*, Raven Press, New York, 327–334, 1989.

149. Hernandez, T. D. and Holling, L. C., Disruption of behavioral recovery by the anti-convulsant phenobarbital, *Brain Research*, 635, 300–306, 1994.

150. Watson, C. W. and Kennard, M. A., The effect of anticonvulsant drugs on recovery of function following cerebral cortical lesions, *Journal of Neurophysiology*, 8(4), 221–231, 1945.

151. Brailowsky, S., Knight, R. T., and Efron R., Phenytoin increases the severity of cortical hemiplegia in rats, *Brain Research*, 376, 71–77, 1986.

152. Schallert, T., Jones, T. A., Weaver, M. S., Shapiro, L. E., Crippens, D., and Fulton, M. A., Pharmacological and anatomic considerations in recovery of function, in S. Hanson and D. M. Tucker (Eds.), *Neuropsychological Assessment: Physical Medicine and Rehabilitation: State of the Art Reviews*, Hanley and Belfus, Philadelphia, 373–393, 1992.

153. Wallace, A. E., Kline, A. E., Montanez, S., and Hernandez, T.D., Impact of the novel anticonvulsant vigabatrin on functional recovery following brain lesion, *Restorative Neurology and Neuroscience*, 14(1), 35–45, 1999.

154. Montañez, S., Kline, A. E., Selwyn, A. P., Suozzin, J. C., Butler, S. E., and Hernandez, T. D., Vigabatrin directed against kindled seizures following cortical insult: Impact on epileptogenesis and somatosensory recovery, *Journal of Neurotrauma*, 18(11), 1255–1266, 2001.

155. Montañez, S., Kline, A. E., Gasser, T. A., and Hernandez, T. D., Phenobarbital administration directed against kindled seizures delays functional recovery following brain insult, *Brain Research*, 860, 29–40, 2000.

156. Brailowsky, S., Knight, R. T., Blood, K., and Scabini, D., Gamma-aminobutyric acid-induced potentiation of cortical hemiplegia, *Brain Research*, 363, 322–330, 1986.

157. Hernandez, T. D. and Schallert, T., Long-term impairment of behavioral recovery from cortical damage can be produced by short-term GABA-agonist infusion into adjacent cortex, *Restorative Neurology and Neuroscience*, 14(1), 323–330, 1990.

158. Schallert, T. and Hernandez, T. D., GABAergic drugs and neuroplasticity after brain injury: Impact on functional recovery, in L. Goldstein (Ed.), *Restorative Neurology: Advances in the Pharmacotherapy of Recovery after Stroke*, Futura Publishing, Armonk, NY, 91–120, 1998.

159. Erdo, S. L., Michler, A., and Wolff, J. R., GABA accelerates excitotoxic cell death in cortical cultures: Protection by blockers of GABA-gated chloride channels, *Brain Research*, 542, 254–258, 1991.

160. Lucas, J. H., Emery, D. G., and Rosenber, L. J., Physical injury of neurons: Important roles for sodium and chloride ions, *Neuroscientist*, 3(2), 89–101, 1997.

161. Chen, Q., Mouler, K., Tenkova, T., Hardy, K., Olney, J. W., and Romano, C., Excitotoxic cell death dependent on inhibitory receptor activation, *Experimental Neurology*, 160(1), 215–225, 1999.

162. Zafra, F., Castren, E., Thoenen, H., and Lindholm D., Interplay between glutamate and gamma-aminobutyric acid transmitter systems in the physiological regulation of brain-derived neurotrophic factor and nerve growth factor synthesis in hippocampal neurons, *Proceedings of the National Academy of Sciences of the United States of America*, 88(22), 10037–10041, 1991.

163. von Monakow, C., Die lokalisation im grosshim und der abbau der funktiondurch kortikale herde, J. F. Bergman, Wiesbaden, Translated and excerpted by G. Harris, 1969, in K. H. Pribram (Ed.), *Moods, States and Mind*, Penguin, London, 27–37, 1941.

164. Boyeson, M. B. and Feeney, D. M., Striatal dopamine after cortical injury, *Experimental Neurology*, 89(2), 479–483, 1985.

165. Hovda, D. A., Sutton, R. L., and Feeney, D. M., Recovery of tactile placing after visual cortex ablation in cat: A behavioral and metabolic study of diaschisis, *Experiential Neurology*, 97(2), 391–402, 1987.

166. Kempinsky, W. H., Experimental study of distal effects of acute focal injury, *Archives of Neurology and Psychiatry*, 79(4), 376–389, 1958.

167. Meyer, J. S., Shinohara, M., Kanda, T., Fukuuchi, Y., Ericsson, A. D., and Kok, N. K., Diaschisis resulting from acute unilateral cerebral infarction, *Archives of Neurology*, 23(3), 241–247, 1970.

168. Deuel, R. K. and Collins, R. C., The functional anatomy of frontal lobe neglect in the monkey: Behavioral and quantitative 2-deoxyglucose studies, *Annals of Neurology*, 15, 521–529, 1984.

169. Glassman, R. B. and Malamut, D. L., Recovery from electroencephalographic slowing and reduced evoked potentials after somatosensory cortical damage in cats, *Behavioral Biology*, 17(3), 333–354, 1976.

170. Hovda, D. A., Metabolic dysfunction, in R. K. Narayan, J. E. Wilberger, and J. T. Povlishock (Eds.), *Neurotrauma*, McGraw-Hill, New York, 1459–1478, 1996.

171. Vespa, P. M., McArthur, D., O'Phelan, K., Glenn, T., Etchepare, M., Kelly, D., Bergsneider, M., Martin, N. A., and Hovda, D. A., Persistently low extracellular glucose correlates with poor outcome 6 months after human traumatic brain injury despite a lack of increased lactate: A microdialysis study, *Journal of Cerebral Blood Flow and Metabolism*, 23(7), 865–877, 2003.

172. Hernández, T. D., Posttraumatic neural depression and neurobehavioral recovery after brain injury, *Journal of Neurotrauma*, 23(8), 1211–1221, 2006.

173. Feeney, D. M., Bailey, B. Y., Boyeson, M. G., Hovda, D. A., and Sutton, R. L., The effects of seizures on recovery of function following cortical contusion in the rat, *Brain Injury*, 1(1), 27–32, 1987.

174. Hamm, R. J., Pike, B. R., Temple, M. D., O'Dell, D. M., and Lyether, B. G., The effect of postinjury kindled seizures on cognitive performance in traumatically brain-injured rats, *Experimental Neurology*, 136(2), 143–148, 1995.

175. Hernandez, T. D. and Schallert, T., Seizures and recovery from experimental brain damage, *Experimental Neurology*, 102(3), 318–324, 1988.

176. Kline, A. E., Montanez, S., Bradley, H. A., Millar, C. J., and Hernandez, T. D., Distinctive amygdala kindled seizures differentially affect neurobehavioral recovery and lesion-induced basic fibroblast growth factor (bFGF) expression, *Brain Research*, 880, 38–50, 2000.

177. Buytaert, K. A., Kline, A. E., Montanez, S., Likler, E., Millar, C. J., and Hernandez, T. D., The temporal patterns of c-Fos and basic fibroblast growth factor expression following a unilateral anteromedial cortex lesion, *Brain Research*, 894, 121–130, 2001.

178. Scott, B. W., Wang, S., Burnham, W. M., De Boni, U., and Wojtowicz, J. M., Kindling-induced neurogenesis in the dentate gyrus of the rat, *Neuroscience Letters*, 248(2), 73–76, 1998.

179. Parent, J. M., Janumpalli, S., McNamara, J. O., and Lowenstein, J. O., Increased dentate granule cell neurogenesis following amygdala kindling in the rat, *Neuroscience Letters*, 247(1), 9–12, 1998.

180. Binnie, C. D., Channon, S., and Marston, D., Learning disabilities in epilepsy: Neurophysiological aspects, *Epilepsia*, 31(Suppl. 4), S2–S8, 1990.

181. Shewmon, D. A. and Erwin, R. J., The effect of focal interictal spikes on perception and reaction time: I. General considerations, *Electroencephalography and Clinical Neurophysiology*, 69(4), 319–337, 1988.

182. Beldhuis, H. J. A., Everts, G. J., Van der Zee, E. A., Luiten, P. G. M., and Bohus, B., Amygdala kindling-induced seizures selectively impair spatial memory: 1. Behavioral characteristics and effects on hippocampal neuronal protein kinase C isoforms, *Hippocampus*, 2(4), 397–410, 1992.

183. Holmes, G. L., Chronopoulos, A., Stafstrom, C. E., Mikati, M., Thurber, S., and Hyde, P., Long-term effects of kindling in the developing brain on memory, learning, behavior and seizure susceptibility, *Epilepsia*, 33(Suppl. 3), 42, S3–S42, 1992.

184. Omrani, A., Ghadami, R. R., Fathi, N., Tahmasian, M., Fathollahi, Y., and Touhidi, A., Naloxone improves impairment of spatial performance induced by pentylenetetrazol kindling in rats, *Neuroscience*, 145(3), 824–831, 2007.

185. Ben-Ari, Y. E., Limbic seizure and brain damage produced by kainic acid: Mechanisms and relevance to human temporal lobe epilepsy, *Neuroscience*, 14(2), 375–403, 1985.

186. Dikmen, S. and Reitan, R. M., Neuropsychological performance in posttraumatic epilepsy, *Epilepsia*, 19(2), 177–183, 1978.
187. Kirby, S. and Sadler R. M., Injury and death as a result of seizures, *Epilepsia*, 36(1), 25–28, 1995.
188. Walker, A. E. and Blumer, D., The fate of World War II veterans with posttraumatic seizures, *Archives of Neurology*, 46(1), 23–26, 1989.
189. Vargha-Khadem, F., Issacs, E., van der Werf, S., Robb, S., and Wilson, J., Development of intelligence and memory in children with hemiplegic cerebral palsy, *Brain*, 115(1), 315–329, 1992.
190. Armstrong, K. K., Sahgal, V., Bloch, R., Armstrong, K. J., and Heinemann, A., Rehabilitation outcomes in patients with posttraumatic epilepsy, *Archives of Physical Medicine and Rehabilitation*, 71(2), 156–160, 1990.
191. Haltiner, A. M., Temkin, N. R., Winn, H. R., and Dikmen, S. S., The impact of posttraumatic seizures on one-year neuropsychological and psychosocial outcome after head injury, *Journal of the International Neuropsychological Society*, 2(6), 494–504, 1996.
192. Vespa, P. M., Prins, M., Ronne-Engstrom, E., Caron, M., Shalmon, E., Hovda, D. A., Martin, N. A., and Becker, D. P., Increase in extracellular glutamate caused by reduced cerebral perfusion pressure and seizures after human traumatic brain injury: A microdialysis study, *Journal of Neurosurgery*, 89(6), 971–982, 1998.
193. Vespa, P., Martin, N. A., Nenov, V., Glenn, T., Bergsneider, M., Kelly, D., Becker, D. P., and Hovda, D.A., Delayed increase in extracellular glycerol with post-traumatic electrographic epileptic activity: Support for the theory that seizures induce secondary injury, *Acta Neurochirurgica*, 81(Suppl.), 355–357, 2002.

3

Neurobehavioral Consequences of Combat-Related Blast Injury and Polytrauma

Jay M. Uomoto, Rhonda M. Williams, and Leigh Anne Randa

CONTENTS

3.1 Introduction

Blast-related traumatic injuries have become a primary health concern for military treatment facilities operated by the Department of Defense (DoD), the Veterans' Health Administration (VHA), and civilian providers who provide health care for U.S. active-duty service members and veterans. The Kevlar body armor used in the current wars provides improved protection from penetrating shrapnel fragments and other material dispersed by high-velocity blast explosions, dramatically increasing the likelihood of survival after blast exposure. Blast exposure, however, can be the source of an array of physiologic, neurocognitive, and psychological disorders in military service members. The goals of this chapter are primarily threefold: (1) to describe common aftereffects of blast exposures in military personnel, with emphasis upon traumatic brain injury (TBI) and the assessment of these problems; (2) to describe the many co-occurring disorders that complicate the medical and psychological symptom picture for those who have had blast exposures and have undergone deployment to war zones; and (3) to discuss the current approach for polytrauma rehabilitation and integrated care for U.S. active-duty service members and veterans who have served in Operation Enduring Freedom (OEF) in Afghanistan and Operation Iraqi Freedom (OIF).

3.2 Traumatic Brain Injuries in Combat Zones

The occurrence of acquired brain injury during war dates back as far as history has been recorded. Blunt head trauma and penetrating head wounds occur from the multiplicity of exposures that can occur in the war zone. For troops deployed who have been engaged in combat since the time of the U.S. Civil War, much has been written and learned about the consequences of injuries sustained in war theaters. A historical review of the concept of "shell shock" by Jones et al.[1] discusses the early phases of battle during World War I being characterized by significant exposures to blast explosions with consequent head and brain injuries. Immediate postconcussion symptoms were present, and persisting symptoms that were not explainable by organic lesions began to be referred to as *shell shock*. The authors go on to describe how the British government awarded pensions for some 32,000 soldiers for shell shock by 1918, and increasing numbers of soldiers were subsequently pensioned for the disorder. As the concept evolved, both physiologic and psychological aspects of shell shock were recognized, much akin to what is ascribed to the phenomenology of postconcussion syndrome.

During World War II, the concept of "war neuroses" was posited by Kurt Goldstein, a German neurologist and psychiatrist who is thought of as one of the founders of modern neuropsychology. He is well known for his work in evaluating and developing early cognitive rehabilitation approaches for soldiers who sustained combat-related TBIs with the publication of his book *Aftereffects of Brain Injuries in War*.[2] During that same time era, Goldstein[3] described "catastrophic behavior" that occurred in soldiers who sustained brain injuries, with anxiety and fear being a root cause of these reactions, that results in the context of being in the battlefield. Goldstein[3] talked about three types of "nervous breakdown due to war conditions," including (1) acute anxiety states, (2) that characterized by conversion symptoms, and (3) exacerbation of previous neuroses by being in the combat war theater. Many of Goldstein's[3] descriptions of these catastrophic reactions are today familiar as symptoms of posttraumatic stress disorder (PTSD). As discussed later in this chapter, the overlap of symptomatology with mild TBI with PTSD and depression may represent the modern equivalent to the shell shock phenomena of past war conflicts.

During the current wars in Afghanistan (initiated in 2001) and Iraq (initiated in 2003), blast exposures and consequent injuries have been a common occurrence. Blast-related injuries in OEF/OIF largely occur as a result of exposure to explosive materials and devices, including bombs, land mines, rocket-propelled grenades (RPGs), mortar rounds, and improvised explosive devices (IEDs). Vehicle-borne IEDs (VBIEDs) involving the packaging of enormous amounts of explosives and other materials that can act as damaging shrapnel are common in this war theater. Explosively formed penetrators or projectiles (EFPs) are particularly menacing new weapons that can pierce vehicle armor. These and other devices can create significant overpressurization waves and secondary damage that can result in the service member experiencing a blast-related TBI. Later in this chapter we describe some of the potential causes of injury secondary to blast injury.

It is recognized that blast exposures can produce multiple injuries, oftentimes simultaneous to the blast event. In an introductory article regarding VHA initiation of the Polytrauma System of Care, Sigford[4] states:

> The first combat-injured "polytrauma" patient was admitted into a U.S. Department of Veterans' Affairs (VA) rehabilitation unit in January 2002. This began a remarkable change in the provision and delivery of rehabilitation services to the combat injured. The commitment of the VA to Abraham Lincoln's famous statement "to care for him who shall have borne the battle and for his widow and his orphan" is nowhere more evident than in the current Polytrauma System of Care. (p. 160)

Sigford[4] goes on to describe the VHA's definition of polytrauma as including "two or more injuries to physical regions or organ systems, one of which may be life threatening, resulting in physical, cognitive, psychological, or psychosocial impairments and functional disability" (p. 160).

Injury to the brain is seen as the "lead impairment" that shapes the nature of polytrauma rehabilitation as inherently interdisciplinary in service delivery, and collaborative with many other service providers. Initially, it was thought that polytrauma would result from a single blast event resulting in moderate to severe TBI along with other system injuries (e.g., traumatic amputation, vision loss, hearing loss, and so forth). As OEF and OIF continues, it has become apparent that the majority of blast injuries result in what in the civilian literature is known as *mild TBI*, often caused by multiple blast exposures with resultant multiple concussions. Cumulative injuries secondary to multiple deployments also characterize the individual with polytrauma.

By definition, most blast-related brain injuries occur in a combat theater, resulting in two main types of injured: persons engaged in the armed forces, and civilians or insurgents wounded in combat. As of March 2009, the DoD reported a total of 3425 killed in action in OIF and 446 killed in action in OEF. According to the RAND Center for Military Policy Research report,[5] approximately 1.64 million U.S. troops have deployed as part of OEF and OIF. The RAND report[5] goes on to describe that, as of October 2007, approximately 300,000 OEF/OIF service members suffer from PTSD and 320,000 sustained a TBI. The President's Commission on Care for America's Returning Wounded Warriors[6] surveyed active duty, reservists, and former military personnel from OEF/OIF and asked if they had been exposed to an event or blast that caused a jolt or blow to the head. The report states:

"59% of active duty and 52% of reserve component and 65% of retired/separated service members had been exposed to such an event."[6, p.8] It should be noted that these reported numbers were generated by survey measures and that exposure to blast does not necessarily translate into that person sustaining a TBI. However, these findings underscore the fact that, at this point in time, there continues to be a need for research that prospectively defines and follows those with blast-related TBI from the point of injury to 1, 3, 5, and 10 years out from these injuries. Currently, the ability to assess the nature of blast events that occur in theaters of combat, as well as early head injury indices, is limited by the nature of war conflicts.

Although we appreciate the importance of blast-related injury globally, the focus of the current chapter is on blast-related brain injury among active-duty service members and veterans of OEF and OIF. Military personnel differ in several important ways from their civilian counterparts. Even in peacetime, rates of TBI are elevated among military personnel. Men in the military have 1.6 times the rate of TBI as their civilian counterparts, whereas women in the military have 2.5 times higher rates of TBI than civilian women.[7] During war, the incidence of TBI increases, with closed head injuries remaining the most prevalent (compared with penetrating head injuries). In a recent study of 2525 soldiers who were 3 to 4 months postdeployment (59% response rate), Hoge et al.[8] found that service members who report mild TBI were more likely to have experienced high combat intensity, be injured in a blast, have multiple blast exposures, be hospitalized during deployment, and be younger males of junior rank.

As noted earlier, RAND researchers estimate that approximately 320,000 of U.S. armed forces personnel deployed since 2002 have suffered a probable TBI during deployment.[5] Among those with brain injury, blasts are the most common cause.[9] Several studies have indicated that IEDs are the leading cause of head, neck, and face injuries[10] in battle, whereas motor vehicle crashes are the leading cause of such injuries outside of combat. Among those injured in OEF and OIF, the proportion of head and neck wounds (30%) is significantly higher than the proportion experienced in World War II, Korea, and the Vietnam War (16%–21%).[11]

3.2.1 Differences between OEF/OIF and Other War Conflicts

The nature of combat characterizing OEF and OIF differs in several significant ways from previous conflicts, which likely contributes to the elevated incidence of brain injury. The first factor that accounts for differences is that, in the current conflicts, unique methods of attack and weaponry are being used by enemy combatants. The current insurgency in Iraq and Afghanistan, has seen the widespread use of the IED, with more than 10,000 such attacks reported in Iraq during 2005 alone, as reported in Ramasamy et al.[12] This latter study reported that of the 100 consecutive causalities sustained by coalition forces in January 2006, 53 of these were the result of IED explosions across 23 incidents. Of note is that 21 of the 23 incidences that resulted in causalities were caused by explosively formed projectiles, known for their high kill rate. In another study, by Holcomb et al.,[13] of the deaths among U.S. Special Forces service members who died between October 2001 and November 2004 ($N = 82$), 43% were caused by explosions, followed by 28% dying from gunshot wounds. According to the U.S. Joint Theater Trauma Registry for injuries accounted for in OEF and OIF between October 2001 and January 2005, blast explosions accounted for 75% of the mechanisms of extremity wounds.[14] Of a total 1566 soldiers, 6609 wounds were recorded; of these, 54% of these soldiers sustained extremity wounds. This figure is noted to be consistent with previous wars (World War II, Korea, Vietnam, Desert

Storm). The previously cited study by Owens et al.[11] also reports on the U.S. Joint Theater Trauma Registry indicating that blasts were the causative mechanism of injury in 79% of troops wounded in action, and IEDs accounted for 38% of all combat injuries and 32% of combat fatalities. Blast injuries are consistently shown to be a primary mechanism of injury in the Global War on Terror.

The second factor contributing to the elevated rates of injury secondary to blast explosions is likely a result of the fact that more soldiers are surviving their injuries today than in previous wars. Kevlar body armor provides improved protection of vital body organs from penetrating shrapnel fragments and other material dispersed by high-velocity over-pressurization waves created by blast explosions. The armor on combat vehicles differs somewhat by vehicle model and purpose, with some vehicles able to survive driving over an IED, and others relatively more vulnerable. Medical support for troops is faster, more mobile, and closer to battle than has historically been the case, providing the ability both to treat and evacuate injured troops rapidly. As a result of improved armor, approximately 10% of those wounded in OEF/OIF sustain lethal war wounds compared with 24% in the Persian Gulf War of 1990 to 1991, 24% in Vietnam, and 30% in World War II.[15]

The third factor contributing to the elevated rates of blast-related injuries are changes in military operations. As described in the RAND report,[5] the conflicts in Iraq and Afghanistan represent the most sustained U.S. combat operations since the Vietnam War. To meet the manpower requirements for such a sustained conflict, troops are being deployed for longer tours, being deployed for multiple tours, and have less recovery time between deployments. These factors can lead to increased physical and psychological stress among troops. In addition, more units from the Army and Navy Reserves and Army National Guard are serving in infantry roles. Because of the nature of operations in Iraq and Afghanistan, it is in these infantry roles that many of the blast-related injuries occur.

3.2.2 Unique Characteristics of Combat-Related Traumatic Brain Injury

There are (at least) two characteristics that make blast-related TBI, especially of "mild" severity, unique from other types of mild TBI. First, blast-related TBI frequently occurs in a complex context, notable for high rates of comorbid physical injuries, the probability of repeated blast exposure and injury, and the physical and psychological stress associated with the theater of combat. Second, the physiologic mechanisms of blast-related TBI may be meaningfully distinct from mild TBI as a result of the blunt trauma mechanisms seen more typically in civilian settings. Blast-related TBIs less frequently result in severe TBI, and many service members returning from the war theater report multiple blast exposures, many that are associated with immediate postconcussive symptomatology, and any one of these concussive events could be considered a mild TBI. However, blast-related mild TBI may differ in outcome from TBI because of the presence of other co-occurring conditions, and thus may moderate predictions of recovery that are commonly associated with the natural recovery from a single civilian mild TBI. The context within which these mild TBIs or multiple concussions occur, along with co-occurring conditions such as combat-related PTSD, depression, chronic multisite pain disorders, and the presence of sleep disorders and fatigue differentiate OEF and OIF blast injury from that seen in the civilian world.

3.2.2.1 A Note on Terminology Used in This Chapter

Mild TBIs are usually classified as injuries resulting in loss of consciousness (LOC) up to 30 minutes and posttraumatic amnesia (PTA) up to 24 hours; for most, recovery is fairly complete and rapid, occurring within 3 months of injury. TBIs of moderate severity, on the other hand, are characterized by LOC of up to 6 hours and PTA ranging from 1 to 7 days, and the typical recovery trajectory is more gradual, more prolonged, and less likely to be characterized by a complete return to baseline function. Note that in this chapter, we interchangeably use the terms *mild TBI* and *concussion,* and we do not differentiate between concussions of different grades. The definition of concussion and mild TBI are defined in the next section.

3.2.2.2 Differences between Combat-Related and Civilian Mild Traumatic Brain Injury

The term *mild traumatic brain injury* has been applied to combat-related and blast-exposure TBI. Significant similarities have been drawn between the sports concussion literature and military concussions. Lew et al.[16] commented on common characteristics among those who have experienced concussive injuries, including signs (e.g., alteration of consciousness, nausea/vomiting, reduced coordination); symptoms (e.g., headache, dizziness, visual changes, tinnitus, and sleep and fatigue problems); and cognitive problems (e.g., disorientation, attention and memory deficits, impaired fluency). These signs, symptoms, and cognitive problems can also be seen in combat-related mild TBI, particularly in those whose injuries may be the result of falls or motor vehicle accidents, during which blunt head trauma occurs, much akin to that seen in civilian injuries. Combat-related mild TBI differs from that in the civilian sector as a result of contextual issues such as the number of concussive events that a service member may sustain within any single deployment, and the number of these events accumulated during the course of multiple deployments. Although many who play sports may incur multiple concussive events, few athletes would be allowed to continue active sports engagement after two, three, or four consecutive concussions within a given season (e.g., in football, the season may extend to 4 to 6 months). Furthermore, there are numerous other exposures that occur in the war theater that typically do not occur in the civilian setting, such as exposure to very high-temperature atmospheres (frequently exceeding 120°F) where dehydration risk exists. Other environmental exposures, such as toxic exposures and depleted uranium may affect the general health status of the service member. Superimposing a mild TBI on other health risks may therefore result in different outcomes and it may not be appropriate to translate the expectation of recovery for a single civilian mild TBI to military personnel who experience multiple blast-related concussions and whose health status may also be affected by other war theater exposures.

Differences between civilian mild TBI and combat-related mild are noted in Table 3.1. For example, for those with persistent postconcussive syndrome in the civilian sector, many may be seeking compensation or have pending litigation. Although many veterans seek service connection for their combat-related illnesses and disorders, many OEF and OIF veterans desire redeployment and wish to rejoin their unit rather than remaining stateside. This may also result, in part, because service members in OEF and OIF are drawn from an all-volunteer military force. When a service member is in the midst of a fire fight, or when mortar rounds are landing nearby, it would be difficult to ascertain information such as a Glasgow Coma Scale score (something that might be assessed by a paramedic or emergency medical technician in the civilian sector); therefore, early head injury index information is often absent when trying to judge the level of injury several months later by retrospective report. If the service member sustains an injury severe enough to be medically assessed in the combat support hospital, early-head injury indices may be obtained and deemed useful for later determinations of TBI diagnoses and rehabilitation. Currently,

TABLE 3.1

Differences between Civilian and Combat-Related Mild TBI

Civilian Mild TBI Characteristics	Combat-Related Mild TBI Characteristics
Single-incident TBI	Multiple concussive events; cumulative injuries
Most occur as a result of a motor vehicle accident, fall, or assault	Blast-related exposures, falls, motor vehicle accidents—sometimes all three mechanisms occur in a single incident
Common to have immediate medical response, emergency medical technician evaluation, hospitalization; prescription of rest with slow reactivation ideal	Immediate medical evaluation in war environment difficult; less opportunity for rest and slow reactivation, superimposed on increased hypothalamic–pituitary–adrenal axis activation
Resolution of neuropsychological symptoms within 1 to 3 months	Co-occurring exposures
Many are in litigation	Desire for redeployment

it is also unclear regarding the extent to which multiple concussion outcomes are affected by the superimposition of a dysregulated hypothalamic–pituitary–adrenal axis secondary to significant sleep deprivation, maintaining high alert levels, and exposure to multiple stressors. These are but a few of the differences between civilian mild TBI and combat-related mild TBI that cautions the health care provider in completing assessments and developing plans of care for these service members. Table 3.1 presents other differences between civilian and combat-related mild TBI.

3.2.3 Classification of Blast-Related Injuries

In order for someone even to be considered as having experienced a mild TBI, he or she must have experienced some event, such as a blast exposure, fall, or blow to the head that constitutes a plausible cause of such injury. According to DePalma et al.,[17] most recent terrorist attacks have involved explosive devices. In Iraq, the use of IEDs has been one of the prime means with which enemy combatants attacked U.S. and coalition troops in OIF. Each explosion creates a blast wind that will travel in excess of 1000 miles per hour. As illustrated by Taber et al.,[18] peak overpressurization of the blast wave will occur fairly immediately after the explosion. This is followed by a negative pressure wave that results in airflow pressure back toward the origin of the explosion. A second, but smaller, pressurization wave can also occur as a third phase of the blast wind process. It should be noted that, depending upon the type and magnitude of the blast explosion, the blast wind can reach a velocity capable of creating a traumatic amputation or eye enucleation. This is just to underscore the pernicious nature of blast wave exposures and the prominent aftereffects on the human body. The physics of a blast exposure is such that the blast wind and overpressurization force will affect the air and fluid-filled organs of the body (e.g., lungs, ear canal, stomach, and colon). The blast wind can be powerful enough to propel a service member a significant distance from the explosion, depending on how close that individual was from the source of the blast. Displacement by the wind can then result in a fall or other blow to the head by being thrown into objects or by having other material fall on the body. Blunt and penetrating wounds to the body can also occur secondary to blast wave exposure. Although Kevlar body armor is protective of ballistic projectiles and shrapnel penetrating injuries in the regions most protected by the body armor (e.g., back, shoulder to waist), the body armor does not protect against the pulmonary overpressure wave effects and potential for pulmonary acute gas embolism.

Blast-related injuries, including those that cause TBI, are categorized into primary, secondary, tertiary, and quaternary types, depending on the mechanisms, according to the Center for Disease Control and Prevention.[19] Table 3.2 provides the classification of blast-related injuries along with examples of such injuries at each level (see also DePalma and coworkers[17] for descriptions and examples). The quinary classification included in Table 3.2 is a recently defined fifth mechanism of blast injury defined by Kluger et al.[20] and Bhatoe.[21]

3.2.4 Clinical and Diagnostic Considerations in Combat-Related Mild Traumatic Brain Injury

In contrast to the presentation of mild TBI in civilian settings, the presentation of troops who sustained blast or combat-related TBI tends to be complicated. Personnel who sustain concussive injuries in combat may be unaware that their brief LOC or altered mental status, in fact, may constitute an injury requiring medical evaluation. Moreover, soldiers with basic combat life support training are taught to assess for and prioritize aid for persons with life-threatening injuries. Transient alterations in mental status are relatively lower priority injuries and are frequently ignored because of the necessity of the situation. Presentation is further complicated by the frequent presence of comorbid physical injuries (polytrauma) that may have been incurred during the same event causing mild TBI, or during the same deployment. For example, in a study of OEF/OIF patients evacuated from combat to Walter Reed Army Medical Center, 28% had a TBI, and of those, 19% had a concomitant amputation.[9] The majority of persons seen with TBI at Walter Reed Army Medical Center had experienced closed head injury (88%), and less than half were mild in severity. In a related vein, the probability of repeated blast exposure and concussion, both prior to and during deployment, must be considered as part of the context in which blast

TABLE 3.2

Classification of Blast-Related Injuries with Examples

Blast-Injury Type	Mechanism	Consequences
Primary	Overpressurization wave	Tympanic membrane rupture, pulmonary injury and "blast lung" effects, ruptures of the viscus and viscus injury, traumatic amputation, eye enucleation/rupture of the eye globe, associated with dyspnea and chest pain after blast exposure, bowel perforation
Secondary	Projectile, fragments, debris	Penetrating wounds, fragment injuries and shrapnel injuries, blunt trauma to the head and body
Tertiary	Displacement by blast wind, structural collapse of buildings and other nearby structures	Blunt and penetrating trauma, acceleration and deceleration forces to the head/brain by being thrown into stationary objects, traumatic amputation, fractures, crush injuries
Quaternary	Explosion-related illnesses and diseases, and other injuries	Burns, asphyxia, toxic exposures and inhalation, worsening of existing diseases (e.g., asthma), exposure to depleted uranium, chemical exposures
Quinary	Absorption of toxic materials	Induction of hyperinflammatory state (hyperpyrexia, sweating, low central venous pressure, positive fluid balance); for example, chlorine gas additive to IED

injury occurs. On interview, it is critical to establish, as accurately as possible, not only the number of concussive events, but, if possible, their dates and relative temporal separation from each other.

Common methods of grading the severity level of blast-related and other combat-related TBI can be applied; however, as noted earlier, such application is done with caution. After the presence of a plausible mechanism of injury is established (e.g., blast wave exposure, including being thrown from the site of the blast with consequent blunt head trauma), the presence of certain immediate symptoms is central to defining initial head injury severity. It is important to note that defining initial head injury severity is separate from determining what may be producing persisting neurobehavioral, physical, and cognitive problems in the active-duty service member or veteran. Although there continues to be discussions regarding uniform definitions of mild TBI,[22] clinicians who are tasked with determining whether or not there is history of TBI by patient self-report, will frequently use the American Congress of Rehabilitation Medicine's definition of mild TBI,[23] the American Academy of Neurology practice parameters on concussion,[24] and screening questions that assist in case identification for consideration of mild TBI developed by the Defense and Veterans Brain Injury Center.[25,26]

Using the American Congress of Rehabilitation Medicine criteria includes identifying a plausible mechanism of injury that results in immediate and transient focal neurologic deficits, including LOC or altered mental status lasting 30 minutes or less and any loss of memory for events immediately before or after the accident (but not exceeding 24 hours). Such information is not readily available in the war theater, and much of this type of information is gathered retrospectively by service member or veteran self-report. Reliance on self-report alone may be insufficient to establish a diagnosis of mild TBI, and extensive information gathering around concussive events is important. Establishing type of explosive device (e.g., IED, VBIED, mortar round, RPG) to which the service member was exposed, how close in proximity that person was to the explosion, the extent to which there was displacement of the body away from the explosion, and whether there was blunt head trauma are important variables to ascertain. Obtaining information regarding immediate symptoms after the explosion, such as dazing or disorientation afterward, may be helpful to know; however, such experiences reported by the service member or veteran may be the result of nonneurologic factors, such as being startled by an explosion and being in the midst of a fire fight, which can be disorienting, stressful, and confusing.

Concussions can be graded by the American Academy of Neurology practice parameters and technically differentiated into three levels of severity. Grade I concussions are characterized by transient confusion, no LOC, and symptoms of mental status abnormalities that resolve within 15 minutes or less. Grade II concussions are also defined as transient confusion and no LOC, but symptoms persist for longer than 15 minutes. Grade III concussions are characterized by LOC up to 30 minutes. All grades of concussion are technically considered to be mild TBI. Again, these variables may be obtained by self-report and are, therefore, less reliable as the sole source of information to determine head injury severity.

A range of postconcussion symptoms can emerge within the first 48 hours of injury. The most common physical symptoms include headache, dizziness, nausea or vomiting, fatigue, noise or light intolerance, and insomnia. These physical symptoms may result in the service member being seen at the combat support hospital, where a diagnosis of concussion may be made. Cognitive complaints are usually evident within 1 to 2 weeks and include memory complaints and poor concentration. Emotional or psychological symptoms, which also emerge within 24 to 48 hours of injury, include depression, anxiety, irritability, or mood lability. These problems may not be readily reported by the active-duty service member for a variety of reasons, including the need and desire to continue to perform his or her duties in theater, potential stigma in reporting psychological symptoms that may arise secondary to postconcussion symptoms, and the belief that symptoms will abate eventually, with the attitude of "pushing through" minor or persisting symptoms.

Symptoms tend to be most apparent immediately after the blast event, with significant variability in the resolution depending upon whether the service member continues to serve in a high-combat-intensity environment, exposure to further blasts or other mechanism of head injury, and the extent to which that service member seeks help for symptoms. Severity of symptoms of mild TBI is also in proportion to the severity of initial injury. For example, a service member might describe being hit by a mortar round that exploded 10 feet away, with no recollection of being thrown several feet from the blast into a concrete barrier, with immediate experiences of being dazed and disorientated. Immediately afterward, that service member may describe having trouble carrying out their duties, or being told by other unit members that cognitive problems (e.g., repeating information, memory problems, difficulty carrying through on tasks) were noticeable after the blast exposure. In this case, the clinician may suspect that a concussion may have occurred. Others might describe being near a VBIED (e.g., 50 yards away) and feeling the overpressurization wave, but did not exhibit any immediate symptoms. The latter scenario is not likely to have produced a concussion. There is no symptom that is unique to or diagnostic of mild TBI in the combat environment. In addition, in the case of the active-duty service member or veteran, co-occurring conditions may complicate the clinical picture; thus, it is difficult to draw direct connections between symptom complex and diagnosis.

3.2.5 Assessment of Blast-Related Traumatic Brain Injury

Beginning in April 2007, the VHA[27] implemented a routine primary screen for TBI. Comprised of the following four questions, the VHA screened for (1) the presence of an event that could plausibly cause TBI (blast or explosion, vehicular accident, fragment wound or bullet wound above the shoulders, fall); (2) any immediate symptoms around the event (losing consciousness or being "knocked out"; being dazed, confused, or "seeing stars"; not remembering the event); (3) beginning of, or worsening, symptoms after the event (memory problems or lapses, balance problems or dizziness, sensitivity to bright light, irritability, headaches, sleep problems); and (4) current problems within the past week (including the same set of symptoms noted in no. 3). Screening positive on all four items automatically triggers a referral for more in-depth evaluation. This next level of evaluation, known as the *TBI Secondary Evaluation*, is conducted by a licensed medical practitioner (MD, DO, PA, ARNP) and is frequently done in tandem with a psychologist (clinical psychologist, rehabilitation psychologist, neuropsychologist). The goal of the TBI Secondary Evaluation is to diagnose the veteran more definitively, including TBI, PTSD, and other co-occurring conditions, and to develop a rehabilitation plan of care.

Diagnosing mild TBI after the fact and against a backdrop of myriad competing plausible etiologic factors is fraught with challenges; yet, it is a typical referral question among providers within the DoD and VHA. The goal of this section is to outline concrete assessment strategies to aid the clinician in differential diagnosis and treatment planning. It is our impression that there is no substitute for an in-depth interview in understanding a possible history of blast injury.

Before outlining the specific components of an interview, we would like to suggest some general factors to consider. First, a brief caveat about interviewing persons who have served in recent combat: Clinicians working with this population are strongly encouraged to obtain some basic familiarity with the unique language used by military personnel so that they can establish credibility and rapport with the patients. For example, familiarity with terms and abbreviations related to rank, job duties, geographic locations, weapons, equipment, operations, and vehicles will greatly enhance the interviewee's comfort and likelihood of obtaining accurate information. Second, it should also be emphasized that the context of the interview is important. Anecdotally, many soldiers have reported to us that they have denied symptoms of TBI in certain interview contexts (e.g., routine postdeployment evaluations) because of fear of this diagnosis interfering with their expedient return home or with future promotions. Thus, it is important to explain the purpose of the evaluation and assess up front any misconceptions or concerns the patient may have about undergoing such assessment. Third, it should be clarified that the domains of assessment (blast event details, immediate and persistent symptoms) need to be evaluated for each and every blast event that occurred. After this is completed, a systematic assessment of the following components can begin.

3.2.5.1 Blast or Injury-Inducing Event

To evaluate for the presence of a blast that could plausibly cause a brain injury, several questions are recommended to appreciate fully the mechanism, including (1) type, size, and estimated amount of explosive; (2) proximity of blast to patient and orientation of patient to the blast (i.e., facing the explosion directly vs. having one's back to it, height and direction of the blast force); (3) protective or buffering layers between patient and explosion (i.e., in a building or vehicle vs. exposed on foot); (4) presence of protective gear (e.g., helmet, protective eyewear, ear plugs); (5) associated secondary, tertiary, quaternary, and quinary mechanisms of injury; and (6) other physical evidence to help gauge force, such as damage to proximal vehicles and buildings, injuries to others nearby, and displacement from the site of the explosion. The clinician should also pinpoint the date of each blast injury, if possible, to allow for evaluation of the effect of cumulative exposure. Without a plausible mechanism of injury or blast event, the diagnosis of TBI cannot be made.

3.2.5.2 Immediate Symptoms after Traumatic Brain Injury in Combat Theater

Although it is critical to evaluate the immediate symptoms of TBI (altered level or LOC, peritraumatic amnesia), this may be difficult to accomplish because patients may be unaware of whether they had a period of LOC and, if so, the duration. This is especially true if the event was not witnessed and patients regain consciousness by the time they were evaluated. Moreover, patients who regain consciousness during a combat situation are frequently immediately forced into action and are unable to assess or attend to any symptoms they may be experiencing in even a cursory way.

When assessing loss of or alteration in level of consciousness, multiple questions and a flexible approach may be beneficial. Obvious questions such as "Did you lose consciousness after this event?" may be difficult for the patient to answer because of amnesia about details of the event or lack of understanding of the true meaning of LOC. Alternative ways of interviewing patients about such events may include having patients describe the event in as much detail as they can remember, including things they heard, saw, experienced, thought, and did. Assessing altered mental status accurately may need to be differentiated from psychological shock or confusion after a blast. To differentiate confusion or shock resulting from trauma, combat, or simply proximity to a large blast, we recommend asking detailed questions to ascertain the degree to which patients are able to provide a continuous detailed account of the event. If they have gaps in memory or periods for which they cannot account, the clinician may be more confident in surmising an altered LOC was likely. Similarly, when assessing posttraumatic amnesia, multiple interview questions may be necessary to truly appreciate breaks in continuous memory. Service members may have retroactively received information about blast events from their fellow soldiers, and this needs to be differentiated from their own memory of the event in real time. Posttraumatic amnesia is strictly defined as the time interval from the impact until the patient is able to form memories for ongoing events continuously. During posttraumatic amnesia, the person is not fully oriented or able to remember information after a period of distraction. Ways to ask about this include things like "Please tell us, moment by moment, what happened after the blast," with repeated requests for more detail, until the examiner is reasonably confident that the time is plausibly and completely accounted for (or clear gaps are identified). The interviewing provider is also encouraged to ask patients about information they received, after the fact, from others who might have witnessed the event.

Responsiveness and behavior immediately after the event, which in the civilian world is often measured by emergency medical technicians and paramedics using the Glasgow Coma Scale (GCS), and reported in the field notes are rarely available. Interviewers are encouraged to ask questions that mirror GCS domains that allow them to appreciate responsiveness and behaviors after the event. For example, one might ask about motor responsiveness (Could you move about voluntarily? Were you able to continue your mission? Did you notice any physical changes in your ability to move?) and verbal responsiveness (Were you able to understand other people immediately after this happened? Could you say what you wanted to say? What, if any, changes did you notice in your ability to talk or understand others?). Some of these direct questions may be unnecessary if patients provide an account of sufficient detail that it is apparent that they were fully responsive and engaged.

3.2.5.3 Postconcussion Symptoms

Signs and symptoms of TBI that typically emerge within 48 hours of injury (or sooner) can include headaches or neck pain; lightheadedness, dizziness, or loss of balance; nausea; insomnia; tinnitus or ringing in the ears; sensitivity to light or sound; difficulty remembering, concentrating, or making decisions; slowness in thinking, speaking, acting, or reading; getting lost or easily confused; and feeling irritable or experiencing changes in mood or personality. The interviewing clinician is encouraged to assess systematically for the presence of these symptoms in the days following the blast injury. Related to this, the interviewing clinician should also inquire about any medical attention that was sought and the outcome of that effort, as well as any other behaviors that were required to cope with symptoms. For example, inquire about the use of over-the-counter medication, the need for extra rest, the need for any compensatory strategies that were identified, whether the soldier has any feedback from superiors or other service members. The clinician is also advised to ask about the effect of the injury on the service member's ability to perform his or her duties in the days and weeks after the event, recognizing that, even though rest or other postconcussion treatment measures may have been indicated medically, these may not have been realistically available options in the combat zone.

3.2.5.4 Assessment of Current Cognitive and Neurobehavioral Symptom Complex

For a majority of civilians, postconcussion symptoms tend to resolve rapidly, with full restoration of preinjury function expected within 3 to 6 months. Those with symptoms that persist beyond 6 months may be experiencing a persistent postconcussive syndrome. It is unknown whether this trajectory is also true for those with blast-related injury whose co-occurring conditions may, in fact, slow or complicate recovery to baseline levels of functioning. As part of the TBI Secondary Evaluation, the VHA uses the Neurobehavioral Symptom Inventory[28] to assess current symptoms. The spectrum of symptoms contained on this questionnaire allows the clinician to probe in greater depth regarding the patient's experience and functional limitations that may be the result of reported symptoms. Clusters of symptoms can be examined on this questionnaire (see the Appendix at the end of this chapter) that can also provide hypotheses regarding potential overlap of concussion and mental health conditions. For example, emotional symptoms that appear on the Neurobehavioral Symptom Inventory may be secondary to the presence of PTSD or depression. It is conceivable that emotional symptoms of concussion could be enhanced by PTSD/depression and, by the same token, the severity and persistence of PTSD/depression may be complicated by the concussion. In summary, the clinical evaluation of the OEF/OIF service member or veteran must take into account not only the individual diagnoses, signs, symptoms, and conditions that are presented but must also appreciate the interactive elements when there are multiple co-occurring conditions. Hence, the term *polytrauma* has been used and is characteristic of this new population of injured military personnel and veterans.

3.3 Co-occurring Disorders and Polytrauma

Combat zones are clearly some of the most stressful and physically demanding arenas in which to carry out operations and to accomplish missions as directed by military command. Herein is where there is significant divergence between civilian settings of TBI and those acquired in combat environments. Active-duty service members are exposed to an array of stressors and traumatic experiences that would be highly atypical in the civilian environment. Many of these experiences occur in less than predictable circumstances. For example, when engaged in a convoy, enemy combatants frequently craft ambushes meant to block convoys and direct U.S. military personnel into danger zones where IEDs or other explosive devices are planted, and where there is great vulnerability for attack by small weapons fire, RPG attack, and mortar rounds. The aftereffect may include civilian casualties, military personnel being killed or seriously injured, and significant trauma associated with experiencing these and other events. Such occurrence may be somewhat random in nature; it is difficult to predict when and where such events will occur. Furthermore, military personnel are tasked with the cleanup of the aftermath, requiring service members to handle human remains and body parts, witness others being injured, and seeing members of their own unit killed or injured. Other combat exposures include being surrounded, ambushed, and overrun by enemy combatants. Caring for wounded individuals, including enemy combatants, civilians, and fellow service members, can add to an already high-stress environment.

In addition to the physical context of blast injury, several salient aspects of the psychosocial environment must be considered. First, exposure to the extreme psychological and physical stress associated with combat can modify baseline physiology at the time of injury and make it difficult to detect postconcussion symptoms, such as irritability and sleep problems. This baseline alteration in physiology may also alter or amplify the actual biochemical events that occur during the acute stages of concussion. Other contextual factors that complicate presentation and assessment include the lack of opportunity to comply with recommended postconcussive care (e.g., rest) in a combat zone and the military cultural context, where fear of stigma, professional repercussions, or stoic norms prevent persons from seeking treatment.

The environment of the battlefield also plays a role in the health of active-duty service members. There are multiple environmental and occupational exposures in the combat theater, both in Iraq and Afghanistan, that can affect the general health condition of the service member (see VHA[27] for medical intake questions for the patient with polytrauma). These can include reactions to the following: smallpox and anthrax vaccinations, antimalaria pills, DEET on the skin, inhalation of trash/feces fumes and smoke, sand and dust exposures, vehicular exhaust, exposures to solvents and paints, acoustic traumas, heat stroke, exposure to blood, contamination from food and water, illness exposure (e.g., tuberculosis), exposures to ionizing radiation and depleted uranium, and exposures to chemical/biologic agents.

3.3.1 Mental Health Conditions and Exposures

Although this book chapter focuses on blast-related TBI, these injuries occur within combat zone environments that are replete with other war theater exposures and stressors that can lead to other non-TBI-related disorders. The mental health outcomes of U.S. military personnel, as well as having been studied by other coalition forces, have been recently studied. The presence of mental health problems as a consequence of participating in combat operations is therefore a complicating factor when describing blast injury consequences. A study by Hoge et al.[31] surveyed three U.S. Army units and one U.S. Marine Corp unit prior to and after deployment to Iraq and Afghanistan, where symptoms of major depression, generalized anxiety, and PTSD were assessed. Greater symptom reports were relatively higher among those deployed to Iraq compared with Afghanistan in 2003. Combat experiences were also reported as a part of this study and Table 3.3 is excerpted from their study, which illustrates some of these combat experiences.[29, p.18]

Higher rates of those meeting screening criteria for a mental disorder occurred after deployment when compared with predeployment levels. These researchers also found that, although many reported mental health problems, only a smaller percentage of those enduring such problems sought help.[29] They go on to note that issues of stigma regarding mental disorders and seeking help for those problems may be responsible for the lower rates of mental health help-seeking despite the presence of significant psychological disorder.

Several comorbid conditions are particularly prevalent among persons with mild TBI, and, because there is considerable overlap between symptoms associated with these various conditions, it is important to conduct an assessment to ensure that the appropriate etiologies are identified. For example, Hoge et al.[29] reported rates of PTSD were 43.9% among soldiers who had a definite LOC, and 27.3% among those who experienced altered mental status. The DoD routinely conducts postdeployment health assessments 3 to 6 months after deployment. The self-assessment portion of this assessment includes four items assessing combat experiences, a two-item screen for depression, a four-item screen for PTSD, and single items assessing suicidal ideation, concerns about excessive aggression, interpersonal concerns, and alcohol use. Another study by Hoge et al.[30] studied a group of 303,905 U.S. Army soldiers and U.S. Marine Corps service members who completed

TABLE 3.3

Combat Experiences of U.S. Military Personnel in OEF and OIF

Combat Experience	U.S. Army, Afghanistan (N = 1962)	U.S. Army, Iraq (N = 894)	U.S. Marines, Iraq (N = 815)
Being attacked or ambushed	58	89	95
Receiving incoming artillery, rocket, or mortar fire	84	86	92
Being shot at or receiving small-arms fire	66	93	97
Being responsible for the death of an enemy combatant	12	48	65
Being responsible for the death of a noncombatant	1	14	28
Seeing dead bodies or human remains	39	95	94
Handling or uncovering human remains	12	50	57
Seeing dead or seriously injured Americans	30	65	75
Knowing someone seriously injured or killed	43	86	87
Participating in demining operations	16	38	34
Seeing ill or injured women or children you were unable to help	46	69	83
Being wounded or injured	5	14	9
Having a close call; was shot or hit, but protective gear saved you	Not included in survey	8	10
Having a buddy shot or hit near you	Not included in survey	22	26
Clearing or searching homes or buildings	57	80	86
Engaging in hand-to-hand combat	3	22	9
Saving the life of soldier or civilian	6	21	19

Source: Hoge, C. W., Castro, C. A., Messer, S. C., McGurk, D., Cotting, D. I., and Koffman, R. L., *New England Journal of Medicine*, 351, 13–22, 2004.

the postdeployment health reassessment between May 2003 and April 2004, upon return from OEF/OIF, including those returning from Bosnia and Kosovo. Of those who met risk criteria for a mental health concern, 19% of those who returned were from OIF, 11.3% from OEF, and 8.5% from other locations. Furthermore, those exposed to combat situations correlated with screening positive for PTSD (on a PTSD screening instrument). Of those who screened positive on the PTSD screening after returning from OIF, 79.6% reported seeing persons being wounded or killed, or had engaged in a combat situation in which that service member discharged a weapon.

Rates of mental health disorders have also been reported by military personnel deployed by the United Kingdom. A study by Turner et al.[31] examined personnel who were evacuated from war zones because of combat-related stress. Tracked from January 2003 to October 2003 (recall that the invasion of Iraq by coalition forces occurred in March 2003), military personnel with psychiatric evacuations were counted. A total of 116 individuals were followed, with the greatest number of psychiatric evacuations occurring during the war compared with prewar and postwar phases of participants' military operation involvement. The top two reasons for psychiatric evacuations were the result of environmental issues (i.e., difficulty coping with the physical conditions in war) and difficulty coping with separating from close family members, spouses, or partners. Presenting symptoms included low mood (78.4%), anxiety (12.0%), and somatic symptoms (3.4%). The greatest majority of the sample was diagnosed (via ICD-10 codes) with adjustment disorder (50.8%), no psychiatric diagnosis (30.2%), acute stress reaction (6.9%), and mild depressive episode (6.0%).

It also appears that exposures either in peacekeeping activities or those associated with combat operations are associated with increased rates of mental health disorders. Sareen and coworkers[32] surveyed 8441 Canadian active military service members to evaluate the relative rates of mental disorder and combat exposures. Interestingly, of those who were exposed to peacekeeping operations, 80.3% were also exposed to combat and 84.2% witnessed atrocities or massacres. Hence, although one's duty may be primarily that of peacekeeping operations, significant stressful combat exposures were experienced by Canadian military personnel. Not surprisingly, those who experienced exposure to combat or witnessed atrocities or massacres reported higher rates of any mental health disorder, with major depression and PTSD being more common.

In a longitudinal assessment of mental health symptoms, 88,235 soldiers completed the postdeployment health assessment and postdeployment health reassessment at least 6 months apart.[33] The authors found that rates of any mental health concerns increased from approximately 18% to 29% during the first 6 months postdeployment among active-duty soldiers, and from 16% to 38% among those from the Reserves or National Guard. Similarly, rates of PTSD increased from 12% to 17% among active-duty soldiers, and from 13% to 23% among reservists. Given that many symptoms of PTSD and mild TBI overlap (i.e., difficulty concentrating, irritability, mood or personality changes, insomnia or sleep difficulties) and that symptoms of mild TBI also overlap with symptoms of depression, it is essential that comorbidities be evaluated concurrently with mild TBI.

3.3.2 Overlap between PTSD and Traumatic Brain Injury Symptomatology

Much is in common between symptoms related to TBI, often referred to as the *postconcussion syndrome*, and those symptoms that are common among those with PTSD and major depression—the latter two being the most common types of mental disorder among U.S. active-duty servicemen and veterans. Furthermore, the literature on postconcussion syndrome also finds that typical symptoms associated with concussion are also shared by healthy control subjects, as well as those with fibromyalgia.[34] Table 3.4 lists typical postconcussion symptoms that may arise from multiple concussion secondary to blast exposures, and denoted within the table are those symptoms that share a common phenomenology with PTSD. This overlap between PTSD, as well as depression-related symptomatology, with the consequences of multiple concussive events, results in a complicated clinical picture in evaluating military personnel and veterans who have been diagnosed both with TBI and PTSD.

Those who are sensitive to noises can be a result of hypervigilance symptoms of PTSD where the service member or veteran may be "on alert status," just as they had been in war theater, despite knowing, rationally, that there is no immediate threat within the home or in their home community. Mood symptoms, such as irritability, temper loss, dysphoria, and sadness or anxiety, are common in those with PTSD and clinical depression. Sleep and fatigue problems are frequently described by those with PTSD secondary to nightmares (that result in less total sleep per night) or hypervigilance during the evening hours and, thus, difficulty falling and staying asleep. Those with chronic sleep deprivation during their deployment in theater may also have marked difficulty readjusting their sleep–wake cycle upon return home. The overlap of PTSD and postconcussion symptoms is well illustrated in a study by Schneiderman et al.[35] who surveyed 2235 OEF/OIF

TABLE 3.4

Overlap of Symptoms between Postconcussive, PTSD, and
Depressive Symptomatology

Postconcussion Symptoms[a]	Overlaps with PTSD/Depression
Headache	
Dizzy/lightheaded	
Nauseous/feeling sick	
Fatigue	X
Extrasensitive to noises	X
Irritable	X
Sad	X
Nervous or tense	X
Temper problems	X
Poor concentration	X
Memory problems	X
Difficulty reading	
Poor sleep	X
Sensitive to light[a]	
Change in taste/smell[a]	

[a] Also frequently listed as postconcussion symptoms.
Source: N. D. Zasler, D. I. Katz, and R. D. Zafonte (Eds.), *Brain Injury Medicine:*
Principles and Practice, Demos Medical Publishing, New York, 2006.

military personnel and found that 12% reported a history consistent with TBI and 11%
screened positive for PTSD. Higher rates of PTSD occurred in those reporting polytrauma
and combat-related mild TBI. Furthermore, the best predictor of postconcussive symptoms was the presence of PTSD, after the overlapping symptoms were extracted from
PTSD scores.

Overlapping symptoms can also account for cognitive problems seen in those with
PTSD and combat-related TBI. However, cognitive problems are not specific to TBI alone.
In a prospective cohort-controlled study by Vasterling et al.,[36] active-duty U.S. Army soldiers ($n = 654$) were compared with nondeployed soldiers ($n = 307$) prior to and after
deployment to OIF on mood and neuropsychological measures. The average length of
deployment was 16.9 months (standard deviation, 3.1 months). Not surprisingly, deployed
soldiers demonstrated compromise in sustained attention, verbal learning and memory,
and visual–spatial memory. In addition, those who were deployed reported increased
negative state affect for confusion and tension. An interesting additional finding was the
fact that, after controlling for deployment-related TBI, stress, and depression symptoms,
these cognitive and mood findings held. These findings point to the presence of cognitive performance decrements secondary to deployment, even without the presence of
known TBI.

To examine the relationship between mild TBI and PTSD symptoms in U.S. military,
Hoge and coworkers[8] documented 2525 soldiers, of whom 4.9% reported injuries with
LOC, 10.3% with altered consciousness, and 17.2% noted other injuries during deployment (i.e., nonhead injury). Those with LOC and altered mental status reported they had
been involved in a blast explosion (79% and 72.7%, respectively). PTSD was associated
with mild TBI in that 43.9% with LOC also met criteria for PTSD. Of those with altered
mental status, 27.3% met PTSD criteria, and this compares with 9.1% with PTSD who
had no injuries. Combat intensity and LOC was significantly associated with PTSD. They

concluded that the data "indicate that a history of mild traumatic brain injury in the combat environment, particularly when associated with loss of consciousness, reflects exposure to a very intense traumatic event that threatens loss of life and significantly increases the risk of PTSD."[8, p.461] Further research and studies that are prospective in nature are needed to better understand the natural recovery and complications associated with combined PTSD and TBI. These data underscore the complicated relationship between the two disorders.

3.3.2.1 Assessment of Co-occurring Mental Health Conditions

A key issue to assist with accurate diagnosis of PTSD symptomatology in those who have experienced blast injury include several well-validated instruments that are available to evaluate PTSD symptoms, and these are recommended for use in conjunction with a clinical interview. A version of the PTSD Checklist (or PCL) that is specific to military experiences (PCL-M) has been developed and validated for this purpose.

More information about briefer screening instruments are available at the National PTSD website[37] and there are numerous other resources that are available to the public, veterans, family members, health care providers, and researchers from that website. For example, posted on this website is the *Iraq War Clinician Guideline*, 2nd edition,[38] that covers topics about the psychiatric treatment of OEF/OIF active-duty service members and veterans, rehabilitation for those who are amputees, military sexual trauma, VA/DoD practice guidelines, selection of assessment instruments for the evaluation of OEF/OIF war veterans coping with traumatic stress, as well as educational materials for family members.

Similarly, there are multiple available inventories to evaluate for symptoms of depressive disorders, including the Patient Health Questionnaire-9 which is a nine-item self-report module from the Primary Care Evaluation of Mental Disorders (or PRIME-MD)[39] that assesses depressive symptom severity and screens for major and minor depressive episodes.

The assessment of combat-related stress is an important variable for returning service members. These measures allow the clinician to understand the breadth and depth of experiences that may be unique to war zone deployment. Furthermore, it helps to define the types of traumatic exposures that may be playing a role in initiating and maintaining mental health problems that arise out of war. It is important that, when assessing the active-duty service member or veteran, what may appear to be the most traumatic event to the clinician may not necessarily be the most traumatic to the service member. Therefore, self-reported questionnaires may be seen as a beginning point to understanding the types and nature of traumatic events that may be fueling PTSD symptoms and, therefore, prolonging functional disability in these individuals. One such instrument, the Combat Experiences Scale (an 18-item dichotomous yes/no response inventory), includes entries such as: While deployed, I went on combat patrols or missions. While deployed, I or members of my unit were attacked by terrorists or civilians. While deployed, my unit engaged in battle in which it suffered casualties. These items will assess not only the array of combat stressors, but also will denote the level of combat intensity that, in previous studies cited in this chapter, has been associated with the presence of PTSD.

Within VHA medical centers and VA community-based outpatient centers, processes are in place to provide mandatory screening for PTSD, Iraq/Afghanistan exposure screening, and TBI screening after a service member separates from the military and becomes a veteran. Throughout each service line with the VHA, clinicians are alerted to these template and interactive screening procedures via the electronic medical chart. Notices show on the electronic chart regarding which screens are due, and clinicians from any discipline who see the veteran within the medical center or VA community-based outpatient center (including primary care physicians, psychologists, mental health clinicians, dentists, nursing staff, and others) have been trained to ask specific questions that, if the screen is positive, initiates further evaluations for conditions of PTSD, suicidal ideology, depression, alcohol abuse, and TBI. These simple screening questions are meant to assess more easily, then to engage more systematically the veteran in a process of comprehensive postcombat care evaluations to develop effective plans of care.

3.3.3 Common Polytrauma Conditions

As noted earlier in this chapter, Owens and colleagues[11] reported on the data gathered through the U.S. Joint Theater Trauma Registry, in which 6609 combat wounds were recorded among 1566 combatants. The largest percentage of these wounds were extremity injuries (54%), followed by abdominal (11%) and facial wounds (10%). Other wounds were distributed among the head, eyes, ears, neck, and thorax. Extremity wounds are high, likely secondary to the protection offered by body armor around vital body organs, but leaving the extremities exposed. Extremity injuries occurred in similar proportions in World War II, Korea, and Vietnam. Wade et al.[10] reported on the U.S. Navy–Marine Corps Combat Trauma Registry data in a retrospective analysis of the period March 1, 2004, to September 30, 2004, in OIF. The focus of this data review was on head, face, and neck injuries, in which the majority of these were facial injuries (65%), again largely attributable to IED explosions. They note that, despite the protection to penetrating head and chest injuries with modern Kevlar body armor, the face is exposed to injury. The authors comment: "Ballistic eye protection is available, but reportedly worn less frequently than other types of body armor at the time of injury. This may be because of the deliberate removal of protective eyewear before the injury event to improve visual acuity while scanning the combat environment."[10, p.839] Polytrauma injuries are characterized by significant problems with chronic musculoskeletal pain, persistent headaches, vision and hearing loss, traumatic amputations, and other problems that are consistent with the previously mentioned injury reporting data.

Chronic pain is prevalent among OEF/OIF veterans as reported in a sample of veterans seeking treatment at a VA medical center by Gironda and coworkers.[40] In this sample, 28% ($n = 219$ of a total 793 whose charts included pain documentation) reported moderate to severe pain intensity. Common diagnoses in this cohort were musculoskeletal and connective tissue disorders for 82% of those whose pain duration was greater than 1 month. Among those with TBI, *headaches* were common in this group of OEF/OIF veterans with polytrauma. A good example of the multiple co-occurring conditions for which the presence of chronic headaches are frequent are findings published by Ruff et al.[41] who found that, of 126 veterans who screened positive on the aforementioned TBI screens, 80 demonstrated neurologic impairments. Those with impairments had a history of multiple blast exposures, higher frequency of headaches (including migraine), more severe chronic pain, PTSD, and sleep disturbances with nightmares. *Migraines* have also been found to be prevalent in U.S. Army soldiers who returned from a 1-year deployment to Iraq.[42] Among this group, 19% were found to screen positive for migraine headaches with another 17% noted to have possible migraines.

Military operations involve the use of an array of weaponry, and war environments are characterized by exposure to explosives and other events (e.g., open fire pits) that can lead to *burns*. Patients in OEF/OIF with burns are treated at the U.S. Army Institute of Surgical Research in San Antonio, Texas. From April 2003 to April 2005, it was found that 55% of burns were caused by IED blasts, followed by 16% resulting from VBIEDs, 15% caused by RPG, 7% secondary to mortar round exposure, and 4% resulting from land mine exposure.[43] Of those casualties, hand and head areas of the body comprised the greatest percentage (80% and 77%, respectively). Burn mechanisms in war theater occur as a direct result of heat from the explosive blast, and from the secondary effect of burning vehicles, clothing, and equipment.

Ocular trauma and perforating globe injuries also occur as a result of blast exposures. Because the eyes are fluid-filled organs, they are therefore vulnerable to damage secondary to the primary overpressurization wave (both positive and negative phases of the blast wind cycle), and to fragment injuries that result from the explosive device and secondary damage.[44–46] In a sample of those admitted to a polytrauma rehabilitation center, and seen at an inpatient optometry clinic ($N = 50$), 18% had one eye enucleated and 8% had bilateral blindness, with 74% self-reporting vision complaints.[47]

Dizziness, *balance*, and *vestibular* disorders occur as a consequence of TBI, and these are also seen after blast exposures. The primary blast overpressurization wave can cause tympanic membrane damage and rupture, and damage to the inner ear canals occurs. In mild TBI, dizziness problems can occur as well[48]; for service members, dizziness problems can be complicated by musculoskeletal injuries acquired in theater. According to Cave et al.,[49] the overpressurization wave creates sensorineural, conductive, and mixed hearing loss damage, as well as fracture to the ossicles. Their study, conducted at the Army Audiology and Speech Center at the Walter Reed Army Medical Center, consisted of examination of OEF and OIF service members seen between April 2003 and August 2005. Close to 60% of the patients evaluated had hearing loss, and 32% had tympanic membrane perforation. Scherer and colleageus[50] studied blast-related traumatic amputees and found that 24% of these patients reported experiencing vertigo or oscillopsia after the blast event, and 51% reported subjective hearing loss. These findings underscore the importance of audiologic and vestibular examinations for those who have been exposed to blasts.

Traumatic amputations are another consequence of blast wave exposures. These occur as a result of the primary blast wind, and occur secondary to limb injuries that lead to eventual amputation of that limb. With the majority of explosions occurring from ground-implanted IEDs, lower extremity amputations tend to be more common. In a retrospective analysis of 8058 military casualties in Iraq and Afghanistan between October 2001 and June 2006, 70.5% of these were listed as having a major limb injury. Of those having had a major limb injury, 7.4% underwent a limb amputation.[51] This is compared with an 8.3% rate of limb amputation during the Vietnam War among those with major limb injury. These rates were judged to be comparable. Facing those who are postamputees of the OEF and OIF conflicts are potential problems with skin breakdown and subsequent surgery, phantom limb pain problems, and possibility of heterotopic ossification. Regarding heterotopic ossification, Potter et al.[52] found that, of a group of 330 patients from OEF/OIF with 373 traumatic and combat-related amputations, heterotopic ossification was identified in 134 (63%) of the 213 residual limbs.

These conditions, and many other residual physical, cognitive, and neurobehavioral problems after blast-related TBI, have altered both military treatment facilities and VHA medical centers to develop comprehensive systems of care for those with polytrauma.

3.4 Polytrauma Rehabilitation and Integrated Care Approaches

The system of care for polytrauma extends from the combat theater to care delivered in VHA facilities and in the community. For example, in Iraq, combat lifesaving is done in the field, with the intention of stabilizing patients sufficiently to transfer them to combat support hospitals, which are 200+-bed hospitals that provide care to troops and Iraqis (including insurgents, police forces, prisoners, and civilians). Average length of stay is less than 3 days, with the goal being stabilization rather than definitive surgical repair. Iraqis receive all of their care in Iraq, whereas wounded troops are typically evacuated rapidly to one of three level IV hospitals (in Kuwait; Rota, Spain; or Landstuhl, Germany). If expected to require more than 30 days of treatment, soldiers are evacuated to the United States, typically to DoD treatment facilities such as Walter Reed Army Medical Center in Washington, DC, and the Brooke Army Medical Center in San Antonio, Texas.[15] From the DoD facilities, patients are typically transferred to a military treatment facility close to their homes, or close to the original post or base from which their unit was deployed. Transition to the VHA may occur after it becomes apparent that the soldier is likely to be discharged from the armed forces because of his or her injuries. A medical boarding process occurs for those deemed to be no longer fit for duty. The DoD and VHA have a memorandum of agreement that allows for active-duty service members to be treated in VHA facilities, and this also facilitates a smoother transition from active duty to veteran/ civilian status.

3.4.1 VHA Polytrauma System of Care

In 2005, the VHA issued a directive to create the polytrauma system of care. In place, up to that time, were the existing Defense and Veterans' Brain Injury Centers (established in 1992 as the Defense and Veterans' Head Injury Program), with locations at the Walter Reed Army Medical Center, Naval Medical Center San Diego, Brooke Army Medical Center/ Wilford Hall Medical Center (San Antonio, Texas), and the VA medical centers located in Tampa, Florida; Minneapolis, Minnesota; Richmond, Virginia; and Palo Alto, California. The VHA polytrauma system of care is a four-tier integrated care network and, as of March 2009, consists of four polytrauma rehabilitation centers, which are the four VA medical centers located in Tampa, Minneapolis, Richmond, and Palo Alto (a fifth polytrauma rehabilitation center in San Antonio, Texas, is under construction), 22 polytrauma network site programs (one per each VHA region known as a *vicinity integrated service network*), 81 polytrauma support clinic teams (which are located at smaller and more local VA medical centers), and 48 polytrauma points of contact (individuals at VA medical centers that are designated as a key contact person to connect patients with the polytrauma system of care and with local resources). This large system of care was put into place in a relatively short period of time and provides a full range of acute, transitional living, postacute, and community/vocational reentry rehabilitation services for OEF/OIF veterans and active-duty service members. Some components of care for those with polytrauma are described in the following sections.

3.4.2 Acute Care

Acute management of concussion is guided by the accumulated wisdom from the sports concussion literature. After a grade I concussion, soldiers should be examined immediately and subsequently monitored every 5 minutes for 15 minutes to ensure that mental status abnormalities or postconcussive symptoms clear within 15 minutes. If this is the case, they may resume duties. After a grade II concussion, it is recommended that soldiers immediately be removed from the situation, examined frequently for 24 to 48 hours for signs of evolving intracranial pathology, and cleared by a physician before resuming duties after a full asymptomatic week of rest and with exertion. After a grade III concussion, soldiers should be emergently treated. Treatment should include a thorough neurologic evaluation, including neuroimaging, if available and indicated. Hospital admission is indicated if any signs of pathology are detected or if mental status remains abnormal. Among athletes, at least 2 weeks of rest is indicated before resuming "play" after a single concussion. In the instance of multiple grade III concussions, a month or longer is indicated before resuming play and should be determined by a physician.

These recommendations are practically impossible to institute in a combat theater. Most soldiers who sustain a concussion in combat immediately reengage in combat activities. In our clinical experience, we have heard numerous soldiers report that they were injured in combat situations and remained under direct fire or ambush for an extended period. Soldiers have reported that, even while clearly dizzy, disoriented, or otherwise experiencing immediate postconcussion symptoms, they have vague memories of continuing to attempt to man their post, fire their weapons, drive their vehicles, or otherwise engage, to the best of their abilities, often for several more hours. Others have reported regaining consciousness in extremely dangerous situations (e.g., outside of a vehicle in fire fights or ambush situations) and having to locate their unit and get to safety independently, despite severe confusion, pain, dizziness, and auditory, visual, and vestibular postconcussion symptoms. In sum, although rest and careful monitoring is the recommended acute treatment for concussion, followed by careful and gradual reengagement in activities, this is possible in only a small minority of combat-related cases.

3.4.3 Postacute Care for Mild Traumatic Brain Injury

For those who have been injured within the past 3 months, the primary treatment is education about expected symptoms, course of recovery, strategies to ensure adequate rest, gradual resumption of normal level of activities, and signs and symptoms to watch for that might indicate additional evaluation or treatment is needed. A brief cognitive–behavioral intervention developed by Ferguson and Mittenberg[53] has been useful to prevent or minimize the longer term impact or persistence of postconcussive symptomatology.

3.4.4 Treatment beyond Six Months

By definition, if a patient is seeking treatment for mild TBI beyond 6 months, they are seeking treatment for postconcussion syndrome. The principal tenet of treatment at this stage is symptom specific. The clinician is advised to treat the primary conditions (i.e., the ones that explain most or all of the symptoms). For example, complaints of ongoing memory or attentional difficulties would warrant consideration of neuropsychological assessment and cognitive rehabilitation therapies as indicated. Complaints of mood symptoms (irritability, depression, or anxiety) would warrant psychologically, behaviorally, or pharmacologically oriented therapies. The presence of a significant comorbid psychiatric condition, such as PTSD or alcohol abuse, would also be a primary focus of intervention, because this would be expected to affect functional improvement. Each of these is discussed in detail later in the chapter.

3.4.5 Treatment of Cognitive Sequelae in Polytrauma

Those that are seen for polytrauma rehabilitation frequently present with cognitive complaints. Such cognitive problems are likely a result of a combination of conditions, including the aftereffects of multiple concussions, presence of PTSD, chronic pain, and sleep disorders. The cognitive problems presented by the patient with blast-related TBI are not significantly different from those TBIs that are the result of nonblast mechanisms, such as motor vehicle accidents, falls, or other blunt head trauma.[54] This study also found a higher rate of PTSD among those with blast-related TBI, again underscoring the complex clinical presentations of this population. If cognitive impairments are identified through a comprehensive polytrauma team evaluation, then engagement of a rehabilitation team, particularly speech–language pathology, occupational therapy, neuropsychology, and vocational rehabilitation might be indicated, with a focus on developing compensatory cognitive strategies and symptoms. In addition, the rehabilitation team can provide TBI education and support to patients and their family. Appropriate treatment can be delivered in individual or group format. Considerable literature exists supporting the efficacy of group-based therapy for individuals who are status–postmild TBI.[55,56] Sample components of group-based cognitive rehabilitation are below.

A group designed to enhance compensatory cognitive skills after mild TBI should address several core components, including attention, memory, and executive function. Sohlberg and Mateer's[57] Clinical Model of Attention is recommended as a foundation for improving attention. Based on this model, the clinician focuses on the development of strategies and environmental supports to change the type of attention required, such as reducing distractions (thus moving from selective attention to sustained or focused attention), breaking tasks into smaller chunks (thus moving from sustained to focused attention), prioritizing and simplifying tasks (thus moving from tasks that require divided or alternating attention to focused or sustained attention), and using external aids (e.g., checklists; alarms; electronic organizers; task-specific devices, such as key hooks, pill box reminders). Several prospective trials have indicated that such strategies are effective in improving day-to-day attentional abilities.[58,59] Group participants should be encouraged to enlist psychosocial support concurrently as an adjunct to all attention strategies, and to become educated about the ways that nonneurocognitive factors (e.g., sleep deprivation, pain, psychological distress) can detract from attentional abilities. To evaluate the effectiveness of such strategies, ongoing self-evaluation in daily function is indicated, rather than formal neuropsychological testing.

To address memory concerns post-TBI, a group should include the development of prospective memory strategies and systems, with emphasis on the selection and refinement of compensatory memory tools. Several prospective studies have indicated that such strategies are effective for persons with mild TBI-related impairments. Cotreatment with speech–language pathology and psychology is often helpful to develop these strategies. Hi-tech tools to aid memory (e.g., digital voice recorders, cell phones) are appealing to the military cohort and have been shown to be effective strategies for aiding prospective memory.[60] Development of memory systems needs to be highly tailored to each individual within the class, and conceptualized as an ongoing "work in progress."

3.4.6 Managing Mood after Traumatic Brain Injury

Among the most prevalent emotional and behavioral issues that affect participants' abilities to utilize compensatory cognitive strategies effectively after TBI are depression,[61] anxiety, anger/frustration, impulsivity, lability, lack of insight, and substance use-related problems.[62] Treatment is needed to address these affective and behavioral dysregulation problems so that compensatory cognitive strategies might be more accessible and feasible, through education, social support, and improved deficit awareness, and through the development of self-monitoring and problem-solving skills. Some practical aspects of leading such a group are summarized in the work by Delmonico et al.[63] To address disability awareness and insight-related problems, a sample exercise involves coaching participants on how to conduct structured interviews with two to three carefully selected people outside of group to solicit feedback. In group, we review this feedback, look for themes, and consider it in light of participants' own experiences and perceptions. Discrepancies in self-perception and reports of others are identified as opportunities to gain insight. In a parallel fashion, several exercises are also taught to inventory participants' "dependable strengths." For example, participants generate a record of situations in which they recently felt successful, effective, or happy, and identify the role that their personality, values, or actions played during each of these situations. When several records are completed, as a group, we look for themes or consistent "dependable strengths."

A combination of techniques can be taught to regulate mood, including strategies to recognize and label alternations in mood state rapidly, strategies to control behavior (and damage) when in emotional crisis (e.g., taking "time outs," increasing distress tolerance, relaxation), and strategies to improve baseline mood and hone coping skills between crises. The strategies taught are largely derived from two schools of thought: a cognitive–behavioral approach, which involves defining "problems" concretely, generating and weighing alternative solutions, and decision making; and a mindfulness approach (from acceptance and commitment therapy).[64] The rationale for utilizing somewhat disparate approaches lies in the fact that different strategies appeal to different group members, and the goal is to provide them with a repertoire of coping skills from which they can choose.

3.4.7 Family Support

In the case of serious injuries, family members frequently assume the burdens of physically caring for their injured family member and advocating for their family member, as well as assuming increased financial, parenting, and house management duties. When injuries include brain injury, mental illness, or other conditions that affect service members' cognitive and psychological function, relationships may evidence strain in the realms of intimacy and relationship satisfaction, secondary traumatization may occur, and increased rates of aggression and intimate partner violence have been reported. As stated in the RAND report, "the effects of post-combat mental and cognitive conditions inevitably extend beyond the afflicted service member … their impairments cannot fail to wear on those with whom they interact and those closest to the service member are most likely to be affected." [5, p.141] Caregivers are at significant risk for increased health and mood problems of their own. When these problems are superimposed upon the existing stresses related to deployment, families are particularly vulnerable and in need of support. Although the RAND report stresses that further research is needed to understand better the causal links and particular risk factors associated with adverse family outcomes, the authors also underscore the importance of offering assistance to caregivers that is accessible and appropriate (RAND Center for Military Health Policy Research).[5]

3.4.8 Importance and Potential Role of Peer Support and Visitation

Since the Vietnam War, the importance of peer support for and by veterans has been critical among approaches to assist veterans with combat-related injuries. The inception and success of the veterans' centers around the United States attests to the need for both professional and peer support for PTSD, as an example. In the polytrauma population, peer visitation (PV) can provide individuals coping with multiple disorders and disability an opportunity to interact with a peer who has survived and managed a similar condition. The effectiveness of peer visitation is well explained by social learning theory.[65] Through observation of successful role models, we increase self-efficacy and learn specific actions and coping strategies. Such increases in efficacy and knowledge can, in turn, engender hope and improve motivation to engage in treatment.

In current practice, peer support is provided in group or one-on-one settings, face-to-face or virtual settings, may or may not involve training for the peer leader, and may or may not be overseen by an organization or allied health professional.[66] Many peer visitor programs are tailored for persons with medical conditions. Some organizations offer nationally based PV programs (e.g., the National Spinal Cord Injury Association and the Amputee Coalition of America), whereas others operate more regionally.[67–70] Although many organizations offer peer visitors, there is great inconsistency in their provision of training, methods of matching of visitors to recipients, and evaluating visits.

Despite the widespread availability of PV programs, empirical support for their efficacy is limited. Of the limited literature available, most is comprised of retrospective qualitative evaluations of peer visits. This literature consistently indicates that recipients find peer support beneficial.[70–73] For example, in one study of a PV program for persons with spinal cord injury, recipients of a PV reported that they perceived PVs as providing a unique type of social support that was more credible, provided more practical and detailed information than is given by clinicians, inspired hope, and relieved distress.[74] In a study of women newly diagnosed with breast cancer and participating in a cancer support service, 53% reported that meeting someone with a similar experience was the most important aspect of the program and 89% said that they would definitely recommend this to others.[75]

The handful of studies that have examined more objective outcomes indicate that continued efforts to develop and evaluate PV are warranted. In one of the few case–control studies published, breast cancer patients who received peer mentorship through the Canadian Cancer Society's Reach to Recovery program reported decreased feelings of isolation, increased optimism for the future, increased knowledge of treatment and coping options, increased coping ability, and improved functional social support and relationships with their doctors compared with case subjects who did not have peer visitors.[72] Participants in this program identified peer knowledge as a key aspect of peer visits; participants were 11 times more likely to report satisfaction with the program if they felt their peer visitor was helpful in answering their questions. Other important aspects of peer visits that have been identified across studies are good peer visitor listening skills,[66] perceived similarity between visitor and patient,[67] and perceived supportiveness of the peer visitor.[72] These latter findings underscore the importance of screening and training peer visitors appropriately. Despite growing program availability and encouraging empirical support, peer support programs are used by a minority (20%–30%) of those who might benefit.[71]

Apropos to OEF/OIF active-duty service members and veterans with polytrauma, application of peer support approaches is found in the Traumatic Brain Injury Model System of Care in Santa Clara, California, which includes a peer support component.[76] Both peer visitors and recipients of peer visitors can be either individuals who have survived an injury or a family member of a person who has survived a brain injury. Although the program has not been empirically evaluated, qualitative data indicate that it is not only possible but ultimately therapeutic for persons with brain injury to provide peer support to more recently injured persons (after they have achieved a significant degree of recovery themselves). Moreci[76] emphasized the importance of thorough initial training as well as ongoing education and programmatic support.

3.5 Conclusions

Each war conflict tends to be characterized by specific types of injuries and, as a consequence, new medical innovations and health care delivery models emerge. Evolving from the concept of "shell shock," we are now applying modern scientific knowledge regarding mild TBI, evidence-based treatments for PTSD, and new models of rehabilitation for combat-related injuries such as the VHA polytrauma system of care to active-duty service members and veterans. Greater awareness of the medical, psychological, and rehabilitation needs by health care providers at military treatment facilities, VHA care systems, and community providers has advanced the efficacy and efficiency to those who have experienced blast-related TBI and polytrauma. As this system of care evolves, a better understanding of the complex set of problems that are presented by OEF/OIF service member and veterans will emerge, despite some of the current controversies that continue to arise with regard to the nature of the disorders presented by this population.[77] Delivering services not only to those with combat-related injuries with polytrauma, but also work toward understanding the needs of and developing effective interventions for family members[78,79] and caregivers will likely characterize continued and lifelong care that is and will expand in VHA facilities.

Research partnerships between the DoD, VHA, and the larger academic community are now occurring to advance the knowledge base regarding the potential unique characteristics of blast exposures and the longer term neurobehavioral and physical consequences of blast injuries. Much remains to be learned, however. For example, recent research is suggesting that blast-related brain dysfunction may be contributed to by stimulating nitric oxide production in the reticular formation and dorsal hippocampal regions, leading to cognitive deficits.[80] Pulmonary blast injury has been studied in animals in which systemic circulatory dysfunction with changes in the medulla oblongata were found,[81] implicating cognitive and regulatory dysfunction. Mismatching of ventilation with pulmonary blood flow that leads to hypoxemia is another mechanism of blast-induced neurotrauma that has been demonstrated in animal models of primary blast injury.[82] Thoracic mechanisms of mild TBI secondary to blast overpressurization wave exposure has been forwarded by Courtney and Courtney,[83] who noted that brain injury may be caused through pressure waves transferred to the brain (affecting brain cells) through thoracic mechanisms.

The role of the neuroendocrine system, both in TBI[84] and PTSD,[85] is likely to gain further attention. Here, the involvement of the hypothalamic–pituitary–adrenal axis may be a common pathway that explains the significant overlap of symptoms in both conditions. Further discoveries in these areas may lead to development of more targeted and efficacious psychopharmacology and neuropharmacology for combat veterans and active-duty service members with polytrauma.

A clearer understanding of the role of neurorehabilitation strategies is emerging for combat-related TBI. In a recent multicenter, randomized, controlled trial conducted by Vanderploeg et al.,[86] cognitive–didactic versus functional–experiential rehabilitation approaches were compared in active-duty service members with TBI. Long-term functional outcomes (independence in living skills, work/school reentry) were similar in both approaches, whereas the cognitive–didactic group fared better with regard to posttreatment cognitive functioning. Further work is needed to develop specific and efficacious neurorehabilitation strategies, of both a compensatory and restorative nature, to address the continuing and growing needs of active-duty service members and veterans who sustain blast injuries and subsequent polytrauma.

Finally, it should be said that effective delivery of care to military personnel and veterans will rely on the ability of the larger organizations and systems of care that are brought to bear to care for these individuals. The interdisciplinary rehabilitation team is the lowest common denominator in polytrauma care, and formulating interventions requires a philosophy of postcombat care that appreciates the significant synthesis of psychological, physical,[87] and existential dimensions of coping and suffering, the latter defined by Cassel[88] as "a specific state of distress that occurs when the intactness or integrity of the person is threatened or disrupted."[p.531] An integrated care approach requires the collaboration of postcombat care and polytrauma rehabilitation teams. Their success in promoting resilience and coping, improving functioning, and facilitating community reintegration such that *the threat to the integrity of the person* is diminished or eliminated will hinge also on partnerships of teams with their surrounding organization and the organization's ability to support and collaborate with postcombat care teams. To this point, Strasser et al.[89] state the following:

> Our "prescription for partnership" represents a progression to a cellular level of the organization, namely, the interdisciplinary team. This partnership needs to be an interactive process in which insights gained at the level of the team integrate with other service providers, senior leadership, and stakeholders in other key organizations . . . . We owe it to our patients and our future patients to critically examine the underpinnings of the rehabilitation process and to incorporate the knowledge gained into new practice strategies and approaches. (p. 180)

Acknowledgment

This material is the result of work supported by resources from the VA Puget Sound Health Care System, Seattle, Washington.

Appendix: Neurobehavioral Symptom Inventory

Please rate the following symptoms with regard to how much they have disturbed you *SINCE YOUR INJURY.*

0 = None—Rarely, if ever, present; not a problem at all

1 = Mild—Occasionally present, but it does not disrupt activities; I can usually continue what I'm doing; doesn't really concern me.

2 = Moderate—Often present, occasionally disrupts my activities; I can usually continue what I'm doing with some effort; I feel somewhat concerned.

3 = Severe—Frequently present and disrupts activities; I can only do things that are fairly simple or take little effort; I feel like I need help.

4 = Very Severe—Almost always present and I have been unable to perform at work, school, or home due to this problem; I probably cannot function without help.

1. Feeling dizzy:
2. Loss of balance:
3. Poor coordination, clumsy:
4. Headaches:
5. Nausea:
6. Vision problems, blurring, trouble seeing:
7. Sensitivity to light:
8. Hearing difficulty:
9. Sensitivity to noise:
10. Numbness or tingling on parts of my body:
11. Change in taste and/or smell:
12. Loss of appetite or increased appetite:
13. Poor concentration, can't pay attention, easily distracted:
14. Forgetfulness, can't remember things:
15. Difficulty making decisions:
16. Slowed thinking, difficulty getting organized, can't finish things:
17. Fatigue, loss of energy, getting tired easily:
18. Difficulty falling or staying asleep:
19. Feeling anxious or tense:
20. Feeling depressed or sad:
21. Irritability, easily annoyed:
22. Poor frustration tolerance, feeling easily overwhelmed by things:

Source: Cicerone, K. D. and Kalmar, K., Persistent postconcussion syndrome: The structure of subjective complaints after mild traumatic brain injury, *Journal of Head Trauma Rehabilitation*, 10, 1–17, 1995.

References

1. Jones, E., Fear, N. T., and Wessely, S., Shell shock and mild traumatic brain injury: A historical review, *American Journal of Psychiatry*, 164(11), 1641–1645, 2007.
2. Goldstein, K., *Aftereffects of Brain Injuries in War*, Grune & Stratton, New York, 1942.
3. Goldstein, K., On so-called war neuroses, *Psychosomatic Medicine*, 5(4), 376–383, 1943.
4. Sigford, B. J., "To care of him who shall have borne the battle and for his widow and his orphan" (Abraham Lincoln): The Department of Veterans Affairs Polytrauma System of Care, *Archives of Physical Medicine and Rehabilitation*, 89(1), 160–162, 2008.

5. Tanielian, T. and Jaycox, L. H. (Eds.), *Invisible Wounds of War: Psychological and Cognitive Injuries, Their Consequences, and Services to Assist Recovery*, RAND Corporation, Santa Monica, CA, 2008.

6. President's Commission on Care for America's Returning Wounded Warriors, *Serve, Support, Simplify: Report of the President's Commission on Care for America's Returning Wounded Warriors*, Washington, DC, 2007.

7. Ommaya, A. K., Ommaya, A. K., Dannenberg, A. L., and Salazar, A. M., Causation, incidence, and costs of traumatic brain injury in the U.S. military medical system, *Journal of Trauma*, 40(2), 211–217, 1996.

8. Hoge, C. W., McGurk, D., Thomas, J. L., Cox, A. L., Engel, C. C., and Castro, C. A., Mild traumatic brain injury in U.S. soldiers returning from Iraq, *New England Journal of Medicine*, 358(5), 453–463, 2008.

9. Walden, D., Military TBI during the Iraq and Afghanistan wars, *Journal of Head Trauma Rehabilitation*, 21(5), 398–402, 2006.

10. Wade, A. L., Dye, J. L., Mohrle, C. R., and Galarneau, M. R., Head, face, and neck injuries during Operation Iraqi Freedom II: Results from the U.S. Navy–Marine Corps Combat Trauma Registry, *Journal of Trauma*, 63(4), 836–840, 2007.

11. Owens, B. D., Kragh, J. F., Wenke, J. C., Macaitis, J., Wade, C. E., and Holcomb, J. B., Combat wounds in Operation Iraqi Freedom and Operation Enduring Freedom, *Journal of Trauma*, 64(2), 295–299, 2008.

12. Ramasamy, A., Harrisson, S. E., Clasper, J. C., and Stewart, M. P. M., Injuries from roadside improvised explosive devices, *Journal of Trauma*, 65(4), 910–914, 2008.

13. Holcomb, J. B., McMullin, N. R., Pearse, L., Caruso, J., Wade, C. E., Oetjen-Gerdes, L., Champion, H. R., Lawnick, M., Farr, W., Rodriquez, S., and Butler, F. K., Causes of death in U.S. Special Operations Forces in the Global War on Terrorism, 2001–2004, *Annals of Surgery*, 245(6), 986–991, 2007.

14. Owens, B. D., Kragh, J. F., Macaitis, J., Svoboda, S. J., and Wenke, J. C., Characterization of extremity wounds in Operation Iraqi Freedom and Operation Enduring Freedom, *Journal of Orthopaedic Trauma*, 21(4), 254–257, 2007.

15. Gawande, A., Casualties of war: Military care for the wounded from Iraq and Afghanistan, *New England Journal of Medicine*, 351(24), 2471–2475, 2004.

16. Lew, H. L., Thomander, D., Chew, K. T. L., and Bleiberg, J., Review of sports-related concussion: Potential for application in military settings, *Journal of Rehabilitation Research and Development*, 44(7), 963–974, 2007.

17. DePalma, R. G., Burris, D. G., Champion, H. R., and Hodgson, M. J., Blast injuries, *New England Journal of Medicine*, 352(13), 1335–1342, 2005.

18. Taber, K. H., Warden, D. L., and Hurley, R. A., Blast-related traumatic brain injury: What's known?, *Journal of Neuropsychiatry and Clinical Neurosciences*, 18(2), 141–145, 2006.

19. Center for Disease Control and Prevention, Blast injuries: Essential facts, Department of Health and Human Services, 2008, www.emergency.cdc.gov/BlastInjuries, accessed March 20, 2009.

20. Kluger, Y., Nimrod, A., Biderman, P., Mayo, A., and Sorkin, P., The quinary pattern of blast injury, *American Journal of Disaster Medicine*, 2(1), 21–25, 2007.

21. Bhatoe, H. S., Blast injury and the neurosurgeon, *Indian Journal of Neurotrauma*, 5(June), 3–6, 2008.

22. Ruff, R. M. and Jurica, P., In search of a unified definition for mild traumatic brain injury, *Brain Injury*, 13(12), 943–952, 1999.

23. American Congress of Rehabilitation Medicine, Definition of mild traumatic brain injury, *Journal of Head Trauma Rehabilitation*, 8(3), 86–87, 1993.

24. American Academy of Neurology, Practice parameter: The management of concussion in sports (summary statement). Report of the Quality Standards Subcommittee, *Neurology*, 48(3), 581–585, 1997.

25. Defense and Veterans Brain Injury Center, Three-question DVBIC TBI screening tool instruction sheet, Washington, DC, 2009, www.dvbic.org/patientcare.php, accessed March 23, 2009.

26. Schwab, K. A., Baker, G., Ivins, B., Sluss-Tiller, M., Lux, W., and Warden, D., The Brief Traumatic Brain Injury Screen (BTBIS): Investigating the validity of a self-report instrument for detecting traumatic brain injury (TBI) in troops returning from deployment in Afghanistan and Iraq, *Neurology*, 66(5)(Suppl. 2), A235, 2006.

27. Lew, H. L., Poole, J. H., Vanderploeg, R. D., Goodrich, G. L., Dekelboum, S., Guillory, S. B., Sigford, B., and Cifu, D. X. Program development and defining characteristics of returning military in a VA Polytrauma Network Site, *Journal of Rehabilitation Research and Development*, 44(7), 1027–1034, 2007.

28. Cicerone, K. D. and Kalmar, K., Persistent postconcussion syndrome: The structure of subjective complaints after mild traumatic brain injury, *Journal of Head Trauma Rehabilitation*, 10(3), 1–17, 1995.

29. Hoge, C. W., Castro, C. A., Messer, S. C., McGurk, D., Cotting, D. I., and Koffman, R. L., Combat duty in Iraq and Afghanistan, mental health problems, and barriers to care, *New England Journal of Medicine*, 351(1), 13–22, 2004.

30. Hoge, C. W., Auchterlonie, J. L., and Milliken, C. S., Mental health problems, use of mental health services, and attrition from military service after returning from deployment to Iraq or Afghanistan, *Journal of the American Medical Association*, 295(9), 1023–1032, 2006.

31. Turner, M. A., Kiernan, M. D., McKechanie, A. G., Finch, P. J. C., McManus, F. B., and Neal, L. A., Acute military psychiatric casualties from the war in Iraq, *British Journal of Psychiatry*, 186(6), 476–479, 2005.

32. Sareen, J., Cox, B. J., Afifi, T. O., Stein, M. B., Belik, S.- L., Meadows, G., and Asmundson, G. J. G., Combat and peacekeeping operations in relation to prevalence of mental disorders and perceived need for mental health care: Findings from a large representative sample of military personnel, *Archives of General Psychiatry*, 64(7), 843–852, 2007.

33. Milliken, C. S., Auchterlonie, J. L., and Hoge, C. W., Longitudinal assessment of mental health problems among active and reserve component soldiers returning from the Iraq War, *Journal of the American Medical Association*, 298(18), 2141–2148, 2007.

34. Iverson, G. L., Zasler, N. D., and Lange, R. T., Post-concussive disorder, in N. D. Zasler, D. I. Katz, and R. D. Zafonte (Eds.), *Brain Injury Medicine: Principles and Practice*, Demos Medical Publishing, New York, 373–403, 2006.

35. Schneiderman, A. I., Braver, E. R., and Kang, H. K., Understanding sequelae of injury mechanisms and mild traumatic brain injury incurred during the conflicts in Iraq and Afghanistan: Persistent postconcussive symptoms and posttraumatic stress disorder, *American Journal of Epidemiology*, 167(12), 1446–1452, 2008.

36. Vasterling, J. J., Proctor, S. P., Amoroso, P., Kane, R., Heeren, T., and White, R. F., Neuropsychological outcomes of Army personnel following deployment to the Iraq War, *Journal of the American Medical Association*, 296(5), 519–529, 2006.

37. National Center for Posttraumatic Stress Disorder, National Center for PSTD home, 2009, http://www.ncptsd.va.gov/ncmain/index.jsp, accessed December 15, 2009.

38. National Center for Posttraumatic Stress Disorder and Walter Reed Army Medical Center, Iraq War Clinician Guide, 2nd ed., 2004, http://www.ptsd.va.gov/professional/manuals/manual-pdf/iwcg/iraq_clinician_guide_v2.pdf, accessed December 15, 2009.

39. Spitzer, R. L., Kroenke, K., and Williams, J. B. W., Validation and utility of a self-report version of the PRIME-MD, *Journal of the American Medical Association*, 282(18), 1737–1744, 1999.

40. Gironda, R. J., Clark, M. E., Massengale, J. P., and Walker, R. L., Pain among veterans of Operations Enduring Freedom and Iraqi Freedom, *Pain Medicine*, 10(7), 339–343, 2006.

41. Ruff, R. L., Ruff, S. S., and Wang, X.- F., Headaches among Operation Iraqi Freedom/Operation Enduring Freedom veterans with mild traumatic brain injury associated with exposures to explosions, *Journal of Rehabilitation Research and Development*, 45(7), 941–952, 2008.

42. Theeler, B. J, Mercer, R., and Erickson, J. C., Prevalence and impact of migraine among U.S. Army soldiers deployed in support of Operation Iraqi Freedom, *Headache*, 48(6), 876–882, 2008.

43. Kauvar, D. S., Wolf, S. E., Wade, C. E., Cancio, L. C., Renz, E. M., and Holcomb, J. B., Burns sustained in combat explosions in Operations Iraqi and Enduring Freedom (OIF/OEF explosion burns), *Burns*, 32(7), 853–857, 2006.

44. Colyer, M. H., Chun, D. W., Bower, K. S., Dick, J. S., and Weichel, E. D., Perforating globe injuries during Operation Iraqi Freedom, *Ophthalmology*, 115(11), 2087–2093, 2008.

45. Weichel, E. D. and Colyer, M. H., Combat ocular trauma and systemic injury, *Current Opinion in Ophthalmology*, 19(6), 519–525, 2008.

46. Weichel, E. D., Colyer, M. H., Ludlow, S. E., Bower, K. S., and Eiseman, A. S., Combat ocular trauma visual outcomes during Operations Iraqi and Enduring Freedom, *Ophthalmology*, 115(12), 2235–2245, 2008.

47. Goodrich, G. L., Kirby, J., Cockerham, G., Ingalla, S. P., and Lew, H. L., Visual function in patients of a polytrauma rehabilitation center: A descriptive study, *Journal of Rehabilitation Research and Development*, 44(7), 929–936, 2007.

48. Hoffer, M. E., Gottshall, K. R., Moore, R., Balough, B. J., and Wester, D., Characterizing and treating dizziness after mild head trauma, *Otology & Neurotology*, 25(2), 135–138, 2004.

49. Cave, K. M., Cornish, E. M., and Chandler, D. W., Blast injury of the ear: Clinical update from the Global War on Terror, *Military Medicine*, 172(7), 726–730, 2007.

50. Scherer, M., Burrows, H., and Pinto, R., Characterizing self-reported dizziness and otovestibular impairment among blast-injured traumatic amputees: A pilot study, *Military Medicine*, 172(7), 731–737, 2007.

51. Stansbury, L., Lalliss, S. J., Branstetter, J. G., Bagg, M. R., and Holcomb, J. B., Amputations in U.S. military personnel in the current conflicts in Afghanistan and Iraq, *Journal of Orthopaedic Trauma*, 22(1), 43–46, 2008.

52. Potter, B. K., Burns, T. C., Lacap, A. P., Granville, R. R., and Gajewski, D. A., Heterotopic ossification following traumatic and combat-related amputations, *Journal of Bone and Joint Surgery*, 89(3), 476–486, 2007.

53. Ferguson, R. J. and Mittenberg, W., Cognitive–behavioral treatment of postconcussion syndrome: A therapists manual, in V. B. Van Hasselt and M. Hersen (Eds.), *Sourcebook of Psychological Treatment Manuals for Adult Disorders*, Springer, New York, 615–635, 1996.

54. Belanger, H. G., Kretzmer, T., Yoash-Gantz, R., Pickett, T., and Tupler, L. A., Cognitive sequelae of blast-related versus other mechanisms of brain trauma, *Journal of the International Neuropsychological Society*, 15(1), 1–8, 2009.

55. Prigatano, G. P., Fordyce, D. J., Zeiner, H. K., Roueche, J. R., Pepping, M., and Case Wood, B., *Neuropsychological Rehabilitation after Brain Injury*, Johns Hopkins University Press, Baltimore, MD, 1985.

56. NIH Consensus Development Panel on Rehabilitation of Persons with Traumatic Brain Injury, Rehabilitation of persons with traumatic brain injury, *Journal of the American Medical Association*, 282(10), 974–983, 1999.

57. Sohlberg, M. M. and Mateer, C. A., *Cognitive Rehabilitation: An Integrated Neuropsychological Approach*, Guilford Press, New York, 2001.

58. Cicerone, K. D., Dahlberg, C., Kalmar, K., Langenbahn, D. M., Malec, J. F., Brequist, T. F., et al., Evidence-based cognitive rehabilitation: Recommendations for clinical practice, *Archives of Physical Medicine and Rehabilitation*, 81(12), 1596–1615, 2000.

59. Cicerone, K. D., Dahlberg, C., Malec, J. F., Langenbahn, D. M., Felicetti, T., Kneipp, S., Ellmo, W., et al., Evidence-based cognitive rehabilitation: Updated review of the literature from 1998 through 2002, *Archives of Physical Medicine and Rehabilitation*, 86(8), 1681–1692, 2005.

60. Gentry, T., Wallace, J., Kvarfordt, C., and Bodisch-Lynch, K., Personal digital assistants as cognitive aids for individuals with severe traumatic brain injury: A community-based trial, *Brain Injury*, 22(1), 19–24, 2008.

61. Seel, R. T., Kreutzer, J. S., Rosenthal, M., Hammond, F. M., Corrigan, J. D., and Black, K., Depression after traumatic brain injury: A National Institute on Disability and Rehabilitation Research Model Systems Multicenter Investigation, *Archives of Physical Medicine and Rehabilitation*, 84(2), 177–184, 2003.

62. Hanks, R. A., Temkin, N., Machamer, J., and Dikmen, S., Emotional and behavioral adjustment issues after traumatic brain injury, *Archives of Physical Medicine and Rehabilitation*, 80(9), 991–999, 1999.

63. Delmonico, R. L., Hanley-Peterson, P., and Englander, J., Group psychotherapy for persons with traumatic brain injury: Management of frustration and substance abuse, *Journal of Head Trauma Rehabilitation*, 13(6), 10–22, 1998.

64. Hayes, S. C. and Smith, S., *Get Out of Your Mind and Into Your Life: The New Acceptance and Commitment Therapy.* New Harbinger Publications, Oakland, CA, 2005.

65. Bandura, A., *Self-Efficacy: The Exercise of Control*, Freeman, New York, 1997.

66. Dunn, J., Stegina, S. K., Rosoman, N., and Millichap, D., A review of peer support in the context of cancer, *Journal of Psychosocial Oncology*, 21(2), 55–67, 2003.

67. Wells, L. M., Schacter, B., Little, S., Shylie, B., and Balogh, P. A., Enhancing rehabilitation through mutual aid: Outreach to people with recent amputations, *Health and Social Work*, 18(3), 221–230, 1993.

68. Davison, K. P., Pennebaker, J. W., and Diskerson, S. S., Who talks? The social psychology of illness support groups, *American Psychologist*, 55(2), 205–217, 2000.

69. Dunn, J., Stegina, S. K., Occhipinti, S., and Willson, K., Evaluation of a peer support program for women with breast cancer: Lessons for practitioners, *Journal of Community and Applied Psychology*, 9(1), 13–22, 1999.

70. Hibbard, M. R., Cantor, J., Charatz, H., Rosenthal, R., Ashman, T., Gundersen, N., Ireland-Knight, L., Gordon, W., Avner, J., and Gartner, A., Peer support in the community: Initial findings of a mentoring program for individuals with traumatic brain injury and their families, *Journal of Head Trauma Rehabilitation*, 17(2), 112–131, 2002.

71. Williams, R. M., Patterson, D. R., Schwenn, C., Day, J., Bartman, M., and Engrav, L. H., Evaluation of a peer consultation program for burn inpatients, *The Journal of Burn Care and Rehabilitation*, 23(6), 449–453, 2002.

72. Ashbury, F. D., Cameron, C., Mercer, S. L., Fitch, M., and Nielsen, E., One-on-one peer support and quality of life for breast cancer patients, *Patient Education and Counseling*, 35(2), 89–100, 1998.

73. Giese-Davis, J., Bliss-Isberg, C., Carson, K., Star, P., Donaghy, J., Cordova, M. J., Stevens, N., Wittenberg, L., Batten, C., and Spiegel, D., The effect of peer counseling on quality of life following diagnosis of breast cancer: An observational study, *Psycho-Oncology*, 15(11), 1014–1022, 2006.

74. Veith, E. M., Sherman, J. E., Pellino, T. A., and Yasui, N. Y., Qualitative analysis of the peer–mentoring relationship among individuals with spinal cord injury, *Rehabilitation Psychology*, 51(4), 289–298, 2006.

75. Rankin, N., Williams, P., Davis, C., and Girgis, A., The use and acceptability of a one-on-one peer support program for Australian women with early breast cancer, *Patient Education and Counseling*, 53(2), 141–146, 2004.

76. Moreci, G., A model system of traumatic brain injury peer support importance, development, and process, *NeuroRehabilitation*, 7(3), 211–218, 1996.

77. Belanger, H. G., Uomoto, J. M., and Vanderploeg, R. D., The Veterans Heath Administration system of care for mild traumatic brain injury: Costs, benefits, and controversies, *Journal of Head Trauma Rehabilitation*, 24(1), 4–13, 2009.

78. Oddy, M. and Herbert, C., Intervention with families following brain injury: Evidence-based practice, *Neuropsychological Rehabilitation*, 13(1 & 2), 259–273, 2003.

79. Rotondi, A. J., Sinkule, J., Balzer, K., Harris, J., and Moldovan, R., A qualitative needs assessment of persons who have experienced traumatic brain injury and their primary family caregivers, *Journal of Head Trauma Rehabilitation*, 22(1), 14–25, 2007.

80. Cernak, I., Wang, Z., Jiang, J., Bian, X., and Savic, J., Cognitive deficits following blast injury-induced neurotrauma: Possible involvement of nitric oxide, *Brain Injury*, 15(7), 593–612, 2001.

81. Cernak, I., Savic, J., Malicevic, Z., Zunic, G., Radosevic, P., Ivanovic, I., and Davidovic, L., Involvement of the central nervous system in the general response to pulmonary blast injury, *Journal of Trauma*, 40(3S), 100S–104S, 1996.

82. Irwin, R. J., Lerner, M. R., Bealer, J. F., Brackett, D. J., and Tuggle, D. W., Cardiopulmonary physiology of primary blast injury, *Journal of Trauma*, 43(4), 650–655, 1997.

83. Courtney, A. C. and Courtney, N. W., A thoracic mechanism of mild brain injury due to blast pressure waves, *Medical Hypotheses*, 72(1), 76–83, 2009.

84. Rothman, M. S., Arciniegas, D. B., Filley, C. M., and Wierman, M. E., The neuroendocrine effects of traumatic brain injury, *Journal of Neuropsychiatry and Clinical Neurosciences*, 19(4), 363–372, 2007.

85. Yehuda, R., Biology of posttraumatic stress disorder, *Journal of Clinical Psychiatry*, 62(7), 41–46, 2001.

86. Vanderploeg, R. D., Schwab, K., Walker, W. C., Fraser, J. A., Sigford, B. J., Date, E. S., Scott, S. G., Curtiss, G., Salazar, A. M., and Warden, D. L., Rehabilitation of traumatic brain injury in active duty military personnel and veterans: Defense and Veterans Brain Injury Center randomized controlled trial of two rehabilitation approaches, *Archives of Physical Medicine and Rehabilitation*, 89(12), 2227–2238, 2008.

87. Jakcupcak, M., Luterek, J., Hunt, S., Conybeare, D., and McFall, M., Posttraumatic stress and its relationship to physical health functioning in a sample of Iraq and Afghanistan War veterans seeking postdeployment VA health care, *Journal of Nervous and Mental Disease*, 196(5), 425–428, 2008.

88. Cassel, E. J., Diagnosing suffering: A perspective, *Annals of Internal Medicine*, 131(7), 531–534, 1999.

89. Strasser, D. C., Uomoto, J. M., and Smits, S. J., The interdisciplinary team and polytrauma rehabilitation: Prescription for partnership, *Archives of Physical Medicine and Rehabilitation*, 89(1), 179–181, 2008.

4

Neurotransmitters and Pharmacology

Ronald A. Browning

CONTENTS

Editor's Note

Pharmacologic treatment of traumatic brain injury (TBI) is complex and still in its infancy as a field of clinical investigation. Patients with TBI have a wide variety of central nervous system (CNS) problems, as well as numerous peripheral disorders (e.g., hypertension, reduced bowel function) that can be addressed pharmacologically. One of the major difficulties in identifying useful medications for TBI patients is the diversity of brain injury encountered in this population. The non-CNS medical problems in TBI patients often require the use of drugs to control hypertension or to increase bowel function, and drugs that affect the autonomic nervous system are commonly used for such disorders. Although this chapter focuses on the medications that are used to alter neurologic or behavioral functions (i.e., those that act on the CNS), neurotransmission in the autonomic nervous system and the drugs that modify it are also described.

4.1 Introduction

Most drugs that are used for an action on the central nervous system (CNS), such as those used in neurology and psychiatry, exert their action by acting at the site where neurons communicate with one another—namely, the synapse. These drugs therefore exert their effect by modifying the process of neurotransmission. The exceptions to this rule are those classes of drugs known as (1) the *local anesthetics,* which prevent nerve conduction by blocking sodium channels and, thereby, alleviating pain; (2) *general anesthetics,* which produce a reversible loss of consciousness by unknown means, although recent evidence suggests these agents can also modify neurotransmission; and (3) some *antiepileptic agents,* which prevent seizures by acting directly on voltage-gated ion channels to alter nerve conduction. It should be noted that some antiepileptic drugs clearly produce their beneficial effects by altering neurotransmission (e.g., diazepam, tiagabine).

Drug classes with a mechanism of action that involves a modification of synaptic neurotransmission include narcotic analgesics (used to alleviate pain), antipsychotic agents (used to treat schizophrenia), antidepressants, antianxiety agents (e.g., diazepam or Valium), some antiepileptic drugs, antispasmodics, and muscle relaxants. In addition, because of the ubiquitous role of the peripheral autonomic nervous system in the regulation of organ system function such as cardiovascular, respiratory, gastrointestinal (GI), nasal congestion, and the like, it is not surprising to find that drugs altering peripheral neurotransmission are used to treat a wide variety of disorders, such as hypertension, heart disease, GI disorders, hiccups, asthma, hay fever, and so forth.

There is some controversy concerning whether chemicals released from neurons should be referred to as *neurotransmitters* or *neuromodulators.* Some authors believe the term *neurotransmitter* should be reserved for those substances that act through ligand-gated ion channels to produce rapid changes in the postsynaptic cell, whereas the slower acting chemicals that act through G-protein-coupled receptors (described later) should be called *neuromodulators.* Others believe that any chemical released from a nerve that causes a change in a nearby cell is a *neurotransmitter,* and this is the terminology rule followed in this chapter. For a more detailed discussion of the definitions of neurotransmitters and neuromodulators, see Cooper et al.[1]

The question of whether a substance functions as a neurotransmitter is not always an easy one to answer and requires extensive experimental testing by neuroscientists. Neurobiologists have set specific criteria that must be fulfilled before a substance is accepted as a neurotransmitter. These criteria were established in the mid 1960s by Werman[2] and, although the original criteria were extremely useful for more than 25 years, they may not be entirely adequate because knowledge of how neurons communicate with one another and with target organs in the periphery has expanded. Indeed, some of the recently discovered signaling molecules, such as the gases nitric oxide and carbon monoxide, and the endogenous lipids anandamide and 2-arachidonoyl glycerol (endocanabinoids), do not fulfill the previously established criteria, yet clearly function as important neural messengers.[2-7]

Nevertheless, there are about seven chemicals that have been well established as neurotransmitters and another 20 to 30 substances that are highly suspected as neurotransmitters or neuromodulators in the nervous system. The seven well-established or classic neurotransmitters include

1. Acetylcholine
2. Norepinephrine

3. Dopamine

4. 5-Hydroxytryptamine (5-HT, serotonin)

5. Gamma-aminobutyric acid (GABA)

6. Glycine

7. Glutamate/aspartate

All have been associated with the action of a drug or group of drugs that exert clinically useful effects (with the possible exception of glycine) on the nervous system. In addition, there are several neuropeptides that serve as neurotransmitters or neuromodulators (i.e., modify the action of the classic neurotransmitters) that have been associated with the action of drugs, and these will be discussed.

To appreciate the physiologic and/or biochemical mechanisms by which drugs alter neurotransmission, one must have an understanding of the events involved in synaptic neurotransmission. Thus, let us begin with a description of the physiology of chemical neurotransmission, and then proceed to discuss the individual neurotransmitters and the drugs that mediate their effects through such neurotransmitters. It should be kept in mind that synaptic transmission is not only important for understanding the action of drugs, but also it is vital for all functions of the nervous system, and it appears to be the site at which learning and memory take place in the CNS (see Chapter 13).

4.2 Chemical Neurotransmission

In the mammalian nervous system (both central and peripheral), the predominant form of communication between two nerves and between nerve and muscle (or nerves and glands) is chemical. Electrical transmission between nerve cells can also occur, but is not easily modified by drugs and will not be considered here. The site at which this chemical transmission occurs is called the *synapse*. From Figure 4.1, it can be seen that the synapse consists of several cellular and subcellular structures. Although synapses can occur at several locations on a neuron that is receiving information from another neuron, the more typical arrangement is that described in Figure 4.1. Thus, the axon terminal of one neuron generally synapses on the cell body (soma or perikaryon called *axosomatic synapses*) or dendrites of another neuron (called *axodendritic synapses*). Axons may also synapse on other axons, especially at the nerve terminals (called *axo-axonic synapses*) and, under unusual circumstances, dendrites may synapse with other dendrites (*dendrodendritic synapses*) or cell bodies may synapse with one another (*soma-somatic synapses*). At the prototypical synapse, the neurotransmitter, which is usually a small, water-soluble organic amine, is synthesized from precursors within the axon terminal, taken up into and stored in a small round or ovoid vesicle, and released from the nerve terminal in a calcium-dependent process when an action potential or nerve impulse reaches the nerve terminal. Indeed, the steps associated with neurotransmission at a chemical synapse are as follows:

Step 1: The first step is the release of the neurotransmitter from its storage site in a vesicle resulting from the arrival of an action potential that, in turn, opens voltage-gated calcium channels and that allows the influx of calcium from the extracellular fluid. The calcium then triggers a release process called *exocytosis*. Exocytosis

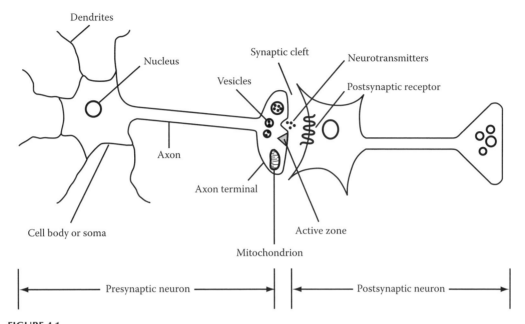

FIGURE 4.1

Drawing of an axosomatic (typical) synapse between two neurons. The neuron synapsing on another neuron is referred to as the *presynaptic* neuron, whereas the neuron receiving the input is called the *postsynaptic* neuron. Various subcellular structures associated with the synapse are labeled. Vesicles contain the neurotransmitter destined for release into the synaptic cleft. The active zone is the site at which vesicles attach to the docking sites just prior to release.

involves fusion of the vesicle membrane with the nerve membrane and the opening of the vesicle into the synaptic cleft (Figure 4.1).[8] Fusion of the vesicle membrane with the nerve terminal membrane requires calcium to enter the nerve through channels that have been opened by the arrival of the action potential. Calcium initiates the fusion process, which requires, in addition to calcium, an interaction of vesicle membrane proteins (called *v-SNARES*) with nerve terminal membrane proteins (called *t-SNARES*). The vesicle membrane then collapses into the nerve terminal membrane. Thus, the vesicle extrudes its contents into the synaptic cleft. The release process is also regulated by receptors found on the nerve terminal (called *presynaptic receptors* or *autoreceptors). It* should be noted that, under special circumstances, neurotransmitters can be released by a calcium-independent process that does not involve exocytosis, but involves a membrane transporter. An example of the latter is the amphetamine-induced release of norepinephrine and dopamine.[8]

Step 2: The next step in neurotransmission involves binding of the neurotransmitter to *receptors* in the postsynaptic membrane and the initiation of postsynaptic events (i.e., a depolarization or a hyperpolarization). Receptors give both neurotransmitters and drugs their selectivity and specificity. The receptors, which are typically membrane proteins or glycoproteins, only recognize and bind chemicals of the "correct" chemical structure. Thus, just as only one key opens a lock, only one chemical structure can initiate postsynaptic events via the receptor. The receptors for neurotransmitters come in two varieties: (1) those that actually form an ion channel in the membrane (such as the nicotinic cholinergic receptor) and mediate rapid events when the transmitter binds (which are called *ligand-gated ion channels,* also referred to as *ionotropic receptors*), or (2) those that are connected to ion channels indirectly via "second messenger" molecules that become activated inside the cell when the transmitter binds to the receptor. In the latter case, the receptor is linked to a guanine nucleotide binding protein (called a *G-protein*), which functions as the link between the receptor protein and the enzymes that synthesize the "second messenger." This class of receptors is referred to as *G-protein-coupled receptors* (GPCR) or *metabotropic receptors*.[8]

The potentials that develop in the postsynaptic cell either move the membrane potential farther from the threshold for triggering an action potential (hyperpolarization) or move it closer to the threshold (depolarization). Hyperpolarization (inhibitory postsynaptic potentials, or IPSPs) results from the opening of chloride or potassium channels in the membrane, allowing chloride to flow in or potassium to flow out. Hyperpolarization, then, inhibits postsynaptic firing. Depolarization (excitatory postsynaptic potentials, or EPSPs) results from the opening of channels that allow both sodium and potassium to flow down their concentration gradients through the same channel. This is different from the sodium-selective channel that is involved in the propagation of the action potential down the axon. If the depolarization is great enough, the threshold for an action potential is reached and an action potential (regenerative, sodium current) is propagated down the axon to initiate more synaptic transmission.

In the CNS, a neuron can only respond in one of two ways: (1) it either reaches threshold and fires an action potential, which in turn propagates information to the next neuron via synaptic transmission, or (2) it is inhibited and does not fire an action potential.

Step 3: The third step of the neurotransmission process consists of the postsynaptic response. The postsynaptic response can consist of an action potential in the neuron, the contraction of muscle, or the secretion of a gland.

Step 4: This step consists of inactivation of the neurotransmitter in the synaptic cleft. The transmitter must be removed from the synaptic cleft in order for the postsynaptic cell to repolarize, which is necessary for the synapse to remain responsive to incoming information. The two most important mechanisms for removing the neurotransmitter from the cleft are (1) reuptake into the neuron from which it was released and (2) enzymatic degradation. In addition, other mechanisms include diffusion away from the cleft and uptake (transport) into other cells (e.g., glial cells, muscle cells in the periphery, or other neurons). Just as the neurotransmitter can be taken up and reused by the cell that released it, the vesicle membrane can be retrieved from the nerve terminal where it fused. Thus, vesicles are also recycled.

It is now clear that there are signaling molecules (which do not meet the criteria of a neurotransmitter) that play a role in fine-tuning synaptic transmission. For example, there is evidence that the release of classic neurotransmitters from axon terminals is modified by a variety of messenger molecules that are synthesized and released from the postsynaptic neuron and diffuse back across the synapse (i.e., backward transmission) to bind to receptors on the presynaptic axon terminal. This phenomenon is referred to as *retrograde signaling* and is the mechanism by which the endocanabinoids (natural agonists for the marijuana receptor) and the gases (e.g., nitric oxide) function as neuromodulators.[9,10]

4.3 Sites Where Drugs Act

Drugs may either facilitate (enhance) or inhibit neurotransmission. Some of the mechanisms by which drugs can facilitate neurotransmission include

- Stimulation of the release of the neurotransmitter into the cleft
- Increased synthesis of the neurotransmitter in the presynaptic terminal
- Prevention of inactivation of the transmitter following release (e.g., blocking reuptake or blocking enzymes of degradation)
- Stimulation of the postsynaptic receptors directly to produce a response (A drug that does this is called an *agonist*.)

Some of the mechanisms by which drugs inhibit neurotransmission include

- Inhibition of the synthesis of the transmitter
- Prevention of transmitter release
- Interference with neurotransmitter storage in the vesicle
- Blocking the neurotransmitter receptor or functioning as an inverse agonist at the receptor

A drug that binds to a receptor, blocking the neurotransmitter action but producing no effect, is called an *antagonist*. A drug that binds to a receptor and produces an effect *opposite* that of the agonist is called an *inverse agonist*. Because of the discovery of inverse agonists, the term *neutral antagonist* is sometimes used to describe a drug that binds to the receptor and produces no effect.[11] Inverse agonists are drugs that bind to GPCRs that have constitutive activity (i.e., a GPCR that is spontaneously active in the absence of any agonist or ligand). The inverse agonist binds to the GPCR and blocks the constitutive activity.[12] In the sections that follow, let us consider the individual neurotransmitters and the drugs that produce clinical effects by altering chemical neurotransmission.

4.4 Acetylcholine

Acetylcholine (ACh) is one of the most widely studied neurotransmitters and one of the oldest, phylogenetically. It was, in fact, the neurotransmitter for which chemical neurotransmission was originally demonstrated, when it was found to be released from nerves innervating the frog heart by Loewi in 1921.[13] It has been most thoroughly studied in the peripheral nervous system where it functions as a neurotransmitter of the motor neurons innervating skeletal muscle (involved in the voluntary control of movement). ACh is also the neurotransmitter of the preganglionic sympathetic and parasympathetic fibers as well as the postganglionic parasympathetic fibers.[14] The response to stimulating parasympathetic nerves innervating various organs in the body is shown in Table 4.1. As you can see, these nerves affect every organ in the body. Drugs that alter neurotransmission at these synapses can have very profound effects.

TABLE 4.1

Organ Response to Parasympathetic Nerve Stimulation

Organ Receiving Innervation	Response to Stimulation	Receptor Type
Eye		
Iris, sphincter	Pupillary constriction (miosis)	Muscarinic
Ciliary muscle	Contraction, near vision	Muscarinic
Heart		
SA node	Decrease in heart rate	Muscarinic
Atrium	Shortens refractory period	Muscarinic
AV node	Slows conduction	Muscarinic
Ventricles	No response, poor innervation	
Vasculature	No parasympathetic innervation, has muscarinic receptors that can respond with vasodilation	Muscarinic
Trachea and bronchioles	Constriction	Muscarinic
Stomach and intestine	Increase in motility, tone, and secretions; relaxation of sphincters	Muscarinic
Urinary bladder		
Detrusor muscle	Contraction, bladder emptying	Muscarinic
Trigone and sphincter	Relaxation	Muscarinic
Sex organs, male	Erection	Muscarinic
Sweat glands	Secretion	Muscarinic
Lacrimal glands	Secretion	Muscarinic
Nasopharyngeal glands	Secretion	Muscarinic

SA, sinoatrial; AV, atrioventricular.

Source: J. G. Hardman, L. E. Limbird, and A. G. Gilman (Eds.), *The Pharmacological Basis of Therapeutics*, McGraw-Hill Medical Publishing, New York, 115, 2001.

ACh is also a neurotransmitter in the CNS where specific pathways have been identified in the brains of primates and other species. Basically, there are two groups of ACh neurons (cell bodies) from which axonal pathways project[14]: (1) those pathways innervating the forebrain (cell bodies in the basal forebrain around the medial septum and nucleus basalis of Meynert) as well as the interneurons in the striatum (basal ganglia) and (2) those innervating the brainstem and diencephalon (cell bodies in the laterodorsal tegmental nucleus and the pedunculopontine tegmental nucleus). Some of the proposed functions of ACh in these CNS pathways are given in Table 4.2, but it is clear that there is much to learn about the intricate details of how ACh regulates such things as learning and memory, sleep, seizures, and emotional states.

TABLE 4.2

Some Proposed Functions of ACh in the CNS

Learning and memory
(cholinergic neurons lost in Alzheimer's disease)
Sleep and arousal states
Body temperatures
Susceptibility to seizures
Affective states (mood)
Cardiovascular function via hypothalamus
Motor disorders (Parkinson's disease)

4.4.1 Synthesis, Storage, Release, and Inactivation of Acetylcholine

Neurons that utilize ACh as a neurotransmitter are referred to as *cholinergic* neurons, and a schematic diagram of such a neuron is shown in Figure 4.2. Acetylcholine is synthesized within cholinergic neurons from the precursor *choline*, which comes from the diet, and/or the breakdown of phospholipids, primarily in the liver.[15] Some of the choline that is taken up into cholinergic neurons for synthesis of ACh comes from the enzymatic degradation of released ACh (Figure 4.2). In fact, about 50% of the choline released as ACh is recaptured by the neuron for the synthesis of more ACh.[1]

Choline is transported into the nerve by a transporter or "carrier" protein in the membrane. This transporter or carrier, referred to as *ChT* by some authors,[16] has a high affinity for choline, which means that it avidly picks up choline from the surrounding area. It has, however, a limited number of transport sites, meaning that it can get filled up or saturated. Increasing the concentration of choline up to the point at which the sites become filled results in a proportional increase in the rate of choline transport. However, after all the transporters are occupied, the rate of transport becomes constant. Theoretically, one should be able to increase the synthesis of ACh by increasing the availability of choline, especially because the enzyme that converts choline to ACh, choline acetyltransferase, is not saturated with substrate (choline).

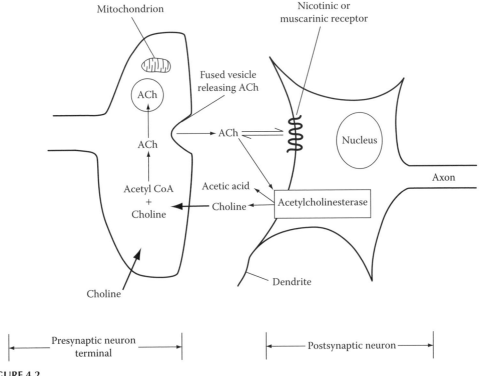

FIGURE 4.2
Drawing of a cholinergic synapse showing the fate of ACh after release into the synaptic cleft. Note that the neuron utilizes choline from two sources: the blood and from what is recycled from the breakdown of released ACh in the synaptic cleft. Acetylcholinesterase associated with the postsynaptic membrane terminates the action of released ACh. Acetyl CoA, acetylcoenzyme A.

A cosubstrate to choline is utilized in the synthesis of ACh. This cosubstrate is called *acetylcoenzyme A* (acetyl CoA). Acetyl CoA derives from pyruvate via the breakdown of glucose and is therefore plentiful inside the neuron.

Experimental studies have established that the rate-limiting factor in the overall synthesis of ACh is the uptake of choline by the neuron.[1,17] Because ACh neurons are lost in Alzheimer's disease, it has been of interest to attempt to increase ACh synthesis in brains of Alzheimer's patients. Although some studies have suggested that this is possible, choline has not been found terribly useful for improving memory in this or other populations.[18] The reason for this may be that the choline uptake transporter saturates and that the intracellular or cytoplasmic choline concentration can only be increased to a limited extent. An additional problem is that choline in the plasma may not be readily available to the neurons in the brain because it has difficulty crossing the blood–brain barrier.[16] There are no known drugs to increase the uptake of choline, although there are experimental drugs that inhibit the uptake of choline and interfere with the synthesis of ACh, such as hemicholinium-3 and triethylcholine, both of which are competitive inhibitors of choline uptake.

Choline can also get into neurons by another mechanism, called *low-affinity uptake*, which may account for the increase in synthesis of ACh that is seen in some peripheral organs following the administration of high doses of choline. Much higher concentrations of choline are required to saturate the transport proteins involved in low-affinity transport.

It has been hypothesized that the selective vulnerability of cholinergic neurons in Alzheimer's disease may be the result of the double role of choline in forming membrane phospholipids and ACh in these neurons, and the selective breakdown of cell membrane to shunt choline into the neurotransmitter, leading to cell membrane damage.[19] If the latter hypothesis is true, treatment with choline may be beneficial. There is evidence that giving choline to rats can increase the release of ACh in the striatum[20] and this effect can apparently be enhanced by caffeine.[21]

The enzyme that catalyzes the synthesis of ACh is choline acetyltransferase, which is found both as a soluble enzyme (nonmembrane bound) in the cytoplasm and as a particulate enzyme (membrane bound) in cholinergic neurons.[1] Most experts believe the soluble form of the enzyme is responsible for the majority of ACh being released from the neuron. The gene responsible for forming choline acetyltransferase is expressed only in cholinergic neurons and this enzyme, therefore, serves as a phenotypic marker for cholinergic neurons. The overall synthetic scheme is given in Figure 4.3.

After ACh is synthesized, it is stored in small, spherical (synaptic) vesicles along with several other constituents, including adenosine triphosphate (ATP) and a protein called

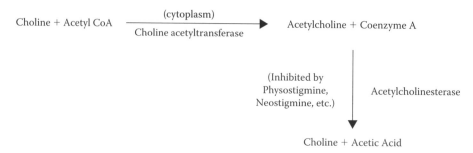

FIGURE 4.3
Synthesis and enzymatic degradation of ACh. ACh is synthesized in the cytoplasm of the nerve terminal where choline acetyltransferase (synthetic enzyme) is found. Acetylcholinesterase (degradative enzyme) is associated with the postsynaptic membrane. Acetyl CoA, acetylcoenzyme A.

vesiculin. The sequestration of ACh within these tiny vesicles serves to protect it from destruction by the enzyme acetylcholinesterase. Uptake into these vesicles is accomplished by vesicular ACh transporter (VAChT), which uses an electrochemical gradient produced by the proton ATPase. The VAChT transports ACh from the cytosol into the vesicle by exchanging two hydrogen ions (protons) for one molecule of ACh.[22] Although there appears to be some ACh in the cytoplasm of the neuron, the vast majority is found within the vesicles from which it is released directly into the synaptic cleft. This is accomplished by the complex process called *exocytosis.*

Exocytosis requires that the vesicle membrane fuse with the neuron membrane and "dump" its contents into the cleft in an all-or-none process. Some of the ACh that is free within the cytoplasm of the neuron may have just been synthesized en route to being taken up by the vesicle membrane transporter[1] (VAChT) for storage within the vesicle. The only drug currently known to interfere with the storage of ACh is vesamicol, which blocks the uptake of ACh into the vesicle and prevents the release of newly synthesized ACh.[16,23]

Considerable electrophysiologic and morphologic evidence indicates that ACh is released from neurons by exocytosis.[1,16] Some toxins are known to inhibit ACh release, including botulinum toxin A.[13] Botulinum toxin A (Botox) is commercially available and can be injected directly into muscles to block ACh release and relax the muscle. It is approved for the treatment of blepharospasm and facial wrinkles.[24]

After ACh has been released from the neuron, it can diffuse to the postsynaptic receptor (a discussion of ACh receptor subtypes is provided later in the chapter) to mediate a response in the postsynaptic neuron. However, it must then be inactivated if the synapse is to remain functional. In the case of ACh, inactivation occurs by *enzymatic destruction* of the neurotransmitter. Almost all other neurotransmitters (except for the peptides) are inactivated by reuptake into a neuron. Thus, ACh is unique among neurotransmitters in terms of the mechanism of inactivation following release into the synaptic cleft.

The enzyme that degrades ACh is called *acetylcholinesterase.* However, several cholinesterases have been found in the body. One of them circulates in plasma and is known as *pseudocholinesterase* or *butyrylcholinesterase,* which hydrolyzes butyrylcholine faster than ACh.[1] Acetylcholinesterase is associated with the synaptic cleft, where it is attached both to the presynaptic and postsynaptic membranes. This enzyme has been shown to exist in several molecular forms that differ in their lipid solubility and in the way they attach to membranes. Several inhibitors of acetylcholinesterase are available and they produce a dramatic increase in the concentration of ACh in the body. Such drugs are widely used in medicine and are discussed next.

4.4.2 Acetylcholine Receptors

Like other neurotransmitters, ACh produces its effects and obtains its selectivity by binding to specific receptors in the postsynaptic cell membrane. These receptors chemically recognize ACh and allow it to interact with specific functional groups in the receptor. Based on the early studies of Dale,[25] which were confirmed and extended by modern biochemical techniques, it is now known that there are two major types of ACh receptors, both of which were first identified in the peripheral nervous system: (1) ACh receptors at which nicotine can mimic the action of ACh are called *nicotinic receptors* and (2) ACh receptors that are activated by the alkaloid muscarine (from mushrooms) are called *muscarinic* receptors. In the peripheral nervous system, the nicotinic receptors are found at the neuromuscular junction (voluntary nerves to skeletal muscle), the autonomic ganglia, and the adrenal medulla, whereas muscarinic receptors are found at the effector organs innervated by the postganglionic parasympathetic fibers (e.g., heart, GI tract, exocrine glands). Both types of ACh receptors have been found in the brain.

4.4.2.1 Nicotinic Receptors

Nicotinic acetylcholine receptors (nAChR) have been widely studied, and most of our knowledge about nicotinic receptors comes from work on electric fish such as the Torpedo, which uses its electric organs to kill prey. It turns out that the high voltage in these fish is generated by ACh receptors, which are highly concentrated in the electric organ. Thus, the electric fish has served as a rich source of nicotinic receptor protein for biochemists to study.

The nicotinic receptor was found to be a ligand-gated ion channel composed of five subunits (termed *alpha, beta, gamma, delta,* and *epsilon*). However, it takes five subunits to form the ion channel, so the channel is formed by two alphas, one beta, one gamma, and one delta subunit.[26] In adult muscle of rats and cows, the epsilon subunit replaces the gamma subunit found in the fetal form of the receptor. The ACh binds to the alpha subunit of the receptor and, because there are two alpha subunits in each receptor, it takes two molecules of ACh to open the channel. The techniques of molecular biology (genetic engineering) have contributed greatly to our knowledge of the nicotinic receptor, as well as to our knowledge of the molecular structure of other receptors. These studies have led to a widely accepted model of the nicotinic receptor at the neuromuscular junction of mammals.

However, the nAChR associated with neurons (e.g., the autonomic ganglia and in the brain) appear to be slightly different from the muscle nicotinic receptor. For example, it has long been known that neuronal nicotinic receptors are not blocked by the classic neuromuscular nicotinic antagonist, *d*-tubocurarine, but are blocked by hexamethonium, another nicotinic antagonist. Moreover, their subunit composition is different from that of the muscle receptors. Indeed, some nAChRs found in brain are homomeric, meaning that they are composed of five identical subunits (e.g., the alpha-7 nAChR). Research on neuronal nicotinic receptors is still quite active and has important bearing on nicotine addiction and Alzheimer's disease, because nicotine has been shown to increase the release of ACh in the cerebral cortex.[27,28] There is also some evidence that nicotinic receptor agonists may be beneficial in restoring memory that has been impaired as a result of Alzheimer's disease. Nicotine may stimulate nAChRs in the hippocampus to have beneficial effects in schizophrenia.[29] A mutant form of the nAChR has been implicated in one heritable form of epilepsy. Neuronal-type nicotinic receptors have also been identified in nonneural cells (e.g., glial cells, endothelial cells, cancer cells), and there is evidence that some of these may play a role in promoting cancer in smokers.[30]

4.4.2.2 Muscarinic Receptors

Muscarinic receptors are thought to make up the majority of the ACh receptors in the mammalian brain. Unlike nicotinic receptors, the muscarinic receptors are linked to G-proteins and second messengers that carry the signal ultimately to produce a response or change in the cell. Based on molecular cloning technology, five subtypes of muscarinic receptor have been identified.[31] The basic chemical structure (i.e., the amino acid sequence) of these muscarinic receptors has been determined. The best described of the muscarinic receptors are the so-called *M1, M2,* and *M3,* which correspond to the m1, m2, and m3 cloned receptors.[32] Inasmuch as the muscarinic receptors are G-protein linked, they mediate their effects through second messengers. Muscarinic receptors may be involved in mediating either excitation or inhibition in the brain, which is usually produced by the opening (inhibition) or closing (excitation) of K^+ channels (i.e., potassium channels).

All G-protein-coupled receptors consist of a polypeptide chain (protein) with seven hydrophobic regions (i.e., areas containing amino acids that are more lipid than water soluble). It has been found that these hydrophobic regions of the molecule correspond to positions where the protein loops (crosses) through the cell membrane. So, these receptors loop back and forth through the membrane seven times and are said to contain *seven membrane-spanning regions*. Other G-protein-coupled receptors with seven membrane-spanning regions include the adrenergic, dopaminergic, and serotonergic receptors (described later in this chapter).

The M2 receptor found in the heart is the one most often involved in inhibition. The M1, M3, and cloned m5 subtypes increase phospholipase C activity via a G-protein called G_q. The activation of phospholipase C by the latter muscarinic receptors and G_q leads to the hydrolysis of phosphatidyl inositol and the formation of diacylglycerol (DAG) or inositol triphosphate (IP_3), which in turn function as second messengers to activate protein kinase C and increase intracellular calcium levels, respectively. M2 and M4 receptors result in the inhibition of adenylate cyclase by acting through a G_i protein and, in addition, may activate (open) K^+ channels directly. These effects can lead to a slowing of the heart, as shown in Table 4.1.[33]

Atropine is a nonselective antagonist for all muscarinic receptors whereas pirenzepine is selective for the M1 receptor, and AFDX 116 and methoctramine are antagonists for the M2 receptor. The release of ACh and other neurotransmitters may be regulated in part by the activation of M2 receptors located on presynaptic nerve terminals.[34]

4.4.3 Clinically Useful Drugs That Alter Cholinergic Neurotransmission

4.4.3.1 Facilitators of Cholinergic Neurotransmission

4.4.3.1.1 Cholinergic Agonists

There are a number of cholinergic agonists (drugs that bind to the receptor and produce a response or mimic the action of ACh), but only the muscarinic agonists find significant clinical usefulness. These drugs are primarily used in ophthalmology to treat glaucoma or to treat bowel and bladder retention postoperatively.

Muscarinic agonists include ACh, which is not used because it is rapidly destroyed by acetylcholinesterase or butyrylcholinesterase; methacholine, which is only partially sensitive to the action of acetylcholinesterase and is available as a diagnostic tool; bethanechol (Urecholine), which is used for bowel and bladder hypofunction; carbachol, which is used to treat glaucoma and has some nicotinic agonist activity as well; and pilocarpine, a naturally occurring alkaloid found in plants, which is a potent muscarinic agonist used to treat glaucoma. Pilocarpine is generally given in eye drops applied topically to the eye.

All these drugs are used for their effect on the peripheral autonomic nervous system rather than the CNS. Presumably, some of these agonists have some difficulty crossing the blood–brain barrier. However, when given in high doses, pilocarpine gets into the brain and causes seizures in experimental animals.[35] Another muscarinic agonist, oxotremorine, seems to produce marked effects on the brain at low doses in that it produces many of the symptoms of Parkinson's disease. Based on the apparent role of the ascending cholinergic neurons in the brain in regulating states of consciousness, it seems possible that cholinergic agonists that enter the brain produce arousal and insomnia. Indeed, even small doses of pilocarpine, given intravenously in cats, have been shown to produce arousal.[33]

There are two therapeutically useful nicotinic agonists for the treatment of tobacco dependence and these include nicotine itself, which is available in patches or gum to treat smokers' dependence, and varenicline (Chantix), which binds to the alpha-4/beta-2 nicotinic receptor and relieves the cravings and withdrawal symptoms.[36] Given the fact that the neuronal nicotinic receptor is damaged by beta amyloid in Alzheimer's disease, it is likely that we will soon see some new nicotinic drugs that are useful in treating this disorder.[37]

4.4.3.1.2 Cholinesterase Inhibitors

Other than agonists, the only drugs used clinically to facilitate cholinergic neurotransmission are the inhibitors of acetylcholinesterase. These include the reversible cholinesterase inhibitors such as physostigmine (Antilirium), neostigmine (Prostigmin), pyridostigmine (Mestinon), and edrophonium (Tensilon) that are used to treat or diagnose myasthenia gravis. Physostigmine crosses the blood–brain barrier whereas others do not, as a result of the fact that they are highly charged molecules. Tacrine (Cognex), donepezil (Aricept), rivastigmine (Exelon), and galantamine (Razadyne) are lipid-soluble, reversible cholinesterase inhibitors that easily reach the brain. These drugs are approved for the treatment of memory and cognitive impairment associated with Alzheimer's disease. There are also several irreversible inhibitors of cholinesterase, such as the organophosphates (e.g., diisopropylfluorophosphate, or DFP), which irreversibly inhibit the enzyme and are used primarily as insecticides. However, some of these are present in eye drops for the treatment of glaucoma. Obviously, the irreversible cholinesterase inhibitors are extremely toxic and are of interest because of their toxicologic effects. They are too dangerous for systemic use.

4.4.3.2 Inhibitors of Cholinergic Neurotransmission

4.4.3.2.1 Muscarinic Antagonist

Alkaloids present in the belladonna plant have long been used as muscarinic antagonists. These include atropine and scopolamine (hyoscine), both of which are nonselective muscarinic antagonists. These drugs readily enter the brain after systemic administration, and some antimuscarinic agents, like benztropine (Cogentin), are used exclusively for their effect on the brain. The latter compound has been used to prevent the parkinsonianlike side effects associated with antipsychotic drugs like Haldol. In the days before H_2 histamine receptor antagonists (e.g., cimetidine) and proton pump inhibitors (e.g., omeprazole), which are among the most commonly used ulcer drugs, atropine and other belladonna alkaloids were used to treat gastric ulcers and other conditions associated with increased GI activity. However, pirenzepine, the M1 selective antagonist, has been found to be better at reducing gastric secretion. A new muscarinic antagonist, ipratropium (Atrovent), is delivered in an aerosol in the treatment of bronchial asthma. Anticholinergic drugs reduce bronchial secretions and cause bronchodilatation, while decreasing GI activity and dilating the pupils. Hence, they are also used by ophthalmologists to dilate the pupils for examination of the retina. When there is hypersecretion of saliva or bronchiolar secretions, as there is during general anesthesia, atropine or other antimuscarinic drugs (e.g., glycopyrrolate) are also used to reduce secretions and to dilate bronchiolar passages.

4.4.3.2.2 Nicotinic Antagonists

Currently, nicotinic antagonists may be divided into two general categories: (1) those that are muscle nicotinic receptor antagonists or so-called *neuromuscular blockers,* such as d-tubocurarine (curare, the South American arrow poison), and (2) the neuronal nicotinic antagonists or so-called *ganglionic blockers*, such as hexamethonium or mecamylamine (Inversine). Neuromuscular and ganglionic blockers interfere with neurotransmission by acting on the postsynaptic nicotinic receptor (ion channel) and binding to it in a competitive or noncompetitive manner to prevent the binding of ACh to the receptor. The drugs that act at the neuromuscular junction to produce muscle paralysis bind directly to the nicotinic receptor, preventing access of ACh. This is also how some of the ganglionic blocking agents work (e.g., mecamylamine, trimethaphan). However, some of the ganglionic blockers (e.g., hexamethonium) enter the ion channel and form a plug, which also effectively interferes with neurotransmission by preventing influx of sodium ions.[38]

The neuromuscular blocking agents are also classified into two types: (1) depolarizing blockers and (2) nondepolarizing blockers. Succinylcholine (Anectine) is the most commonly used and best-known depolarizing blocker. It binds to the nicotinic receptor at the neuromuscular junction and produces a depolarization of the membrane, which remains in persistent depolarization for a long time, rendering the synapse nonfunctional. After a period of time, the neuromuscular block actually converts to a competitive-type block, which is called *phase II*. Giving a cholinesterase inhibitor will not antagonize the action of a depolarizing blocker, and in fact, may make the block worse. On the other hand, *d*-tubocurarine, gallamine, vecuronium, and pancuronium are competitive neuromuscular blockers that compete with ACh for the receptor. Thus, administering a cholinesterase inhibitor (e.g., physostigmine or neostigmine) can reverse the block produced by competitive antagonists such as *d*-tubocurarine. All neuromuscular blockers and most ganglionic blockers have a charged nitrogen atom and, therefore, do not get into the brain when injected systemically. In fact, if they are injected into the cerebrospinal fluid, they typically cause seizures. Mecamylamine, on the other hand, is a secondary amine that can enter the brain. Ganglionic blockers are used to lower blood pressure during removal of tumors of the adrenal gland, and neuromuscular blockers are used to relax muscles during endoscopic examinations, surgery, and electroconvulsive shock therapy.

4.4.4 Cholinergic Drugs in the TBI Patient

There is evidence of changes in ACh neurotransmission following TBI. Immediately following injury, there appears to be a hyperfunction of the cholinergic system, which lasts 15 minutes to 4 hours. During this time, administration of antimuscarinic drugs has been shown in animal studies to enhance the recovery of function.[39] This is followed by a period of cholinergic hypofunction during which administration of cholinergic agonists can reduce cognitive deficits. Thus, cholinesterase inhibitors such as those used in Alzheimer's disease (e.g., tacrine, donepezil, rivastigmine, or galantamine) may be beneficial for improving memory in TBI patients. Indeed, donepezil was found to improve memory in two TBI patients.[40] Clearly, more extensive clinical trials are warranted and should be undertaken. It has been found that TBI causes a loss of alpha-7 nAChRs in brain, and that treatment with dietary choline in rats subjected to TBI can restore the nAChRs and protect against memory loss, as well as reduce inflammation and cell loss.[41] It may be time to examine the effects of dietary choline supplements on recovery of function in humans with TBI. Indeed, various forms of choline, such as cytidine-5'-diphosphate choline have shown to improve cognitive deficits following TBI in rats.[42]

4.5 Norepinephrine

Norepinephrine is one of three endogenous chemicals known as *catecholamines* that function as neurotransmitters in the mammalian nervous system. The other two are epinephrine, which is a neurotransmitter in brain but a hormone in the periphery, and dopamine, which is a neurotransmitter in brain. Norepinephrine is the neurotransmitter of the sympathetic postganglionic fibers of the autonomic nervous system, where it is involved in such things as increasing heart rate, constricting blood vessels or raising blood pressure, reducing GI motility, and dilating pupils (see Table 4.3 for the response of various organs to sympathetic nerve stimulation). There are some exceptions to the rule that all postganglionic sympathetic nerves are "adrenergic" (i.e., use norepinephrine as a transmitter)—namely, those postganglionic fibers going to sweat glands and those going to certain blood vessels in lower mammals, which use ACh as a transmitter.

The finding that catecholamines form fluorescent compounds in tissue exposed to formaldehyde gas greatly facilitated the mapping of such neurons in the brain. The technique known as *fluorescence histochemistry* was developed by Falk and Hillarp in Sweden in the early 1960s.[43]

TABLE 4.3

Organ Response to Sympathetic Nerve Stimulation

Organ Receiving Innervation	Response to Stimulation	Receptor Type
Eye		
Iris, radial muscle	Dilation (mydriasis)	Alpha-1
Iris, ciliary muscle	Relaxation of far vision	Beta-2
Heart		
SA node	Increase in heart rate	Beta-1
Atrium	Increase in contractility	Beta-1
AV node	Increased conduction velocity	Beta-1
Ventricle	Increased contractility	Beta-1
Vasculature		
Skin and mucosa	Constriction	Alpha-1
Skeletal muscle	Constriction, dilation	Alpha-1, Beta-2
Cerebral	Constriction	Alpha-1
Abdominal viscera	Mostly constriction, some dilation	Alpha-1, Beta-2 for dilation
Trachea and bronchioles	Relaxation	Beta-2
Stomach and intestine	Decrease in motility, tone, and secretion; contraction of sphincters	Alpha-1, Alpha-2 Beta-2
Urinary bladder		
Detrusor muscle	Relaxation	Beta-2
Trigone and sphincter	Contraction	Alpha-1
Sex organ, male	Ejaculation	Alpha-1
Sweat glands	Localized secretion (palms of hands)	Alpha-1
Lacrimal glands	Slight secretion	Alpha-1
Nasopharyngeal glands	No direct innervation	—

SA, sionatrial; AV, atrioventricular.

Source: J. G. Hardman, L. E. Limbird, and A. G. Gilman (Eds.), *The Pharmacological Basis of Therapeutics*, McGraw-Hill Medical Publishing, New York, 115, 2001.

The noradrenergic neurons in the brain are found in one of two systems: (1) the locus ceruleus system and (2) the lateral tegmental system. A description of these two systems is beyond the scope of this chapter, but can be found in an excellent review by Moore and Bloom.[44] Histochemical studies showed that the noradrenergic axons have a very widespread distribution, reaching essentially all levels of the neuraxis. For example, neurons in the nucleus locus ceruleus of the pons innervate everything from the cerebral cortex to the spinal cord. The diffuse nature of noradrenergic innervation allows this system to have global influences on brain function. The norepinephrine system in the brain has been implicated in a wide variety of functions including anxiety, affective states (mood), arousal, rapid eye movement sleep, aggression, pain perception, pleasure experience, seizures, and endocrine function.

4.5.1 Synthesis, Storage, Release, and Inactivation of Norepinephrine

Neurons that synthesize and use norepinephrine as a neurotransmitter are referred to as *adrenergic* neurons or *noradrenergic* neurons. Norepinephrine is synthesized in postganglionic sympathetic neurons and in neurons of the brain from tyrosine, an amino acid that is formed from phenylalanine in the liver. Phenylalanine is referred to as an essential amino acid because it must be supplied in the diet. Tyrosine is transported into adrenergic neurons by a high-affinity uptake transporter.[45] Once inside the neuron, tyrosine is converted to norepinephrine by the reactions shown in Figure 4.4.

The rate-limiting enzyme in the overall synthesis of catecholamines (both norepinephrine and dopamine) is tyrosine hydroxylase, which is found in the cytoplasm of the neuron. This enzyme utilizes molecular oxygen and tyrosine as substrates and requires iron and tetrahydrobiopterin as cofactors. Under most conditions, the concentration of tyrosine in the neuron saturates the enzyme. Thus, increasing the tyrosine concentration will not enhance the rate of norepinephrine synthesis.[46] However, under conditions of increased utilization (e.g., stress), it may be possible to increase the rate of norepinephrine synthesis by administering tyrosine.[46]

The second step in the pathway, the conversion of DOPA (dihydroxyphenylalanine) to dopamine, requires aromatic-L-amino acid decarboxylase, which uses pyridoxal phosphate (vitamin B6) as a cofactor (Figure 4.4).

The third step in the pathway utilizes dopamine-β-hydroxylase (DBH) to convert dopamine to norepinephrine. DBH is a copper-containing enzyme that uses ascorbic acid as a cofactor and is located in the membrane of the storage vesicle. Thus, as dopamine is actively

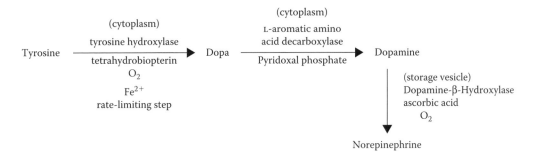

FIGURE 4.4
Synthesis of norepinephrine in the adrenergic nerve terminal. This diagram shows the enzymes and cofactors required for synthesis, as well as their location (see parentheses) within the neuron.

transported into the vesicle, it gets converted to norepinephrine.[1] Apparently, there is some soluble DBH inside the vesicle that is coreleased with norepinephrine. Inhibition of DBH should reduce the levels of norepinephrine without affecting the levels of dopamine. In the adrenal medulla and in some neurons of the brain, norepinephrine is converted to epinephrine by the enzyme phenylethanolamine-N-methyltransferase, which is found in the cytoplasm of cells.[13] Synthesis of norepinephrine within a neuron is regulated by a wide variety of factors, including the intracellular concentration of norepinephrine and the firing rate of the neuron.

Once synthesized, the catecholamines (norepinephrine, dopamine, and epinephrine in the brain) are stored in both small (200–300 Å) or large (500–1200 Å) membrane-bound vesicles. Inside the vesicle, norepinephrine is stored in a complex with ATP, as shown in Figure 4.5. Norepinephrine is actively transported into the vesicle from the surrounding cytoplasm by an ATP–Mg^{++}-dependent process.[47] The transporter responsible for uptake into the vesicle is known as the *vesicular monoamine transporter* (VMAT). Uptake of norepinephrine into the vesicle by VMAT is inhibited by the drug reserpine, which ultimately leads to the depletion of the tissue content of norepinephrine.

The release of norepinephrine from nerve terminals occurs when the terminal is depolarized by the incoming action potential. This results in the opening of voltage-dependent Ca^{2+} channels and triggers the process of exocytosis, similar to the release of ACh described earlier. The sites at which drugs can act to alter neurotransmission at a noradrenergic synapse are shown in Figure 4.5.

Many drugs can facilitate the release of norepinephrine from nerve endings to increase the concentration in the synaptic cleft and the postsynaptic receptors. These include the amphetamines (Adderall) and methylphenidate (Ritalin), which stimulate the release of norepinephrine and dopamine by a Ca^{2+}-independent mechanism that does not involve exocytosis.

After release of norepinephrine into the synaptic cleft and interaction with the postsynaptic receptors, neurotransmitter action is terminated primarily by reuptake into the presynaptic terminal from which it was released. This is carried out by a protein called the *norepinephrine transporter* (NET).[1,46] NET transports norepinephrine along with sodium (cotransporter), a process that is inhibited by antidepressants and cocaine, but not by drugs like reserpine, which inhibit VMAT. The molecular characteristics of NET have been studied in great detail and the chemical structure of this protein has been determined from cloning experiments.[48] Although reuptake has been shown to be the major process responsible for terminating the action of norepinephrine, enzymatic degradation also takes place via the enzymes monoamine oxidase (MAO) and catechol-O-methyltransferase (COMT).

MAO, which is present in the outer membrane of the mitochondrion, is involved in the intraneuronal degradation of free norepinephrine that is present in the cytoplasm of neurons. The MAO that is found in human and rat brain is present in two forms that are referred to as *type A* and *type B,* based on the fact that they have different substrate specificity and different sensitivity to specific inhibitors. For further discussion of the different types of MAO, see Cooper et al.[1] COMT is present in most cells of the body and takes care of the extraneuronal metabolism of catecholamines (norepinephrine and dopamine) before they reach the urine.[1,46]

Drugs that act as inhibitors of MAO cause elevations in the intraneuronal content of catecholamines (norepinephrine and dopamine) as well as serotonin and eventually enhance the concentration of neurotransmitter reaching the receptors. MAO inhibitors are used as antidepressant drugs. COMT inhibitors are used in the treatment of Parkinson's disease to

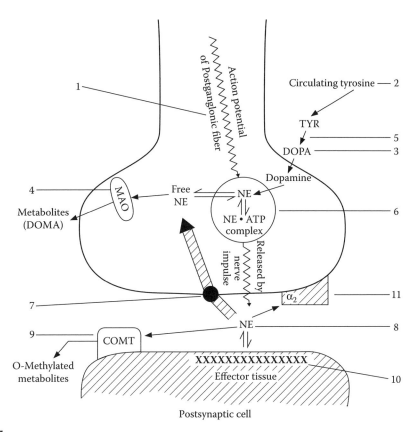

FIGURE 4.5

Drawing of adrenergic (sympathetic) neuron terminal synapsing on an effector organ in the peripheral autonomic nervous system. This also serves as a model for adrenergic synapses in the CNS. The numbers shown indicate the sites where drugs are known to act to modify neurotransmission. 1, some drugs (e.g., guanethidine and bretylium) inhibit release by blocking the propagation of the action potential (essential for release) into the nerve terminal; 2, under conditions of stress, it may be possible to increase norepinephrine (NE) synthesis by increasing the concentration of circulating tyrosine (i.e., by administering tyrosine); 3, a more effective way to increase dopamine and norepinephrine synthesis is to administer L-DOPA because it bypasses the rate-limiting step involving tyrosine hydroxylase; 4, inhibitors of monoamine oxidase (MAO) (e.g., tranylcypromine) act at site 4 to prevent the degradation of norepinephrine; 5, inhibitors of tyrosine hydroxylase (e.g., alpha-methyltyrosine) act here to block synthesis of norepinephrine; 6, drugs that interfere with the storage of norepinephrine (e.g., reserpine) act on the vesicle and eventually deplete the neuron on norepinephrine; 7, drugs that block reuptake (e.g., cocaine and tricyclic antidepressants) act to increase the concentration of norepinephrine in the synapse; 8, norepinephrine in the synaptic cleft can act as an agonist on the postsynaptic receptors, as can other agonists for alpha or beta receptors; 9, inhibitors of catechol-*O*-methyltransferase (COMT) can increase the availability of norepinephrine for agonist action; 10, norepinephrine, as well as other directly acting agonists, initiates a response (however, antagonists can also act here to block the response); 11, presynaptic alpha-2 (α_2) receptors decrease the release of norepinephrine when these receptors are activated by norepinephrine or drugs such as clonidine. TYR, tyrosine.

reduce the metabolism of levodopa and enhance its action. The metabolic products resulting from the action of COMT and MAO on norepinephrine and dopamine are shown in Figure 4.6. These products represent clinically important metabolites that can be measured in cerebrospinal fluid or urine to provide an index of how the catecholamine systems have been altered by disease or drug treatment.[46]

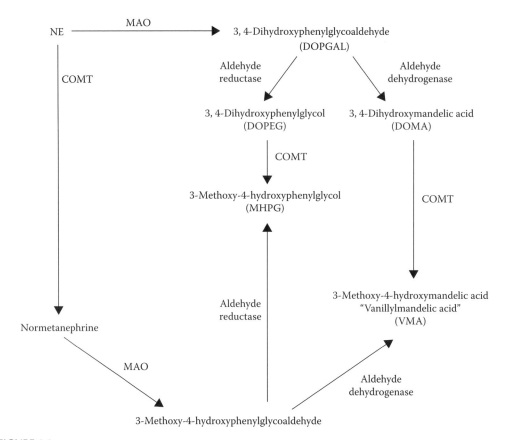

FIGURE 4.6
Enzymatic degradation of norepinephrine (NE) by monoamine oxidase (MAO) and catecholamine-*O*-methyl-transferase (COMT).

4.5.2 Norepinephrine Receptors

Norepinephrine receptors (adrenoceptors) mediate the effects of norepinephrine. Adrenoceptor subtypes that respond to norepinephrine include alpha-1, alpha-2, and beta-1. Beta-2 receptors have a lower affinity for norepinephrine, but have a high affinity for epinephrine and are involved in mediating some of the effects of the latter neurotransmitter or hormone. Specific agonists and antagonists exist for each receptor, and some of these are described later in this chapter. Norepinephrine can also activate beta-3 receptors found in fat cells to enhance lipolysis, but these are not considered here.

In recent years, a great deal of information has been gained about the molecular nature of the adrenoceptors, both in terms of their coupling to second messenger systems (so-called *signal transduction mechanisms*) and their chemical structure. Each receptor is known to be an integral membrane protein with seven transmembrane-spanning regions and a molecular weight of 64,000 to 80,000 Da.[49]

Unlike the nicotinic cholinergic receptor, which is intimately associated with an ion channel and produces ultrarapid effects, the adrenoceptors mediate their effects through GPCRs like the muscarinic ACh receptor.[13,46] Both beta-1 and beta-2 adrenoceptors are linked to adenylate cyclase in the membrane by a G_s (stimulatory G) protein which is activated by a combination between the receptor protein and an adrenergic agonist. The alpha subunit of the G_s protein with gaunosine triphosphate (GTP) bound to it can then interact with adenylate cyclase and activate it, leading to the conversion of ATP to cyclic adenosine monophosphate (cAMP). The latter can, in turn, activate various protein kinases that are involved in the phosphorylation (i.e., the addition of a phosphate group or PO_4-) of various proteins that regulate membrane ion transport to alter membrane potentials (Figure 4.7).

The alpha-2 adrenoceptors, which are usually located presynaptically (Figure 4.5), also mediate their effect on membrane potential through a G-protein and adenylate cyclase activity, but unlike the beta receptors, the alpha-2 receptor is linked to a G_i protein, which causes an inhibition of adenylate cyclase and a reduction in the amount of cAMP (and, presumably, a reduction in protein phosphorylation) in the neuron.

The alpha-1 adrenergic receptor mediates its action through another second messenger system that is linked to the receptor by a G_q protein. The second messengers produced when an agonist binds to the alpha-1 receptor are actually metabolites of phosphoinositide breakdown mediated by phospholipase C and include IP_3 and DAG, as was the case for certain muscarinic receptors described earlier. IP_3 causes the release of Ca^{2+} from intracellular storage sites and Ca^{2+} can then activate protein kinases to produce phosphorylation of membrane proteins (Figure 4.7). DAG activates protein kinase C, which in turn phosphorylates various proteins to mediate various cellular responses of alpha-1 agonists.[1,50]

Three subtypes of alpha-1 receptors (e.g., α_{1a}, α_{1b}, α_{1d}) and three subtypes of alpha$_2$ receptors (α_{2a}, α_{2b}, and α_{2c}) have been identified.[51] There are also three subtypes of beta receptor (β_1, β_2, and β_3). Selective agonists and antagonists are available for alpha-1, alpha-2, beta-1, and beta-2 receptors, and these drugs are primarily used for their effects on the peripheral autonomic nervous system, especially in the area of cardiovascular disease. Chronic treatment with agonists or antagonists can result in compensatory changes in the sensitivity and/or receptor number of adrenergic receptors. Such changes appear to be carried out by enzymes that phosphorylate the receptor (i.e., receptor kinases).[51]

4.5.3 Clinically Useful Drugs That Alter Noradrenergic Neurotransmission

4.5.3.1 Facilitators of Noradrenergic Neurotransmission

4.5.3.1.1 Adrenergic Agonists

Adrenergic agonists are also referred to as *direct-acting sympathomimetic amines* and they are classified as either alpha or beta agonists. There are both alpha-1 and alpha-2 agonists available, but many are nonselective. Norepinephrine (Levophed), itself, is available and is an agonist for alpha-1, alpha-2, and beta-1 receptors, whereas epinephrine is an agonist for all adrenergic receptors. **Phenylephrine** is an alpha$_1$ agonist that is used in nose drops (Neo-Synephrine) as a nasal decongestant, where it acts to vasoconstrict the mucosal blood vessels and reduce congestion. Other alpha agonists that are predominantly alpha-1 selective include methoxamine and metaraminol. Clonidine (Catapres) is an alpha-2 agonist used as an antihypertensive agent because of its action on the brain, where stimulation of alpha-2 receptors presumably decrease the activity of the peripheral sympathetic nervous system. Other alpha-2 agonists include guanfacine and guanabenz.

Isoproterenol (Isuprel) is a beta agonist that stimulates both beta-1 and beta-2 receptors and has been used as a bronchodilator because of the beta-2 receptors in the bronchioles that mediate bronchiolar relaxation (Table 4.3). Indeed, most of the beta agonists are used for the treatment of diseases that are associated with bronchoconstriction, such as asthma. Selective beta-2 agonists are also available and have the advantage of not causing cardiac stimulation when used in asthma. These include metaproterenol (Metaprel), terbutaline

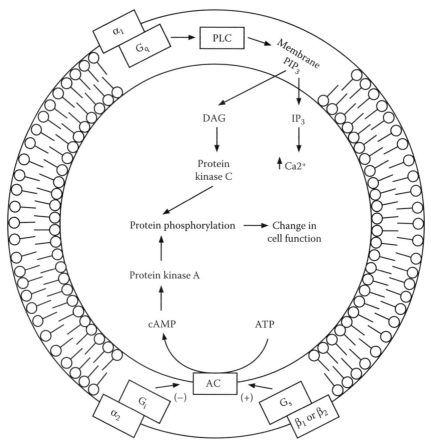

FIGURE 4.7
Diagram of second messenger (signaling) system linked to alpha- and beta-adrenergic receptors in a cell (neuron or effector cell) containing such receptors. The alpha-1 (α_1) receptor is linked by a G-protein (G_q) to phospholipase C (PLC), which, when activated (by agonist binding to the α_1 receptor), leads to the breakdown of phosphatidylinositol 4,5-bisphosphate (PIP_2) to form two second messengers (diacylglycerol [DAG] and inositol triphosphate or [IP_3]). DAG activates protein kinase C, which can in turn phosphorylate proteins, including those in ion channels, whereas IP_3 causes an increase in intracellular calcium by releasing it from various stores. The calcium can activate calcium/calmodulin-dependent protein kinase, which can phosphorylate other proteins. Beta-1 (β_1) and beta-2 (β_2) receptors act through a G_s protein to stimulate adenylyl cyclase (AC), leading to an increase in the formation of cAMP, which can activate protein kinase A to increase the phosphorylation of various proteins. Note that the alpha-2 (α_2) receptor acts through a G_1 protein (inhibitory G-protein) which leads to inhibition of adenylyl cyclase and a decrease in the intracellular concentration of cAMP. As can be seen here, protein phosphorylation is the major mechanism by which receptors act through signal transduction to alter cell function.

(Brethine), and albuterol (Proventil). There are no highly selective beta$_1$ agonists available. However, dopamine and dobutamine (Dobutrex) are used for their ability to stimulate beta-1 receptors in the heart to increase cardiac output in states of shock or heart failure.

4.5.3.1.2 *Drugs That Block Norepinephrine Reuptake*

Inasmuch as reuptake (via NET) is the major mechanism for inactivating released norepinephrine, drugs that block this process have a marked ability to facilitate noradrenergic neurotransmission. The classic example of a drug that does this is cocaine. Cocaine, however, also blocks dopamine and serotonin reuptake. Many of the antidepressant drugs (so-called *tricyclic antidepressants*) are potent and selective inhibitors of norepinephrine uptake and, presumably, mediate some of their beneficial effects in depression via this mechanism.[52] Selective norepinephrine uptake inhibitors include desipramine (Norpramin), protriptyline (Vivactil), nortriptyline (Aventyl), maprotiline (Ludiomil), and atomoxetine (Strattera). All of these are used to treat depression, except for atomoxetine, which is used to treat attention deficit hyperactivity disorder. Side effects of these drugs include their ability to increase heart rate and blood pressure as a result of peripheral effects on the cardiovascular system. At plasma concentrations that exceed the recommended level, these drugs can also lower the seizure threshold and may precipitate seizures. However, therapeutic plasma levels have been shown to exert anticonvulsant effects in experimental animals.

4.5.3.1.3 Drugs That Increase Norepinephrine Release

Several drugs are available to increase the release of norepinephrine (as well as dopamine in CNS) from nerve endings. The mechanism by which this is accomplished is not entirely clear. However, it appears to involve the release of norepinephrine from a nonvesicular pool that does not require calcium and does not involve exocytosis. The current hypothesis is that these drugs are taken up by the uptake transporter for norepinephrine, bringing the carrier to the inside of the neuron, where norepinephrine can bind to it for exchange transport. Such drugs also interfere with the uptake of norepinephrine by vesicles, increasing the cytoplasmic concentration of norepinephrine and making more available for reverse transport.[13] Drugs that facilitate the release of norepinephrine include amphetamine, dextroamphetamine (Dexedrine), methamphetamine (Desoxyn), and methylphenidate (Ritalin). These drugs also increase the release of dopamine from nerve terminals, which is believed to be responsible for many of their effects and is discussed later.

Amphetamine is the racemic mixture of D- and L-amphetamine. Dextroamphetamine is three to four times more potent in stimulating the CNS than is L-amphetamine. One commercial product contains a mixture of amphetamine and dextroamphetamine (Adderall). All amphetamine analogues have powerful cardiovascular stimulating effects that lead to an increase in blood pressure and the work of the heart. The CNS stimulating effects of amphetamine on arousal and locomotor activity are dependent on newly synthesized norepinephrine or dopamine, because these effects are blocked by alpha methyltyrosine, a tyrosine hydroxylase inhibitor used to block norepinephrine synthesis.[38]

The amphetamines, as a group, are used to suppress appetite in the treatment of obesity and to treat narcolepsy (a sleep disorder) and attention deficit hyperactivity disorder. These drugs are regulated as controlled substances because of their abuse potential. High doses can produce a psychosis that is indistinguishable from an acute paranoid schizophrenic syndrome. Moreover, it has been shown, in both rats and nonhuman primates, that repeated injections of methamphetamine can produce neurotoxicity leading to the loss of both dopamine and serotonin-containing neurons in the brain.[53–56] The mechanism responsible for this neurotoxicity remains unknown, although several hypotheses have been proposed.

4.5.3.1.4 Drugs That Decrease the Enzymatic Degradation of Norepinephrine

Norepinephrine is degraded intraneuronally by the enzyme MAO, as indicated earlier. Inhibiting this enzyme should eventually increase the concentration of norepinephrine in the synaptic cleft. Several MAO inhibitors are used clinically as antidepressants. These include tranylcypromine (Parnate), phenelzine (Nardil), and isocarboxazid (Marplan). Some MAO inhibitors are being used to prevent further deterioration of Parkinson's disease. One drug in the latter category is selegiline (deprenyl, Eldepryl), which is selective for MAO-B. Patients on MAO inhibitors cannot eat foods containing tyramine (a potent norepinephrine releaser), such as cheese. Normally, tyramine is metabolized by MAO in the intestine, but this enzyme is inactive in patients on an MAO inhibitor. Tyramine reaching the circulation causes a hypertensive crisis with very dangerous consequences. Thus, individuals taking MAO inhibitors must avoid foods containing tyramine, such as wine, beer, cheese, and other fermented products.

4.5.3.2 Inhibitors of Noradrenergic Neurotransmission

4.5.3.2.1 Adrenoceptor Antagonists

There have long been available drugs that are selective antagonists of either alpha or beta adrenergic receptors. Now, we have drugs that are even selective for a specific subtype of alpha or beta receptor. The main advantage of a subtype selective antagonist is that it will have fewer side effects. Nonselective alpha antagonists include phenoxybenzamine and phentolamine, whereas nonselective beta antagonists include propranolol (Inderal), sotalol, and pindolol. Of interest for the treatment of hypertension are the alpha-1 selective antagonists, prazosin (Minipress) and terazosin (Hytrin). Beta-1 selective antagonists are useful because they can be used to reduce blood pressure, stop cardiac arrhythmias, or prevent subsequent heart attacks with minimal effects on bronchiolar smooth muscle. Metoprolol (Lopressor), atenolol (Tenormin), acebutolol (Sectral), and esmolol (Brevibloc) are all currently marketed beta-1 selective antagonists used to treat cardiovascular disorders.

4.5.3.2.2 Inhibitors of Norepinephrine Release

Some drugs are selectively taken up into noradrenergic nerve terminals and then prevent the release of norepinephrine, apparently by blocking the invasion of the action potential into the terminal (i.e., a local anestheticlike effect). Drugs in this category are referred to as *adrenergic neuronal blocking agents* and include guanethidine (Ismelin), guanadrel (Hylorel), and bretylium. Initially, these drugs cause a transient release of norepinephrine, prior to the inhibition of release. When used chronically, guanethidine also has a reserpine-like effect (discussed in the next section) by interfering with norepinephrine storage and depleting the neurons of norepinephrine. Such drugs are primarily used as antihypertensive agents. However, bretylium is now used exclusively to treat cardiac arrhythmias.

4.5.3.2.3 Inhibitors of Norepinephrine Storage

Reserpine is the classic drug for inhibiting the storage of catecholamines (norepinephrine, epinephrine, and dopamine) and serotonin (see the following text). Reserpine binds to the vesicle membrane and interferes with the uptake of monoamines into the vesicle, rendering the vesicle nonfunctional. When norepinephrine cannot be stored in the vesicle, it is not protected and is degraded by MAO. Thus, reserpine leads to a depletion of the norepinephrine from the nerve terminals. It is primarily used in combination with other drugs as an antihypertensive agent.[57]

4.5.3.2.4 Inhibitors of Norepinephrine Synthesis

There are two sites within the norepinephrine synthetic pathway where drugs can be used to block synthesis: (1) the tyrosine hydroxylase step (which is the rate-limiting enzyme) and (2) the dopamine β hydroxylase step. The latter is more selective and can be accomplished with the drug disulfiram (Antabuse) or its active metabolite diethyldithiocarbamate.

Unfortunately, these drugs inhibit many other enzymes and have many side effects. The most common way to interfere with synthesis of norepinephrine is to inhibit tyrosine hydroxylase with α-methyltyrosine (metyrosine, Demser®). However, this drug also blocks the synthesis of epinephrine and dopamine and is, therefore, not very selective.

4.5.4 Noradrenergic Drugs in the TBI Patient

There is considerable evidence that enhancing noradrenergic neurotransmission in the CNS has beneficial effects on recovery of function after TBI in animal studies.[58–62] Moreover, interference with noradrenergic neurotransmission (e.g., using alpha adrenoceptor antagonists) was found to retard the recovery of motor function in rats after head injury.[63] Because of these findings, Feeney et al.[59] have put forth the norepinephrine hypothesis of recovery. Consistent with this hypothesis is the finding that amphetamines, when paired with physical therapy, have been shown to enhance recovery following stroke.[64,65]

These findings indicate that drugs that enhance norepinephrine neurotransmission (e.g., *d*-amphetamine, tricyclic antidepressants) facilitate recovery following TBI. However, more clinical studies are needed because most of the data has been obtained in animals.

4.6 Dopamine

Although dopamine can be found in the peripheral nervous system in such places as the carotid body and sympathetic ganglia, it is of interest primarily for its neurotransmitter role in the CNS, where it is involved in a wide variety of functions from regulating motor function (basal ganglia) to inhibiting the release of prolactin from the pituitary gland. Most of the dopamine neurons in the brain have their cell bodies either in the midbrain (e.g., substantia nigrum and ventral tegmental area), where they are involved in the regulation of emotional states or motor activity (e.g., substantia nigra dopamine is lost in Parkinson's disease) or the hypothalamus, where it is involved in regulating endocrine function.[1] Thus, there are three major dopaminergic pathways in the CNS: (1) the nigrostriatal pathway (which projects from the substantia nigra to the striatum and is important in Parkinson's disease), (2) the mesocortical/mesolimbic system (which projects from the ventral tegmental area of the midbrain to the limbic system and the cerebral cortex, playing a role in psychiatric disorders), and (3) the tuberoinfundibular pathway (which projects from the arcuate nucleus of the hypothalamus to the median eminence of the pituitary stalk and regulates endocrine function).

4.6.1 Synthesis, Storage, Release, and Inactivation of Dopamine

Dopamine is an intermediate compound in the synthesis of norepinephrine and is, in fact, the immediate precursor of norepinephrine (see Figures 4.4 and 4.8). Thus, the synthesis is identical to that of norepinephrine up through the formation of dopamine, but does not proceed to norepinephrine because dopaminergic neurons lack the enzyme dopamine-β-hydroxylase. As was the case with norepinephrine synthesis, tyrosine hydroxylase is the rate-limiting enzyme in the synthetic pathway and, if one wants to block synthesis, this is the enzyme to block.

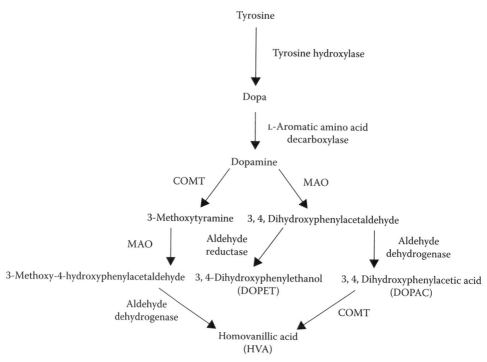

FIGURE 4.8
Synthesis and degradation of dopamine. Note that homovanillic acid is the major metabolite.

Dopamine synthesis is regulated somewhat differently than is norepinephrine synthesis. This is largely because dopaminergic neurons have autoreceptors on the dopamine nerve terminal that regulate both synthesis and release, whereas norepinephrine neurons have autoreceptors (which are α_2) that regulate release only.[1] However, like norepinephrine, the intracellular concentration of dopamine can regulate synthesis through end-product inhibition. Again, tyrosine hydroxylase is normally saturated with tyrosine, so that administering tyrosine is not an effective way to enhance the synthesis of dopamine. However, DOPA decarboxylase is not saturated with substrate, and synthesis of dopamine can be increased by the administration of DOPA, given as *levodopa,* which is now the drug of choice in the treatment of Parkinson's disease. In Parkinson's disease, the nigrostriatal dopaminergic pathway degenerates and the administration of levodopa helps replace the dopamine in the striatum.

Dopamine is stored in vesicles in a manner similar to that of norepinephrine in a complex with ATP. Several soluble proteins called *chromogranins* are also present in the dopamine storage vesicle. The release of dopamine from nerve terminals, like that of norepinephrine, is triggered by the arrival of an action potential. Release occurs by a process of exocytosis and, therefore, is calcium dependent. The release of dopamine is apparently reduced by a negative feedback mechanism when excess dopamine in the synaptic cleft interacts with presynaptic receptors (autoreceptors). Activation of autoreceptors on the cell body reduces the firing rates of dopaminergic neurons.[1] All dopaminergic autoreceptors are believed to be of the D_2 or D_3 subtype (see Section 4.6.2).

Dopamine is inactivated following release by a high-affinity uptake transporter called the *dopamine transporter* (DAT), which transports it back into the neuron from which it was released. This is an energy-requiring process that is dependent on sodium and is similar to norepinephrine reuptake. As is the case with norepinephrine and most other neurotransmitters, DAT has been cloned and found to be a member of a large family of transporter proteins that have 12 membrane-spanning regions. Indeed, much is known about the molecular characteristics of DAT.[66]

Although reuptake into the neuron from which it was released is the primary mechanism for terminating the physiologic effects of released dopamine, it may also undergo enzymatic metabolism similar to norepinephrine. Thus, both MAO and COMT can convert dopamine to inactive compounds according to the schema shown in Figure 4.8. Moreover, the resulting metabolites 3, 4-dihydroxyphenylacetic acid and homovanillic acid (Figure 4.8) are often used as indices of the rate of dopamine turnover in the CNS. Antipsychotic drugs (neuroleptics) that block dopamine receptors increase the concentration of dopamine metabolites in CSF and in brain.[1]

4.6.2 Dopamine Receptors

Two subtypes of dopamine receptors (D_1 and D_2) were originally identified and described using receptor binding techniques.[67] However, using molecular cloning techniques, five dopamine receptors have been identified and all of them, including the new ones (D_3, D_4, and D_5), are now classified as either D_1-like or D_2-like receptors.[68–71] The D_1-like include the D_1 and D_5 receptors, whereas the D_2 like include D_2, D_3, and D_4 receptors. The D_1-like receptors appear to mediate their effects through a G_s protein that activates adenylate cyclase and increases cAMP, whereas the D_2-like receptors appear to be negatively coupled to adenylate cyclase, producing an inhibition of the latter through a G_i protein. All the dopamine receptors (D_1, D_2, D_3, D_4, and D_5) structurally are typical GPCRs.

There is considerable sequence homology (similar sequence of amino acids in the protein) between the various dopamine receptors as well as between these receptors and other members of this family, such as the beta-1 and muscarinic receptors.[68] The D_3 receptor appears to represent both an autoreceptor and postsynaptic receptor and is found in limbic areas of brain.[68] For older so-called *typical antipsychotic* drugs, there is a high correlation between their clinical potency and their D_2 receptor blocking action. However, clozapine is much more potent at blocking D_4 receptors and has fewer motor side effects than the other antipsychotic drugs. Moreover, clozapine is effective at alleviating the symptoms of schizophrenia in some patients who are refractory to other antipsychotic drugs. Because of these differences, clozapine and newer antipsychotic drugs are referred to as *atypical antipsychotics*. In general, the functions of most subtypes of dopamine receptor are unknown; D_1 receptors have only been found postsynaptically, but D_2 receptors occur either pre- or postsynaptically and autoreceptors are usually of the D_2 subtype. The use of D_1 and D_2 agonists has shown that activation of both receptors may be necessary for expression of certain dopamine functions. Although the atypical antipsychotic drugs, such as clozapine and olanzapine, have a low affinity for the D_2 dopamine receptor, it appears that blockade of this receptor subtype is still important in their action.

The dopamine neurons have been implicated in the abuse of stimulants such as cocaine and amphetamine. Mesolimbic dopaminergic neurons have also been implicated in addiction to alcohol, opioids, and nicotine. It has been proposed that variations in the gene for the D_2 receptor may contribute to interindividual differences in vulnerability to alcoholism and polysubstance abuse.[72]

4.6.3 Clinically Useful Drugs That Alter Dopamine Neurotransmission

4.6.3.1 Facilitators of Dopaminergic Neurotransmission

4.6.3.1.1 Dopamine Agonists

Dopamine, itself, does not cross the blood–brain barrier and, therefore, cannot be used for effects on the CNS. However, dopamine is used intravenously for its effects on the cardiovascular system, where it acts on beta-1 receptors in the heart to increase contractility and on dopamine receptors in the renal vasculature to cause vasodilation. Because of the latter two actions, dopamine is used to treat various forms of shock. Apomorphine is a nonselective dopamine agonist that does get into the brain and has been used to treat such things as Parkinson's disease. However, it is poorly absorbed from the gut and must be administered parenterally. Apomorphine (Apokyn) is now available in an injectable form (subcutaneous) for the rescue from the "off phenomenon" in patients with advanced Parkinson's disease.[73] When apomorphine is used in patients, it is given with an antiemetic (trimethobenzamide or Tigan). This is because apomorphine achieves high concentrations in the chemoreceptor trigger zone in the area postrema of the medulla oblongata, which leads to nausea and vomiting unless an antiemetic is given first. Other nonselective dopamine agonists include bromocriptine (Parlodel), which has long been used to treat endocrine disorders, such as hyperprolactinemia, where it acts in the anterior pituitary gland to inhibit the release of prolactin. Bromocriptine is also now recommended for the treatment of Parkinson's disease. Pergolide (Permax) is another dopamine agonist[1] that, along with bromocriptine, has been used in Parkinson's disease. However, bromocriptine and pergolide, which are ergot alkaloids, are not used much because of possible heart valve damage. Only bromocriptine remains on the market in the United States.

Several nonergot dopaminergic agonists have been introduced for the treatment of Parkinson's disease in recent years. These include ropinirole (Requip), a D_2 selective agonist; pramipexole (Mirapex), a D_1 and D_2; and rotigotine (Neupro).

4.6.3.1.2 Drugs That Increase the Synaptic Concentration of Dopamine by Acting Indirectly

Drugs that increase the synaptic concentration of dopamine by acting indirectly include the indirectly acting agents, such as amphetamine and methylphenidate (Ritalin), which increase the release of dopamine into the synaptic cleft, the dopamine reuptake inhibitors (GBR 12909, amphetamine, nomifensine, benztropine, amantadine), and the drugs that increase dopamine synthesis (levodopa). Note that some drugs have more than one action. For example, amphetamine and amantadine increase the release of dopamine from nerve endings as well as prevent the inactivation by reuptake.

4.6.3.1.3 Drugs That Block Enzymatic Degradation of Dopamine

Like other catecholamines, dopamine is degraded by MAO and COMT (see Figure 4.8). Therefore, MAO inhibitors can increase the synaptic concentration of dopamine. Selegiline (Eldepryl; described previously), as well as rasagiline (Azilect), is now being used to treat Parkinson's disease because it may prevent the enzymatic degradation of dopamine and may prevent the formation of neurotoxins that destroy dopaminergic neurons and arrest the progression of the disease.[74,75] All the MAO inhibitors described earlier in the section on norepinephrine will also prevent the enzymatic degradation of dopamine. Two COMT inhibitors have recently become available for the treatment of Parkinson's disease. These include tolcapone (Tasmar) and entacapone (Comtan), which block the conversion of levodopa to 3-*O*-methyldopa and increase the amount of levodopa that gets converted to dopamine in the brain.[76]

The COMT inhibitors can reduce the "wearing off" symptoms in patients treated with levodopa/carbidopa. It should be noted that tolcapone has been removed from the market in Canada because of three fatalities resulting from hepatotoxicity. However, it remains on the market in the United States with a black box warning.

4.6.3.2 Inhibitors of Dopaminergic Neurotransmission

4.6.3.2.1 Drugs That Interfere with Dopaminergic Neurotransmission

In this category, we have just two groups of drugs: (1) the receptor antagonists or blockers and (2) the drugs that interfere with storage (e.g., reserpine). As would be expected, the only ones that provide selective effects on dopaminergic neurotransmission are the receptor blockers, because reserpinelike drugs interfere with the storage of all monoamines. We will, therefore, consider only the dopamine antagonists here.

Antagonists of dopamine receptors are primarily used as antipsychotic drugs (also called *neuroleptics*) to treat schizophrenia. The fact that essentially all the drugs effective in schizophrenia are dopaminergic antagonists has led to the hypothesis that schizophrenia is caused by too much dopamine at certain synapses—a hypothesis that has been difficult to prove. Essentially, all the dopamine antagonists block D_2 receptors, but D_1 and D_4 receptors may be affected by certain drugs. The atypical antipsychotic drugs, unlike the older (typical) drugs, appear to have a low affinity for the D_2 receptor and have a higher affinity for the D_3 or D_4 receptor. The latter drugs are also effective antagonists at the 5-HT_{2A} receptor.[77] A list of the dopamine antagonists is given in Table 4.4.

Dopamine antagonists have many side effects because they block dopamine receptors not only in the limbic system, which regulates emotion, but also in the basal ganglia, where loss of dopamine function causes parkinsonianlike symptoms, and in the pituitary, where they cause endocrine-related side effects. Metoclopramide (Reglan) is a dopamine antagonist used for its peripheral effects and its effects on the chemoreceptor trigger zone (which is outside the blood–brain barrier) to prevent nausea and vomiting. Although it

TABLE 4.4

Dopamine Receptor Antagonists (Blockers)

Chemical Class	Examples of Drugs	Receptor Type
Phenothiazines	Chlorpromazine	D_1 and D_2
	Thioridazine	
	Perphenazine	
Thioxanthenes	Chlorprothixene	D_2
Butyrophenones	Haloperidol (Haldol)	Some selectivity for D_2
Dihydroindoles	Molindone	D_2
Dibenzodiazepines	Clozapine (Clozaril)	D_4 (?)
Substituted benzamides	Metoclopramide (Reglan)	D_2
	SCH23390	Selective for D_1
Atypical antipsychotics	Clozapine (Clozaril)	D_2, D_4, 5-HT_{2A}
	Risperidone (Risperdal)	D_2, D_4, 5-HT_{2A}
	Olanzapine (Zyprexa)	D_2, D_4, 5-HT_{2A}
	Quetiapine (Seroquel)	D_2, D_4, 5-HT_{2A}
	Ziprasidone (Geodon)	D_2, D_4, 5-HT_{2A}

Source: J. G. Hardman, L. E. Limbird, and A. G. Gilman (Eds.), *The Pharmacological Basis of Therapeutics*, McGraw-Hill, New York, 485, 2001.

penetrates the brain poorly, some does reach the basal ganglia, which can cause some parkinsonianlike side effects. All the D_2 dopamine receptor antagonists have antiemetic properties, but only some (e.g., metoclopramide and prochlorperazine [Compazine]) are approved for such use.

4.6.4 Dopaminergic Drugs in the TBI Patient

Several reports in recent years suggest that enhancing dopaminergic neurotransmission may be beneficial to patients with TBI. Improving dopaminergic function appears to be useful for two types of deficits in these patients. First, some TBI patients display parkinsonianlike symptoms; second, dopaminergic agents may improve arousal and the ability to focus attention on the task at hand, and generally improve cognitive ability.[78] The latter effect may be mediated through the prefrontal cortex, but the level (regulated by dose) of dopamine receptor stimulation may be critical.[78] Just as L-DOPA (levodopa) is effective in Parkinson's disease, it may help similar symptoms in patients with TBI. The combination of L-DOPA with a peripheral decarboxylase inhibitor will reduce the metabolism of L-DOPA in the periphery and increase the amount that actually reaches the brain. Thus, the combination of levodopa and carbidopa (a decarboxylase inhibitor) is often used. Sinemet (a mixture of L-DOPA and carbidopa) has, in fact, been used successfully in some patients with TBI.[79,80] There is also some evidence from animal studies that treatment with dopamine agonists (e.g., ropinirole) can either reduce or reverse the motor and cognitive deficits produced by brain injury.[81]

A variety of dopamine agonists are also available and may have an advantage because they do not depend on intact dopaminergic neurons. The dopaminergic agonists include such things as the ergot derivatives (e.g., bromocriptine) and nonergot agonists (e.g., ropinirole) described earlier. The antiviral drug amantadine may be considered as an indirect-acting agonist. There is some evidence that these drugs can reduce fatigue, distractibility, and bradykinesia; and improve attention, concentration, and purposeful movement in TBI patients.[82,83]

The use of dopamine antagonists can be advantageous in controlling the symptoms of psychosis, but could impair motivation. The role of dopamine neurons in motivation and reward, as well as in addiction, is well established.[14] Thus, blocking dopamine receptors could reduce motivation. Perhaps it would be possible to enhance motivation with a dopamine reuptake inhibitor like bupropion (Wellbutrin, Zyban). There is one report that shows that bupropion improved restlessness in a TBI patient.[84]

4.7 5-Hydroxytryptamine (Serotonin)

5-Hydroxytryptamine or serotonin (5-HT) is an indolamine that is found both in the periphery and in the CNS. About 90% of the 5-HT in the body is found in the GI tract (in enterochromaffin cells and neurons of the myenteric plexus), whereas 8% of the 5-HT of the body is found in platelets, and only 2% is found in the brain.[1] It is, however, the 2% in the brain that receives most of the attention, and this is the fraction we will focus on. Nevertheless, there are 5-HT receptors throughout the body and many side effects of serotonergic drugs used for an action in the CNS are mediated via the peripheral effects. Sometimes, the serotonergic drugs are used clinically for their peripheral effects, such as the use of 5-HT_3 antagonists for the treatment of irritable bowel syndrome.

Within the brain, 5-HT is localized in neurons that express the gene for tryptophan hydroxylase (TPH). Extensive mapping of serotonergic neurons in the CNS of the rat has been performed using fluorescence histochemistry and immunocytochemistry. In general, the cell bodies of the serotonergic neurons are located along the midline of the brainstem in what are called *raphe nuclei*. Originally, nine separate groups of 5-HT cell bodies were described by Dahlstrom and Fuxe,[85] but more recently, other cell groups have been detected in the area postrema (vomiting area) and in the caudal locus ceruleus, as well as in the interpeduncular nucleus.[1] Like the noradrenergic neurons, the serotonergic neurons have a widespread distribution innervating essentially all areas of the CNS from the cerebral cortex to the spinal cord. The more caudal cell groups (B1–B3) primarily innervate the brainstem and spinal cord, whereas the rostral cell groups (B6–B9) innervate the forebrain. A detailed description of the neuroanatomy of serotonergic neurons has been provided by Molliver.[86]

4.7.1 Synthesis, Storage, Release, and Inactivation of Serotonin

The amino acid precursor for 5-HT synthesis is tryptophan, which is an essential amino acid supplied in the diet. Tryptophan, like tyrosine, is a neutral amino acid that also gains entry into the brain by the large neutral amino acid transporter. Thus, plasma tryptophan will compete with other neutral amino acids, such as tyrosine and phenylalanine, for transport into the brain, which means that the concentration of brain tryptophan will be determined not only by the concentration of tryptophan in plasma but also by the plasma concentration of other neutral amino acids.[1,87] Once in the extracellular fluid of the brain, tryptophan is transported into the serotonergic neurons by a high-affinity and a low-affinity transport system where it can then be converted to 5-HT by a two-step reaction (Figure 4.9), with each step being catalyzed by a different enzyme.[88]

The rate-limiting step in the overall conversion of tryptophan to serotonin is the first step, which is catalyzed by TPH (Figure 4.9) and results in the conversion of tryptophan to 5-hydroxytryptophan (5-HTP). Like tyrosine hydroxylase, TPH is a cytoplasmic mixed-function oxidase that requires molecular oxygen and a reduced pteridine as cofactors. It should also be noted that a membrane-associated form of TPH has been found, indicating that some of the enzyme may be membrane bound. Two isoforms of TPH (TPH1 and TPH2) have been identified. TPH2 is the one that is expressed primarily in brain.[89] Various inhibitors of TPH have been identified, the best known of which is parachlorophenylalanine, which has been used experimentally to study the function of 5-HT.

Inasmuch as the Km of TPH (50–120 μM) is higher than the concentration of brain tryptophan (30 μM), the enzyme is not saturated with tryptophan, which means that increasing the concentration of brain tryptophan can increase the synthesis of 5-HT and lead to higher brain levels of serotonin.[88,90] Thus, it has been found that dietary manipulations of tryptophan can change the brain concentration of serotonin. The 5-HTP formed by the action of TPH2 on tryptophan is immediately converted to 5-HT (serotonin) by the action of L-aromatic amino acid decarboxylase, the same enzyme that converts DOPA to dopamine in catecholaminergic neurons. The decarboxylation of 5-HTP, like that of DOPA, requires pyridoxal phosphate as a cofactor. Inasmuch as the decarboxylation takes place in the cytoplasm, the resulting 5-HT must then be transported into vesicles for storage (see the following text).

The rate of 5-HT synthesis appears to be regulated by the rate of neuronal firing. The latter control over 5-HT synthesis appears to be exerted on TPH by a Ca^{2+}-dependent phosphorylation of the rate-limiting enzyme.[90]

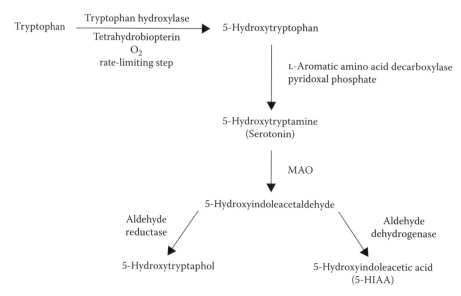

FIGURE 4.9

Synthesis and degradation of 5-hydroxytryptamine (serotonin) in the CNS. Note that 5-HIAA is the major metabolite.

Serotonin, like the catecholamines, is stored in membrane-bound synaptic vesicles inside nerve terminals.[91] These vesicles have been shown to take up serotonin from the cytoplasm via the same VMAT (VMAT-2) that transports catecholamins.[92–94] Release of 5-HT, like that of other neurotransmitters, appears to occur by exocytosis in a calcium-dependent manner.[91] However, certain drugs, such as *p*-chloroamphetamine, are believed to release serotonin from the cytoplasmic pool rather than the vesicular pool,[95] and there is some evidence that the depolarization mediated release by neurons can involve either vesicular or cytoplasmic pools.[96] The available evidence suggests that 5-HT is stored in the vesicles in a complex with ATP and perhaps a serotonin-binding protein.[91]

The release of 5-HT from nerve endings is also regulated via a negative feedback mechanism through serotonin autoreceptors located on the presynaptic (serotonergic) nerve terminals. The evidence indicates that these 5-HT autoreceptors are of the 5-HT_{1B} subtype (see the following text).[90]

Mechanisms similar to those of catecholamine inactivation (described earlier) have been shown to occur for serotonin inactivation. Thus, both reuptake into the neuron from which it was released and MAO may be involved in the inactivation of 5-HT following its action in the synaptic cleft. A high-affinity, sodium-dependent, energy-dependent (requires ATP) uptake of 5-HT has been demonstrated in experimental studies,[87] and reuptake into serotonergic terminals appears to function as the primary inactivation mechanism for removing released serotonin from the synaptic cleft. The serotonin uptake transporter known as *SERT* has been cloned and widely studied.[1,94] There is much interest in determining whether genetic variability in SERT is associated with various psychiatric disorders. Indeed, the importance of SERT in psychiatric disease is supported by studies showing major antidepressants, such as fluoxetine (Prozac), sertraline (Zoloft), or paroxetine (Paxil), exert their effects by inhibiting SERT and thereby enhancing the action of serotonin. Additionally, molecular studies in mice lacking the SERT gene (referred to as *SLC5A4*) show an important role of SERT in behavioral states.[97]

As indicated earlier, the uptake of serotonin by SERT can be followed by degradation by MAO to form 5-hydroxyindoleacetic acid (5-HIAA). Many investigators have suggested that brain or CSF levels of 5-HIAA can be used as an index of serotonin turnover and utilization.[98] From Figure 4.8, it can be seen that 5-hydroxytryptophol can also be formed by the action of MAO on serotonin in brain, although the major metabolite is 5-HIAA.[90]

Serotonin has been implicated in various psychiatric disorders including depression, anxiety disorders, and depression associated with suicide. Indeed, it is not always easy to determine what changes in 5-HT are important because they may involve opposing alterations in different subnuclei of the raphe (serotonergic neurons).[99] However, it is clear that reducing serotonergic neurotransmission in some areas of brain can precipitate depressive episodes in some patients, whereas restoring a downregulated 5-HT neurotransmission can alleviate depression in some patients.[100]

4.7.2 Serotonin Receptors

In the past 15 years, there has been an explosion of information about the 5-HT receptor. The 5-HT receptor family has become very large, with at least 14 distinct receptor subtypes, all of which have been cloned. These include the 5-HT$_1$ subfamily (including 5-HT$_{1A}$, 5-HT$_{1B}$, 5-HT$_{1D}$, 5-ht$_{1E}$, and 5-ht$_{1F}$), the 5-HT$_2$ subfamily (including 5-HT$_{2A}$, 5-HT$_{2B}$, and 5-HT$_{2C}$), the 5-HT$_3$ subfamily, as well as the individual 5-HT$_4$, 5-ht$_5$, 5-HT$_6$, and 5-HT$_7$ receptors. The lower case designation (e.g., 5-ht) is used for receptors for which no known function has yet been established.[101,102]

The 5-HT$_1$ subfamily is negatively coupled to adenylate cyclase through a G$_i$ protein similar to the alpha-2 adrenergic receptor and, when activated, produces a decrease in the adenylate cyclase activity. The 5-HT$_2$ subfamily, consisting of 5-HT$_{2A, 2B}$, and $_{2C}$, is linked to phospholipase C and the phosphoinositide second messenger system through a G$_q$ protein similar to the alpha-1 adrenergic receptor. 5-HT$_4$, 5-HT$_6$, and 5-HT7 are positively coupled with adenylate cyclase through a G$_s$ protein similar to the beta adrenergic receptors.[101] The intracellular signaling system for the 5-ht$_5$ (5-ht$_{5A}$ and $_5$-ht$_{5B}$) receptors has not been determined. There are no clinically used drugs that act on the 5-HT$_5$, 5-HT$_6$ or 5-HT$_7$ receptors. However, we are likely to see such drugs in the future.

The 5-HT$_3$ family was originally identified in the periphery.[103] These receptors are unique among the monoamine receptors in that, instead of being G-protein-linked receptors, they are ligand-gated ion channels similar to the nicotinic ACh receptor. The 5-HT$_3$ receptor is a nonselective cation channel that allows Na$^+$ and K$^+$ to enter the cell when 5-HT is bound to it. Thus, the 5-HT$_3$ receptor produces excitation when activated. Originally, the 5-HT$_3$ receptor was identified primarily by its affinity for specific agonists and antagonists,[103,104] but it has now been cloned.[105] Indeed, at least two subtypes of 5-HT3 receptors have now been identified (known as 3A and 3B) and there may be others. These subtypes differ in the protein subunit composition, much like the nicotinic ACh receptor or the GABAA receptor.[106] The 5-HT$_3$ receptors are present in the area postrema and autonomic afferent nerves, where they play a role in promoting nausea and vomiting. Indeed, the 5-HT$_3$ antagonists ondansetron (Zofran), granisetron (Kytril), alosetron (Lotronex), and dolasetron (Anzemet) are widely used to treat the nausea and vomiting associated with cancer chemotherapy. Alosetron has been approved for the treatment of diarrhea associated with irritable bowel syndrome. It is likely that, in the future, we will see 5-HT$_3$ antagonists used in the treatment of psychiatric disorders as drugs that are more selective for subtypes of the receptor become available.

4.7.3 Clinically Useful Drugs That Alter Serotonergic Neurotransmission

4.7.3.1 Facilitators of Serotonergic Neurotransmission

4.7.3.1.1 Drugs That Increase the Synthesis and/or Release of 5-HT

Because the rate-limiting enzyme, TPH2, is not saturated with tryptophan, it is possible to increase the synthesis of 5-HT by administering tryptophan. However, a number of factors affect the amount of tryptophan that actually gets into the brain, such as the ratio of tryptophan to other neutral amino acids in the plasma that compete with tryptophan for transport into the brain, and the concentration of free fatty acids in the plasma that compete with tryptophan for binding to plasma proteins.

Tryptophan administration has apparently been used in the treatment of depression, but its effectiveness has been questioned. It is also possible to increase the release of 5-HT from nerve terminals with fenfluramine, a drug that was marketed as an appetite suppressant (anorexiant) to treat obesity. Fenfluramine is no longer on the market in the United States because of toxicities associated with pulmonary hypertension and damaged heart valves. It was one of the ingredients in Fen-Phen used to treat obesity.

4.7.3.1.2 Drugs That Are 5-HT Agonists

The availability of agonists highly selective for specific subtypes of 5-HT receptors is low. Serotonin, itself, does not cross the blood–brain barrier, and many of the other agonists are hallucinogenic. However, there are three partial agonists for $5-HT_{1A}$ receptors (ipsapirone, gepirone, and buspirone) that are being used for the treatment of anxiety. Of these, buspirone (BuSpar) is the only one approved for use in the United States in the treatment of anxiety. Sumatriptan (Imitrex), zolmitriptan (Zomig), naratriptan (Amerge), almotriptan (Axert), eletriptan (Relpax), frovatriptan (Frova®), and rizatriptan (Maxalt®) are agonists for the $5-HT_{1D}$ and $5-HT_{1B}$ receptors, and are used widely for the treatment of migraine headache. The latter are believed to act by increasing cerebral vascular constriction during the vasodilatory phase of a migraine headache.[107,108]

4.7.3.1.3 Drugs That Block the Reuptake or Prevent Enzymatic Degradation of 5-HT

It is clear that the most common way to increase serotonergic neurotransmission, clinically, is to use a reuptake blocker. The ones approved for clinical use include fluoxetine (Prozac), sertraline (Zoloft), paroxetine (Paxil), citalopram (Celexa), escitalopram (Lexapro), fluvoxamine (Luvox), and clomipramine (Anafranil)—the first five of which are used as antidepressants, and the last two (fluvoxamine and clomipramine) are used for obsessive–compulsive disorder. In addition to their use in obsessive–compulsive disorder, the 5-HT reuptake inhibitors can be used to suppress appetite, although they are not approved for this use. MAO, described earlier in Section 4.5, can also be used to enhance serotonergic neurotransmission because they will prevent the degradation of this amine as well.[1] However, the MAO inhibitors are not selective and could result in an increase in the synaptic content of norepinephrine, dopamine, and 5-HT.

4.7.3.2 Inhibitors of Serotonergic Neurotransmission

There are few drugs clinically available for interfering with serotonergic neurotransmission, and these fall into one of two categories: (1) drugs that interfere with storage of 5-HT and (2) drugs that block 5-HT receptors. The drugs that interfere with the storage of 5-HT are the same drugs that do this to norepinephrine and dopamine—namely, reserpine or tetrabenazine. The only one used clinically is reserpine, which is used to treat hypertension.

A side effect of reserpine is depression with suicidal tendency, which apparently results from the depletion of brain norepinephrine and 5-HT.

There is a host of experimental drugs that block 5-HT receptors, but only a few are currently available for clinical use. These include methysergide (Sansert), a nonselective (broad spectrum) 5-HT antagonist that is used to prevent the onset of migraine headaches, and selective 5-HT_3 antagonists ondansetron (Zofran) and granisetron (Kytril), which are used to treat nausea and vomiting along with the other 5-HT3 antagonists described in Section 4.7.2. Given the plethora of 5-HT receptors and the rate at which new ones are being discovered, it is clear that the drug companies have a difficult road ahead; however, it is also clear that a wide variety of new and, it is hoped, selective 5-HT antagonists will be available in the near future.

Serotonin has been implicated in a wide variety of functions including anxiety, sleep states, pain perception, affective states (depression), food intake, thermoregulation, seizures, vomiting, neuroendocrine functions, and blood pressure. New drugs to treat disorders of these functions may well come from selective agents for modifying serotonergic neurotransmission.

4.7.4 Serotonergic Drugs in the TBI Patient

The role of 5-HT in brain injury and the recovery of function after injury is not clear. Studies done in animal models of TBI suggest that 5-HT synthesis increases after TBI and that this is associated with a decrease in local cerebral glucose utilization in the cerebral cortex.[109] Moreover, inhibition of 5-HT synthesis with *p*-chlorophenylalanine was found to reduce cerebral blood flow changes, cerebral edema, and cell injury following TBI in animals.[110] Such findings suggest that 5-HT contributes to the damage after TBI. However, several studies show that drugs that increase the concentration of 5-HT at its receptors in brain enhance recovery of function after TBI. For example, an agonist for the 5-HT_{1A} receptor has been shown to reduce learning deficits in rats following TBI.[111] The antidepressant fluoxetine has also been shown to facilitate cognitive function in rats following TBI.[112] Fluoxetine has also been found to reduce obsessive–compulsive disorder in TBI patients.[113] The antidepressant effects of selective serotonin reuptake inhibitors are also seen in TBI patients, just as they are in the noninjured population. Thus, it would appear that enhancing serotonergic neurotransmission is beneficial in TBI patients. However, more studies are needed before definitive conclusions can be reached regarding the use of serotonergic drugs for TBI patients. There is evidence that 5-HT enhances the expression of brain-derived neurotrophic factor (BDNF) and that BDNF promotes the growth of 5-HT neurons. These two signaling molecules seem to interact to enhance neuronal plasticity and prevent neurodegeneration.[114] Thus, 5-HT may facilitate recovery of brain function after injury via increasing BDNF. There is evidence that this may also play a role in the antidepressant effects of selective serotonin reuptake inhibitors.

4.8 Gamma Aminobutyric Acid

GABA is one of two amino acids (the other being glycine) that function as major inhibitory neurotransmitters in the mammalian brain. GABA is present in essentially all areas of the brain and has been implicated in the mechanism of action of several antiepileptic drugs, as well as in the action of hypnotics (sleeping aids), anesthetics, and antianxiety drugs. The concentration of GABA in the brain is much higher than that of the monoamine neurotransmitters. Studying the neurotransmitter role of GABA and other amino acids has not been easy for researchers because these amino acids also play a metabolic role and are structural components of proteins. Thus, within the neuron, there is both a metabolic and a neurotransmitter pool of GABA. Determining whether one is dealing with the metabolic pool or the neurotransmitter pool of GABA is crucial, but not always easy.

GABAergic neurons are widely distributed throughout the brain and spinal cord. In most areas of the brain, GABAergic neurons are short interneurons (inhibitory interneurons) rather than long projection cells. However, some GABAergic pathways have been mapped and these include the pathway from the striatum (caudate) to the substantia nigra and another from the globus pallidus to the substantia nigra. The Purkinje cells of the cerebellum are also GABAergic and some of these project to the lateral vestibular nucleus in the medulla oblongata.[115]

4.8.1 Synthesis, Storage, Release, and Inactivation of GABA

GABA is synthesized from glutamic acid by the enzyme glutamic acid decarboxylase (L-glutamate decarboxylase, GAD), which serves as a biochemical marker for GABA ergic neurons.[116] The glutamate is formed from glucose via the glycolytic pathway and the Krebs cycle.[116,117] Pyruvate, formed from glucose, enters the Krebs cycle as acetyl CoA and is converted to alpha ketoglutarate, the first component of the "GABA shunt," which leads to the synthesis of GABA (Figure 4.10).[117]

The GABA shunt represents an alternative pathway between two intermediates of the Krebs cycle. In this shunt, alpha ketoglutarate is converted to glutamic acid in a transamination reaction involving GABA-alpha ketoglutarate transaminase. Some authorities have suggested the transamination of alpha ketoglutarate to glutamate may involve the enzyme aspartate amino transferase, which is coupled to the conversion of aspartic acid to oxaloacetic acid.[118,119] The glutamate is then converted to GABA by GAD.

GABA is degraded by GABA-transaminase (GABA-T), which converts it to succinic semialdehyde. During this process, a molecule of GABA can be broken down only if a molecule of precursor is formed (Figure 4.10).[116] The succinic semialdehyde is then converted to succinic acid by the enzyme succinic semialdehyde dehydrogenase, returning the shunt to the Krebs cycle (Figure 4.10).

Released GABA may also enter the glutamine loop. In the latter case, the GABA is taken up by glial cells where it is converted back to glutamate by a reverse transamination involving GABA-T. The glia cannot convert glutamate to GABA because they lack GAD, but they convert the glutamate to glutamine with glutamine synthetase. The newly formed glutamine can be transported out of the glial cells and into the GABAergic nerve endings where it can be converted back to glutamate by glutaminase. This provides another mechanism by which neurons can conserve GABA.[116]

GAD and GABA-T can be manipulated pharmacologically. Both enzymes require pyridoxal phosphate (vitamin B6) as a cofactor, but the subcellular location of the enzymes differs for the two. GAD is a soluble enzyme found in cytoplasm and GABA-T is a mitochondrial enzyme.

It turns out that there are two types of GAD, each of which is formed from a different gene. The two types of GAD are referred to as GAD_{65} and GAD_{67}.[105,120] These forms differ in molecular weight, amino acid sequence, interaction with pyridoxal phosphate, and expression in different parts of the brain. GAD_{65} appears to be localized to nerve terminals to a

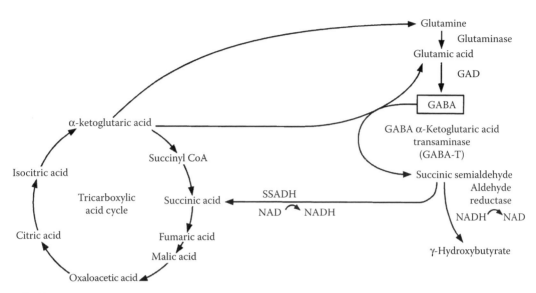

FIGURE 4.10
Synthesis and degradation of GABA via the "GABA shunt" of the tricarboxylic acid (Krebs) cycle. Note that glutamate is a precursor of GABA. SSADH, succinic semialdehyde dehydrogenase. NAD, nicotinamide adenine dinucleotide; NADH, reduced form of NAD.

greater extent than GAD_{67}, and it seems to be involved in the synthesis of GABA that is packaged in synaptic vesicles, whereas GAD_{67} appears to be associated with the synthesis of nonvesicular GABA.[121] The significance of this is not clear.

There is some controversy over whether GAD is saturated with glutamate. Some authorities suggest that it is[116] whereas others[120] suggest that it is not. However, all investigators agree that there is no evidence that GABA synthesis is controlled by the availability of glutamate, which should be the case if GAD is unsaturated with substrate. Of interest is the finding that GAD is the target of antibodies present in people who later develop insulin-dependent diabetes mellitus (type 1 diabetes). In these patients, the antibody that destroys the beta islet cells of the pancreas is directed at GAD.[122,123]

GABA-T is also a pyridoxal phosphate-dependent enzyme that has been purified to homogeneity and was shown to have a molecular weight of about 109,000 daltons. The availability of alpha ketoglutarate may regulate the tissue levels of GABA. Variations in the concentration of alpha ketoglutarate could be responsible for the postmortem changes in GABA levels that are known to occur. For example, when respiration stops, the dependence of the Krebs cycle on respiration results in a marked decline in the availability of alpha ketoglutarate and the consequent reduction in GABA-T activity, which depends on alpha ketoglutarate for transamination. However, GABA synthesis can still occur from glutamate via GAD, which is an anaerobic enzyme.[116]

GABA and other amino acid neurotransmitters are stored in and released from synaptic vesicles via exocytosis. However, both a vesicular and a cytoplasmic pool of GABA exist within the neuron, and release occurs in both a Ca^{2+}-dependent and Ca^{2+}-independent manner.[124] Thus, a nonvesicular release of GABA has been found (see the following text).[99]

As has been demonstrated for the uptake of norepinephrine and 5-HT into synaptic vesicles, GABA may be taken up into synaptic vesicles by a Na^+-independent mechanism that is driven by a proton gradient maintained by Mg^{++}-ATPase.[125] Evidence also suggests that GABA is released from both a vesicular and a cytoplasmic fraction.[126] The cytoplasmic release may involve an exchange transporter between cytoplasmic and extracellular compartments. The latter exchange system seems to be coupled to a Na^+ transporter.[124]

After release from nerve endings, high-affinity uptake by neurons and glial cells is believed to be responsible for terminating the neurotransmitter action of GABA because no rapid enzymatic destruction system similar to that for ACh has been identified. The plasma membrane transporter responsible for GABA uptake requires extracellular sodium and chloride ions. Two sodiums and one chloride ion are cotransported with each molecule of GABA.[105,127,128] The high-affinity uptake transporter of GABA is capable of moving GABA against a concentration gradient and, generally, concentrates the amino acid three to four orders of magnitude higher in the intracellular compartment than in the extracellular compartment.

High-affinity uptake of GABA and excitant amino acid (EAA) into neurons and *glial cells* has also been demonstrated by several laboratories.[129] The operation of the glial transporter is similar to the neuronal transporter and is in the direction of net uptake.

Four distinct plasma membrane GABA transporters have been cloned. These are referred to as *GAT-1, GAT-2, GAT-3,* and *BGT-1.*[130] Such findings suggest a much greater heterogeneity of GABA transporters than was expected, and the significance of this heterogeneity is still unknown. Although it was hoped that these could be localized to either neurons or glia, this is not the case. However, some regions of the brain appear to contain a predominance of one type of transporter over another.[130] Of interest is the finding that certain drugs (e.g., hydroxynipecotic acid) appear to inhibit the glial vs. the neuronal transporter preferentially,[105] although the pharmacology of these transporters is still being determined.

4.8.2 GABA Receptors

Two subtypes of GABA receptor have been described in detail and are referred to as $GABA_A$ and $GABA_B$ receptors. The $GABA_A$ receptor has been more thoroughly investigated and is a ligand-gated ion channel that functions as a channel for the chloride ion.[131,132] This receptor is usually placed in a gene superfamily that also includes the nicotinic ACh receptor, $5\text{-}HT_3$ receptor, and the glycine receptor. This gene superfamily is sometimes called the *cys-loop family,* which distinguishes it from the excitatory amino acid ligand-gated channel family of receptors.[121] $GABA_A$ receptors are stimulated by GABA, muscimol, and isoguvacine and are blocked by the convulsants bicuculline (competitive antagonist) and picrotoxin (noncompetitive antagonist). The $GABA_A$ receptor is a heteropentamer composed of five polypeptide subunits forming the chloride ion channel in the cell membrane.

Molecular cloning has indicated that there are 19 different but closely related polypeptide subunits, any five of which (in combination) can form a $GABA_A$ receptor. These include six different alpha, three beta, three gamma, one delta, one epsilon, one theta, one pi, and three rho subunits. Like the nicotinic ACh receptor, each subunit has four membrane-spanning regions, one of which is believed to contribute to the walls of the ion channel. Scientists often use cells that do not normally express (contain) GABA receptors, like the *Xenopus* oocyte. By adding the genes for the GABA receptor to these cells, they can cause them to express GABA receptors, the function of which can then be studied. By examining recombinant receptors in *Xenopus* oocytes, it is possible to determine the importance of each subunit. It appears that although GABA-regulated chloride conductance, which is inhibited by bicuculline and picrotoxin, can be obtained with the expression of alpha and beta subunits only, full benzodiazepine sensitivity is only obtained if the neurons contain the alpha, beta, and the $gamma_2$ subunits.[133] Thus, recombinant receptors containing α, β, and γ_2 subunits most closely resemble GABA$_A$ receptors found in brain and which specific type α and β subunits are present determines the various affinities for drugs, such as benzodiazepines. The resulting heteropentameric chloride channel must contain at least two alpha and two beta subunits because, as was true of the nicotinic ACh receptor, it takes two molecules of GABA to open the channel, and the GABA binding sites are at the interface of an α and β subunit. The GABA-gated chloride channel also contains binding sites for other ligands (drugs) that allosterically modulate (positively or negatively) the channel. These include a binding site for benzodiazepines, barbiturates, intravenous anesthetics (e.g., propofol), and anesthetic steroids. Benzodiazepines bind to the interface of an α and γ subunit.[121]

The GABA$_B$ receptor is insensitive to bicuculline, 3-aminopropanesulfonic acid, and isoguvacine, but has a weak sensitivity to muscimol and is stereospecifically sensitive to (–)baclofen (Lioresal). The GABA$_B$ receptor, unlike the GABA$_A$ receptor, is a G-protein-coupled receptor linked to a second messenger system like the muscarinic–cholinergic and the adrenergic receptors. Thus, GABA$_B$ receptors are seven transmembrane proteins. However, it has recently been found that there are two subunits of this receptor (R1 and R2) and, to be functional, they seem to form a dimer (two proteins can form a dimer) or heterodimer of R1 and R2 subunits.[121] Most of the early studies suggested that GABA$_B$ receptors were primarily presynaptic receptors involved in inhibiting the release of neurotransmitters; however, it is now clear that they may also mediate postsynaptic inhibition as well.[134,135] Basically, two membrane effects have been attributed to the GABA$_B$ receptors: (1) a decrease in Ca^{2+} conductance (usually a presynaptic effect leading to decreased neurotransmitter release) and (2) an increase in K$^+$ conductance (usually leading to postsynaptic hyperpolarization), as occurs in hippocampal pyramidal cells following the application of baclofen. It has been suggested that the reason for the different effects may be related to the fact that GABA$_B$ receptors are linked to different channels in different locations. Thus, they are probably linked via second messengers to Ca^{2+} channels on presynaptic terminals and to K$^+$ channels at postsynaptic sites.[135] The second messengers to which GABA$_B$ receptors have been suggested to be linked are cAMP (decreased) and phosphatidyl inositols.

The classic agonist for GABA$_B$ receptors is (–)baclofen. A number of studies have been carried out with baclofen to assess the function of GABA$_B$ receptors. However, one difficulty with the use of baclofen is that it crosses the blood–brain barrier rather poorly.[135]

A third subtype of GABA receptor, called the *GABA$_C$* receptor, has recently been identified on the basis of its lack of sensitivity to bicuculline and baclofen, and its sensitivity to *cis*-4-aminocrotonic acid (agonist). These receptors were first discovered in the retina, but have now been found in retina, cerebellum, optic tectum, hippocampus, and spinal cord. GABA$_C$ receptors form a chloride channel from five rho subunits and are, therefore, referred to as *homomeric channels*.[105,136] Although many known drugs act on GABA$_A$ and GABA$_B$ receptors, we have no useful pharmacologic agents for the GABA$_C$ receptor.

4.8.3 Clinically Useful Drugs That Alter GABAergic Neurotransmission

4.8.3.1 Facilitators of GABAergic Neurotransmission

4.8.3.1.1 GABA Agonists

Several experimental drugs are used as agonists for the GABA$_A$ receptor including muscimol, tetrahydroisoxazolopyridinol (THIP), and isoguvacine. In fact, there are no clinically approved drugs that act as GABA$_A$ agonists per se. However, the benzodiazepines are allosteric modulators of the GABA$_A$ receptor that, when bound to their high-affinity site on the GABA$_A$ receptor, enhance the binding of GABA to its binding site and increase the frequency of chloride channel opening. The benzodiazepines are, by far, the most popular clinically used drugs with a mechanism of action that involves the GABA$_A$ receptor. The latter compounds have a wide variety of uses, including the treatment of anxiety, seizures, insomnia, and muscle spasms. The benzodiazepines bind with high affinity to a site on the chloride channel and enhance the inhibitory action of GABA.

Benzodiazepines used to treat anxiety include diazepam (Valium), oxazepam (Serax), alprazolam (Xanax), and lorazepam (Ativan). Those used as antiepileptic drugs include diazepam, clonazepam (Klonopin), and nitrazepam. Benzodiazepines used as hypnotics include flurazepam (Dalmane), temazepam (Restoril), triazolam (Halcion), and quazepam (Doral). There are now several novel benzodiazepine receptor agonists that, chemically, are not classified as benzodiazepines, but that bind to the same binding site as benzodiazepines on the GABA/chloride channel.[137] These novel agents are now widely used as hypnotic drugs (sleeping pills) to treat insomnia and include zolpidem (Ambien), zaleplon (Sonata), and eszopiclone (Lunesta). In addition, all these drugs have muscle-relaxing properties, but diazepam is, probably, most commonly used for this purpose.

There is another major class of drugs that act as positive allosteric modulators of the GABA$_A$ chloride channel. These are the barbiturates such as phenobarbital, pentobarbital, and secobarbital. The barbiturates are widely used as hypnotic agents (sleeping pills) and as adjuncts to anesthetics during surgery. Moreover, some barbiturates find important use as antiepileptic drugs (e.g., phenobarbital and primidone [Mysoline]). Barbiturates bind to a different site on the chloride channel than do the benzodiazepines, and they increase the duration of channel open time, rather than the frequency of opening.

GABA$_B$ receptors also mediate inhibition in the nervous system through the action of G-proteins and second messengers. Baclofen (Lioresal) is a GABA$_B$ receptor agonist that has long been used to treat spasticity in patients with multiple sclerosis or other neurologic diseases.

4.8.3.1.2 Drugs That Block GABA Degradation

There are a whole host of compounds used experimentally to block GABA-T, but only one of these is used clinically and that is gamma vinyl-GABA or vigabatrin, which is used as an antiepileptic drug in Europe but has not been approved for use in the United States.[138,139] Vigabatrin is an irreversible GABA transaminase inhibitor that has been shown to be of value in some drug-refractory epileptic patients. Valproic acid (Depakene) has also been shown to elevate brain GABA levels by inhibiting GABA-T.[140] Valproic acid is used to treat a variety of seizure types including absence and generalized tonic–clonic seizures. Whether the action of valproic acid in epilepsy is primarily the result of an enhancement of the action of GABA is not known, because it has another important effect that is probably responsible for its effect in tonic–clonic seizures—namely, it blocks sodium channels in a frequency- and voltage-dependent fashion.[138]

4.8.3.2 Inhibitors of GABAergic Neurotransmission

4.8.3.2.1 Drugs That Block GABA Receptors

There are several GABA antagonists available for experimental use. However, because all the GABA$_A$ antagonists are convulsants, they currently have no clinical use. The classic GABA$_A$ antagonist is bicuculline, but picrotoxin is also an antagonist. Saclofen and phaclofen are GABA$_B$ antagonists that are being used in experimental animals to help deduce the functional importance of the GABA$_B$ receptor. There are also a group of experimental compounds that bind to the benzodiazepine binding site on the chloride channel and cause a reduction in the effectiveness of GABA. The latter compounds, of which beta-carboline-3-carboxylic acid (and other beta carbolines) is an example, are called *inverse agonists*. Clearly, the GABA antagonists and the inverse benzodiazepine agonists are proconvulsant and have no clinical use in medicine. However, it is possible that such drugs may be developed for use in the TBI patient (described in the next section).

4.8.4 GABAergic Drugs in the TBI Patient

GABA is the major inhibitory neurotransmitter in brain and, therefore, changes in GABAergic neurotransmission can have major consequences. In general, anything that reduces GABA neurotransmission can cause seizures and would be detrimental to the patient. Indeed, loss of GABAergic neurons following TBI may be responsible for post-traumatic epilepsy. However, immediately following TBI in animals, it appears that GABA release is increased.[141]

The increase in GABA release may represent a compensatory attempt to reduce seizures in the injured region. However, other studies have found a decrease in benzodiazepine receptor binding that may also reflect a reduction in GABA receptor function because the benzodiazepine binding site is on the same chloride channel as the GABA binding site (see Section 4.8.2).[142]

Drugs that facilitate GABAergic neurotransmission are widely used in TBI patients. For example, $GABA_B$ agonists, such as baclofen, are used to treat spasticity, whereas benzodiazepines, such as clonazepam and diazepam, are used to suppress seizures and anxiety. In general, however, drugs that facilitate neurotransmission at $GABA_A$ receptors (e.g., benzodiazepines, barbiturates, and some antiepileptics) may impair memory and cognition, and could ultimately retard recovery of intellectual function in TBI patients. Thus, it is not surprising to see that an inverse benzodiazepine agonist (MDL 26479, suritozole) that lacks proconvulsant or anxiogenic effects has been shown to reduce cognitive deficits in rats following TBI.[143]

4.9 Glycine

Glycine has the simplest chemical structure of any amino acid and it is not an essential component of the diet. It is believed to function as a neurotransmitter in spinal cord interneurons (e.g., Renshaw cell, which mediates recurrent inhibition) and in the brainstem.[1] Like GABAergic synapses, all of the glycinergic synapses appear to be inhibitory. The inhibition also seems to be mediated through a ligand-gated chloride channel that, as indicated earlier, places these receptors in a common family with the nicotinic ACh, $GABA_A$, and $5\text{-}HT_3$.

The anatomic distribution of glycinergic neurons has not been extensively mapped. However, the concentrations of glycine found in the spinal cord (dorsal and ventral horn), medulla, and pons are higher than in other CNS regions. Neuronal pathways suggested to be glycinergic include spinal interneurons, a corticohypothalamic pathway, reticulospinal projections from the raphe and reticular formation, brainstem afferents to the substantia nigra, cerebellar Golgi cells, and retinal amacrine cells.[115,144]

4.9.1 Synthesis, Storage, Release, and Inactivation of Glycine

Glycine is synthesized from glucose via the glycolytic pathway to produce 3-phospho-glycerate and 3-phosphoserine, which forms serine. Serine (the immediate precursor of glycine) is converted to glycine by the enzyme serine hydroxymethyltransferase, which is found in the mitochondria. Radioactive tracer studies show that most of the glycine in brain is made from serine.[118] Serine hydroxymethyltransferase requires tetrahydrofolate, pyridoxal phosphate, and manganese ion for activity.[116]

Glycine appears to be abundant in the CNS and it is not clear what factors, if any, are rate limiting in the overall synthesis. Moreover, it is not clear whether neurons utilizing glycine as a neurotransmitter must synthesize it *de novo* or whether they accumulate existing glycine.[1] Serine hydroxymethyltransferase is inhibited by pyridoxal phosphate inhibitors, which also interfere with GABA synthesis and degradation. Enzymatic degradation of glycine can occur via a glycine cleavage system, which is also located in the mitochondria, mainly of astrocytes.[121] Genetic mutations in the proteins of the glycine cleavage system can cause metabolic disorders known as *nonketotic hyperglycinemias*.[145]

Glycine is packaged into vesicles from which it is released. The evidence suggests that glycine uptake into vesicles (like that of GABA and glutamate) is driven by an electro-chemical proton gradient generated by an ATP-dependent proton pump (ATPase) located in the synaptic vesicle membrane. Kish et al.[146] have found that the glycine vesicle transporter has a different substrate specificity from that of the GABA uptake system and a different regional distribution in the brain, suggesting they are in separate neurons. The likelihood that there is both vesicular and cytoplasmic release of glycine, as there appears to be for GABA (see Section 4.8.1), remains very high.

After its release into the synaptic cleft, glycine is primarily inactivated by reuptake into the terminal of the releasing neuron or by uptake into glial cells. Glycine reuptake is carried out by a glycine transporter in the membrane. The Na^+ and Cl^- electrochemical gradients assist in the movement of glycine against its concentration gradient.[145] Two glycine membrane transporters have been identified by molecular cloning: GLYT-1 and GLYT-2. It appears that GLYT-1 is found in both neurons and glial cells, whereas GLYT-2 is localized to neurons. Both transporters are expressed in the hindbrain, whereas GLYT-1 can also be found in forebrain areas even though there are few, if any, glycinergic terminals. Because glycine also functions as a coagonist with glutamate at NMDA receptors (described in the following section and in Section 4.10), there is speculation that the GLYT-1 transporter might regulate glutamate receptor function in forebrain areas.[145] Selective inhibitors of the glycine transporter are not yet available, but could become useful drugs in the future. It has been suggested that GLYT-1 is the glial transporter, whereas GLYT-2 is the neuronal transporter, but this remains somewhat controversial.[1]

4.9.2 Glycine Receptors

As indicated earlier, the glycine receptor is a member of a superfamily of ligand-gated ion channels in which the ligand binding site and the ion channel are in the same molecule. In this regard, the glycine receptor, like that of the nicotinic ACh and $GABA_A$ receptors, has been classified as an ionotropic receptor.[115] The glycine receptor, which consists of five subunits forming a chloride channel (i.e., is a pentamer), has been cloned.[147] Two polypeptide subunits (α and β) have been shown to form a quasisymmetric pentameric chloride ion channel.[121]

Like the nicotinic ACh and GABA receptors, the subunits of the glycine receptor have four hydrophobic membrane-spanning regions (M1–M4). Three alpha and two beta subunits are often responsible for forming the ion channel.[148]

The glycine receptor is associated with a 93-kD protein, called *gephyrin*, which associates with the intracellular domain of the beta subunit. Gephyrin is believed to function as an anchoring protein that connects the membrane receptor protein with the protein tubulin in the cytoplasm.

Strychnine is the classic glycine antagonist, and radioactive strychnine was originally used to map the distribution of glycine receptors in the CNS. The strychnine binding site is on the 48-kDa subunit, which is where glycine also binds.[148]

Glycine also has an action at a strychnine-insensitive receptor that has been linked to the NMDA excitatory amino acid receptor.[116] This is a high-affinity site that appears to increase the action of glutamate at its NMDA receptor.[149] This strychnine-insensitive glycine binding site has a widespread distribution in brain, which corresponds to the distribution of the NMDA receptors. Thus, glycine, in submicromolar concentrations, appears to enhance the action of EAA neurotransmitter glutamate at the NMDA receptor (described later) by functioning as a coagonist.[149] In this regard, it appears to be analogous to the interaction between the GABA receptor and the benzodiazepine binding site. The strychnine-insensitive glycine binding site (NMDA receptor) also appears to have an endogenous antagonist. The tryptophan metabolite, kynurenic acid, is an antagonist of the glycine binding site on the NMDA receptor. However, 7-cholorkynurenic acid is a more selective and more potent antagonist and is now being widely used to study this glycine receptor.[149]

4.9.3 Clinically Useful Drugs That Alter Glycinergic Neurotransmission

Currently, there are no clinically available drugs with a mechanism of action that is mediated through glycinergic neurotransmission. However, there is an experimental drug called *milacemide* that is believed to increase glycine levels in the brain and is being tested as an anticonvulsant agent in experimental animals. Thus, we may have drugs available to enhance glycinergic neurotransmission in the future.

As far as antagonists are concerned, strychnine, which is a convulsant drug, was once used to treat a variety of disorders, as well as being a potent poison. This agent no longer finds any medical use. As indicated earlier, glycine appears also to bind to a site on the NMDA receptor (the so-called *strychnine-insensitive receptor*) to enhance the excitatory effects of glutamate or aspartate. Thus, at this site, glycine is proconvulsant. Currently, there is considerable interest among drug companies to explore the use of strychnine-insensitive glycine antagonists (e.g., 7-chlorokynurenic acid) as potential antiepileptic drugs and it is conceivable that we will see such agents available in the future. The ability of glycine to enhance the excitatory effects of glutamate may stem from its ability to block NMDA receptor desensitization.[1]

4.9.4 Glycinergic Drugs in the TBI Patient

As indicated earlier, there are no drugs currently available that modulate glycine neurotransmission. However, the drug milacemide, which increases glycine levels in brain, may eventually be useful as an anticonvulsant. The antagonist at the strychnine-insensitive glycine receptor (7-chlorokynurenic acid) may also prove to be useful in the future. There is currently no information on whether glycinergic drugs would be useful in the TBI patient.

4.10 L-Glutamic Acid

The major excitatory neurotransmitter in the CNS is glutamic acid or glutamate. Aspartate is also plentiful and may function as an amino acid neurotransmitter, but glutamate has been more widely studied and is considered to be the most important excitatory transmitter. Glutamate and aspartate are sometimes referred to as the *excitant amino acids*. Glutamate is found in higher concentrations than any other free amino acid in the CNS, being three or four times higher than aspartate and six times higher than GABA.[150] The role of glutamate as an excitatory neurotransmitter continues to be the subject of intense investigation, in part because of glutamate's abundance and importance in so many neural pathways, and in part because of studies implicating it in such pathologic conditions as epilepsy, postanoxic cell loss, and neurotoxicity. It has been suggested that 80% to 90% of the of the synapses in the mammalian brain use glutamate as a neurotransmitter.[151,152] It has also been estimated that the repolarization of membranes depolarized by glutamate uses about 80% of the brain's energy expenditure.[152]

So, glutamatergic neurons are found throughout the CNS. There are, however, some specific pathways that have been mapped using lesion and biochemical analyses. These include the well-known corticostriate pathway from the cerebral cortex to the striatum, as well as many other corticofugal pathways.[115] In addition, the perforant pathway, from the entorhinal cortex to the dentate gyrus of the hippocampus, contains a heavy glutamatergic component, as do the Schaffer collaterals from CA3 to CA1 of hippocampus.[115] The dorsal horn of the spinal cord has a high concentration of glutamate, which disappears after cutting the primary sensory afferents, indicating that glutamate is an important neurotransmitter of the primary afferents.

4.10.1 Synthesis, Storage, Release, and Inactivation of Glutamate

Glutamate is a nonessential amino acid that does not cross the blood–brain barrier. Therefore, it must be synthesized in the brain.[115] However, unlike most other neurotransmitters, the synthesis of glutamate is far from straightforward. This problem arises, in part, because glutamate plays many roles in the brain and is available from many sources. For example, in addition to its neurotransmitter role, it is an important component of protein and peptide (e.g., glutathione) synthesis.[153] It also functions as an amino group acceptor to detoxify ammonia in the brain, and it is the immediate precursor of GABA for GABA synthesis. Glutamate can be synthesized from several sources, but it is not always clear which one contributes most to the neurotransmitter pool.[1]

Some investigators have suggested that the main pathways contributing to the transmitter pool of glutamate are from glucose via the Krebs cycle intermediates or from glutamine by the enzyme glutaminase (in the mitochondria). Although both glucose and glutamine are readily converted to glutamate, the pool derived from glutamine is preferentially released,[118] suggesting that this may be more important. However, *in vivo* studies using ^{14}C–glucose and ^{14}C–glutamine showed that released glutamate was derived equally from glucose and glutamine.[154]

The two main routes of synthesis are shown in Figure 4.11. Glial cells also play a role in the synthesis of glutamate.[155] The latter cells actively accumulate glutamate by a sodium-dependent process after its release and convert the glutamate to glutamine by the enzyme glutamine synthetase. The glutamine can be transported out of glial

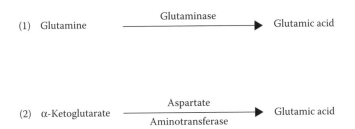

FIGURE 4.11
Two pathways that can synthesize glutamic acid in the brain. The glutamine and α-ketoglutarate pathways are primarily responsible for synthesizing glutamate in nerve terminals.

cells and into glutamatergic terminals, where it is converted back to glutamate by glutaminase. This appears to be one of the mechanisms by which the neurotransmitter is recycled.

After glutamate is synthesized in the neuron, it is transported into the synaptic vesicles via a transporter. The vesicular glutamate transporter protein is apparently the same transporter that moves inorganic phosphate ions across the cell membrane, but the one found in synaptic vesicles of glutamatergic neurons has been called *VGLUT1*.[156] Three VGLUTs have now been cloned.[152] Glutamate is released from neurons in a calcium-dependent manner by exocytosis.[145]

High-affinity uptake across the cell membrane is responsible for terminating the synaptic actions of glutamate and is a sodium-dependent, high-affinity transporter that has been studied in synaptosomes and brain slices. It does not distinguish between L-glutamate, L-aspartate, and D-aspartate.[153,157,158] This transporter has an uneven brain regional distribution consistent with a role in neurotransmission. However, glial cells also possess a high-affinity uptake for glutamate and aspartate, which is believed to play an important role in terminating the action of the EAA neurotransmitters following their release from nerve endings, as was discussed earlier for GABA. Indeed, it has been shown that some glial cells possess receptors for glutamate that, when activated, lead to a transient increase in intracellular calcium (i.e., a Ca^{2+} wave) that may pass from one glial cell to another and function as a form of intercellular communication.[159] Molecular cloning studies have revealed at least four different high-affinity Na^+-dependent glutamate transporters, three of which are found in rat brain.[145] These are referred to as *GLAST* (glutamate–aspartate transporter), *GLT-1* (glutamate transporter 1), and *EAAC1* (excitatory amino acid carrier 1). GLAST is expressed only in astrocytes, whereas GLT-1 is expressed in neurons and glial cells and EAAC1 is expressed in neurons. These transporters are believed to be responsible for the majority of the glutamate inactivation in the CNS.[145] The human homolog of these rat transporters are designated as *excitatory amino acid transporters* (EAATs) and are referred to as *EAAT-1, EAAT-2* and *EAAT-3*.[1,152]

4.10.2 Excitatory Amino Acid Neurotransmitter Receptors

The EAA receptors (i.e., receptors for glutamate and aspartate) have been actively investigated during the past 20 years and are still among the most vigorously targeted areas of research by drug companies seeking new compounds for epilepsy, stroke, psychiatric disorders, and degenerative brain disease (e.g., Alzheimer's disease) and memory loss.

As with other neurotransmitter receptors, the EAA receptors are either ligand-gated channels (ionotropic receptors) or G-protein-coupled receptors (metabotropic receptors).

The ionotropic glutamate receptors are ion channels for sodium, potassium, and calcium similar to the nicotinic ACh, GABA, and glycine receptors. These channels are opened by glutamate and various synthetic chemicals with a similar structure. Three subtypes of ionotropic glutamate receptors have been identified, originally based on the chemicals that activate them: (1) N-methyl-D-aspartate, or NMDA, receptor; (2) α-amino-3-hydroxy-5-methyl-4-isoxazole propionic acid, or AMPA, receptor; and (3) kainate receptor. Separate families of genes have been identified for each of these ionotropic receptor subtypes.[145] In the past, these receptors were separated into NMDA and non-NMDA because of the antagonists that blocked either the NMDA or non-NMDA (AMPA, kainate) receptors. A variety of protein subunits that comprise the EAA receptors have been identified through molecular cloning. The subunits for the NMDA receptor are referred to as *NR1, NR2A, NR2B, NR2C,* and *NR2D,* whereas those for the AMPA receptor are designated as *GluR1* through *GluR4.* The protein subunits that form the kainate receptor include *GluR5* through *GluR7* and *KA1* and *KA2.*[145]

Of the ligand-gated EAA receptor channels, the NMDA receptor is unique in that it is voltage dependent (as well as ligand dependent), requiring some depolarization of the membrane to remove a Mg^{++} block within the ion channel.[150] The NMDA receptor also has several functional subcomponents with discrete binding domains, which make it similar to the $GABA_A$–benzodiazepine receptor complex.[151] In this regard, glycine has a binding site on the NMDA receptor and has been shown to facilitate the excitatory action of NMDA receptor agonists.[144,151,160] The latter has often been referred to as a *strychnine-insensitive* glycine binding site (see Section 4.9.2). Thus, glycine appears to be a coagonist at the NMDA receptor and there are now some selective antagonists for this glycine site (e.g., 7-chlorokynurinate). The NMDA receptor is also unique in that it conducts calcium, as well as sodium, into the cell.

The agonist binding site on the NMDA receptor has several selective competitive antagonists (e.g., 2-amino-5-phosphonovalerate, or AP5; 2-amino-7-heptanoate, or AP7; and 2-carboxypiperazin propyl-1-phosphonic acid, or CPP). In addition, some noncompetitive antagonists of the NMDA receptor have been discovered. These apparently bind to a site within the ion channel to inhibit neurotransmission. The latter compounds include such drugs as phencyclidine (PCP), ketamine (Ketalar), and MK-801 (dizocilpine).[145,151] The EAA receptors (especially the NMDA receptor) are believed to be important in learning and memory (see Chapter 13), which is believed to be mediated through their role in long-term potentiation (LTP).[150] Indeed, the NMDA receptor may be the primary receptor responsible for LTP. The distribution of the NMDA and non-NMDA glutamate (AMPA and kainate) receptors has been extensively mapped in the rat brain using radioactive ligands and autoradiography.[151]

However, excessive amounts of EAAs in the brain are believed to be responsible for excitotoxicity (leading to neuronal death) and seizures mediated through the ionotropic EAA receptors. The latter effect has led to the interest in EAA antagonists in neuropathologic states such as those following stroke.[151] EAAs have also been shown to play a role in post-TBI,[161] and the neuropathology may be the result of the excitotoxic effects of EAAs released after injury.

AMPA receptors can be blocked selectively by the quinoxaline diones such as 6-nitro-7-sulphamobenzo-quinoxaline 2,3-dione (or NBQX). There are no selective antagonists at the kainate receptor except, perhaps, the experimental drug LY294486.

Eight different metabotropic glutamate receptors have now been cloned, which are designated as mGluR1 through mGluR8. Like other G-protein-coupled receptors, these have seven membrane-spanning regions, but are larger (i.e., contain more amino acids) than most other G-protein-coupled receptors. The mGluRs are classified into three groups based on amino acid sequence homology, signal transduction mechanisms, and pharmacology: Group I includes mGluR1 and mGluR5, group II includes mGluR2 and mGluR3, and group III includes mGluR4, mGluR6, mGluR7, and mGluR8.[162] Several of the mGluRs are located on presynaptic nerve terminals and seem to decrease neurotransmitter release. Depending on which transmitter is released, an agonist for the mGluR can produce either excitation or inhibition.[145] Currently, there are no clinically approved drugs that act on the mGluRs, but selective antagonists for group I, group II, and group III have been identified and it is likely that some of these drugs will be available for clinical use in the future. Group I mGluRs are linked to a G_q protein, leading to activation of the phosphatidylinositol pathway (described earlier), whereas groups II and III appear to signal through the Gi/Go proteins, leading to a decrease in cAMP.[162]

4.10.3 Clinically Useful Drugs That Alter Excitant Amino Acid Neurotransmission

4.10.3.1 Drugs That Enhance the Action of Glutamate

Basically, there are no clinically useful drugs that are known to enhance the action of excitant amino acids. Indeed, those that are available for experimental studies in animals (e.g., glutamate, kainate, ibotenic acid, and so forth) are all convulsants, which also cause excitotoxic lesions of neuronal cell bodies. Cycloserine and drugs developed for the treatment of tuberculosis are weak partial agonists at the NMDA receptor, and there is some evidence that these drugs have antipsychotic effects that can be used to treat schizophrenia. Whether agents that selectively enhance LTP in the hippocampus can be developed without the dangers of killing neurons remains to be determined.

4.10.3.2 Drugs That Inhibit the Action of Glutamate

Several glutamate receptor antagonists are available for experimental work in animals and some of these have been described earlier. However, currently there is only one available for clinical use (memantine, or Namenda) that is touted as being an NMDA receptor antagonist, although there are other drugs on the market that have some minor glutamate receptor antagonistic action (e.g., felbamate and amantadine) along with other effects. Glutamate receptor antagonists are of interest for treating such disorders as epilepsy, postischemic brain syndrome, and post-TBI. Moreover, such drugs are believed to have some potential in various neurodegenerative diseases such as Huntington's chorea, Alzheimer's disease, Fredrick's ataxia, and stroke. Indeed, memantine, an NMDA receptor antagonist, is used to treat Alzheimer's disease. Thus, the search for new glutamate receptor blockers continues to be active research. One disappointing aspect of this work has been the psychoticlike side effects that have accompanied the testing of some NMDA antagonists in humans.

It is of interest to note that the widely used drug dextromethorphan (marketed as a cough suppressant) has also been shown to antagonize experimental seizures in animals and has been found to have some NMDA antagonist properties.[163–165] Because of all the modulatory sites on the NMDA receptor, several drugs are known to have some antagonist effects on this receptor via a modulatory site. For example, phencyclidine (PCP, angel dust) and ketamine act as noncompetitive antagonists of the NMDA receptor and have psychotomimetic effects at low doses and function as dissociative anesthetics at higher doses. Although both are still used in veterinary medicine, only ketamine is currently used in humans, where it is mainly used as a pediatric anesthetic. Both are considered drugs of abuse in humans.[145]

4.10.4 Glutamatergic Drugs in the TBI Patient

Glutamate and other excitatory amino acids have long been known to produce excitotoxic damage to neurons and glial cells, and are believed to play a role in producing brain damage in the hours immediately following TBI.[166,167] Indeed, it has been suggested that the EAAs contribute to CNS damage in a variety of neurologic disorders such as epilepsy, stroke, and other neurodegenerative diseases.[168] Moreover, animal and human studies using microdialysis have shown the extracellular levels of glutamate are increased immediately following TBI.[168] Therefore, treatment with glutamate antagonists during the early hours following TBI should limit the damage and facilitate recovery.

Most of the evidence suggests that the NMDA subtype of glutamate receptor is responsible for the neuronal damage because of the increase in intracellular calcium that follows the opening of this channel. Calcium, in high concentrations, can damage and kill cells.[14] Thus, administration of NMDA antagonists immediately following injury has been shown to improve recovery in rats. The hallucinogen PCP, an NMDA antagonist, was found to attenuate long-term neurobehavioral deficits in rats receiving TBI.[168] Clearly, more studies are needed in this area.

Because glutamate is involved in normal cognitive processing and in learning and memory, and because it appears that glutamate release is decreased chronically after the initial increase, it seems reasonable that NMDA agonists might improve cognitive function in the chronic phase following TBI. Because too much glutamate receptor activation can lead to seizures and neuron cell death, moderate or controlled activation of NMDA receptors would seem to be more useful. In this regard, the chronic administration of D-cycloserine, an NMDA partial agonist acting at the glycine site, has been shown to improve cognitive function in rats following TBI.[169] It is of interest that D-cycloserine is an approved drug for the treatment of tuberculosis and, therefore, is available for human use. In addition, aniracetam, an AMPA receptor-positive allosteric modulator has also been shown to enhance cognition in a rat model of TBI.[143] However, aniracetam is not a clinically approved drug in the United States. These animal studies suggest that weeks or months after the injury, it may be beneficial to augment glutamate neurotransmission. Metabotropic glutamate agonists may also turn out to be useful in this regard. Clearly, drugs acting on glutamate receptors can have profound effects in TBI patients and should provide some new therapeutic tools in the future.

4.11 Peptide Neurotransmitters

Until 1960, ACh and the monoamines were the only well-recognized neurotransmitters. Then GABA and the amino acids were identified as neurotransmitters in the 1960s and 1970s. The amine and amino acid neurotransmitters are sometimes referred to as the *classic* neurotransmitters. However, from 1975 to 1990, there was an explosion in the number of candidate neurotransmitters largely resulting from the discovery of various peptides that may function as neurotransmitters. Many of these neuroactive peptides (neuropeptides) were first discovered as hormones and were then found also to be present in neurons within the CNS. Another common finding was that many of the neuroactive peptides were also found in the gut, where they served as GI hormones (e.g., cholecystokinin).

Although one finds that the peptide neurotransmitters are not classified in any consistent manner, a common approach used by authors is based on localization. For example, peptide neurotransmitters have been grouped into the following categories: (1) the gut–brain peptides, (2) the pituitary peptides, and (3) the hypothalamic-releasing hormones.[170]

There are far too many candidate peptide neurotransmitters to cover here. Moreover, there are no clinically useful drugs to affect their action, except in the case of the opioid peptides, which mediate their effects through the receptors on which morphine and other potent narcotic analgesics act. Therefore, we will restrict this discussion to the opioid peptides.

However, substance P is also of interest because it was the first peptide neurotransmitter isolated from horse gut and brain by Von Euler and Gaddam,[171] although it was 40 years later before its structure was determined. Substance P is of interest because, although there are no clinically available drugs to modify its action, it is the neurotransmitter of some primary sensory afferent fibers carrying pain sensation (i.e., C-fibers) and it can be released from such nerve terminals by the active ingredient in chili peppers (i.e., capsaicin).[172,173] Moreover, neurons containing opioid peptides appear to synapse on the terminals of substance P containing neurons in the dorsal horn of the spinal cord. Substance P is one of a group of interesting peptides known as *tachykinins* for which three receptors have been cloned and new antagonists are being developed.[1] There has been interest in tachykinin antagonists for the treatment of depression and anxiety, and several of these drugs have undergone clinical trials for depression.[1,174] The value of tachykinin antagonists as antidepressants has been unimpressive, but they do appear to have considerable value as antiemetics in cancer chemotherapy.[174]

4.11.1 Opioid Peptides as Neurotransmitters

The first discovered opioid peptides were the pentapeptides (containing five amino acids), leucine–enkephalin and methionine–enkephalin, which were isolated by Hughes et al.[175] Although there may be other families of opioid peptides, currently interest is focused on three separate families of opioid peptides, each derived from a separate gene family.[176] These include (1) the enkephalins (pentapeptides derived from a proenkephalin precursor), (2) the endorphins (e.g., β-endorphin, a 31 amino acid containing peptide derived from proopiomelanocortin, or POMC), and (3) the dynorphins (8–13 amino acid containing peptides derived from a prodynorphin precursor). Three other endogenous opioid peptides have more recently been discovered and are known as orphanin FQ, endomorphin-1, and endomorphin-2. Much current research is focused on whether the endormorphins are selective mu agonists, but because there is relatively little known about the edomorphin peptides, we will focus our discussion on the enkephalins, endorphins, and dynorphins. Orphanin FQ, also known as nociceptin, has effects opposite those of morphine and is referred to as pronociceptive (see Section 4.11.3).

Extensive maps of the enkephalin-, endorphin-, and dynorphin-containing neurons in the rat brain have been obtained using immunocytochemistry, but these will be only briefly described here (see Khachaturian et al.[177] for more detail). In general, the enkephalinergic neurons are short interneurons widely distributed throughout the neuraxis. A high density of enkephalinergic neurons is found in the basal ganglia, cerebral cortex, amygdala, hippocampus, and in such brainstem areas as the periaqueductal gray, interpeduncular nucleus, parabrachial nucleus (concerned with respiration), and the nucleus tractus solitarius, as well as in the dorsal horn of the spinal cord.

The dynorphinlike immunoreactivity follows the distribution of the enkephalinergic neurons fairly closely and also appears to be found mostly in short local neurons (interneurons) rather than in long projection fibers. Thus, the enkephalin and dynorphin systems appear to be anatomically contiguous. The endorphin-containing neurons are, however, different in that they tend to be long projection neurons that arise from the arcuate nucleus of the hypothalamus. Another area containing a high density of endorphin-containing (POMC) cell bodies is the pituitary gland from which β-endorphin is presumably released into the blood. However, the precursor of β-endorphin, POMC, is also the precursor for adrenocorticotrophic hormone and melanocyte stimulating hormone (α-MSH). Thus, depending on where in its structure POMC is cleaved by enzymes, one gets different biologically active peptides. It is little wonder, then, that the endorphins are intimately related to the endocrine system and are apparently released during stress.

4.11.2 Synthesis, Storage, Release, and Inactivation of Opioid Peptides

The synthesis of any peptide involves transcription of the information in the genetic code of DNA (the gene) into messenger RNA (mRNA), and the translation of the message in mRNA into the appropriate sequence of amino acids in the peptide chain to form a functionally important peptide or protein. A detailed description of protein synthesis is clearly beyond the scope of this chapter (refer to a basic textbook of biochemistry for more detail).

As indicated earlier, there are three families of opioid peptides derived from different genes that lead to the synthesis of precursor proteins from which the neuroactive peptide is cleaved by the action of enzymes. Thus, proenkephalin, prodynorphin, or POMC can be synthesized in the cell body of a cell that expresses these genes.

After the peptide precursors are formed, they are usually sent to the Golgi apparatus where they are packaged into membrane-bound vesicles and then transported to the nerve terminals by axoplasmic transport. At the axon terminal, the opioid peptides are stored in vesicles from which they are released by exocytosis.[115] However, currently, the mechanisms of peptide packaging, storage, and release are poorly understood. It is important to note that peptides cannot be synthesized at nerve terminals and must be made in the cell body and transported to the terminal for release, making them much more expensive in terms of energy expenditure.

After the opioid or any other neuroactive peptide is released from a neuron, it is apparently degraded by peptidases (enzymes) and cannot be recaptured by reuptake. Thus, utilization of peptides is less efficient than that for the classic neurotransmitters and is, again, a more energy-expensive process. Moreover, after they are used, it will take a significantly longer time to replace them at the nerve terminal than it does for the classic transmitters.[115,178]

Another interesting aspect of peptide neurotransmitters is that they appear to be costored in neurons with other neurotransmitters, either other peptides or the classic neurotransmitters. Examples of a classic transmitter coexisting in a neuron with a peptide include (1) serotonin and substance P, (2) dopamine and cholecystokinin, and (3) ACh together with vasoactive intestinal polypeptide. In some neurons, the classic transmitter and the peptide may even be stored within the same vesicle (e.g., 5-HT and substance P).[178] However, in most cases, they are stored in separate vesicles that are referred to as *large, dense core vesicles*, which may be three times larger in diameter than the vesicles in which classic neurotransmitters are stored, and they appear dark (dense core) in electron micrographs of synapses.[174,179] Interestingly, the vesicles in which neuropeptides are stored are not found at the "active zone" of the nerve terminal where classic neurotransmitters dock and fuse during exocytoses. Instead, they are found in a separate pool that typically is remote from the active zone and seems to require a lower concentration of calcium for release. These large, dense core vesicles seem to undergo exocytosis only after prolonged stimulation of the nerve.[174,179]

4.11.3 Opioid Receptors

Opioid receptors were known to exist long before the discovery of the opioid peptides. Indeed, it was the discovery of opioid receptors using radioactive ligands that led to the search for the endogenous peptides by Hughes and Kosterlitz.[170] The distribution of opioid receptors was mapped before the distribution of the peptides. The opioid receptors are now divided into three main subtypes: (1) mu (μ) receptors, (2) delta (δ) receptors, and (3) kappa (κ) receptors, although some authors include the sigma (σ) receptors as a fourth subtype.

Mu receptors appear to be the primary receptors involved in mediating analgesia and, therefore, have a high affinity for morphine and related drugs. The endorphins have a higher affinity for mu receptors than for any other opiate receptor subtypes. Indeed, the rank-order potency of agonists for opioids binding to the mu receptor is β-endorphin > morphine > met-enkephalin > leu-enkephalin > dynorphin.

The mu receptor is believed to be a 65-kDa protein with a widespread distribution in the CNS.[180] The density of mu receptors is high in striatum, amygdala, cortex, periaqueductal gray regions of midbrain, and thalamus.[181] Mu receptors are also found in the periphery. The mu receptor is a G-protein-linked receptor that is negatively coupled with cAMP (i.e., a G_i protein) and is involved in mediating hyperpolarization by opening K^+ channels.[181]

The use of mu agonists can alleviate the opiate withdrawal syndrome. Beta-endorphin is probably the naturally occurring ligand for the mu receptor, although morphine and its analogues appears to mediate most of their effects through the mu receptor. Naloxone (Narcan) is a potent antagonist of the mu opioid receptor.

The delta receptor binds leu-enkephalin with a greater affinity than met-enkephalin, β-endorphin, or morphine. Thus, the enkephalins are believed to be the natural ligands for the delta receptor.[154] The distribution of delta receptors corresponds closely to the distribution of enkephalin neurons and, like the mu receptors, are linked to adenylate cyclase in a negative fashion via a Gi protein.[180] Naloxone is a less potent antagonist at delta receptors than it is at mu receptors, so that higher concentrations of naloxone are required.

The kappa opioid receptors bind ketocyclazocine with high affinity. The latter compound, along with pentazocine, bremazocine, and butorphanol, is a kappa receptor agonist. The density of kappa receptors is highest in the spinal cord and brainstem, and the dynorphins are believed to be the naturally occurring agonists for these receptors. Naloxone can act as an antagonist at kappa receptors, but it is less potent than at mu receptors. Kappa agonists cannot alleviate the symptoms of opioid withdrawal. However, stimulation of kappa receptors can alleviate pain, especially viscerally mediated chemical pain.[180] Dynorphin is believed to be the natural agonist for the kappa receptor, and dynorphin levels are increased immediately following TBI. Indeed, kappa agonists may increase neurologic deficits when administered following TBI (see Section 4.11.5). A major goal of opioid research has long been to find analgesic drugs with the efficacy of opioids, but that do not produce tolerance, dependence, and addiction. It was believed that gaining an understanding of what causes tolerance would help accomplish this goal. Unfortunately, understanding the mechanism of tolerance to these drugs has been very elusive. Studies showing changes in receptor number following chronic narcotic treatment have not been very revealing, although changes in second messengers (i.e., receptor signaling cascade) have been observed. Recently, much interest in receptor trafficking between an intracellular form and the membrane form have begun to show that the number of receptors in the cell do change, but that they move from the membrane into the cell where agonists do not stimulate. These studies are beginning to identify the mechanisms of receptor desensitization and downregulation, and have already shown differences between mu and delta receptor mechanisms in terms of how phosphorylation plays a role.[181–184]

More recently, a new receptor related to the opioid receptors was cloned. Because it had a high degree of homology (similarity) to other opioid receptors, but was unresponsive to endogenous opioid peptides (enkephalins, endorphins, dynorphins), it was referred to as an orphan receptor. More recently, a novel endogenous peptide for the orphan receptor was isolated and sequenced. This peptide appeared to have antiopioid effects (i.e., cause pain) when bound to the orphan receptor. Thus, it was named *nociceptin/orphanin FQ*. Now, there appears to be a family of these peptides and they all bind to G-protein-coupled receptors (i.e., G_i/G_o).[174,185] The functional significance of the nociceptin/orphanin FQ system is not known, but there is interest in developing antagonists for these receptors because they could be useful in the treatment of pain.

4.11.4 Clinically Useful Drugs That Alter Opioid Neurotransmission

4.11.4.1 *Drugs That Enhance Opioidergic Neurotransmission*

4.11.4.1.1 Opioid Agonists

A comprehensive discussion of the pharmacology of opioid agonists and antagonists has been provided by Gutstein and Akil[186] and is beyond the scope of this chapter. The agonists are the only available drugs for enhancing opioidergic neurotransmission. These are the narcotic analgesics used to treat severe pain, such as that occurring postoperatively. Morphine is the prototypical drug in this class and has been around since 1806. It is a natural constituent of opium powder, but can now be made in the chemistry laboratory. Meperidine (Demerol) is a synthetic analogue of morphine widely used in hospitals for postoperative pain. Both of these are primarily mu agonists, but also have some agonist activity at delta and kappa receptors. Codeine, the *o*-methyl analogue of morphine, has similar properties, but is a weaker agonist. Indeed, codeine is metabolized to morphine in the body. Pentazocine (Talwin) is a kappa agonist and a mu antagonist, and butorphanol (Stadol) has similar properties. Pentazocine was originally marketed as a nonnarcotic analgesic, but this error was eventually corrected. Buprenorphine (Buprenex) is a long-acting partial mu agonist. The latter drugs are sometimes referred to as *mixed agonist–antagonists*.

Opioid analgesics have many side effects, not the least of which is respiratory depression, which can kill the patient in overdose. These drugs are also very useful to suppress the cough reflex and are commonly added to cough mixtures (syrups).

4.11.4.2 *Drugs That Inhibit Opioidergic Neurotransmission*

4.11.4.2.1 Opioid Antagonists

Naloxone (Narcan) is a pure opioid antagonist that is used to treat life-threatening overdoses of opioid analgesics. It functions as an antagonist at mu, delta, and kappa receptors, but must be given by injection. The administration of 0.4 to 0.8 mg intravenously or intramuscularly can reverse the effects of mu opioid agonists in humans and will precipitate a withdrawal syndrome in addicted individuals.[186] Naltrexone (Trexan) is also a pure narcotic antagonist with greater oral efficacy and a longer duration of action, allowing it to be administered orally. Naltrexone is approved for the treatment of alcoholism where it apparently reduces craving.

4.11.5 Opioids in the TBI Patient

An increase in dynorphin has been demonstrated following TBI in an animal model of brain injury,[187] and kappa receptor agonists have been shown to increase neurologic deficits after experimentally induced spinal cord injury in rats. Moreover, kappa antagonists have been found to reverse deficits associated with spinal cord injury.[188] Kappa agonists may, in fact, facilitate neuronal damage via an action through glutamate, because NMDA antagonists were found to reverse the neurotoxicity associated with dynorphin in the spinal cord injury model.[189]

Although activation of kappa receptors appears to enhance neurologic damage, activation of mu and delta opioid receptors may be neuroprotective rather than neurotoxic.[190] Thus, it appears that, immediately following injury, administering a kappa antagonist or a mu agonist could be beneficial in reducing neurologic damage associated with TBI. However, more research is needed to determine the appropriate timing and dose needed to reduce neurologic deficits.

Other uses of opioids in the TBI patient obviously includes their use as analgesics to alleviate pain while recovering from multiple injuries. However, when using opioids as analgesics, it is important for practitioners to be cognizant of possible detrimental effects that can also occur. Knowledge of the specific receptors on which the drugs act and the selection of specific mu or delta agonists may prevent such detrimental effects.

4.12 Summary

The preceding pages provide considerable detail concerning the process of neurotransmission in the nervous system. It is clear that this is a major form of communication between neurons and the principal site of controlling neuronal function. It is also clear that neurotransmission is the principal target for drugs that affect the nervous system. Although it is impossible to provide a concise summary of the broad array of topics covered in this chapter, the editor felt that some type of summary of the clinically relevant drugs showing the neurotransmitters through which they exert their action would be useful for the busy practitioner, and I fully agree. Therefore, an Appendix is provided at the end of this chapter to summarize these relationships and to give the reader a quick mechanism for linking the drugs to the neurotransmitters. It should be noted, however, that, in the interest of space, we have only included those drugs discussed in this chapter. Although they represent some of the more popular ones in use today, they are by no means the only ones available. Practitioners of rehabilitation, as well as other specialties in medicine, must be aware that pharmacology is a constantly changing field, with new drugs being introduced every day. It is hoped that this chapter also provides a foundation that allows you to appreciate and understand the mechanism of action of new (undiscovered) drugs that will be introduced in the future.

Appendix: Summary of Relationship between Therapeutically Used Drugs and Various Neurotransmitters

Drug Name	Brand Name[a]	Neurotransmitter	Receptor	Drug Action
Acebutolol	Sectral	Norepinephrine	Beta-1	Beta-1 receptor blocker
Acetylcholine	Miochol (ophthalmic)	ACh	Nicotinic and muscarinic–cholinergic	Agonist for muscarinic and nicotinic receptors
Albuterol	Proventil	Epinephrine (hormone)	Beta-2	Beta-2 receptor agonist
Almotriptan	Axert	Serotonin	$5\text{-HT}_{1D/1B}$	Serotonin 1D/1B receptor agonist
Alosetron	Lotronex	Serotonin	5-HT_3	Blocks 5-HT_3 receptors
Alpha-methyltyrosine (metyrosine)	Demser	Dopamine; norepinephrine	—	Blocks synthesis of dopamine and norepinephrine
Alprazolam	Xanax	GABA	Benzodiazepine-GABA_A complex	Agonist for benzodiazepine receptor
Amantadine	Symmetrel	Dopamine	—	Increases release and blocks reuptake of dopamine
Amphetamine	Obetrol	Dopamine, norepinephrine	—	Increases release and blocks reuptake of norepinephrine and dopamine
Apomorphine	Apomorphine HCl	Dopamine	D_1 and D_2 dopamine	Agonist for D_1 and D_2 receptors
Atenolol	Tenormin	Norepinephrine	Beta-1	Blocks beta-1 receptors
Atomoxetine	Strattera	Norepinephrine	—	Norepinephrine uptake blocker
Atropine	Atropine Sulfate	ACh	Muscarinic–cholinergic	Blocks muscarinic receptors
Baclofen	Lioresal	GABA	GABA_B	Agonist for GABA_B receptors
Benztropine	Cogentin	ACh	Muscarinic–cholinergic	Blocks muscarinic receptors
Bethanechol	Urecholine	ACh	Cholinergic–muscarinic	Agonist for muscarinic receptor
Botulinum toxin A	Botox	ACh	—	Blocks release of ACh
Bretylium	Bretylium Tosylate	Norepinephrine	—	Blocks release of norepinephrine
Bromocriptine	Parlodel	Dopamine	Dopamine (D_1, D_2, and so on)	Nonselective dopamine receptor agonist
Buprenorphine	Buprenex	β-endorphin, enkephalin	Opioid (mu)	Partial agonist for mu receptor and a kappa antagonist
Bupropion	Wellbutrin, Zyban	Dopamine	—	Blocks reuptake of dopamine
Buspirone	BuSpar	Serotonin (5-HT)	5-HT_{1a}	Partial agonist for 5-HT_{1a} receptor
Butorphanol	Stadol	β-endorphin, enkephalin	Opioid (kappa)	Kappa agonist and mu antagonist

Capsaicin	Zostrix-HP	Substance P	—	Depletes C-fibers (pain fibers) of Substance P, used as topical analgesic
Carbachol	Isopto Carbachol	ACh	Muscarinic–cholinergic, nicotinic–cholinergic	Muscarinic and nicotinic agonist
Chlorpromazine	Thorazine	Dopamine	Dopamine D_2	Blocks dopamine receptors
Cimetidine	Tagamet	Histamine (not covered in this chapter)	H_2, histamine receptors	H_2 blocker
Citalopram	Celexa	Serotonin	—	Blocks serotonin reuptake
Clomipramine	Anafranil	Serotonin	—	Blocks serotonin reuptake
Clonazepam	Klonopin	GABA	Benzodiazepine–$GABA_A$ complex	Facilitates action of GABA
Clonidine	Catapres	Norepinephrine	Alpha-2	Alpha-2 agonist
Clozapine	Clozaril	Dopamine	Dopamine D_4	D_4 antagonist
Cocaine	Cocaine HC1	Norepinephrine, dopamine	—	Blocks reuptake of norepinephrine and dopamine
Codeine	Found in many cough syrups and analgesics containing acetaminophen	Opioid	β-endorphin, enkephalin	Agonist for mu and delta opioid receptors
d-tubocurarine	Tubocurarine chloride	ACh	Nicotinic–cholinergic	Nicotinic receptor blocker
Desipramine	Norpramin	norepinephrine	—	Blocks norepinephrine reuptake
Dextroamphetamine	Dexedrine	Norepinephrine, dopamine	—	Increases release of norepinephrine and dopamine and blocks reuptake
Dextromethorphan	Found in many cough syrups (e.g., Robitussin-DM)	Glutamate	NMDA	Blocks glutamate NMDA receptor
Diazepam	Valium	GABA	Benzodiazepine-$GABA_A$ complex	Agonist for benzodiazepine receptor
Disulfiram	Antabuse	Norepinephrine	—	Blocks synthesis of norepinephrine
Dobutamine	Dobutrex	Norepinephrine	B_1 adrenergic receptor	Agonist for B_1 receptors
Dolasetron	Anzemet	Serotonin	$5-HT_3$	Blocks $5-HT_3$ receptors
Donepezil	Aricept	ACh	—	Blocks enzymatic breakdown of ACh
Edrophonium	Tensilon	ACh	—	Cholinesterase inhibitor, prevents degradation of ACh

(continued)

Drug Name	Brand Name[a]	Neurotransmitter	Receptor	Drug Action
Eletriptan	Relpax	Serotonin	$5\text{-HT}_{1D/1B}$	Agonist for $5\text{-HT}_{1D/1B}$ receptor
Entacapone	Comtan	Norepinephrine, dopamine	—	Blocks enzymatic breakdown of norepinephrine and dopamine by blocking COMT
Escitalopram	Lexapro	Serotonin	—	Blocks serotonin reuptake
Esmolol	Brevibloc	Norepinephrine	B_1	Blocks B_1 receptor
Eszopiclone	Lunesta	GABA	Benzodiazepine–GABA complex	Facilitates the action of GABA
Fenfluramine	Pondimin	Serotonin	—	Increases the release of serotonin
Fluoxetine	Prozac	Serotonin	—	Blocks reuptake of serotonin
Flurazepam	Dalmane	GABA	Benzodiazepine–$GABA_A$ complex	Facilitates the action of GABA
Fluvoxamine	Luvox	Serotonin	—	Blocks serotonin reuptake
Frovatriptan	Frova	Serotonin	$5\text{-HT}_{1D/1B}$	Agonist for $5\text{-HT}_{1D/1B}$ receptor
Galantamine	Razadyne	ACh	—	Blocks enzymatic breakdown of ACh
Gallamine	Flaxedil	ACh	Nicotinic–cholinergic	Blocks nicotinic receptors at neuromuscular junction
Glycopyrrolate	Robinul	ACh	Muscarinic	Blocks muscarinic receptors
Granisetron	Kytril	Serotonin	5-HT_3	Blocks 5-HT_3 receptors
Guanabenz	Wytensin	Norepinephrine	Alpha-2	Alpha-2 agonist
Guanadrel	Hylorel	Norepinephrine	—	Blocks the release of norepinephrine
Guanethidine	Ismelin	Norepinephrine	—	Blocks the release of norepinephrine
Guanfacine	Tenex	norepinephrine	Alpha-2	Alpha-2 agonist
Haloperidol	Haldol	Dopamine	Dopamine D_2	Blocks dopamine receptors
Ipratropium	Atovent	ACh	Muscarinic–cholinergic	Muscarinic blocker
Isocarboxazid	Marplan	Norepinephrine, dopamine, serotonin	—	Inhibits degradative enzyme (MAO)
Isoproterenol	Isuprel	Norepinephrine	B_1 and B_2	Agonist for all beta receptors
Ketamine	Ketalar	Glutamate	NMDA	Noncompetitive blockers of NMDA receptor
L-DOPA and carbidopa	Sinemet	Dopamine	—	Increases synthesis of dopamine
Levodopa	Larodopa	Dopamine	—	Increases synthesis of dopamine

		GABA	Benzodiazepine–GABA$_A$ complex	
Lorazepam	Ativan	GABA	Benzodiazepine–GABA$_A$ complex	Agonist for benzodiazepine receptor
Maprotiline	Ludiomil	Norepinephrine	—	Norepinephrine reuptake inhibitor
Mecamylamine	Inversine	ACh	Nicotinic–cholinergic	Blocks neuronal nicotinic receptors
Memantine	Namenda	Glutamate	NMDA	Blocks NMDA receptors
Meperidine	Demerol	β-endorphin, enkephalin	Opioid (mu)	Agonist for mu opioid receptors
Metaproterenol	Metaprel	Norepinephrine	Beta-2	Selective agonist for beta-2 receptor
Metaraminol	Aramine	Norepinephrine	Alpha-1	Agonist for alpha-1 receptors
Methacholine	Provocholine	ACh	Muscarinic–cholinergic	Agonist for muscarinic receptors
Methamphetamine	Desoxyn	Norepinephrine and dopamine	—	Increases release of norepinephrine and dopamine
Methoxamine	Vasoxyl	Norepinephrine	Alpha-1	Agonist for alpha-1 receptor
Methylphenidate	Ritalin	Dopamine and norepinephrine	—	Increases release of dopamine and norepinephrine
Methysergide	Sansert	Serotonin	Serotonin	Nonselective serotonin receptor blocker
Metoclopramide[b]	Reglan	Dopamine, serotonin	Dopamine D$_2$, 5-HT$_3$	Blocks dopamine D$_2$ and 5-HT$_3$ receptors
Metoprolol	Lopressor	Norepinephrine	Beta-1	Blocks beta-1 receptors
Molindone	Moban	Dopamine	Dopamine D$_2$	Blocks dopamine receptors
Morphine	Morphine Sulfate	β-endorphin	Mu opioid	Agonist for mu receptor
Naloxone	Narcan	β-endorphin, enkephalin	Opioid	Nonselective opioid receptor blocker
Naltrexone	Trexan	β-endorphin, enkephalin	Opioid	Nonselective opioid receptor blocker
Naratriptan	Amerge	Serotonin	5-HT$_{1D/1B}$	Serotonin receptor 1B/1D agonist
Neostigmine	Prostigmin	ACh	—	Blocks degradation of ACh by cholinesterase
Nicotine	Nicoderm (patch), Nicorette (gum)	ACh	Nicotinic–cholinergic	Agonist for nicotinic receptor
Nitrazepam	Mogadon	GABA	Benzodiazepine–GABA$_A$ complex	Agonist for benzodiazepine receptor
Norepinephrine	Levophed	Norepinephrine	Alpha-1, alpha-2, beta-1	Agonist for adrenergic receptors
Nortriptyline	Aventyl	Norepinephrine	—	Blocks reuptake of norepinephrine
Olanzapine	Zyprexa	Dopamine, serotonin	Dopamine D$_{3/4}$, 5-HT$_{2A}$	Blocks dopamine and serotonin receptors
Ondansetron	Zofran	Serotonin	5-HT$_3$	Blocks 5-HT$_3$ receptor

(continued)

Drug Name	Brand Name[a]	Neurotransmitter	Receptor	Drug Action
Oxazepam	Serax	GABA	Benzodiazepine–GABA$_A$ complex	Agonist for benzodiazepine receptor
Pancuronium	Pavulon	ACh	Nicotinic–cholinergic (at neuromuscular junction)	Blocks nicotinic receptor
Paroxetine	Paxil	Serotonin	—	Blocks serotonin reuptake
Pentazocine	Talwin	β-endorphin, enkephalin	Mu opioid, kappa opioid	Mu antagonist, kappa agonist
Pentobarbital	Nembutal	GABA	GABA$_A$	Facilitates action of GABA
Pergolide	Permax	Dopamine	Dopamine D$_1$ and D$_2$	Agonist for D$_1$ and D$_2$ receptors
Perphenazine	Trilafon	Dopamine	Dopamine D$_2$	Blocks dopamine receptors
Phenelzine	Nardil	Norepinephrine, dopamine, serotonin	—	Blocks MAO to prevent degradation of monoamine transmitters
Phenobarbital	Luminal	GABA	GABA$_A$	Facilitates action of GABA$_A$
Phenylephrine	Neo-Synephrine	Norepinephrine	Alpha-1	Alpha-1 agonist
Phenoxybenzamine	Dibenzyline	Norepinephrine	Alpha-1, alpha-2	Irreversibly blocks alpha-1 and alpha-2 receptors
Phentolamine	Regitine	Norepinephrine	Alpha-1, alpha-2	Reversibly blocks alpha-1 and alpha-2 receptors
Physostigmine	Eserine Sulfate	ACh	—	Blocks enzymatic breakdown of ACh
Pilocarpine	Pilocarpine HC1	ACh	Muscarinic–cholinergic	Muscarinic agonist
Pindolol	Visken	Norepinephrine	Beta-1 and beta-2	Blocks beta adrenergic receptors
Pirenzepine	Gastrozepine	ACh	M1 muscarinic	Blocks M1 receptors
Pramipexole	Mirapex	Dopamine	Dopamine D$_1$, D$_2$	Agonist for dopamine receptors
Prazosin	Minipress	Norepinephrine	Alpha-1	Blocks alpha-1 receptor
Primidone	Mysoline	GABA	GABA$_A$	Facilitates action of GABA$_A$
Prochlorperazine	Compazine	Dopamine	Dopamine D$_1$ and D$_2$	Blocks D$_1$ and D$_2$ receptors
Propranolol	Inderal	Norepinephrine	Beta-1 and beta-2	Blocks beta-1 and beta-2 receptors
Protriptyline	Vivactil	Norepinephrine	—	Blocks reuptake of norepinephrine
Pyridostigmine	Mestinon	ACh	—	Blocks enzymatic breakdown of ACh
Quazepam	Doral	GABA	Benzodiazepine–GABA$_A$ complex	Agonist for benzodiazepine receptor
Quetiapine	Seroquel	Dopamine, serotonin	Dopamine D$_{3/4}$, 5-HT$_{2A}$	Blocks dopamine and serotonin receptors
Rasagiline	Azilect	Dopamine	—	Inhibits MAO type B
Reserpine	Serpasil	Norepinephrine, dopamine, serotonin	—	Blocks storage of monoamine transmitter and depletes nerves

Risperidone	Risperdal	Dopamine, serotonin	Dopamine $D_{3/4}$, 5-HT_{2A}	Blocks dopamine and serotonin receptors
Rivastigmine	Exelon	ACh	—	Blocks enzymatic breakdown of ACh
Rizatriptan	Maxalt	Serotonin	5-$HT_{1D/1B}$	Serotonin receptor 1B/1D agonist
Ropinirole	Requip	Dopamine	Dopamine D_1, D_2	Dopamine receptor agonist
Rotigotine	Neupro	Dopamine	Dopamine D_1, D_2, and D_3	Agonist for dopamine receptors
Scopolamine (hyoscine)	Isopto Hyoscine	ACh	Muscarinic–cholinergic	Muscarinic blocker
Secobarbital	Seconal	GABA	$GABA_A$	Facilitates action of $GABA_A$
Selegiline	Eldepryl	Dopamine	—	Inhibits MAO type B, which degrades dopamine
Sertraline	Zoloft	Serotonin	—	Serotonin reuptake inhibitor
Sotalol	Betapace	Norepinephrine	Beta-1 and beta-2	Beta-1 and beta-2 blocker
Succinylcholine	Anectine	ACh	Nicotinic–cholinergic (at neuromuscular junction)	Nicotinic receptor blocker
Sumatriptan	Imitrex	Serotonin	5-HT_{1D}	Agonist for 5-HT_{1D} receptors
Tacrine	Cognex	ACh	Nicotinic and muscarinic–cholinergic	Cholinesterase inhibitor, partial agonist at muscarinic receptors
Temazepam	Restoril	GABA	Benzodiazepine–$GABA_A$ complex	Agonist for benzodiazepine receptor
Terazosin	Hytrin	Norepinephrine	Alpha-1	Alpha-1 blocker
Terbutaline	Brethine	Norepinephrine	Beta-2	Agonist at beta-2 receptor
Thioridazine	Mellaril	Dopamine	Dopamine D_2	Blocks dopamine receptors
Tiagabine	Gabitril	GABA	—	Blocks GABA uptake
Tolcapone	Tasmar	Norepinephrine, dopamine	—	Blocks enzymatic breakdown of norepinephrine and dopamine by blocking COMT
Tranylcypromine	Parnate	Norepinephrine, serotonin, dopamine	—	Inhibits degradation of monoamines by MAO
Triazolam	Halcion	GABA	Benzodiazepine–$GABA_A$ complex	Agonist for benzodiazepine receptor
Trimethaphan	Arfonad	ACh	Nicotinic–cholinergic (at autonomic ganglia)	Blocks nicotinic receptor
Valproic acid	Depakene	GABA	—	Increases synthesis and blocks degradation of GABA

(continued)

Drug Name	Brand Name[a]	Neurotransmitter	Receptor	Drug Action
Varenicline	Chantix	ACh	Nicotinic–cholinergic in brain	Partial agonist for nicotinic receptor
Vecuronium	Norcuron	ACh	Nicotinic–cholinergic (at neuromuscular junction)	Blocks nicotinic receptor
Zaleplon	Sonata	GABA	Benzodiazepine receptor on GABA channel	Agonist for benzodiazepine receptor
Ziprasidone	Geodon	Dopamine, serotonin	Dopamine $D_{3/4}$, $5\text{-}HT_{2A}$	Blocks dopamine and serotonin receptors
Zolmitriptan	Zomig	Serotonin	$5\text{-}HT_{1D/1B}$	Serotonin receptor 1B/1D agonist
Zolpidem	Ambien	GABA	Benzodiazepine receptor on GABA channel	Agonist for benzodiazepine receptor

[a] Includes only one example of a brand name.

[b] See Table 4.4 for other dopamine receptor antagonists.

ACh, acetylcholine; GABA, gamma aminobutyric acid; 5-HT, 5-hydroxytryptamine; MAO, monoamine oxidase; NMDA, N-methyl-D-aspartate.

References

1. Cooper, J. R., Bloom, F. E., and Roth, R. H., *The Biochemical Basis of Neuropharmacology*, 8th ed., Oxford University Press, New York, 2003.
2. Werman, R., Criteria for identification of a central nervous system transmitter, *Comparative Biochemistry and Physiology*, 18(4), 745–766, 1966.
3. Snyder, S. H. and Bredt, D. S., Biological roles of nitric oxide, *Scientific American*, 266(5), 68–71, 1992.
4. Kiss, J. P. and Vizi, E. S., Nitric oxide: A novel link between synaptic and nonsynaptic transmission, *Trends in Neurosciences*, 24(4), 211–215, 2001.
5. Barañano, D. E., Ferris, C. D., and Snyder, S. H., Atypical neural messengers, *Trends in Neurosciences*, 24(2), 99–106, 2001.
6. Wilson, R. I. and Nicoll, R. A., Endocannabinoid signaling in the brain, *Science*, 296(5568), 678–682, 2002.
7. Nicoll, R. A. and Alger, B. E., The brains own marijuana, *Scientific American*, 291(6), 68–75, 2004.
8. Rang. H. P., Dale, M. M., Ritter, J. M., and Flower, R. J., *Rang & Dale's Pharmacology*, 6th ed., Churchill Livingstone/Elsevier, Philadelphia, PA, 2007.
9. Alger, B. E., Retrograde signaling in the regulation of synaptic transmission: Focus on endocannabinoids, *Progress in Neurobiology*, 68(4), 247–286, 2002.
10. Schlicker, E. and Kathmann, M., Modulation of transmitter release via presynaptic cannabinoid receptors, *Trends in Pharmacological Science*, 22(11), 565–572, 2001.
11. Costa, T. and Cotecchia, S., Historical review: Negative efficacy and the constitutive activity of G-protein-coupled receptors, *Trends in Pharmacological Science*, 26(12), 618–624, 2005.
12. Bond, R. A. and Ijzerman, A. P., Recent developments in constitutive receptor activity and inverse agonism, and their potential for GPCR drug discovery, *Trends in Pharmacological Science*, 27(2), 92–96, 2006.
13. Westfall, T. C. and Westfall, D. P., Neurotransmission: The autonomic and somatic motor nervous systems, in L. L. Brunton, J. S. Lazo, and K. L. Parker (Eds.), *The Pharmacological Basis of Therapeutics*, 11th ed., McGraw-Hill Medical Publishing, New York, 137–181, 2006.
14. Kandel, E. R., Schwartz, J. H., and Jessell, T. M., *Principles of Neural Science*, 4th ed., McGraw-Hill, New York, 2000.
15. Blusztajn, J. K. and Wurtman, R. J., Choline and cholinergic neurons, *Science*, 221(4611), 614–620, 1983.
16. Taylor, P. and Brown, J. H., Acetylcholine, in G. J. Siegel, R. W. Albers, S. T. Brady, and D. L. Price (Eds.), *Basic Neurochemistry*, 7th ed., Lippincott-Raven, New York, 185–209, 2006.
17. Collier, B., Kwok, Y. N., and Welner, S. A., Increased acetylcholine synthesis and release following presynaptic activity in a sympathetic ganglion, *Journal of Neurochemistry*, 40(1), 91–98, 1983.
18. Johns, C. A., Greenwald, B. S., Mohs, R. C., and Davis, K. L., The cholinergic treatment strategy in aging and senile dementia, *Psychopharmacology Bulletin*, 19(2), 185–197, 1983.
19. Wurtman, R. J., Choline metabolism as a basis for the selective vulnerability of cholinergic neurons, *Trends in Neurosciences*, 15(4), 117–122, 1992.
20. Koshimura, K., Miwa, S., Lee, K., Hayashi, Y., Hasegawa, H., Hamahata, K., Fujiwara, M., Kimura, M., and Itokawa, Y., Effects of choline administration on *in vivo* release and biosynthesis of acetylcholine in the rat striatum as studied by *in vivo* brain microdialysis, *Journal of Neurochemistry*, 54(2), 533–539, 1990.
21. Johnson, D. A., Ulus, I. H., and Wurtman, R. J., Caffeine potentiates the enhancement by choline of striatal acetylcholine release, *Life Sciences*, 51(20), 1597–1601, 1992.
22. Prado, M. A., Reis, R. A., Prado, V. F., de Mello, M. C., Gomez, M. V., and de Mello, F. G., Regulation of acetylcholine synthesis and storage, *Neurochemistry International*, 41(5), 291–299, 2002.

23. Marshall, I. G. and Parsons, S. M., The vesicular acetylcholine transport system, *Trends in Neurosciences*, 10(4), 174–177, 1987.

24. Abramowics, M. (Ed.), Botulinum toxin (BOTOX Cosmetic) for frown lines, *Medical Letters*, 44(W113A), 47–48, 2002.

25. Dale, H. H., The action of certain esters and ethers of choline and their relation to muscarine, *Journal of Pharmacology and Experimental Therapeutics*, 6(2), 147–190, 1914.

26. Taylor, P., Agents acting at the neuromuscular junction and autonomic ganglia, in L. L. Brunton, J. S. Lazo, and K. L. Parker (Eds.), *The Pharmacological Basis of Therapeutics*, 11th edition, McGraw-Hill, New York, 217–236, 2006.

27. Beani, L., Bianchi, C., Nilsson, L., Nordberg, A., Romanelli, L., and Sivilotti, L., The effect of nicotine and cytisine on 3H-acetylcholine release from cortical slices of guinea-pig brain, *Archives of Pharmacology*, 331(2–3), 293–296, 1985.

28. Richard, J., Araujo, D. M., and Quirion, R., Modulation of cortical acetylcholine release by cholinergic agents in an *in vivo* dialysis study, *Society for Neuroscience Abstracts*, 15(2), 1197, 1989.

29. Lisman, J. E., Coyle, J. T., Green, R. W., Javitt, D. C., Benes, F. M., Heckers, S., and Grace, A. A., Circuit-based framework for understanding neurotransmitter and risk gene interactions in schizophrenia, *Trends in Neurosciences*, 31(5), 234–242, 2008.

30. Egleton, R. D., Brown, K. C., and Dasgupta, P., Nicotinic acetylcholine receptors in cancer: Multiple roles in proliferation and inhibition of apoptosis, *Trends in Pharmacological Sciences*, 29(3), 151–158, 2008.

31. Hulme, E. C., Birdsall, N. J., and Buckley, N. J., Muscarinic receptor subtypes, *Annual Review of Pharmacology and Toxicology*, 30, 633–673, 1990.

32. Browning, R. A., Overview of neurotransmission: Relationship to the action of antiepileptic drugs, in C. L. Faingold and G. Fromm (Eds.), *Drugs for Control of Epilepsy: Actions on Neuronal Networks Involved in Seizure Disorders*, CRC Press, Boca Raton, FL, 23–56, 1992.

33. Brown, J. H. and Taylor, P., Muscarinic receptor agonists and antagonists, in L. L. Brunton, J. S. Lazo, and K. L. Parker (Eds.), *The Pharmacological Basis of Therapeutics*, 11th edition, McGraw-Hill, New York, 183–200, 2006.

34. Lapchak, P. A., Araujo, D. M., Quirion, R., and Collier, B., Binding sites for [3H] AF-DX 116 and effect of AF-DX 116 on endogenous acetylcholine release from rat brain slices, *Brain Research*, 496(1–2), 285–294, 1989.

35. Turski, L., Ikonomidou, C., Turski, W. A., Bortolutto, Z. A., and Cavalheiro, E. A., Review: Cholinergic mechanisms and epileptogenesis. The seizures induced by pilocarpine: A novel experimental model of intractable epilepsy, *Synapse*, 3(2), 154–171, 1989.

36. Drugs for tobacco dependence, *Treatment guidelines from the Medical Letter*, 6(73), 61–66, 2008.

37. Dani, J. A. and Bertrand, D., Nicotinic acetylcholine receptors and nicotinic cholinergic mechanisms of the central nervous system, *Annual Review of Pharmacology and Toxicology*, 47, 699–729, 2007.

38. Clark, W. G., Brater, D. C., and Johnson, A. R., *Medical Pharmacology*, 13th ed., Mosby-Year Book, St. Louis, MO, 1992.

39. Lyeth, B. G., Dixon, C. E., Jenkins, L. W., Hamm, R. J., Alberico, A., Young, H. F., Stonnington, H. H., and Hayes, R. L., Effects of scopolamine treatment on long-term behavioral deficits following concussive brain injury to the rat, *Brain Research*, 452(1–2), 39–48, 1988.

40. Taverni, J. P., Seliger, G., and Lichtman, S. W., Donepezil medicated memory improvement in traumatic brain injury during post acute rehabilitation, *Brain Injury*, 12(1), 77–80, 1998.

41. Guseva, M. V., Hopkins, D. M., Scheff, S. W., and Pauly, J. R., Dietary choline supplementation improves behavioral, histological, and neurochemical outcomes in a rat model of traumatic brain injury, *Journal of Neurotrauma*, 25(8), 975–983, 2008.

42. Kokiko, O. N. and Hamm, R. J., A review of pharmacological treatments used in experimental models of traumatic brain injury, *Brain Injury*, 21(3), 259–274, 2007.

43. Falck, B., Hillarp, N. A., Thieme, G., and Torp, A., Fluorescence of catecholamines and related compounds condensed with formaldehyde, *Journal of Histochemistry and Cytochemistry*, 10(3), 348–365, 1962.

44. Moore, R. Y. and Bloom, F. E., Central catecholamine neuron systems: Anatomy and physiology of the norepinephrine and epinephrine systems, *Annual Review of Neuroscience*, 2, 113–168, 1979.

45. Kuhar, M. J., Couceyro, P. R., and Lambert, P. D., Catecholamines, in G. J. Siegel, B. W. Agranoff, S. K. Fisher, R. W. Albers, and M. D. Uhler (Eds.), *Basic Neurochemistry: Molecular, Cellular, and Medical Aspects*, 6th ed., Lippincott-Raven, Philadelphia, 242–261, 1999.

46. Feldman, R. S., Meyer, J. S., and Quenzer, L. F., *Principles of Neuropsychopharmacology*, Sinauer Associates, Sunderland, MA, 1997.

47. Bogdanski, D. F., Norepinephrine uptake dependent upon apparent Mg^{++}–ATPase activity and proton transport in storage vesicles in axoplasm, *Synapse*, 2(4), 424–431, 1988.

48. Graham, D. and Langer, S. Z., Minireview: Advances in sodium-ion coupled biogenic amine transporters, *Life Sciences*, 51(9), 631–645, 1992.

49. O'Dowd, B. F., Lefkowitz, R. J., and Caron, M. G., Structure of the adrenergic and related receptors, *Annual Review of Neuroscience*, 12, 67–83, 1989.

50. Minneman, K. P., Alpha 1-adrenergic receptor subtypes, inositol phosphates, and sources of cell Ca^{2+}, *Pharmacological Reviews*, 40(2), 87–119, 1988.

51. Insel, P. A., Seminars in medicine of the Beth Israel Hospital, Boston. Adrenergic receptors: Evolving concepts and clinical implications, *New England Journal of Medicine*, 334(9), 580–585, 1996.

52. Baldessarini, R. J., Drugs and the treatment of psychiatric disorders, depression, and anxiety disorders, in J. G. Hardman, L. E. Limbird, and A. G. Gilman (Eds.), *The Pharmacological Basis of Therapeutics*, 10th edition, McGraw-Hill, New York, 447–483, 2001.

53. Bakhit, C., Morgan, M. E., Peat, M. A., and Gibb, J. W., Long-term effects of methamphetamine on the synthesis and metabolism of 5-hydroxytryptamine in various regions of the rat brain, *Neuropharmacology*, 20(12A), 1135–1140, 1981.

54. Ricaurte, G. A., Schuster, C. R., and Seiden, L. S., Long-term effects of repeated methylamphetamine administration on dopamine and serotonin neurons in the rat brain: A regional study, *Brain Research*, 193(1), 153–163, 1980.

55. Ricaurte, G. A., Seiden, L. S., and Schuster, C. R., Further evidence that amphetamines produce long-lasting dopamine neurochemical deficits by destroying dopamine nerve fibers, *Brain Research*, 303(2), 359–364, 1984.

56. Axt, K. and Molliver, M. E., Immunocytochemical evidence for methamphetamine-induced serotonergic axon loss in the rat brain, *Synapse*, 9(4), 302–313, 1991.

57. Westfall, D. P., Antihypertensive drugs, in C. R. Craig and R. E. Stitzel (Eds.), *Modern Pharmacology with Clinical Applications*, 5th ed., Little, Brown, Boston, 235–252, 1997.

58. Feeney, D. M. and Sutton, R. L., Pharmacotherapy for recovery of function after brain injury, *Critical Reviews in Neurobiology*, 3(2), 135–197, 1987.

59. Feeney, D. M. and Sutton, R. L., Catecholamines and recovery of function after brain damage, in G. G. Stein and B. A. Sabel (Eds.), *Pharmacological Approaches to the Treatment of Brain and Spinal Cord Injury*, Plenum Publishing, New York, 121–142, 1988.

60. Feeney, D. M., Mechanisms of noradrenergic modulation of physical therapy: Effects on functional recovery after cortical injury, in L. B. Goldstein (Ed.), *Restorative Neurology: Advances in Pharmacotherapy for Recovery After Stroke*, Futura Publishing, Armonk, NY, 35–78, 1998.

61. Goldstein, L. B., Basic and clinical studies of pharmacologic effects on recovery from brain injury, *Journal of Neural Transplantation and Plasticity*, 4(3), 175–192, 1993.

62. McIntosh, T. K., Novel pharmacologic therapies in the treatment of experimental traumatic brain injury: A review, *Journal of Neurotrauma*, 10(3), 215–261, 1993.

63. Feeney, D. M. and Westerberg, V. S., Norepinephrine and brain damage: Alpha noradrenergic pharmacology alters functional recovery after cortical trauma, *Canadian Journal of Psychology*, 44(2), 233–252, 1990.

64. Crisostomo, E. A., Duncan, P. W., Propst, M. A., Dawson, D. V., and Davis, J. N., Evidence that amphetamine with physical therapy promotes recovery of motor function in stroke patients, *Annals of Neurology*, 23(1), 94–97, 1988.

65. Goldstein, L. B., Effects of amphetamines and small related molecules on recovery after stroke in animals and man, *Neuropharmacology*, 39(5), 852–859, 2000.

66. Giros, B. and Caron, M. G., Molecular characterization of the dopamine transporter, *Trends in Pharmacological Sciences*, 14(2), 43–49, 1993.

67. Creese, I., Sibley, D. R., and Leff, S. E., Agonist interactions with dopamine receptors: Focus on radioligand-binding studies, *Federation Proceedings*, 43(13), 2779–2784, 1984.

68. Sokoloff, P., Giros, B., Martres, M. P., Bouthenet, M. L., and Schwartz, J. C., Molecular cloning and characterization of a novel dopamine receptor (D_3) as a target for neuroleptics, *Nature*, 347(6289), 146–151, 1990.

69. Van Tol, H. H., Bunzow, J. R., Guan, H. C., Sunahara, R. K., Seeman, P., Niznik, H. B., and Civelli, O., Cloning of the gene for a human dopamine D_4 receptor with high affinity for the antipsychotic clozapine, *Nature*, 350(6319), 610–614, 1991.

70. O'Dowd, B. F., Structures of dopamine receptors, *Journal of Neurochemistry*, 60(3), 804–816, 1993.

71. Seeman, P. and Van Tol, H. H., Dopamine receptor pharmacology, *Trends in Pharmacological Sciences*, 15(7), 264–270, 1994.

72. Uhl, G., Blum, K., Noble, E., and Smith S., Substance abuse vulnerability and D_2 receptor genes, *Trends in Neurosciences*, 16(3), 83–88, 1993.

73. Apomorphine (Apokyn) for advanced Parkinson's disease, *Medical Letter on Drugs and Therapeutics*, 47(1200), 7–8, 2005.

74. Drugs for Parkinson's disease, *Treatment Guidelines from The Medical Letter*, 5(62), 89–94, 2007.

75. Rasgiline (Azilect) for Parkinson's disease, *Medical Letter on Drugs and Therapeutics*, 48(1249/1250), 97–99, 2006.

76. Standaert, D. G. and Young, A. B., Treatment of central nervous system degenerative disorders, in L. L. Brunton, J. S. Lazo, and K. L. Parker (Eds.), *The Pharmacological Basis of Therapeutics*, McGraw-Hill, New York, 207, 2006.

77. Baldessarini, R. J. and Tarazi, F. I., Pharmacotherapy of psychosis and mania, in L. L. Brunton, J. S. Lazo, and K. L. Parker (Eds.), *The Pharmacological Basis of Therapeutics*, McGraw-Hill, New York, 461–500, 2006.

78. Seamans, J. K. and Yang, C. R., The principal features and mechanisms of dopamine modulation in the prefrontal cortex, Progress in Neurobiology, 74(1), 1–58, 2004.

79. Lal, S., Merbitz, C. P., and Grip, J. C., Modification of function in head-injured patients with Sinemet, *Brain Injury*, 2(3), 225–233, 1988.

80. Eames, P., The use of Sinemet and bromocriptine, *Brain Injury*, 3(3), 319–322, 1989.

81. Medico, M., DeVivo, S., Tomasello, C., Grech, M., Nicosia, A., Castorina, M., D'Agata, M. A., Rampello, L., Lempereur, L., and Drago, F., Behavioral and neurochemical effects of dopaminergic drugs in models of brain injury, *European Neuropsychopharmacology*, 12(3), 187–194, 2002.

82. Zafonte, R. D., Lexell, J., and Cullen, N., Possible applications for dopaminergic agents following traumatic brain injury: Part I, *Journal of Head Trauma Rehabilitation*, 15(5), 1179–1182, 2000.

83. Zafonte, R. D., Lexell, J., and Cullen, N., Possible applications for dopaminergic agents following traumatic brain injury: Part II, *Journal of Head Trauma Rehabilitation*, 16(1), 112–116, 2001.

84. Teng, C. J., Bhalerao, S., Lee, Z., Farber, J., Morris, H., Foran, T., and Tucker, W., The use of bupropion in the treatment of restlessness after a traumatic brain injury, *Brain Injury*, 15(5), 463–467, 2001.

85. Dahlstrom, A. and Fuxe, K., A method for the demonstration of monoamine containing nerve fibers in the central nervous system, *Acta Physiologica Scandinavica*, 60(3), 293–294, 1964.

86. Molliver, M. E., Serotonergic neuronal systems: What their anatomic organization tells us about function, *Journal of Clinical Psychopharmacology*, 7(6 Suppl.), 3S–23S, 1987.

87. Gershon, M. D., Biochemistry and physiology of serotonergic transmission, in J. M. Brookhart, V. Mountcastle, and E. Kandel (Eds.), *Handbook of Physiology: The Nervous System I*, American Physiological Society, Washington, DC, 573, 1977.

88. Wurtman, R. J., Hefti, F., and Melamed, E., Precursor control of neurotransmitter synthesis, *Pharmacological Reviews*, 32(4), 315–335, 1981.
89. Shishkina, G. T., Kalinina, T. S., and Dygalo, N. N., Up-regulation of tryptophan hydroxylase-2 mRNA in the rat brain by chronic fluoxetine treatment correlates with its antidepressant effect, *Neuroscience*, 150(2), 404–412, 2007.
90. Green, J. P., Histamine and serotonin, in G. J. Siegel, B. W. Agranoff, R. W. Alberts, and P. B. Molinoff (Eds.), *Basic Neurochemistry*, Raven Press, New York, 253, 1989.
91. Sanders-Bush, E. and Martin, L. L., Storage and release of serotonin, in N. N. Osborne (Ed.), *Biology of Serotonergic Transmission*, Wiley, New York, 95, 1982.
92. Halaris, A. E. and Freedman, D. X., Vesicular and juxtavesicular serotonin: Effect of lysergic acid diethylamide and reserpine, *Journal of Pharmacology and Experimental Therapeutics*, 203(3), 575–586, 1977.
93. Maynert, E. W., Levi, R., and deLorenzo, A. J. D., The presence of norepinephrine and 5-HT in vesicles from disrupted nerve-ending particles, *Journal of Pharmacology and Experimental Therapeutics*, 144(3), 385–392, 1964.
94. Iversen, L., Neurotransmitter transporters and their impact on the development of psychopharmacology, *British Journal of Pharmacology*, 147(Suppl. 1), S82–S88, 2006.
95. Adell, A., Sarna, G. S., Hutson, P. H., and Curzon, G., An *in vivo* dialysis and behavioural study of the release of 5-HT by p-chloroamphetamine in reserpine-treated rats, *British Journal of Pharmacology*, 97(1), 206–212, 1989.
96. Kuhn, D. M., Wolf, W. A., and Youdim, M. B. H., Review: Serotonin neurochemistry revisited: A new look at some old axioms, *Neurochemistry International*, 8(2), 141–154, 1986.
97. Murphy, D. L., Fox, M. A., Timpano, K. R., Moya, P. R., Ren-Patterson, R., Andrews, A. M., Holmes, A., Lesch, K. P., and Wendland, J. R., How the serotonin story is being rewritten by new gene-based discoveries principally related to SLC6A4, the serotonin transporter gene, which functions to influence all cellular serotonin systems, Neuropharmacology, 55(6), 932–960, 2008.
98. Reinhard, J. F. and Wurtman, R., Relation between brain 5-HIAA levels and the release of serotonin into brain synapses, *Life Sciences*, 21(12), 1741–1746, 1977.
99. Lowry, C. A., Hale, M. W., Evans, A. K., Heerkens, J., Staub, D. R., Gasser, P. J., and Shekhar, A., Serotonergic systems, anxiety, and affective disorder: Focus on the dorsomedial part of the dorsal raphe nucleus. *Annals of the New York Academy of Sciences*, 1148, 86–94, 2008.
100. Cowen, P. J., Serotonin and depression: Pathophysiological mechanism or marketing myth?, *Trends in Pharmacological Sciences*, 29(9), 433–436, 2008.
101. Hoyer, D., Hannon, J. P., and Martin, G. R., Molecular, pharmacological, and functional diversity of 5-HT receptors, *Pharmacology, Biochemistry, and Behavior*, 71(4), 533–554, 2002.
102. Barnes, N. M. and Sharp, T., A review of central 5-HT receptors and their function, *Neuropharmacology*, 38(8), 1083–1152, 1999.
103. Richardson, B. P. and Engel, G., The pharmacology and function of 5-HT$_3$ receptors, *Trends in Neurosciences*, 9, 424–428, 1986.
104. Schmidt, A. W. and Peroutka, J., 5-Hydroxytryptamine receptor "families," The *FASEB Journal*, 3(11), 2242–2249, 1989.
105. Nestler, E. J., Hyman, S. E., and Malenka, R. C., *Molecular Neuropharmacology: A Foundation for Clinical Neuroscience*, McGraw-Hill, New York, Ch. 9, 2001.
106. Jensen, A. A., Davies, P. A., Bräuner-Osborne, H., and Krzywkoski, K., 3B but which 3B and that's just one of the questions: The heterogeneity of human 5-HT3 receptors, *Trends in Pharmacological Sciences*, 29(9), 437–444, 2008.
107. Drugs for the treatment of migraine, *Treatment Guidelines from the Medical Letter*, 6(67), 17–22, 2008.
108. Ferrari, M. D. and Saxena, P. R., Clinical and experimental aspects of sumatriptan in humans, *Trends in Pharmacological Sciences*, 14(4), 129–133, 1993.
109. Pappius, H. M., Significance of biogenic amines in functional disturbances resulting from brain injury, *Metabolic Brain Disease*, 3(4), 303–310, 1988.

110. Sharma, H. S., Winkler, T., Stålberg, E., Mohanty, S., and Westman, J., p-Chlorophenylalanine, an inhibitor of serotonin synthesis reduces blood–brain barrier permeability, cerebral blood flow, edema formation, and cell injury following trauma to the rat brain, *Acta Neurochirurgica*, 76 (Suppl.), 91–95, 2000.

111. Kline, A. E., Yu, J., Horváth, E., Marion, D. W., and Dixon, C. E., The selective 5-HT(1A) receptor agonist repinotan HCl attenuates histopathology and spatial learning deficits following traumatic brain injury in rats, *Neuroscience*, 106(3), 547–555, 2001.

112. Wilson, M. S. and Hamm, R. J., Effects of fluoxetine on 5-HT1A receptor and recovery of cognitive function after traumatic brain injury in rats, *American Journal of Physical Medicine and Rehabilitation*, 81(5), 364–372, 2002.

113. Stengler-Wenzke, K. and Müller, U., Fluoxetine for OCD after brain injury, *American Journal of Psychiatry*, 159(5), 872, 2002.

114. Mattson, M. P., Maudsley, S., and Martin, B., BDNF and 5-HT: A dynamic duo in age-related neuronal plasticity and neurodegenerative disorders, *Trends in Neurosciences*, 27(10), 589–594, 2004.

115. McGeer, P. L., Eccles, J. C., and McGeer, E. G., *Molecular Neurobiology of the Mammalian Brain*, 2nd ed., Plenum Press, New York, 1987.

116. Olsen, R. W. and DeLorey, T. M., GABA and glycine, in G. J. Siegel, B. W. Agranoff, R. W. Albers, S. K. Fisher, and M. D. Uhler (Eds.), *Basic Neurochemistry*, 6th ed., Lippincott-Raven, New York, 335, 1999.

117. Obata, K., Biochemistry and physiology of amino acids neurotransmitters, in J. M. Brookhart, V. Mountcastle, and E. Kandel (Eds.), *Handbook of Physiology: The Nervous System I*, American Physiological Society, Washington, DC, 625, 1977.

118. Bradford, H. E., *Chemical Neurobiology*, W. H. Freeman, New York, 1986.

119. Meldrum, B., GABA and other amino acids, in H. H. Frey and D. Janz (Eds.), *Antiepileptic Drugs, Handbook of Experimental Pharmacology*, Vol. 74, Springer-Verlag, Berlin, 153, 1985.

120. Martin, D. L. and Rimvall, K., Regulation of gamma-aminobutyric acid synthesis in the brain, *Journal of Neurochemistry*, 60(2), 395–407, 1993.

121. Olsen, R. W. and Betz, H., GABA and glycine, in G. L. Siegel, R. W. Albers, S. T. Brady, and D. L. Price (Eds.), *Basic Neurochemistry, Molecular, Cellular and Medical Aspects*, 7th ed., Elsevier, Boston, 291–301, 2006.

122. Tobin, A. J., Molecular biological approaches to the synthesis and action of GABA, *Seminars in Neuroscience*, 3(3), 183–190, 1991.

123. Kaufman, D. L. and Tobin, A. J., Glutamate decarboxylases and autoimmunity in insulin-dependent diabetes, *Trends in Pharmacological Sciences*, 14(4), 107–109, 1993.

124. Nicholls, D. G., Release of glutamate, aspartate, and gamma-aminobutyric acid from isolated nerve terminals, *Journal of Neurochemistry*, 52(2), 331–341, 1989.

125. Fykse, E. M., Christensen, H., and Fonnum, F., Comparison of the properties of gamma-aminobutyric acid and l-glutamate uptake into synaptic vesicles isolated from rat brain, *Journal of Neurochemistry*, 52(3), 946–951, 1989.

126. De Belleroche, J. S. and Bradford, H. F., On the site of origin of transmitter amino acids released by depolarization of nerve terminals in vitro, *Journal of Neurochemistry*, 29(2), 335–343, 1977.

127. Erecińska, M., Wantorsky, D., and Wilson, D. F., Aspartate transport in synaptosomes from rat brain, *Journal of Biological Chemistry*, 258(15), 9069–9077, 1983.

128. Wheeler, D. D. and Hollingsworth, R. G., A model of GABA transport by cortical synaptosomes from the Long-Evans rat, *Journal of Neuroscience Research*, 4(4), 265–289, 1979.

129. Erecinska, M., The neurotransmitter amino acid transport systems: A fresh outlook on an old problem, *Biochemical Pharmacology*, 36(21), 3547–3555, 1987.

130. Borden, L. A., GABA transporter heterogeneity: Pharmacology and cellular localization, *Neurochemistry International*, 29(4), 335–356, 1996.

131. Barnard, E. A., Darlison, M. G., and Seeburg, P., Molecular biology of the GABA$_A$ receptor: The receptor/channel superfamily, *Trends in Neurosciences*, 10(12), 502–509, 1987.

132. Olsen, R. W. and Tobin, A. J., Molecular biology of GABA$_A$ receptors, The *FASEB Journal*, 4(5), 1469–1480, 1990.

133. Sieghart, W., GABA$_A$ receptors: Ligand-gated Cl-ion channels modulated by multiple drug-binding sites, *Trends in Pharmacological Science,* 13(12), 446–450, 1992.

134. Matsumoto, R. R., GABA receptors: Are cellular differences reflected in function?, *Brain Research, Brain Research Reviews,* 14(3), 203–225, 1989.

135. Bowery, N., GABA$_B$ receptors and their significance in mammalian pharmacology, *Trends in Pharmacological Sciences,* 10(10), 401–407, 1989.

136. Bormann, J. and Feigenspan, A., GABA$_C$ receptors, *Trends in Neurosciences,* 18(12), 515–519, 1995.

137. Trevor, A. J. and Way, L. Sedative–hypnotic drugs, in B. G. Katzung (Ed.), *Basic and Clinical Pharmacology,* 10th ed., New York, McGraw Hill, 347–362, 2007.

138. Rogawski, M. A. and Porter, R. J., Antiepileptic drugs: Pharmacological mechanisms and clinical efficacy with consideration of promising developmental stage compounds, *Pharmacological Reviews,* 42(3), 223–286, 1990.

139. Brodie, M. J., Do we need any more new antiepileptic drugs?, *Epilepsy Research,* 45(1–3), 3–6, 2001.

140. Rho, J. M. and Sankar, R., The pharmacologic basis of antiepileptic drug action, *Epilepsia,* 40(11), 471–483, 1999.

141. Nilsson, P., Hillered, L., Pontén, U., and Ungerstedt, U., Changes in cortical extracellular levels of energy-related metabolites and amino acids following concussive brain injury in rats, *Journal of Cerebral Blood Flow and Metabolism,* 10(5), 631–637, 1990.

142. Sihver, S., Marklund, N., Hillered, L., Långström, B., Watanabe, Y, and Bergström, M., Changes in mACH, NMDA, and GABA$_A$ receptor binding after lateral fluid-percussion injury: *In vitro* autoradiography of rat brain frozen sections, *Journal of Neurochemistry,* 78(3), 417–423, 2001.

143. Kokiko, O. N. and Hamm, R. J., A review of pharmacological treatments used in experimental models of traumatic brain injury, *Brain Injury,* 21(3), 259–274, 2007.

144. Feldman, R. S., Meyer, J. S., and Quenzer, L. E., *Principles of Neuropsychopharmacology,* Sinauer Associates, Sunderland, MA, Ch. 10, 1997.

145. Nestler, E. J., Hyman, S. E., and Malenka, R. C., *Molecular Neuropharmacology: A Foundation for Clinical Neuroscience,* 2nd ed., McGraw-Hill, New York, Ch. 5, 2009.

146. Kish, P. E., Fischer-Bovenkerk, C., and Ueda, T., Active transport of γ-aminobutyric acid and glycine into synaptic vesicles, *Proceedings of the National Academy of Sciences of the United States of America,* 86(10), 3877–3881, 1989.

147. Greeningloh, G., Rienitz, A., Schmitt, B., Methfessel, C., Zensen, M., Beyreuther, K., Gundelfinger, E. D., and Betz, H., The strychnine-binding subunit of the glycine receptor shows homology with nicotinic acetylcholine receptors, *Nature,* 328(6127), 215–220, 1987.

148. Langosch, D., Thomas L., and Betz, H., Conserved quaternary structure of ligand-gated ion channels: The postsynaptic glycine receptor is a pentamer, *Proceedings of the National Academy of Sciences of the United States of America,* 85(19), 7394–7398, 1988.

149. Thomson, A. M., Glycine modulation of the NMDA receptor/channel complex, *Trends in Neurosciences,* 12(9), 349–353, 1989.

150. Dingledine, R. and McBain, C. J., Glutamate and aspartate, in G. J. Siegel, B. A. Agranoff, R. W. Albers, S. K. Fisher, and M. D. Uhler (Eds.), *Basic Neurochemistry,* 6th ed., Lippincott-Raven, New York, 315–333, 1999.

151. Monaghan, D. T., Bridges, R. J., and Cotman, C. W., The excitatory amino acid receptors: Their classes, pharmacology, and distinct properties in the function of the central nervous system, *Annual Review of Pharmacology and Toxicology,* 29, 365–402, 1989.

152. Hassel, B. and Dingledine, R., Glutamate, in G. J. Siegel, R. W. Alber, S. T. Brady, and D. L. Price (Eds.), *Basic Neurochemistry: Molecular, Cellular and Medical Aspects,* 7th ed., Academic Press, Boston, 267–290, 2006.

153. Fonnum, F., Glutamate: A neurotransmitter in mammalian brain, *Journal of Neurochemistry,* 42(1), 1–11, 1984.

154. Ward, H. K., Thanki, C. M., and Bradford, H. F., Glutamine and glucose as precursors of transmitter amino acids: *Ex vivo* studies, *Journal of Neurochemistry,* 40(3), 855–860, 1983.

155. Robinson, M. B. and Coyle, J. T., Glutamate and related acidic excitatory neurotransmitters: From basic science to clinical application, *The Federation of American Societies for Experimental Biology Journal*, 1(6), 446–455, 1987.

156. Bellocchio, E. E., Reimer, R. J., Fremeau, R. T., Jr., and Edwards, R. H., Uptake of glutamate into synaptic vesicles by an inorganic phosphate transporter, *Science*, 289(5481), 957–960, 2000.

157. Balcar, V. J. and Johnston, G. A., The structural specificity of the high affinity uptake of L-glutamate and L-aspartate by rat brain slices, *Journal of Neurochemistry*, 19(11), 2657–2666, 1972.

158. Snyder, S. H., Young, A. B., Bennett, J. P., and Mulder, A. H., Synaptic biochemistry of amino acids, *Federation Proceedings*, 32(10), 2039–2047, 1973.

159. Cornell-Bell, A. H., Finkbeiner, S. M., Cooper, M. S., and Smith, S. J., Glutamate induces calcium waves in cultured astrocytes: Long-range glial signaling, *Science*, 247(4941), 470–473, 1990.

160. Lehmann, J., Randle, J. C. R., and Reynolds, I. J., Meeting report: Excitatory amino acid receptors, *Trends in Pharmacological Sciences*, 11(1), 1, 1990.

161. Faden, A. I., Demediuk, P., Panter, S. S., and Vink, R., The role of excitatory amino acids and NMDA receptors in traumatic brain injury, *Science*, 244(4906), 798–800, 1989.

162. Ozawa, S., Kamiya, H., and Tsuzuki, K., Glutamate receptors in the mammalian central nervous system, *Progress in Neurobiology*, 54(5), 581–618, 1998.

163. Faingold, C. L. and Meldrum, B. S., Excitant amino acids in epilepsy, in M. Avoli, P. Gloor, P. Kostopoulos, and R. Naquet (Eds.), *Generalized Epilepsy: Cellular, Molecular, and Pharmacological Approach*, Birkhauser, Boston, 102, 1990.

164. Feeser, H. R., Kadis, J. L., and Prince, D. A., Dextromethorphan, a common antitussive reduces kindled amygdala seizures in the rat, *Neuroscience Letters*, 86(3), 340–345, 1988.

165. Leander, J. D., Rathbon, R. C., and Zimmerman, D. M., Anticonvulsant effects of phencyclidine-like drugs: Relation to N-methyl-D-aspartic acid antagonism, *Brain Research*, 454(1–2), 368–372, 1988.

166. Olney, J. W., Ho, O. L., and Rhee, V., Cytotoxic effects of acidic and sulfur-containing amino acids on the infant mouse central nervous system, *Experimental Brain Research*, 14(1), 61–76, 1971.

167. Olney, J., Price, M., Salles, K. S., Labruyere, J., and Frierdich, G., MK-801 powerfully protects against N-methyl aspartate neurotoxicity, *European Journal of Pharmacology*, 141(3), 357–361, 1987.

168. McIntosh, T. K., Juhler, M., and Wieloch, T., Novel pharmacologic strategies in the treatment of experimental traumatic brain injury, *Journal of Neurotrauma*, 15(10), 731–769, 1998.

169. Temple, M. D. and Hamm, R. J., Chronic, postinjury administration of D-cycloserine, an NMDA partial agonist, enhances cognitive performance following experimental brain injury, *Brain Research*, 741(1–2), 246–251, 1996.

170. Snyder, S. H., Brain peptides as neurotransmitters, *Science*, 209(4460), 976–983, 1980.

171. Von Euler, U. S. and Gaddam, J. H., An unidentified depressor substance in certain tissue extracts, *Journal of Physiology*, 72(1), 74–87, 1931.

172. Krieger, D. T. and Martin, J. B., Brain peptides: Part 2, *New England Journal of Medicine*, 304(16), 944–951, 1981.

173. Otsuka, M. and Yanagisawa, M., Does substance P act as a pain transmitter?, *Trends in Pharmacological Sciences*, 8(12), 506–510, 1987.

174. Nestler, E. J., Hyman, S. E., and Malenka, R. C., *Molecular Neuropharmacology, A Foundation for Clinical Neuroscience*, 2nd ed., McGraw-Hill, New York, Ch. 7, 2009.

175. Hughes, J., Smith, T. W., Kosterlitz, H. W., Fothergill, L. A., Morgan, B. A., and Morris, H. R., Identification of two related pentapeptides from the brain with potent opiate agonist activity, *Nature*, 258(5536), 577–580, 1975.

176. Jaffe, J. H. and Martin, W. R., Opioid analgesics and antagonists, in A. G. Gilman, T. W. Rall, A. S. Nies, and P. Taylor (Eds.), *Goodman and Gilman's The Pharmacological Basis of Therapeutics*, Pergamon Press, New York, 485, 1990.

177. Khachaturian, H., Lewis, M. E., Schafer, M. K. H., and Watson, S. J., Anatomy of the CNS opioid systems, *Trends in Neurosciences*, 8(3), 111–119, 1985.

178. Krieger, D. T., Brain peptides: What, where, and why?, *Science*, 222(4627), 975–985, 1983.
179. Mains, R. E. and Eipper B. A., Peptides, in G. J. Siegel, R. W. Albers, S. T. Brady, and D. L. Price (Eds.), *Basic Neurochemistry, Molecular, Cellular and Medical Aspects*, 7th ed., Academic Press, Boston, 317–332, 2006.
180. Simon, E. J., Opioid receptors and endogenous opioid peptides, *Medical Research Reviews*, 11(4), 357–374, 1991.
181. Civelli, O., Machida, C., Bunzow, J., Albert, P., Hanneman, E., Salon, J., Bidlack, J., and Grandy, D., The next frontier in the molecular biology of the opioid system: The opioid receptors, *Molecular Neurobiology*, 1(4), 373–391, 1987.
182. Bailey, C. P., Smith, F. L., Kelly, E., Dewey, W. L., and Henderson, G., How important is protein kinase C in μ-opioid receptor desensitization and morphine tolerance?, *Trends in Pharmacological Sciences*, 27(11), 558–565, 2006.
183. Cahill, K. M., Holdridge, S.V., and Morinville, A. Trafficking of delta-opioid receptors and other G-protein-coupled receptors: Implications for pain and analgesia, *Trends in Pharmacological Sciences*, 28(1), 23–31, 2007.
184. Zhang, X., Bao, L., and Guan, J. S., Role of delivery and trafficking of δ-opioid peptide receptors in opioid analgesia and tolerance, *Trends in Pharmacological Sciences*, 27(6), 324–329, 2006.
185. Henderson, G. and McKnight, A. T., The orphan opioid receptor and its endogenous ligand–nociceptin/orphanin FQ, *Trends in Pharmacological Sciences*, 18(8), 293–300,1997.
186. Gutstein, H. B. and Akil, H., Opioid analgesics, in J. G. Hardman, L. E. Limbird, and A. G. Gilman (Eds.), *The Pharmacological Basis of Therapeutics*, 10th edition, McGraw-Hill, New York, 569–619, 2001.
187. McIntosh, T. K., Head, V. A., and Faden, A. I., Alterations in regional concentrations of endogenous opioids following traumatic brain injury in the cat, *Brain Research*, 425(2), 225–233, 1987.
188. Faden, A. I., Sacksen, I., and Noble, L. J., Opiate-receptor antagonist nalmefene improves neurological recovery after traumatic spinal cord injury in rats through a central mechanism, *Journal of Pharmacology and Experimental Therapeutics*, 245(2), 742–748, 1988.
189. Isaac, L., O'Malley, T., Ristic, H., and Stewart, P., MK-801 blocks dynorphin A(1–13)-induced loss of the tail-flick reflex in the rat, *Brain Research*, 531(1–2), 83–87, 1990.
190. Lyeth, B. G. and Hayes, R. L., Cholinergic and opioid mediation of traumatic brain injury, *Journal of Neurotrauma*, 9(Suppl. 2), S463–S474, 1992.

5

Neuropharmacologic Considerations in the Treatment of Vegetative State and Minimally Conscious State Following Brain Injury

Deborah Lynne Doherty

CONTENTS

5.1 Introduction

The treatment of individuals with prolonged disorders of consciousness following trauma or other insults to the brain remains a challenge. This chapter reviews definitions of low arousal states, the neurophysiology of consciousness, the pathophysiology of alterations of consciousness, and the basic underlying neurotransmitter functions that may be affected by injury. Neurotransmitter systems provide a potential target for pharmacologic manipulation. The goal of drug treatment is to improve arousal and attention, thereby facilitating neurologic recovery. Medications that may be useful in the treatment of disorders of consciousness will be reviewed and organized by the neurotransmitter systems through which they exert their effects. Although still in its infancy, our understanding of neurotransmitter interactions and cognitive function will serve as the foundation upon which novel drug therapies will someday be developed.

5.2 Definitions of Coma, Vegetative State, and Minimally Conscious State

Recovery from traumatic and nontraumatic brain injury is characterized by gradual emergence from coma. Depending upon the severity of the underlying brain damage, patients may transition from coma to vegetative state, to minimally conscious state, and ultimately to good recovery. However, individuals may also plateau at any point along this continuum.

Coma is a state in which the patient is neither awake nor aware.[1] Comatose patients demonstrate no meaningful interaction with the environment. No purposeful movement is observed. No command following is seen. The eyes remain closed even in the presence of noxious stimulation, and no sleep–wake cycles are observed. After traumatic brain injury, coma is typically a self-limited condition that evolves to vegetative state or higher levels of consciousness.

The term *vegetative state* was first introduced by Jennett and Plum[2] in 1972. It is defined as a condition of unconsciousness devoid of cognitive content and characterized by wakefulness without awareness. The individual in vegetative state demonstrates eye opening and gradually develops sleep–wake cycles. Spontaneous, nonpurposeful motor activity may be seen. Vegetative patients cannot comprehend language, nor can they communicate. Evidence of reproducible, purposeful responses to visual, auditory, tactile, or noxious stimuli are absent.[3] Roving eye movements and brief, unsustained visual tracking may be observed. One of the first signs of emergence from vegetative state is the appearance of sustained visual pursuit.

Minimally conscious state (MCS) is a condition in which meaningful responses are observed, although on an inconsistent basis. MCS is a relatively new clinical diagnosis that requires behavioral evidence of meaningful interaction. This may include command following, motor responses such as reaching for an object, intelligible verbalization, or the use of gestures to communicate.[4] MCS is sometimes misdiagnosed as vegetative state, because verification of meaningful responses can be difficult in patients who exhibit daily fluctuations in consciousness and who have meager available motor repertoires with which to follow commands.[5,6] Serial examinations over time and the use of a reliable standardized neurobehavioral rating scale are therefore recommended to improve diagnostic accuracy.[7]

However, even in the absence of behavioral evidence of consciousness, willful patterns of cortical activation have been demonstrated on functional magnetic resonance imaging (fMRI) in a small number of traumatically brain injured patients, indicative of some degree of awareness and cognition in patients who appeared vegetative. This finding suggests that fMRI may be a useful adjunct in distinguishing vegetative state from MCS.[8]

5.3 Neurophysiology of Arousal and Consciousness

Consciousness is a state of awareness dependent upon adequate arousal mechanisms, functioning selective attention, and the ability to perceive and interpret sensory information from the world around us. Arousal, the foundation of consciousness, depends upon multiple connections between the ascending reticular activating system (ARAS) and the cortex via subcortical relay stations. The ARAS originates in the brainstem and exerts its effects on higher cortical centers by way of collateral projections through the thalamus, posterior hypothalamus, and basal forebrain. The brainstem ARAS is comprised of several distinct nuclei that rely on a number of different neurotransmitters to activate rostral brain regions. Thus, redundancy is built into the systems that support our most basic of cognitive functions.

Dorsal projections from the brainstem ARAS reach the thalamus. The thalamus serves as the main relay and filtering station for ascending sensory information. Without the thalamus, most sensory input would not reach the cortex. Activation of the thalamic nuclei by cholinergic and glutaminergic fibers of the ARAS facilitates transmission of sensory input to higher cortical regions. The thalamic nuclei have both afferent and efferent connections with the cerebral cortex and brainstem. The thalamic reticular nucleus, in particular, is involved in the process of sensory gating. Gating of the stream of sensory data allows attention to be selectively focused on some aspects of sensory input and not others. The ascending pathways from the thalamus to the primary sensory areas of the cerebral cortex are predominantly glutaminergic. From the primary sensory areas, collateral connections proceed to the sensory association areas, where information is processed, interpreted, and consciously experienced.

The projections from the ventral ARAS modulate basal forebrain activation via catecholaminergic, glutaminergic, and cholinergic neurotransmission. Projections from the hypothalamus to the basal forebrain facilitate arousal through the release of histamine and orexin. The basal forebrain is located on the medial and ventral surface of the cerebral hemispheres. It acts as a ventral extrathalamic relay station between the ARAS and the cerebral cortex. The afferent connections from the basal forebrain to the cerebral cortex can be conceptualized as the most rostral part of the ARAS. These pathways mediate arousal and attention through both cholinergic and gamma aminobutyric acid (GABA)-ergic neurotransmission. Finally, additional connections with the limbic system, as well as regions involved in memory and executive function, allow us to interact with our environment in a genuinely meaningful way.

5.4 Neuroanatomic Substrates of Disorders of Consciousness

Given the widespread regions involved in the maintenance of arousal and attention, persistent disorders of consciousness may be the result of diverse pathology within the central nervous system. Injury may be seen in any part of the neuronal network important for arousal, including bilateral damage to the cerebral cortex, thalami, or subcortical white matter, or damage to the tegmentum of the rostral pons and midbrain.

Adams et al.[9] undertook a detailed neuropathologic study of the brains of 49 patients who remained in vegetative state until their deaths 1 month to 8 years after an acute brain insult. Although diffuse axonal injury was sometimes seen, the more common findings in this study were damage to the major relay nuclei of the thalamus or the subcortical white matter tracks. A few cases were identified in which the cerebral cortex and the brainstem were both of normal appearance. The authors concluded that damage to the thalamus essentially severed the connections between any preserved functioning cortex and other cortical or subcortical regions, resulting in vegetative state. Interestingly, neuropathologic studies of individuals in minimally conscious state have shown less consistent thalamic involvement, indicative of relative sparing of corticothalamic connections.[10]

Damage to the tegmentum of the brainstem, an area comprising part of the ARAS, may also result in loss of consciousness. In a retrospective study of magnetic resonance images (MRIs) from 47 patients with brainstem stroke, Parvizi and Damasio[11] found that all patients who remained comatose had lesions either in the pons alone or in the upper pons and midbrain. Lesions were bilateral in seven of nine cases. These findings suggest that lesions confined to the upper pons can cause coma in humans, even in the absence of damage to the midbrain. Parvizi and Damasio[11] excluded cases with lesions in the hypothalamus, basal forebrain, or bilateral cerebral cortex, because dysfunction in these sites can also impair consciousness.

Patrick et al.[12] examined the MRI patterns of brain damage in 17 children and adolescents (average age, 15 years) who remained at a Rancho Los Amigos level of III or less for at least 30 days following traumatic brain injury. Brainstem injury alone was strongly associated with the observed low response state with a predicted probability of .81. The combination of injury to the brainstem, basal ganglia, and thalamus increased the likelihood of a persistent low response state to .95.

5.5 Functional Neuroimaging in Disorders of Consciousness

Positron emission tomography and functional MRI (fMRI) data have been analyzed in patients in vegetative state and minimally conscious state in the presence of auditory stimulation or noxious sensory stimulation.[13–16] These imaging techniques have identified functioning islands of preserved cerebral cortex in patients in vegetative state. Because active areas of the brain require more oxygen, fMRI demonstrates these areas as hot spots. Coleman et al.[17] used fMRI to determine whether patients in vegetative state retain some aspects of language comprehension. Indeed, some evidence of activation of the primary auditory cortex was noted in response to spoken language. However, the authors conceded that these findings did not imply actual language comprehension or consciousness. For conscious awareness of speech to occur, language must be "heard" in the auditory primary cortex, recognized in the auditory association cortex, and finally, comprehended in Wernicke's area. Laureys et al.[18] found that, although auditory primary cortices are activated by auditory stimulation in the patient in vegetative state, the higher order association areas were not. They concluded that these functional disconnections preclude the integrated processing necessary for understanding, reflection, and awareness. Consistent with this view is the finding of some improvement in the disrupted connections between thalamic nuclei and their projections to the prefrontal and cingulate cortical regions in patients who have recovered consciousness.

5.6 Prognosis of Vegetative State

In 1994, the Multi-Society Task Force on Persistent Vegetative State (PVS)[19] performed a retrospective analysis of available outcome data for individuals who remained in a vegetative state for 1 month or more following either traumatic or nontraumatic injuries to the brain. The prognosis for recovery was found to be directly related to the duration of vegetative state and its cause.

Outcome data were available for 434 adult patients who had sustained traumatic brain injuries. Of those still in vegetative state 1 month after injury, 52% went on to recover consciousness by 1 year posttrauma. Of those still in vegetative state at 3 months following traumatic brain injury, 35% recovered consciousness by 1 year. The likelihood of recovery by 1 year postinjury fell to 16% for those who were still in a vegetative state at 6 months.

The Multi-Society Task Force on PVS[19] also examined the available outcome data for 169 adult patients who remained in vegetative state at 1 month after nontraumatic brain injuries, such as anoxia. Of those still in vegetative state 30 days after a nontraumatic brain injury, the chance of recovering consciousness at 1 year was only 15%. Among those still in vegetative state at 3 months postinsult, only 7% improved by 1 year. No patient who remained in vegetative state at 6 months recovered consciousness by 1 year.

Given the decreasing probability of recovery from vegetative state of increasing duration and the difference in prognosis associated with the cause of vegetative state (traumatic vs nontraumatic), the Multi-Society Task Force on PVS[19] suggested that the adjective *permanent* be applied to the term *vegetative state* 12 months after traumatic brain injury and 3 months after nontraumatic brain injury. The term *persistent* is applied when the duration of vegetative state exceeds 30 days.[20] However, the use of the terms *persistent vegetative state* and *permanent vegetative state* are the subject of some controversy as a result of rare cases of late recovery. The Aspen Group has proposed that the terminology *vegetative state* be used, accompanied by its duration and causes.[21]

Prognosis for recovery from vegetative state corresponds not only to the duration of vegetative state but also to age (with older patients having a poorer prognosis) and initial Glasgow Coma Scale score and likely corresponds to the findings on imaging studies discussed in the preceding sections of this chapter.

5.7 Enhancing the Potential for Recovery from Vegetative and Minimally Conscious States

5.7.1 Establish a Baseline of Neurologic Function

The patient's medical history must be thoroughly reviewed and careful serial examinations must be undertaken to document a neurologic baseline. Giacino et al.[22] have outlined a thoughtful approach to the assessment of the patient with a disorder of consciousness.

The assessment of arousal and cognitive content is but a part of a complete physical and neurologic examination. Cranial nerves should be evaluated because their function is a reflection of brainstem integrity. Muscle tone and abnormal posturing should be assessed. Severe spasticity or rigidity may preclude visible limb movement. In patients with disorders of consciousness, strength is inferred from observed spontaneous movement because formal manual muscle testing is not possible. Be aware of contractures that may limit movement. The patient's response to noxious stimulation should be assessed, and reflexes (normal and pathologic) should be noted.

When establishing a baseline of cognitive function, some general principals should be observed. All evaluations should be conducted in an environment free of competing stimuli. A period of observation at the outset of the evaluation is warranted to determine the frequency of spontaneous, nonpurposeful movement prior to evaluating the patient's ability to respond. Commands should be short, clear, and given at a time of day when the patient is typically most alert. Requests should target responses that are within the patient's available motor repertoire. Sufficient time should be allowed for an individual with slowed central processing to respond. Eye blinks are notoriously difficult to interpret because the average individual blinks spontaneously more than five times per minute. To optimize the chances of command following, requests should be repeated and one may wish to add visual demonstration to verbal requests. If it is difficult to determine whether an observed motor response is random, a simple command such as "Stop moving" or "Keep still" can be given. Limited cognitive endurance/attention should be considered. Most patients with disorders of consciousness will saturate relatively quickly and prolonged examinations are unlikely to elicit a patient's best performance.

Multistep instructions, which may include if/then and yes/no components, are significantly more difficult for patients to understand than simple one-step commands. During the early stages of recovery, patients generally have severe memory deficits, including impairments in working memory. When if/then requests are made, the patient may be unable to hold the first part of the command in working memory. As a result, they may follow the instruction given at the end of the sentence. For example, when asked, "If you are a man, then raise one finger," the female patient may proceed to move the designated body part, unrelated to any if/then or yes/no communicative intent. When assessing an individual's ability to accurately answer yes/no questions, it is essential to select simple questions that do not rely on the patient's impaired short-term memory as well as questions to which the clinician knows the answer.

When attempting to determine whether a patient has emerged from vegetative state, one should keep in mind that the first signs of recovery include the appearance of sustained visual fixation and tracking as well as localization to auditory or tactile stimuli. Thus, these are the goal behaviors for individuals in vegetative state. An examination targeting more complex behaviors may overlook these important emerging signs of meaningful interaction.

For those in MCS, recovery is contingent upon improvements in sustained attention and arousal. More accurate, reliable, and consistent command following, communication, and/or object discrimination will generally be seen as patients improve beyond MCS.[6]

Standardized rating scales should be used to assist in the evaluation of patients with disorders of consciousness. The Western Neuro Sensory Stimulation Profile, the JFK Coma Recovery Scale–Revised, and the Coma/Near-Coma Scale have all been used with some success.[5,7,23,24]

5.7.2 Rule Out Treatable Causes of Failure to Improve

Before considering the off-label prescription of activating medication, the physician should rule out treatable causes of the patient's failure to improve. This workup should include a noncontrast computed tomographic scan of the brain, neuroendocrine screening, an electroencephalogram, basic laboratory testing for the treatable causes of dementia, an assessment of the patient's general nutrition, and a review of the patient's sleep habits to diagnose possible disruptions in restorative sleep.

5.7.2.1 *Intracranial Complications*

Intracranial complications can impede recovery. A noncontrast computed tomographic brain scan is the screening test of choice to rule out the delayed development of complications such as hydrocephalus. Ventricular dilatation occurs in a large percentage of patients after severe brain injury, either as the result of cerebral atrophy, hydrocephalus, or both. Hydrocephalus can, therefore, present a diagnostic challenge, especially when it is superimposed on severe brain injury with some degree of associated encephalomalacia. In the awake and alert patient, the classic triad of dementia, ataxia of gait, and incontinence may be readily apparent. However, patients who are vegetative or minimally conscious are more difficult to evaluate. The physician should maintain a high index of suspicion in patients who have risk factors for the development of hydrocephalus, including a history of subarachnoid hemorrhage, intraventricular extension of blood, skull fractures (especially depressed skull fractures), and meningitis.[25] Hydrocephalus is generally treated with surgical placement of a ventriculoperitoneal shunt. In uncertain cases, a confirmatory test such as a cisternogram or lumbar tap test may be considered.[26] However, no single test or combination of tests has proven to be entirely accurate in predicting shunt responsiveness. Untreated, hydrocephalus will cause progressive neurologic decline in awake and alert patients. In vegetative patients, untreated hydrocephalus can preclude neurologic recovery. In those patients who fail to improve following shunt placement, a nuclear medicine shunt study can rule out suboptimal shunt function.

5.7.2.2 *Endocrine Dysfunction*

Endocrine dysfunction is also associated with traumatic brain injury. Kelly et al.[27] found that approximately 40% of patients with moderate or severe head injuries sustained post-traumatic pituitary hormonal insufficiency. The sodium and water abnormalities associated with posterior pituitary dysfunction (diabetes insipidus and syndrome of inappropriate antidiuretic hormone) are typically readily apparent to the general practitioner. However, the signs and symptoms of anterior pituitary dysfunction are frequently masked by the patient's neurologic deficits. Therefore, screening should include morning serum cortisol, free T_3, free T_4, thyroid-stimulating hormone, insulin-like growth factor (IGF-1), follicle-stimulating hormone, luteinizing hormone, testosterone (in men) or estradiol (in women), and prolactin levels. Because IGF-1 may lack adequate sensitivity, a provocative test such as an arginine infusion study may be warranted. If levels are abnormal or there is a high index of suspicion, the patient may be referred to an endocrinologist for further evaluation. Outcome may be optimized by the identification and treatment of pituitary dysfunction.[28]

5.7.2.3 *Subclinical Seizure Activity*

Subclinical seizure activity can preclude emergence from vegetative state. Seizures and nonconvulsive status epilepticus can be diagnosed electroencephalographically. After electroencephalographic confirmation, anticonvulsant treatment should be provided. Elimination of previously unrecognized ongoing seizure activity may markedly improve an individual's level of arousal and attention.

5.7.2.4 Laboratory Testing

Laboratory testing to screen for the abnormalities associated with reversible dementias may be useful. These tests include a vitamin B_{12} level, folate level, rapid plasma reagin, and thyroid-stimulating hormone. In the presence of abnormal liver function, one may consider checking a serum ammonia level, serum copper level, and ceruloplasmin. For the most part, these dementias are easy to diagnose and treat. Left untreated, however, they can negatively affect an individual's ability to improve neurologically.

5.7.2.5 Malnutrition

Malnutrition and an associated catabolic state may render patients less able to demonstrate robust neurologic recovery. Many patients with disorders of consciousness present to rehabilitation hospitals or long-term care facilities with a history of significant weight loss and laboratory indices consistent with malnutrition. Attention to adequate nutrition is a basic tenet of care of the brain-injured patient.

5.7.2.6 Sleep Disturbance

Sleep is closely linked to brain function. Mounting evidence supports the role of sleep in learning, memory, and neural plasticity.[29–32] Efforts should be made to normalize disturbed sleep–wake cycles. In addition, adequate time for restorative naps during the day should be scheduled.

5.7.3 Eliminate or Reduce Sedating Medications

Pharmacologic intervention should first focus on identifying and reducing or eliminating potentially sedating medication when possible. In a classic study by Temkin et al.,[33] the prescription of anticonvulsant therapy provided no reduction in the incidence of posttraumatic seizures beyond the first 7 days following acute severe head trauma. When continued anticonvulsant therapy is necessary, several issues warrant consideration. Trimble et al.[34,35] have demonstrated that anticonvulsant drug selection, blood levels, and combination drug therapy (polytherapy) have an effect on cognitive function. Higher drug levels, even within the therapeutic range, are associated with an increased incidence of adverse cognitive effects. Polytherapy is generally associated with greater impairment on neuropsychological testing than monotherapy.

Of the older anticonvulsant drugs, phenytoin (Dilantin) may have a larger negative effect on cognition than valproic acid (Depakote, Depakene). Among the newer generation anticonvulsants, evidence points to greater cognitive impairment with topiramate (Topamax) and zonisamide (Zonegran).[36–38] Gualtieri and Johnson[39] examined the differential cognitive effects of carbamazepine (Tegretol), oxcarbazepine (Trileptal), lamotrigine (Lamictal), topiramate, and valproic acid in 159 patients with bipolar disorder. Lamotrigine and oxcarbazepine were found to have the least negative effect on cognition. In a separate study, levetiracetam (Keppra) was found to have no effect on neuropsychological test performance across several cognitive domains in patients with focal epilepsy.[40]

In an uncontrolled preliminary study of the effect of lamotrigine on recovery from severe traumatic brain injury, 13 patients who remained at Rancho Los Amigos levels I to III for an average of 87.5 days after injury were switched from another anticonvulsant to lamotrigine.[41] Compared with the rehabilitation unit's general experience with similar patients, a trend toward improved outcomes, as evidenced by a greater percentage of home discharges, was observed. Given the small size of the study, lack of a control group, and treatment during a phase of spontaneous neurologic recovery, no firm conclusions can be drawn about the effect of switching to lamotrigine for facilitation of recovery.

Animal studies have demonstrated that a number of drugs may exert a positive or negative influence on the recovery of function following brain injury or stroke.[42–44] In a seminal study by Feeney et al.,[45] a single dose of d-amphetamine (which increases levels of the neurotransmitters norepinephrine and dopamine) was given 24 hours after unilateral motor cortex ablation in the rat. When coupled with the opportunity for training, a measurable and enduring improvement in motor recovery was documented, compared with injured control animals who did not receive d-amphetamine. Interestingly, animals who received a single dose of d-amphetamine, but who were restrained in cages too small to allow significant locomotion, did not show this facilitation of motor recovery. The investigators also found that the administration of a single dose of the dopamine receptor blocker haloperidol within 24 hours of unilateral motor cortex injury markedly slowed recovery of motor skills in the rat, even if an opportunity for training was allowed. This study elegantly demonstrated that medications can facilitate or inhibit motor recovery.

Goldstein[44] makes the case that neural plasticity and recovery from traumatic brain injury may be modulated by drugs that affect neurotransmitter systems. The weight of available experimental evidence supports avoiding medications that are dopamine or norepinephrine antagonists. This includes neuroleptics, metoclopramide (Reglan), and prochlorperazine (Compazine). Neuroleptic medications may prolong the period of posttraumatic amnesia.[46,47] Prazosin (Minipress) and terazosin (Hytrin) may inhibit noradrenergic neurotransmission via selective blocking of alpha-1 receptors. The alpha-2 selective adrenergic receptor agonist, clonidine (Catapres), has been found to inhibit motor recovery in animal models when given acutely after injury.[44] This alpha-2 agonist suppresses the release of norepinephrine from postganglionic sympathetic nerves. (See Chapter 4 in this text for a detailed discussion of commonly used medications and their effects on neurotransmitter systems.)

5.8 Pharmacologic Intervention to Enhance Arousal and Responsiveness

Medications that are prescribed to facilitate recovery from vegetative state and minimally conscious state are thought to exert their effects through the modulation of neurotransmitter systems. Our understanding of these systems is still evolving, and current research does not offer sufficient clinical evidence to support specific treatment recommendations. Nevertheless, empiric use of activating medication may be beneficial in the treatment of individuals with disorders of consciousness. The drugs used to facilitate neurologic recovery in these patients are generally well-known medications that are being used off-label. A discussion of herbal medications is outside the scope of this chapter.

Off-label prescribing is the physician practice of prescribing a drug for a purpose different from that for which it is approved by the Food and Drug Administration (FDA). It should be noted that the prescription of each of the medications to be discussed here for brain injury-induced disorders of consciousness is considered off-label. Legally, any approved product may be used for purposes other than that for which it has received FDA approval.[48] In other words, off-label prescribing is not illegal. Because there are no approved drugs for the treatment of certain diseases such as disorders of consciousness, and because the discovery of novel therapeutic applications of existing medications proceeds faster than the historically slow FDA review process, off-label use may reflect state-of-the-art treatment or even the standard of care. Physicians may wish to inform patients or their representatives of the intent to use a medication off-label.[49] As with all informed consent, the risks and benefits of both the proposed treatment and its alternatives should be discussed. If the intent of drug treatment is to provide potential patient benefit, it is not considered experimental and therefore approval of an institutional review board is not necessary. If, on the other hand, the drug is being prescribed to test a theory, then the intervention should be considered an experiment and institutional review board approval is recommended.

The rationale for neurotransmitter augmentation relates to known disturbances in neurotransmitter systems following brain injury. Immediately following brain trauma, acute neuroexcitation releases neurotransmitters, and the measured levels of glutamate, dopamine, norepinephrine, and acetylcholine are elevated. However, during the chronic phase, beginning more than 24 hours after injury and lasting for weeks to months, these neurotransmitter systems may be functionally depressed.[43] In theory, pharmacologic intervention may be able to normalize the equilibrium of neurotransmitter systems that have been altered by trauma.

Arciniegas and Silver[50] proposed that medication choices should be based on the hypothesized link between the neurotransmitter systems and the targeted cognitive process. Thus, posttraumatic impairments in arousal would be expected to be sensitive to catecholaminergic, cholinergic, histaminergic, and/or glutaminergic augmentation.

5.8.1 Catecholaminergic Neuromodulation

Dopamine and norepinephrine both fall under the category of catecholamine neurotransmitters. Each has been studied in the context of improving cognitive function after brain injury. Dopaminergic neurons are found in the hypothalamus and the substantia nigra of the midbrain, whereas noradrenergic neurons are primarily located in the locus ceruleus and lateral tegmentum of the brainstem. These neurons contribute to the ARAS and have been implicated in the maintenance of arousal and attention.

5.8.1.1 Dopaminergic Neuromodulation

5.8.1.1.1 Sinemet

Sinemet, a preparation of carbidopa and levodopa, increases dopamine synthesis presynaptically. In 1988, Lal et al.[51] explored the use of Sinemet for 12 patients who had sustained either traumatic brain injuries or hypoxic ischemic brain injuries. Sinemet was found to exert a favorable effect on measures of alertness, memory, posture, and speech.

Patrick et al.[52] studied 10 children (mean age, 13.7 years) who were 30 days or more posttraumatic brain injury. One of a variety of dopaminergic agents (either methylphenidate, pramipexole, amantadine, bromocriptine, or levodopa) was prescribed. The slope of the patients' premedication recovery curve was used for comparison against the rate of change observed on medication. A trend toward greater improvement over time was documented, using the Western Neuro Sensory Stimulation Profile, when the children were prescribed a dopaminergic drug. The authors concluded that dopamine-enhancing medications may accelerate recovery in children with reduced responsiveness. This small study was under-taken during the period of spontaneous recovery, within the first 3 to 4 months postinjury, making generalization of these results difficult.

Matsuda et al.[53] subsequently investigated the effect of dopaminergic augmentation in three patients who remained in persistent vegetative state after traumatic brain injury. All three patients had MRI evidence of high-intensity lesions within the dopaminergic pathway of the dorsolateral midbrain. In addition, all three exhibited physical findings consistent with parkinsonism, including rigidity, akinesia, and/or tremor. Rapid recovery within 1 to 4 weeks after initiation of Sinemet was seen in all patients.

Case 1 was a 14-year-old boy who had sustained a traumatic brain injury with an initial Glasgow Coma Scale score of IV. He remained in a vegetative state at 3 months postinjury, at which point benserazide/levodopa 25/100 mg twice daily was prescribed. Nine days later, he began to localize by turning his eyes toward voices. Twenty days after the initiation of levodopa, he was able to follow commands. One year later, he was able to walk to high school independently, and the medication was discontinued.

Case 2 was a 27-year-old man who had sustained a traumatic brain injury with an initial Glasgow Coma Scale score of IV. He remained in a vegetative state at 1 year postinjury, at which time levodopa was prescribed. Eight days later, he began to show evidence of visual tracking. Twenty-five days later, the medication was changed to benserazide/levodopa. At that point, he began to communicate yes and no via eye blinks. Ten months after the start of the medication (22 months after his injury), he began to use a word processor to communicate. One year after the drug was started, he was able to write, "I want to eat sushi and drink beer!"

Case 3 was a 51-year-old gentleman status posttraumatic brain injury with an initial Glasgow Coma Scale score of VI. Seven months after trauma, he remained in vegetative state. It was at this time that carbidopa/levodopa was initiated in a dose of 10/100 mg three times daily. Four days after the start of treatment, he was able to follow simple verbal commands for the first time. Two months after the medication was started, his tracheostomy tube was weaned and he was able to speak and state his name and address correctly. The authors concluded that levodopa treatment should be considered for patients with signs of parkinsonism and MRI findings of lesions in the dopaminergic pathways from the substantia nigra or tegmentum of the brainstem.

Levodopa works presynaptically and therefore requires relatively intact dopaminergic neurons to exert its effect. Matsuda et al.[54] contended that one should select a specific dopaminergic agent based on whether the drug acts presynaptically or postsynaptically, using neuroimaging studies to help guide drug selection. For example, if there is only incomplete damage to the substantia nigra or tegmentum, levodopa may be effective.[54] In the absence of contraindications, this drug is a reasonable choice to facilitate neurologic recovery in patients who have plateaued in vegetative or minimally conscious state.

When levodopa is administered alone, it is rapidly decarboxylated in the peripheral tissue so that only a small portion is left to cross the blood–brain barrier. The addition of carbidopa inhibits the inactivation of peripheral levodopa. Sinemet, which is a combination of levodopa and carbidopa, is FDA approved for use in Parkinson's disease and parkinsonian syndrome. Its use to facilitate improved alertness for brain-injured patients is off-label. The mean time to peak concentration of levodopa after a single dose of Sinemet is 0.5 hours. The plasma half-life of levodopa in the presence of carbidopa is approximately 1.5 hours. Extended-release preparations are available, such as Sinemet CR, which release the drug over a 4- to 6-hour period. Peak concentrations of levodopa are reached approximately

2 hours after a single dose of Sinemet CR 50/200. However, the bioavailability of levodopa from Sinemet CR is not has high as that in Sinemet. Therefore, the total daily dose of levodopa necessary to produce a clinical response is usually higher when using the sustained-release formulation.

Because of the risk of insomnia, it may be preferable to administer Sinemet two to three times per day, with the last dose given in the late afternoon. There are no specific guidelines regarding its use in vegetative state and minimally conscious state, and there is wide variation in how this drug is prescribed. It is estimated that 70 to 100 mg daily of carbidopa is necessary to saturate peripheral dopa decarboxylase. Therefore, patients who are receiving less than this amount of carbidopa may be more likely to experience nausea and vomiting. Upward titration of the dose should proceed carefully while observing for the possibility of side effects. Because patients with disorders of consciousness are unable to communicate that they are nauseated, gastric residuals should be carefully checked. If gastric residuals consistently exceed 70 to 100 mL, the dose should be decreased and/or a preparation with more carbidopa should be considered (i.e., changing from a single 25/250 [25 mg carbidopa and 250 mg levodopa] tablet to two tablets of 25/100 each).

Sinemet should be administered cautiously to patients with a history of myocardial infarct and/or atrial, nodal, or ventricular arrhythmias. Because of the possibility of adverse cardiac effects, it may be prudent to obtain an electrocardiogram (EKG) prior to the initiation of Sinemet, and to check a follow-up EKG a few days into treatment. Malignant melanoma and narrow-angle glaucoma are contraindications to use of this drug. Sinemet may also increase the possibility of an upper gastrointestinal hemorrhage in patients with a history of peptic ulcer disease. The most common adverse reactions seen with Sinemet are nausea, dyskinesias, and other involuntary movements. Psychosis may be seen in high-level patients on rare occasion. Neuroleptic malignant syndrome has been reported in association with rapid dose reductions or withdrawal of Sinemet. Sinemet should not be used with nonselective monoamine oxidase (MAO) inhibitors. Orthostatic hypotension may be observed when Sinemet is added to a drug regimen including antihypertensive medication, and adjustment of the dose of the antihypertensive drug or drugs may be necessary. The concommitant use of tricyclic antidepressants and Sinemet may rarely cause hypertension and dyskinesia.

Drugs that are dopamine receptor antagonists may reduce the effectiveness of Sinemet. Although Reglan may improve gastric emptying and thus increase bioavailability of Sinemet, its action as a dopamine receptor antagonist may adversely affect Sinemet's therapeutic efficacy.

5.8.1.1.2 *Amantadine Hydrochloride*

Originally designed as an antiviral medication, amantadine (Symmetrel) has been explored as an agent to facilitate recovery following severe traumatic brain injury. Amantadine enhances dopaminergic neurotransmission both pre- and postsynaptically. It facilitates dopamine release and blocks its reuptake presynaptically. Amantadine also increases the number of postsynaptic dopaminergic receptors and potentially alters their configuration. In addition, amantadine may help restore the balance between glutaminergic and dopaminergic neurotransmitter systems through its role as an *N*-methyl-*D*-aspartate (NMDA) antagonist. The NMDA receptor is one of several glutamate receptors.

In a single case design study by Zafonte et al.,[55] amantadine was prescribed to a 36-year-old man 5 months following a traumatic brain injury. His initial Glasgow Coma Scale score was III. His best performance prior to drug administration included only visual fixation and tracking. The dose of amantadine was gradually increased to 400 mg per day.

Neurologic improvements were subsequently noted, including command following. When the amantadine dose was reduced, a sharp deterioration in the patient's level of functioning was observed. With reinstitution of amantadine at a total daily dose of 400 mg, the patient went on to make significant progress in his rehabilitation program. He ultimately became independent in basic self-care and ambulation using a cane. Eight months after the injury, amantadine was discontinued and the patient maintained his neurologic gains. Thus, the authors suggest that amantadine may have a role in the treatment of patients in minimally conscious state.

In an 8-week, prospective, double-blind, randomized trial, Patrick et al.[56] assessed the effectiveness of the dopamine agonists amantadine and pramipexole (Mirapex) on the neurologic recovery of 10 children and adolescents who were at or below a Rancho Los Amigos level of III for at least 1 month following traumatic brain injury. The mean age of study participants was 16.7 years. Six of the 10 children were prescribed amantadine and four were prescribed pramipexole. Overall, the weekly rate of change, as measured with the Coma/Near-Coma Scale, Western Neuro Sensory Stimulation Profile, and Disability Rating Scale, was significantly better for those children who were prescribed a dopamine agonist medication than those who were not. No significant difference in efficacy was seen between the two drugs.

Meythaler et al.[57] conducted a double-blind, randomized pilot study to assess the effectiveness of amantadine in improving neurologic recovery following traumatic brain injury. A consistent trend toward more rapid functional improvement was demonstrated when amantadine was started within the first 3 months of injury. This study did not include patients in vegetative state. Although the results were promising, methodologic limitations of the study preclude drawing firm conclusions regarding the efficacy of amantadine in this setting.

Hughes et al.[58] studied 123 adults who remained at a Rancho level III or below when amantadine was prescribed at approximately 6 weeks postinjury. There were 28 patients who received amantadine and 95 who served as control subjects. Although amantadine was found to be safe, it had no measurable effect on either the duration of unconsciousness or the likelihood of recovery. However, significant spontaneous neurologic improvement probably occurred during the time that this study was conducted, making drug effect potentially difficult to detect.

Kraus et al.[59] evaluated the effect of amantadine in 22 traumatically brain-injured adults, the majority of whom were more than 1 year postinjury. The investigators hypothesized that amantadine would exert its effect in the prefrontal cortex. Neuropsychological testing demonstrated significant improvements in executive function, and analysis of positron emission tomographic data revealed a corresponding measurable increase in left prefrontal cortex glucose utilization.

Amantadine is approved for use in the prophylaxis and treatment of infection caused by various strains of influenza A virus. Amantadine is also used to treat parkinsonism and drug-induced extrapyramidal reactions. Its use for disorders of consciousness associated with brain injury is considered off-label.

Peak plasma concentration is achieved between 2 and 4 hours after oral administration. The half-life of amantadine averages 24 hours or less.

The most common adverse reactions associated with amantadine are nausea, dizziness, and insomnia. Because patients with disorders of consciousness are unable to complain of nausea, it is prudent to monitor gastric residuals in those individuals on tube feeding. If gastric residuals exceed 70 to 100 mL, the dose should be decreased or the drug should be discontinued to reduce the risk of emesis and aspiration. Less frequently reported are depression, anxiety, irritability, confusion, anorexia, dry mouth, constipation, diarrhea, ataxia, orthostatic hypotension, peripheral edema, headache, somnolence, lability, and fatigue. Rare instances of reversible liver enzyme abnormalities have been reported in patients receiving amantadine. It may cause mydriasis and should not be given to patients with untreated angle closure glaucoma. Furthermore, amantadine should not be discontinued abruptly because of the possibility of triggering neuroleptic malignant syndrome, especially if the patient is receiving neuroleptics concurrently. When given with triamterene/hydrochlorothiazide (Dyazide), an increase in blood levels of amantadine may occur, increasing the likelihood of adverse effects. Because of the possibility of adverse cardiac effects, it may be prudent to obtain an EKG prior to the initiation of amantadine and to check a follow-up EKG a few days into treatment.

Adult dosing may start at 50 mg once daily. The dose can be increased to a maximum of 400 mg per day, generally given in divided doses of 200 mg twice daily. An improvement in arousal may be apparent at doses of 100 mg twice daily. The dose should be reduced in patients with renal disease and in individuals age 65 and older.

5.8.1.1.3 Bromocriptine

Bromocriptine (Parlodel) is a nonselective dopamine receptor agonist that works post-synaptically primarily at D2 and less so at D1 receptor sites. Bromocriptine may have an advantage over other dopaminergic drugs that work presynaptically, in that it does not rely on intact dopaminergic neurons. Bromocriptine affects dopamine receptor sites directly. Therefore, if dopaminergic neurons are so severely damaged that no amount of presynaptic activation will result in sufficient dopamine release across the synaptic junction, then a direct dopamine agonist such as bromocriptine should be considered.

In a small study evaluating the effect of bromocriptine on recovery from vegetative state, Passler and Riggs[60] found that five adult patients who were in vegetative state for more than 30 days showed greater recovery of physical and cognitive function compared with patients described in previous outcome studies reported in the literature. However, the small sample size and the prescription of medication during a time of spontaneous recovery prohibits drawing firm conclusions from this study.

A double-blind, placebo-controlled, crossover design study with 24 high-level patients demonstrated that bromocriptine improved performance on tasks of executive function subserved by the prefrontal region, but it had no effect or a negative effect on working memory.[61] The effect of bromocriptine on working memory was subsequently evaluated by Gibbs and D'Esposito[62] using fMRI. Decreased activity during memory encoding was observed, suggesting that excess dopaminergic stimulation may result in impaired working memory encoding.

Bromocriptine is approved for use in the treatment of Parkinson's disease, hyperprolactinemia, and acromegaly. Its prescription for disorders of consciousness following brain injury is considered off-label use. Bromocriptine is generally started at 2.5 mg once daily. The dose can be increased gradually every few days as tolerated until an optimal response is seen. Adverse effects are more likely if the dose exceeds 20 mg daily.

Contraindications to the prescription of bromocriptine include uncontrolled hypertension and sensitivity to any ergot alkaloid. Use during pregnancy or the postpartum period is not recommended.

As with Sinemet, bromocriptine should be prescribed with caution to patients with a history of myocardial infarct and/or atrial, nodal, or ventricular arrhythmia. Because of the possibility of adverse cardiac effects, it may be prudent to obtain an EKG prior to the initiation of bromocriptine and to check a follow-up EKG a few days into treatment.

Adverse reactions include nausea, headache, dizziness, vomiting, fatigue, hypotension, and insomnia. The incidence of adverse effects is highest at the beginning of treatment and, as noted, with doses in excess of 20 mg daily. Blood pressure should be monitored closely during the first few days of drug administration.

5.8.1.1.4 Combination Dopaminergic Therapy

Kraus and Maki[63] assessed combined amantadine and carbidopa/levodopa therapy in the treatment of a 50-year-old woman with frontal lobe syndrome 5 years after her traumatic brain injury. Treatment with amantadine reduced some but not all of her symptoms. The addition of carbidopa/levodopa resulted in significant additional improvements. The robust effect of combined dopaminergic treatment was attributed to the differential effect of each agent on pre- and postsynaptic dopaminergic activity as well as on the role of amantadine as an NMDA glutamate receptor antagonist. These findings may have implications for the use of combination therapy in patients with disorders of consciousness.

I have found the combination of amantadine and Sinemet to be particularly powerful in improving the alertness of patients with disorders of consciousness (pers. obs.). However, more research is needed before any specific treatment regimen can be recommended.

5.8.1.2 Noradrenergic Neuromodulation

Stimulants such as methylphenidate (Ritalin), amphetamines (Dexedrine and Adderall), and atomoxetine (Strattera) have effects on arousal, attention, processing speed, distractibility, memory, and mood in healthy people. Therefore, their usefulness in the treatment of the cognitive deficits seen after brain injury has been the subject of much interest. However, their potential for exacerbating the tachycardia so frequently seen in the acute stages of recovery following brain injury may limit the patient's ability to tolerate these drugs. In addition, tricyclic antidepressants, which modulate several neurotransmitters including norepinephrine, have been explored as potential beneficial agents in the treatment of brain injury.

5.8.1.2.1 Methylphenidate

Methylphenidate (Ritalin) works presynaptically to increase the release of both dopamine and norepinephrine, thereby facilitating catecholaminergic neurotransmission. Thus, methylphenidate requires relatively intact catecholaminergic neurons to exert its presynaptic effect.

Methylphenidate is approved for the treatment of attention deficit hyperactivity disorder (ADHD) and narcolepsy. Its prescription for disorders of consciousness following brain injury is considered off-label.

Plenger et al.[64] studied the effect of methylphenidate on recovery from traumatic brain injury. They concluded that methylphenidate enhanced the rate of recovery but not the ultimate outcome following brain trauma. However, limitations of this study included small sample size, high dropout rate, and administration of the drug during the period of spontaneous recovery.

In two separate studies by Whyte et al.,[65,66] methylphenidate appeared to improve processing speed in awake and alert brain-injured patients. More recently, Martin and Whyte[67] assessed the effect of methylphenidate on patients in either vegetative state or minimally conscious state with disappointing results. In their rigorous single-subject, crossover design trials, methylphenidate had no effect on the level of arousal in either vegetative or minimally conscious state. In addition, no improvement in the accuracy of responses was observed in minimally conscious patients. Thus, the promising results of methylphenidate trials in higher level patients did not generalize to this patient population. However, the impact of methylphenidate in combination with medication that targets different aspects of neurotransmitter systems has not been systematically studied.

Methylphenidate is generally started at a dose of 5 mg twice daily. The dose can be increased gradually until an optimal response is achieved or intolerance develops. The usual dose prescribed in the rehabilitation setting is between 10 mg and 20 mg twice per day. Peak effect is observed between 30 minutes to 2 hours after drug administration. The duration of drug effect is approximately 3 to 6 hours. Generally, the first tablet is given upon awakening, with additional doses given at 4- to 6-hour intervals. To reduce the likelihood of insomnia, drug administration should be avoided in the evening. Longer acting preparations are available.

Adverse effects include insomnia, headache, nervousness, and anorexia. Modest increases in heart rate and blood pressure may be observed. Contraindications to the prescription of methylphenidate include serious structural cardiac abnormalities, cardiomyopathy, coronary heart disease, serious arrhythmias, and glaucoma. Use in pregnant or breast-feeding women and in individuals on MAO inhibitors should be avoided.

5.8.1.2.2 Amphetamines

Dextroamphetamine (Dexedrine) and Adderall (a mixture of dextroamphetamine and racemic amphetamine) work presynaptically to increase the levels of both norepinephrine and dopamine. Thus, amphetamines require relatively intact catecholaminergic neurons to exert their effect. In addition, amphetamines inhibit the reuptake of serotonin, increasing available serotonin, a monoamine neurotransmitter that normalizes mood and sleep and reduces nociception. Despite the promising results seen in Feeney's[45] rat model of amphetamine-enhanced motor recovery, at this time, no compelling evidence exists that definitively supports the use of amphetamines for disorders of consciousness.

Amphetamines are approved for the treatment of narcolepsy and ADHD, and as a short-term adjunct to calorie restriction and behavior modification for the management of obesity. The prescription of amphetamines for disorders of consciousness following brain injury is considered off-label use.

Amphetamines are typically started at a dose of 5 mg twice per day. The dose may be raised by 5 to 10 mg at weekly intervals until an optimal response is achieved or intolerance develops. The usual adult dose varies between 10 mg and 20 mg twice per day in the rehabilitation setting. Peak effect is observed between 30 minutes and 60 minutes after drug administration. Typically, the first tablet is given upon awakening, with additional doses given at 4- to 6-hour intervals. To reduce the likelihood of insomnia, drug administration should be avoided in the evening. Extended-release preparations are available.

Amphetamines are contraindicated in the presence of advanced arteriosclerosis, heart failure, recent myocardial infarction, serious cardiac structural abnormalities, coronary artery disease, cardiac arrhythmias, cardiomyopathy, moderate to severe hypertension, hyperthyroidism, agitated states, and glaucoma, and in individuals with known hypersensitivity to sympathomimetic amines. Pregnant or breast-feeding women and individuals on MAO inhibitors should avoid taking amphetamines. Although a history of drug abuse is a relative contraindication, this may be a moot point for patients with disorders of consciousness. Serious cardiovascular effects can be seen if amphetamines are administered with tricyclic antidepressants, resulting from marked increases in the concentration of the amphetamine. Adverse effects include hypertension, palpitations, tachycardia, dizziness, psychosis, insomnia, dyskinesia, headaches, tremor, dryness of the mouth, anorexia, weight loss, urticaria, and impotence.

5.8.1.2.3 Atomoxetine

Atomoxetine (Strattera) is a selective norepinephrine reuptake inhibitor that is approved for use in the treatment of ADHD. Atomoxetine may also increase levels of dopamine and acetylcholine. Its prescription for disorders of consciousness following brain injury is considered off-label use.

Murdock and Hamm[68] assessed the effect of atomoxetine given within 24 hours of moderate traumatic brain injury in rats. They found that the atomoxetine-treated animals had measurably less cognitive deficits than saline-treated animals. However, in a separate experiment, it was found that if atomoxetine treatment was delayed for 10 days after brain trauma and provided on days 11 through 29 after injury, the treated animals developed greater cognitive impairment. Therefore, it is clear that the timing of drug administration may influence its potential impact on the central nervous system.[43]

There are no clinical studies evaluating the efficacy of atomoxetine for prolonged disorders of consciousness following traumatic brain injury. However, Ripley[69] asserts that, theoretically, this norepinephrine reuptake inhibitor may be useful if added to agents that affect different aspects of the catecholaminergic neurotransmitter systems.

Strattera should not be taken with an MAO inhibitor or within 2 weeks of discontinuing an MAO inhibitor. Use of Strattera is contraindicated in the presence of narrow-angle glaucoma. Liver function should be monitored while on Strattera and dosage adjustment is recommended for patients with liver disease. Uncommon allergic reactions including angioneurotic edema, urticaria, and rash have also been reported in patients taking Strattera. Because Strattera can increase blood pressure and heart rate, it should be used with caution in patients with hypertension, tachycardia, or cardiovascular disease. Orthostatic hypotension and urinary retention have also been described. The dose of atomoxetine may need to be reduced when the drug is administered with paroxetine (Paxil), fluoxetine (Prozac), and quinidine.

Adverse events in patients treated with Strattera include dyspepsia, nausea, vomiting, fatigue, reduced appetite, dizziness, insomnia, urinary retention, and mood swings. Aggression, irritability, somnolence, and vomiting are generally the main reasons for discontinuation of the drug.

5.8.1.2.4 Tricyclic Antidepressants

Tricyclic antidepressants including desipramine (Norpramin), protriptyline (Vivactil), doxepin (Sinequan), imipramine (Tofranil), amitriptyline (Elavil), and nortriptyline (Pamelor) are FDA approved for the treatment of depression, panic disorder, obsessive–compulsive disorder, ADHD, migraine headaches, eating disorders, and bipolar disorder. Tricyclic antidepressants may affect widespread neurotransmitter systems. These drugs selectively block norepinephrine reuptake, thereby increasing available norepinephrine in the central nervous system. Tricyclic antidepressants may also inhibit the reuptake of serotonin, thereby potentiating its effects. In addition, tricyclic antidepressants exhibit significant anticholinergic and antihistaminergic properties.

Reinhard et al.[70] examined the effects of tricyclic antidepressants in three brain-injured patients. Case 1 was a 27-year-old man in a minimally conscious state 6 months postinjury. He was started on amitriptyline 50 mg daily, and within several days, he began to verbalize and respond to yes/no questions. By 7 months postinjury, he was able to begin gait training. When the amitriptyline was discontinued, his level of responsiveness deteriorated and his verbalizations ceased. With reinstatement of the drug, he once again improved. Case 2 was a 23-year-old woman at a Rancho Los Amigos level III, 2 months postinjury. Desipramine was started and gradually increased to a total daily dose of 50 mg. Following administration of the drug, she began to follow commands. Three months later, the desipramine was gradually discontinued, and the patient became lethargic. When the drug was resumed, once again there was a rapid improvement in her level of alertness and function. Case 3 was a 26-year-old man who remained in a minimally conscious state for 19 months. He was prescribed desipramine, 75 mg daily. Four days later, he began to verbalize single words for the first time. Within months, he was able to communicate effectively. When the desipramine was discontinued several months later, there was no deterioration in his level of function. In all three cases, there was a close temporal relationship between the neurologic improvement and the prescription of a tricyclic antidepressant. In two of the three cases, the level of arousal deteriorated when the drug was withdrawn, and improved when the drug was resumed, supporting the contention that the tricyclic antidepressant was responsible for the change in neurologic status.

Tricyclic antidepressants may be administered once a day because of their long half-life. Most adverse effects reflect the anticholinergic and central nervous system properties of this class of drugs. Thus, in the population of patients with disorders of consciousness, the primary relevant concerns include urinary retention, gastroesophageal reflux with possible aspiration of stomach contents, and lowering of seizure threshold. Although drowsiness is common, some patients may demonstrate restlessness and insomnia. The presence of glaucoma, cardiovascular disease, or the concomitant administration of MAO inhibitors are contraindications to use of tricyclics.

In addition, drug interactions may be serious. Sympathomimetic medication, such as amphetamines, should not be given with tricyclic antidepressants because of the possibility of fatal pressor and cardiac effects. Coadministration of tricyclics with levodopa may delay gastric emptying of levodopa, allowing for its inactivation. Caution should also be exercised when prescribing tricyclic antidepressants to patients on thyroid medication.

5.8.2 Glutamatergic Neuromodulation

One of the important excitatory neurotransmitters in the central nervous system is L-glutamic acid (glutamate). Glutamate is synthesized in the brain and it serves not only as an excitatory amino acid neurotransmitter, it is also the precursor of GABA. In the hours immediately after traumatic brain injury, glutamate is responsible for some degree of excitotoxic brain damage. Following injury, excess glutamate is associated with increased seizure risk. However, because glutamate is involved in normal cognitive processes, there may be a place for modulation of this neurotransmitter to improve cognitive function in chronic brain injury.

5.8.2.1 Modafinil

Modafinil (Provigil) is a central nervous system stimulant that is pharmacologically distinct from other stimulants. Modafinil likely exerts its effects through several neurotransmitters, including the catecholaminergic and serotonergic systems. In addition, modafinil may reduce GABA release and increase the release of glutamate.[71]

Lin et al.[72] used immunocytochemistry techniques to differentiate the potential brain neuronal targets for amphetamine, methylphenidate, and modafinil-induced wakefulness in the cat. Amphetamines and methylphenidate administration caused increased activity in widespread areas of the cortex, including the caudate nucleus and medial frontal cortex. However, cats treated with modafinil demonstrated activity in the anterior hypothalamus, hippocampus, and amygdala. Because of its relatively unique mechanism of action among the activating medications, modafinil may have a place either as a single agent or in combination therapy with other activating drugs if monotherapy is ineffective.

Modafinil treatment of 10 brain-injured outpatients with excessive daytime sleepiness was described by Teitelman.[73] Moderate to marked improvements in subjective feelings of wakefulness and well-being were reported. Formal neuropsychological testing was not performed.

Modafinil is approved for use in narcolepsy, obstructive sleep apnea/hypopnea syndrome, and shift work sleep disorder. Although modafinil has been used in the treatment of states of hypoarousal following brain injury, its use for disorders of consciousness is considered off-label.

Peak plasma concentration occurs roughly 2 to 4 hours after each dose. Because the primary route of modafinil elimination is via metabolism through the liver, the dose should be reduced in patients with severe liver disease.

Serious rashes have been reported in patients taking modafinil, and this requires prompt discontinuation of the drug. Multiorgan hypersensitivity reactions, with diverse signs and symptoms, including fever and rash with other organ system involvement, have been reported. Psychiatric symptoms may develop in association with modafinil and may necessitate discontinuation of the drug. Insomnia has been reported as well. Modafinil has not been evaluated in patients with a recent history of myocardial infarct or unstable angina. Modafinil should not be used in patients with a history of left ventricular hypertrophy or mitral valve prolapse syndrome.

Adverse effects associated with modafinil include headaches, nausea, vomiting, nervousness, rhinitis, diarrhea, back pain, anxiety, insomnia, dizziness, and dyspepsia. Because patients with disorders of consciousness are unable to communicate that they are nauseated, gastric residuals should be carefully checked. If gastric residuals consistently exceed 70 to 100 mL, the dose should be decreased or the drug should be discontinued to avoid emesis and aspiration.

The recommended dose of modafinil is 200 mg once daily. Although doses have been prescribed up to 400 mg per day, there is no compelling evidence to suggest that a higher dose confers additional benefit. Patients with severe liver disease should receive a reduced dose of modafinil.

Modafinil may affect the elimination of diazepam, propranolol, and phenytoin, necessitating their possible dose reduction. Modafinil may cause increased blood levels of tricyclics in some patients. However, no significant change in pharmacokinetics has been identified when modafinil is prescribed with either amphetamines or methylphenidate.

5.8.3 Gamma Aminobutyric Acid Neuromodulation

GABA is a major inhibitory neurotransmitter. Medications such as diazepam (Valium), lorazepam (Ativan), and baclofen (Lioresal) facilitate GABA neurotransmission.

5.8.3.1 Benzodiazepines

Benzodiazepines reduce spasticity and suppress seizures with generally negative effects on memory and overall cognition. Nevertheless, there are isolated case reports of recovery from poorly responsive states following administration of Valium. A 45-year-old Wisconsin man, in a vegetative state for 8 years, reportedly improved significantly after being injected with Valium for a routine dental procedure.[74] When medicated, he was able to talk and perform complicated mathematical calculations. How benzodiazepines may produce this paradoxic effect is unknown. They may work by reducing abnormal tone to the point that patients, who were previously dominated by severe spasticity, can demonstrate volitional movement to command. Alternatively, benzodiazepines may temporarily abort subclinical seizure activity. Referring to cases of very late emergence from vegetative state, Wijdicks[75] raises the question of recovery versus discovery. He suggests that "miracle cases" of late recovery may in fact represent late discovery of existing neurologic function that had previously gone unrecognized.

5.8.3.2 Zolpidem (Ambien)

Zolpidem facilitates GABA neurotransmission. It is a nonbenzodiazepine hypnotic of the imidazopyridine class. Benzodiazepines bind nonselectively to all omega receptor subtypes of the $GABA_A$ receptor complex. Zolpidem, however, stimulates GABA neurotransmission by selectively binding to only omega 1 receptors.

Clauss and Nel[76] studied the effect of Zolpidem on three patients who had been in vegetative state for at least 3 years. Prior to drug administration, the patients' Rancho Los Amigos levels ranged from I to II and their Glasgow Coma Scale scores were between VI and IX. All three patients regained transient awareness and the ability to follow commands and communicate for up to 4 hours after drug administration. One hour after drug administration, Rancho Los Amigos levels increased to between V and VII, and Glasgow Coma Scale scores ranged from X to XV. It is noteworthy that all of the patients who emerged from vegetative state did so within 1 hour on the first day that the drug was administered. However, all three patients returned to vegetative state daily when the effect of the medication subsided. Clauss and Nel[76] postulated that brain injury triggers a state of dormancy of normal unaffected brain tissue called *diaschisis* and that the symptoms exhibited by brain-injured patients are the result of a combination of damaged brain tissue as well as dormant brain tissue. Reversal of diaschisis and neurodormancy was proposed to explain the drug effect. In a separate study of four brain-injured patients, three were found to have poor tracer uptake in the areas of brain damage as well as in undamaged areas of the cerebellum, consistent with cerebellar diaschisis.[77] After Zolpidem administration, cerebral perfusion in the areas of brain injury improved measurably, and the cerebellar diaschisis was completely reversed. Thus, to the extent that GABA receptor-based diaschisis contributes to the persistence of impaired consciousness, Zolpidem may be an effective treatment.

Zolpidem is available in 5-mg and 10-mg tablets. It has been approved for the short-term treatment of insomnia. Use for disorders of consciousness is considered off-label. The initial dose for adults with disorders of consciousness or patients with hepatic insufficiency is 5 mg. The dose of Zolpidem may be increased but should not exceed 10 mg. Peak concentration is typically achieved 1 to 2 hours after oral administration. It is short acting, with a half-life of up to 4 hours. The most common adverse effects are dizziness, drowsiness, and diarrhea.

5.8.4 Cholinergic Neuromodulation

Medications that facilitate cholinergic neurotransmission are strongly associated with their impact on arousal and memory, particularly in patients with dementia. Cholinergic neurotransmission has also been found to be partly responsible for some aspects of attention and may improve signal to noise processing in the cortex.[78]

Activation of the thalamus, through the cholinergic projections of the ARAS, facilitates transmission of sensory input to higher cortical regions. The ventral projections from the brainstem ARAS modulate basal forebrain activation via catecholaminergic, glutaminergic, and cholinergic neurotransmission. In turn, the pathways from the basal forebrain to the cerebral cortex mediate arousal and attention through cholinergic and GABAergic systems. The cholinergic neurons of the forebrain and hippocampus are particularly susceptible to damage during head trauma as a result of their location near the bony prominences of the skull.

After a state of cholinergic hyperactivity seen in acute traumatic brain injury, the chronic phase of recovery is associated with reduced cholinergic activity.[79] Some aspects of brain injury-induced cognitive impairments in attention and memory have been attributed to this posttraumatic disruption of cholinergic function.[80,81]

The drugs most commonly used to increase the concentration of acetylcholine at cholinergic synapses are cholinesterase inhibitors, which reduce the breakdown of acetylcholine. This class of drugs includes donepezil (Aricept), galantamine (Reminyl), rivastigmine (Exelon), and tacrine (Cognex).

Zhang et al.[82] examined the effects of donepezil on memory and attention in 18 brain-injured patients who were able to participate in neuropsychological testing. The mean time since injury was 4.6 months and the average Glasgow Coma Scale score, measured between 24 and 48 hours of injury, was IX. In a 24-week, randomized, placebo-controlled, double-blind crossover trial, this pilot study demonstrated improved scores on tests of both sustained attention and short-term memory. These improvements were maintained through the final testing, which was performed 14 weeks after the medication had been terminated. The authors hypothesized that this lasting drug effect might be attributable to long-term alteration of the cholinergic system. Khateb et al.[83] studied the effects of donepezil on 10 patients whose head injury had occurred at least 6 months previously. Although the study did not include a control group, significantly improved performance in divided attention, learning, and speed of processing was documented on the drug. Walker et al.[84] retrospectively examined the effects of donepezil during the acute inpatient rehabilitation of 36 patients with moderate to severe brain injuries. Patients were enrolled in this study within 90 days of injury. No differences were seen between the treatment group and a matched control group in outcome, as measured by the Functional Independence Measure Cognitive Total Score and rehabilitation length of stay. However, there was a trend toward a greater rate of improvement in global cognitive functioning if patients were started on donepezil early during their inpatient rehabilitation program. The authors suggested that perhaps the measurement tools used in this pilot study may have been too crude to detect subtle improvements in cognition. At this time, there are no controlled studies examining the effect of cholinergic modulation on recovery from vegetative state or minimally conscious state.

For the treatment of dementia of the Alzheimer's type, the recommended initial dosage of donepezil is 5 mg daily. The dose may be increased to a maximum of 10 mg daily. As with the other medications reviewed in this chapter, the use of this drug is considered off-label when prescribed for disorders of consciousness.

Cholinesterase inhibitors should be used with caution in patients with bradycardia or cardiac conduction abnormalities and in patients with asthma or obstructive pulmonary disease. Common side effects include nausea, vomiting, diarrhea, fatigue, insomnia, muscle cramping, and anorexia.

5.8.5 Histaminergic Neuromodulation

Histamine, which is synthesized in the hypothalamus, may have a role in maintaining arousal. Supporting this contention are recent animal studies that demonstrate that histidine decarboxylase knockout mice are unable to remain awake when high task vigilance is required.[85] Furthermore, narcoleptic dogs have been found to have a histamine deficiency.[86] The interaction between histaminergic and other neurotransmitters systems is the subject of considerable research at this time.[87] Although no histaminergic agents are available as yet, this neurotransmitter holds great promise for future use in the treatment of disorders of consciousness.

5.9 Conclusion

The neural construct of consciousness involves multiple overlapping anatomic pathways and diverse neurotransmitter systems. How chronic neurotransmitter dysfunction affects receptor sensitivity or produces adaptive changes in other neuronal systems is largely unknown. Augmentation of a single neurotransmitter system may have far-reaching effects on other neurochemical networks.

Patients with disorders of consciousness may have a range of underlying neuroanatomic and neurochemical alterations. However, currently we are unable to identify precisely which neurotransmitter systems are functionally depressed in individual patients. As our ability to detect these unique differences among patients improves, the term *disorders of consciousness* will likely be replaced with more exact diagnoses that reflect the distinct anatomic and neurochemical systems involved. These advances will hopefully allow new and effective therapeutic agents to be developed to improve the lives of brain injury survivors.

References

1. Plum, F. and Posner, J., *The Diagnosis of Stupor and Coma*, 3rd ed., F. A. Davis, Philadelphia, PA, 1982.
2. Jennett, B. and Plum, F., Persistent vegetative state after brain damage: A syndrome in search of a name, *Lancet*, 1(7753), 734–737, 1972.
3. Multi-Society Task Force on PVS, Medical aspects of the persistent vegetative state (Pt. 1 of 2), *New England Journal of Medicine*, 330(21), 1499–1508, 1994.
4. Giacino, J. T. and Kalmar, K., Diagnostic and prognostic guidelines for the vegetative and minimally conscious states, *Neuropsychological Rehabilitation*, 15(3–4), 166–174, 2005.
5. Childs, N. L., Mercer, W. N., and Childs, H. W., Accuracy of diagnosis of persistent vegetative state, *Neurology*, 43(8), 1465–1467, 1993.
6. Giacino, J. T., Kalmar, K., and Whyte, J., The JFK Coma Recovery Scale–Revised: Measurement characteristics and diagnostic utility, *Archives of Physical Medicine and Rehabilitation*, 85(12), 2020–2029, 2004.
7. Schnakers, C., Vanhaudenhuyse, A., Giacino, J., Ventura, M., Boly, M., Majerus, S., Moonen, G., and Laureys S., Diagnostic accuracy of the vegetative and minimally conscious state: Clinical consensus vs. standardized neurobehavioral assessment, *BMC Neurology*, 9(35), 2009.

8. Monti, M. M., Vanhaudenhuyse A., Coleman, M. R., Boly, M., Pickard, J. D., Tshibanda, L., Owen, A. M., and Laureys, S., Willful modulation of brain activity in disorders of consciousness, *New England Journal of Medicine*. DOI: 10.1056/NEJMoa0905370, 2010.

9. Adams, J. H., Graham, D. I., and Jennett, B., The neuropathology of the vegetative state after an acute brain insult, *Brain*, 123(Pt. 7), 1327–1338, 2000.

10. Jennett, B., Adams, J. H., Murray, L. S., and Graham, D. I., Neuropathology in vegetative and severely disabled patients after head injury, *Neurology*, 56(4), 486–490, 2001.

11. Parvizi, J. and Damasio, A. R., Neuroanatomical correlates of brainstem coma, *Brain*, 126(Pt. 7), 1524–1536, 2003.

12. Patrick, P. D., Mabry, J. L., Gurka, M. J., Buck, M. L., Boatwright, E., and Blackman, J. A., MRI patterns in prolonged low response states following traumatic brain injury in children and adolescents, *Brain Injury*, 21(1), 63–68, 2007.

13. Schiff, N. D., Ribary, U., Moreno, D. R., Beattie, B., Kronberg, E., Blassberg, R., Giacino, J., et al., Residual cerebral activity and behavioral fragments can remain in the persistently vegetative brain, *Brain*, 125(Pt. 6), 1210–1224, 2002.

14. Laureys, S., Faymonville, M. E., Degueldre, C., Fiore, G. D., Damas, P., Lambermont, B., Janssens, N., et al., Auditory processing in the vegetative state, *Brain*, 123(Pt. 8), 1589–1601, 2000.

15. Laureys, S., Faymonville, M. E., Peigneux, P., Damas, P., Lambermont, B., Del Fiore, G., Degueldre, C., et al., Cortical processing of noxious somatosensory stimuli in the persistent vegetative state, *NeuroImage*, 17(2), 732–741, 2002.

16. Owen, A. M., Coleman, M. R., Menon, D. K., Johnsrude, I. S., Rodd, J. M., Davis, M. H., Taylor, K., and Pickard, J. D., Residual auditory function in persistent vegetative state: A combined PET and fMRI study, *Neuropsychological Rehabilitation*, 15(3–4), 290–306, 2005.

17. Coleman, M. R., Rodd, J. M., Davis, M. H., Johnsrude, I. S., Menon, D. K., Pickard, J. D., and Owen, A. M., Do vegetative patients retain aspects of language comprehension? Evidence from fMRI, *Brain*, 130(Pt. 10), 2494–2507, 2007.

18. Laureys, S., Faymonville, M. E., Luxen, A., Lamy, M., Franck, G., and Maquet, P., Restoration of thalamocortical connectivity after recovery from persistent vegetative state, *Lancet*, 355(9217), 1790–1791, 2000.

19. The Multi-Society Task Force on PVS, Medical aspects of the persistent vegetative state (Pt. 2 of 2), *New England Journal of Medicine*, 330(22), 1572–1579, 1994.

20. The Quality Standards Subcommittee of the American Academy of Neurology, Practice parameters: Assessment and management of patients in the persistent vegetative state (summary statement), *Neurology*, 45(5), 1015–1018, 1995.

21. Giacino, J. T., Zasler, N. D., Katz, D. I., Kelly, J. P., Rosenberg, J. H., and Filley, C. M., Development of practice guidelines for assessment and management of the vegetative and minimally conscious states, *Journal of Head Trauma Rehabilitation*, 12(4), 79–89, 1997.

22. Giacino, J. T., Ashwal, S., Childs, N., Cranford, R., Jennett, B., Katz, D. I., Kelly, J. P., et al., The minimally conscious state: Definition and diagnostic criteria, *Neurology*, 58(3), 349–353, 2002.

23. Ansell, B. J. and Keenan, J. E., The Western Neuro Sensory Stimulation Profile: A tool for assessing slow-to-recover head-injured patients, *Archives of Physical Medicine and Rehabilitation*, 70(2), 104–108, 1989.

24. Rappaport, M., Dougherty, A. M., and Kelting, D. L., Evaluation of coma and vegetative states, *Archives of Physical Medicine and Rehabilitation*, 73(7), 628–634, 1992.

25. Beryl, B. and Black, P. M., Posttraumatic hydrocephalus, *Neurosurgery*, 15(2), 257–261, 1984.

26. Doherty, D., Post-traumatic hydrocephalus, *Physical Medicine and Rehabilitation Clinics of North America*, 3(2), 389–405, 1992.

27. Kelly, D. F., Gonzalo, I. T., Cohan, P., Berman, N., Swerdloff, R., and Wang, C., Hypopituitarism following traumatic brain injury and aneurysmal subarachnoid hemorrhage: A preliminary report, *Journal of Neurosurgery*, 93(5), 743–752, 2000.

28. Urban, R. J., Harris, P., and Masel, B., Anterior hypopituitarism following traumatic brain injury, *Brain Injury*, 19(5), 349–358, 2005.

29. Dang-Vu, T. T., Desseilles, M., Peigneux, P., and Maquet, P., A role for sleep in brain plasticity, *Pediatric Rehabilitation*, 9(2), 98–118, 2006.

30. Walker, M. P., Issues surrounding sleep-dependent memory consolidation and plasticity, *Cellular and Molecular Life Sciences*, 61(24), 3009–3015, 2004.

31. Ferrara, M., Iaria, G., De Gennaro, L., Guariglia, C., Curcio, G., Tempesta, D., and Bertini, M., The role of sleep in the consolidation of route learning in humans: A behavioural study, *Brain Research Bulletin*, 71(1–3), 4–9, 2006.

32. Rauchs, G., Bertran, F., Guillery-Girard, B., Desgranges, B., Kerrouche, N., Denise, P., Foret, J., and Eustache, F., Consolidation of strictly episodic memories mainly requires rapid eye movement sleep, *Sleep*, 27(3), 395–401, 2004.

33. Temkin, N. R., Dikmen, S. S., Wilensky, A. J., Keihm, J., Chabal, S., and Winn, H. R., A randomized, double-blind study of phenytoin for the prevention of post-traumatic seizures, *New England Journal of Medicine*, 323(8), 497–502, 1990.

34. Trimble, M. R., Anticonvulsant drugs and cognitive function: A review of the literature, *Epilepsia*, 28(Suppl. 3), S37–S45, 1987.

35. Thompson, P. J. and Trimble, M. R., Anticonvulsant serum levels: Relationship to impairments of cognitive functioning, *Journal of Neurology, Neurosurgery, and Psychiatry*, 46(3), 227–233, 1983.

36. Thompson, P. J., Baxendale, S. A., Duncan, J. S., and Sander, J. W., Effects of topiramate on cognitive function, *Journal of Neurology, Neurosurgery, and Psychiatry*, 69(5), 636–641, 2000.

37. Mula, M., Trimble, M., Thompson, P., and Sander, J. W., Topiramate and word-finding difficulties in patients with epilepsy, *Neurology*, 60(7), 1104–1107, 2003.

38. Goldberg, J. F. and Burdick, K. E., Cognitive side effects of anticonvulsants, *Journal of Clinical Psychiatry*, 62(Suppl. 14), 27–33, 2001.

39. Gualtieri, C. T. and Johnson, L. G., Comparative neurocognitive effects of 5 psychotropic anticonvulsants and lithium, *Medscape General Medicine*, 8(3), 46–55, 2006.

40. Meador, K. J., Cognitive effects of levetiracetam versus topiramate, *Epilepsy Currents*, 8(3), 64–65, 2008.

41. Showalter, P. E. and Kimmel, D. N., Stimulating consciousness and cognition following severe brain injury: A new potential clinical use for lamotrigine, *Brain Injury*, 14(11), 997–1001, 2000.

42. Kokiko, O. N. and Hamm, R. J., A review of pharmacological treatments used in experimental models of traumatic brain injury, *Brain Injury*, 21(3), 259–274, 2007.

43. Goldstein, L. B. and Davis, J. N., Clonidine impairs recovery of beam-walking after a sensorimotor cortex lesion in the rat, *Brain Research*, 508(2), 305–309, 1990.

44. Goldstein, L. B., Neuropharmacology of TBI-induced plasticity, *Brain Injury*, 17(8), 685–694, 2003.

45. Feeney, D. M., Gonzalez, A., and Law, W. A., Amphetamine, haloperidol, and experience interact to affect the rate of recovery after motor cortex injury, *Science*, 217(4562), 855–857, 1982.

46. Rao, N., Jellinek, H. M., and Woolfton, D. C., Agitation in closed head injury: Haloperidol effects on rehabilitation outcome, *Archives of Physical Medicine and Rehabilitation*, 66(1), 30–34, 1985.

47. Mysiw, W. J., Bogner, J. A., Corrigan, J. D., Fugate, L. P., Clinchot, D. M., and Kadyan, V., The impact of acute care medications on rehabilitation outcome after traumatic brain injury, *Brain Injury*, 20(9), 905–911, 2006.

48. Center for Drug Evaluation and Research (CDER), U.S. Food and Drug Administration, Oncology tools: A short tour, 2003, http://www.fda.gov/cder/cancer/tour.htm.

49. Beck, J. M. and Azari, E. D., FDA, off-label use, and informed consent: Debunking myths and misconceptions, *Food and Drug Law Journal*, 53(1), 71–104, 1998.

50. Arciniegas, D. B. and Silver, J. M., Pharmacotherapy of posttraumatic cognitive impairments, *Behavioral Neurology*, 17(1), 25–42, 2006.

51. Lal, S., Merbitz, C., and Grip, J. C., Modification of function in head-injured patients with Sinemet, *Brain Injury*, 2(3), 225–233, 1990.

52. Patrick, P. D., Buck, M. L., Conaway, M. R., and Blackman, J. A., The use of dopamine-enhancing medications with children in low-response states following brain injury, *Brain Injury*, 17(6), 497–506, 2003.

53. Matsuda, W., Matsumura, A., Komatsu, Y., Yanaka, K., and Nose, T., Awakenings from persistent vegetative state: Report of three cases with parkinsonism and brain stem lesions on MRI, *Journal of Neurology, Neurosurgery, and Psychiatry*, 74(11), 1571–1573, 2003.
54. Matsuda, W., Komatsu, Y., Yanaka, K., and Matsumura, A., Levodopa treatment for patients in persistent vegetative or minimally conscious states, *Neuropsychological Rehabilitation*, 15(3–4), 414–427, 2005.
55. Zafonte, R. D., Watanabe, T., and Mann, N. R., Amantadine: A potential treatment for the minimally conscious state, *Brain Injury*, 12(7), 617–621, 1998.
56. Patrick, P. D., Blackman, J. A., Mabry, J. L., Buck, M. L., Gurka, M. J., and Conaway, M. R., Dopamine agonist therapy in low-response children following traumatic brain injury, *Journal of Child Neurology*, 21(10), 879–885, 2006.
57. Meythaler, J. M., Brunner, R. C., Johnson, A., and Novack, T. A., Amantadine to improve neurorecovery in traumatic brain injury-associated diffuse axonal injury: A pilot double-blind randomized trial, *Journal of Head Trauma Rehabilitation*, 17(4), 300–313, 2002.
58. Hughes, S., Colantonio, A., Santaguida, P. L., and Paton, T., Amantadine to enhance readiness for rehabilitation following severe traumatic brain injury, *Brain Injury*, 19(14), 1197–1206, 2005.
59. Kraus, M. F., Smith, G. S., Butters, M., Donnell, A. J., Dixon, E., Yilong, C., and Marion, D., Effects of the dopaminergic agent and NMDA receptor antagonist amantadine in cognitive function, cerebral glucose metabolism, and D2 receptor availability in chronic traumatic brain injury: A study using positron emission tomography (PET), *Brain Injury*, 19(7), 471–479, 2005.
60. Passler, M. A. and Riggs, R. V., Positive outcomes in traumatic brain injury–vegetative state: Patients treated with bromocriptine, *Archives of Physical Medicine and Rehabilitation*, 82(3), 311–315, 2001.
61. McDowell, S., Whyte, J., and D'Esposito, M., Differential effect of a dopaminergic agonist on prefrontal function in traumatic brain injury patients, *Brain*, 121(Pt. 6), 1155–1164, 1998.
62. Gibbs, S. E. and D'Esposito, M., A functional MRI study of the effects of bromocriptine, a dopamine receptor agonist, on component processes of working memory, *Psychopharmacology (Berl)*, 180(4), 644–653, 2005.
63. Kraus, M. and Maki, P., The combined use of amantadine and L-dopa/carbidopa in the treatment of chronic brain injury, *Brain Injury*, 11(6), 455–460, 1997.
64. Plenger, P. M., Dixon, C. E., Castillo, R. M., Frankowski, R. F., Yablon, S. A., and Levin, H. S., Subacute methylphenidate treatment for moderate to moderately severe traumatic brain injury: A preliminary double-blind placebo-controlled study, *Archives of Physical Medicine and Rehabilitation*, 77(6), 536–540, 1996.
65. Whyte, J., Hart, T., Schuster, K., Fleming, M., Polansky, M., and Coslett, H. B., Effects of methylphenidate on attentional function after traumatic brain injury: A randomized, placebo-controlled trial, *American Journal of Physical Medicine and Rehabilitation*, 76(6), 440–450, 1997.
66. Whyte, J., Vaccaro, M., Grieb-Neff, P., and Hart, T., Psychostimulant use in the rehabilitation of individuals with traumatic brain injury, *Journal of Head Trauma Rehabilitation*, 17(4), 284–299, 2002.
67. Martin, R. T. and Whyte, J., The effects of methylphenidate on command following and yes/no communication in persons with severe disorders of consciousness: A meta-analysis of n-of-1 studies, *American Journal of Physical Medicine and Rehabilitation*, 86(8), 613–620, 2007.
68. Murdock, W. M. and Hamm, R. J., Chronic Atomoxetine Treatment Improves Cognition Following Lateral Fluid Percussion in Rats, Poster session presented at the annual meeting of the National Neurotrauma Society, St. Louis, MO, 2006.
69. Ripley, D. L., Atomoxetine for individuals with traumatic brain injury, *Journal of Head Trauma Rehabilitation*, 21(1), 85–88, 2006.
70. Reinhard, D. L., Whyte, J., and Sandel, M. E., Improved arousal and initiation following tricyclic antidepressant use in severe brain injury, *Archives of Physical Medicine and Rehabilitation*, 77(1), 80–83, 1996.

71. Ferraro, L., Antonelli, T., Tanganelli, S., O'Connor, W. T., Perez de la Mora, M., Mendez-Franco, J., Rambert, F. A., and Fuxe, K., The vigilance-promoting drug modafinil increases extracellular glutamate levels in the medial preoptic area and the posterior hypothalamus of the conscious rat: Prevention by local GABAA receptor blockade, *Neuropsychopharmacology*, 20(4), 346–356, 1999.

72. Lin, J. S., Hou, Y., and Jouvet, M., Potential brain neuronal targets for amphetamine-, methylphenidate-, modafinil-induced wakefulness, evidenced by c-fos immunocytochemistry in the cat, *Proceedings of the National Academy of Sciences of the United States of America*, 93(24), 14128–14133, 1996.

73. Teitelman, E., Off-label uses of modafinil, *American Journal of Psychiatry*, 158(8), 1341–1342, 2001.

74. Doctors puzzled by man's recovery from vegetative state. *The Fargo-Moorhead Forum*, 1990, A17.

75. Wijdicks, E. F., Minimally conscious state vs. persistent vegetative state: The case of Terry (Wallis) vs. the case of Terri (Schiavo), *Mayo Clinic Proceedings*, 81(9), 1155–1158, 2006.

76. Clauss, R. and Nel, W., Drug induced arousal from the permanent vegetative state, *NeuroRehabilitation*, 21(1), 23–28, 2006.

77. Clauss, R. P. and Nel, W. H., Effect of zolpidem on brain injury and diaschisis as detected by 99mTc HMPAO brain SPECT in humans, *Arzneimittel-Forschung*, 54(10), 641–646, 2004.

78. Freo, U., Pizzolato, G., Dam, M., Ori, C., and Battistin, L., A short review of cognitive and functional neuroimaging studies of cholinergic drugs: Implications for therapeutic potentials, *Journal of Neural Transmission*, 109(5–6), 857–870, 2002.

79. McIntosh, T. K., Juhler, M., and Wieloch, T., Novel pharmacologic strategies in the treatment of experimental traumatic brain injury: 1998, *Journal of Neurotrauma*, 15(10), 731–769, 1998.

80. Masanic, C. A., Bayley, M. T., VanReekum, R., and Simard, M., Open-label study of donepezil in traumatic brain injury, *Archives of Physical Medicine and Rehabilitation*, 82(7), 896–901, 2001.

81. Arciniegas, D., Adler, L., Topkoff, J., Cawthra, E., Filley, C. M., and Reite, M., Attention and memory dysfunction after traumatic brain injury: Cholinergic mechanisms, sensory gating, and a hypothesis for further investigation, *Brain Injury*, 13(1), 1–13, 1999.

82. Zhang, L., Plotkin, R., Wang, G., Sandel, M. E., and Lee, S., Cholinergic augmentation with donepezil enhances recovery in short-term memory and sustained attention after traumatic brain injury, *Archives of Physical Medicine and Rehabilitation*, 85(7), 1050–1055, 2004.

83. Khateb, A., Ammann, J., Annoni, J. M., and Diserens, K., Cognition-enhancing effects of donepezil in traumatic brain injury, *European Neurology*, 54(1), 39–45, 2005.

84. Walker, W., Seel, R., Gibellato, M., Lew, H., Cornis-Pop, M., Jena, T., and Silver, T., The effects of donepezil on traumatic brain injury acute rehabilitation outcomes, *Brain Injury*, 18(8), 739–750, 2004.

85. Parmentier, R., Ohtsu, H., Djebarra-Hannas, Z., Valatx, J. L., Watanabe, T., and Lin, J. S., Anatomical, physiological, and pharmacological characteristics of histidine decarboxylase knock-out mice: Evidence for the role of brain histamine in behavioral and sleep–wake control, *Journal of Neuroscience*, 22(17), 7695–7711, 2002.

86. Nishino, S., Fujiki, N., Ripley, B., Sakurai, E., Kato, M., Watanabe, T., Mignot, E., and Yanai, K., Decreased brain histamine content in hypocretin/orexin receptor-2 mutated narcoleptic dogs, *Neuroscience Letters*, 313(3), 125–128, 2001.

87. Blandina, P. and Passani, M. B., Central histaminergic system interactions and cognition, in E. D. Levine (Ed.), *Neurotransmitter Interactions and Cognitive Function*, Birkhauser, Verlag/Switzerland, 149–163, 2006.

6

Diagnosis and Management of Balance Disturbances Following Traumatic Brain Injury

Peter S. Roland and Patti Blau

CONTENTS

6.1 Introduction

The complaint of vertigo is not the only symptom of vestibular injury. Other symptoms may include imbalance (dysequilibrium); visual complaints (double vision, blurriness); or nausea. Complaints that may or may not be symptoms of vestibular injury per se, but often accompany a vestibular lesion after a head injury include headache, irritability, oversensitivity to sounds and/or lights, and decreased attention and concentration span. These symptoms are often seen as a psychological response following a head injury and are not related to organic damage.

Only after a complete evaluation can the process of treatment begin. Treatment may include exercise, medication, and/or a surgical procedure.

A counselor can be crucial in dealing with adjustment to any disability, including balance dysfunction. The counseling process should include patient education about the extent of the lesion and its consequences. Patient education is critical to help bring under control a process that otherwise might lead to a degree of disability not warranted by the lesion itself.

Recovery from head injury is now recognized to be a complex process that progresses over many months. The patient recovering from a head injury is frequently afflicted with more than a single area of difficulty or dysfunction. Many of these areas are the focus of specific chapters in this book. Such problem areas frequently cross disciplinary boundaries and, in practical clinical situations, symptoms outside the specialty area of the primary caregiver may receive less than adequate attention. Comprehensive care is, therefore, improved when the head-injured patient is served by multidisciplinary team members whose efforts are orchestrated by a designated coordinator. Review of the literature suggests that dizziness or disequilibrium following a head injury represents an area that requires considerably more attention and postinjury rehabilitation than it has received to date.

6.1.1 Demographics

Although previous investigations are few in number, the evidence presented by available studies argues powerfully that postconcussive balance disturbance is the primary cause of very substantial morbidity and long-term disability. Indeed, Healy[1] asserted in the *New England Journal of Medicine* that "cochlear and vestibular dysfunction represent the largest group of delayed complications of head injury."[2]

Berman and Fredrickson[3] evaluated 321 head injury patients within the Canadian Workman's Compensation System. Forty percent of this group complained of postinjury vertigo and, of those complaining of vertigo, 50% had objective electronystagmographic (ENG) findings of organic dysfunction. When the 140 patients with complaints of vertigo were evaluated 5 years after injury, only 14% had returned to their preaccident or equivalent work. Forty-six percent of this group had not returned to any work at all. Vertigo, together with headache, was of prime importance in determining long-term work status. Although no long-term studies exist for U.S. populations, because social, cultural, and compensation variables are quite similar, it seems reasonable to extrapolate these results to the United States.

Rantanen et al.[4] evaluated 41 patients within several days of head injury. Sixty percent complained of vertigo. When eye movement was evaluated by physical examination alone (even with Frenzel lenses), only 20% had observable nystagmus. However, when ENG was performed with eyes closed, nystagmus was detectable in more than 60%. Elimination of "visual fixation," by eye closure, releases pathologic nystagmoid eye movement in a significant percent of injured people, and Rantanen et al.[4] emphasize that formal ENG evaluation is important in the objective evaluation of postinjury patients complaining of dizziness.

Saito et al.[5] evaluated 22 patients who complained of dizziness after head injury. All had positional nystagmus on ENG. Eleven had ENG findings suggestive of central nervous system (CNS) injury. Of the 11 patients with ENG findings suggestive of CNS injury, only four recovered in 2 months or less and four were still not recovered after 3 months. Patients with ENG indicators of peripheral vestibular dysfunction recovered much more quickly. By differentiating between central and peripheral pathology, ENG was helpful in establishing a prognosis.

Tuohimaa[6] carefully studied 82 patients who had sustained only "mild" head injuries (duration of unconsciousness less than 2 hours or not at all) and compared them with a matched control group. Seventy-eight percent of the postinjury patients complained of vertigo. Central ENG disturbances were observed immediately after injury in 60% of the patients, but the incidence fell to 12% at 6 months after injury. The incidence of persistent central ENG changes increased with increasing age of the head-injured patient. Tuohimaa's[6] group of patients demonstrated a dramatic impairment in the ability to suppress nystagmus by deliberate visual fixation. He argues that diminished fixation suppression indicates that reduced central inhibition is a frequent consequence of mild head injury. The incidence of both spontaneous and positional nystagmus was significantly higher in patients with mild head injury immediately after injury than in normal control subjects.

Grimm and colleagues[7] studied 102 patients with mild craniocervical trauma who experienced positional vertigo. This group displayed a set of symptoms often referred to as *postconcussion syndrome*. More than 95% of these patients experienced disequilibrium and 70% from vertigo. Headache, memory loss, tinnitus, nausea, confusion, clumsiness, alteration of subjective visual perception, and stiff neck were all present in more than 50% of this group of patients. Their conclusion that all these patients had a perilymphatic fistula is highly controversial, but their work does highlight the importance of balance disturbance in patients with even mild head injury. Moreover, they have documented well the pattern of characteristic symptomatology found so frequently after head injury.

Vartiainen et al.[8] examined 199 children after blunt head trauma. Fifty percent had positional or spontaneous nystagmus and 50% had central ENG disturbances. The incidence of abnormalities dropped rapidly after 2 to 8 years, but was somewhat higher in the peripheral group (18%) than in the central group (12%). Clinically, when compared with adults, a much lower percentage of these children (1.5%) remained symptomatic at 2 to 8 years.

Evatar et al.[9] evaluated 22 children ages 6 to 18 years for posttraumatic vertigo. Children with hearing loss were excluded. Five pathologically distinct etiologies were identified, including posttraumatic migraine ($n = 5$), seizure disorders ($n = 4$), postconcussion syndrome ($n = 4$), whiplash injury ($n = 4$), posttraumatic neurosis ($n = 5$). Their work emphasizes the variety of processes that can produce posttraumatic disequilibrium and emphasizes the value of objective ENG testing in distinguishing among various etiologies.

Hoffer et al.[10] evaluated a series of individuals ($N = 72$) with posttraumatic benign paroxysmal positional vertigo (BPPV), who became asymptomatic most rapidly and returned to work most quickly. At the other end of the spectrum were patients with "spatial disorientation." On average, these individuals did not return to work for 15 weeks and were symptomatic for up to 40 weeks.

6.2 Anatomy and Physiology of the Vestibular System

The anatomy of the vestibular system is complex and, especially in its ramifications within the CNS, poorly understood. Anatomically speaking, one may divide the vestibular system into four parts: (1) the peripheral vestibular end organ enclosed within the bony labyrinthine capsule; (2) the vestibular nerve; (3) the brainstem vestibular nuclei together with their vestibulo-ocular, vestibulocerebellar, vestibulospinal radiations, and feedback loops; and (4) the vestibular cortex (Figure 6.1).

6.2.1 Vestibular End Organ

The *labyrinth* (inner ear) consists of a folded, fluid-filled tube (membranous labyrinth or endolymphatic space) that lies within the bony labyrinthine capsule. The membranous labyrinthine is suspended in and cushioned by a second fluid compartment (perilymphatic space). Anteriorly, within the bony labyrinth, is the spirally shaped cochlea, the organ of hearing. Posteriorly, are the three semicircular canals. Between the cochlea and semicircular canals is a central chamber, the vestibule, which contains the utricle and saccule (Figure 6.2).

The two inner fluids are chemically distinct. Endolymph (like intracellular fluid) contains a relatively high concentration of potassium and a relatively low concentration of sodium. Perilymph (like extracellular fluid) contains much sodium, but relatively little potassium. The difference in electrolyte composition between these two fluids is essential in maintenance of the resting electrical potential, which is critical for normal functioning of the receptor cells.

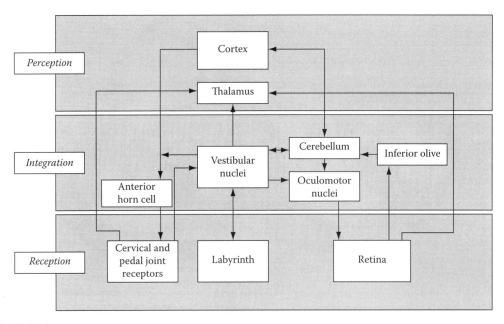

FIGURE 6.1

Conceptual schema of the vestibular system. This subdivides the various components of the vestibular system into a vertically oriented hierarchy with receptor organs at the bottom and perception at the top. Lateral organization distinguishes between various different receptors at the lowest level and brainstem nuclei at the higher levels. A fully functional vestibular system requires coordination and integration of sensory receptor information. Plasticity of the vestibular system arises from the fact that deficiencies in information provided by receptors can be compensated for at the integrative or perceptive level by reorganizing input from residual receptors. (From Brown, J. J., *Neurologic Clinics*, 8(2), 209–224, 1990. With permission.)

The composition of endolymph is thought to be regulated by a vascular structure within the lateral wall of the endolymphatic duct called the *stria vascularis*. The production and composition of endolymph may therefore be altered by conditions and substances that alter blood flow, vascular permeability, or systemic fluid balance. Perilymph is, at least partially, an ultrafiltrate of spinal fluid. The perilymphatic space is connected with the subarachnoid cerebrospinal fluid space via the cochlear aqueduct. Changes within the subarachnoid space may alter the perilymphatic compartment. Increased intracranial pressure produced by disease or by straining may be transmitted to the perilymphatic space and may produce chronic or acute perilymphatic hypertension. Chemicals, toxins, and viral and bacterial infectious agents may all pass from the cerebrospinal fluid to the perilymph via the cochlear aqueduct.

Alterations in the chemical composition, relative volumes, or mixing of the inner ear fluids may incapacitate both the vestibular and hearing end organ. Depending upon the anatomic extent and severity of the alteration, various combinations of balance disturbance, hearing loss, aural fullness, and tinnitus may result.

The common sensory receptor within the inner ear is the *hair cell*. Its function is to translate fluid motion into a pattern of neuronal electrical discharge. The labyrinthine fluids first translate both head acceleration and sound waves into fluid movement. Movement of fluid across the stereocilia of receptor hair cells deflects the stereocilia and changes the resting rate of discharge in the nerve attached to the hair cell (Figures 6.3 and 6.4). Movement in one direction may increase the rate of discharge; movement in the opposite

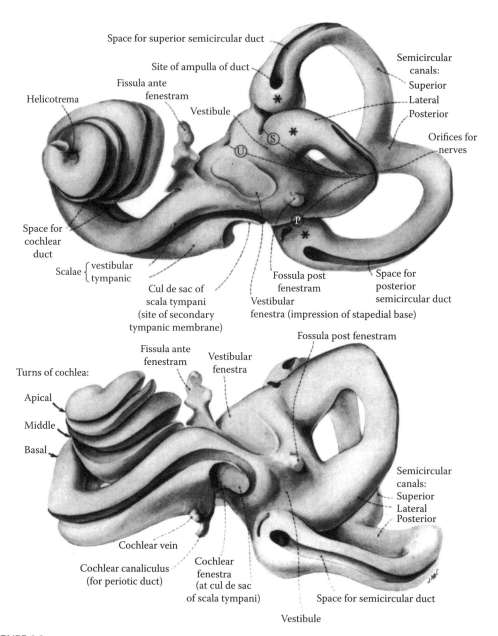

FIGURE 6.2
The labyrinth is seen from the lateral position (top) and from below (bottom). The bony labyrinth has been opened to show the position of the membranous endolymphatic duct. Asterisks indicate the cupular dilatations of the semicircular canals. S, saccule; U, utricle. (From Lindermann, H. H., *Studies on the Morphology of Sensory Regions of the Vestibular Apparatus*, Springer-Verlag, New York, 1969. With permission.)

direction may decrease the rate of discharge. It is this change in rate of neuronal activity that is processed by the CNS into conscious and subconscious information about spatial orientation and sound.

The vestibular end organ consists of five separate structures, each with its own specialized sensory epithelium. The three semicircular canals are at right angles to each

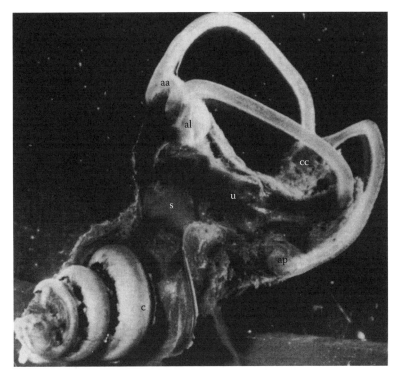

FIGURE 6.3

This is an actual microdissection. The bone has been completely removed leaving only the membranous endo-lymphatic duct system. The microdissection is oriented in approximately the same position as the top drawing in Figure 6.2. aa, cupula of the superior canal; al, cupula of the lateral semicircular canal; ap, cupula of the poste-rior semicircular canal; c, cochlea; cc, crus communis; s, saccule; u, utricle. (From Lindermann, H. H., *Studies on the Morphology of Sensory Regions of the Vestibular Apparatus*, Springer-Verlag, New York, 1969. With permission.)

other—one in the horizontal, one in the sagittal, and one in the coronal plane. The receptor organ of the semicircular canals is the *crista ampullaris* (Figure 6.5). Each crista consists of a group of hair cells, the stereocilia of which protrude into a dilated portion of the membranous labyrinth called the *ampulla*. The stereocilia of the hair cells are embedded in a gelatinous matrix that fills the ampulla. Head acceleration in the plane of the semicircular canals results in the bending of stereocilia resulting from iner-tial lag in the movement of endolymph. The same "bending" event occurs when head movement is stopped because the endolymph will "keep going" for a few milliseconds after the head comes to a complete rest. The semicircular canals therefore respond exclusively to angular acceleration. They do not respond to constant velocity—only to changes in velocity. This distinction is important. After constant velocity is achieved, the sense of motion is eliminated. A pilot in a rolling airplane may, absent visual clues, lose all sense of rotation if the rotation continues at constant velocity for more than a few seconds.

The saccule and utricle are the two otolithic end organs. They sense linear acceleration and static tilt. They are gravity sensitive and maintain the ability to distinguish "up" from "down." Each otolithic end organ consists of an out-pouching of the endolymphatic duct on one wall of which rests a collection of hair cells called the *macula*. The hair cells are covered with a gelatinous matrix in which are embedded crystals of calcium carbonate called *otoconia*. The otoconia (Figure 6.6) are acted upon by gravitational forces as well as

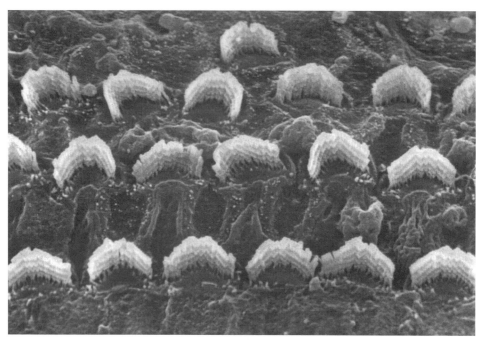

FIGURE 6.4
Scanning electron micrograph of stereocilia on outer hair cells of the human cochlea. Original magnification approximately ×1200. (Courtesy of C. Gary Wright, PhD.)

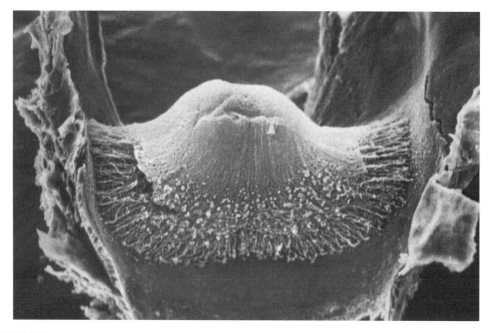

FIGURE 6.5
Crista ampullaris of the lateral semicircular duct of the vestibular apparatus. The structure in the central portion of this scanning electron micrograph is the gelatinous cupula into which the stereocilia on the surface of the crista project and which stimulates the receptor cells in response to angular acceleration. Original magnification approximately ×200. (Courtesy of C. Gary Wright, PhD.)

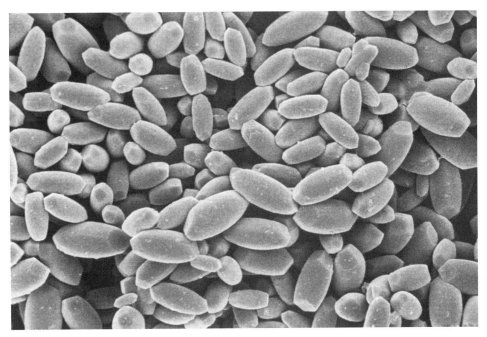

FIGURE 6.6
Scanning electron micrograph of calcium carbonate otoconia from the human saccule. The otoconia provide the necessary mass for stimulation of vestibular hair cells in the saccular and utricular neuroepithelia. Original magnification approximately ×2000. (Courtesy of C. Gary Wright, PhD.)

linear acceleration. A change in head position alters the direction in which the otoconia are pulled by gravity and bends the stereocilia of the macular hair cells in that direction. Thus, any change in head position produces a sense of head movement. Because resting head position produces constant otoconial displacement and stereociliar "bending," the otolithic organs are also sensitive to static "tilt" and help maintain orientation to "up and down."

6.2.2 Vestibular Nerve

Information from the vestibular labyrinth is carried to the brainstem by the vestibular nerve. The superior vestibular nerve carries fibers originating from the superior and horizontal semicircular canals, utricle, and a small portion of the saccule. The inferior vestibular nerve carries fibers originating from the posterior semicircular canal and from most of the saccule. Within the internal auditory canal, the superior and inferior vestibular nerves join together, first with each other, and then with the auditory nerve, and form a single cochleovestibular nerve. The facial nerve also travels through the temporal bone within the internal auditory canal in close proximity to the vestibular and auditory nerves. The vestibulocochlear nerve crosses the subarachnoid spinal fluid space to the brainstem, where the vestibular fibers synapse within the vestibular nuclei. The anterior inferior cerebellar artery, or one of its branches, is often closely associated with the vestibulocochlear nerve, either within the internal auditory canal or within the subarachnoid space between the temporal bone and the brainstem.

6.2.3 The Central Vestibular System

The first-order vestibular neurons that constitute the vestibular nerves synapse with one or more of the four brainstem vestibular nuclei. The neurons from one labyrinth will often synapse within the vestibular nuclei on both sides of the head, thus providing bilateral representation of the vestibular system even at the brainstem level. The wide-ranging ramifications of the vestibular system within the CNS are very complex and poorly understood. Four principal areas can then be conceptually distinguished, even if they cannot always be precisely anatomically delineated: vestibulo-ocular, vestibulospinal, vestibulo-cerebellar, and vestibulocortical.

Vestibulo-ocular connections form the basis of the vestibulo-ocular reflex (VOR).[11–13] Each semicircular canal has an elaborate pattern of both direct and indirect synaptic connections to the ocular motor nuclei that control eye movements. The vestibular nuclei on each side are connected to the ocular motor nuclei of both eyes in such a way that stimulation of each semicircular canal can produce eye movements in the plane of that canal (i.e., stimulation of the horizontal semicircular canal can produce horizontal eye movement). These complicated connections are responsible for the production of nystagmus. Stimulation of one labyrinth produces slow movement of the eyes in the opposite direction from the direction of head movement and of roughly equal magnitude. Eye movement continues until a predetermined amount of lateral deviation is reached. Ocular centers within the brain are able to recognize that no further eye movement is appropriate. To prevent "pinning" of the eyes in extreme lateral gaze, the eyes are returned to the neutral "straight ahead" position from which lateral deviation can begin again. The eye movement perceived by an observer, therefore, is of slow lateral deviation followed a very "quick" return movement that, in turn, is followed by another slow movement phase. The rapid return phase is a *saccade*. Saccades are the mechanism of eye movement utilized during volitional change of focus when we "look around." Saccades may occur with speeds of up to 800 degrees per second. During each saccade, reflex brainstem activity suppresses vision so that the visual field is prevented from constant "jumping." Because the fast phase of nystagmus is a saccade, vision is suppressed as it occurs. Because this is not true of the "slow" phase, which is controlled by the labyrinth, some patients will complain that their visual field "jumps" in the direction opposite to slow phase when they have nystagmus. Because the slow phase of nystagmus is about equal to but in the opposite direction of head movement, it appears to be a mechanism that reflexively permits retention of visual fixation during head movement or when falling.

6.2.3.1 Vestibulocerebellar

There are extensive direct and indirect descending (efferent) and ascending (afferent) pathways between the midline cerebellar nuclei (principally the vermis and fastigial nucleus) and the brainstem vestibular nuclei and associated integrative centers. These extensive connections permit precise modulation of equilibrium, both at rest and during complex body movements. Because most of the pathways discussed have a pattern of inhibitory connections as complex as the excitatory ones, brainstem centers subserving the vestibular system are capable of making very fine discriminations and executing highly precise adjustments of movement and balance.

6.2.3.2 Cortical Projections

The vestibular system (via the thalamus) projects onto the superior temporal gyrus near the auditory cortex. Stimulation of this cortical area can produce a sense of movement often described as "spinning." Input from proprioceptive and visual centers is integrated to produce the final conscious "sensation." Occasionally, epileptiform discharges or neoplasms produce "vertigo" by direct stimulation of these areas of cerebral cortex.

6.3 Pathophysiology: Specific Disease Processes

Although the pathophysiologic mechanisms of posttraumatic vertigo are frequently obscure, several specific injuries with reasonably well-described mechanisms are recognized.

6.3.1 Temporal Bone Fracture

Because the largest portion of the skull base is made up of the temporal bone, most basilar skull fractures involve some portion of the temporal bone. Such fractures are loosely categorized into two types: longitudinal and transverse. Longitudinal fractures are more common, and fortunately, are accompanied by a low incidence of fracture into the labyrinthine capsule and facial nerve paralysis. Transverse temporal bone fractures are less common (5%–10% of temporal bone fractures) but are much more likely to fracture into the labyrinthine capsule, despite the fact that the labyrinthine bone is the hardest bone found anywhere within the human body.[14] When fracture lines extend into the labyrinthine capsule, complete ipsilateral hearing loss and total ablation of ipsilateral vestibular function is the rule. If normal vestibular function is retained in the contralateral ear, then, following several days of overwhelming rotational vertigo with nausea and vomiting, normal functioning will likely return. The rate of improvement depends on the presence or absence of associated injuries and on the age of the injured subject. Younger patients recover at a much faster rate than older patients. An individual in his 20s may be expected to be able to ambulate unassisted in 3 to 4 days. He may be able to resume fairly demanding activities like bicycle riding and ladder climbing in 3 to 4 weeks. (Ultimately, clinical recovery in this age group is usually complete, although subtle testing will continue to uncover abnormalities of the vestibular system.) The pattern of recovery will be quite different in more elderly persons. It will be slower. A person who is in his 60s or 70s may not be able to ambulate unassisted for several weeks and may be able to perform demanding tasks only after several months. Recovery of fine balance skills may never be complete in the older person. Although vestibular rehabilitation therapy will hasten recovery in the younger individual, many younger patients will do well without a formal rehabilitation program. The outcome in persons older than 40, even if the vestibular loss is an isolated disability, may depend critically on the early implementation of a comprehensive, individualized rehabilitation program. This may also be so in younger patients if the vestibular injury is accompanied by other motor, sensory, or neurologic deficits.

6.3.2 Perilymphatic Fistulas

Head injury may produce rupture of the membranes that seal the inner ear and prevent escape of perilymphatic fluid into the middle ear space (Figure 6.7). When perilymph is removed from the labyrinth, inner ear function is degraded. A combination of otologic symptoms may result and symptoms may fluctuate in complex ways that are difficult for

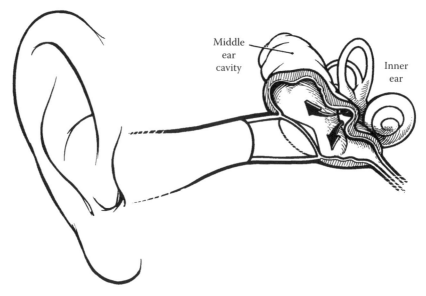

FIGURE 6.7
Diagrammatic representation of a perilymph fistula. Perilymph can escape from either the oval window (upper arrow) or round window (lower arrow). Because the amount of fluid is extraordinarily small, the patient has no subjective sense of fluid within his middle ear space.

the patient to explain. In obvious cases, trauma is accompanied (or followed within a few minutes) by rapid, severe hearing loss; loud, roaring tinnitus; and severe rotational vertigo. Vertigo is often incapacitating and accompanied by visceral autonomic symptoms (sweating, pallor, nausea, vomiting). Even cursory examination will demonstrate marked instability and nystagmus. Audiometric evaluation reveals sensorineural hearing loss. Platform posturography will confirm disequilibrium with a vestibular pattern and the platform fistula test will be positive. Vertigo and, to a lesser degree, tinnitus and hearing loss are sometimes exacerbated by straining or Valsalva maneuver. Repair of the fistula by grafting the round and oval windows often produces immediate and complete elimination of vertigo. Infrequently, hearing will be improved as well.

Unfortunately, many perilymph fistulas do not manifest themselves in this straightforward manner.[7,15] Onset of symptoms may be delayed for several days, or the acute phase may be masked by more serious injuries in other areas. Rotational vertigo may be entirely absent and disequilibrium may be mild, vague, and episodic. Hearing loss, tinnitus, and aural fullness may come and go unpredictably. Such protean and elusive symptomatology has led to controversy. Opinions differ widely among credible otologists about how frequently perilymph fistulas occur, what types of injuries and forces produce them, and what sorts of ancillary symptoms (headache, concentration defects, phobias, and impaired mentation) accompany them. Although one might hope that middle ear exploration could resolve this controversy by establishing the actual frequency with which perilymph fistulas occur, it has not. The average human inner ear contains only 70 μL perilymph and therefore even relatively rapid leaks will, in absolute terms, be quite small. Even with magnification, leaks involving only 5% to 10% of the perilymph will be difficult to see in an operative field where local anesthetics have been injected, irrigating fluids have been used, and where there is even minimal bleeding.

Because no reliable method of proving the absence or presence of perilymph fistula is yet available, reliable incidence and prevalence figures do not exist. Currently, considerable effort at the national level is being expended to clarify the perilymph fistula controversy, but at this time, it remains unresolved.

6.3.3 Posttraumatic Ménière's Syndrome

In 1861, Prosper Ménière described a syndrome of episodic rotational vertigo accompanied by tinnitus and fluctuating neurosensory hearing loss. A sense of aural fullness or pressure is now also considered an important part of this syndrome. Attacks generally last 15 to 100 minutes and are followed by several hours of asthenia, nausea, and disequilibrium. When no cause (i.e., syphilis, acoustic tumor, or viral labyrinthitis) can be established, the syndrome is idiopathic and may be termed *Ménière's disease*. Histopathologic evidence demonstrates that this syndrome arises as a consequence of excess amounts of endolymph that produce distension of the endolymphatic space. Both Ménière's syndrome and perilymph fistula share a common factor: The ratio of endolymph to perilymph is altered in the same direction (relative excess of endolymph compared with perilymph); although, in Ménière's, it results from excess endolymph whereas in perilymph fistula it results from loss of perilymph. While in their typical or classic presentations, these conditions are clinically separable; in their atypical manifestations, they are indistinguishable. Ménière's disease may, like perilymph fistula, manifest as a highly variable and changing combination of aural fullness, disequilibrium, hearing loss, and tinnitus. No physical finding, laboratory test, or radiographic or audiometric study can definitively separate these two conditions. Although uncommon, the development of Ménière's syndrome after traumatic brain injury (posttraumatic Ménière's syndrome) is well established and not rare.[16] It usually appears weeks or months (perhaps even years) after the original injury. Diagnosis depends on history, documentation of fluctuating neurosensory hearing loss, positive electrocochleography and/or positive dehydration audiometry.

Treatment for Ménière's syndrome, whether idiopathic or posttraumatic, should begin with attempted medical management. Surgical intervention should be limited to patients who fail aggressive medical therapy. Rigorous adherence to a salt-restricted diet (2000 mg daily) and diuretic therapy are the mainstays of medical treatment. A vestibular suppressant should be added during symptomatic periods. If aggressive medical management is inadequate or poorly tolerated, then consideration should be given to one of the many surgical options available.

6.3.4 Benign Paroxysmal Positional Vertigo

Traumatic injury may dislodge otoconia from the macula of the saccule or utricle. Two hypotheses have been developed to explain how dislodged otoconia can produce the clinical phenomenon of BPPV. The *cupulolithiasis* theory proposes that these loose otoconia migrate and become attached to the ampulla of the semicircular canal.[17] The additional mass added to the ampulla makes it gravity sensitive. Consequently, cupular deflection occurs with a variety of head movements, not only as a result of angular acceleration.

The *canalithiasis* theory proposes that otoconia are floating freely in the endolymphatic fluid of the vestibule. Provocative positioning results in displacement of these mobile otoconia into the fluid of the semicircular canal, producing unilateral movement of labyrinthine fluid, cupular deflection, and a sensation of movement.[18,19] BPPV may arise from a combination of these two mechanisms.

BPPV is a common cause of vertigo.[20,21] Many cases are idiopathic, but this entity is often seen after upper respiratory infection, trauma, Ménière's disease, surgery, otologic infection, and in combination with other inner ear disorders. Twenty percent of patients with traumatic head injury present with bilateral involvement.[22] Posttraumatic BPPV appears to have characteristics and outcomes different than the idiopathic form and may be dependent on the nature and severity of the injury. Consequently, resolution may be more difficult with greater chance of reoccurrence.[23–25]

BPPV classically presents with intense, brief, rotary vertigo, which occurs when rolling from side to side while in the supine position (such as in bed). The rotary sensation itself typically lasts for about 30 seconds, but patients frequently describe a second component consisting of persistent dysequilibrium. BPPV will cause vertigo and nystagmus with the following characteristic features:

- Latency of onset, usually 2 to 6 seconds
- Short duration, usually less than 30 seconds
- Reversibility
- Fatigability
- Direction

BPPV constitutes a specific pathophysiologic entity with characteristic videonystagmography/electronystagmography (VNG/ENG) findings and should not be confused with other disorders mimicking BPPV.[26,27]

Prior to assessing the patient in provoking positions, one must determine whether the patient is a candidate for treatment. Contraindications to performing the Dix-Hallpike test and subsequent treatment include a history of recent neck trauma, cervical spine instability including atlantoaxial and occipitoatlantal instability, cervical myelopathy and radiculopathy, syncope, history of neck surgery, severe osteoporosis, and rheumatoid arthritis.[28] The patient's neck should be assessed for pain and mobility to determine whether modifications to the testing positions need be made by using the side-lying test, cervical collar, or tilt table.

BPPV can be diagnosed during the physical examination. For Dix-Hallpike testing for the posterior and anterior semicircular canals, the patient starts in the sitting position with head turned 45 degrees horizontally. The patient is then rapidly moved into a supine position with the head hanging over the edge of the table.[13] When this maneuver is performed to the affected side, then vertigo and nystagmus may be induced after a latency of a few seconds and may continue for less than 30 seconds, after which it will disappear. If the patient is returned rapidly to the sitting position, the nystagmus may reappear (again, with a brief latency), beating this time in the opposite direction (reversibility). The response fatigues quickly and repeated Dix-Hallpike maneuvers will eliminate the phenomenon within a few repetitions at most. The side-lying test can be substituted for the Dix-Hallpike when the patient has limited passive or active range of motion of the neck. During this examination, the patient sits on the edge of the table with the head rotated 45 degrees away from the tested side. The patient is quickly moved to the right or left side-lying position to evaluate the presence of nystagmus.[29–31]

The roll test is used to identify horizontal canal BPPV. The patient lies supine with the head flexed 20 degrees.[32–34] Characteristic nystagmus is produced by quickly rolling the head to one side for no longer than 1 minute. The head is slowly rolled back to midline and then quickly rolled to the opposite side. Casani et al.[35] identified three variants: bilateral geotropic nystagmus, bilateral ageotropic nystagmus that may switch into bilateral geotropic, and bilateral ageotropic nystagmus that is persistent and does not switch. VNG/ENG evaluation is always helpful and frequently essential in clarifying and documenting these classic characteristics.[36]

Most cases of BPPV are self-limited, resolving over a 2- to 6-month period. There are three different bedside treatments for BPPV: the canalith repositioning treatment (CRT), the liberatory maneuver, and Brandt-Daroff habituation exercises.[31,37–41] Each has specific indications, but CRT is the most widely used because it is well tolerated by patients and is easy to perform. Modifications of these treatments have been proposed depending upon the canal involved and other medical comorbities.[31,42–44] Long-term follow-up studies for canal repositioning procedures for BPPV indicate that treatments discussed earlier are effective and longlasting.[45–51] A review of randomized controlled studies can be found in Tusa and Herdman,[52] and Pinder.[53]

The choice of treatment techniques depends on which canal is involved as well as the identification of whether one presumes canalithiasis or cupulolithiasis (Table 6.1). Brandt-Daroff exercises are reserved for residual complaints following maneuvers. The most common form of BPPV has been reported in the posterior semicircular canal and is the canalithiasis type. This treatment involves a four-position cycle in which the patient

TABLE 6.1

Characteristic Nystagmus Patterns for BPPV and Treatment

Type of Pathology	Provocation Test	Nystagmus Pattern	Duration	Treatment
R PSC canalithiasis	R Dix-Hallpike	Upbeating and torsional; downward ear	<1 min	R CRT
R PSC cupulolithiasis	R Dix-Hallpike	Downbeating and torsional; downward ear	>1 min	R liberatory; head turned L
L PSC canalithiasis	L Dix-Hallpike	Upbeating and torsional; downward ear	<1 min	L CRT
L PSC cupulolithiasis	L Dix-Hallpike	Upbeating and torsional; downward ear	>1 min	L liberatory: head turned R
R ASC canalithiasis	R Dix-Hallpike	Downbeating and torsional; downward ear	<1 min	R CRT
R ASC cupulothiasis	R Dix-Hallpike	Downbeating and torsional; downward ear	>1 min	R liberatory; head turned R
L ASC canalithiasis	L Dix-Hallpike	Downbeating and torsional; downward ear	<1 min	L CRT
L ASC cupulothiasis	L Dix-Hallpike	Downbeating and torsional; downward ear	>1 min	L liberatory; head turned L
R HSC canalithiasis	R head turn, supine	R horizontal geotropic	R > L	Bar-B-Que roll to L Appiani to L side FPP R → L
R HSC cupulothiasis	R head turn, supine	R horizontal apogeotropic	R > L	Modified Brandt-Daroff to R
L HSC canalithiasis	L head turn, supine	L horizontal geotropic	L > R	Bar-B-Que roll to R Appiani to R side FPP L → R
L HSC cupulothiasis	L head turn, supine	L horizontal apogeotropic	L > R	Modified Brandt-Daroff to L

ASC, anterior semicircular canal; CRT, canalith repositioning treatment; FPP, forced prolonged position; HSC, horizontal semicircular canal; L, left; PSC, posterior semicircular canal; R, right.

Source: Modified from Herdman, S. J. and Tusa, R. J., *Diagnosis and Treatment of Benign Paroxysmal Positional Vertigo*, ICS Medical Corporation, Schaumburg, IL, 1999.

is taken through a series of head positions to move the head around the debris (Figure 6.8). At each position, the operator should pause until induced nystagmus approaches termination. Reversal of nystagmus during the second portion of the maneuver suggests that debris is moving back toward the cupula, and has been identified as a factor predicting poor response by Parnes and Price-Jones.[54] Hain et al.[55] reported that mastoid

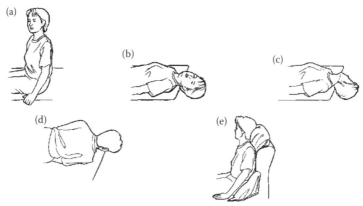

(a) Turn head 45 deg to the left

(b) Lie down with the head hanging 20 deg down over the edge of the bed. Keep head rotated 45 deg to left. Stay in this position for 20 secs or until dizziness stops, whichever is longer.

(c) While keeping the head tilted back 20 deg, rotate head such that it is 45 deg to right. Stay in this position for 20 secs or until dizziness stops, whichever is longer.

(d) Roll over onto right shoulder and rotate head such that it is 45 deg down. Stay in this position for 20 secs or until dizziness stops, whichever is longer.

(e) Slowly sit straight up with head still rotated to the right. Straighten head and stay in an upright position for 20 minutes.

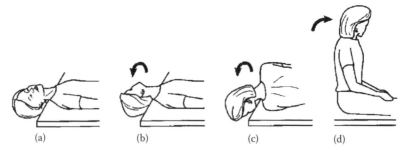

(a) Turn head 45 deg to the right and lie down with the head hanging 20 deg over the edge of the bed. Stay in this position for 20 secs or until dizziness stops, whichever is longer.

(b) While keeping the head tilted back 20 deg, rotate head such that it is 45 deg to the left. Stay in this position for 20 secs or until dizziness stops, whichever is longer.

(c) Roll over onto left shoulder such that head is 45 deg down. Stay in this position for 20 secs or until dizziness stops, whichever is longer.

(d) Slowly sit straight up with head still rotated to the left. Straighten head and stay in an upright position for 20 minutes.

FIGURE 6.8
Canalith repositioning maneuver for left-sided (top) and right-sided (bottom) BPPV. Handouts given to patients for canalith repositioning treatment for posterior semicircular canal BPPV. (From Tusa, R. J. and Herdman, S. J., *Audiological Medicine*, 3(1), 57–62, 2005. With permission.)

oscillation during CRT does not significantly affect recurrence rates in patients followed for 5.25 years and therefore is not routinely used, except in patients who do not show any response to the maneuver.[31] The use of soft cervical collars is no longer advocated, unless a patient requests one.[31,56] Finally, several studies investigated the need for post-treatment restrictions and found there was no difference between subjects that were instructed to stay upright for 48 hours and those without restrictions.[52,56,57] Herdman and Tusa[31] recommend, however, that patients remain in the upright position for 20 minutes after a maneuver.

The liberatory maneuver also developed as a single-treatment approach for canalithiasis is typically used today for both cupulolithiasis and canalithiasis (Figure 6.9).[38] Levrat et al.[58] reported a 90% resolution of symptoms after four sessions. This is an

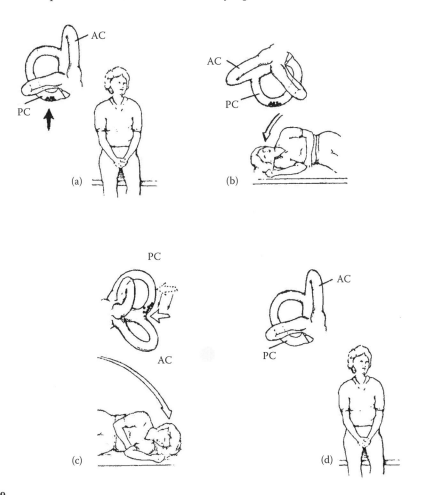

FIGURE 6.9
Liberatory maneuver for treatment of posterior semicircular canal for right-sided BPPV. (a) The patient sits on the examination table sideways and the head is rotated 45 degrees toward the unaffected side. (b) The patient is then moved quickly onto the affected side (parallel to the plane of the affected posterior canal) until the head is hanging down 20 degrees. (c) After 1 minute, the patient is rapidly moved through the initial sitting position to the opposite side with the head still positioned 45 degrees toward the unaffected side (the nose will now be angled 45 degrees down toward the floor). (d) The patient holds the position for 1 minute and then moves slowly to a sitting position. Arrows indicate position and movement of debris. AC, anterior canal; PC, posterior canal. (From S. J. Herdman and R. T. Tusa (Eds.), *Vestibular Rehabilitation*, 3rd ed., 233–260, 2007. With permission.)

awkward manipulation, especially in the elderly population, and is used primarily for cupulolithiasis.

Brandt-Daroff habituation exercises require the patient to sit on the edge of the bed and move repeatedly into the provoking side-lying position several times per day. Recovery is reported in approximately 95% of patients but often requires several weeks to 6 months.[19,31,40] Patient compliance issues make CRT preferable to the Brandt-Daroff exercises (Figure 6.10).

Treatment for horizontal canal BPPV is based on identifying its subtypes by observing the nystagmus pattern.[34,35] In unilateral canalithiasis, the nystagmus is geotropic (beats toward the undermost ear) and fatigues, whereas, in cupulolithiasis, the nystagmus is apogeotropic (beats away from the undermost ear) and persists. Nystagmus will occur in both directions but is greater on the involved side (the treatment side). The Bar-B-Que roll treatment consists of 360-degree rotation toward the unaffected side (Figure 6.11). Variations to the Bar-B-Que maneuver have been reported.[34,35,59] Appiani et al.[60] reported success using a different approach to canalithiasis by having the patient sitting on the edge of the bed and quickly lying down on the *unaffected* side for 2 minutes (Figure 6.12). Other researchers have advocated a forced prolonged position (FPP).[61] In the FPP treatment, the patient lies on the *affected* ear, followed by a 45-degree downward rotation of the head. This position is

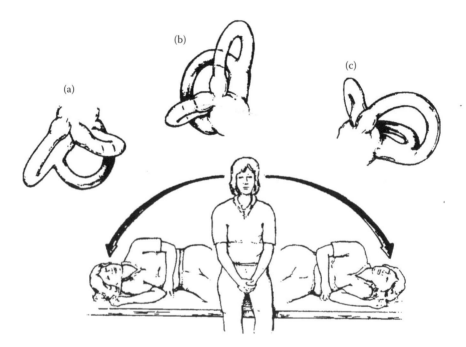

FIGURE 6.10
Brandt-Daroff exercise. (a) The patient is sitting and turns her head 45 degrees toward the unaffected side and then rapidly moves into the side-lying position. The patient stays in that position until nystagmus or the sensation of vertigo stops. (b) The patient sits up and remains in that position until sensation of vertigo ceases. (c) The patient then turns her head 45 degrees to the affected side and moves rapidly into the opposite side-lying position and remains in that position until symptoms (if present) stop. She then sits up. Each position is held for 30 seconds or more, depending upon the presence of symptoms. The entire exercise sequence is repeated until vertigo is diminished. The exercise should be repeated every 3 hours until the patient is symptom free for 2 consecutive days. (From Herdman, S. J., *Neurology Report*, 20(3), 46–53, 1996. With permission.)

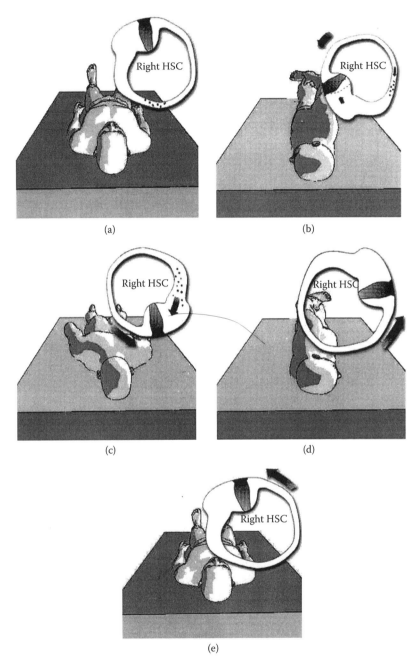

FIGURE 6.11

Bar-B-Que roll for right-sided horizontal semicircular canal positional vertigo (geotropic nystagmus) undergoing the Bar-B-Que maneuver. (a) The patient lays down supine. (b) A 90-degree rotation of the head and trunk are made toward the unaffected side. (c) A further 90-degree rotation is performed and the patient is now lying prone. (d) After a third 90-degree turn, the patient is now on the affected side. (e) The patient is turned to the supine position (original starting position) and sits up. Positions (b), (c), and (d) are held for 15 seconds or until dizziness stops. The movement of the right semicircular canal with the relative shifting of otoconial debris is shown (top right). (From Casani, A. P., et al., *Laryngoscope*, 112(1), 172–178, 2002. With permission.)

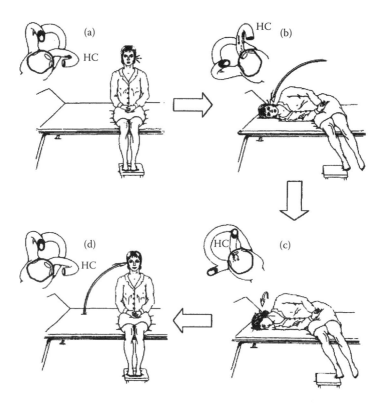

FIGURE 6.12
Liberatory maneuver for geotropic left horizontal canal (BPPV). (a) The patient is sitting sideways on the treatment table looking straight ahead. (b) The patient quickly lays on the unaffected side. (c) The head is quickly turned 45 degrees downward. (d) The patient returns to the sitting position. Positions (b) and (c) are held for 2 minutes each. Arrows indicate the position of the debris within the canal during the different stages of the maneuver. (From Appiani, G. A., et al., *Otology & Neurotology*, 22, 66–69, 2001. With permission.)

held for 2 minutes before sitting up. Casani et al.[35] reported using the Bar-B-Que roll prior to performing the FPP.

For patients who demonstrate apogeotropic nystagmus (cupulolithiasis), Casani and investigators[35] report 75% remission of symptoms in nine patients with a modified Semont maneuver. During this maneuver, the patient quickly lies down on the *affected* side, followed by a passive 45-degree downward rotation of the head. This position is also maintained for 2 minutes before sitting up.

Treatment for anterior semicircular canal BPPV of the canalithiasis type is determined by observing downbeating and torsional nystagmus in the Dix-Hallpike position. Because the posterior canal and the opposite anterior canal are in the same plane of excitation, one has to determine whether the nystagmus pattern is consistent with the downward ear or the opposite upward ear. According to Herdman,[62] if the downside ear is affected, the torsional component will beat in the same direction as the posterior semicircular canal on the same side (i.e., toward the same downside ear). If the nystagmus pattern is beating in a downward direction with the torsional component beating toward the upside ear, the opposite anterior semicircular canal is implicated. Performing a Dix-Hallpike test to the opposite side should confirm the affected side. If canalithiasis is suspected, one would perform the same treatment that is described for the posterior semicircular canal. If cupulolithiasis is suspected, the liberatory maneuver is modified so that the patient is sitting on the side of the bed with the head rotated 45 degrees toward the involved side. He is moved quickly toward the affected side, nose is down, and remains there for 1 minute. The patient is then quickly moved through the sitting position to the opposite side with head remaining in the initial 45-degree position, nose up. After maintaining that position for 1 minute, the patient sits up slowly to the sitting position.[31]

Several complications following CRT have been described.[26,52] Postural instability, although improved after treatment, may persist in patients following maneuvers.[41,52,63] This appears to be more common in the elderly and in patients with preexisting problems. Other complications include conversion of posterior canal BPPV to anterior or horizontal canal BPPV, stiff neck or neck pain, and severe nausea that may require premedication prior to the treatment.

In general, approximately 80% to 85% of patients with BPPV will experience remission of vertigo with just one episode of repositioning.[19,37] Many patients with BPPV, however, have persistent balance problems lasting several weeks after resolution of the episodic vertigo.[63,64] Because head injury patients may have additional physical, cognitive, and behavioral dysfunction, symptoms related to BPPV may be persistent and disabling, with delay in returning to work.[65] An exercise program directed by a physical or occupational therapist is recommended for those patients.[52]

The role of medications in the treatment of BPPV is limited to vestibular suppressants and antiemetics. Benzodiazepines (such as diazepam and alprazolam) are effective vestibular suppressants, but have sedative side effects and must, therefore, be used with caution. Promethazine is a commonly used antiemetic that is available in oral and intravenous formulations but may also cause sedation. Cases refractory to repositioning maneuvers have been successfully treated surgically with posterior semicircular canal occlusion.[54,66] The first published reports of posterior semicircular canal occlusion were in 1990 by Parnes and McClure.[67] This procedure is based on the theory of cupular deflection and endolymph displacement. The goal of the technique is to occlude the semicircular canal, thereby creating a closed, fluid-filled space and causing the cupula to become fixed. During this procedure, a mastoidectomy is performed and the posterior semicircular canal is punctured. Various materials including bone dust, bone wax, fibrin glue, and fascia may then be used to occlude the semicircular canal. Labyrinthectomy, vestibular neurectomy, and singular neurectomy are further surgical options that have largely been replaced by posterior semicircular canal occlusion.

6.3.5 Labyrinthine Concussion

Labyrinthine concussion is an imprecise term that subsumes a variety of symptoms, complaints, and, possibly, etiologies. Generally, it is assumed that the injury arises from bleeding within the labyrinthine capsule, but mechanical membrane disruption caused by acceleration and deceleration effects may also occur.[14,15] Diagnosis depends on detecting objective vestibular abnormalities in the vestibular laboratory. ENG testing is the most frequently helpful, and pathologic positional nystagmus is the most common abnormality. Unilateral weakness on ENG testing occurs less commonly, but is compelling when identified. Platform posturography showing reduced function with a vestibular pattern is confirmatory. Sinusoidal harmonic acceleration may show asymmetry with or without phase lag, depending on the extent of the injury and the degree of compensation.

Symptoms may include vertigo and disequilibrium with or without hearing loss, tinnitus, or aural fullness. Recovery depends upon the extent of the injury and the presence or absence of associated abnormalities. Often, recovery is complete within a few weeks. When recovery is slow, vestibular rehabilitation can hasten its arrival and often improve the final outcome. If unilateral weakness can be demonstrated on ENG, consideration should be given to surgical ablation of the injured labyrinthine end organ.

6.3.6 Posttraumatic Vascular Loop

From time to time, head injury may displace one of the posterior fossa intracranial vessels and cause it to come to rest against the eighth cranial nerve in the cerebellopontine angle. Generally, the anterior inferior cerebellar artery or one of its branches is involved. Vascular compression of the cochleovestibular nerve produces a characteristic syndrome. The afflicted individual is overwhelmed by an almost constant, severe positional vertigo often associated with visceral symptoms. Although actual severity may vary over a fairly wide range, the patient is frequently not able to function. Motion usually results in marked exacerbation of symptoms. Unilateral tinnitus and hearing loss may accompany the vestibular symptoms, but are frequently absent. Diagnosis depends on the presence of typical abnormalities seen during auditory brainstem response audiometry. Specifically, changes in interpeak latency suggestive of cochlear–vestibular nerve pathology will be noted. Radiographic demonstration of the juxtaposition of the nerve to the vessel is helpful, but not essential. When present, surgical decompression is curative.

6.3.7 Cervicogenic Dizziness

Because cervical position sense receptors in joint capsules and deep cervical muscle stretch receptors provide information to the CNS about the orientation of the head in space, musculoskeletal abnormalities of the neck and cervical spine may result in "dizzy" or "swimming sensations.[68–73]

Altered cervical proprioceptive input and/or pain may be associated with disturbed standing balance, limited cervical range of motion, muscle spasm, and/or occipital region headache in persistent whiplash injuries.[74,75] Sensory mismatch between vestibular and proprioceptive inputs may produce dizziness and imbalance.[72]

Most common, cervicogenic dizziness is associated with flexion–extension injuries that may lead to myofascial pain dysfunction syndromes involving either the lateral or posterior cervical muscles. Because cervical proprioception is not the most important sensory modality subserving equilibrium, disorders of the cervical musculoskeletal system usually produce symptomatology that is relatively mild. Patients typically complain of a vague disquiet and uneasiness about their balance. They resist free movement and frequently use support structures (wall, handrails, and so forth). "Spinning" is not experienced and falls do not, in fact, occur, although patients are ever fearful that they *will* fall. Frequent headaches occur commonly.

One of the major difficulties in identifying this problem remains the lack of a specific and sensitive test that clearly identifies this diagnosis.[74,76,77] The duration and frequency of symptoms lasting from minutes to hours as well as the onset of dizziness related to pain or head movements are important to identify in the history.

Physical examination will generally detect muscle spasms and tenderness resulting in restricted cervical motion and pain. Tenderness is frequently focal and of the "trigger point" variety.[77] Common focal points are the spinous process of the seventh cervical vertebrae and along the posterior nuchal line, where the posterior cervical muscles insert into the periosteum of the skull or at the insertion of the sternocleidomastoid and splenius capitis muscles into the mastoid tip.

One method to differentiate symptoms of dizziness or pain between vestibular, cervical, or a combination of the two is to perform provocation tests of body-on-head rotations while the examiner holds the head still (cervical component) with the patient sitting on a rolling chair. This would be followed by moving the head and body en bloc (vestibular component).[78]

Aggressive physical therapy and anti-inflammatory and muscle relaxant medications must be combined regularly for several weeks to achieve relief.[79–81] Limited use of cervical collars are recommended for 1 to 2 hours daily to allow muscle spasm and pain to diminish. Gentle range-of-motion exercises, gentle manual traction, and acupressure may be utilized. Cotreatment with or referral to a vestibular rehabilitation therapist will improve the ability to use a variety of strategies for postural stability.

6.3.8 Central Vertigo

Dizziness and disequilibrium originating within the nervous system and not from the labyrinth or eighth nerve is a relatively common component of posttraumatic head injury. Vertigo, which arises within the CNS itself, is accompanied more often by other cranial neuropathies and neurologic deficits than peripheral vertigo. Dysarthria, dysphagia, ocular motor deficits, numbness and tingling in the extremities, and focal motor weakness are common.[14,82–87] A significant number of these individuals have been severely injured so that they have been in prolonged coma. Many have significant long tract signs. Involvement of the cerebellum produces "dizziness" and disequilibrium only in the standing position and when attempting to walk.[88] Ambulation may be severely impaired and is no better with eyes open than with eyes closed. Subjective rotational vertigo is notably absent. Excessive postural sway may be noted, whereas strategies to minimize this may lead to decreased neck and trunk mobility combined with a wide base of support.[89] Nystagmus will also be as vigorous with eyes open as with eyes closed. Indeed, nystagmus may be so pronounced as to be apparent from several feet away, but when queried, the patient will often deny subjective vertigo.

Computerized assessment of postural sway indicates patients with traumatic brain injury rely more on visual cues to decrease sway than healthy subjects.[90] Prolonged motor latency following support surface perturbations are also observed.[91]

Frequently, disorders of balance are recognized relatively late in the rehabilitation of these individuals. Early in treatment, other injuries are more apparent and need to be addressed more urgently. As consciousness returns, mentation improves, motor weakness resolves, and efforts can be directed toward beginning ambulation and resuming normal activities. It may be when such retraining is begun and proceeds poorly that balance disturbance is first recognized.

The pathophysiology of central balance disturbance remains unclear. Olsson[14] has demonstrated punctate hemorrhage and degeneration within the vestibular nuclei of head-injured guinea pigs.

Much evidence of central involvement comes from VNG/ENG evaluation. Many investigators have shown a high incidence of central VNG/ENG findings in the head-injured population. Tuohimaa[6] has argued cogently that VNG/ENG findings imply that vestibular dysfunction may be the result of impaired cortical inhibition and not solely the result of disruption of brainstem nuclei or pathways. Subjective vertigo from stimulation or injury to the temporal cortical projections of the vestibular system is uncommon, but may occur as a component of a seizure disorder.

There are no medical or surgical methods for managing central vestibular injury. Indeed, the presence of a central component is frequently cited as a cause for the reduced effectiveness of eighth nerve section in head injury patients even when a clearcut peripheral component is present. Vestibular rehabilitation will continue to be the mainstay of treatment for patients who have a significant central component, although recovery is often protracted, with symptoms persisting years after the injury.[92–95] Medical and surgical treatment may be of significant ancillary assistance when there is a concomitant peripheral vestibular injury.

6.4 Clinical Evaluation

6.4.1 Patient History

An adequate history is frequently the key to both diagnosis and management of vestibular disorders. This can be a difficult undertaking in the individual recovering from brain injury. However, every effort should be made to elicit as much information as possible even though this may be taxing to the evaluator.

Questions about premorbid leisure activities can give important information regarding physical impairment, including vestibular injury. Did the patient return to sports and leisure after his injury and, if not, why not? Are there any close relatives or friends able to substantiate this information?

Does the patient's direct family report any changes regarding the patient's participation in the family circle? Specifically, are there complaints regarding balance (e.g., in darkness or with leisure activities)? Has the patient become less physically active at all? Are there any complaints of visual or auditory overstimulation that can be associated with a vestibular lesion?

When balance dysfunction is present, it should first be established whether the patient is experiencing a subjective sense of vertigo or disequilibrium. Individuals with central dysfunction and cerebellar disorders, although clearly impaired by balance dysfunction, may have no associated sense of disequilibrium or vertigo. When present, such sensations are frequently referred to as feeling *dizzy*. It is astonishing how frequently this term may remain unclarified and ill defined even though treatment persists for months. It is critical to clarify, in as much detail as possible, what the individual means by the term *dizzy*. Often, the patient will protest that he is unable to elucidate the experience further, but if pressed, this is almost never the case and important information can almost always be obtained with perseverance. *Vertigo* is a technical term that refers to the illusion of movement when no movement is, in fact, present. The most obvious example of such a sensation is the sense of rotation when one is still. However, a sense that one is falling, when one is not falling, or the sense that one is "veering" when one is not, also constitute an illusion of movement when none is present. These sensations are appropriately subsumed under the term *vertigo*. It will turn out that a goodly number of patients do not have an illusion of movement even when they use the term *dizzy*. Such patients may be referring to a sense of lightheadedness, giddiness, a vague feeling of nausea, a sense that they are walking on air, a feeling of being "closed in," weakness, disorientation, or a general sense of "confusion."

After clarifying the character of the dizzy sensation, it is crucial to determine whether the sensation is invariably present or present only episodically. If present episodically, then how frequently and for how long it persists are important data to be gathered. Whether the symptoms are always of the same severity needs to be ascertained and, if the severity is variable, then a search for exacerbating or remitting factors needs to be made. The relationship of the symptoms to movement is crucial. Many patients either have their symptoms only in certain head or body positions, or the act of moving into certain positions precipitates symptomatic episodes. The patient should be questioned regarding whether there is any relationship between his symptoms and diet, exercise, or situational stress. One should determine whether the symptoms are reliably reproduced in a given place. Individuals suffering from anxiety disorders, for example, will frequently have their symptoms very reliably "place associated.[96,97] They may experience symptoms in open places or closed places, or in church or in the car. When symptoms are closely linked to a specific place or situation, organic vestibular dysfunction is improbable. On the other hand, certain types of visual stimuli will reliably produce symptoms in patients with vestibular disease. Complex geometric patterns and rapid movement in the peripheral visual field are two such common stimuli. A surprising number of patients will complain of disequilibrium when shopping in the grocery store because of the rapid movement of the high, grocery-laden shelves in their peripheral visual field as they move down the aisle.

A search for associated symptoms should be made. The patient must be carefully queried regarding the presence or absence of dysarthria, dysphagia, visual change, numbness or tingling in the extremities or around the mouth, and focal motor weakness. Patients should be questioned about the presence or absence of headache and syncopal episodes. Moreover, it would be important to assess the patient's perceived level of disability and impact on quality of life as one method of determining the overall impairment, treatment plan, and improvement after therapies.

The Dizziness Handicap Inventory (DHI), a self-report measure, has been shown to be a sensitive measure of subtle changes in balance after concussion.[98,99] Whitney et al.[100] concluded that items on a newly developed subscale of the DHI may assist in screening for BPPV. The Activities Specific Balance Confidence Scale, another questionnaire that measures an individual's confidence in performing different tasks that challenge balance, has been found to correlate with the DHI in assessing perceived problems in patients with vestibular dysfunction.[101]

6.4.2 Physical Examination

A complete neurotologic examination must be performed. It should start with close examination of the external auditory canals and tympanic membranes. Such an examination will not only determine the stigmata of temporal bone fracture or serious head injury, but also the more mundane findings of middle ear effusion, cholesteatoma, or tympanic membrane perforation. It must always be remembered that the traumatically brain-injured individual is not immune to the commonplace afflictions of everyday life. The pneumatic otoscope should be utilized to ensure adequate tympanic membrane mobility. A complete cranial nerve examination is mandatory. Eye movement abnormalities should be noted prominently because they will affect interpretation of the ENG. Similarly, evaluation of the facial nerve must be compulsive because it travels so closely with the vestibular nerve that it is an invaluable localizing sign. Evaluation of hearing is compelling for the same reasons and should include the Rinne and Weber tests, as well as a complete audiometric battery. Abnormalities of the lower cranial nerves, including swallowing dysfunction and disorders of voice, may indicate significant brainstem injury.

Coordination is evaluated using standard tests of cerebellar function, such as the fingertip-to-nose test; test for dysdiadochokinesia and rebound phenomenon, which are performed for the upper extremities; and the heel–shin maneuver for the lower extremities. Cerebellar ataxia in gait comprises a widened base of support, an irregular step length, and weaving from side to side. Vestibular dysfunction can also result in an ataxic gait quite similar to the one described here, but does not result in positive cerebellar tests. Gait and station should be evaluated using the Romberg test and tandem gait as well as heel and toe walking. A severely disabled individual might not be able to perform some of these tests, in which case these tests will have to be omitted.

6.4.2.1 *Clinical Testing*

Clinical evaluation of the head injury patient suspected of vestibular dysfunction will have to go beyond the administration of a few clinical tests because, in addition to the suspected vestibular dysfunction, other symptoms of CNS injury might compromise overall physical functioning. Also, clinical vestibular tests are not pathognomonic for specific lesions but are indicators. Routinely, several functional vestibular tests are performed. If any is positive, a vestibular lesion should be suspected. The temporal association of head injury and onset of dizziness is critical to ascertain. In addition, the vestibular patient will not always be able to clearly discuss/communicate the changes that are a result of the vestibular injury.

The clinician will decide which tests to administer based on the patient's history and system review. Provocation of specific deficits can be done if the patient's history indicates a specific lesion. A good example is the Dix-Hallpike maneuver done when a patient's complaints are suspect for BPPV. The examination of a brain-injured individual is comprised of the patient's history, musculoskeletal assessment (including postural alignment), cervical and upper quadrant screening, neuromuscular screening (including strength testing), somatosensory screening, visual perception, and cardiorespiratory deconditioning. Medication review, functional ability, activity level, and report of health status provide the clinician with an understanding of environmental and societal issues affecting the patient's recovery.

6.4.3 Eye Movements

Observation for spontaneous nystagmus should be performed with Frenzel lenses or with a video infrared camera to prevent fixation by a lighted environment. Observed nystagmus can help separate peripheral from central vestibular disorders. Gaze-evoked nystagmus, a sign of a brainstem problem, assesses the patient's ability to demonstrate stable conjugate eye deviations away from the primary position. An ocular tilt reaction (skew eye deviation) assesses for misalignment of the eyes secondary to otolith dysfunction. Misalignment may result in complaints of diplopia, vertigo, or oscillopsia. Subtle misalignments may be detected by alternately covering each eye while having the patient fixate on a distant object. If movement is noted in one eye after covering the other, an ocular misalignment is present. Misalignment, which is variable in different fields of gaze, may be the result of an abnormality of an extraocular muscle. Obvious misalignment in a patient with no complaints likely represents long-standing strabismus. Vertical misalignment is associated with brainstem or cerebellar lesions. Three different types of eye movement should be assessed: vergence, saccades, and smooth pursuit. Vergence movements can be elicited by asking the patient to follow a finger toward and away from the nose; these movements are normally slow and smooth. Abnormal oscillation is suggestive of a functional disorder. Saccades are evaluated by having the patient fixate alternately on two stationary targets. Velocity, accuracy, and initiation time of the saccades should be assessed; any abnormality points to a central etiology. Smooth pursuit movements are assessed by having the patient track a target, such as a pen, without head movement. Asymmetry in horizontal smooth pursuit movement is suggestive of CNS pathology. Mild impairment, however, may be seen in the elderly or as a side effect of medications. Only very gross abnormalities can be detected on physical examination. Subtle dysfunction, which is much more common, can only be detected by electro-oculography.

6.4.3.1 Vestibulo-ocular Reflex Testing

Several bedside tests may be used to evaluate the VOR. These are based on the premise that a unilateral reduction of the VOR will cause motion of the visual surround during head movements (oscillopsia), primarily with movements toward the affected ear. A bilateral hypofunction/loss results in oscillopsia with all head movements.

The head thrust test assesses the doll's-eye reflex and is performed by rapidly rotating the patient's head to midline from an initial position 30 degrees off midline. This is performed with the patient maintaining fixation on a target and is considered positive if the eyes have to make a saccade to refixate. The test is less sensitive in detecting incomplete versus complete loss of vestibular function. Maintaining the head in a pitched 30-degree down angle and performing unpredictable timing and direction of thrusts, however, appears to improve sensitivity.[102]

Testing visual acuity during head movements (dynamic visual acuity) is another method of assessing the VOR. Initially, static visual acuity is assessed by asking the patient to read the lowest line on the Snellen chart. Then the patient's head is rotated horizontally through a 60-degree arc at a frequency of 1 to 2 cycles per second while testing visual acuity. Normal individuals lose one line of acuity. Patients with a unilateral loss of vestibular function may lose two to four lines; those with bilateral loss may lose five to six lines.

Head shaking-induced nystagmus may be elicited by passively or actively rotating the patient's head at a high frequency for 10 to 20 seconds with eyes closed and then stopping abruptly. Patients with severe unilateral vestibular loss will have nystagmus with the initial slow phase directed toward the affected side and a subsequent reversal phase directed toward the unaffected side. Bilateral vestibular hypofunction and acute unilateral hypofunction do not produce nystagmus after head shaking.

6.4.3.2 Positional Testing

Tests for positional nystagmus help to separate peripheral from central pathology and often localize peripheral pathology. Positional nystagmus is assessed by placing the patient in each of the upright, supine, right-ear-down, and left-ear-down positions for at least 30 seconds and observing for nystagmus. Nystagmus that lasts longer than 1 minute and changes direction typically indicates central pathology. Positional nystagmus that lasts longer than 1 minute but does not change direction can be seen in peripheral or central disorders. Transitory nystagmus that lasts less than 1 minute is usually described as positional nystagmus and indicates peripheral pathology (usually BPPV).

TABLE 6.2

Characteristics of Central and Peripheral Positioning Nystagmus

Characteristic	Central	Peripheral
Latency	None	2–15 seconds
Duration	30–120 seconds	5–30 seconds
Fatigability	+/−	+
Vertigo	Absent	Present
Fixation	No suppression	Suppression
Direction	Vertical, horizontal	Horizontal, rotary
Characteristic	Direction changing	Direction fixed

The Dix-Hallpike maneuver is the most commonly performed positional test and is used to examine for BPPV.[103] The test is performed by starting with the patient in the seated upright position with the head turned 30 degrees toward the examiner. The patient's head is held between the examiner's hands, and the patient is rapidly moved into the supine position, with head extended 30 degrees over the edge of the table. The patient's eyes are observed for nystagmus as this position is held for at least 30 seconds before returning to the upright position. This maneuver is then repeated for the opposite ear, with the head turned in the opposite direction. The direction of the nystagmus is specific to the involved semicircular canal. In general, in canalithiasis, peripheral nystagmus has a latency period, short duration, and fatigability. However, in cupulolithiasis, constant nystagmus and vertigo may be present for more than 1 minute. Nystagmus that persists, often vertical and not present in the seated position, may indicate a central positional vertigo (Table 6.2).

The Motion Sensitivity Quotient (MSQ)[91] is a subjective rating of the patient's perception of symptoms as he actively undergoes 16 different positions or movements that have been adapted from work by Norre (Table 6.3).[104] Based on these findings, patients will be given specific exercises based on principles of habituation for remediation of their symptoms. This approach works well with chronic unilateral vestibular hypofunction and has been reported to decrease sensitivity and duration of symptoms as quickly as 2 weeks; however, in the head injury population, it may take as long as 6 months or more.[91,105,106]

6.4.3.3 Balance Assessments

Testing for balance deficits should include a range of tests that assess sitting balance, static standing, self-initiated movements, altering sensory cues, and gait activities. Table 6.4 provides a list and references of common balance and gait tools used in clinical practice. These tests may indicate balance can be affected by a vestibular deficit, but also by generalized weakness, dyscoordination, spasticity, rigidity, impaired vision, or lack of sensation. However, a vestibular deficit can be expected when any of the following indicators of vestibular involvement are present:

- Difficulty with any balance task that either limits or excludes vision. An example of the first is the sharpened Romberg with eyes closed. Vestibular patients rely heavily on visual input to compensate for the loss of (reliable) vestibular information. When this is denied in a testing situation, they score poorly.

- Difficulty with postural adjustment with static balance tests such as single leg stance or the sharpened Romberg test. The tests require a period of 30 seconds for a normal score. Normal subjects can adjust smoothly to balance disturbance.

TABLE 6.3

Motion Sensitivity Quotient Test for Assessing Movement- and Position-Related Dizziness

Baseline Symptoms	Intensity[a] (0–5)	Duration[b] (0–3)	Total Score[c]
1. Sitting → supine			
2. Supine → left side			
3. Left → right side			
4. Supine → sitting			
5. Left Dix-Hallpike			
6. Return to sitting			
7. Right Dix-Hallpike			
8. Return to sitting			
9. Sitting → nose to left knee			
10. Return to upright position			
11. Sitting → nose to right knee			
12. Return to upright position			
13. Sitting: Head rotation five times			
14. Sitting: Head flexion/extension five times			
15. Standing: Turn 180 degrees right			
16. Standing: Turn 180 degrees left			

[a] Intensity: 0, no symptoms; 5, severe symptoms.
[b] Duration: 1 point, 5 to 10 seconds; 2 points, 11 to 30 seconds; 3 points, ≥30 seconds.
[c] Total Motion Sensitivity Quotient (MSQ) $= \dfrac{\text{No. of Provoking Positions} \times \text{Score}}{2048} \times 100$

MSQ score: mild, 0 to 10 points; moderate, 11 to 30 points; severe, 31 to 100 points.
Source: Modified from Smith-Wheelock, M., Shepard, N. T., and Telian, S. A., *American Journal of Otology*, 12(3), 218–225, 1991.

Vestibular patients can perceive gravitational effects sometimes, but not accurately, and therefore overcorrect, ultimately leading to a loss of balance or excessive weaving.

- Difficulty with performing multiple tasks in varied sensory contexts increases postural sway under all sensory conditions and slows reactions times, resulting in loss of balance, depending upon the age of the patient or the severity of the injury.

Dynamic functional skills are important to assess because postural control is highly complex and multidimensional. In the Fukuda stepping test,[107] patients march in place for 50 steps with eyes open and closed and arms extended. Normal subjects move forward less than 50 cm and turn less than 30 degrees.[108] Patients with bilateral or uncompensated unilateral deficits may be identified, but not those with other sensory deficits or musculoskeletal deficits. Marked variability in rotation by the same individual makes this test unreliable.[108]

The Functional Reach Test and the Berg Balance Test are two additional performance-based measures of balance that have been widely used as screens for balance deficits and predicting risk of falls in the elderly.[109,110] Both have good interrater reliability, especially in the elderly population and are widely used to assess patients with balance deficits. However, caution should be used in predicting falls in the neurologic population because

TABLE 6.4

Clinical Balance Tests

Clinical Tests	Time	Score	Norms Available	Reference
Performance based				
Reach tests: functional reach			√	109
Berg Balance Scale		_/56	√	110
Gait				
Dynamic gait index (20 feet)		_/24	√	115–117
Self-selected gait velocity (7.62 m)			√	126
Functional gait assessment (20-foot walkway)		_/30	√	122
Three-minute walk test (524-foot indoor course)			√	111

little insight into quality of movements used to accomplish balance and underlying impairments can be gleaned from most performance tests.[111]

When posturography is not available, the influence of sensory interactions can be assessed with the Clinical Test for Sensory Interaction of Balance[112] and is based on the concepts developed by Nashner.[113] This technique originally used medium density foam 24 × 24 inch and a Japanese lantern with vertical stripes placed inside to produce inaccurate visual and surface orientation inputs. This test has been modified to exclude conditions 3 and 6, which were not sufficiently sensitive to detect visual motion sensitivity.[114]

Frequently, patients with symptomatic dizziness and disequilibrium display diminished arm swing, rigid trunk, widened based of support, decreased stride length, and reduced gait speed during initial observations in the clinic. The severity of these deviations depends upon the underlying conditions and acuteness of the disorder. Moreover, imbalance during ambulation may be observed in varied environments depending upon lighting, surface, distractions, or head movements. Demanding gait tasks combined with cognitive and secondary tasks or obstacle courses may yield further insight into functional problems the patient may be experiencing and the need for assistive devices.[115–118]

The Dynamic Gait Index is commonly used to assess abnormal gait in patients with vestibular dysfunction as well as fall risk in seniors.[117,119,120] The scale has eight tasks (total of 24 points) with varying activities that require walking at different speeds, with head movements, around obstacles, up and down stairs, and making quick turns. Nineteen points or less is predictive of falls. It is an inexpensive and simple clinical tool to administer but should be used with caution in patients with vestibular disorders. Investigators report good reliability in total Dynamic Gait Index scores, but individual items demonstrate moderate to poor reliability.[120,121] Several other mobility tests are available but beyond the scope of this chapter.[122–124]

Gait speed has been correlated with function and disability,[114,125] and patients with vestibular deficits will exhibit slower speeds than age-matched normal subjects.[121] Self-selected walking speeds are indicative of an individual's confidence, and functional mobility and normative values are available for adults age 20 to 79 years.[126] However, Moseley et al.[127] studied patients after head injury and found that gait speed established in the clinic during functional tests such as the 6-minute walk decreased during ambulation in the community in complex environments, indicating that additional tests need to reflect the demands in real-life situations. Shumway-Cook and Woollacott[111] advocate the Three-Minute Walk Test over a 524-foot indoor carpeted course that has a 15-inch walking path. Patients walk at their preferred speed, making four different turns. Scoring includes the distance walked in 3 minutes and the number of times the patient moves outside the 15-inch path. Gait deviations are common in patients with symptomatic dizziness and imbalance and can be further delineated when patients walk under varying conditions such as firm and altered surfaces, with head movements, and in varied lighting environments.

The balance assessments described previously provide the clinician with information about balance abilities in the patient with a head injury. Evaluation of more dynamic tasks that involve interactions of cognitive processing, visual processing, and dual tasks are challenging and perhaps more sensitive to problems the patient encounters in the community Each test described has its strengths and weaknesses, and the clinician must determine the most appropriate to use for each patient. None of these tests is pathognomonic for a particular type of vestibular lesion, but the entire evaluation can give strong indicators of vestibular dysfunction that can be clarified by an in-depth laboratory evaluation. A vestibular evaluation by an otolaryngologist specializing in vestibular dysfunction is often requested.

6.4.4 Laboratory Evaluation

6.4.4.1 Auditory Testing

Because the vestibular system and auditory system are so closely interrelated, both at the level of the labyrinth, the eighth cranial nerve, and within the brainstem, complete audiometric testing is essential in the evaluation of any patient with balance disturbance. This should include a formal audiogram that tests pure tone reception at octave intervals from 125 Hz (cycles per second) to 8000 Hz. Both air conduction and bone conduction should be tested. Speech discrimination scores should be obtained and the speech reception threshold measured. If inconsistent or ambiguous information is developed within the pure tone audiogram or speech testing, then this information should be confirmed or expanded using auditory brainstem response audiometry.[128] The initial pure tone evaluation should be accompanied by immittance testing, which measures not only tympanic membrane compliance, but also assists in identification of ossicular disarticulation and assesses the stapedius reflex at several frequencies. Stapedius reflex testing is sensitive to a variety of different sorts of retrocochlear pathology. Abnormalities of stapedius reflex testing, if not explained by known difficulties, should be considered indications for further evaluation with auditory brainstem response audiometry or radiographic imaging. Based on the history and the pure tone audiogram, further evaluation with electrocochleography, vestibular testing, middle latency response evaluation, or central auditory testing can be considered.[85,129,130] The results of auditory testing should be consistent with the results of tuning fork tests as determined during the physical examination. If there are inconsistencies between these test results, these inconsistencies need to be resolved.

6.4.4.2 The Electronystagmogram

Nystagmus is the only sign on physical examination uniquely linked to the vestibular system. Therefore, the ENG plays a crucial and pivotal role in evaluating the vestibular system. The ENG offers a number of advantages. First and foremost, it is capable of detecting nystagmus with eyes closed. The vast majority of peripheral nystagmus is effectively suppressed by visual fixation and will not be apparent to the examiner with the patient's eyes open. Frenzel lenses are thick 20-diopter lenses used to assist in the detection of nystagmus on physical examination. These lenses make the detection of pathologically significant nystagmus easier in two ways. First, they prevent visual fixation by the patient because they make it virtually impossible to see anything but light. Second, they magnify the cornea and iris when the examiner views the patient's globe through the Frenzel glasses. Frenzel lenses will permit the detection of clinically significant nystagmus that would be otherwise inapparent. But even with Frenzel lenses, about half of pathologically significant nystagmus will be missed.[131,132]

The ENG is capable of detecting subtle abnormalities of both volitional and reflex eye movement controlled at the brainstem and even higher levels. These abnormalities cannot be detected by any other method. Their detection can be the most significant and easily documented evidence for brainstem dysfunction.

An additional advantage to the ENG is the ability of this testing method to test each labyrinthine end organ separately. No other clinical test of vestibular function permits unequivocal isolation of one labyrinth from its contralateral partner.

The ENG produces a permanent objective record of labyrinthine function. Such a record can be reviewed months or years after it was made and compared with new tracings to determine the evolution of a pathologic process or to document improvement.

There are some disadvantages to the ENG. The stimulus is not physiologic and stimulus intensity is subject to a variety of variables only partially under the examiner's control. These include the shape and nature of the external auditory canal, the size of the tympanic cavity, and the thickness and position of the tympanic membrane. The test requires a compulsive and meticulous examiner who is willing to recalibrate equipment before every examination, remove any cerumen impeding the flow of air/water into the canal, and ensure good contact between the electrodes and the skin. A first-rate ENG technician will also interact with the patient in a tactful, compassionate, and sympathetic fashion. Not only is this an intrinsically desirable end in itself, but it will also encourage maximum effort from the patient and procure the most consistent and reliable tracings.

Electronystagmography requires relatively intact extraocular muscle function. Thus, individuals with certain intrinsic abnormalities of the extraocular muscles or paresis of cranial nerves III, IV, or VI may generate tracings that are uninterpretable.

Electronystagmography is, perhaps, more properly termed *electro-oculography*. Although generally used to measure and detect nystagmus in the evaluation of individuals with vertigo, the test actually measures the movement of the globe within the orbit. The positively charged cornea and the negatively charged retina together create a dipole with a movement that can be detected when electrodes are placed around the orbits. The testing apparatus is calibrated so that eye deviations to the right produce an upward deflection and eye deviations to the left produce a downward deviation of the pen. In the vertical channel, upward eye movements create an upward deviation of the pen and downward movements produce a downward movement of the pen. The system is calibrated so that each degree of eye movement produces a 1-mm deflection of the pen. The system needs to be recalibrated before each test.

The complete ENG consists of a set of seven different subtests: the saccade test, the gaze test, the tracking test, the optokinetic test, the positional test, the Dix-Hallpike maneuver, and the bithermal caloric test. The saccade test is usually done first because the system can be calibrated at the same time the test is performed. With lights on, patients are instructed to look back and forth between two spots located on the wall directly in front of them without moving their head. An arbitrary distance of about 6 feet is selected so that patients eyes move about twenty degrees in the horizontal and vertical planes as they look back and forth, as directed, between spots. The spots on the wall are then selected to produce a 20-mm pen deflection. The speed and accuracy with which these movements are produced is inspected and measured. Normal individuals can perform this test with great rapidity and with very high degrees of accuracy. Brainstem dysfunction produces well-recognized abnormalities including systematic "overshoot" and "undershoot." These abnormalities may occur in one or in both directions of gaze.

Gaze testing is performed by having the patient look straight ahead and then thirty degrees to the right, left, up, and down. Gaze in these positions is maintained for at least 20 seconds with eyes open, then an additional 20 seconds with eyes closed. Any nystagmus present during these sustained eye deviations is recorded. Gaze nystagmus can arise from both central and peripheral vestibular pathology as well as a consequence of normal variations such as end point nystagmus or congenital nystagmus (Figure 6.13). Frequently, one can distinguish between various etiologies by carefully examining the eye position in which the nystagmus occurs and the morphology of typical nystagmoid beats. Nystagmus that occurs with eyes open and disappears with eyes closed is reliably attributed to CNS pathology.

Sinusoidal tracking or pursuit testing is also performed in a lighted room. Patients are asked simply to track visually an object moving back and forth in front of their visual field. This may be a ball suspended on a string from the ceiling or a sophisticated computer-driven light bar. Normal individuals can track such sinusoidal motions with amazing accuracy. A variety of possible abnormalities can be detected (Figure 6.14). Certain of these are characteristic of CNS (particularly brainstem) pathology and others may simply represent the superimposition of peripherally induced nystagmus on the tracing.

Optokinetic testing is performed by moving a series of alternating black and white stripes in front of the patient's visual field. This reliably induces nystagmus in normal

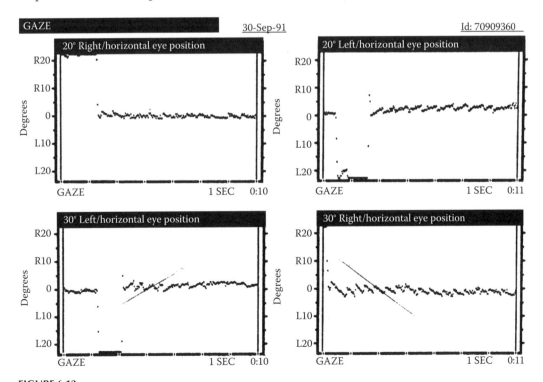

FIGURE 6.13
Gaze nystagmus is present in all gaze positions. It is most obvious in the 30-degree left and right deviations (lower tracings) than in the upper 20-degree eye deviation tracings.

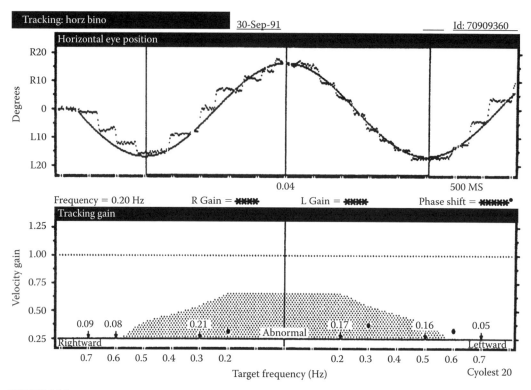

FIGURE 6.14
Horizontal tracking is illustrated in this computerized electronystagmographic tracing. Most subjects can follow a sinusoidal pattern very accurately. This patient follows it in a steplike "saccadic" fashion that is usually pathognomonic for CNS pathology.

individuals. Typically, the stripes are moved first to the right and then to the left in front of the patient's visual fields at 20 degrees per second and then 40 degrees per second. Comparisons are then made between the resulting tracings. Several possible abnormalities can occur. Optokinetic nystagmus can be effectively and normally induced in one direction, but not in the other. Occasionally, the system breaks down under stress and individuals whose optokinetic nystagmus is normal at lower speeds produce abnormal optokinetic nystagmus when the speed is increased. Virtually all abnormalities of optokinetic testing arise from central pathology, most commonly within the brainstem.

Positional testing is important not only to document pathologic eye movements in patients whose chief complaint is positional nystagmus, but also because abnormal test results occur in individuals who complain of nonpositionally related disequilibrium and vertigo. The test is performed by examining ENG tracings produced in four positions: with the patient sitting up looking straight ahead, with the patient lying supine looking straight ahead, with the right ear down, and with the left ear down. Not only does the tracing need to be examined for the presence of nystagmus produced in one position or another, but in patients with preexisting spontaneous nystagmus, a record needs to be carefully examined to determine whether positional changes produce any alteration in the underlying nystagmus pattern. A large variety of different patterns of positional nystagmus have been detected. These include direction-fixed and direction-changing varieties. Among direction-changing varieties are those that beat consistently away from the ground (ageotropic) and those that beat consistently toward the ground (geotropic).

Although direction-fixed nystagmus is more characteristic of peripheral disorders, and direction-changing nystagmus is more characteristic of central disorders, so many exceptions to these rules have been identified that it is not possible to make definitive statements about the etiologic significance of particular positional patterns.[133–135] An exception is the individual in whom the direction of the nystagmus changes while in a single head position. Such a pattern is invariably associated with CNS pathology.

An objective record of fistula testing can be made using the ENG and the impedance bridge. To accomplish this, the immitance probe is placed into first one ear and then the other. The pressure in the external auditory canal is varied between +200 mm Hg and –200 mm Hg. The ENG is then examined for induced nystagmus. Each ear is tested separately. A positive test result is identified by the production of nystagmus associated with a change in pressure on the tympanic membrane. In some cases, the nystagmus can seem to change direction as the pressure changes from positive to negative. One would expect that the patient's subjective symptoms of vertigo, with or without nausea, will be induced during the presence of nystagmoid eye movements in positive tests. The results of the ENG fistula test can then be compared (when available) to platform fistula test results.[12,86,105]

Dix-Hallpike testing is a test of position*ing* nystagmus. In this test, the patient is rapidly moved from a sitting position to the supine position with first the right ear and then the left ear down. The test is specifically designed to identify benign paroxysmal positional nystagmus. The test is positive when, after a latency of 2 to 15 seconds, bursts of torsional horizontal–rotary and upbeating nystagmus lasting 5 to 30 seconds are observed.

The response fatigues rapidly, so that when the maneuver is repeated, the response will be much less vigorous. Usually, several repetitions in rapid succession are sufficient to eliminate any detectable response whatsoever. Positive Dix-Hallpike testing is classically associated with canalithiasis. Canalithiasis is a not uncommon consequence of blunt head injury. Because the response fatigues rapidly, Dix-Hallpike testing should precede other forms of positional testing. If it follows conventional positional testing, the expected response may actually have been inadvertently "fatigued out" by the previous positioning maneuvers.

Bithermal caloric testing permits quantification of the "strength" of the response obtained from each labyrinth separately. Although the strength of the bithermal caloric response is generally assumed to represent the activity of the individual labyrinth as a whole, it is important to remember that, in actuality, only the horizontal semicircular canal is stimulated. Careful evaluation of patients and comparison of ENG and sinusoidal harmonic acceleration (SHA) responses clearly demonstrate that it is possible to have residual function in the superior and posterior semicircular canals even when no response can be generated using bithermal caloric testing in the horizontal canal.

The test depends on the production of convection currents within the horizontal semicircular canal. Warmed and cooled air or water is systematically irrigated through the external auditory canal. This produces a raising or lowering of the temperature of the tympanic membrane and produces a temperature change within the middle ear space. As air is cooled or heated in the middle ear space, that portion of the horizontal semicircular canal that protrudes effectively into the middle ear space is also cooled or warmed. Because the nonexposed portions of this canal do not suffer the same temperature change, convection currents are produced within the endolymphatic space of the horizontal semicircular canal. This fluid movement will produce cupular deflection, discharges within the vestibular nerve, and nystagmus, which can be measured. Thermal stimuli reliably produce nystagmus in a specific direction. Cold water will produce nystagmus with its fast component away from the irrigated ear. Warm stimuli, on the other hand, will produce nystagmus with the fast component toward the stimulated ear. A useful pneumonic for these relationships is COWS (cold opposite warm same). The simplest clinical application of this principle is seen in the utilization of ice-water caloric examination that can be performed at the bedside or in the emergency department. Ice-water calorics are performed by putting 10 to 20 mL ice water into the external auditory canal. This will produce an extremely vigorous response in normal individuals with easily detected gross nystagmus away from the irrigated ear. Unfortunately, nausea and vomiting often accompany such intense stimulation. The vigorous response produced by ice-water caloric examination is poorly accepted by patients and, therefore, current testing protocols use stimuli that produce a less violent response. When water is used, the temperature is usually adjusted to 30°C for the cool irrigation and 44°C for the warm irrigation. If air is chosen as the stimulating medium, then temperatures of 24°C and 50°C are generally utilized. Understanding the mechanics of the test makes it obvious that certain types of ear pathology invalidate or change test results. An individual with a unilateral tympanic perforation can be expected to have a much more vigorous response on the perforated side than on the intact side because the irrigant will pass through the perforation and stimulate the horizontal semicircular canal directly. Individuals with stenoses, mass lesions, or other types of obstruction of the external auditory canal can be expected to produce little or no response on the affected side. This, however, does not mean that the examination should not be performed. It means that interpreters must be aware of the condition and make their interpretation in light of the existing pathologic process. Should, for example, an individual have no response in an ear with a perforated tympanic membrane, the perforation does not invalidate the pathologic finding. Indeed, the presence of the perforation makes one even more secure that this labyrinth lacks appropriate physiologic function.

Normal individuals produce a fairly typical nystagmus response to caloric irrigation. There is generally a latency of 20 to 30 seconds followed by the onset of nystagmus, which rapidly peaks in intensity at 60 to 90 seconds. The response then gradually diminishes over the next 3 to 4 minutes. To compare one labyrinth to the other, it is crucial that comparisons of nystagmoid response be made between peak responses for each irrigation. This is done by examining the tracing and picking out the strongest beats on each irrigation. Three or four of these beats should be measured and then averaged to obtain a typical "peak" response. The magnitude of the response is quantified in terms of *eye speed* in degrees per second. One should note that this is a different measurement than the assessment of *total amplitude* of the response. Very large deviations can be obtained at slow speeds. A variety of calculations can then be made to assess labyrinthine integrity. The most useful measurement is one that detects unilateral weakness. This measurement compares the total response from the right ear to the total response from the left ear using the formula below when all the responses are measured in degrees per second:

$$\frac{(RW + RC) - (LC + LW)}{(RW + RC + LC + LW)} \times 100 = \text{Percent Unilateral Weakness}$$

where RW is right warm, RC is right cool, LC is left cool, and LW is left warm. Using this formula, negative values indicate weakness on the right and positive values indicate weakness on the left. Convention dictates that the weakness is expressed according to the weaker side in absolute magnitude (i.e., one would say that there is a left unilateral weakness of 28%).

Most practitioners utilize a 20% difference between ears as the threshold for abnormality. Some examiners, however, use a more stringent 25% or 30% difference.

In addition to evaluating the strength of an individual labyrinth, one can also compare the total strength of all beats in one direction to all the beats in another (i.e., compare the strengths of right-beating nystagmus to that of left-beating nystagmus). To make such a calculation, one uses the following formula:

$$\frac{(RW + LC) - (RC + LW)}{(RW + LC + RC + LW)} \times 100 = \text{Percent Directional Preponderance}$$

where RW is right warm, LC is left cool, RC is right cool, and LW is left warm.

When there is an apparent preference for the eyes to beat in the right or left direction, this is referred to as a *direction preponderance.* As a general rule, directional preponderances are a reflection of spontaneous nystagmus. Although directional preponderances can occur in the absence of spontaneous nystagmus, one should be suspicious that there has been some technical error in the irrigations whenever directional preponderance occurs in the absence of spontaneous nystagmus. The significance of directional preponderance when not associated with spontaneous nystagmus remains unclear and, for that reason, some evaluators do not make this calculation.

An important part of the caloric examination is the test for visual fixation suppression. At some point, when the induced nystagmoid response is still brisk, patients should be asked to open their eyes. Eye opening should produce a marked reduction in the intensity of nystagmus (Figure 6.15). Indeed, the strength of the response should be reduced by at least 60%. When this is not the case, CNS pathology is implied.

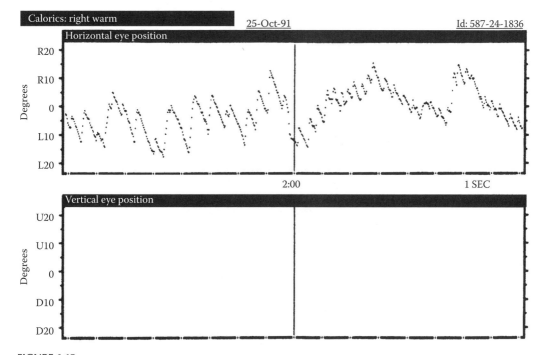

FIGURE 6.15
ENG tracing taken from a patient with a CNS tumor. The right warm caloric is shown. At the vertical bar in the middle of the tracing, the patient was asked to open his eyes and fixate on a mark on the wall. Visual fixation produced only a very slight decrease in the velocity of his nystagmus. Failure of visual fixation is as reliable sign of CNS pathology.

6.4.5 Computed Sinusoidal Harmonic Acceleration

An alternative method of assessing the VOR utilizes a motorized chair to produce a back-and-forth (sinusoidal) movement (Figure 6.16). In response to such movement, the VOR will induce compensatory eye movements in the opposite direction to body movement. These eye movements can be measured and compared with the rotational stimulus. Because the stimulus that initiates the VOR is, in this case, mechanically generated by a chair in which the patient sits, it can be very precisely and accurately controlled. One advantage of SHA is that the stimulus can be determined with much greater precision than can the thermal effects utilized to generate a caloric response in conventional ENG. An additional advantage of SHA is that the stimulus is physiologic. That is, the sort of rotational movement used to generate a response in the VOR arc is qualitatively and quantitatively like many of the stimuli encountered in everyday movement. Generally speaking, most movements performed during ambulation are a bit quicker, but certainly the stimuli used to generate a response utilizing the motorized chair are basically normal. This same characteristic (of providing a physiologic stimulus), which constitutes a principle advantage of SHA, is also responsible for one of its principle disadvantages compared with conventional ENG. By necessity, both labyrinths are stimulated simultaneously and it is not possible to collect data from one side alone.

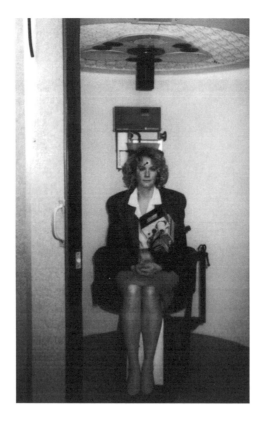

FIGURE 6.16
A rotational chair. The subject is seated in the chair and is seen through the open door. With the door closed, the patient will be in complete darkness. The subject can be monitored from outside the booth by infrared photography. Electrodes are placed in the appropriate positions for monitoring of the induced VOR.

The patient is tested at five separate rotational speeds measured in cycles per second (Hertz). Typical rotational speeds are 0.01 Hz/second, 0.02 Hz/second, 0.04 Hz/second, 0.08 Hz/second, and 0.16 Hz/second. Three separate characteristics of the VOR response are determined for each frequency of rotation.[132,136–138]

6.4.5.1 Phase

It is reasonably appropriate and much easier to understand phase relationships as synonymous with latency. Because the SHA uses a rotational stimulus, it happens that relationships usually characterized as latency can be appropriately described as phase relationships. Suffice it to say that abnormalities of phase (latency) represent changes in how long after the start of the stimulus, the compensatory eye movement occurs. It so happens in SHA (as in many other neurodiagnostic tests) that changes in latency are relatively reliable and sensitive indicators of pathologic disturbance of function, and most peripheral vestibular disorders (e.g., severe viral labyrinthitis, Ménière's disease, traumatic ablation) have been associated with abnormalities of phase. It is quite typical in these cases for the phase abnormality to be more pronounced at lower frequencies and to return toward normal at the higher frequencies. In fact, if phase abnormalities are the same or worse at higher frequencies, then central dysfunction should be suspected. The data are presented by comparing the patient's response to established norms. As a rule, any response more than two standard deviations from normal is considered pathologic. After injury has occurred, phase generally remains abnormal indefinitely. Adaptation and compensation do not eliminate phase abnormalities.

6.4.5.2 Gain

Another parameter of the VOR evaluated at each frequency during SHA is the magnitude of the induced eye movement compared with the magnitude of the rotational stimulus. This comparison is referred to as *gain*. If the eye movements induced by a given rotation (in degrees per second), were exactly the same as the magnitude of the chair rotation (in degrees per second) then the gain would be said to be 1.0. If the induced eye movements were twice as large as the initial movement of the chair, the gain would be 2.0, and if they were half as large, the gain would be 0.5. Not surprisingly, the amount of gain depends on the velocity of rotation. Very slow rotational movements induce relatively small eye movements; typical gains for 0.01-Hz stimuli are 0.5. As the speed of rotation increases, the amount of eye movement similarly increases. It increases faster than the rotational speed so that, at 0.16 Hz, normal gains are in the 0.7 range.

Patients with bilateral vestibular weakness have abnormal gains and, generally speaking, the abnormality is more pronounced at the lower frequencies. As the frequency of rotation is increased, the amount of gain tends to return toward normal, even in patients with bilateral vestibular hypofunction. When gain is very low, there is insufficient vestibular input to provide meaningful data and, with very low gains, one should not interpret abnormalities of phase or symmetry. Low gains will occasionally occur in response to acute labyrinthine lesions when the cerebellum deliberately suppresses output from the vestibular nuclei. However, very low gains are more usually a consequence of chronic bilateral vestibular weakness. Patients with central vertigo will occasionally show increased gain as a result of the absence of descending inhibition.

6.4.5.3 Symmetry

Asymmetric responses are a manifestation of directional preponderance or "bias." That is to say, if there is asymmetry to the right, right-beating nystagmus is always greater than left beating, regardless of the stimulus. The most obvious examples are situations in which there is spontaneous nystagmus to one side. If the patient at rest has 10 degrees of right-beating nystagmus, then his right-beating responses to rotational stimuli will be enhanced by 10 degrees per second but his left-beating responses will be reduced by 10 degrees per second. Thus, when examining the response to rotational stimuli, it appears that the individual's eyes "prefer" to beat toward the right. Acute peripheral lesions frequently have significant asymmetries associated with them. If the lesion is peripheral, then one would expect a phase abnormality to be apparent as well. With classic unilateral vestibular injury, marked phase and symmetry abnormalities are present during the first several weeks or months. With the passage of time and the development of compensation, the asymmetry tends to disappear, but the phase lag will remain. Some types of central disorders will have associated with them variable low-level asymmetries (Figure 6.17). Rotary chair testing has a number of advantages that make it a useful addition to the armamentarium of vestibular testing:

- The stimulus is precisely controlled and physiologic.
- The test is quite sensitive and very repeatable. Test variability is minimized.
- It produces an objective, quantified assessment of vestibular function.

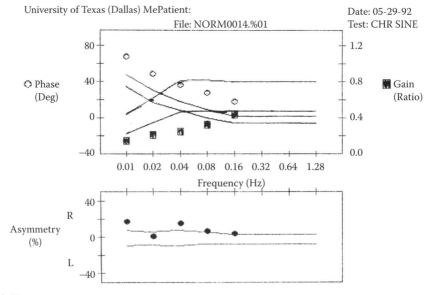

FIGURE 6.17

Summary of diagnostic information obtained from SHA. In this patient, there is a significant phase lag. The circles are shown above the lines, indicating that they are significantly outside the usual standard deviation. In the bottom graph, one can see a mild asymmetry to the right. However, the small squares indicating gain on the upper tracing are less than two standard deviations from the norm, indicating a bilateral weakness. In the face of such reduced gain, it is not possible to interpret phase or symmetry changes accurately. These tracings are from a patient after head injury with significant reduced bilateral vestibular function. ENG evaluation showed no response to warm- or coldwater irrigations bilaterally.

- In many cases, elimination of asymmetry can document compensation and adaptation.
- Generally speaking, it is well accepted by patients and produces less subjective discomfort than ENG.

There are some disadvantages associated with SHA:

- Both labyrinths are stimulated simultaneously.
- The test is relatively expensive and requires fixed equipment installation.
- It was initially thought that asymmetry data could not be utilized to identify the side of lesion. Recently, Hamid[139] documented convincingly that asymmetry is reliably toward the side of the lesion when *phase abnormalities are present.* In the absence of phase abnormalities, asymmetry has no localizing value whatsoever. If additional centers are able to confirm this observation, then the role for SHA testing will be considerably enhanced.

6.4.6 Vestibular Autorotation Testing

The VOR is the dominant mechanism for gaze stabilization during locomotion. Because other ocular control systems are relatively insensitive above 2 Hz, high-frequency vestibular autorotation testing (VAT) was developed to isolate the VOR for testing. VAT uses high-frequency (2–6 Hz) active head movements to stimulate the horizontal and vertical VOR to produce measurable eye movements that can be used to calculate gain and phase.[140]

Patients are fitted with a rotational sensor (on a head strap) and conventional electrooculographic electrodes during testing. They are then instructed to move their heads in synchrony with computer-generated auditory tones, with an interval ranging from 0.5 Hz to 6 Hz. Gain and phase data are collected from the last 12 seconds of the test at higher frequencies (2–6 Hz).

Advantages of VAT over SHA include the ability to test both horizontal and vertical VOR gains and phases in the most clinically relevant frequency range. Saadat et al.[141] compared the results of VAT with alternate bilateral bithermal calorics and found that many patients with normal caloric test results had abnormal VAT results. This emphasizes the fact that cognitive processes or competing ocular motor systems can influence the VOR at low frequencies but are ineffective at higher frequencies. They recommend VAT as an adjunct to traditional vestibular testing.

In 1994, Murphy[142] evaluated 120 patients with vestibular dysfunction using both ENG and VAT. He noted that ENG continued to demonstrate abnormal vestibular responses in patients with permanent labyrinthine injury, even after central compensation. VOR results often normalized after compensation. In this series, ENG was determined to be the most useful initial study in the evaluation of patients with probable peripheral vestibular dysfunction. Certain diagnoses (such as trauma and nondescript dizziness, which is not easily determined to be peripheral) were best evaluated initially with VAT.

In short, ENG and VAT provide valuable complimentary information in the evaluation of vertigo. ENG allows localization of peripheral vestibular dysfunction without information about central compensation. VAT examines the VOR in the clinically relevant frequency range and provides information about central compensation, although it does not allow localization of the injury.

6.4.7 Computerized Dynamic Visual Acuity Test (DVAT)

DVAT may be sensitive to acute changes after a mild concussion when patterns of performance are evaluated.[99] Computerized DVAT has been found to identify central compensation in patients with unilateral and bilateral vestibular dysfunction, but should not be used to diagnose these problems.[143]

6.4.8 The VEMP Test: Vestibular Evoked Myogenic Potential

VEMP testing provides diagnostic information about the function of the saccule, inferior portion of the vestibular nerve, and brainstem. It is based on the vestibulocollic reflex. The vestibulocollic reflex is a fairly short reflex arc between the saccule and the sternocleidomastoid muscle. Stimulation of the saccule normally results in relaxation of the sternocleidomastoid. Unilateral stimulation is achieved by using high-intensity sound. The position of the saccule in the vestibule exposes the saccule to acoustic stimulation. Specifically, the response pathway is from the saccule to the lateral vestibular nucleus via the inferior vestibular portion of cranial nerve XIII, then to the sternocleidomastoid muscle.

VEMP is one of the few clinically available tests of otolith function and, consequently, is appropriate for any patient in need of differential vestibular site of lesion testing. Abnormal findings for the VEMP have been reported in Ménière's disease, vestibular schwannomas, vestibular neuronitis, semicircular canal dehiscence syndrome, viral labyrinthitis, sudden neurosensory hearing loss, multiple sclerosis, lower brainstem stroke, and spinal cerebellum degeneration.

To perform the test, subjects must be able to turn their head sufficiently to contract the sternocleidomastoid muscle. A weakness of the test is that it requires sustained and repeatable contraction of the sternocleidomastoid. If the sternomastoid muscle is not contracted, then the reflex-induced relaxation of that muscle cannot be detected. One way to ensure relatively uniform sternocleidomastoid contraction is to monitor ENG activity in the muscle during head turning.

If the amplitude of the VEMP is asymmetric between ears and one side is enhanced with a lower threshold, superior semicircular canal dehiscence syndrome is suggested. If the VEMP is asymmetric between ears with one side reduced or absent, it is a nonlocalizing abnormality, which suggests saccular and/or inferior vestibular nerve involvement. VEMP latency can also be measured, and a prolonged response is nonlocalizing abnormality suggestive or neurologic involvement.

6.4.9 Dynamic Visual Acuity Testing

DVAT can be utilized as a "bedside" test of the integrity of the VOR. The VOR produces reflexive ocular movement in a direction opposite to head movement. This allows the retinal image to remain stable during head movement. DVAT assesses the adequacy of the VOR by determining how much residual acuity changes with head movement.

In its simplest form, a Snellin chart is utilized to determine the subject's visual acuity. The visual acuity determination is then repeated with subjects moving their head back and forth at a rate of about 1 to 2 cycles per second. If his visual acuity degrades more than two lines on the Snellin chart, the subject probably has an abnormal VOR. A variety of much more sophisticated computerized versions of DVAT is available. Gottshall et al.[99] have shown that computerized DVAT and objective findings on DVAT testing correlate well with symptomatic improvement.

6.4.10 Dynamic Platform Posturography

The development of dynamic platform posturography has been an important addition to the armamentarium in evaluating individuals with disorders of balance (Figure 6.18). The use of dynamic platform posturography directly assesses the individual's ability to maintain balance in a variety of circumstances. It is thus capable of assessing not only vestibular function but also contributions to balance from the visual and proprioceptive systems. Dynamic platform posturography assesses changes in the subject's center of gravity in response to a variety of stimuli in different test conditions. Movement of the center of gravity around a fixed point is termed *sway*. Sway can be measured in both the anterior–posterior and in the lateral planes. Excessive sway can occur at rest in a variety of circumstances but occurs most frequently in response to deliberate perturbations.[144–146]

6.4.10.1 Sensory Organization Testing and Motor Coordination Testing

The amount of sway produced in response to six different situations is recorded. The different test conditions are designed either to eliminate information normally utilized in maintaining equilibrium or to subvert the system by providing inaccurate information. Movement of the patient's center of gravity is assessed in the following situations:

- Sensory Test Condition 1: The patient stands on the platform with eyes open.

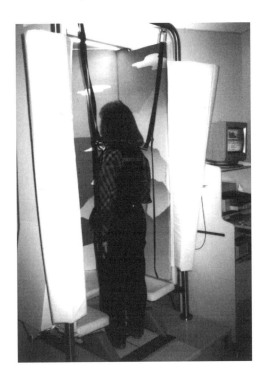

FIGURE 6.18
Neurocom7 dynamic platform posturography. The patient is standing on a moveable platform within the visual surround. Safety straps prevent injury from falling. Sway is monitored in response to a variety of different sensory test conditions.

- Sensory Test Condition 2: The patient stands on the platform with eyes closed. This test condition eliminates vision as a source of information in maintaining balance.

- Sensory Test Condition 3: The patient stands on the platform with eyes open; however, when the patient sways, the amount of movement made is exactly compensated for and mimicked by the movement of the visual surround. The patient will stay exactly the same distance from the visual surround regardless of the movement the body makes. Thus, vision will provide inaccurate information regarding where he is in space relative to the visual surround. In short, in this test condition, the patient's visual system will "lie" to him. This is a more stressful situation than the mere absence of visual information produced in sensory test condition 2. This condition is termed *sway-referenced vision* (i.e., the visual surround is "referenced" to the amount of sway the patient has).

- Sensory Test Condition 4: The patient stands on the platform with eyes open. Each swaying motion the patient produces is now exactly compensated for by a similar movement in the platform on which he is standing. This is a condition analogous to sensory test condition 3, except that in this condition, it is the patient's lower extremity proprioceptive system that is "lying" to him. This is referred to as *sway-referenced support*.

- Sensory Test Condition 5: This condition is exactly the same as sensory test condition 4. There is sway-referenced support, but the patient is asked to keep his eyes closed. This functionally produces a situation in which the patient's lower extremities are lying to him, and his visual system is providing no helpful information. Theoretically, his balance is now dependent on vestibular function.

- Sensory Test Condition 6: The patient stands on the platform with eyes open, but both vision and support are sway referenced. That is to say, each sway excursion is matched both by compensatory movement in the platform and in the visual surround. Thus, both the patient's visual and proprioceptive systems are "lying" to him. In this condition, balance is determined solely by the intact vestibular system, which must overcome false information from the visual and proprioceptive systems.

If patients do not perform well during the first trial, they are allowed two additional chances during which to improve their performance. "Learning" is frequent and many patients will be able to develop a normal response given two or three tries. However, if when compared with statistical norms, the patients' center of gravity shows abnormal excursions (i.e., sway), they are considered to have "failed" that test condition.

As it turns out, different types of pathology produce different patterns of dysfunction on dynamic platform posturography. Not surprisingly, vestibular disorders are reliably associated with very poor performance in conditions 5 and 6, when compensatory mechanisms are crippled by the test conditions. Patients who are overly dependent on vision tend to perform very poorly under test conditions 3 and 6. Patients who are visually dependent and also have vestibular abnormalities tend to do poorly on conditions 3, 5, and 6. If conditions 4, 5, and 6 are abnormal, it suggests that the patient is quite dependent on somatosensory input to maintain balance. Additional combinations and patterns can be correlated with different sorts of abnormalities. Patients with functional disorders or patients who are malingering frequently produce as bad or worse results on the easier conditions than on the harder ones.

An important contribution of dynamic platform posturography is the ability of this test to determine what sort of "strategy" the patient is utilizing to recover his balance. While standing still, the platform is suddenly "jerked" and the patient response is assessed. Several forward and several backward perturbations (jerks) are evaluated. Well-functioning, normal individuals tend to move their center of gravity around their ankles in response to impending disequilibrium. The use of movement about the hips or "hip strategy" is maladaptive and counterproductive. Fortunately, vestibular rehabilitation may be able to redirect patients' efforts and reorient their strategy from hip to a more effective ankle strategy.

In addition to assessing the sensory modalities utilized to maintain and correct balance, dynamic platform posturography is able to characterize, in part, the motor response generated after perturbations. The length of time it takes for the muscle response to occur is measured and is called *latency*. In actual clinical situations, it turns out that abnormalities of latency are almost always associated with extravestibular CNS pathology. The strength "symmetry" is measured. This simply assesses the amount of strength utilized in each leg to retain balance. In normal persons, equal amounts of strength will be utilized in each leg during the process of balance recovery. Once again, in the absence of obvious peripheral or orthopedic problems (e.g., peripheral muscle atrophy, unilateral hip disease), abnormalities of symmetry also reflect CNS disorders. The size of the response is also measured. If minor induced external perturbations produce very large compensatory excursions, large sway oscillations are induced.

Dynamic platform posturography is useful not only in the diagnosis but also in the assessment of risk and in rehabilitation. Not surprisingly, patients who perform poorly on platform posturography are at greater risk for falling than patients who perform normally. Specific pattern abnormalities in sensory organization and movement coordination testing correlate even more closely with risk for falling. However, a study by O'Neill et al.[147] reported that changes on the sensory organization test were not predictive of changes in functional performance in patients with peripheral vestibular hypofunction, and they concluded that this test must be used in conjunction with other tests, such as gait examinations, to assess balance and functional changes.

Mallinson and Longridge[148] studied subjects who were chronically dizzy at least 2 years after whiplash and mild head injury. They reported that posturography was able to delineate the type of injury (i.e., head injury or whiplash) by the compensatory strategy. An understanding of what sort of compensatory mechanisms the patient is using in response to balance perturbations can be helpful in guiding vestibular rehabilitation therapy. Patients who are overly dependent on vision can be given tasks to enhance their ability to utilize vestibular and proprioceptive information. Persons utilizing a maladaptive hip strategy, for example, can be redirected to a more appropriate ankle strategy (Figure 6.19).

6.4.10.2 *Platform Fistula Testing*

Dynamic platform posturography can be used to generate a sensitive test for perilymphatic fistula. In this test, pressure is applied to the external auditory canal. This increase or decrease (i.e., "negative" pressure) is transmitted to the tympanic membrane, middle ear space, and, if a fistula is present, the inner ear. When perilymph fistula is present, abnormal sway will be generated by these pressure changes. Using the acoustics impedance bridge to quantify changes in external auditory canal pressure and the dynamic platform to quantify both anterior posterior and lateral sway in response to such pressure changes, a sensitive assessment for perilymph fistula can be developed.

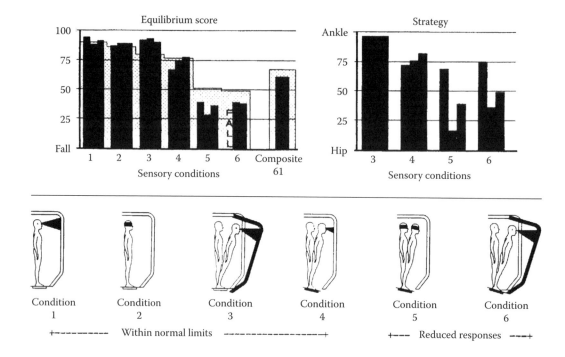

Interpretation/recommendation:

   Reduced responses on conditions 5 and 6 are consistent with a deficiency in the vestibular system.

FIGURE 6.19
Six different sensory organization test conditions are monitored and the patient's performance is compared with statistically valid norms. A typical summary form is illustrated here. This patient had an acute unilateral vestibular lesion resulting in a very poor performance in sensory organization test conditions 5 and 6.

6.5 Vestibular Rehabilitation

The clinical rehabilitation process of the brain-injured individual can be much more complicated than the rehabilitation of an individual with vestibular dysfunction only. Cognitive impairment with decreased attention span, inability to concentrate, and poor frustration tolerance can discourage the patient as well as the therapist. Furthermore, patients present with a wide spectrum of central neurologic impairments affecting different subsystems of the CNS. These impairments demonstrate themselves with symptoms of upper motor neuron lesion (spasticity, weakness); rigidity; and dyscoordination. Given these complicated circumstances added to the vestibular dysfunction, the task at hand is very difficult at least. It is necessary to develop a treatment philosophy and to explain this philosophy to the patient each time circumstance dictates the need for more comprehension or motivation.

   Vestibular rehabilitation depends on two important characteristics of the vestibular system: redundancy and plasticity.[84] Redundancy occurs principally at the receptor level. That is, there are several sensory systems that process information about the body's position in space and relay that information to the CNS. These include the vestibular system, the visual system, muscle stretch and position sense receptors in the lower extremities, and muscle stretch and position sense receptors in the cervical area.

The last two are generally subsumed under the single heading of the somatosensory or proprioreceptive system, but in fact they often function quite independently of each other. The visual and vestibular systems are themselves redundant in the sense that the system has two separate sides. When information from one side is eliminated, the system can function using the intact contralateral side alone. Data received from all the available sensory receptors is initially processed in the brainstem, where decisions are made on a reflex basis. Details of this process remain obscure, but it appears that most of the processing is done in or close to the vestibular nuclei with significant input from both the cerebellar nuclei and descending cortical projections. The ability of sensory receptor information to be evaluated, emphasized, deemphasized, or changed at this level is the principle feature of the vestibular system allowing for progressive modification or *plasticity*.[149]

One way plasticity can be achieved is by the systematic "substitution" of sensory input from one receptor cell system for another. For example, individuals with bilateral vestibular weakness come to utilize visual information more intensively for maintenance of balance and equilibrium. *Habituation* is an additional mechanism for compensation, although its exact physiologic basis remains unclear. Despite its elusive electroneurophysiologic basis, it is clear that constant exposure to situations that produce unpleasant and counterproductive stimulation will reduce or eliminate the unpleasant response.

An instructive example of neuroplasticity is the response of the CNS to acute unilateral labyrinthine ablation. In the circumstance of abrupt and devastating injury to one inner ear (e.g., temporal bone fracture), the afflicted individual will immediately experience rapid, violent rotation with massive visceral autonomic outflow producing intense diaphoresis, weakness, nausea, and vomiting. This effect is a consequence of asymmetry at the level of the vestibular nuclei. Vestibular nuclei connected to the intact labyrinth are continuing to receive normal sensory input and continue to respond in an appropriate way. Cells in the vestibular nuclei connected to the affected side now no longer receive stimulation from the ablated labyrinth and are "silent." Initial adaptation to this injury occurs within several hours to a couple of days and consists of marked inhibition of those cells still connected to the intact labyrinth. Control of this process occurs in the cerebellum and is accomplished via afferent cerebellobulbar fibers.[150] This response has been termed by McCabe[151] the *cerebellar clamp* because it diminishes activity in normally functioning vestibular cells. By reducing function in the normal intact cells, the level of imbalance between the nonfunctioning cells and intact cells is reduced and the symptoms of disequilibrium, nausea, vomiting, and rotational vertigo are reduced. This response has been documented in acute vestibular lesions using SHA where, occasionally, within a day or two after ablative vestibular procedures, a marked decrease in gain can be documented on SHA testing. Over time, those vestibular nuclei originally connected to the now-nonfunctioning labyrinth will develop a spontaneous rate of discharge. As spontaneous activity develops in these neurons, inhibition of the "clamped" normal vestibular nerve cells by the cerebellum is reduced. As individuals regain normal activity and as they are exposed to situations challenging the vestibular system, they will slowly regain normal function. This series of events is an excellent example of neuroplasticity in the vestibular system.[152,153]

Data from patients and animals with acute unilateral vestibular ablation as well as from other types of studies suggest that "relearning" is an important characteristic of vestibular compensation. Stressing the system by having the individual engage in activities that produce disorienting or discomforting symptoms is an important stimulus for compensation and rehabilitation.

Vestibular rehabilitation capitalizes on the natural plasticity of the vestibular system.[154] A good vestibular rehabilitation program should both extend and accelerate the normal process of physiologic adaptation to injury.

Because of the wide variety of possible separate injuries and the almost infinite possible combinations of different sorts of injuries, we believe that each vestibular rehabilitation program needs to be specifically tailored to a particular individual's needs. This is particularly true when dealing with head-injured patients because they will almost always have significant concomitant deficits outside the vestibular system. We believe that this is best accomplished by a physical or occupational therapist who has made a special study and gained experience in managing vestibular injuries. Such an individual will be best qualified to create programs that take into consideration all the patient's deficits and potential assets.

Propedeutic to developing a program for rehabilitation, vestibular rehabilitation therapists need to make their own assessment.[149,154] At first glance, this would appear to be redundant, but in fact, it is not. The assessment made by the rehabilitation expert will not only review the history, physical, and laboratory findings already obtained by physicians and other health care professionals, but will make a detailed assessment of specific situations that induce vertigo (e.g., elevators, crowded stores, driving), assess the severity on a quantitative scale, and do a detailed assessment of the affect of both position and positioning. Sixteen separate positions and movements can be separately assessed, and each position or movement can be rated for intensity, duration, and presence of nystagmus and/or dizziness. The patient's history and type of complaint dictate how much positional testing is required. A separate evaluation of eye, head coordination, and gaze stabilization is made, as well as a separate and detailed assessment of postural control, both in the sitting and standing positions. Gait is evaluated separately.

Whenever making an assessment for vestibular rehabilitation, it is important to determine whether there are other areas of difficulty outside the vestibular system that may affect rehabilitative strategies. This is clearly especially important in the head-injured area.

A complete evaluation of the musculoskeletal system needs to be made to determine whether there are any coexisting difficulties or deficits. Reduction in strength is common in the head-injured patient. Such reduced muscle strength may be secondary to muscle atrophy from coma or inactivity, or may be secondary to direct neural injury. It may, therefore, be generalized or may affect only a specific body part. Restricted range of motion should be determined. Range of motion is frequently reduced in the extremities secondary to orthopedic extremity injuries and may then be limited to a specific body part. Many patients will have associated back injuries. The effects of cervical spine injuries especially need to be taken into consideration. Patients with significant cervical spine injuries will either have had surgery or prolonged periods of neck immobilization. Many, if not all, of these patients will have disordered somatosensory feedback from cervical muscle stretch and joint position sense receptors.

The presence of pain will frequently limit movement. The nature of the pain, its severity, what movements provoke it, and which positions relieve it, all need to be detailed as part of the initial assessment.

Some musculoskeletal abnormalities, especially those involving the cervical spine and neck musculature, may actually be secondary to the vestibular disorder itself. Individuals prone to vertigo and disequilibrium will limit head and trunk movements to avoid symptoms. Over time, these limitations of movement may cease to be volitional and require specific consideration.

The presence or absence of associated neurologic injuries also needs to be addressed. Such injuries may limit or prohibit motor control. These abnormalities may be subtle and manifest only on sophisticated testing as increased response latencies, or may be quite blatant in the form of spasticity or paralysis. Such disorders may arise out of injury to either the peripheral nervous system or the CNS. Special note should be made of injuries to the extraocular muscle system. Inability to move and position the eyes appropriately may have a significant effect on balance and equilibrium, and certainly can be expected to complicate a proposed program of vestibular rehabilitation.

In addition, and perhaps particularly important in head injuries, is injury to the cortical, subcortical, and brainstem areas. Such injuries may produce abnormalities of sensory selection, gaze control, and perceived stability. It is probable that some of the abnormal oculovestibular reflex (production of vertigo secondary to repetitive rapid movement in the visual field) seen in head-injured patients also occurs at this level. Oftentimes, sophisticated neuropsychiatric testing will have documented abnormalities of memory, perception, and cognitive processing, which are frequently associated with head-injured cortical dysfunction.

Any or all of these associated difficulties may contribute to the patient's symptomatology, and require specific and special consideration when a vestibular rehabilitation program is being designed.[155,156] Clearly, individuals with significant associated visual deficits will need management different from those who have associated spastic hemiparesis. Many patients requiring vestibular therapy and especially the head-injured patient will have experienced significant deconditioning and will require directed programs to improve both muscle strength and general aerobic conditioning.

6.5.1 Vestibular Rehabilitation Process

The process of rehabilitation consists of several parts:

1. Vestibular adaptation
2. Substitution of other strategies
3. Mechanical dispersion (CRT)
4. Desensitization (habituation)
5. Balance retraining
6. Cardiorespiratory endurance training or conditioning

6.5.2 Vestibular Adaptation

Adaptation describes the ability of the vestibular system to make long-term changes in the neuronal response to input. The signal that induces adaptation is the movement of a visual image across the retina, referred to as *retinal slip*. The brain adapts by increasing the gain of the vestibular responses. This can be accomplished using two simple exercises that are designed to increase progressively the gain of the vestibular system by inducing retinal slip. In one exercise, patients are instructed to maintain visual fixation on a stationary object while moving their head back and forth (VOR in phase). A second exercise uses a moving target, with the target and the head moving in opposite directions while maintaining fixation (VOR out of phase).[157]

6.5.3 Substitution

Substitution exercises aim to enhance other strategies for balance (such as postural stability and gaze) in patients with severe bilateral loss of vestibular function.[158] Unfortunately, no other mechanism can completely compensate for the loss of vestibular function, and most patients will continue to have some instability and oscillopsia while pursuing daily activities.

6.5.4 Mechanical Dispersion

See Section 6.3.4.

6.5.5 Desensitization (Habituation)

Peripheral lesions produce hypersensitivity to movement, with dizziness and nausea as common complaints. Patients are particularly sensitive to specific angular or linear acceleration and deceleration.[104] Habituation, the reduction in symptoms through repetitive sensory stimulation of provoking positions or movements, presumably occurs through central mechanisms. Desensitization is accomplished by giving the patient a variety of positional exercises designed to reproduce his vertiginous symptoms.[106] Up to four movements are repeated two or three times until the symptoms are ameliorated, which may take 4 weeks for a decrease in intensity. Usually, the exercises are performed for 2 months. It is important for the patient to rest after each movement to prevent summation of symptoms. The simplest (although often effective) habituation exercises are those first used by Cooksey.[159] We use them on a limited basis, depending upon the client (Table 6.5). A variety of more sophisticated techniques has been developed.[39,150,160,161] It is important to explain to the patient that to get less sensitive to these complaints, it is necessary to provoke them. With repetition of the prescribed exercise, sensitivity to these movements will subside (Table 6.3).

Journals are used to illustrate progress over a period of time. They are good tools for motivation for the patient and give the clinician information regarding the patient's compliance and effectiveness of the program.

6.5.6 Balance Retraining

Balance retraining with any vestibular lesion will always start at a level that the patient is independently able to perform. It is very important to stress the issue of independence with rehabilitative exercise, as this will build confidence. Modifications to programs for the head-injured client may need to provide greater supervision in tasks, physical assistance to accommodate motor problems such as spasticity, and increased time required to achieve stated goals. Cognitive impairments, behavioral problems, and judgment deficits require increased vigilance by the therapist during treatment sessions. Repetition of balance exercises, during the session as well as for an agreed period of time after the session, also helps build confidence because the exercises will become easier to perform and can be performed quicker.

Simplicity of design will enhance both repetition and independence. Obstacle courses are good exercise, but in the beginning of the rehabilitation process, they may increase patients' sense of frustration rather than a feeling of accomplishment.

Functionality of the exercise is important; nothing will frustrate the balance-impaired subject more than exercise that has no bearing in daily life. And realistically, do we improve a person's ability to balance if we teach him to stand on one leg? Patients' functional deficits need to be identified. Examples of deficits might include the instability patients encounter while shopping for groceries. Such a task involves multiple types of head movements as

TABLE 6.5

Cawthorne-Cooksey Exercises

Begin in a sitting position
Lay flat on your back
Roll to the left side
Roll to the right side
Back flat
Sit up
Now stand
Turn to the right
Turn to the left
Sit again
Put your nose on your left knee
Place your right ear on your right shoulder
Nose to right knee
Left ear on left shoulder
While sitting
Turn your head counterclockwise
Now turn it clockwise
Repeat while bending forward
Repeat while going from a sitting to an erect standing position
Repeat as you move your head forward
Repeat as you move your head backward
In a sitting position
Hang your head between your legs, turning to the left
Sit
Hang your head, turning to the right
Sit
Hang your head in the middle, between your legs
Sit

Cawthorne-Cooksey exercises have been used since the 1940s as effective treatment for vertigo and disequilibrium. Patients are asked to select the six exercises from the list that provoke the most severe symptoms and are then asked to perform these six selected exercises for 10 minutes twice a day.

well as making sure they do not collide with other shoppers. Moreover, patients have to be able to anticipate obstacle courses, judge distances, and perhaps respond quickly to changes in tasks. Patients will need to practice such "real-life" situations in simple contexts prior to adding more complexity in the visual environment or surface orientations.[118,162] With the development of simulator-based virtual reality environments or activity-based exercises in rehabilitation (Sony Eyetoy, Play 2 on a PlayStation 2), patients with vestibular disorders, including postconcussive head injury, are exposed to engaging environments that are safe, motivating, and repetitive.[163–167] Furthermore, augmented feedback with visual and auditory cues provide clients with knowledge of results about their position in space, motor skill, and so on, to allow mastery of the task before progressing to more difficult combinations. Patients become involved in synthetic environments that have been developed to control for specific variables, such as a moving visual scene causing retinal slip, and habituation to specific conditions that cause dizziness, anxiety, and imbalance. In addition, the feasibility of low-cost virtual reality systems allow for self-directed practice on a regular basis in the home.

The treatment approach with balance retraining is not identical for peripheral or central lesions; however, the philosophy remains the same. The difference is that we expose our centrally affected patients to the same exercise longer during a treatment session and for a longer period of time. (The time that is necessary until they can move to more complex balance activities.)

6.5.6.1 Central Vestibular Lesions

Central vestibular lesions are hard to deal with because they do not respond to desensitization exercises as described in the previous group. Central vestibular pathology gives rise to complaints that cannot be specifically provoked by certain movements or positions, but form a more steady ingredient in the activities of daily life of a patient.[155,161,168] A diagnosed central lesion does therefore require a somewhat different approach. The diagnosis "central lesion" does not exclude the possibility of adaptation of the CNS. The expectation, however, is that rehabilitation will be less complete and usually take a longer period of time.

We still implement a program based on angular and linear acceleration and deceleration, but we use more repetitions per session, usually at a lower speed, and maintain the program for 6 to 12 weeks. The effects of such an approach are (1) a decrease in vestibular symptoms, (2) an increase in self-confidence, and (3) the patient becoming more physically active.

6.5.7 Cardiorespiratory Endurance Training or Conditioning

Cardiorespiratory endurance training is even more crucial to these patients because physical reconditioning will enhance self-confidence and esteem, which will impart overall motivation. The vestibularly impaired patient experiences difficulty with balance, or nausea and dizziness, when moving about and, therefore, becomes less active, no matter the premorbid lifestyle.[169] As a consequence, all our patients experience deconditioning and sometimes undesirable weight gain as a result.

Ideally, patients are started on the Schwinn Air Dyne bicycle with a modified Cooper test to get baseline information on the level of conditioning. This stationary bike provides a gentle form of exercise, which rarely triggers vestibular complaints. Patients are encouraged to maintain a pace that will elevate their heart rate to a level appropriate for their gender and age group (target heart rate). Resting heart rate, postexercise heart rates (immediately after stopping and 5 minutes thereafter), and resting blood pressure are monitored. The less change in heart rate and the fast recovery to resting rate indicates a better fitness level (Figure 6.20).

Not all our patients can be motivated to participate in such a rigorous exercise routine, and they are asked to participate in another form of endurance exercise. Most patients can be motivated to participate in some form of cardiorespiratory training, and it is best to engage patients in a form of training that has their full motivation because it will increase the possibility of overall success of the rehabilitation process. Therefore, in addition to the use of the Schwinn Air Dyne bicycle, we use treadmills, swimming pools, walking groups, stair climbers, or anything else that will increase the activity level of our vestibular patients. Walking activities are important because the stationary bicycle does not improve postural and gait stability.

A number of variables will influence the overall outcome. First and foremost is compliance. Our current program of vestibular rehabilitation requires the patient to spend 15 minutes twice a day in specifically directed exercises that are advanced on a weekly or biweekly basis. We believe a typical program will require 8 to 12 weeks. Poor compliance is common in individuals with multiple deficits and they generally do less well. Poor compliance may result because patients have had serious central nervous injury that impairs motivation and cognition or because they have associated musculoskeletal or sensory injuries that make it impossible for them to perform the most helpful sorts of exercises. In many of these patients, two to three rehabilitation programs will be in progress simultaneously, which may overwhelm their ability. Individuals with central dysfunction improve at a much slower rate and may never achieve the same improvement as those who have peripheral receptor level disorders. Age is another variable that works against rapid recovery.

There is objective evidence to support the usefulness of vestibular rehabilitation.[170–173] In a 1998 report, Cowand et al.[174] used the DHI to study retrospectively a group of 37 patients undergoing vestibular rehabilitation, and found a significant improvement in test scores of 78% of patients posttreatment. Telian et al. have evaluated the outcome in 98 patients with a variety of different vestibular problems.[106,161,175] Some patients were excluded because of disease process, but all had to meet one of the following criteria: (1) positional or motion-provoked vertigo, (2) abnormalities of sensory organization testing or abnormal recovery strategies, and (3) abnormal chair/ENG findings. After a 10- to 15-week program performed at home, 87% of patients reported significant subjective improvement and 83% had objective improvement in disability ratings. Thirty-one percent of the patients were completely asymptomatic at the time a follow-up evaluation was performed. Ten percent were worse. Half of these had unequivocal progressive unilateral vestibular injuries and underwent deafferentation surgical procedures.

Horak et al.[176] studied the relative effectiveness of vestibular rehabilitation, general conditioning exercises, and vestibular suppressant medication on dizziness and imbalance in patients with chronic vestibular symptoms. They found that all methods reduced dizziness, but that only vestibular rehabilitation improved postural stability. A 1995 report from Shepard and Telian[177] analyzed the benefits of customized versus generic vestibular rehabilitation therapy programs and found that a superior level of vestibular compensation was

Cardiorespiratory endurance

Clearance for fitness program obtained:
    From——————————————— (M.D.) Date————————————

Resting blood pressure:————————————————————————————

Resting heart rate:————————————————————————————————

Target heart rate for M/F—————————————— Age————————————
    Formula   Men   205 - 1/2 age × .8
               Women   220 - age × .8

12 Minute cooper air-dyne bicycle:
    Distance————————————————————————————————————
    Post exercise heart rate——————————————————————————
    5 Minute recuperating heart rate————————————————————

Fitness category:

FIGURE 6.20
The cardiorespiratory endurance table is used on a weekly basis to evaluate cardiovascular fitness improvements.

achieved in the patients undergoing customized rehabilitation. After 3 months of therapy, only the group performing customized vestibular rehabilitation exercises had a significant reduction in dizziness during daily activities, improvement in postural stability, reduction in motion sensitivity, and a decrease in asymmetry of vestibular function. Patients receiving generic vestibular rehabilitation improved only in static postural stability.

An unsupervised program of Cawthorne-Cooksey exercises is not as effective as a customized, supervised program of vestibular adaptation exercises. Each patient with vestibular dysfunction after traumatic brain injury should, therefore, be independently evaluated in the context of his or her unique cognitive and vestibular symptoms.

6.6 Summary

In summary, vestibular rehabilitation is an effective way of utilizing the natural plasticity of the CNS to compensate for vestibular dysfunction. Specifically, it is useful to improve postural and balance control, eliminate vertigo and disequilibrium, and reduce the effects of visually provoked stimuli. Although most patients achieve improvement, only about one third achieve complete elimination of symptomatology. It is useful to present these techniques to the patient as methods for managing and controlling symptoms rather that eliminating them. Vestibular rehabilitation needs to be integrated into an overall plan that takes into consideration all of the patient's deficits, as well as assets and abilities. Those therapists whose priority is improvement in balance and elimination of vertigo need constantly to coordinate with the patient's multidisciplinary team leader to achieve a maximally effective overall rehabilitation strategy for the posttraumatically brain-injured individual.

References

1. Healy, G. B., Hearing loss and vertigo secondary to head injury, *New England Journal of Medicine*, 306(17), 1029–1031, 1982.
2. Pearson, B. W. and Barber, H. O., Head injury: Some otoneurologic sequelae, *Archives of Otolaryngolosy*, 97(1), 81–84, 1973.
3. Berman, J. M. and Fredrickson, J. M., Vertigo after head injury: A five year follow-up, *Journal of Otolaryngology*, 7(3), 237–245, 1978.
4. Rantanen, T., Aantaa, E., Salmivalli, A., and Meurman, O. H., Audiometric and electronystagmographic studies of patients with traumatic skull injuries, *Acta Oto-laryngologica*, 224(Suppl.), 256, 1966.
5. Saito, Y., Ishikawa, T., Makiyama, Y., Hasegawa, M., Shigihara, S., Yasukata, J., Ishiyama, E., and Tomita, H., Neuro-otological study of positional vertigo caused by head injury, *Auris Nasus Larynx*, 13(Suppl. 1), S69–S73, 1986.
6. Tuohimaa, P., Vestibular disturbances after acute mild head injury, *Acta Oto-laryngologica*, 359(Suppl.), 3–67, 1978.
7. Grimm, R. J., Hemenway, W. G., Lebray, P. R., and Black, F. O., The perilymph fistula syndrome defined in mild head trauma, *Acta Oto-laryngologica*, 464 (Suppl.), 1–40, 1989.
8. Vartiainen, E., Karjalainen, S., and Karja, J., Vestibular disorders following head injury in children, *International Journal of Pediatric Otorhinolaryngology*, 9(2), 135–141, 1985.

9. Evatar, M., Bergtraum, M., and Randel, R. M., Post traumatic vertigo in children: A diagnostic approach, *Pediatric Neurology*, 2(2), 61–66, 1986.
10. Hoffer, M. E., Balough, B. J., and Gottshall, K. R., Posttraumatic balance disorders, *International Tinnitus Journal*, 13(1), 69–72, 2007.
11. Baloh, R. W. and Honrubia, V., *Clinical Neurophysiology of the Vestibular System*, F. A. Davis, Philadelphia, 1990.
12. Barber, H. O. and Stockwell, C. W., *Manual of Electronystagmography*, Mosby, St. Louis, MO, 1980.
13. Stockwell, C. W., *ENG Workbook*, Pro-Ed, Austin, TX, 1983.
14. Olsson, J. E., Blunt trauma of the temporal bone, Presented at the American Academy of Otolaryngology–Head and Neck Surgery meeting, September 1986, San Antonio, Texas.
15. Hughes, G. B., *Textbook of Clinical Otology*, Thieme-Stratton, New York, 1988.
16. Clark, S. K. and Rees, T. S., Post-traumatic endolymphatic hydrops, *Archives of Otolarynogology*, 103(12), 725, 1977.
17. Schuknecht, H. F., Cupulolithiasis, *Archives of Otolaryngology*, 90(6), 765–778, 1969.
18. Hall, S. F., Ruby, R. R., and McClure, J. A., The mechanics of benign paroxysmal vertigo, *Journal of Otolaryngology*, 8(2), 151–158, 1979.
19. Gianoli, G. J., DDX: Fluctuating vestibular disease, in J. A. Goebel (Ed.), *Practical Management of the Dizzy Patient*, Lippincott Williams & Wilkins, Philadelphia, 235–250, 2001.
20. Nedzelski, J. M., Barber, H. O., and McIlmoyl, L., Diagnoses in a dizziness unit, *Journal of Otolaryngology*, 15(2), 101–104, 1986.
21. Caruso, G. and Nuti, D., Epidemiological data from 2270 PPV patients, *Audiological Medicine*, 1(3), 7–11, 2005.
22. Fetter, M., Vestibular system disorders, in S. J. Herdman (Ed.), *Vestibular Rehabilitation*, 3rd ed., F. A. Davis, Philadelphia, 2007.
23. Gordon, C. R., Levite, R., Joffe, V., and Gadoth, N., Is posttraumatic benign paroxysmal positional vertigo different from the idiopathic form?, *Archives of Neurology*, 61(10), 1590–1593, 2004.
24. Cho, C. H., Lee, J. H., Kim, J. H., Kim, D. K., and Kim, D. Y., The analysis of post-traumatic BPPV, *Otolaryngology–Head and Neck Surgery*, 135(2S), 246, 2006.
25. Katsarkas, A., Benign paroxysmal positional vertigo (BPPV): Idiopathic versus post-traumatic, *Acta Oto-Laryngology*, 119(7), 745–749, 1999.
26. Herdman, S. J., Blatt, P. J., and Schubert, M. C., Vestibular rehabilitation of patients with vestibular hypofunction or with benign paroxysmal positional vertigo, *Current Opinion in Neurology*, 13(1), 39–43, 2000.
27. Tusa, R. J., Differential diagnosis mimicking BPPV, in S. J. Herdman (Ed.), *Vestibular Rehabilitation*, 3rd ed., F. A. Davis, Philadelphia, 2007.
28. Humphriss, R. L., Baguley, D. M., Sparkes, V., Peerman, S. E., and Moffat, D. A., Contraindications to the Dix-Hallpike manoeuvre: A multidisciplinary review, *International Journal of Audiology*, 42(3), 166–173, 2003.
29. Cohen, H. S., Side-lying as an alternative to the Dix-Hallpike test of the posterior canal, *Otology & Neurotology*, 25(2), 130–134, 2004.
30. Cohen, H. S. and Murphy, E. K., An augmented liberatory maneuver for benign paroxysmal positional vertigo for patients who are difficult to move, *Otolaryngology–Head and Neck Surgery*, 136(2), 309–310, 2007.
31. Herdman, S. J. and Tusa, R. J., Physical therapy management of benign positional vertigo, in S. J. Herdman (Ed.), *Vestibular Rehabilitation*, 3rd ed., F. A. Davis, Philadelphia, 2007.
32. McClure, J. A., Horizontal canal BPV, *Journal of Otolaryngology*, 14(1), 30–35, 1985.
33. Baloh, R. W., Jacobson, K., and Honrubia, V., Horizontal semicircular canal variant of benign positional vertigo, *Neurology*, 43(12), 2542–2549, 1993.
34. White, J. A., Coale, K. D., Catalano, P. J., and Oas, J. G., Diagnosis and management of lateral semicircular canal benign paroxysmal positional vertigo, *Otolaryngology–Head and Neck Surgery*, 133(2), 278–284, 2005.

35. Casani, A. P., Vannucci, G., Fattori, B., and Berrettini, S., The treatment of horizontal canal positional vertigo: Our experience in 66 cases, *Laryngoscope*, 112(1), 172–178, 2002.

36. Yakinthou, A., Maurer, J., and Mann, W., Benign paroxysmal positioning vertigo: Diagnosis and therapy using video-oculographic control, *Journal for Oto-Rhino-Laryngology, Head and Neck Surgery*, 65(5), 290–294, 2003.

37. Epley, J. M., The canalith repositioning procedure: For treatment of benign paroxysmal positional vertigo, *Otolaryngology–Head and Neck Surgery*, 107(3), 399–404, 1992.

38. Semont, A., Freyss, G., and Vitte, E., Curing the BPPV with a liberatory maneuver, *Advances in Oto-Rino-Laryngology*, 42, 290–293, 1988.

39. Brandt, T. and Daroff, R. B., Physical therapy for benign paroxysmal positional vertigo, *Archives of Otolaryngology–Head and Neck Surgery*, 106(8), 484–485, 1980.

40. Ford-Smith, C. D., The individualized treatment of a patient with benign paroxysmal positional vertigo, *Physical Therapy*, 77(8), 848–855, 1997.

41. Herdman, S. J., Tusa, R. J., Zee, D. S., Proctor, L. R., and Mattox, D. E., Single treatment approaches to benign paroxysmal positional vertigo, *Archives of Otolaryngology–Head and Neck Surgery*, 119(4), 450–454, 1993.

42. Cohen, H. S., Kimball, K. T., and Stewart, M. G., Benign paroxysmal positional vertigo and comorbid conditions, *Journal for Oto-Rhino-Laryngology and Its Related Sepcialities,* 66(1), 11–15, 2004.

43. Cohen, H. S. and Kimball, K. T., Effectiveness of variations on the Epley maneuver for BPPV, *Otolaryngology–Head and Neck Surgery*, 131(2), 107, 2004.

44. Chiou, W. Y., Lee, H. L., Tsai, S. C., Yu, T. H., and Lee, X. X., A single therapy for all subtypes of horizontal canal positional vertigo, *Laryngoscope*, 115(8), 1432–1435, 2005.

45. Prokopakis, E. P., Chimona, T., Tsagournisakis, M., Christodoulou, P., Hirsch, B. E., Lachanas, V. A., Helidonis, E. S., Plaitakis, A., and Velegrakis, G. A., Benign paroxysmal positional vertigo: 10-Year experience in treating 592 patients with canalith repositioning procedure, *Laryngoscope*, 115(9), 1667–1671, 2005.

46. Steenerson, R. L., Cronin, G. W., and Marbach, P. M., Effectiveness of treatment techniques in 923 cases of benign paroxysmal positional vertigo, *Laryngoscope*, 115(2), 226–231, 2005.

47. Woodworth, B. A., Gillespie, M. B., and Lambert, P.R., The canalith repositioning procedure for benign positional vertigo: A meta-analysis, *Laryngoscope*, 114(7), 1143–1146, 2004.

48. Wietske, R., Bruintjes, P., Osstenbrink, P., and van Leeuwen, R. B., Efficacy of the Epley maneuver for posterior canal BPPV: A long term, controlled study of 81 patients, *Ear, Nose, and Throat Journal*, 84(1), 22–25, 2005.

49. Chang, A. K., Schoeman, G., and Hill, M., A randomized clinical trial to assess the efficacy of the Epley maneuver in the treatment of acute benign positional vertigo, *Academic Emergency Medicine*, 11(9), 918–924, 2004.

50. Cohen, H. S. and Jerabek, J., Efficacy of treatments for posterior canal benign paroxysmal positional vertigo, *Laryngoscope*, 109(4), 584–590, 1999.

51. Richard, W., Bruintjes, T. D., Oostenbrink, P., and van Leeuwen, R. B., Efficacy of the Epley maneuver for posterior canal BPPV: A long-term, controlled study of 81 patients, *Ear, Nose, and Throat Journal*, 84(1), 22–25, 2005.

52. Tusa, R. J. and Herdman, S. J., BPPV: Controlled trials, contraindications, post-manoeuvre instructions, complications, imbalance, *Audiology Medicine*, 3(1), 57–62, 2005.

53. Pinder, M. H., The Epley (canalith repositioning) manoeuvre for benign paroxysmal positional vertigo, *Cochrane Database of Systematic Reviews*, 2, CD003162.

54. Parnes, L. S. and Price-Jones, R. G., Particle repositioning maneuver for benign paroxysmal positional vertigo, *Annals of Otology, Rhinology & Laryngology*, 102(5), 325–331, 1993.

55. Hain, T. C., Helminski, J. O., Reis, I. L., and Uddin, M. K., Vibration does not improve results of the canalith repositioning procedure, *Archives of Otolaryngology–Head and Neck Surgery*, 126(5), 617–622, 2000.

56. Nuti, D., Nati, C., and Passali, D., Treatment of benign paroxysmal positional vertigo: No need for postmaneuver restrictions, *Otolaryngology–Head and Neck Surgery*, 122(3), 440–444, 2000.

57. Andreoli, S. M. and Devaiah, A., Posture restrictions in benign paroxysmal positional vertigo, *Otolaryngology–Head and Neck Surgery*, 137(2), 258, 2007.

58. Levrat, E., van Melle, G., Monnier, P., and Maire, R., Efficacy of the Semont maneuver in benign paroxysmal positional vertigo, *Archives of Otolaryngology–Head and Neck Surgery*, 129(6), 629–633, 2003.

59. Lempert, T. and Tiel-Wilck, K., A positional maneuver for treatment of horizontal-canal benign positional vertigo, *Laryngoscope*, 106(4), 476–478, 1996.

60. Appiani, G. C., Catania, G., and Gagliardi, M., A liberatory maneuver for the treatment of horizontal canal paroxysmal positional vertigo, *Otology and Neurotology*, 22(1), 66–69, 2001.

61. Vannucchi, P., Giannoni, B., and Pagnini, P., Treatment of horizontal semicircular canal benign paroxysmal positional vertigo, *Journal of Vestibular Research*, 7(1), 1–6, 1997.

62. Herdman, S. J., Advances in the treatment of vestibular disorders, *Physical Therapy*, 77(6), 602–618, 1997.

63. Blatt, P. J., Georgakakis, G. A., Herdman, S. J., Clendaniel, R. A., and Tusa R. J., The effect of the canalith repositioning maneuver on resolving postural instability in patients with benign paroxysmal positional vertigo, *American Journal of Otology*, 21(3), 356–363, 2000.

64. Kollen, L., Bjerlemo, B., and Moller, C., Evaluation of treatment in benign paroxysmal positional vertigo (BPPV), *Advances in Physiotherapy*, 8(3), 106–115, 2006.

65. Motin, M., Keren, O., Groswasser, Z., and Gordon, C. R., Benign paroxysmal positional vertigo as the cause of dizziness in patients after severe traumatic brain injury: Diagnosis and treatment, *Brain Injury*, 19(9), 693–697, 2005.

66. Shaia, W. T., Zappia, J. J., Bojrab, D. I., LaRouere, M. L., Sargent, E. W., and Diaz, R. C., Success of posterior semicircular canal occlusion and application of the dizziness handicap inventory, *Otolaryngology–Head and Neck Surgery*, 134(3), 424–430, 2006.

67. Parnes, L. S. and McClure, J. A., Posterior semicircular canal occlusion for intractable benign paroxysmal positional vertigo, *Annals of Otology, Rhinology & Laryngology*, 99(5 pt 1), 330–334, 1990.

68. Chester, J. B., Whiplash, postural control, and the inner ear, *Spine*, 16(7), 716, 1991.

69. Fitz-Ritson, D., Assessment of cervicogenic vertigo, *Journal of Manipulative and Physiological Therapeutics*, 14(3), 193–198, 1991.

70. Galm, R., Rittmeister, M., and Schmitt, E., Vertigo in patients with cervical spine dysfunction, *European Spine Journal*, 7(1), 55–58, 1998.

71. Treleaven, J., Jull, G., and Sterling, M., Dizziness and unsteadiness following whiplash injury: Characteristic features and relationship with cervical joint position error, *Journal of Rehabilitation Medicine*, 35(1), 36–43, 2003.

72. Brandt, T. and Bronstein, A. M., Cervical vertigo, *Journal of Neurology, Neurosurgery & Psychiatry*, 71(1), 8–12, 2001.

73. Heikkilä, H. V. and Wenngren, B. I., Cervicocephalic kinesthetic sensibility, active range of cervical motion, and oculomotor function in patients with whiplash injury, *Archives of Physical Medicine and Rehabilitation*, 79(9), 1089–1094, 1998.

74. Wrisley, D. M., Sparto, P. J., Whitney, S. L., and Furman, J. M., Cervicogenic dizziness: A review of diagnosis and treatment, *Journal of Orthopaedic & Sports Physical Therapy*, 30(1), 755–766, 2000.

75. Treleaven, J., Jull, G., and Lowchoy, N., Standing balance in persistent whiplash: A comparison between subjects with and without dizziness, *Journal of Rehabilitation Medicine*, 37(4), 224–229, 2005.

76. Brown, J. J., Cervical contribution to balance: Cervical vertigo, in A. Berhoz, P. P. Vidal, and W. Graf (Eds.), *Head and Neck Sensory Motor System*, Oxford University Press, New York, 1992.

77. Clendaniel, R. A. and Landel, R., Non-vestibular diagnosis and imbalance: Cervicogenic dizziness, in S. J. Herdman (Ed.), *Vestibular Rehabilitation*, 3rd ed., F. A. Davis, Philadelphia, 2007.

78. Travell, J. G. and Simons, D. G., *Myofascial Pain and Dysfunction: The Trigger Point Manual*, Williams & Wilkins, Baltimore, 1983.

79. Karlberg, M., Johansson, R., Magnusson, M., and Fransson, P. A., Dizziness of suspected cervical origin distinguished by posturographic assessment of human postural dynamics, *Journal of Vestibular Research*, 6(1), 37–47, 1996.

80. Reid, S. A. and Rivett, D. A., Manual therapy treatment of cervicogenic dizziness: A systematic review, *Manual Therapy*, 10(1), 4–13, 2005.

81. Schenk, R., Coons, L. B., Bennett, S. E., and Huijbregts, P.A., Cervicogenic dizziness: A case report illustrating orthopaedic manual and vestibular physical therapy comanagement, *Journal of Manual and Manipulative Therapy*, 14(3), E56–E68, 2006.

82. Barber, H. O. and Sharpe, J. A., *Vestibular Disorders*, Year Book Medical Publishers, Chicago, 1988.

83. Baloh, R. W., *The Essentials of Neurology*, F. A. Davis, Philadelphia, 1984.

84. Brown, J. J., A systematic approach to the dizzy patient, *Neurology and Clinical Neurophysiology*, 8(2), 209–224, 1990.

85. DeWeese, D. D., Differential diagnosis of dizziness and vertigo, in M. M. Paparella, D. D. Shumrick, J. L. Gluckman, and W. L. Meyerhoff (Eds.), *Otolaryngology*, W. B. Saunders, Philadelphia, 1991.

86. Rudge, P., Central causes of vertigo, in M. R. Dix and J. D. Hood (Eds.), *Vertigo*, Wiley, New York, 321, 1984.

87. Vesterhauge, S., Clinical diagnosis of vestibular disorders. A system approach to dizziness, *Acta Otolaryngology*, 460(Suppl.), 114–121, 1988.

88. Allison, L., Imbalance following traumatic brain injury in adults: Causes and characteristics, *Neurology Report*, 23(1), 13–18, 1999.

89. Carr, J. H. and Sheperd, R. B., *Physiotherapy in Disorders of the Brain*, Aspen Publishers, London, 1989.

90. Wober, C., Oder, W., Kollegger, H., Prayer, L., Baumgartner, C., Wöber-Bingöl, C., Wimberger, D., Binder, H., and Deecke, L. Posturographic measurement of body sway in survivors of severe closed head injury, *Archives of Physical Medicine and Rehabilitation*, 74(11), 1151–1156, 1993.

91. Smith-Wheelock, M., Shepard, N. T., and Telian, S. A., Physical therapy program for vestibular rehabilitation, *American Journal of Otology*, 12(3), 218–225, 1991.

92. Pfaltz, C. R. and Kamath, R., Central compensation of vestibular dysfunction, I: peripheral lesions, *Advances in Oto-Rhino-Laryngology*, 32(6), 335–349, 1970.

93. Berman, J. M. and Fredrickson, J. M., Vertigo after head injury: A five year follow-up, *Journal of Otolaryngology*, 7(3), 237–245, 1978.

94. Tangerman, P. T. and Wheeler, J., Inner ear concussion syndrome: Vestibular implications and physical therapy treatment, *Topics Acute Case Trauma Rehabil*, 1(1), 72–83, 1986.

95. Shepard, N. T., Telian, S. A., Smith-Wheelock, M., and Raj, A., Vestibular and balance rehabilitation therapy, *Annals of Otology, Rhinology & Laryngology*, 102(3 Pt 1), 198–205, 1993.

96. Jacob, R. G., Furman, J. M., Durrant, J. D., and Turner, S. M. Panic, agoraphobia, and vestibular dysfunction, *American Journal of Psychiatry*, 153(4), 503–512, 1996.

97. Jacob, R. G., Woody, S. R., and Clark, D. B., Discomfort with space and motion: A possible marker of vestibular dysfunction assessed by the situational characteristics questionnaire, *Psychopathol Behav Assoc*, 15(4), 299–324, 1993.

98. Jacobson, G. P. and Newman, C. W., The development of the Dizziness Handicap Inventory, *Archives of Otolaryngology–Head and Neck Surgery*, 116(4), 424–427, 1990.

99. Gottshall, K., Drake, A., Gray, N., McDonald, E., and Hoffer, M. E., Objective vestibular tests as outcome measures in head injury patients, *Laryngoscope*, 113(10), 1746–1750, 2003.

100. Whitney, S. L., Marchetti, G. F., and Morris, L. O., Usefulness of the Dizziness Handicap Inventory in the screening for benign paroxysmal positional vertigo, *Otology and Neurotology*, 26(5), 1027–1033, 2005.

101. Powell, L. E. and Myers, A. M., The Activities-specific Balance Confidence (ABC) Scale, *Journal of Gerontology: Biological Sciences*, 50A(1), M28–M34, 1995.

102. Schubert, M. C., Tusa, R. J., Grine, L. E., and Herdman, S. J., Optimizing the sensitivity of the head thrust test for identifying vestibular hypofunction, *Physical Therapy*, 84(2), 151–158, 2004.

103. Dix, M. R. and Hallpike, C. S., The pathology, symptomatology and diagnosis of certain common disorders of the vestibular system, *Proceedings of the Royal Society of Medicine*, 45(6), 341–354, 1952.

104. Norre, M. E., Treatment of unilateral vestibular hypofunction, in W. J. Oosterveld (Ed.), *Otoneurology*, Wiley, New York, 23, 1984.

105. Shepard, N. T. and Telian, S. A., Balance disorders, in J. T. Jacobson and J. L. Northern (Eds.), *Diagnostic Audiology*, Pro-Ed, Austin TX, 1991.

106. Shepard, N. T., Telian, S. A., and Smith-Wheelock, M., Habituation and balance training therapy: A retrospective review, *Neurology and Clinical Neurophysiology*, 8(2), 459–475, 1990.

107. Fukuda, T., The stepping test: Two phases of the labyrinthine reflex, *Acta Oto-Laryngologica*, 50(2), 95–108, 1959.

108. Norre, M. E., Forrez, G., and Beckers, A., Functional recovery of posture in peripheral vestibular disorders, in B. Amblard, A. Berthoz, and F. Clarac (Eds.), *Posture and Gait: Development, Adaptation, and Modulation*, Elsevier, Amsterdam, 1988.

109. Duncan, P. W., Weiner, D. K., Chandler, J., and Studenski, S., Functional reach: A new clinical measure of balance, *Journal of Gerontology*, 45(6), M192–M197, 1990.

110. Berg, K. O., Wood-Dauphinee, S. L., Williams, J. I., and Maki, B., Measuring balance in the elderly: Validation of an instrument, *Canadian Journal of Public Health*, 83(Suppl. 2), S7–S11, 1992.

111. Shumway-Cook, A. and Woollacott, M., *Motor Control: Translating Research into Clinical Practice*, 3rd ed., Lippincott, Williams & Wilkins, Baltimore, 2007.

112. Shumway-Cook, A. and Horak, F. B., Assessing the influence of sensory interaction of balance: Suggestion from the field, *Physical Therapy*, 66(10), 1548–1550, 1986.

113. Nashner, L. M., Black, F. O., and Wall, C., Adaptation to altered support and visual conditions during stance: Patients with vestibular deficits, *Journal of Neuroscience*, 2(5), 536–544, 1982.

114. Shumway-Cook, A., Assessment and management of the patient with traumatic brain injury and vestibular dysfunction, in S. J. Herdman (Ed.), *Vestibular Rehabilitation*, 3rd ed., F. A. Davis, Philadelphia, 2007.

115. Shumway-Cook, A., Gruber, W., Baldwin, M., and Liao, S., The effect of multidimensional exercises on balance, mobility, and fall risk in community-dwelling older adults, *Physical Therapy*, 77(1), 46–57, 1997.

116. Shumway-Cook, A., Woollacott, M., Kerns, K. A., and Baldwin, M., The effects of two types of cognitive tasks on postural stability in older adults with and without a history of falls, *Journal of Gerontology: Biological Science*, 52(4), M232–M240, 1997.

117. Shumway-Cook, A., Baldwin, M., Polissar, N. L., and Gruber, W., Predicting the probability for falls in community-dwelling older adults, *Physical Therapy*, 77(8), 812–819, 1997.

118. Shumway-Cook, A. and Woollacott, M., Attentional demands and postural control: The effect of sensory context, *Journal of Gerontology: Biological Sciences*, 55(1), M10–M16, 2000.

119. Whitney, S. L., Hudak, M. T., and Marchetti, G. F., The dynamic gait index relates to self-reported fall history in individuals with vestibular dysfunction, *Journal of Vestibular Research*, 10(2), 99–105, 2000.

120. Wrisley, D. M., Walker, M. L., Echternach, J. L., and Strasnick, B., Reliability of the dynamic gait index in people with vestibular disorders, *Archives of Physical Medicine and Rehabilitation*, 84(10), 1528–1533, 2003.

121. Hall, C. D. and Herdman, S. J., Reliability of clinical measures used to assess patients with peripheral vestibular disorders, *Journal of Neurologic Physical Therapy*, 30(2), 74–81, 2006.

122. Wrisley, D. M., Marchetti, G. F., Kuharsky, D. K., and Whitney, S. L., Reliability, internal consistency, and validity of data obtained with the functional gait assessment, *Physical Therapy*, 84(10), 906–918, 2004.

123. Winograd, C. H., Lemsky, C. M., Nevitt, M. C., Nordstrom, T. M., Stewart, A. L., Miller, C. J., and Bloch, D. A., Development of a physical performance and mobility examination, *Journal of the American Geriatrics Society*, 42(7), 743–749, 1994.

124. Collen, F. M., Wade, D. T., Robb, G. F., and Bradshaw, C. M., The Rivermead Mobility Index: A further development of the Rivermead Motor Assessment, *International Disability Studies*, 13(2), 50–54, 1991.

125. Guralnik, J. M., Simonsick, E. M., Ferrucci, L., Glynn, R. J., Berkman, L. F., Blazer, D. G., Scherr, P. A., and Wallace, R. B., A short physical performance battery assessing lower extremity function: Association with self-reported disability and prediction of mortality and nursing home admission, *Journal of Gerontology*, 49(2), M85–M94, 1994.

126. Bohannon, R. W., Comfortable and maximum walking speed of adults aged 20–79 years: Reference values and determinants, *Age Ageing*, 26(1), 15–19, 1997.

127. Moseley, A. M., Lanzarone, S., Bosman, J. M., van Loo, M. A., de Bie, R. A., Hassett, L., and Caplan, B., Ecological validity of walking speed assessment after traumatic brain injury: A pilot study, *Journal of Head Trauma Rehabilitation*, 19(4), 341–348, 2004.

128. Glasscock, M. E., Jackson, C. G., and Josey, A. F., *The ABR Handbook: Auditory Brainstem Response*, Thieme Medical Publishers, New York, 1987.

129. Ruth, R., Lambert, P., and Ferraro, J., Electrocochleography: Methods and clinical applications, *American Journal of Otology*, 9(Suppl.), 1–11, 1988.

130. Vermeersch, H., Meyerhoff, W. L., and Boothby, R., Vertigo, in *Diagnosis and Management of Hearing Loss*, W. B. Saunders, Philadelphia, 1985.

131. Coats, A. C., *Electronystagmography, Physiological Measures of the Audio-Vestibulary System*, Academic Press, New York, 1975.

132. Jacobson, G. P. and Newman, C. W., Rotational testing, *Seminars in Hearing*, 12(3), 199–225, 1991.

133. Baloh, R. W., Konrad, H. R., and Honrubia, V., Vestibulo-ocular function in patients with cerebellar atrophy, *Neurology*, 25(2), 160–168, 1975.

134. Baloh, R. W., Honrubia, V., and Jacobson, K., Benign positional vertigo: Clinical and oculographic features in 240 cases, *Neurology*, 37(3), 371–378, 1987.

135. Barber, H. O., Positional nystagmus especially after head injury, *Laryngoscope*, 74(7), 891–944, 1964.

136. Baloh, R. W., Honrubia, V., Yee, R. E., and Jacobson, K. M., Rotational testing: An overview, in H. O. Barber and J. A. Sharpe (Eds.), *Vestibular Disorders*, Year Book Medical Publishers, Chicago, 1988.

137. Cyr, D. G., Moore, G. F., and Moller, C. G., Clinical application of computerized dynamic posturography, *ENTechnology*, September (Suppl.), 36–47, 1988.

138. Hirsh, B. E., Computed sinusoidal harmonic acceleration, *Ear Hearing*, 7(3), 198–203, 1986.

139. Hamid, M. A., Determining side of vestibular dysfunction with rotary chair testing, *Otolaryngology–Head and Neck Surgery*, 105(1), 40–43, 1991.

140. O'Leary, D. P. and Davis, L. L., High-frequency autorotational testing of the vestibulo-ocular reflex, *Neurology and Clinical Neurophysiology*, 8(2), 297–312, 1990.

141. Saadat, D., O'Leary, D. P., Pulec, J. L., and Kitano, H., Comparison of vestibular autorotation and caloric testing, *Otolaryngology–Head and Neck Surgery*, 113(3), 215–222, 1995.

142. Murphy, T. P., Vestibular autorotation and electronystagmography testing in patients with dizziness, *American Journal of Otology*, 15(4), 502–505, 1994.

143. Herdman, S. J., Tusa, R. J., Blatt, P., Suzuki, A., Venuto, P. J., and Roberts, D. Computerized dynamic visual acuity test in the assessment of vestibular deficits, *American Journal of Otology*, 19(6), 790–796, 1998.

144. Balzer, G. K., Clinical contributions of dynamic platform posturography, *Seminars in Hearing*, 12(3), 238, 1991.

145. Hunter, L. L. and Balzer, G. K., Overview and introduction to dynamic platform posturography, *Seminars in Hearing*, 12(3), 226, 1991.

146. Mirka, A. and Black, F. O., Clinical application of dynamic posturography for evaluating sensory integration and vestibular dysfunction, *Neurology and Clinical Neurophysiology*, 8(2), 351, 1990.

147. O'Neill, D. E., Gill-Body, K. M., and Krebs, D. E., Posturography changes do not predict functional performance changes, *American Journal of Otology*, 19(6), 797–803, 1998.

148. Mallinson, A. I. and Longridge, N. S., Dizziness from whiplash and head injury: Differences between whiplash and head injury, *American Journal of Otology*, 19(6), 814–818, 1998.

149. Dix, M. R., Rehabilitation of vertigo, in M. R. Dix and J. D. Hood (Eds.), *Vertigo,* Wiley, New York, 1984.

150. Katsarkas, A., Electronystagmographic (ENG) findings in paroxysmal positional vertigo (PPV) as a sign of vestibular dysfunction, *Acta Oto-Laryngologica*, 111(2), 193–200, 1991.

151. McCabe, B. F., Vestibular physiology: Its clinical application in understanding the dizzy patient, in M. M. Paparella, D. A. Shumrick, J. L. Gluckman, and W. L. Meyerhoff (Eds.), *Otolaryngology,* W. B. Saunders, Philadelphia, 911, 1991.

152. Dichgans, J., Bizzi, E., Morasso, P., and Tagliasco, V., Mechanisms underlying recovery of eye–head coordination following bilateral labyrinthectomy in monkeys, *Experimental Brain Research*, 18(5), 548, 1973.

153. Fetter, M. and Zee, D. S., Recovery from unilateral labyrinthectomy in the rhesus monkey, *Journal of Neurophysiology*, 59(2), 370, 1998.

154. Norre, M. E., Rationale of rehabilitation treatment for vertigo, *American Journal of Otolaryngology*, 8(1), 31, 1987.

155. Shumway-Cook, A. and Horak, F. B., Rehabilitation strategies for patients with vestibulary deficits, *Neurology and Clinical Neurophysiology*, 8(2), 441, 1990.

156. Shumway-Cook, A. and Horak, F. B., Vestibular Rehabilitation: An exercise approach to managing symptoms of vestibular dysfunction, *Seminars in Hearing*, 10(1) 196–207, 1989.

157. Zee, D. S., Vestibular adaptation, in S. J. Herdman (Ed.), *Vestibular Rehabilitation*, 3rd ed., F. A. Davis, Philadelphia, 2007.

158. Keshner, E. A., Postural abnormalities in vestibular disorders, in S. J. Herdman (Ed.), *Vestibular Rehabilitation*, 3rd ed., F. A. Davis, Philadelphia, 2007.

159. Cooksey, F. S., Rehabilitation in vestibular injuries, *Proceedings of the Royal Society of Medicine*, 39(5), 273, 1946.

160. Hecker, H. C., Haug, C. O., and Herdon, J. W., Treatment of the vertiginous patient using Cawthorne's vestibular exercises, *Laryngoscope*, 84(11), 2065, 1974.

161. Telian, S. A., Shepard, N. T., Smith-Wheelock, M., and Kemink, J. L., Habituation therapy for chronic vestibular dysfunction: Preliminary results, *Otolaryngology–Head and Neck Surgery*, 103(1), 89, 1990.

162. Patla, A. E., Mobility in complex environments: Implications for clinical assessment and rehabilitation, *Neurology Report*, 25(3), 82–90. 2001.

163. Pavlou, M., Lingeswaran, A., Davies, R. A., Gresty, M. A., and Bronstein, A. M., Simulator based rehabilitation in refractory dizziness, *Journal of Neurology*, 251(8), 983–995, 2004.

164. Whitney, S. L., Sparto, P. J., Hodges, L. F., Babu, S. V., Furman, J. M., and Redfern, M. S., Responses to a virtual reality grocery store in persons with and without vestibular dysfunction, *CyberPsychology and Behavior*, 9(2), 152–156, 2006.

165. Thornton, M., Marshall, S., McComas, J., Finestone, H., McCormick, A., and Sveistrup, H., Benefits of activity and virtual reality based balance exercise programmes for adults with traumatic brain injury: Perceptions of participants and their caregivers, *Brain Injury*, 19(12), 989–1000, 2005.

166. Whitney, S. L., Sparto, P. J., Brown, K. E., Furman, J. M., Jacobson, J. L., and Redfern, M. S., The potential use of virtual reality in vestibular rehabilitation: Preliminary findings with the BNAVE, *Neurology Report*, 26(2), 72–78, 2002.

167. Flynn, S., Palma, P., and Bender, A., Feasibility of using the Sony PlayStation 2 Gaming Platform for an individual poststroke: A case report, *Journal of Neurologic Physical Therapy*, 31(4), 180–189, 2007.

168. Norre, M. E. and Beckers, A. M., Vestibular habituation training, *Archives of Otolaryngology–Head & Neck Surgery*, 114(8), 883, 1988.

169. Herdman, S. J. and Whitney, S. L., Interventions for the patient with vestibular dysfunction, in S. J. Herdman (Ed.), *Vestibular Rehabilitation*, 3rd ed., F. A. Davis, Philadelphia, 2007.

170. Whitney, S. L. and Rossi, M. M., Efficacy of vestibular rehabilitation, in N. T. Shepard and D. Solomon (Eds.), *The Otolaryngologic Clinics of North America: Practical Issues in the Management of the Dizzy and Balance Disorder Patient*, W. B. Saunders, Philadelphia, 2000.

171. Cohen, H., Vestibular rehabilitation reduces functional disability, *Otolaryngology–Head and Neck Surgery*, 107(5), 638–643, 1992.

172. Keim, R. J., Cook, M., and Martini, D., Balance rehabilitation therapy, *Laryngoscope*, 102(11), 1302, 1992.

173. Telian, S. A., Shepard, N. T., Smith-Wheelock, M., and Hoberg, M., Bilateral vestibular paresis: Diagnosis and treatment, *Otolaryngology–Head and Neck Surgery*, 104(1), 67–71, 1991.

174. Cowand, J. L., Wrisley, D. M., Walker, M., Strasnick, B., and Jacobson, J. T., Efficacy of vestibular rehabilitation, *Otolaryngology–Head and Neck Surgery*, 118(1), 49–54, 1998.

175. Telian, S. A., Shepard, N. T., Smith-Wheelock, M., and Kemink, J. L., Habituation therapy for chronic vestibular dysfunction: Preliminary results, *Otolaryngology–Head and Neck Surgery*, 103(1), 89–95, 1990.

176. Horak, F. B., Jones-Rycewicz, C., Black, F. O., and Shumway-Cook, A., Effects of vestibular rehabilitation on dizziness and imbalance, *Otolaryngology–Head and Neck Surgery*, 106(2), 175–180, 1992.

177. Shepard, N. T. and Telian, S. A., Programmatic vestibular rehabilitation, *Otolaryngology–Head and Neck Surgery*, 112(1), 173–182, 1995.

7

Visual Dysfunction Following Traumatic Brain Injury

Ronald L. Morton

CONTENTS

7.1 Introduction

Individuals sustaining traumatic brain injury (TBI) often sustain other injuries in tandem with injury to the brain. Injuries involving the face, neck, back, torso, and extremities are commonly associated with TBI. Frequently, these injuries are readily diagnosed and treated because they are easily evidenced when the person presents at the emergency room.

Less obvious injuries, however, can be overlooked during lifesaving endeavors—in particular, those involving systems that are more difficult to evaluate thoroughly, such as the vestibular or visual systems. This chapter focuses on deficits commonly observed in the visual systems of people with TBI. The purpose of the chapter is to provide a review of the neuroanatomy of vision and illustrate the relationship of commonly observed visual–perceptual and visual–motor deficits following TBI to neuroanatomic structures. Visual system dysfunction following TBI is fairly common and can be quite subtle or relatively frank. Bontke et al.[1] found the overall incidence of cranial nerve injury, for example, in persons hospitalized following TBI to be 19%. Cranial nerve VII was most frequently injured (9%), whereas cranial nerves III (6%) and VI (6%) followed.[1] The visual system has not been long regarded as one that can respond to treatments that are other than compensatory (i.e., lenses) or surgical in nature. That the visual system can respond to treatments that impact visual–perceptual and/or visual–motor skills is a relatively recent concept as applied to acquired neurologic damage. The visual system functions as a primary sensory receptor for motor, social, cognitive, communicative, and emotive functions. As such, the visual system is highly integrated with many neural functions other than simply sight. Visual system disorders, then, require a fair amount of attention in the person with TBI and should be considered an integral part of the rehabilitation program. Remediation of visual–perceptual and visual–motor disorders can enhance function in all of the aforementioned areas as well as reduce the likelihood of reinjury and enhance maximal functional improvement.

7.2 Anatomic Considerations

7.2.1 Retina

To appreciate fully the complexities of the visual system, one must recognize that visual integration is not just a cortical process. Rather, visual integration begins peripherally in the visual receptor fields of the retinas.[2]

The fact that visual processing starts in the retina may seem strange until it is recalled that the eye is actually an outpouching of the brain from early during embryologic development.[3,4] Figure 7.1 depicts the organization of the photoreceptors, bipolar cells, and ganglion cells. Photoreceptors, when stimulated, pass information to adjacent bipolar cells that, in turn, differentially affect firing of the ganglion cells. Linear and crossconnections of ganglion and adjacent bipolar cells is demonstrated by the fact that the adjacent bipolar cells increase the firing rate of ganglion cells when certain conditions are met.

For example, if a spot of light lands on one photoreceptor while adjacent photoreceptors remain nonilluminated, the stimulated photoreceptor will fire at a higher rate compared with the rate at which it will fire when all surrounding photoreceptors are simultaneously illuminated. These patterns of illuminated and nonilluminated photoreceptors were referred to by Werblin and Dowling[5] as on-center and off-surround groups.

On-center and off-surround groups may be joined in such combinations as to form units sensitive to stimuli in the environment of particular spatial orientations. These include, for example, vertical, horizontal, and diagonal lines or edges. Stimuli that are thus organized are relayed to the cortex via the optic tract. The processing of visual stimuli continues, via the optic tract, to be further processed in the lateral geniculate bodies, the occipital cortex, and associated cortices receiving radiations from the primary occipital areas.

As a normal individual gazes upon an object, the image is registered simultaneously in both the right and left retinas. Each retina, however, is situated slightly differently in orientation to the object, thus producing a slightly different image to the brain from each retina.[6] This can be demonstrated by gazing at an object and alternately closing one eye, then the other. The object appears to move as a result of the fact that the image registered is different because of the distance separating the eyes and the slight difference in angular

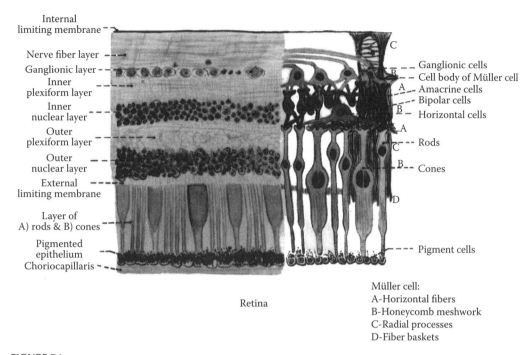

Müller cell:
A-Horizontal fibers
B-Honeycomb meshwork
C-Radial processes
D-Fiber baskets

Retina

FIGURE 7.1
Eye anatomy. (From W. Jacobson, Jr. (Ed.), *The Eye* (chart). Copyright 1979, 1981, 1986 by Anatomical Chart Co., Skokie, IL. With permission.)

orientation of each eye to the object. Stereopsis, which is the ability to visualize the dimension of depth, arises from the fusing of these two separate images by the sensory system[6] and, consequently, plays a major role in several visual perceptual skills.

7.2.2 Optic Tract Organization and Lesion Characteristics

Knowledge of organization of the optic tract is of great importance in determination of site of lesion from visual deficits presented. Lesions at different points in the optic tract will be demonstrated by pathognomonic visual deficits.[4] In the days prior to computed tomographic scanning and magnetic resonance imaging (MRI), the localization of injury was dependent upon knowledge of anatomic relationships. Knowing the proximity of motor and sensory pathways adjacent to the visual pathways allowed determination of site of lesion based upon the constellation of signs and symptoms. Localization of the site of lesion or injury can assist in further diagnosis, determination of etiology, and likely systemic sequelae.

Each retina must direct its information toward the cortex and does so via the optic nerve. The information passes from the ganglion cells, located in each retina, posteriorly via the optic nerve to the optic chiasm. Figure 7.2 illustrates how, at the optic chiasm, right and left visual space are segregated with the contribution of each hemiretina passed to a single corresponding lateral geniculate body, the specific thalamic relay nucleus for the visual pathway.[7] Right visual space images upon the nasal retina of the right eye and the temporal retina of the left eye. At the chiasm, the optic fibers of the nasal retina of the right eye cross to the left to join the optic fibers of the temporal retina of the left eye. The temporal fibers of the left eye continue uncrossed in the optic tract beyond the chiasm and find their

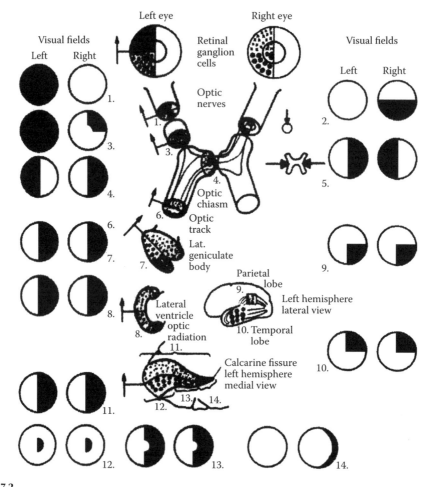

FIGURE 7.2

Visual pathway and resultant field defects. (From Jones, L. T., Reeh, M. J., and Wirtschafter, J. D., *Ophthalmic Anatomy: A Manual with Some Clinical Application*, American Academy of Ophthalmology, San Francisco, CA, 1970. With permission.)

way to the lateral geniculate body on the left. Thus, the left lateral geniculate body receives information from the right visual space from both eyes.

Information from the upper retinal fibers (nasal crossed, temporal uncrossed) passes through the corresponding lateral geniculate body and continues in a portion of the optic tract known as the *geniculocalcarine tract* until it projects to the primary visual cortex (cuneate gyrus, area 17) of the occipital lobe.[8] The geniculocalcarine tract courses through the parietal lobe; a lesion involving the geniculocalcarine tract on the right would result in an inferior contralateral quadranopsia (Figure 7.2, item 9).

Information from the nasal lower retina, however, after crossing over at the optic chiasm to join the temporal lower retinal fibers, leaves the lateral geniculate body and courses into the temporal lobe (Figure 7.3) in a band of fibers known as *Meyer's loop*.[8] These fibers terminate in the lingual gyrus of the occipital lobe. A lesion involving Meyer's loop on the right would cause a contralateral left superior quadranopsia (Figure 7.2, item 10).

Bitemporal hemianopsia (Figure 7.2, item 4), for example, results from a lesion that involves the optic chiasm—in particular, the fibers that cross from the nasal field of each

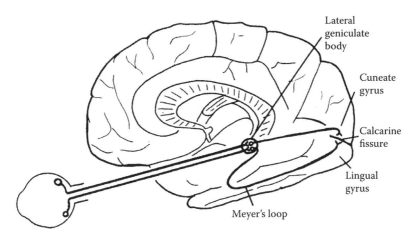

FIGURE 7.3
Meyer's loop. (From Willis, W. D. and Grossman, R. G., *Medical Neurobiology: Neuroanatomical and Neurophysiological Principles Basic to Clinical Neuroscience*, 2nd ed., C.V. Mosby, St. Louis, MO, 1977. With permission.)

retina, serving temporal visual space, to the lateral geniculate body of the contralateral side of the brain. Pituitary hormone dysfunction may be associated with this visual system deficit as a result of the proximity of the optic chiasm to the pituitary gland. Binasal hemianopsia (Figure 7.2, item 5), on the other hand, would implicate a lesion of the lateral aspects of the optic chiasm involving the uncrossed temporal fibers from the nasal fields of each retina. In this instance, carotid disease may be involved.

The primary visual cortex is made up of the region of the cortex immediately surrounding the calcarine fissure, extending anteriorly toward the splenium of the corpus callosum.[9] This area is known as the *calcarine cortex*. Lesions involving selective portions of the calcarine fissure and occipital pole can likewise present with specific visual field defects. Figure 7.2, item 12, depicts an occipital pole lesion-induced central scotoma. A lesion at the midportion of the calcarine fissure or of fibers to this area would result in a contralateral homonymous hemianopsia with macular sparing (Figure 7.2, item 13). Lastly, a lesion involving the anterior portion of the calcarine fissure results in a contralateral temporal crescentic field deficit (Figure 7.2, item 14).

7.2.3 Oculomotor and Brainstem Organization

Discussion of the visual system must include a review of the oculomotor system and its innervation. Oculomotor deficits following brain injury can result in misalignment of the eyes that, in turn, may be reported by the person as double vision, blurred vision, impaired eye–hand coordination, impaired tracking during reading, and so on. Misalignment of the eyes can also lead to cortical image suppression with resultant perceptual deficits that will impact therapeutic performance, balance, coordination, and safety.

Perhaps the most common oculomotor dysfunction seen is that of esophoria. In this condition, the lateral rectus of one eye is weakened, presumably as a result of injury to the corresponding cranial nerve VI nucleus or pathway. These people may report blurred or double vision, although they may also accommodate to misaligned images via cortical suppression of the image from one eye. Careful evaluation may turn up additional subtle impairments of other extrinsic muscle innervations. Suffice it to say that innervational deficits resulting in complete or partial motor paralysis of the

TABLE 7.1

Cranial Nerve Innervation

Cranial Nerve	Muscle Innervated	Brainstem Nucleus
III	Pupilloconstrictor and ciliary muscles	Edinger-Westphal
	Superior, inferior, and medial rectus	Oculomotor
	Inferior oblique	
	Levator palpebra	
IV	Superior oblique	Trochlear
VI	Lateral rectus	Abducens

corresponding extrinsic muscles are prevalent following TBI and require careful delineation and treatment.

The six extrinsic muscles of the eye[10] are innervated by three cranial nerves as listed in Table 7.1. Cranial nerve III is responsible for innervation of the superior rectus, medial rectus, inferior rectus, and inferior oblique. The superior rectus rotates the eye upward when the eye is abducted; however, when the eye is adducted, this muscle moves the superior part of the eye toward the medial wall of the orbit (intorsion). The medial rectus rotates the eye nasally. The inferior rectus rotates the eye downward when the eye is in abduction and extorts the eye when in adduction. The inferior oblique elevates the eye when the eye is adducted and extorts the eye during abduction.

Cranial nerve IV innervates the superior oblique, which is responsible for eye depression during eye adduction and intorts the eye during abduction (Figure 7.4). Cranial nerve VI innervates the lateral rectus, which produces temporally directed rotation of the eye.

The nuclei of cranial nerves III, IV, and VI are found in the brainstem, ranging from the midbrain to the pons.[11] Figure 7.5 shows the nuclei of cranial nerve III located inferior to the superior colliculus and lateral to midline on either side. The axons innervating the four

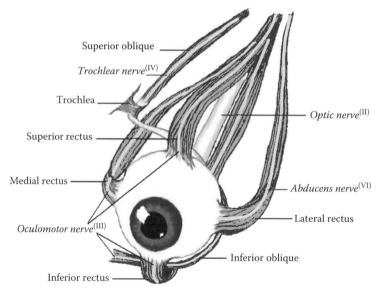

FIGURE 7.4
Musculature of the eye and cranial nerve innervation.

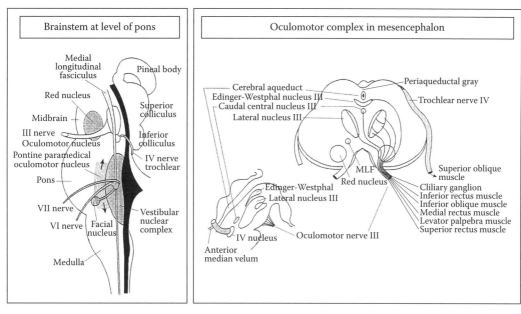

FIGURE 7.5
Brainstem and nuclei and oculomotor complex in mesencephalon cutaneous. MLF, medial longitudinal fasciculus.

extrinsic muscles of the eye innervate ipsilateral muscles, except for the superior rectus, which may project contralaterally.[2]

The nucleus of cranial nerve IV is located below the inferior colliculus. Innervation of the superior oblique muscles is contralateral in nature. Finally, the cranial nerve VI nucleus is located in the pons. Its axons remain ipsilateral as they innervate the lateral rectus muscles.

These three cranial nerves are interrelational in function. The medial longitudinal fasciculus (MLF) comprises the major projection system allowing such interrelation (Figure 7.5).[2] Vestibular projections influencing eye movement connect to these cranial nerves via the MLF and account for a good portion of the MLF. The vestibular projections arise mainly from the superior and medial vestibular nuclei. These interconnections between vestibular and ocular nuclei are responsible for coordination of head/eye movements and the production of nystagmus following vestibular overstimulation.

Cranial nerves III, IV, and VI receive afferents from the retina, the frontal and occipital lobes, the vestibular nuclei, and the superior colliculus. There may be reticular projections as well.[2]

The nucleus of the oculomotor nerve, cranial nerve III, is located dorsally within the midbrain beneath the aqueduct of Sylvius connecting the third and fourth ventricles. The nuclear complex represents a collection of subnuclei that have specific identifiable functions. Most dorsally, the levator complex is a midline structure that supplies both third cranial nerves. Rostrally, the Edinger-Westphal nucleus is a paired structure that sends parasympathetic signals to the sphincter muscles of the pupil via the ciliary ganglion and the muscles of accommodation of the ciliary body (Figure 7.6). The medial complex, which lies most ventrally, has been shown to contain three subnuclei that play variable roles in medial rectus functions. One of these subsets may receive input from the mesencephalic reticular formation, firing in response to retinal temporal disparity that indicates a near target. The

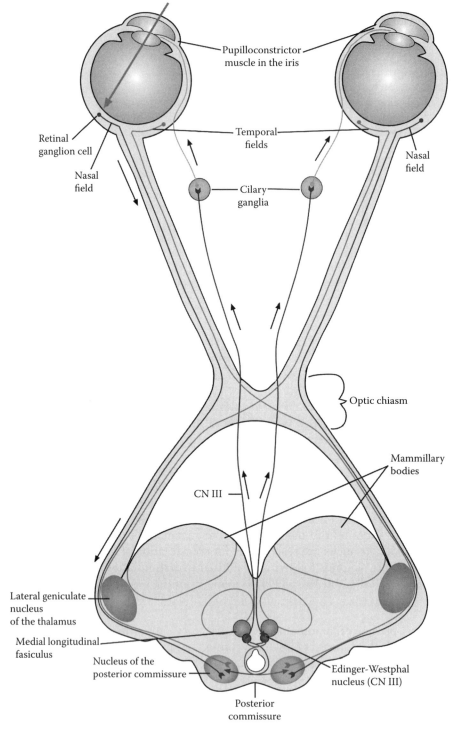

FIGURE 7.6
Edinger-Westphal nucleus and ciliary ganglion.

inferior rectus subnucleus lies dorsally and rostrally. The inferior oblique subnucleus lies laterally between the inferior rectus subnucleus and the more ventral medial rectus subnucleus. Fibers exit ventrally along with the fibers destined to innervate the medial rectus, inferior rectus, and the pupil and ciliary body. The superior subnucleus, which lies along the midline, is unique in that the fibers cross within it before exiting ventrally with the fibers destined for the levator and superior rectus. Cranial nerve III runs slightly oblique to the tentorial edge parallel to the posterior communicating artery. Pupillary fibers are usually found to run on the medial surface of the nerve where they are particularly sensitive to compression and potential inflammation. The most medial aspect of the temporal lobe, the uncus, which is located just above the tentorium and the subarachnoid third cranial nerve, may be forced through the tentorial notch with a supratentorial mass lesion or hemorrhage, and stretch the third cranial nerve against the superior cerebellar artery, resulting in abnormality. As can be seen from the relationships in Figure 7.5, with the sixth cranial nerve tethered as it exits the brainstem and prior to entering Dorello's canal, an axial movement of the brainstem can result in stretching or damage to cranial nerve VI. The fourth cranial nerve is not pivoted as tightly but is exposed to the tentorium, which sweeps around it and so an anterior–posterior movement or swelling of the brain can push on cranial nerve IV and damage that as well during its exposed, long course outside the brainstem.

The fourth cranial nerve lies within the gray matter in the dorsal aspect of the caudal midbrain, just below the aqueduct of Sylvius, contiguous with the rostral third cranial nerve nucleus (Figure 7.7). The intra-axial portion of cranial nerve IV runs dorsally around the periaqueductal gray to cross within the anterior medullary vellum below the pineal gland. The fourth cranial nerve is the only cranial nerve exiting on the dorsal surface of the brain and brainstem. It has the longest unprotected intracranial course and lies just under the tentorial edge, where it is easily damaged by closed head trauma. Just below the

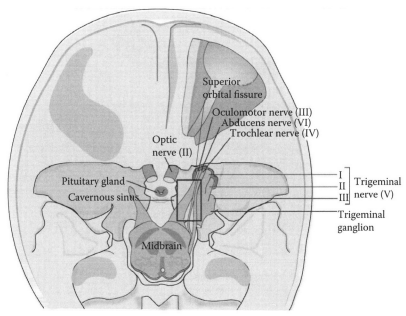

FIGURE 7.7
Course of cranial nerves through the cranial vault.

anterior tentorial insertion, cranial nerve IV enters the posterior lateral aspect of the cavernous sinus just underneath cranial nerve III, runs forward within the lateral wall of the cavernous sinus, then enters the superior orbital fissure just outside the annulus of Zinn, and crosses over the optic nerve down to the superior oblique muscle.

The sixth cranial nerve originates in the dorsal caudal pons just beneath the fourth ventricle, surrounded by looping fibers of the seventh cranial nerve. The nucleus contains the primary motor neurons and interneurons across from the contralateral medial longitudinal fasciculus to reach the third cranial nerve nucleus for coordination. Pathology affecting the sixth cranial nerve nucleus produces an ipsilateral gaze palsy. The axons exit the nucleus, travel ventrally and slightly laterally, medial to the superior olivary nucleus, to exit on the ventral surface of the caudal pons. After exiting the brainstem, the sixth cranial nerve runs rostrally within the subarachnoid space and over the surface of the clivus from the area of the cerebellopontine angle to the posterior superior portion of the posterior fossa. The nerve pierces the dura and travels forward to lie free within the cavernous sinus but runs parallel to the horizontal segment of the carotid artery within the cavernous sinus (Figure 7.7). It enters the supraorbital fissure through the Annulus of Zinn to enter and innervates the lateral rectus muscle.

7.2.4 Frontal Eye Fields

The frontal lobe contains two regions that are also of importance in oculomotor control. Much of what we know about these fields arises from studies with monkeys. The frontal eye field (FEF), the supplementary eye field, and the dorsolateral prefrontal cortex are primarily implicated in saccadic control mechanisms (Figure 7.8). Two specific types of neurons are found in the FEF: movement-related neurons and visual–movement neurons.

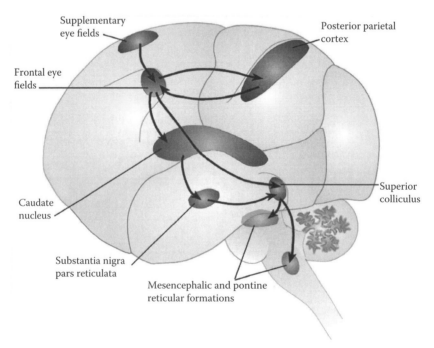

FIGURE 7.8
Frontal and supplementary eye fields of the frontal lobe.

Movement-related neurons fire during all saccades regardless of whether the saccade is directed for the purpose of target location. These neurons fire only when the saccades are relevant to the organism's behavior and project to the superior colliculus. Electrical stimulation of a unilateral FEF will cause a saccade to the movement field of the neuron that has been stimulated. Bilateral stimulation to the FEFs causes vertical nystagmus. Visual–movement neurons are implicated in visually guided saccades. They are active in both visual- and movement-related activity.[12]

Saccadic movements that are involved in cognitive processing appear to be located in the supplemental eye field and the dorsolateral lateral prefrontal cortex. Saccades to a part of a target involve the supplementary eye field whereas saccades to a remembered target involve the dorsolateral lateral prefrontal cortex.[12]

Persons with damage to the FEF may have difficulty suppressing a saccade to a visual target to which they are attending. Parietal neurons implicated in attentional processing send a signal to the superior colliculus, whereas the signal arising from the FEF (which should suppress the saccade by inhibiting the stimulus sent to the superior colliculus) fails to do so.[12]

Eye movements in mammals occur largely in coordination with cognitive function. Direction of eye movement involves cortical centers that communicate with the superior colliculus to effectuate eye movement.[12]

7.2.5 Pupillary Responses

Pupil size is modulated by both the sympathetic nervous system with its dilator fibers and the parasympathetic system with its constrictor fibers. Pupils are normally of equal size, but differences of less than 1 mm may be present in as much as 20% of the normal population. Pathologic anisocoria is caused by lesions either of the sympathetic or parasympathetic pathways or by local iris disease, such as tumors or scar adhesions.

Sympathetic impulses to the eye originate in the hypothalamus. They are transmitted along the spinal cord, synapsing in the lateral gray columns. They exit the cord via preganglionic fibers at C8 to T2 and travel upward in the sympathetic chain to synapse in the superior cervical ganglia, lying at the level of C1 and C2. Nonmyelinated, postganglionic fibers form a plexus around the common carotid artery with vasomotor fibers to the face and the external carotid artery. The internal carotid artery carries sympathetic nerves through the cavernous sinus, where the fibers join the nasociliary branch of cranial nerve V. From the nasociliary nerve, they travel into the eye to the radial dilator muscle fibers in the pupils, resulting in dilation.

Parasympathetic preganglionic axons originate in the Edinger-Westphal nucleus of the third cranial nerve (medulla), where they produce a simultaneous and bilateral response in each third nerve through intraneuronal connections. The parasympathetic preganglionic axons run forward in the third nerve and pass through the inferior division of the anterior aspect of the cavernous sinus to the ciliary ganglion for synapse on their way via the short ciliary nerves into the annular constrictor pupillary fibers. The output of the Edinger-Westphal nucleus represents the summation of the input from both the right and left eyes via a certain set of the ganglion cells, some of which cross in the chiasm, along with the other visual fibers through the optic tract and lateral geniculate body on their way to synapse at the Edinger-Westphal nucleus.

This summation, at the Edinger-Westphal nucleus, allows one to elicit a relative afferent pupillary defect—a different pupil size in response to a monocle light stimulus. This reaction is caused by an asymmetry of conduction in the afferent visual system, either at the retina or optic nerve, specifically in the area anterior to the lateral geniculate body. To illustrate, when a traumatic optic atrophy causes the loss of a significant number of ganglion cell axons, the conduction of a light stimulus to the Edinger-Westphal nucleus is diminished and a larger pupil will result (i.e., 5 mm) rather than the small pupil resulting from full stimulation (i.e., 3 mm). Therefore, as a light is swung[13] from the normal side, with 3-mm pupils in both eyes, to the affected side, the pupils will dilate to 5 mm.

7.2.6 Visual Fields

An understanding of visual field integrity is of key importance in accurate diagnosis of visual deficits and their neurologic correlates in the person with TBI.[14] Visual field is measured in degrees and the center of fixation is used as a zero referent. Visual field extends to approximately 90 degrees in all directions. Decreasing sensitivity is found the farther out the stimulus is from center. Targets in the less sensitive periphery must be larger and brighter to be seen.

Two types of measurement devices are available for delineation of visual fields. Devices can be categorized as *kinetic* or *static*, depending upon whether the stimulus moves or is stationary. The Goldmann Perimeter is a kinetic device in which the stimulus presented is a spot of light of specific size and intensity that is moved toward the center of fixation until the person reports seeing it. The Humphrey Perimeter is a static device that measures visual field by increasing the brightness of a spot at a fixed location until the person sees it. These two devices have been demonstrated to be fairly accurate and reliable in tests of both a neurologically and nonneurologically impaired population. Goldmann fields have been shown to be 97% reliable whereas Humphrey fields were 91% reliable.[15]

Diplopia fields are evaluated using the Goldmann Perimeter. The person's eye is not patched, as they would be for peripheral field testing. The person is positioned at the machine so that the fixation light is aligned between the person's eyes. A light is introduced. The person follows this light from the center outward and informs the examiner when it breaks into a double image. Thus, a specific map of the person's diplopia is made and can be tracked as treatment progresses. It should be noted that the vast majority of diplopia can be accounted for as a result of acquired paresis or palsy of one or more of the extraocular muscles.[16]

Visual fields can also be evaluated by "confrontation," which requires no elaborate devices. Confrontation testing is performed by movement of the examiner's finger or a red bottle cap slowly into the person's visual field, with central visual fixation, until the stimulus is viewed. Although not a precise system of measurement, confrontation testing can reliably demonstrate certain visual field deficits in the absence of more elaborate testing.[16] Fading of the color red in the field periphery can be an early sign of visual field depression.

7.3 Examination

Examination of the person with TBI should first establish best corrected visual acuity, if at all possible. This can be difficult to establish as a result of problems the person may have in cooperating with the evaluation. Communication problems may be lessened by using the services of a speech pathologist or family member familiar with the communication deficits of a given person.

The face should be examined for lacerations, scars, or foreign bodies. Check the lids for position, remembering that cranial nerve III is responsible for palpebral elevation and cranial nerve VII for closure via the orbicularis muscles.[17] These motor systems should be evaluated for weakness. Skin sensation should be checked in distributions of cranial nerve V (Figure 7.9), possibly manifesting as anesthesia or abnormal sensation, as well as associated motor functions that can manifest as paresis of mastication.[18] Head and neck positioning should be carefully evaluated because compensatory head tilts are quite common as a result of diplopia and the person's attempt to compensate for same.[6]

Following any facial neuropathy, including a traumatic crush injury, regenerating axons may reinnervate muscles different from those originally served. Such aberrant regeneration can cause synkinetic movements. In this situation, the involved facial muscle may remain weak. Axons originally destined for the orbicularis muscle may reinnervate lower facial muscles, and each blink may cause a twitch in the corner of the mouth or dimpling of

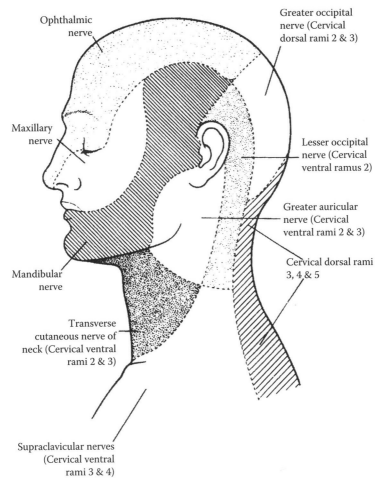

FIGURE 7.9
Distribution of cranial nerve V. (From Warwick, R. and Williams, P. L., *Gray's Anatomy*, 35th ed. Churchill Livingstone, New York, 1973. With permission.)

the chin. Conversely, movement in the lower face, such as pursing the lips or chewing, may invoke involuntary lid closure. Other disorders of aberrant facial innervation include lacrimation invoked by chewing, as in crocodile tears, in which fibers originally supplying the mandibular and sublingual glands reinnervate the lacrimal gland by way of the greater superficial petrosal nerve. This is commonly seen following severe proximal seventh cranial nerve injury and may be accompanied by decreased reflex tearing and decreased taste from the anterior two thirds of the tongue. Another example is a Marcus Gunn jaw-winking syndrome characterized by eyelid elevation with jaw movement caused by an anomalous communication between the trigeminal (pterygoid) and oculomotor (levator) nerves.

The testing of different subsets of the seventh cranial nerve such as salivation, lacrimation, and sensation may help to localize a lesion (e.g., sugar/vinegar on the anterior two thirds of the tongue to test taste). Cutaneous sensation can be evaluated along the posterior aspect of the external auditory canal and tympanic membrane. All functions of cranial nerve VII may be involved if the lesion is relatively proximal from the cerebellar pontine angle to the geniculate ganglia, whereas more distal lesions may affect only certain functions, depending on their location. Testing should include functions of cranial nerves V, VI, and VIII, because this may help further localize the cause of seventh cranial nerve palsy.

7.3.1 Ocular Examination

Examination of the anterior structures of the eye is facilitated by magnification and illumination ranging from penlight and bifocals to slit-lamp examination. Slit-lamp examination allows greater detail to be viewed, as well as better assessment of the depth of any foreign body lodging or scar tissue. The anterior chamber, thus examined, may show blood or inflammatory debris.

Examination of the pupil can provide clues as to the integrity of cranial and optic nerve functions. The responsiveness of a pupil to light and accommodative stimuli can provide information regarding the integrity of the pupillary nerve fibers between the lateral geniculate body, the Edinger-Westphal nucleus (part of the nucleus of cranial nerve III in the medulla of the brainstem), and the sympathetic and parasympathetic nerves, which innervate the dilators and constrictors of the pupil. Thus, a relative afferent pupillary defect may imply optic nerve lesion, traumatic vascular insult, an inflammatory process, or multiple sclerosis.

As shown in Figure 7.10, behind the pupil is the lens.[2] The lens may be affected by trauma in a number of ways, including penetration by a foreign body, laceration of the globe, blunt trauma to the globe, electrical injury, chemical injury, or concussion. Any of these injuries can result in a loss of lens clarity and result in cataract formation. Cataracts may become dense enough to limit visual acuity significantly and may interfere with the rehabilitative process. In this circumstance, surgical intervention may be required. It is important to note that cataract formation can be accelerated by some tranquilizers or steroids.

Opacities of the ocular media, such as a dense cataract, are usually not sufficient to produce an afferent pupillary defect. However, very dense vitreous hemorrhage or dense amblyopia may be sufficient, although it is usually indicative of pathologic lesion in the afferent visual system. This can be correlated with an asymmetric loss of visual field, central acuity, color saturation, or subjective brightness. It should be noted, also, that monocular diplopia can arise from media opacities that cause splitting of the image.[6]

The diagram in Figure 7.11 shows that the intact right eye causes more firings of the central nucleus with light stimulating that side. As the light stimulus is moved to the left side,

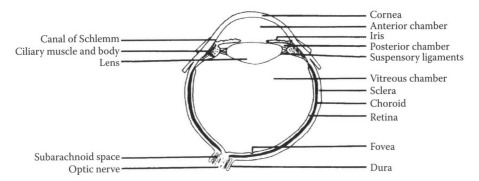

FIGURE 7.10
Major components of the human eye. (From Willis, W. D. and Grossman, R. G., *Medical Neurobiology: Neuroanatomical and Neurophysiological Principles Basic to Clinical Neuroscience*, 2nd ed., C. V. Mosby, St. Louis, MO, 1977. With permission.)

relatively less stimulus is received at the nucleus, resulting in less tone at the constrictor fibers. The result is a larger pupillary aperture. Thus, as the light stimulus is moved from the intact right eye to the affected left eye, the pupils will dilate as the swinging flashlight crosses to the affected side. This is called a *positive swinging flashlight test* or a *left Marcus Gunn pupil*. This is an apparent paradox, with a pupil dilating as it is struck by light, as the light moves from the position determined by the intact right side (i.e., a 3-mm pupil) to the affected left side (i.e., a 5-mm pupil).

Trauma may extend to the posterior segment of the eye. As such, injuries can include retinal breaks, tears, or detachment in which the retina separates from its underlying supportive

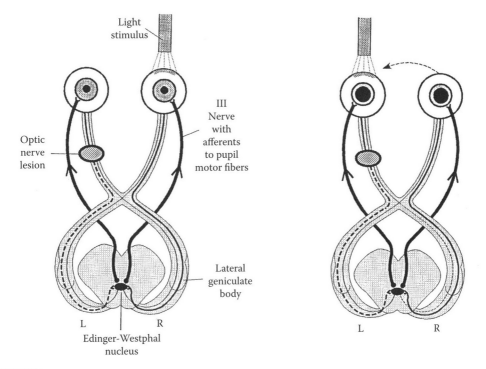

FIGURE 7.11
Anatomy of pupillary defect.

tissues, losing function, and ultimately causing wrinkling and scarring. Hemorrhage may occur and it is possible for there to be contusion to the optic nerve itself.

7.3.2 Extraocular Motility: Peripheral and Central Dysfunction

The extraocular muscles of the eye are responsible for aligning the eyes, enabling them to be pointed at the same object, and moving the eyes to different positions of gaze in a manner that allows the continuous perception of a single image. The movement of each eye is managed by six muscles and is controlled by three cranial nerves. Therefore, between the two eyes, there are 12 muscles and six cranial nerves involved. Any of these muscles or nerves can be adversely affected following injury, resulting in interference with the alignment and tracking of the eyes. Injuries such as direct contusion to the orbit or fracture of the orbit can cause injury to the muscle or nerve complex. Mechanical entrapment of a muscle can occur or bony fragments from an orbital fracture can impinge cranial nerves.

The course of the cranial nerves from the brainstem to the orbit makes them subject to contusion injuries. In particular, cranial nerve VI exits from the ventral side of the brainstem and ascends the bone along the base of the skull. It enters the superior orbital fissure of the orbit on its way to the lateral rectus muscle. Cranial nerve IV exits from the dorsal side of the brainstem and sweeps around to the sides. It also passes through the superior orbital fissure to innervate the superior oblique. Blunt head trauma, with the associated violent shaking of the brain, can cause the dura along the dorsal aspect of the brain to impinge on the nerve as it exits and crosses the dorsum of the brain. The result is a fourth nerve palsy that manifests in the person as the inability to rotate the eye downward during adduction and a loss of intorsion during abduction.

In addition to lesions that can affect individual cranial nerves and muscles, resulting in misalignment, there is also coordination that occurs between various cranial nerve motor nuclei in a tract in the brainstem known as the *medial longitudinal fasciculus* (MLF). The MLF serves as a coordination and integration center between the third, fourth, and sixth cranial nerve motor nuclei. As an example, when people look straight ahead but then wish to turn their gaze to the right, several things must happen in a coordinated fashion. First, the firing rate of the right lateral rectus muscle via the sixth motor nucleus must increase as must the firing rate for the left medial rectus muscle, mediated by the third motor nucleus on the left side. At the same time, a relative inhibition or decrease in the firing rate of the right medial rectus muscle and the left lateral rectus muscle must occur, leading to a deviation of the eyes to the right. A lesion in the brainstem involving the MLF would interfere with the coordination of these four motor nuclei and coordination of eye and/or head movements might subsequently be impaired.

Eye movements must be coordinated with changes in head position or acceleration of the body in any plane that might stimulate the vestibular apparatus. The vestibular apparatus is mediated through the eighth cranial nerve, which has projections into the lateral gaze center located adjacent to the sixth motor nucleus on the ipsilateral side. The right horizontal gaze center fires directly into the adjacent right sixth motor nerve nucleus for its contribution to conjugate deviation of the eyes.

This can be contrasted to a request for a volitional turning of the eyes to the right. Compliance with such a request would require involvement of the left frontal premotor area, which feeds posteriorly in the white tracts and projects to the right horizontal gaze center. Consequently, an injury to the frontal lobe or its conduction path to the horizontal gaze center could adversely affect the ability of a person to turn the eyes voluntarily from one side to the other. At the same time, vestibular input to the lateral gaze center may remain intact. The doll's head maneuver, wherein the head is rotated by the examiner to one side and the normal response is such that the eyes deviate to the opposite side, can be utilized to test the integrity of pathways from the vestibular nuclei to the lateral gaze center.

Horizontal and vertical gaze systems are located in different anatomic locations and tend to function independently of each other (Figure 7.12). Therefore, each should be examined separately to check for impairment. Also, it is important to note if a person can hold steady gaze in the primary or eccentric positions in the presence of any type of nystagmus.

Horizontal gaze palsy with an inability to make a conjugate ocular movement to one side may result from either pontine or supranuclear lesions. Evaluation by the doll's head maneuver or caloric stimulation[16] to the external auditory meatus allows differentiation of a lower pontine lesion from one of the supranuclear pathway, which would cause a loss of saccadic gaze in the direction opposite the site of lesion A (Figure 7.13). Input from the intact hemisphere causes ocular deviation toward the site of the lesion. If the person is unable to look toward that gaze direction by either a voluntary or tracking movement, but can deviate the eyes to the involved side during a doll's head rotation, this demonstrates that the lower pontine reflexes are intact and that the lesion is in the supranuclear pathway.

The vertical gaze centers are divided above and below the aqueduct of Sylvius anterior to the motor nuclei of cranial nerve III. The vertical gaze centers can also be selectively injured. Damage to the dorsal vertical nerve nucleus will affect the ability to initiate upgaze beyond midline, allowing horizontal gaze to be preserved with smooth pursuits and saccades intact (Parinaud's syndrome).

Vertical gaze palsies caused by a lesion of the upper midbrain in the area of the superior colliculus can result in three signs known, collectively, as *Parinaud's syndrome* or *dorsal midbrain syndrome.* This is comprised of a loss of vertical gaze ability and pupillary light

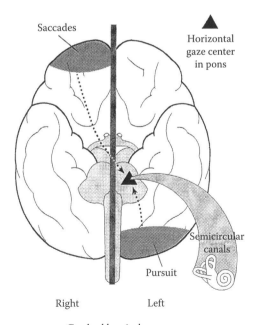

FIGURE 7.12
Inputs to horizontal gaze center.

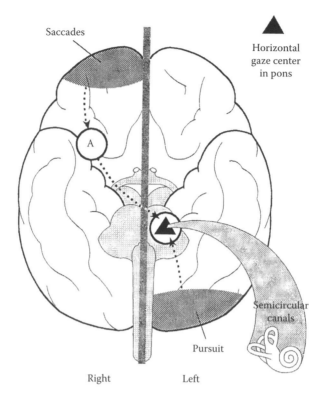

Saccades

Horizontal
gaze center
in pons

A

Semicircular
canals

Pursuit

Right   Left

Cerebral hemispheres

FIGURE 7.13
Supranuclear lesion.

reflex, with preservation of near reflex and the presence of an eye movement disorder called *convergence retraction nystagmus.* Convergence retraction nystagmus is triggered by an upward saccade, either voluntary or in response to a downward-rotating optokinetic drum, which causes simultaneous firing of both the medial and lateral rectus muscles, resulting in convergence and retraction of globes into the orbit. Examination of the pupil shows light/near dissociation with normal to mild dilation of pupils and poor or absent light response; but, with an accommodative target, the pupil will constrict to a near reaction. A person with this condition has the ability to make rapid horizontal saccades, but abilities for voluntary up and down gaze are lost and the person attempts a head posture change to compensate. A doll's head rotation may show that vertical movement can be produced with vestibular input when pontine reflexes are intact and only a supranuclear pathway lesion is present.

Early lesions in the region of the posterior commissure can affect upgaze preferentially, particularly vertical saccades. Lesions can press on the midbrain aqueduct leading to hydrocephalus and papilledema. A lateral extension of such a lesion can involve the optic radiation, whereas a posterior extension of a lesion can produce ataxia from cerebellar compression. Pineal tumors are the most common of such lesions, although emboli, vasculitis, arteriovenous malformations, or arteriosclerosis may also be causal factors. An upper midbrain cerebrovascular accident (CVA), by branches from the posterior cerebral artery, can also result in impairment of vertical gaze with retraction of both upper eyelids, called *Collier's sign.* These symptoms usually recover over 2 to 3 weeks.

As has been stated, ocular deviation or misalignment can result from cranial nerve palsies. Deviation is often initially incomitant or variable in different directions of gaze. There is often more deviation in looking to the side of the affected muscle than when looking away from its field of action. This condition may resolve in time, with return to normal function, or the condition may become more comitant, or even and consistent, in the different fields of gaze. Sequential measurements are used to study the deviation in nine cardinal positions. Via sequential measurements, the examiner can more readily make determinations about whether function is returning to normal or whether deviation is becoming more comitant.

When ocular deviation is relatively even in primary and reading gaze, prisms can be used to move the image optically to compensate for the mechanical misalignment. Press-on prisms can be applied to the person's glasses, resulting in increased comfort and resumption of the ability of the person to see binocularly. Press-on prisms may be changed at will, unlike ground-in prisms. As the person's divergence reduces, the amount of prism can also be diminished to maintain alignment and keep fusional vergence drive active as an aid to further rehabilitation.

7.3.3 Nystagmus

Ocular stability, the maintenance of fixation and alignment on a target, is the result of multiple input paths in a carefully balanced feedback loop. Elements of the feedback loop include a visual stimulus and output from the occipital cortex, vestibular system input, and proprioceptive information arising from head and neck position A decrease or imbalance in any of these systems can lead to spontaneous ocular movements and the failure of the compensatory mechanisms. These spontaneous eye movements may be asymptomatic. However, they can be of sufficient amplitude to result in diminished acuity that people may interpret as blurring or a decrease in vision. Occasionally, people with certain types of nystagmus can complain of oscillopsia or the sensation of the world moving. Because nystagmus may be associated with ocular misalignment, people should be quizzed with regard to whether they do or do not have double vision. Likewise, vestibular dysfunction may be associated with nystagmus, so a problem with hearing or tinnitus and trouble with balance and vertigo may be associated. This subject is dealt with further in Chapter 6 in this volume.

Depending on the degree of movement associated with nystagmus, simple observation may be sufficient or additional magnification and illumination may be needed, either with direct ophthalmoscope or during ophthalmoscopy. It is possible to get very precise oculomotor recordings with an electro-oculogram or other device that will describe the movements and their characteristics with regard to waveforms and velocities. Clinicians should note the amplitude and frequency of the movements, the direction of the gaze that induces nystagmus, and all points where the nystagmus is least evident. The movements are commonly recorded with arrows to designate the fast phase of the eye movement, both in terms of direction and in terms of amplitude. The movement most commonly consists of a slow drift to the eye, followed by a corrective saccade, as in a jerk nystagmus. For instance, a right-jerk nystagmus would have a slow movement to the left with a fast movement to the right. Pendular nystagmus is relatively symmetric in that there is not an identifiable slow phase and it shows relatively equal amplitude in speed in separate directions. Nystagmus may be horizontal, vertical, or have a torsional or rotatory component.

In the early onset category, congenital nystagmus is usually recognized during the first few months of life. There is often a family history and the acuity may be good. People with congenital nystagmus are not bothered by the eye movements. In young children, it is important to detect any impairment of visual tracking or optic atrophy. The presence of either should encourage neuroimaging because congenital nystagmus most often occurs in isolation but may be seen in conditions such as albinism, achromatopsia, Leber's congenital amaurosis, and aniridia. The nystagmus is almost always conjugate and horizontal. It may be continuous or intermittent. It may appear as jerk or pendular in character. Null points are common and the person may adopt a head turn or posture in an attempt to improve vision. Visual fixation often amplifies the nystagmus, which is not the case with peripheral vestibular nystagmus. Two characteristic signs are reversal of the normal pattern of optic kinetic nystagmus in which the slow phase of the eye movement moves in the opposite direction of the rotation of the drum and in electronystagmography when a pattern is observed in which the velocity of slow phase movement increases exponentially with distance from fixation. Nystagmus is also associated with 15% of people having a strabismus. It is abolished by sleep, and in addition to being accentuated by fixation, it is diminished by convergence.

Latent nystagmus is another form that appears early in life and is a horizontal jerk nystagmus that is seen in conditions of monocular viewing. The fast phase tends to be toward the viewing eye, away from the occluded eye. The uncovered eye tends to drift toward midline. Its fast phase reverses each time the eye is alternately covered. To obtain the best acuity, one must blur the nontested eye with a plus lens or other filter and not simply occlude the eye, which will unleash the nystagmus and result in greater optical blurring. Latent nystagmus is very commonly associated with esotropia. Another variation is manifest latent nystagmus in which the characteristics of latent nystagmus are present even when both eyes are open. Both these forms of nystagmus are typically benign.

An important subset is a monocular nystagmus in childhood. This is typically vertical and relatively small in amplitude. The eye may have an afferent pupillary defect, optic atrophy, or decreased vision and is commonly associated with chiasmal glioma. A spasmus nutans may resemble a monocular nystagmus of childhood. It consists of a nystagmus in both eyes that is intermittent, horizontal, low amplitude, rapid, and often dysconjugate. There may be associated head nodding and/or an abnormal head posture. It can be monocular and, thus, would be confused with the more ominous monocular nystagmus of childhood and, therefore, also warrants neuroimaging. It typically is spontaneously resolved after several years.

In the category of acquired nystagmus, the first is gaze-evoked nystagmus, in which people have difficulty in maintaining eccentric gaze. The eye drifts back toward the center and a corrective saccade to reposition the eyes more peripherally is required. Thus, the fast phase is in the direction of the gaze. It is caused by an imbalance in the neural integrator located in the nucleus propositus hypoglossi adjacent to the medial vestibular nucleus in the pontomedullary junction that is responsible for matching neural activity to maintain eyes in the eccentric position. The nystagmus is often symmetric right to left. Advanced age is the most common cause, although metabolic and toxic etiologies are more common in younger adults, either from ethanol or anticonvulsant drugs. Whenever gaze-evoked nystagmus is asymmetric, it can be presumed that there is a lesion of the brainstem or the cerebellum. Perhaps stroke, demyelination, or tumor has asymmetrically affected the vestibular nuclei. Gaze-evoked nystagmus may occur in normal subjects at the extremes of gaze and this should be assessed by examining the stability of fixation at roughly 40 to 50 degrees from primary position.

Disassociated nystagmus may result from lesions of the MLF, causing nystagmus of only the abducting eye when the gaze is directed to the side opposite the lesion. The person is often diplopic because of the limited adduction of the ipsilateral eye. It may be associated with demyelinating disease in younger people or vascular insufficiency in more advanced age. Most acquired jerk nystagmus in primary position is the result of asymmetric vestibular input, which may be related to peripheral pathology affecting the vestibular end organ, semicircular canals, or the vestibular nerves or to the central pathology affecting the vestibulocerebral connection. Because tonic input regarding eye position is mostly vestibular, which feeds directly to the contralateral horizontal gaze center located in the sixth cranial nerve nucleus, asymmetric loss of input results in a conjugate ocular drift. The correcting fast phase is away from the affected side. Peripheral vestibular lesions are typically not discrete and affect all three semicircular canals in the otolith organs. This results frequently in mixed (horizontal, torsional, and vertical) nystagmus. The horizontal component often dominates. Visual fixation tends to dampen the peripheral nystagmus. This can be seen by observing the fundus with direct ophthalmoscope while the alternate eye is covered and uncovered to see the difference in amplitude that fixation on a distant target has on the nystagmus. A peripheral nystagmus is often accompanied by tinnitus, hearing loss, and vertigo or disequilibrium.

Central nystagmus, in which the fast component is directed toward the side of gaze, is relatively common, often secondary to medications, such as anticonvulsants, sleeping aids, sedatives, and antianxiety medications, or alcohol. Visual fixation has little effect on central vestibular nystagmus. Bruns nystagmus is a characteristic form of vestibular nystagmus associated with cerebellar pontine angle tumors. Initially, the vestibular nerve is affected; the eyes drift toward the side of the lesion with corrective phase in the opposite direction. As the lesion enlarges, the ipsilateral brainstem is compressed, causing problems in maintaining ipsilateral eccentric gaze. As the person looks to the side of the lesion, the fast phase changes direction to ipsilateral, beating more slowly and with a coarser amplitude.

Some forms of nystagmus and nonnystagmus saccadic oscillations are highly correlated with lesions and are useful for localization within the central nervous system. Downbeat nystagmus results from defective vertical gaze holding; the eyes tend to drift up and a corrective downward saccade is generated. The presumed mechanism is asymmetric loss of the tonic input from the anterior semicircular canals, resulting in an upward drift of the eyes. Downward nystagmus is almost always present in primary position. People may report difficulty in reading and may report oscillopsia. Structural lesions are present in approximately 50% of people. An Arnold-Chiari malformation, in which the cerebellar tonsils herniate through the foramen magnum and compress the cervical medullary junction, is the most common structural etiology. Differential diagnosis includes angioma, cerebellar hemangiomas in the foramen magnum, and demyelination disease. Stroke, cranial trauma, drugs (alcohol, lithium, antiseizure medications), syrinx of the brainstem or upper cervical spinal cord, brainstem encephalitis, or nutrition are some of the etiologies to be considered.

Upbeat nystagmus may be present in primary position or only in upgaze. It is commonly associated with lesions of the anterior cerebellar vermis. Common causes include demyelination, stroke, cerebellar degeneration, and tobacco smoking.

Seesaw nystagmus is a variety of vertical nystagmus that is dysconjugate—as one eye moves up, the other eye moves down. The upward-moving eye also intorts while the downward-moving eye extorts. This occurs with lesions around the diencephalon. Craniopharyngioma is the most common cause. Other parasellar tumors and trauma may produce seesaw nystagmus. There is an associated afferent system pathology, including bitemporal visual field defects.

Periodic alternating nystagmus may be congenital or acquired and is characterized by an oscillation of cycles of horizontal movements of approximately 4 minutes. The nystagmus beats in one direction for 2 minutes, slows, then reverses to the other side for the next 2 minutes. It is most common in posterior fossa disease, especially of the cerebellum. Common causes include multiple sclerosis, cerebellar degeneration, and Arnold-Chiari malformation. Etiology is thought to be in the vestibulocerebellum and is manifest as a shifting in the null point.

Pendular nystagmus of both a vertical and horizontal component may be oblique (if the components are in phase) or circular or elliptical (if they are out of phase). It is not localizing and is usually acquired in association with multiple sclerosis.

Microsaccadic refixation movements are an abnormal eye movement resulting from inappropriate saccade. Most common is square-wave oscillations, which indicate a small movement away from, and then back to, fixation. The smaller movements are a normal effect of aging. Larger amplitude oscillations may occur in people with progressive supranuclear palsy, cerebellar disease, or multiple sclerosis.

Ocular flutter is a horizontal small-amplitude, high-frequency movement. Opsoclonus or high-frequency multiple direction movements (or saccadomania) are associated with a burst of saccades released from the pons without the normal latency between consecutive saccades. Neoplastic etiology must be excluded in these people. In children, neuroblastoma is a primary consideration. In adults, small cell carcinoma of the lung and cancer of the breast or ovaries must be ruled out. These eye movements may be an early sign of cancer.

Convergence retraction nystagmus commonly occurs as part of a dorsal midline Parinaud syndrome (which includes absent upgaze, light-near dissociation, and Collier's lid retraction). Anomalous eye movements result from a cocontraction of the horizontal extraocular muscles on attempted upgaze. It is best elicited by having the person follow a downward-rotating optokinetic nystagmus drum.

Ocular bobbing is a rare sign in which rapid downward movement of both eyes is followed by a slow return of the eye position to midline. The person is usually comatose or has severely compromised mental status, usually from bilateral pontine infarction or hemorrhage. These lesions ablate the paramedian pontine reticular formation on both sides, thus horizontal movements are lost. Severe metabolic disturbances may, in the absence of structural lesions, cause ocular bobbing with possible later recovery.

The last form of nystagmus to consider is *voluntary* nystagmus. It is typically horizontal in direction, appears as a relatively high-frequency convergent saccades, and can rarely be maintained for longer than 20 seconds. Although it can be induced volitionally in many normal subjects, occasionally, it may not be consciously generated and can distress people because of oscillopsia.

7.4 Learning and Therapy

One model for learning and memory includes repetition. Repetitive use of a synaptic connection causes a broadening and flattening of the end plates with a decrease in resistance across the synaptic gap and a preference for using that synapse over adjacent pathways that have not been so facilitated.[19] Learning has been shown to affect dendritic spine formation.[20] These concepts are anatomically supportive of many standard teaching methods from repetition of spelling lists and multiplication tables to rehearsing a speech to learn a pattern of words.

Repetition may also serve as a foundation for retraining a person with TBI in whom preferred pathways may have been damaged, resulting in an initial inability to perform an old, remembered task. The inherent complexity of the central nervous system may be advantageous in that there seems to be alternate pathways available for bypass of damaged areas and establishment of new circuits or series of synapses that will allow one to perform old tasks in perhaps new ways. Therapy can be thought of as a means of helping to identify some of these previously unused or little used pathways and, through repetition and building upon prior skills, developing new ways of performing old tasks.

7.4.1 Case History 1

A 32-year-old man sustained postconcussion syndrome after being struck in the head by a falling pallet. Initially, he presented with complaints of diplopia and blurry vision. On evaluation, he was noted to have eight prism diopters of exophoria at near and distance, with some difficulty on upgaze. Cogwheeling of saccades was present. It was noted on screening and confrontation fields testing that temporal constriction in the right eye was present. Recommendation was made for saccadic exercises, such as the vertical swinging ball, and convergence exercises. At the next visit, exophoria was decreased to six prism diopters and saccades had improved with therapy.

Two months later, exophoria remained about the same and saccades had ceased cogwheeling on left-to-right gaze and had greatly improved on right to left gaze. The individual continues with vision therapy and has graduated to exercises that are more difficult for him, such as the color bead sorting tray.[21]

7.4.2 Case History 2

A 42-year-old man sustained blunt head trauma from metal pipe. Initially, he presented with complaint of decreased vision. On examination, acuity was correctable to 20/25– in the right eye, 20/20 in the left eye. No strabismus was noted. Saccades were slowed, with difficulty moving eyes left to right, and slight exophoria on upgaze. Pursuit was jerky. Worth four-dot testing revealed partial suppression with left eye. Visual fields, on confrontation, were constricted bilaterally. Recommendations were for pursuit and saccadic exercises, and the individual was started on swinging ball exercise.

Two months later, saccades were greatly improved, with almost no cogwheeling. Approximately 6 months after the initial examination, the individual was started on Ritalin for impaired speed of processing. Immediately, he began to complain of more difficulty with tracking, and decreased vision. On examination, smooth pursuit had become very jerky, as were saccades. Best corrected acuity had decreased to 20/30– in the right eye and 20/40– in the left eye. He discontinued Ritalin 3 months later and was evaluated after 2 weeks, noting vision still decreased. Smooth pursuits and saccades were still jerky. Acuity had increased to 20/20– in each eye, with difficulty. Final evaluation was done 4 months later. Acuity was 20/20 in each eye, best corrected. Smooth pursuits were improved, but still jerky, and suppression was noted in the left eye via Worth four-dot testing.

7.4.3 Case History 3

A 31-year-old man sustained a closed head injury with intracerebral hemorrhaging after a motorcycle versus car accident. Initially, he presented with 20/20 vision, best corrected, bilaterally. Six prism diopters of exophoria with 10 prism diopters of left hyperphoria was noted on primary gaze. There was vertical nystagmus on abduction and large lag on abduction. Smooth pursuits were jerky. Recommendations were for saccadic and smooth pursuit exercises, such as the Marsden ball, color bead sorting tray, and accommodative flexibility exercises. Four diopters of prism were applied to his glasses via press-on prism.

Six months later, with prism, exophoria was decreased to two prism diopters. Vertical nystagmus had improved, as had saccades. He started the bead sorting tray exercises on a vertical orientation and vertical door jamb reading.[21]

7.4.4 Case History 4

A 31-year-old Hispanic man sustained right cavernous fistula after motor vehicle versus pedestrian injury. His chief complaint was that he was unable to move his eyes laterally to the right. On examination, visual acuity was 20/70-2 right and 20/60-1 left, without correction. Extraocular motility was with restriction to midline with limitation of abduction of the right eye. There was injection and dilation of the vessels, especially temporally on the right eye, similar to venous congestion. Auscultation revealed a bruit that seemed louder on the right side.

The man was sent for MRI of the brain, which was not able to be completed as a result of movement even after 2 mg Versed. A "very high-flow" clotted cavernous fistula was confirmed upon second MRI, and cerebral/carotid angiogram was performed under general anesthesia. Surgical intervention, by placement of three balloons in the right carotid fistula to close it, was performed. The man showed a 25- to 30-prism diopter right esotropia that did not resolve after the cavernous fistula surgery. He was still only able to just achieve midline with maximum effort, but had no abduction. Recommendation was for a muscle transposition procedure to obtain alignment in primary gaze. This would require several surgeries to achieve the best result and, even so, would not allow for full range of motion.

Most therapy consists of taking a task, breaking it down into smaller steps, teaching, learning, and repeating each one of the steps, and linking them into larger and larger groups until, finally, a more complex behavior can be performed. Because the goal of therapy is to minimize disabilities and maximize abilities, this retraining process is the key at the heart of the things that we do.

First, the systems or subsystems that have been adversely affected, what things a person is unable to do, and what things the person can do to a limited extent must be determined. Next, a means of working from what the person can do in an additive fashion to allow him or her to regain as much skill as possible must be devised. For example, in treating diplopia, the first temptation might be simply to patch the more severely affected eye to relieve the symptom of diplopia. Although this does relieve the immediate symptom, it does very little toward rehabilitation or establishing these alternate pathways that were discussed earlier. Therefore, the act of putting a patch on the eye temporarily blocks the symptom but does not approach a solution to the problem, which is mistracking of the eyes.

A preferred plan would be to determine whether there is any position of gaze in which the individual does not see double. Treatment would incorporate prisms in glasses to move the images into alignment to allow the person to continue to use both eyes at the same time. The goal would be to enlarge the area of single vision through a series of training exercises. These exercises encourage the movement of the eyes and stimulate the utilization of existing or new pathways to allow smooth tracking of an object or to acquire its fixation and maintain it in good alignment. Treatment may start by using a large amount of prism in the glasses, perhaps a plastic press-on prism so that it can be easily changed as the individual improves with time with therapy, to keep encouraging the person to move ahead. The areas of first concern should be primary gaze (straight-ahead gaze) and slight downgaze in a reading position. These may require two different sets of glasses with two different amounts of prisms.

Programs of visual therapy require coordination of efforts between the physician and the therapist. The physician conducts serial repetitive measurements to determine baseline alignment and to provide comparison with previous measurements to monitor progression. The therapist makes suggestions in consultation with the physician regarding what therapies might best improve the individual's condition, keeping in mind tolerance, strengths, and any other concomitant difficulties. As long as progress is being made, it should be encouraged and allowed to proceed.

It may take many months for damaged neural tracts to repair themselves or for compensation to occur within the neurologic system. Nerve repair proceeds at a slow pace. At some point, the ophthalmologic measurements may plateau and the individual may show no further progress. Depending upon the nature of the deficit at that time, one may consider surgical intervention to realign the eyes in a more central and aligned position. Visual therapy may play a role in stimulating binocular vision, either preoperatively in preparation for surgery or postoperatively in an attempt to stabilize the alignment that has been achieved by mechanical movement of the muscles. Once again, small bits of prism may be utilized to complete the alignment process and then be gradually weaned away as fusional amplitudes increase over time.

A number of people have shown rather dramatic improvement in areas that traditional medicine will tell us should not have improved. Some, who initially could not tolerate things moving near their heads because it gave them a feeling of extreme discomfort, developed a tolerance for having a ball swinging in a circle around their head as they tracked it back and forth. Others needed a program geared specifically to their areas of difficulty, such as working from near to far as they changed their fixation. With time and repeated efforts, they developed an increased facility in this regard. Still other people who had specific difficulties in their saccadic tracking systems were able, with simple repetitive exercises such as door jamb reading, to demonstrate increased facility. This was reported both subjectively, in that they felt they could do the exercises more quickly, more easily, and with less fatigue, and also objectively, in that their examination scores showed improvement over time. It is important to understand that (1) the therapist must realize that the person can get better and (2) the person must be willing to undergo a fairly rigorous and sometimes uncomfortable therapeutic process to develop the synaptic relays necessary for improved function.

7.5 Summary

Detailed understanding of the visual system is necessary for accurate diagnosis of visual disorders following TBI. It should be understood that surgical and therapeutic interventions exist to ameliorate some visual system dysfunction. Rehabilitation of treatable visual system deficits should be undertaken as a regular component of comprehensive rehabilitation following TBI.

References

1. Bontke, C. F., Lehmkuhl, L. D., Englander, J., et al., Medical complications and associated injuries of persons treated in the traumatic brain injury model systems programs, *Journal of Head Trauma Rehabilitation*, 8(2), 34–46, 1993.
2. Willis, W. D. and Grossman, R. G., *Medical Neurobiology: Neuroanatomical and Neurophysiological Principles Basic to Clinical Neuroscience*, 2nd ed., C.V. Mosby, St. Louis, MO, 1977.
3. Cook, C. S., Ozanics, V., and Jakobiec, F. A., Prenatal development of the eye and its adnexa, in *Duane's Foundations of Clinical Ophthalmology*, vol. 1, rev., Tasman, W. and Jaeger, E. A., Eds., J. B. Lippincott, Philadelphia, 1992.
4. Wirtschafter, J. D., Ophthalmic neuroanatomy: The visual pathway, in *Ophthalmic Anatomy: A Manual with Some Clinical Applications*, Jones, L. T., Reeh, M. J., and Wirtschafter, J. D., Eds., American Academy of Ophthalmology and Otolaryngology, Rochester, MN, 1970, 161.
5. Werblin, F. S. and Dowling, J. E., Organization of the retina of the mudpuppy. Necturus maculosus: II. Intracellular recording, *Journal of Neurophysiology*, 32(3), 339, 1969.
6. Neger, R. E., The evaluation of diplopia in head trauma, *Journal of Head Trauma Rehabilitation*, 4(2), 27, 1989.
7. Jones, L. T., Reeh, M. J., and Wirtschafter, J. D., *Ophthalmic Anatomy: A Manual with Some Clinical Applications*, American Academy of Ophthalmology, Rochester, MN, 1970.
8. Glaser, J. S., Anatomy of the visual sensory system, in *Duane's Clinical Ophthalmology*, vol. 2, rev., Tasman, W. and Jaeger, E. A., Eds., J. B. Lippincott, Philadelphia, 1992.
9. Sadun, A. A. and Glaser, J. S., Anatomy of the visual sensory system, in *Duane's Foundations of Clinical Ophthalmology*, vol. 1, rev., Tasman, W. and Jaeger, E. A., Eds., J. B. Lippincott, Philadelphia, 1992.
10. Eggers, H. M., Functional anatomy of the extraocular muscles, in *Duane's Foundations of Clinical Ophthalmology*, vol. 1, rev., Tasman, W. and Jaeger, E. A., Eds., J. B. Lippincott, Philadelphia, 1992.
11. Pedersen, R. A., Abel, L. A., and Troost, B. T., Eye movements, in *Duane's Foundations of Clinical Ophthalmology*, vol. 1, rev., Tasman, W. and Jaeger, E. A., Eds., J. B. Lippincott, Philadelphia, 1992.
12. Goldberg, M. E., The control of gaze, in *Principles of Neural Science*, 4th ed., Kandel, E. R., Schwartz, J. H., and Jessell, T. M., Eds., McGraw-Hill, New York, 2000, 782–800.
13. Levitan, P., Pupillary escape in disease of the retina or optic nerve, *Archives of Ophthalmology*, 62(5), 768, 1959.
14. Glaser, J. S. and Goodwin, J. A., Neuro-ophthalmologic examination: The visual sensory system, in *Duane's Clinical Ophthalmology*, vol. 2, rev., Tasman, W. and Jaeger, E. A., Eds., J. B. Lippincott, Philadelphia, 1992, 1–26.
15. Beck, R. W., Bergstrom, T. J., and Lichter, P. R., The clinical comparison of visual field testing with a new automated perimeter: The Humphrey field analyzer and the Goldmann perimeter, *Ophthalmology*, 92(1), 77, 1985.
16. Glaser, J. S., Neuro-ophthalmologic examination: General considerations and special techniques, in *Duane's Clinical Ophthalmology*, vol. 2, rev., Tasman, W. and Jaeger, E. A., Eds., J. B. Lippincott, Philadelphia, 1992, 1–16.
17. Smith, C. H. and Beck, R. W., Facial nerve, in *Duane's Foundations of Clinical Ophthalmology*, vol. 1, rev., Tasman, W. and Jaeger, E. A., Eds., J. B. Lippincott, Philadelphia, 1992.
18. Beck, R. W. and Smith, C. H., Trigeminal nerve, in *Duane's Foundations of Clinical Ophthalmology*, vol. 1, rev., Tasman, W. and Jaeger, E. A., Eds., J. B. Lippincott, Philadelphia, 1992, 1–16.
19. Schubert, D., The possible role of adhesion in synaptic modification, *Trends in Neurosciences*, 14(4), 127, 1991.
20. Black, J. E. and Greenough, W. T., Developmental approaches to the memory process, in *Learning and Memory: A Biological View*, 2nd ed., Martinez, J. L., Jr. and Kesner, R. P., Eds., Academic Press, San Diego, 1991, 61–91.
21. Richman, J. E. and Cron, M. T., *Guide to Vision Therapy*, Bernell Corporation, South Bend, IN, 1988.

8

Disruptions in Physical Substrates of Vision Following Traumatic Brain Injury

Richard E. Helvie

CONTENTS

8.1 Introduction

The topic of visual dysfunction following traumatic brain injury (TBI) is an enormous subject to cover in one chapter. TBI and the visual system are both complex, and before embarking on this challenge, it is important to have a basic understanding of each subject to appreciate fully their interrelationship and subsequent visual sequelae.

8.1.1 Traumatic Brain Injury

TBI has had limited funding and has been called a "silent epidemic" in the United States. However, with the advent of the Iraq War and the increased media coverage of sports concussion, the public is becoming better informed about the medical consequences of TBI and the long-term side effects on neurologic functioning. Severe and, sometimes, mild TBI can develop into catastrophic neurologic management problems. Surprisingly, because of the difference in biomechanics, women are more prone to concussion than men because, in general, of their smaller heads and thinner necks, the latter of which prevents the shearing forces impacting the brain.

The Center for Disease Control and Prevention estimates the incidents of TBI, including concussion (mild TBI), to be between 1.6 and 3.8 million cases per year, and many are unreported. One million people are seen in the emergency room or hospitalized per year for TBI. A total of 5.3 million children and adults are living with residual disability from TBI.[1]

TBI can result from closed head injury, penetrating head injury, or a combination of both. Penetrating head injuries can involve any part of the brain; closed head injury is always diffuse. The current classification of TBI is divided into *mild, moderate,* and *severe* categories. This classification, however, is thought to be inadequate. Mechanisms of acute brain injury are caused by acceleration, rotational, and blunt trauma forces. The pathophysiology of these injuries is related to focal, multifocal, diffuse axonal injury (DAI), and hypoxic damage. This involves both the gray matter and the white matter. The gray matter (neurons) has its electrical discharge disrupted, revving up its metabolism, in addition to the other cells with which it is interconnected by white matter tracks. An initial secondary chemical cascade results in which there is a heightened physiologic demand with increased glucose metabolism that cannot be met because of inadequate energy production, the latter compounded by loss of autoregulation with resultant decreased blood flow. This results in both cell damage and death. The hallmark pathophysiologic abnormality of TBI is DAI, or involvement of the white matter, the connect between gray matter structures, because of shearing forces. Midline brain structures are most vulnerable to DAI, including the subcortical white matter, corpus callosum, and rostral brainstem—all critical linkages for the operational visual system.

Because of the global, as well as focal, nature of brain injury, the function of primary sensory brain areas and their association areas is adversely affected. One such function is vision—a primary sensory modality. Individuals who sustain TBI often present with other vital injuries in addition to the brain, which can involve the face, back, torso, extremities, or internal organs. Frequently, these injuries are readily addressed and treated early because they are easily evidenced when the patient presents to the emergency room. Less obvious injuries, including those to the vestibular and visual systems, can be overlooked during lifesaving endeavors and early during recovery from TBI. Frequently, these deficits are not appreciated until later in the hospital course or until after the patient has been discharged home. These visual problems are important to diagnosis because it is now well accepted that improvement can be maximized with remedial rehabilitation and not just compensatory treatment (glasses).[2]

8.1.2 Vision

Vision is the process of discovery from images that allows us to interact and navigate the environment. Unlike a camera, our visual system has the ability to create a three-dimensional image and compensate for the changing spectral components of a light source. Vision is a complicated function in which various frequencies of light are absorbed and processed by the photoreceptors in the retina. These light rays are derived from the physical properties of objects and surfaces. This information is processed by serial and parallel systems to produce representations in space. Objects can be recognized by various physical attributes such as construction, shape, color, size, weight, texture, and detail, in addition to their movement and location in space. This includes both stationary and moving objects, writing, written language, including mathematics and music, and faces. Visual perception is creative, transferring two-dimensional patterns of light on the retina into a coherent and stable interpretation of a three-dimensional, visual world. This information is integrated with other sensory modalities, such as touch and sound, combined with information about past events, and modulated by attention. This complex visual process is best appreciated by understanding its anatomic and functional organization. The goal of the remaining portion of this chapter is to present a systematic approach to this complex process that can serve as a guide to understanding vision, thereby allowing proper diagnosis and appropriate treatment for visual deficits following TBI to maximize visual recovery.

8.2 Basic Terminology

Prior to discussing the visual system, it is important to understand basic terminology. *Visual reception* refers to the reception of the primary visual signal or input into the system. This begins in the retina and is carried out by an afferent system to the primary visual cortex. *Visual attention* is a filtering system in which certain stimuli are earmarked at the expense of others. This is executed by excitatory inhibitory mechanisms. It is necessary, because the brain does not have the computational capacity to attend to the vast stimuli in the environment that are simultaneously presented to it. This process also includes the ability to maintain focus that will allow a coherent stream of thought. A *sensation* refers to the reception, filtering, and early analysis of internal/external stimuli resulting in a conscious experience. *Visual perception* requires not only reception and filtering, but higher order analysis of physical attributes in which discrimination and pattern recognition functions are engaged to categorize visual information. This information is then compared with percepts in other sensory modalities and with experiential memories and goals. *Perceptions* are the primary awareness of the world in that it processes and represents all sensory inputs in space, giving meaning to them. This involves the entire continuum of behavior.

8.3 General Brain Anatomy

There are four major anatomic components of the brain—the *cerebral hemispheres*, the *diencephalon*, the *brainstem*, and the *cerebellum*. The cerebral hemispheres are divided into four lobes—*occipital*, *parietal*, *temporal*, and *frontal*—all of which are involved in vision. The occipital lobes are involved with visual reception and early processing; the parietal lobes with processing of motion and location; the temporal lobes with object recognition, memory, and emotional valence; and finally, the frontal lobes with complex higher visual cognition and action plans. The frontal lobes are not considered a single functional entity. The frontal lobes have three major subdivisions—the *premotor area*, the *motor area*, and the *prefrontal areas*. The motor and premotor areas serve as units, whereas the prefrontal cortex is much more complicated, requiring further divisions. The frontal lobes form a sophisticated, integrative system, resulting in processing vision as well as primary sensory modalities, resulting in higher visual cognition and action plans. The brain is composed of both gray matter and white matter. *Gray matter* consists of a vast number of interconnected neurons that fill the cerebral cortex and subcortical nuclei. Pertinent subcortical structures involved in vision function include the *hippocampus, amygdala, pulvinar, lateral geniculate body, superior colliculus,* and *ascending reticular activating system,* the latter a diffuse body of brainstem nuclei. The white matter provides the fibers that connect the neurons of the gray matter. These fibers contain bundles of axons covered with myelin. When diffuse axonal injury occurs, it predominantly impacts white matter structures.

Gray matter and white matter differ significantly in their pattern of development. The entire compliment of brain neurons are formed before birth, beginning development early during gestation.[3] Gray matter remains relatively constant in volume throughout adult life. *White matter* refers to groups of myelinated axons that link gray matter structures. These connections are classified as *cortical–cortical, cortical–subcortical,* and *subcortical–cortical.* There are various terms to describe them, including *fasciculus, tract, funiculus, lemniscus, peduncle,* and *bundle.* White matter does not begin to form until the middle trimester of gestation and is only partially complete at birth—even at 2 years of age, it is only 90% complete.[4] As opposed to gray matter, white matter volume fluctuates at different times throughout life. The remainder of myelination requires many years to complete, with some studies showing it can continue up to the sixth decade.[5] The myelination process proceeds from caudal to rostral structures or from phylogenetically older to newer parts of the brain. Figure 8.1 shows the sequence of myelination in the human brain that, in many ways, reflects the

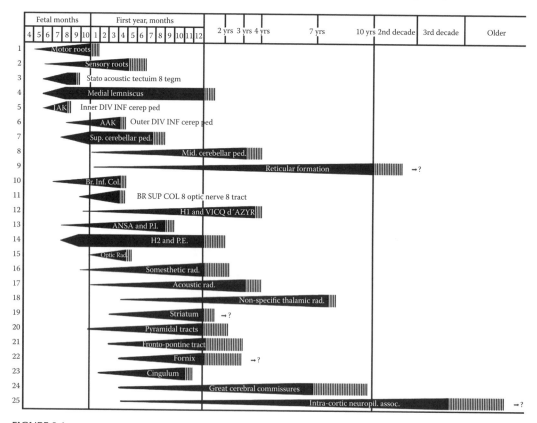

FIGURE 8.1

The sequence of myelination in the human brain. (From Filley, C. M., *The Behavioral Neurology of White Matter,* Oxford University Press, New York, p. 34, 2001. With permission.)

functional maturity of vision and other systems. The atrophy noted on magnetic resonance images in patients following TBI represents mainly the loss of white matter.

The neocortex is a six-layer ribbon covering the cerebral hemispheres. Each cortical area has columns of cells that have a similar structure and function that distinguishes itself from other brain regions. The neocortex is gray matter, although it contains a high percentage of white matter (cortical–cortical connections). More than 100 billion neurons reside in the neocortex, and 70% of those in the central nervous system, of which 75% are in the cortical association areas.[6] Seventy percent of the sensory input to the brain involves vision. It is not surprising, in the rhesus monkey, which provides an excellent model of the human visual system, that more than 50% of the neocortex is involved in visual function.[7] Researchers have identified more than 300 intracortical pathways linking more than 30 different cortical areas involved in visual function, seven of which are considered visual association areas.[8] There is vast networking between the neocortex and subcortical structures, several of which are essential for vision. Important subcortical structures include the hippocampus for memory, the amygdala for emotion, the pulvinar for visual attention, the lateral geniculate body for reception, and the brainstem structures, including the superior colliculus, reticular activating system, gaze centers, and ocular motor cranial nerve nuclei, the functions of which are discussed later in this chapter.

8.4 Anatomic Divisions of the Visual System

The visual system can be divided anatomically into three divisions—the *optical*, the *primary*, and the *secondary visual systems*—and are briefly discussed in the following sections.

8.4.1 Optical System

The purpose of the optical system is to present a clear and undistorted image on the retina. Three primary conditions must be in place for this to occur. The first is a refractory system provided by the cornea and crystalline lens, which converges parallel light rays from distant objects to a specific focus point on the retina. The second involves accommodation that diverges light rays from near objects to the same point focus on the retina. The third component is a transparent ocular media, the nonrefractory space occupied by the aqueous and the vitreous, to project a clear focus on the retina.

8.4.2 Primary Visual System

The primary visual system is involved in the reception of the visual information. This system originates in the retina and involves the optic nerve, optic chiasm, optic tract, and various subcortical structures, eventually terminating in the primary visual cortex. As noted, visual function begins in the retina. Unlike other sensory peripheral end organs, the retina is an extension of the central nervous system. Light enters the eye and is focused both by the cornea and the lens, then passes to the photoreceptors of the retina. There is an area in the retina called the *fovea*, where the cell bodies of the more proximal layers are shifted to the sides, enabling the visual image to be received in its least distorted form. The center of the fovea is called the *foveola*, where the most accurate visual reception occurs. The anatomy of the photoreceptor layer consists of *cones* and *rods*. Cones are closely packed in the center of the fovea, reaching 200,000 cones/mm². This drops off exponentially from the center of the fovea. The cones are responsible for day vision, high visual acuity, and color. There are no rods in the fovea because they are distributed bilaterally in the periphery. They are responsible for night vision and low visual acuity and are achromatic. Thus, for the highest resolution of the visual image to occur, it is mandatory that the fovea be targeted on the visual stimuli.

The retina has three major functional classes of neurons. The *photoreceptors* lie in the outer nuclear layer; *interneurons*, which are the bipolar, horizontal, and amacrine cells, lie in the inner nuclear layer; and *ganglion cells* lie in the ganglion cell layer (Figure 8.2). Photoreceptors, bipolar cells, and horizontal cells make synaptic connections with each other in the outer plexiform layer. The bipolar, amacrine, and ganglion cells make contact in the inner plexiform layer. Information flows vertically from photoreceptor to bipolar cells to ganglion cells, as well as laterally from horizontal cells in the outer plexiform layer and amacrine cells in the inner layer (Figure 8.2). The receptive fields of ganglion cells correspond to patches of receptors laying immediately beneath them. Therefore, a lesion deep within the retina causes a visual field defect with a shape that corresponds exactly to the shape of the lesion. The absorption of light by visual pigments in the photoreceptors triggers a cascade of chemical events that results in the production of electrical energy. The process is called *phototransduction*. This visual information is transmitted in the form of electrical signals by the photoreceptors to the ganglion cells. Modification of the signals occurs as a result of the interneuron cells altering the electrical signals by incorporating different temporal and spatial patterns of light stimulation in the retina.

More than 22 types of ganglion cells exist in the primate,[9] but only three types appear to be involved in visual perception in that they connect to the lateral geniculate body.[10] These

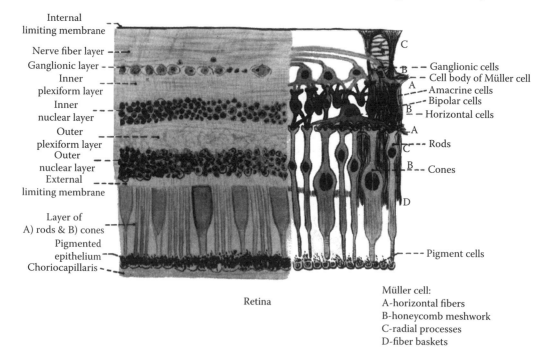

FIGURE 8.2
Layers of the retina. (From W. Jacobson, Jr. (Ed.), *The Eye* (chart). Anatomical Chart Co. Wolters Kluwer Health, Lippincott Williams & Wilkins, 2009. With permission.)

three subsets are termed the *magno-*, *parvo-*, and *koniocellular* types, the former two being most important in human vision. The parvo cells have small receptive fields, respond to high spatial and slow temporal frequency, and are involved in detail. The magno cells have large receptive fields, respond to low spatial and fast temporal frequency, and are involved in low-contrast and large-contour analysis. Of these two subsets of ganglion cells, 80% are parvo cells, whereas the remaining 20% are magno cells. The magno and parvo cells monitor peripheral and central vision, respectively, because of their location in the retina.

Ganglion cells have a concentric visual receptive field with a center surround organization with antagonistic excitatory and inhibitory regions. These cells fall into two classes based on their different response to a small spot of light presented at its center, creating on-center and off-center cells. A functional segregation of ganglion cells occurs in relationship to the size of the receptive fields and light responsiveness to a small spot of light, the latter of which evaluates changes in contrast. The axons of these ganglion cells converge toward the optic disk where they emerge from the eye as the optic nerve. In the superficial retina, between the ganglion cells and the optic nerve, the topography turns horizontal, according to the geography of the axons of the retinal cells. Therefore, a lesion involving this area causes a visual field defect with a configuration that is based on the configuration of the axonal bundles as they sweep across the retinal surface. As the nerve fibers pass through the sclera, a sheathlike structure called the *lamina cribosa* is formed. Because there are no end organs of sight at the optic disk, a blind spot is produced in the field of vision.

Each optic nerve contains retinotopic maps representing both the heminasal and hemitemporal visual space of its companion eye. The optic nerve passes posteriorly through the orbit and enters the cranial cavity through the optic foramen and joins its fellow of the opposite side to form the optic chiasm. At the optic chiasm, a partial decussation of fibers from the two sides takes place. Fibers from each eye destined for either side of the brain are sorted out and rebundled, forming the optic tracts that carry visual information from the contralateral visual fields of each eye.

Each optic tract, in turn, partially encircles the cerebral peduncle and passes to three significant subcortical structures: the *pretectum*, the *superior colliculus*, and the *lateral geniculate body* (Figure 8.3). The majority of the axons of each optic tract proceeds to the lateral geniculate body located in the thalamus. Within the optic tract, these fibers have not yet approximated each other; thus, a lesion in this area will cause an incongruous visual field defect. Ninety percent of the retinal axons terminate in this structure. Conversely, only 10% of the axons that terminate in this nucleus are received from the retina, whereas 90% is received from other areas, predominantly the cerebral cortex. This suggests that the retinogeniculate connection is the driver and the corticogeniculate link is the modulator. Without the retinogeniculate pathway, perception is lost, except under limited conditions referred to as *blindsight* or *unconscious vision*.

As the optic tract enters the lateral geniculate body, there is a continuation of the retinotopic representation of the contralateral visual field. In humans, the lateral geniculate nucleus contains six layers of cell bodies separated by intralaminar layers of white matter or axons. The layers are numbered from one to six, ventral to dorsal. The two most ventral layers of the nucleus are known as the *magnocellular layers* because their main retinal input is from the M-ganglion cells. The four most dorsal layers are known as *parvocellular layers* and receive input from the P-ganglion cells. Both the magno cell and parvo cell layers include the same concentric fields with on- and off-center cells that were present in the ganglion cells in the retina. Furthermore, axonal fibers in the ipsilateral and contralateral eyes are segregated in the layers of the lateral geniculate body. Layers 1, 4, and 6 of the terminal of axons from the contralateral eye, whereas layers 2, 3, and 5 contain

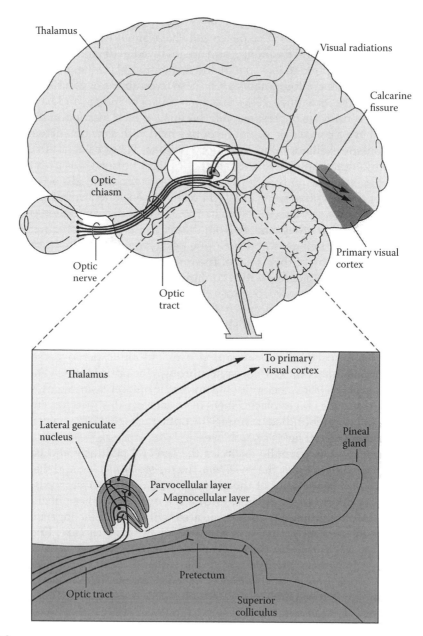

FIGURE 8.3
Route of optic tract to lateral geniculate body, pretectum, and superior colliculus. (From E. R. Kandel, J. H. Schwartz, and T. M. Jessell (Eds.), *Principles of Neural Science*, 4th ed., McGraw-Hill, p. 527, 2000. With permission.)

axons from the ipsilateral eye. Although each layer does contain retinotopic maps, the retinal space is not represented isometrically as the foveal region, which occupies less than 10% of the retinal surface but projects to 50% of the surface area of the lateral geniculate body.

The axons in the magnocellular and parvocellular cells exit the lateral geniculate nucleus grouped separately to form the origin of the M and P pathways. Collectively, this white matter tract is called the *optic radiation*. After exiting the lateral geniculate nucleus, the optic radiation sweeps around the lateral ventricle to terminate in the primary visual cortex, continuing to transmit visual information from the contralateral visual field. The fibers representing the inferior half of the retina are located more ventral than those representing the superior portion of the retina. Those axons representing the inferior retinal input end beneath the calcarine fissure, whereas those representing superior retinal input terminate above the calcarine fissure. A small portion of fibers of the optic tract diverges to the midbrain, whereas the majority connect with the lateral geniculate body.

The divergent fibers from the optic tract project to two areas: the pretectum and the superior colliculus (Figure 8.3). The pretectal group projects to the pretectal nucleus, with cells that project both to the ipsilateral accessory oculomotor nucleus and to the contralateral accessory oculomotor nucleus via the posterior commissar.

Preganglionic neurons in both accessory ocular motor nuclei send axons out of the brainstem in the ocular motor nerve to innervate with the ciliary ganglion. This ganglion contains the postganglionic neurons and innervates the smooth muscles of the papillary sphincter that constricts the pupil. Pupillary reflexes are clinically important because they indicate the functional state of both the afferent and efferent pathways.

The remaining portion of the divergent fibers from the optic tract terminates in the superior colliculus. This is also a nuclear structure of alternating gray and white matter layers. These retinotectal fibers project into its superficial layers conveying, again, a map of the contralateral space. The superficial layers also receive visual input from the visual cortex, whereas cortical input from other sensory modalities projects to deeper layers. Under the control of these cortical connections, multisensory and spatial integration occurs. Thus, cortical control is necessary to process more than one modality at any specific time.[11] The superior colliculus, under the control of the frontal eye field, generates and controls eye and head movements. The superficial layers are the origin of the connection linking the pulvinar, which in turn projects to the cerebral parietal cortex, which is the neural network responsible for the orientation of visual attention.

In addition to the traditional primary visual system, an accessory optic system exists in humans. The accessory optic system is defined as all optic fibers from the contralateral retina that do not terminate in the lateral geniculate body, pretectal nucleus, or superior colliculus. This system involves the processing of retinal, nonvisual (image) information. The retinohypothalamic tract in humans is, clinically, an important structure in this system.[12] This tract transmits photic information from the retina to the suprachiasmic nucleus in the hypothalamus, where circadian rhythms are generated. Most retinal ganglion cells that project to the suprachiasmic nucleus express the photopigment melanopsin.[13] This tract leaves the retina via the optic nerve and exists in the optic chiasm en route to the suprachiasmic nucleus. The clinical significance of other tracts in the accessory optic system in humans has not been precisely delineated.

8.4.3 Secondary Visual System

The secondary visual system is more complex, requiring knowledge of its anatomic and functional organization to understand its operation. It is important to conceptualize the brain as a modular unit to appreciate the anatomy and function of the secondary visual system. The organizational blueprint of the brain begins with the *neocortex*, a six-layered mantle covering the cerebral hemispheres. Different areas of the cortex are distinguished from each other based on variations in their cellular layers.

Each cortical area has columns of cells that are similar in structure and function called *modules*. The primary visual cortex in the occipital lobe is an example of such a module because of its modular structure, with arrangements of columns of cells with a specific function of vision. There are several other primary sensory areas in the brain besides the primary visual cortex. These areas include the *primary auditory cortex* in the temporal lobe, the *primary somatosensory cortex* in the parietal lobe, and the *gustatory* and *olfactory cortices* in the temporal and parietal lobes, respectively. Each primary sensory cortex projects its specific sensory modality to its surrounding association area, such as the primary visual cortex to the visual association areas via cortical–cortical connections, creating a unimodal association cortex. These different sensory association cortices communicate with each other via convergence of their unimodal fibers to multimodal association cortices.

There are three multimodal association cortices—the *posterior*, the *anterior*, and the *limbic association areas*, although the latter two are also classified as supramodal. The posterior multimodal association center involves the posterior parietal lobe, especially the angular gyrus. This area allows percepts of different sensory modalities to be temporally and spatially integrated. This area is crucial for language function. It is noted in Figure 8.4 that connections exist between the visual association areas and all three of these areas, that being the posterior multimodal association area and anterior and limbic supramodal association areas. The anterior association area is located in the prefrontal area and allows visual percepts to be incorporated into various higher cortical functions by determining which of the unimodal and multimodal inputs from the other parts of the brain should be attended at any specific time. This allows for the conversion of percepts to concepts. The limbic association cortices serves as a supervisory system that processes emotions and feelings that interface between the inner self and the external world, in addition to subserving memory. These supramodal systems can transcend processing the interface of vision between the inner self and the external world with the use of experience and inference. In essence, this means that what you know influences what you see. These systems are operational even in the absence of sensory stimulation or action in the immediate present. These areas are shown in Figure 8.5.

The different cortical nodes of primary, unimodal, multimodal, and supramodal cortices are interconnected among themselves, but how are they connected with subcortical structures such as the hippocampus, amygdala, pulvinar, and superior colliculus to create vision? These linkages are carried out by numerous white matter axonal pathways in the

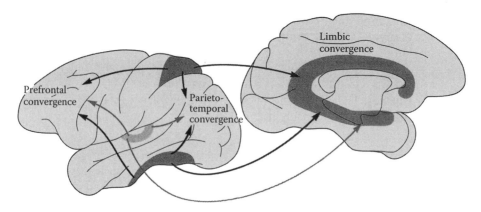

FIGURE 8.4
Visual association cortex connections to the anterior, posterior, and limbic multimodal association cortices. (From E. R. Kandel, J. H. Schwartz, and T. M. Jessell (Eds.), *Principles of Neural Science*, 4th ed., McGraw-Hill, p. 355, 2000. With permission.)

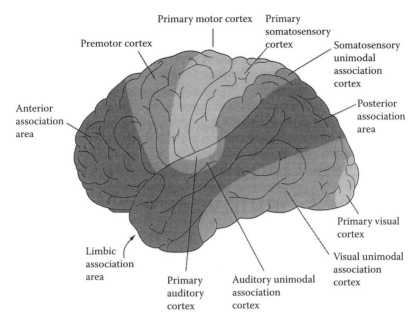

FIGURE 8.5
Different association cortices. (From E. R. Kandel, J. H. Schwartz, and T. M. Jessell (Eds.), *Principles of Neural Science*, 4th ed., McGraw-Hill, p. 350, 2000. With permission.)

subcortical white matter. These pathways, again, consist of large groups of myelinated axons grouped together, which have been identified as fasciculus, bundles, or tracts. These "wires" are multidirectional; they can converge or diverge from lower to higher processing centers, they can be collateral or spread out on the same level, or they can be recurrent or project from higher to lower visual areas.

The organization of brain white matter fiber tracts can be divided into *association fibers*, *commissural fibers*, and *subcortical fibers*.[14] The association fibers can be either *local, neighborhood*, or *long association fibers*. Local association fibers, such as U-fibers, connect to adjacent gyri, neighborhood fibers are directed to nearby cortical regions, and long association fibers travel in discrete bundles to distant cortical areas in the same hemisphere. Commissural fibers interconnect the cerebral hemispheres and subcortical fibers connect the cortex to the subcortical areas or vice versa. Pertinent long association fibers include the *superior longitudinal fasciculus I, superior longitudinal fasciculus II, frontal–occipital fasciculus, inferior longitudinal fasciculus, uncinate fasciculus, arcuate fasciculus*, and the *cingulum bundle* (Figure 8.6). The superior longitudinal fasciculus I is involved in higher order control of body-centered action and initiation of motor activity. It connects the superior parietal lobe where body-centered maps exist with the prefrontal motor areas. The superior longitudinal fasciculus II is involved in spatial attention, connecting the inferior parietal lobe with posterior prefrontal cortices. The frontal–occipital fasciculus is involved in visuospatial processing, connecting the dorsal and medial extrastriate and caudal posterior parietal cortices with the dorsolateral prefrontal cortex. The inferior longitudinal fasciculus connects the ventral temporal lobe with the posterior parahippocampal gyrus, mediating object discrimination, face and object recognition, and object memory. The uncinate fasciculus is involved in processing novel information and understanding emotional aspects of various sensory input, connecting the medial temporal area with the frontal orbital area. The arcuate fasciculus links the caudal superior temporal gyrus with dorsal prefrontal area 8, mediating

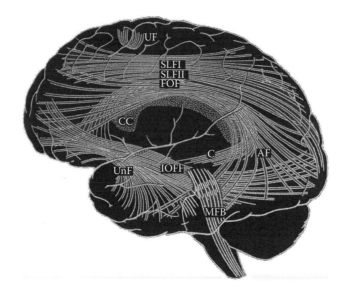

FIGURE 8.6
Major white matter tracts of the brain. CC, corpus callosum; UnF, uncinate fasciculi; IOFF, inferior fronto occipital fasciculus; UF, U-fibers; SLFI, superior longitudinal fasciculus I; SLFII, superior longitudinal fasciculus II; FOF, fronto-occipital fasciculas; AF, arcuate fasciculus; C, cingulum; MFB, medical forebrain bundles. (From C. M. Filley, *The Behavioral Neurology of White Matter*, Oxford University Press, p. 23, 2001. With permission.)

language function. The cingulum bundle connects the caudal cingulate gyrus with parahippocampal and hippocampal areas involved in motivation and emotional aspects of behavior, as well as spatial working memory. The three commissural fiber systems are the *corpus callosum*, the *anterior commissure*, and the *hippocampal commissures*. These commissures allow for functional coordination across hemispheres in processing information in the visual domain. Subcortical fiber systems include the internal capsule, which sends fibers to the thalamus, pons, and other brainstem structures, as well as the sagittal striatum and internal capsule of the posterior brain region, which includes the optic radiation.

The various connections between gray matter structures via fasciculus form distributed neural networks or systems designed to carry out a specific function. These are nicely outlined in Filley's textbook on the *Behavioral Neurology of White Matter*.[15] Table 8.1[15, p.251] shows the arousal, orienting, and spatial attention networks of attention, visuospatial ability, and recognition networks involved in the function of vision, language, memory, emotion, and personality networks. It is important to have knowledge of the structural–functional correlations to understand vision and, in general, behavioral neurology. In summary, there is a multitude of neural assemblies that occur in the brain that are widely anatomically distributed, yet functionally and structurally integrated to serve a specific domain.[16]

8.5 Functional Organization of the Visual System

8.5.1 Principles

The five principles governing the organization of the functional visual system are clearly outlined in the book by Kandel et al.,[17] *Principles of Neural Science*. The first principle states the visual system involves several brain regions that carry out different types of brain processing.

TABLE 8.1

Distributed Neural Networks

Domain	Gray Matter Structures	Connecting Tracts
Arousal	Reticular activating system	Medial forebrain bundle
	Thalamus	Thalamocortical radiations
	Cerebral cortex	Fronto-occipital (right)
Visual orientation	Superior colliculus	Collicular–pulvinar
	Pulvinar	Pulvinar–cortical
	Postparietal lobe	
Spatial attention	Parietal lobe (right)	Superior longitudinal fasciculus II (right)
	Prefrontal lobe (right)	Cingulum (right)
	Cingulate gyrus (right)	
Visuospatial ability	Parietal lobe (right)	Fronto-occipital fasciculus (right)
	Frontal lobe (right)	
Higher order control of body centered action	Superior parietal lobe	Superior longitudinal fasciculus I
	Premotor areas	
Recognition	Temporal lobes	Inferior longitudinal fasciculus
	Occipital lobes	
Language	Broca's area	Arcuate fasciculus (left)
	Wernicke's area	Extreme capsule (left)
Memory	Medial temporal lobe	Fornices
	Diencephalon	Mamillothalamic tracts
	Basal forebrain	Septohippocampal tracts
Emotions and personality	Temporolimbic system	Medial forebrain bundles
	Orbitofrontal cortices	Uncinate fasciculi

Source: Filley, C. M., *The Behavioral Neurology of White Matter,* Oxford University Press, New York, p. 34, 2001. With permission.

The second principle is that identifiable pathways exist, linking the same components in approximately the same location in every brain. Third, every part of the brain projects in an orderly fashion onto the next, creating topographic maps. That is to say, the retina is continuing to be represented topographically throughout successive stages of processing, allowing a neural map of visual information for the receptive fields to be reformed at sequential levels in the brain. Fourth, the visual functional system is hierarchically organized, passing from lower to higher processing centers. In addition, however, there is parallel processing to help connect the numerous visual areas. The fifth principle of the functional organization of the visual system is that one side of the brain controls the other side of the body. These are simple principles that help to explain how the anatomic functional correlates create vision.

8.6 Functional Components of the Visual System

8.6.1 Reception

Visual reception is the ability to see, focus, hold the focus, and project the signal in its purest form to the primary visual cortex. This requires a focused optical image on a retina, healthy eyes, and an intact primary visual system, including convergence and accommodation. It is dependent upon full visual fields for perception. Objects for viewing are selected in the cerebral cortex. To examine objects in the environment, we have to move the fovea to target these stimuli. This requires intact ocular motor skills to keep the eye still when the image is still and to stabilize the image when the object moves in the world or when the head itself moves. This system is carried out by the gaze system.

The gaze system has two components: the *oculomotor system* and the *head movement system*. The oculomotor system contains synchronized supranuclear and intranuclear components. There are six supranuclear neural systems that keep the fovea on target, each controlled by the cortex and with its own individual substrate. The *saccadic eye system* directs the fovea from one object of interest to another, *smooth pursuits* hold the image of a moving target on the fovea, the *vergence system* acts to move the eyes in opposite directions so the image of a single object in space is placed on the fovea, the *vestibulo-ocular* holds images still on the retina during brief head movements driven by signals from the vestibular system, the *optokinetic* holds the head still during sustained head rotation, and finally, a *fixation system* holds the fovea in place on a stationary target. Eye movements are conjugate with all these neural systems except vergence, where they are dysconjugate. These complex supranuclear networks result in eye movement, taking the coordinating efforts of whole muscle groups. Therefore, no one muscle is involved in disorders of the supranuclear system, and diplopia is rarely a complaint. The higher cortical centers that control gaze specify only a desired change in eye position as determined by visual information of the desired environmental stimulus. These signals are transmitted to various brainstem structures where motor programming occurs, integrating the motor nuclei of cranial nerves III, IV, and VI with the horizontal and vertical centers specifying eye position and velocity. The vertical gaze center is located in the mesencephalic reticular activating system and the horizontal gaze center is in the pontine reticular formation. Misalignment of the two visual axes with complaints of diplopia usually results with lesions involving the infranuclear portion of the gaze system, including cranial nerves III, IV, or VI, or the myoneural junction or extraocular muscles they innervate. The infranuclear ocular motor system is a simple motor system requiring the coordination of 12 muscles to move the eyes. These muscles are well known and rotate the eye in the orbit by abduction, adduction, elevation, depression, intorsion, and extorsion. Visual reception will be faulty with supranuclear lesions, resulting in gaze palsies. Intranuclear lesions result in diplopia.

In addition, through multisensory integration, movements of the head help position the fovea on a target in the visual field. Some of these neural systems for specific gaze function are more well delineated than others. Figure 8.7 shows the cortical pathways for saccadic eye movements in the monkey.

8.6.2 Attention

Attention is a modular process that allows us to be aware of our environment. It is mandatory because the brain does not have the capacity to process all stimuli presented to it at any specific time. This refers not only to visual, but to all other sensory stimuli as well. To interact adaptively and selectively with the environment, the cerebral cortex requires the functional integrity of all cortical and subcortical visually related structures.

The term *attention* can be used to describe a variety of phenomena. It comprises different processes and is involved in diffuse cognitive function. *Simple attention* refers to being either alert or aroused to respond to stimuli. *Sustained attention* describes one's ability to focus on related stimuli while ignoring irrelevant stimuli. *Selective attention* is the process

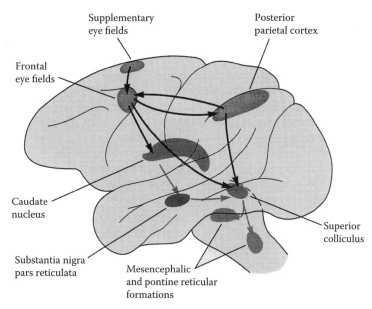

FIGURE 8.7
Cortical pathways for saccadic eye movements in the monkey. (From E. R. Kandel, J. H. Schwartz, and T. M. Jessell (Eds.), *Principles of Neural Science*, 4th ed., McGraw-Hill, p. 793, 2000. With permission.)

that picks out salient stimulus at the exclusion of others. *Divided attention* refers to mandatory focus and arousal over a period of time on more than one task. From one perspective, attention can be divided into different focuses: *spatial attention,* in which stimuli are selected based on their position in space; *object-based attention,* in which stimuli are selected based on identity; *selection-based attention,* in which visual working memory selects items to be remembered; and *executive-based attention,* in which attention is involved in the choosing of paths or behavior that an observer will perform.

What are the neural networks that mediate attention? Devinsky and D'Esposito,[18] in their textbook *Neurology of Cognitive and Behavioral Disorders,* provide a simplistic approach to this question (Figure 8.8). Figure 8.8 shows the three neural networks—the *alerting arousal system,* the *orienting system,* and the *selective attentional network*—all of which interconnect and function in a seamless fashion.

The alerting system is a total subcortical unit involved in bottom-up attention. Structures involved in this system include different brainstem structures comprising the ascending reticular activating system, the medial forebrain bundle, septal nuclei, and thalamus. The locus ceruleus is a brainstem nucleus involved in norepinephrine production, which stimulates the thalamus. The mesolimbic and mesostriatal systems produce dopamine and the medial forebrain bundle is involved with acetylcholine production. These neurotransmitters stimulate the thalamus and the limbic system, which then activates the cortex for arousal and alerting. The prototype clinical example of a disorder affecting this system is delirium.

The orienting network, in regard to vision, is a mixed cortical/subcortical system. Visual orientation involves eye movements that direct peripheral stimuli into foveal view and covert attentional shifts without eye or head movement. There are three major structural components of this system in addition to their interlocking pathways. The superior colliculus is a mesencephalic nucleus involved in detecting novel visual stimuli, targeting location for attentional shifts, and hyperreflexive orienting to the ipsilateral field. The pulvinar,

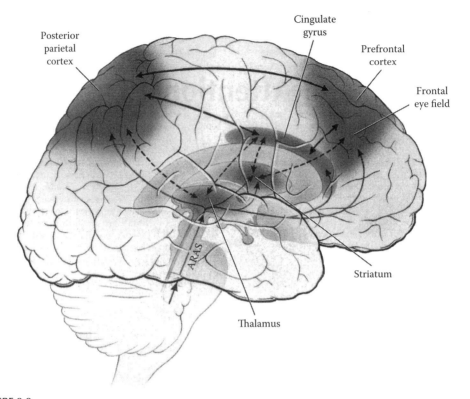

FIGURE 8.8
Functional anatomic networks of attention. ARAS, ascending reticular activating system. (From O. Devinsky and M. D'Esposito, *Neurology of Cognitive and Behavioral Disorders*, Oxford University Press, p. 104, 2004. With permission.)

a large thalamic nucleus, restricts input to selective sensory regions, such as vision, filters out irrelevant stimuli, assists in covert orienting, and facilitates response to a clued target. The posterior parietal area is the cortical component of this system, disengaging attention from present focus in the orienting neural circuit.

The selective attentional network is a totally cortical circuit. Much of its function is mediated by the superior longitudinal fasciculus II. This system has several specialized components, each with numerous interconnections. The posterior parietal cortex is also involved in this system, disengaging attention from present focus. The right side has the greatest effect, mostly disengaging from location; the left side has the least effect, mostly disengaging from objects. The superior parietal lobe is responsible for voluntary shifts of attention, the frontal eye fields generate volitional saccades, the premotor cortex is involved in motor intention based on all sensory inputs, the dorsolateral frontal cortex is involved with working memory and self-monitoring based on all sensory inputs, and the anterior cingulate cortex is responsible for motivation, exploratory behavior, and attention to action. Clinical symptoms of a disorder of this neural circuit can be manifested by lesions of any of its components or interconnections. A prototype disorder of this system is neglect. The cognitive control of attention is carried out by either endogenous, voluntary top-down control, which is goal oriented, or exogenous, automatic (reflexive) bottom-up control, which is stimulus driven.

At the level of cortical hierarchy for perception, the attentional selectivity of information processing is subject to control both from below and from above, with one usually dominating over the other in any specific moment. From below, the cortical networks for the primary and secondary visual association cortices are subject to the structure of visual stimulation in its spatial temporal context from the retina. The saliency and novelty of stimuli enable them to be selected against competition because these features are more likely to be detected and selected by autonomic, unconscious bottom-up processing as opposed to a stimulus embedded in a clutter or in a monotone pattern. This bottom-up control is epitomized by the pop-out phenomena (which is characterized by a preattentive processing that is executed speedily and in parallel in the primary and visual association cortices).[19] This is an example of unconscious attention at work in the cerebral cortex and, as such, bottom-up preattentive processing is subject to top-down control. The supramodal cortices further analyze visual stimuli based on past experience, inference, relevance, and emotion that gives meaning to what is seen and makes a plan for action. Attention directs automatic bottom-up processing, ascending from lower to higher levels in percept formation, whereas top-down processing modulates activity in the supramodal anterior and limbic association cortices, giving meaning to the visual information from the posterior cortices and the subcortical systems. In summary, by using top-down and bottom-up attentional processing, there is a simultaneous binding of different neural networks in time to allow the visual information to be integrated with other sensory stimuli, emotion, and experience to result in the desired behavior or goals. Therefore, the brain decodes patterns of experience into concepts, then in turn, shapes the nature of our perceptions.

The master control of the attentional system is unknown, but probably the prefrontal association cortex is the most important area, although recent reference[20,21] has been made to the claustrum and precuneus as possibly serving this vital function. The prefrontal cortex has reciprocal connections to all cortical and subcortical structures. An analogy would be that this area serves as a switching operator of trains, determining which trains run together on which tracks at any specific time, comparing the related tracks and trains with axonal connections to different structures to bind together at any specific moment to accomplish a desired behavior. This is based on resource allocation of the system exciting some systems while inhibiting others. This is a dynamic process, readjusting to new stimuli, resulting in different nerve assemblies turning off and on. It would seem logical that the repetitive use of some assemblies make them stronger with use and others would be weakened with disuse. Which assemblies are used would be dependent upon their efficiency and processing stimuli. This determines what is included or excluded in the visual receptive fields.

8.6.3 Higher Visual Processing

Early and rudimentary analysis of visual inputs begins in the retina and continues as it is projected to the primary visual cortex. As noted in the previous section, much of visual processing is automatic and unconscious. Higher cortical processing begins in the primary visual cortex and becomes progressively more complex as information travels on to visual association areas and then on to higher cortical centers. The primary visual cortex, V1, is called the *striate cortex*; visual association areas are the *extrastriate cortex*. V1 is densely packed, containing 250 million neurons receiving connections from 1.25 million geniculate neurons.

V1 is a six-layer structure with column organization located in the caudal occipital lobe between the pial surface and the white matter. It contains alternating vertical columns of cells, orientation, and ocular dominance columns with blobs in peg-shaped patches in the upper layers. Cell types in each module have specific functions. Orientation cells respond to a specific axis of orientation, blobs that activate initial color processing, and ocular dominant cells in binocular integration. The magno- and parvocellular pathways remain anatomically segregated as they enter the primary visual cortex through sublayers 4Ca and 4Cb, and then are distributed above and beneath to other layers, to simple and then complex cells.

A major change in the orientation cells' receptive fields occurs outside layer 4 in that the receptive field enlarges and becomes elongated as opposed to being concentric. This changes its maximum response from a spot of light to a bar of light. Despite these changes, the receptive fields of the orientation cells are similar to the ganglion cells in the retina in that they still specify retinal position and have antagonistic excitatory inhibitory zones.

Simple cell response to orientation is related to a specific axis in its visual field. Complex cells monitor several simple cells and react to a specific axis of orientation without regard to their visual field location. Complex cells project to hypercolumns of cells outside the primary visual cortex that respond to all lines of orientation from a represented region in the visual field. These are, in turn, interconnected by lateral networks that bring together all data from positions of the visual field—in other words, put all the pieces of the puzzle together to interlock all lines of orientation to create a representation. In summary, the poorly outlined visual image based on changes of contrast is projected from the retina to the primary visual cortex, is deconstructed into short lines of various orientation by simple and complex cells, and is then reconstructed by the hypercolumns of cells. This is an unconscious event. The blobs are again involved in the early complex function of color perception and the ocular-dominant cells in binocular visual integration as they receive vision from both eyes. The primary visual cortex has extensive output. Tracts leave layer 5 from the superior colliculus, pons, and pulvinar, and from layer 6 to the lateral geniculate body. The magnocellular pathway forms the dorsal stream as it exits layer 4. The parvocellular pathway exits layers 2 and 3 as the ventral stream.

Outside, surrounding the primary visual cortex, there have been seven identified and numbered areas in the visual association cortices in addition to an area that represents the perception of faces (Figure 8.9). V2 lies adjacent to V1 and is the largest numbered association cortex area containing cells that respond to all major visual modalities. It has multiple connections, some reciprocal to V1, V3, and prefrontal sensory and motor areas, and is involved in a higher order analysis than V1. V1 and V2 are involved in early perception, responding to color and form. Signals are assembled here before being sent on to other areas. V3 is adjacent to V2 and its function is motion, form (especially shape of objects in motion), and depth perception, in addition to form analysis at lower contrast. The ventral area of V4 is involved in color perception, the dorsal area with size estimation, and with line orientation. V5 is located in the lateral convexity near the junction of the temporal, parietal, and occipital lobes, responding maximally to motion detection. V6 has not been precisely localized in humans and it is thought to be involved in self-motion, three-dimensional features, target selection, and visual search.[18] V8 is the primary area for color perception. Facial perception is a function of the medial lower temporal area, as noted in Figure 8.9.

How are all these areas interconnected among themselves and with other cortical and subcortical structures? There are two modes for processing visual information: a serial hierarchical system and a parallel, or nonhierarchical, system. The hierarchical system is based on a sequential transfer of visual information from the lower to the higher levels of perception, being reorganized at each level with advanced abstraction occurring. There are, however, numerous feedback systems that assist in the perception of the representation. As noted earlier, there are multiple areas representing visual function in the cortex.

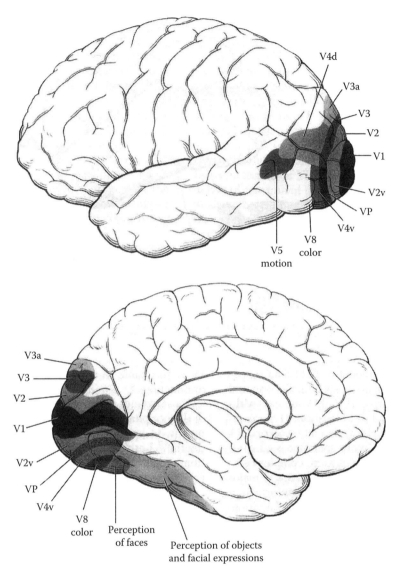

FIGURE 8.9

Principal visual areas in humans. (From O. Devinsky and M. D'Esposito, *Neurology of Cognitive and Behavioral Disorders*, Oxford University Press, p. 125, 2004. With permission.)

Cortical connectivity between these areas does not fit well into a serial processing system. It is best explained by a parallel system in which cortical visual associations have multiple and, sometimes, reciprocal connections among themselves and other structures. This multiplicity of connections explains the feedback or top-down processing from higher to lower centers in a nonduplicated manner for detail and awareness. This is opposed to bottom-up processing in which tiny pieces of information are received at the retina and constructed into a visual image. *Top-down processing*, again, refers to the influence of the supramodal and multimodal cortex structures upon bottom-up visual information.

The primary parallel systems that exit the primary visual cortex have connections with the posterior association cortices and the anterior and limbic association areas. This parallel system is called the *ventral and dorsal streams*.[10] Although the mechanism is not clear, the information in these two streams is bound together by attentional mechanisms. Gamma electroencephalographic synchrony is implicated in this binding of conscious content.[22] One hypothesis is that the ventral and dorsal stream subserve object recognition and spatial processing respectively, the so-called "what" and "where" pathways.[23] Another hypothesis proposes the distinction is between processing for recognition and processing for action or guidance of response to stimuli.[24] Like all theoretical constructs, the view of extrastriate function is simplified and is considered as a guide to understanding visual processing.

The ventral stream or the inferior occipital fasciculus originates in V1, projects to V2, then to V4, and on to specific inferior temporal cortical areas, the angular gyrus, and limbic structures. This pathway to the "what" system is initially involved in processing the visual attributes of the image, including color, shape, construction, size, weight, texture, and detail. The ventral stream connects with the language network, resulting in the recognition of words, naming, and the ability to read. The ventral stream connects with limbic association areas creating visual memory and emotional relevance to the visual input.

The dorsal stream begins in V1 and projects through V2 to V3 to V5. From V5, the pathway continues to additional areas in the parietal and superior temporal cortex. It connects the latter areas to the motor association and anterior association areas representing visuospatial ability, including location of objects in space and visual motor integration. Visuospatial abilities are represented in both hemispheres, but the right is more involved than the left in this domain. This system is critical for representing and attending to space. The dorsal stream specializes in spatial perception in several ways. The visual field representation in individual dorsal stream areas is universally broader than that found in the ventral stream areas. Neurons and several dorsal stream areas are specialized for detection and analysis of moving stimuli, and are sensitive to the depth at which a stimulus appears relative to an individual.

Space is a modality without a known primary sensory organ and is the most complex of sensory representations. There is no evidence of a single explicit topographic representation of space. Evidence points to multiple representations of space in a variety of coordinate frames, which are linked to separate output systems designed to guide specific motor effectors. These reference frames are *viewer centered*, in which locations are represented relative to the observer, and *allocentric*, in which locations are represented in reference frames independent of the observer. The viewer-centered reference frame is the traditional approach of describing the structures involved in vision. Allocentric reference frames include object centered and environment centered. Space is represented predominantly in the parietal lobe. Space is integrated with information from retinal coordinates that are dependent upon an intact attentional system to appreciate space. Space is three-dimensional, having horizontal, vertical, and radial axes, and is further divided into near or peripersonal and far or extrapersonal space. These different divisions of space are coded differently in the brain and are not determined only by hand-reaching distance, but are also dependent on how the brain represents the extension of the body space.[25] The function of the "where" system is the visuospatial analysis of location and movement of objects in space. The function of the "how" system is related to visually guided movements toward objects. The parietal cortex houses a structural body map that refers to a representation of the shape and contours of the human body, in general, and to one's own body, in particular. This representation defines a detailed plan of the body surface and boundaries between body parts that are coded, which interact with spatial maps, which articulate with the motor system. This body representation is divided into different coordinates including *eye centered*, *head centered*, and *body centered*, which form the viewer-centered reference frame for space. This guides reaching movements in the upper extremities and helps to guide navigation in the environment, the latter by a complex system of projections to the frontal eye field, which in turn commands the superior colliculus, where further multisensory/spatial/motor integration occurs. The latter is termed *body schema*, which refers to an active online reproduction of one's own body in space that is derived from multisensory input.[26] This system provides a level three-dimensional representation of the body in space that directs the motor system for action.

Visual control of walking is mediated by the body schema representation. A person perceives the visual direction of the destination with respect to the body and walks in that direction. Steering is based on optic flow, the pattern of visual motion as the person's focus expands in the direction of the walk. Optic flow is measured by the motion neuron sensors in the medial superior temporal lobe.

Visual imagery is a significant part of mental life and it is thought that it is actually an offshoot of our capacity for activating mirror neurons. The mirror neuron system is an observation execution matching system with a main role that has been postulated to the understanding of action. In humans, the neural circuitry for mirror neurons involves the inferior frontal gyrus, the adjacent premotor cortex, and the rostral part of the inferior parietal lobe. This system is connected with the superior temporal sulcus, which provides a higher ordered visual description of the observed action. It allows our social brain to perceive the intention and goal action of others and links these perceptions to the priming of our motor system to engage in the same action and feelings. Identical cortical and subcortical structures are used in visual mental imagery as in the perception of environmental stimuli.[27] Therefore, it is not uncommon for patients with TBI to have problems in these cognitive areas.[18]

8.7 Classification of Visual Defects

Visual defects occur commonly after TBI in view of the extensive networking and multifaceted functions of the visual systems. Humans are highly reliant on vision for spatial orientation and environmental interaction. Lesions involving the primary visual system can be easily localized and accurately diagnosed by medical providers. However, abnormalities involving the secondary visual system are much more complex and difficult to localize and, in general, are more poorly appreciated and difficult to recognize. These deficits are discussed in the remainder of this chapter, as are their relationships to the components of the functional visual system—reception, attention, and higher cortical processing.

8.7.1 Reception

In the receptive system, any impairment in visual input will result in decreased visual sensory ability. Lesions in the eye, retina, or optic nerve will result in decreased visual acuity. Bilateral lesions of the primary visual system can result in primary blindness. Visual field defects, such as scotoma or incomplete or complete homonymous hemianopsia, will impair visual function. Cortical blindness is caused by bilateral lesions of the optic radiations or V1 or primary visual cortex. It differs from primary blindness in that the pupillary light reflex is preserved because of the sparing of the fiber connections of the optic tract to the midbrain. Optokinetic nystagmus is absent. This is differentiated from conversion blindness when pupillary light responses and optokinetic nystagmus are spared. Blindness or unconscious vision is caused by a lesion involving V1 in which a severe contralateral visual field defect exists. These patients do not respond discriminately to movements or flashing stationary light because of preserved rudimentary processing of visual input. This low-level vision is explained by either intact connections of the retino-tectal tract to the superior colliculus or aberrant retrogeniculate connections to the extrastriate visual cortex.

Gaze system abnormalities can result in strabismus or nonstrabismus binocular visual disorders, in addition to problems with visual scanning and gaze palsies. A recent article by Ciuffreda et al.[28] cites a high frequency of ocular motor dysfunction following TBI. Convergence insufficiency was found in about 40%, some type of ocular motor dysfunction in 60% to 85%, cranial nerve palsy in 33%, and accommodative dysfunction in 20%. The frequency of occurrence of dysfunction in all ocular motor areas tested was much higher when compared with the non-TBI patient group.[28]

8.7.2 Attention

The classic defect resulting from dysfunction of the visual attentional system is *visual neglect*, or the inability to attend or orient to the contralateral space. Visual neglect can be classified as either personal or extrapersonal, or viewer-, object-, or environmental-centered disorders. Possible mechanisms causing neglect include orientation of attention toward objects (attributes) laying on the ipsilateral side of space, defects in reorienting attention toward the contralateral side of space, or a nonlateralized defect in rapidly dealing with visual sensory events. The right hemisphere is dominant for spatial attention and mediates attention directed toward both the right and left hemispace, whereas the left hemisphere mediates only the right hemispace. This explains why right-side neglect resolves early and why left-side neglect is more severe, the latter usually a result of a right parietal lesion. Because of the widespread distribution of the attentional system, lesions involving different anatomic areas can result in neglect, including the right and left parietal areas, right and left dorsal lateral frontal areas, right and left medial frontal areas, right and left striatum, right thalamus, and white matter of the internal capsule and hemisphere.[29–31]

Neglect is not a result of any coexistent visual field defect because many patients with homonymous hemianopsias do not have neglect syndromes and many with neglect do not have homonymous hemianopsia. In a recent article studying a large group of patients who sustained posterior cerebral artery infarctions, the severity of neglect was greater after a right posterior cerebral infarction, even in the acute stages of the posterior cerebral infarct.[32] Visual field defects from an isolated right occipital lesion did not cause contralateral neglect unless there was injury not only to the occipital lobe but to the splenium of the corpus callosum.

It can be difficult to differentiate unilateral visual neglect from homonymous hemianopsia. Common tests used in this determination include double simultaneous visual stimulation tests as well as constructional tests. The most commonly used constructional tests include the line cancelation test, letter cancelation test, line bisection test, figure copying, and picture interpretation. The left hemifield, for example, can be tested in a dark room with a small penlight. Patients with neglect will detect the left-side stimulus; those with hemianopsia will not. *Asimultanagnosia* is characterized by the inability to see more than one object at a time not attributable to primary visual field defects. It is explained by the inability to shift visual attention and narrowing effective visual fields and is caused by posterior parietal lesions. This is a form of bilateral visual neglect, with lesions at different sites involving different spatial axes. The Navon letter test is a simple screening test to evaluate this function. *Visual anosognosia* is an attentional defect resulting in a disorder of body schema—our awareness of our body and the spatial relationship of our body parts to each other and the environment.

8.7.3 Higher Cortical Processing

Disorders of higher cortical visual processing can be caused by disconnections involving either the ventral or dorsal stream. Conditions involving the ventral stream can be classified as *visual–visual, visual–verbal,* and *visual–limbic* disconnections. Disruptions in connectivity involving the dorsal stream are more difficult to group but can be broken down to *spatial–spatial, spatial–motor,* and *body spatial*. Visual–visual disconnects result in agnosia. *Agnosia* refers to the clinical condition in which the patient is able to perceive visual stimuli and has efficient language capacity to name the stimuli, but recognition is lost. These conditions involve the loss of recognition of familiar faces, places, color, object feature, and object identify. These are termed, respectively, *aprosopagnosia, topographagnosia, color agnosia, visual apperceptive,* and *associative agnosia.* Apperceptive visual agnosia is the condition in which the patient cannot distinguish one form from another, whereas visual associative visual agnosia is a disturbance of visual recognition with intact visual perception. Loss of connectivity between visual–verbal system results in pure alexia, color, and object anomia. *Visual anomia* is defined as the inability to name objects, although they are perceived. *Visual amnesia* and *hypoemotionality* are related to the loss of linkage of the visual to limbic area. Spatial–spatial disconnects result in vision neglect in which the dorsal stream loses its ability to attend to the contralateral visual space. Body spatial disorientation occurs when the dorsal stream loses input with the structural body map, resulting in finger agnosia, right/left disorientation, and dressing disorder. Egocentric disorders are a form of body spatial disconnects resulting in a loss of orientation of self to localizations of objects in the environment. Primary visual motor disconnects result in defects involving visually guided movements and volitional redirection of gaze. Sequelae of visual disconnects involving the ventral and dorsal stream to the anterior association area and limbic association area results in problems with visual spatial imagery, visual organization, mental figure rotation, design generation, and recognition of embedded figures, all involving higher cortical cognition. The right brain is more involved in visuospatial skills and interpersonal relevance, and lesions in this area can result in problems with territorial boundaries, such as interpersonal space and interpreting proper social signaling, such as smiling or frowning.

8.8 Summary

TBI remains an unappreciated epidemic in the United States. It is the leading cause of death and disability among young adults. Children are particularly vulnerable to TBI because, during childhood, portions of the brain are still myelinating and so patients not only have to recover from the deficit but be able to layer on additional learning to ensure normal development. This is the cause of the saying that children "mature into their deficits." TBI can be a cause of a catastrophic injury, resulting in life-long physical, cognitive, and emotional deficits resulting in a huge emotional burden on families and a financial burden on society.

Visual input accounts for 70% of all sensory information being processed by the brain.[33] Therefore, visual–spatial and visual–perceptual deficits are commonly a sequelae of TBI. The frontal and anterior temporal poles are most frequently damaged because of the way the brain is positioned in the skull, butting up against the jagged bony edges of the anterior and middle fossas. The hallmark pathophysiologic abnormality of TBI is diffuse axonal injury resulting from shearing forces. The supramodal areas—that is, the anterior and limbic association cortices—occupy these areas, and all the major cortical fasciculi project to these areas. Midline brain structures are most vulnerable to diffuse axonal injury, including the subcortical white matter, corpus callosum, and rostral brainstem—the latter explaining the vulnerability of the magnocellular systems. Other structures, such as cranial nerves III, IV, and VI, and the eye, can be damaged. This is a very simple explanation of the frequent occurrence of visual–spatial and visual–perceptual deficits following TBI, in addition to other cognitive problems in the area of memory, attention, and executive function. It is imperative that residual disorders of primary and secondary visual systems be diagnosed early and be treated both appropriately and aggressively to promote proper brain plasticity that will result in the maximal recovery of visual function.

References

1. Thurman, D., Alverson, C., Dunn, K., Guerrero, J., Sniezek, J. Traumatic brain injury in the United States: A public health perspective, *Journal of Head Trauma Rehabilitation*, 14(6), 602–615, 1999.
2. Suter, P. S., Rehabilitation and management of visual dysfunction following traumatic brain injury, in M. J. Ashley (Ed.), *Traumatic Brain Injury: Rehabilitative Treatment and Case Management*, 2nd ed., CRC Press, Boca Raton, FL, 2004, 209–249.
3. Notle, J., *The Human Brain: An Introduction to Its Functional Anatomy*, 4th ed., C. V. Mosby, St. Louis, MO, 1998.
4. Byrd, S. E., Darling, C. F., and Wilczynski, M. A., White matter of the brain: Maturation and myelination on magnetic resonance in infants and children, *Neuroimaging Clinics of North America*, 3, 247–266, 1993.
5. Benes, F. M., Turtle, M., Khan, Y., and Farol, P., Myelination of a key relay zone in the hippocampal formation occurs in the human brain during childhood, adolescence, and adulthood, *Archives of General Psychiatry*, 51(6), 477–484, 1994.
6. Nauta, W. J. H. and Feirtag, M., *Fundamental Neuroanatomy*, W. H. Freeman, New York, 1986.
7. Van Essen, D. C., Functional organization of the primate visual cortex, in A. Peters and E. G. Jones (Eds.), *Cerebral Cortex*, vol. 3, Plenum Press, New York, 1985, 259–329.
8. Felleman, D. J. and Van Essen, D. C., Distributed hierarchical processing in the primate cerebral cortex, *Cerebral Cortex*, 1(1), 1991, 1–47.
9. Rodieck, R. W. and Watanabe, M., Survey of the morphology of macaque retinal ganglion cells that project to the pretectum, superior colliculus, and parvicellular laminae of the lateral geniculate nucleus, *The Journal of Comparative Neurology*, 338(2), 289–303, 1993.
10. Dacey, D. M., Physiology, morphology, and spatial densities of identified ganglion cell types in primate retina, in CIBA Foundation Symposium, *Higher-Order Processing in the Visual System—Symposium No. 184*, John Wiley & Sons, Hoboken, NJ, 1994, 12–28.
11. Holmes, N. P. and Spence, C., Multisensory integration: Space, time, and superadditivity, *Current Biology*, 15(18), R762–R764, 2005.

12. Dai, J., Van der Vliet, J., Swaab, D. F., and Buijs, R. M., Human retinohypothalamic tract as revealed by in vitro postmortem tracing, *Journal of Comparative Neurology*, 397(3), 357–370, 1998.

13. Gooley, J. J., Lu, J., Chou, T. C., Scammell, T. E., and Saper, C. B., Melanopsin in cells of origin of the retinohypothalamic tract, *Nature Neuroscience*, 4(12), 1165, 2001.

14. Schmahmann, J. D. and Pandya, D. N., *Fiber Pathways of the Brain*, Oxford University Press, New York, 2006.

15. Filley, C. M., *The Behavioral Neurology of White Matter*, Oxford University Press, New York, 2001.

16. Mesulam, M. M., Large scale neurocognitive networks and distributed processing for attention, language, and memory, *Annals of Neurology*, 28(5), 597–613, 1990.

17. Kandel, E. R., Schwartz, J. H., and Jessell, T. M., *Principles of Neural Science*, 4th ed., McGraw-Hill, New York, 2000.

18. Devinsky, O. and D'Esposito, M., *Neurology of Cognitive and Behavioral Disorders*, Oxford University Press, New York, 2004.

19. Fuster, J. M., *Cortex and Mind*, Oxford University Press, New York, 2005.

20. Cavanna, A. E., The precuneus and consciousness, *CNS Spectrums*, 12(7), 545–552, 2007.

21. Crick, F. C. and Koch, C., What is the function of the claustrum?, *Philosophical Transactions of the Royal Society B*, 360(1458), 1271–1279, 2005.

22. Hameroff, S. R., The entwined mysteries of anesthesia and consciousness: Is there a common underlying mechanism?, *Anesthesiology*, 105(2), 400–412, 2006.

23. Ungerleider, L. G. and Miskin, M., Two cortical visual systems, in D. J. Ingle, M. A. Goodale, and R. J. W. Mansfield (Eds.), *Analysis of Visual Behavior*, MIT Press, Cambridge, MA, 1982, 549–586.

24. Milner, A. D. and Goodale, M. A., *The Visual Brain in Action*, Oxford University Press, New York, 1996.

25. Berti, A. and Frassinetti, F., When far becomes near: Remapping of space by tool use, *The Journal of Cognitive Neuroscience*, 12(3), 415–420, 2000.

26. Gallanger, S., Body schema and intentionality, in J. L. Bermudez, A. J. Marcel, and N. Eilan, *The Body and the Self*, MIT Press, Cambridge, MA, 1995, 226–244.

27. Kosslyn, S. M., Pascual-Leone, A., Felician, O., Camposano, S., Keenan, J. P., Thompson, W. L., Ganis, G., Sukel, K. E., and Alpert, N. M., The role of area 17 in visual imagery: Convergent evidence from PET and rTMS, *Science*, 284(5411), 167–170, 1999.

28. Ciuffreda, K. J., Kapoor, N., Rutner, D., Suchoff, I. B., Han, M. E., and Craig, S., Occurrence of oculomotor dysfunctions in acquired brain injury: A retrospective analysis, *Optometry*, 78(4), 155–161, 2007.

29. Heilman, K. M., Watson, R. T., and Valenstein, E., Neglect and related disorders, in K. M. Heilman and E. Valenstein (Eds.), *Clinical Neuropsychology*, 3rd ed., Oxford University Press, 1993, 279–336.

30. Healton, E. B., Navarro, C., Bressman, S., and Brust, J. C., Subcortical neglect, *Neurology*, 32(7), 776–778, 1982.

31. Meilman, K. M. and Valenstein, E., Frontal lobe neglect in man, *Neurology*, 22(6), 660–664, 1972.

32. Park, K. C., Lee, B. H., Kim, E. J., Shin, M. H., Choi, K. M., Yoon, S. S., Kwon, S. U., et al., Deafferentation–disconnection neglect induced by posterior cerebral artery infarction, *Neurology*, 66(1), 56–61, 2006.

33. Kaas, J. H., Changing concepts of visual cortex organization in primates, in J. W. Brown (Ed.), *Neuropsychology of Visual Perception*, Lawrence Erlbaum Associates, Hillsdale, NJ ,1989, chap. 1.

9

Rehabilitation and Management of Visual Dysfunction Following Traumatic Brain Injury

Penelope S. Suter

CONTENTS

9.1 Introduction

The two million neurons carrying information from the eyes provide approximately 70% of the sensory input to the brain. Because of this, the visual system gives us enormous leverage to make changes in neurologic systems, and with appropriate therapeutic guidance, can often be the keystone of recovery.

This chapter surveys the nonsurgical rehabilitative services available to provide effective treatment of brain-injured patients with visual sequelae. It should be a useful reference for those who deal with these patients in intensive rehabilitative environments, as well as for primary care professionals who sometimes find these patients in their care when a rehabilitative hospital or center is not accessible. It may also be useful to both novice and experienced vision care providers working in the area of traumatic brain injury (TBI) rehabilitation.

The basic structure of this chapter remains the same as in previous editions. However, in addition to updating the scientific and clinical references, a number of topics have been added or expanded upon. Many of the therapeutic approaches used with TBI patients were developed for other special needs vision patient populations. For this reason, much of the information provided here is applicable not only to the TBI patient, but also to other patients who have sustained organic insult to the brain. For the same reason, although they may lack specific experience with TBI patients, vision care professionals who practice other forms of vision therapy will often be able to provide appropriate rehabilitation for TBI patients who have visual dysfunction—given a few additional concepts that are specific to the brain-injured population.[1]

9.2 Physical Substrates of Vision

The physical substrates of vision are covered in depth in Chapter 7 of this volume, and only a brief overview is given here. In the rhesus monkey, which provides an excellent model of the human visual system, more than 50% of the neocortex is involved in visual processing.[2] To date, researchers have described approximately 305 intracortical pathways linking 32 different cortical areas implicated in visual function; 25 of these are regarded as either predominantly or exclusively involved in visual function, and seven are considered visual association areas.[3] The ganglion cells traveling from the retinas represent approximately 70% of all sensory input fibers to the brain. Subcortical substrates are involved in binocular coordination, visual attention, integrating multi-modal stimuli, and perceptual coherence. In addition to multiple subcortical areas, every lobe of the cortex is involved in visual processing (reviewed by Kaas[4]). The occipital lobe contains primary visual cortex for initial processing of vision as contour, contrast, and depth. The inferior temporal lobe is involved in object identification, the middle temporal area in motion processing, and the parietal lobe in processing for spatial orga-nization and visual attention.[4,5] The frontal eye fields and adjacent areas of the frontal and prefrontal lobes are involved in motor planning and initiation of self-directed eye movements, as well as visual search (Figure 9.1).[6] In addition, simple visual awareness requires interactions between primary visual cortex, posterior parietal cortex, and fron-tal eye fields. Input from the limbic system (especially the cingulate gyrus) may mediate motivational relevance of the external stimulus, guiding sustenance of attentional acti-vation in the visual system.[7]

Considering this, *visual rehabilitation* becomes a sweeping term, which ranges from reha-bilitation of the eye and surrounding structures, to rehabilitation and management of sen-sory processing, organization of sensory input from the eye into visual percepts, and use of these percepts to support cognitive or behavioral functions. Visual dysfunction may affect the ability to carry out daily tasks such as reading, driving, walking, and function-ing in the workplace. Diagnosis and rehabilitation of the eye, eyelids, extraocular muscles

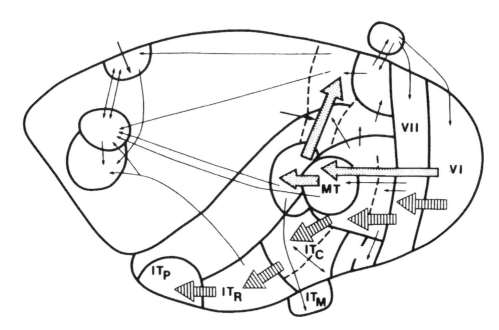

FIGURE 9.1
Areas of visual cortex (VI, VII) and some of the ipsilateral cortical connections in visual cortex of the owl monkey. The arrows indicate two major cortical pathways of visual processing. The superior path (dotted arrows) to the posterior parietal lobe (PP) via the middle temporal (MT) area supports "where" processing. The inferior path (hatched arrows) to the temporal lobe (IT) supports "what" processing. (Adapted from Kaas, J. H., *Neuropsychology of Visual Perception,* Lawrence Erlbaum Associates, Hillsdale, New Jersey, 1989. With permission.)

and surrounding bony structure, and eye movement and eye-teaming disorders, as well as the higher visual functions such as visual perception, spatial organization, visual memory, and the ability to integrate visual information with other modalities, all fall under the umbrella of visual rehabilitation. Multiple professionals may be involved and considerable networking or case management provides for the most effective care.

9.3 The Multidisciplinary Approach

Two types of eye doctors are frequently required in management of the visual consequences of TBI: the ophthalmologist and the optometrist. In general, their roles may be considered analogous to the computer equivalents of hardware and software repair persons, respectively. The ophthalmologist will often be needed to provided medical/surgical treatment of the hardware or anatomic and physiologic aspects of the visual system before the optometrist can provide rehabilitation of the software or functional aspects of the visual system.

Ophthalmologists are trained to diagnose and manage damage to the eye and surrounding structures as well as to diagnose lesions of the visual pathways and ocular–motor system. They sometimes prescribe exercises for eye movement disorders that are often performed with the assistance of an occupational therapist. Occasionally, an ophthalmologist will work with an orthoptist, an ophthalmologically trained therapist, to remediate eye-teaming disorders such as strabismus. However, ordinarily, ophthalmologists are mostly concerned with providing the medical/surgical support required during early rehabilitation, or with later surgical intervention if spontaneous recovery and therapy fail to produce an acceptable result with a traumatic strabismus.

Neuro-ophthalmologists are ophthalmologists who have specialized in diagnosis and treatment of neurologic dysfunction of the visual system. They are more likely to have some experience with rehabilitating the visual software or application of nonsurgical or pharmacologic therapies than general ophthalmologists.

Optometrists specializing in vision therapy and/or rehabilitation are trained in diagnosis and nonsurgical treatment of more complex fixation, eye movement, or eye teaming (i.e., binocular) disorders, as well as perceptual dysfunctions in the visual system. Usually, the treatment of such disorders is performed with the assistance of a vision therapy technician under the doctor's supervision. In an inpatient or rehabilitation center outpatient situation, occupational therapists working under a doctor's supervision or prescription will sometimes assist the patient with vision therapy for perceptual and sensorimotor dysfunctions, or less complex eye movement and eye-teaming dysfunctions. They may also assist with teaching new living skills to compensate for residual vision deficits.

Optometrists specializing in low vision assessment are trained in prescribing low vision aids for patients with reduced visual acuity, and "field expanders," which may be required for patients with visual field defects. These doctors will often work with, or refer to, a low vision rehabilitation specialist, frequently called an *orientation and mobility specialist*, who can assist in teaching the patient new living and mobility skills to cope with his or her acquired visual deficit.

Vestibular system damage may cause nystagmus, vertigo, and imbalance, and/or may obstruct normal fixation and pursuit. In such a case, referral for vestibular workup to a professional equipped to perform eye movement recordings for diagnosis and to make rehabilitative recommendations may be helpful. Neuropsychological examination may help to give a broader perspective on visual–perceptual dysfunctions. Finally, as with other types of rehabilitation following a TBI, visual rehabilitation may be significantly enhanced by the assistance of a counselor or psychotherapist to assist patients in understanding their new limitations and the need to rehabilitate, as well as managing emotional sequelae that can interfere with effective rehabilitation.

9.4 Prevalence and Impact of Visual Dysfunction in TBI Patients

Because of the multifaceted nature of visual dysfunction and the broad distribution of visual functional areas in the brain, many, if not most, TBI patients experience some sort of visual dysfunction. When using visual symptoms to relate the dysfunction to the injury, clinicians must be aware that there are two common circumstances in which symptoms may appear weeks or months following the injury. The first is related to the fact that functional levels tend to change rapidly following brain injury. For instance, patients will report that they have no difficulty reading, but when queried whether they have read since their injury, they will state that they have not because they have been doing other things. Often they are unable to read and do not realize it because their rehabilitation and activities of daily living have been at much more basic levels. As the patient's level of functional competence increases, so do the functional demands, and new symptoms arise. The second common circumstance in which new visual symptoms arise in the months following the injury is when medications related to managing injury-related manifestations are changed, because many medications commonly prescribed following brain injury have visual side effects.[8] These are also "injury-related" symptoms, because the medications are necessitated by the injury.

Transient changes in refractive error, most often in a myopic direction, which may last for months or years, are common after TBI.[9–11] Accommodative (i.e., focusing) dysfunctions are also common[12,13] and may interfere with reading, fine depth discrimination, and rehabilitative therapies that are performed at near point. Near point tasks, as well as balance, orientation, mobility, and daily living skills may be affected by visual field defects and binocular disorders, as well as by dysfunctions in visual–spatial neglect (inattention), visual perception, and spatial organization.[11,13–15] Binocular disorders can cause postural changes as the patient finds ways either to maintain fusion or to enhance suppression of one eye by tilting or turning the head or torso.

It is often the case with TBI patients that eye-care professionals, untrained in diagnosing more subtle visual and ocular–motor dysfunctions, may dismiss patient complaints of headache, dizziness, inability to concentrate, blurred vision, fatigue, light sensitivity, or inability to read as resulting from emotional or other nonvisual etiologies. Although many of these symptoms may have nonvisual causes, a careful assessment of the visual system will often reveal the physiologic or perceptual difficulty underlying the patient's complaint.[16] Gaetz and Weinberg[17] have demonstrated deficits in visual event-related cortical potentials (VECPs) in patients with persistent symptoms from TBIs classified as mild head injuries or concussions. They conclude that patients with postconcussive symptoms frequently have persistent brain damage that cannot be visualized using computed tomography or magnetic resonance imaging (MRI), but can be elucidated using visual and auditory event-related potential techniques. Lachapelle et al.[18] reached similar conclusions in another VECP study of patients with TBI. This group later extended this research to the mild TBI population, and demonstrated changes in VECPs to visual texture and visual cognitive paradigms; latency changes in the VECP following mild TBI correlated with vocational outcome.[19]

Schlageter et al.[20] found that 59% of TBI patients admitted to an acute rehabilitation center had eye movement or eye-teaming dysfunctions. *Therefore, it is important that the TBI patient be examined by an eye-/vision-care provider who has a special interest in the area of neuro-rehabilitative, or therapeutic vision care.* (See the Appendix for a partial list of organizations that can provide educational materials or lists of member doctors who practice in this area.) Cohen et al.[21] found convergence insufficiency (i.e., difficulty pulling the eyes inward, as is necessary for binocular fixation on near targets) in approximately 40% of TBI inpatients with recent injuries and follow-up patients 3 years postinjury. In the follow-up group, convergence insufficiency was positively correlated with duration of coma, dysphasia, cognitive disturbances, and failure to find placement in nonsupported work situations. Lepore[22] examined 60 patients with TBI and resultant strabismus. Among the 51 patients with nuclear or infranuclear findings, fourth cranial nerve palsies were the most common (39%), followed by third nerve palsies (33%), sixth nerve palsies (14%), combined palsies (10%), and restrictive ophthalmopathy (4%). Convergence insufficiency was the most common supranuclear dysfunction. Similarly, in 114 patients referred to an ocular–motor clinic for visual disturbances following motor vehicle accidents, Fitzsimons and Fells[23] noted fourth nerve palsy in 36%, third nerve palsy in 25%, and multiple diagnoses in 25%. Aberrant regeneration was noted in 78% of third nerve palsies. Ciuffreda et al.[24] reviewed records of ambulatory patients, 160 with TBI and 60 with cerebrovascular accident with associated vision symptoms. This group found accommodative and vergence deficits were most common in the group with TBI, and strabismus and cranial nerve palsies were most common in the group with cerebrovascular accident. Ocular–motor dysfunction was found in more than 85% of both groups.

Padula and Argyris[25] have identified a constellation of visual deficits that they have termed *posttrauma vision syndrome*. These deficits may include high exophoria or exotropia, convergence insufficiency, accommodative insufficiency, and ocular–motor dysfunction. Common symptoms include double vision or a perception of motion in stationary objects or printed material, blurred near vision, photophobia, eyestrain, and headache. Furthermore, clinicians and researchers have described visual–motor dysfunctions related to judgments of egocentric visual midline shifts following brain injury. These shifts create symptoms including dizziness and balance problems similar to those created by vestibular dysfunction. Padula et al.[26] demonstrated that the amplitude of the VECP is decreased in posttrauma vision syndrome, and that application of binasal patches, or low amounts of bases in prism cause a significant increase in visual event-related potentials.

Groswasser et al.[27] reported bilateral visual field defects in 14% of severe TBI patients. Ocular–motor defects in these patients were associated with poor recovery as defined by return to work or school. Bilateral visual field defects were more common in the poor recovery group, but this finding was not significant. A 15-year follow-up study of U.S. Vietnam veterans with penetrating head injuries showed that visual field loss and visual memory loss were negatively correlated with return to work.[28] In an assessment of successful versus unsuccessful TBI clients in a supported employment program, Wehman et al.[29] evaluated the functional limitations of those clients rated most difficult and least difficult to maintain in employment. The two areas of functional limitations that were significantly different between these groups were visual impairment and fine motor impairment. Najenson et al.[30] found that performance on the Raven Matrices Test, which is heavily loaded for visual–spatial performance, was highly correlated with successful performance in the rehabilitated TBI patient's working life. McKenna et al.[15] examined the incidence of visual–perceptual impairment in patients with severe TBI, and found, using the Occupational Therapy Adult Perceptual Screening Test, visual–spatial neglect in 45% of their sample. Visual–spatial neglect is frequently underdiagnosed in the brain injury population because the patient is unaware of the deficit, and it may or may not be concurrent with a motor neglect that cues the clinician into realizing that there is a problem.

Lastly, as reviewed by Murray et al.,[31] non-"neglect" types of attentional deficits in TBI patients have been considered in terms of information processing models rather than in terms of constructs such as sustained attention or distractibility. Shum et al.[32] provide evidence for a four-step sequential information processing model in which attentional processes are considered as the sequential stages of (1) feature extraction, (2) identification, (3) response selection, and (4) motor adjustment. Children who sustained severe TBI showed significant impairment on complex choice reaction time tasks designed to test each of these processing stages compared with age- and gender-matched control subjects. Based on these findings, diagnosis and treatment of these primary processing disorders may be the most direct approach to treating attention disorders in TBI patients.

9.5 Therapeutic Intervention: What and Why?

9.5.1 Plasticity and Flexibility in the Adult Visual System

The amazing flexibility in modification of the vestibular–ocular reflex (VOR), as well as the visual–perceptual apparatus, has been demonstrated in normal adults by the application of inverting prisms.[33] Initially, when wearing these prisms, the world appears upside down and backward, but with continued prism wear, the VOR reverses and visual perception reverts to normality. More recently, pre- and posttherapy functional MRI[34] and voxel-based morphometry analysis of high-resolution MRI[35] studies with adults have demonstrated changes in cortex activity and cortical connectivity consistent with the rehabilitation techniques used. Substantial neural plasticity is present in other areas of the adult visual system, as demonstrated by orthoptic therapy remediation of amblyopia and strabismus in adults.[36–38] Freed and Hellerstein[39] have demonstrated that the visual evoked potentials (VEPs) of adults with mild TBI frequently normalize following application of vision rehabilitation techniques, in contrast to VEPs of matched participants who do not receive vision rehabilitation. In the non-TBI population, vision therapy has proved effective for treatment of many visual disorders, such as accommodative dysfunctions, eye movement disorders, nonstrabismic binocular dysfunctions such as convergence insufficiency, strabismus, nystagmus, amblyopia, and some visual–perceptual disorders in both adults and children.[40–42] Most of these visual disorders may be suddenly acquired with a brain injury.

9.5.2 Remediation of Ocular–Motor and Binocular Disorders Following TBI

Vision therapy has also been applied successfully to remediation of vision disorders secondary to brain injury.[43–48] Ron[49] studied six patients with ocular–motor dysfunctions resulting from TBI, such as saccadic dysmetria and decreased optokinetic nystagmus gain. Both saccades and optokinetic nystagmus normalized more rapidly with training compared with control patients, and gains were maintained after cessation of treatment. Convergence insufficiency and strabismus have also been successfully remediated with vision therapy in brain trauma patients.[44,46,50] In an experiment to test the practicality of applying therapy to vision deficits in a short-term acute care rehabilitation setting, Schlageter et al.[20] failed to show statistically significant improvements from repeated baseline measures on pursuits and saccades in six TBI patients who received between 2 hours and 6 hours of therapy. However, when quality of eye movements was graphed against treatment, the slope increased (showing faster improvement) during therapy for both saccades and pursuits, compared with the baseline period. Although the occupational therapists and speech pathologists who administered the therapy were trained in a number of therapy techniques for saccades and pursuits, it became apparent during the study that "establishing a hierarchy of progressively more difficult exercises required a significant amount of training,"[20, p.447] and they may have found even better results had they used staff trained in orthoptic or vision therapy. Because of multiple demands on patient time in the acute care setting, treatment for visual disorders will generally not be completed in this setting. However, progress can be made, and visual dysfunction should be considered when making recommendations for the patient at discharge from acute care.

When surgical intervention is required for remediation of a residual posttraumatic strabismus, patterns of eye movement and teaming must be relearned. Fitzsimons and Fells[23] report that, among 92 TBI patients who had extraocular muscle surgery, 50% required more than one surgery, and 30% more than two. Of these patients, 52% had satisfactory outcomes as defined by a satisfactory field of single binocular vision with tolerable diplopia (i.e., double vision) when shifting gaze to the sides. Another 27% had moderate outcomes defined as suppression or diplopia with the ability to ignore one image comfortably. Finally, 22% had persistent troublesome diplopia necessitating occlusion. Their success rates may have been even better had they used functional therapy in conjunction with surgery. Pre- and postsurgical application of therapy can be a useful adjunct to surgery in encouraging fusion, expanding the range of binocular gaze, and eliminating diplopia. *Unfortunately, it is common that the professionals who treat strabismus are dichotomized into those practitioners who apply surgery and those who apply functional therapies, rather than having the two work as a team.* Those who apply surgery alone rely on the existing visual system to relearn binocular fusion without any guidance. Often, this does not occur. Those who apply therapy alone risk not offering their patients the full range of services to assist in the best possible outcome. As more eye-/vision-care professionals begin to treat TBI patients, hopefully an integrated approach will become more widely accepted.

9.5.3 Management of Other Visual Dysfunctions Following TBI

In patients with visual loss as measured by decreased visual acuity or visual field, low vision devices, such as magnifiers, special telescopes (some of which may be spectacle mounted) or "field-expanding" devices, can be applied. As our population ages, more research and development has gone into rehabilitation for these types of visual loss, which are frequent sequelae of stroke and age-related eye disease. Therapy for homonymous hemianopia has been shown to increase speed and breadth of visual search, and to improve both objective and subjective measures of visual abilities on activities of daily living, including, in some cases, partial recovery of visual field loss.[51,52] Therapy for visual–spatial neglect can be similarly effective.[53] Researchers at the Massachusetts Eye and Ear

Infirmary have documented the effectiveness of using a multidisciplinary team including ophthalmologists, optometrists, occupational therapists, and social workers in increasing patients' functional ability during visual rehabilitation.[54]

Therapies for perceptual dysfunctions other than visual–spatial neglect have been previously applied in non-TBI populations by some educators, optometrists, psychologists, and neuropsychologists. Development of computerized therapies for perceptual deficits have made perceptual rehabilitation more accessible and applicable by other therapists, including occupational therapists. Because perception is dependent on reception, it is advisable to test for and remediate or manage any sensory visual deficits prior to testing for perceptual dysfunction other than neglect. Current evidence (reviewed by Gianutsos and Matheson[55]) generally supports the efficacy of perceptual therapy following brain injury, although one must be aware that substantial spontaneous recovery occurs during the first 6 months following the injury.

9.5.4 When to Treat

The timing of therapeutic intervention has been a controversial issue. Patients who are diplopic should have vision examinations as soon as possible after they are medically stabilized. Appropriate application of prism, cling patches, or partial patching (discussed later) during the early weeks postinjury can give the patient some relief of symptoms as well as prevent maladaptations that must be trained away later. Application of either specialized patches or prisms during these early weeks requires frequent reevaluation and adjustment to keep pace with spontaneous resolution of visual defects.

Although there is evidence that some visual defects, such as muscle palsies and pareses, may spontaneously recover up to 12 months postinjury,[56] other evidence shows that, in general, untreated brain-injured persons do not spontaneously recover from binocular disorders, such as convergence insufficiency.[21] The decision about when to intervene is most appropriately determined by factors other than the hope of spontaneous recovery.

During the initial 3 months postinjury, a rapid resolution may occur in many visual defects as edema in the brain diminishes. After this time, although spontaneous resolution may still be ongoing, it is likely to be slower, and unwanted compensatory mechanisms (such as suppression) set in. Furthermore, in patients who are struggling with such deficits as orientation problems or diplopia, failure to address these difficulties in a timely manner may lead to depression and a poor attitude toward rehabilitation when it is finally offered. Patients who are left to their own devices after the acute phase of medical rehabilitation is completed will find ways to survive with remaining deficits—often in ways that are not positive adaptations. Follow-up studies in untreated TBI patients show that they generally do not make continued functional progress and they may even decline in function over the long run.[55]

Even with the most careful diagnosis, one cannot always tell which patients are going to respond to treatment. In the areas of ocular–motor and binocular dysfunction following TBI, reevaluation on a monthly basis can be used to determine whether the patient is making progress. If therapy has been consistent and intensive and no progress is being made, then compensatory measures should be prescribed. Gianutsos[57] suggests that, during cognitive rehabilitation, intensive rehabilitation with an initial goal of restoration of function should be applied for 6 months. If no progress is made, then a different approach should be tried. This seems to be a good rule for visual–perceptual and visual–memory rehabilitation, with the modification that some compensatory strategies are often applied immediately to help the patient function while pursuing therapy.

9.6 A Useful Model for Organizing Visual Rehabilitation

Moore[58] has emphasized the importance of considering functional units in the brain, taking into account contemporary metabolic maps that show brain function, rather than thinking of the brain as it has been mapped during the past century into discrete compartments associated with individual functions. Although it is necessary to have an understanding of the neuroanatomy of the visual system to help formulate an appropriate diagnosis, knowing the neurons does not provide an adequate basis for guiding therapy. It is equally important to have a working model of visual performance to guide rehabilitation efforts and higher order visual testing. Neuropsychological models of information processing or even of reading will often begin with a box labeled *visual input* or *sensory input*. Exposure to such models may give the nonvision specialist the impression that visual input and its involvement in information processing is discrete and simple enough to fit into such a box. Working without a model of visual processing may encourage attempts to rehabilitate splinter skills, such as convergence, in cases when a more holistic approach is necessary to get the patient reading again or reoriented in space. Many therapy-oriented optometrists use a model of visual processing similar to that developed by Cohen and Rein[59] and shown in Figure 9.2. Figure 9.3 represents a simplified model that may help the practitioner keep the big picture in mind during testing and treatment.

9.6.1 Sensory Input/Reception

Visual system input, or reception, is dependent on formation of a focused optical image on the retina, healthy eyes, and healthy, intact pathways to primary visual cortex. Accommodation (the internal focusing of the eye mediated by the ciliary muscle) and

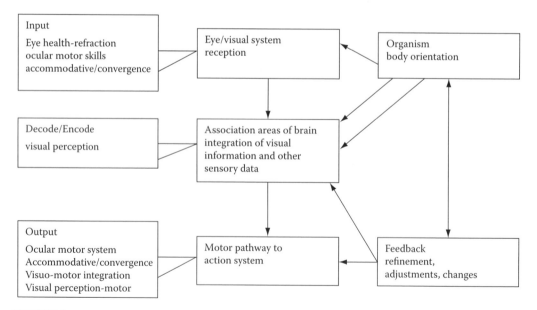

FIGURE 9.2
A model of visual function developed by Cohen and Rein, similar to that used by many optometrists to help guide vision therapy. (From Cohen, A. H. and Rein, L. D., *Journal of the American Optometric Association*, 63, 534, 1992. With permission.)

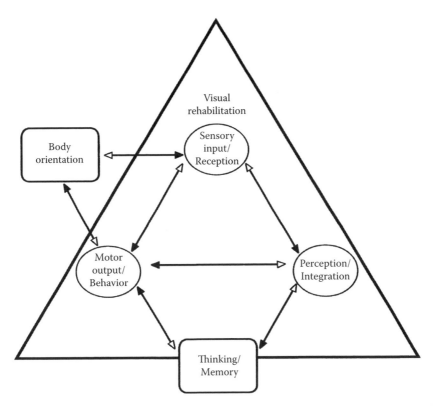

FIGURE 9.3
A modified model for guiding rehabilitation of the visual system. Functions within each processing area (circles) are as delineated in the original model by Cohen and Rein.[59] Visual processes fall within the triangle. Closed head arrows indicate the major direction of information flow. Note that all arrows are bidirectional; information flow is bidirectional in most known pathways in the visual system[2] and other bidirectional influences are explained in the text.

vergence (the ability to make disjunctive or inward and outward movements of the eyes) are also an important part of getting visual input to the visual cortex without confusion. These two functions are tied together by neural feedback loops. As one expends accommodative effort (trying to focus closer), the accommodative effort drives convergence, pulling the eyes inward. As accommodation is relaxed, the eyes diverge, or relax outward, as for viewing distant targets. There is a similar, but lower, amplification loop from convergence to accommodation; as one exerts convergence effort, it drives accommodation. It should be obvious that a disruption in the balance between these two interacting systems—accommodative–convergence and convergence–accommodation—can cause serious dysfunction in eye teaming and focusing. There are useful models of such disturbances[60] reviewed by Ciuffreda.[61]

Visual reception is also dependent on ocular–motor skills—that is, full range of motion of the extraocular muscles, the ability to fixate the target of regard, track it, if desired, or saccade to another target efficiently and accurately. These abilities are dependent on feedback from areas that monitor head and body orientation and movement, as well as those areas that monitor feedback from the ocular–motor drivers. Reception ends at primary visual cortex, where the initial binocular combination of input from the two eyes occurs to allow for fusion and stereopsis. The input is processed as color, contour, contrast, and depth.

9.6.2 Perception/Integration

Visual perception and integration are dependent on intact neural communication within visual processing areas and pathways between these processing areas, as well as intact reception. Current trends in cognitive neuroscience implicate recurrent processing in primary visual cortex (i.e., feedback from higher cortical processing areas to primary processing areas) as critical in awareness of visual input or visual perception.[62,63] Not only does damage to lower visual processing areas decrease activity in higher processing areas through loss of feed forward (e.g., occipital to parietal and parietal to frontal areas), but damage to higher processing areas decreases activity in lower level processing areas through loss of feedback connections.[7]

Integration of visual information is also dependent on pathways to and from processing areas mediating other sensory and motor functions. Much of the cerebral cortex is involved in visual processing, with close to 300 intracortical pathways between the visual areas. Therefore, it is important to maintain a holistic model of the functions of this stage of processing so that one can test for and address functional loss with some guidance from available topographic details of the injury.

The major functions of this stage in the model are organization of space and motion, form perception, and object recognition,[59,64] as well as integration of vision with the other senses and motor system input. Visual awareness is also included here. Interfaces with thinking and memory processes are not in the original model (Figure 9.2) but should be added at this stage in a bidirectional manner, as in the modified model in Figure 9.3. Our percepts feed into our memories and influence how we think, and our thinking and memories influence our perceptions and behaviors.

Two major concurrent vision processing streams proceed forward from the occipital cortex: the dorsal "where" stream to the parietal lobe and the ventral "what" stream to the temporal lobe (Figure 9.1). The dorsal "where" stream mainly carries information originating from magnocellular ganglion cells. This stream is first identified, anatomically, at the lateral geniculate nucleus, where large magnocellular ganglion cells are segregated from the smaller parvocellular ganglion cells. Magno cells are, in general, sensitive to large contours, lower contrast, and faster temporal frequencies, and are retinotopically distributed more peripherally than parvo cells (reviewed by Bassi and Lemkuhle[65]). Some magno cells are color sensitive, but at least half are insensitive to color.[66] The magno system is preserved, in a relatively segregated manner, through primary visual cortex, and then as the dorsal stream to the middle temporal area for motion processing, ultimately ending in the posterior parietal cortex for cortical processing of object localization and visual attention. Parvo cells, in general, transmit more slowly than magno cells and are more sensitive to color, high contrast, and detailed stimuli; they are the origin of the information carried in the ventral stream. The ventral stream ultimately traverses to the inferior temporal cortex and is involved in object perception (discussed later). The cortical dorsal and ventral streams maintain both separate and interactive functions. "Where" the object is and "what" the object is must be integrated to make sense of the world. However, research shows that it is possible to interfere selectively with memory for either "what" or "where."[67] Also, it can be demonstrated, electrophysiologically, that spatial attention has a different effect on each of these two pathways.[68]

More recently, Milner and Goodale[69] have developed and refined a description of the dorsal and ventral streams based on their output, rather than the input to the systems (reviewed in 2008). They present evidence that the dorsal stream provides for visually guided action and programming of the movements involved in those actions, and the ventral stream provides for perception and planning (separate from programming movement). Destruction of the dorsal stream creates optic ataxia, or the inability to program reaching for objects, whereas destruction of the ventral stream creates loss of object perception and planning, such that one might reach accurately, but grasp the wrong portion of an object to use it because the patient does not know visually what the object is.

In addition to the cortical dorsal stream, an extrageniculate, "ambient" midbrain visual system[70,71] processes information both directly from the retina and from the striate cortex to organize orientation in ambient space. Organization of space and motion by both the cortical dorsal stream and the midbrain ambient system requires interpretation of reception from visual sensory substrates, ocular–motor drivers, and from substrates reporting body orientation and motion to ascertain the spatial location of objects in relation to ourselves. This analysis allows us to determine whether we are moving, the external stimulus is moving, or some combination of both. The midbrain system is faster than the cortical magno system and mediates much of our survival-level orienting, head movement, and saccadic eye movement. It is also involved in perceptual coherence. The information from the different senses arrives at the brain with different latencies, both resulting from external differences (think of the lag between lightning and thunder, but at much shorter distances), and internal differences in neural transmission times from receptor organs.[72] The information from various senses associated with a single event must be matched together, largely coordinated in the superior colliculus.

Feedback from both accommodation and convergence helps localize objects in depth.[73] Form perception and object recognition require figure–ground segregation, form constancy, visual closure, and some processing of spatial relationships. These functions interact with visual reception in that the ability to perform these functions may be limited by visual field loss or degraded visual acuity, contrast sensitivity, or fixation.

Cross-modality integration is dependent on intact pathways to and from the neural substrates mediating the other senses, as well as subcortical and cortical processing to make matches between them. Object perception includes integration with the visual input of information about the object from our other sensory modalities.

Visual awareness, although most often taken for granted by rehabilitation professionals, is surprisingly often disrupted in TBI and other pathology of the visual system. Patients with neural damage to the visual system are often unaware that there has been any change in their function. It is only when one demonstrates to them, on a visual field printout, a line bisection or cross-out test for visual neglect or a processing speed test that their performance is grossly subnormal that they begin to understand that there is a visual deficit.

Considering the covert nature of many visual deficits following brain injury, it becomes clear how such a pervasive system as the visual system can be so frequently ignored in the rehabilitation setting because neither patients nor practitioners may be aware that the patient's symptoms are visual in origin. Those systems that traditionally receive the most rehabilitation effort tend to be those that are overt in nature (e.g., language reception and expression, vestibular dysfunction, and motor dysfunction), even though the representation in the brain (and therefore the impact of TBI) is often considerably less for these systems than for the visual system.

9.6.3 Motor Output/Behavior

Organization of body movements in relation to visual targets is mediated, most directly, by the posterior parietal areas and angular gyrus. Three major pathways connect these areas with the motor areas: one via intracortical connections, one via the basal ganglia, and one via the cerebellum.[74] Individual functions of these three pathways are not well understood.

The percepts of our visual world that we construct during reception and perception are used to guide further motor activity, both within the visual system and in visually guided motor activity, such as mobility or eye–hand coordination. These percepts direct our ocular–motor activity and eye pointing. They influence the frontal lobe areas, which generate executive commands for voluntary eye movements, so that we may regard objects at will rather than in a purely stimulus-driven manner. They are involved in direction of the next movement, whether for perception or for action. In short, these visual percepts and the resultant thought processes dependent on them are the foundations for much of the everyday behavior of a sighted person.

9.6.4 Visual Thinking/Memory

Much of our thinking and memory is processed as part of the visual processing stream. Visualization of complex problems or forms is one method of problem solving and organizing that does not require language. Although visual thinking, in general, is typically addressed by education in the rehabilitation setting, the skill of visualization—the ability to generate and manipulate endogenous images—is typically addressed by visual rehabilitation providers. Memory is a concept with which every person is familiar, and yet it is poorly understood. Memory has both short-term and long-term components. In neuropsychology, long-term memory is often subdivided into procedural, perceptual representation, semantic memory, and episodic memory.[75] Short-term, or working, visual memory is encoded and stored separately from auditory and haptic memories[76] and can be broken down into spatial memory (thought to be processed by the magno stream) and object memory (thought to be processed by the parvo stream).[68] Rehabilitation of visual memory most often involves rehabilitation of visual aspects of working memory as well as the ability to transfer this information to long-term perceptual representations.

9.7 Assessment and Rehabilitation of the Visual System

9.7.1 Assessment and Rehabilitation of Sensory Input/Reception

In the rehabilitation setting, testing and treatment of visual dysfunction has traditionally centered on the higher order perceptual disorders, tending to ignore reception.[77] It is important to keep in mind that many of the higher order visual abilities are dependent on sensory input and ocular–motor functions involved in reception.

9.7.1.1 Eye Movements

Eye movements can be classified into those that shift the direction of gaze (i.e., saccades, smooth pursuits, and vergences) and those that hold the direction of gaze steady (i.e., the vestibular driven, optokinetic, cervical–ocular, and fixation mechanisms).[78,79] Vergences are discussed later in Section 9.7.1.2. Optokinetic nystagmus (OKN) may be used in testing and therapy for other visual dysfunctions, but deficits in OKN are not generally considered and rehabilitated in the TBI population as visual deficits. This may be because detection of deficits in OKN requires more sophisticated eye movement monitoring than is available in most vision practices.

9.7.1.1.1 Saccades

Saccades are the fast eye movements one makes to change the object of fixation; the eyes seem to jump from one target to another. They are the movements that take us from word to word in reading and from object to object in driving. Saccades, during reading, may be affected in a bottom-up manner (that is, the eye movement controllers have been damaged) or in a top-down manner (that is, the ability to comprehend text has been damaged, causing more regressions and less accurate fixations as a result of poor guesses about what is coming next).[80] Patients with acquired primary saccadic dysmetria (i.e., saccades that overshoot or undershoot the target) will often complain of slow and inaccurate reading.

Voluntary saccades, which allow us to change our gaze at will, and stimulus-generated or reflexive saccades, when we correct our gaze or saccade to a target that has attracted our gaze, are controlled, in part, by separate brain centers and should be addressed separately. It is also important to assess the ability to inhibit saccades to peripheral targets. This may be a function of the fixation mechanism discussed later. Simple observation while the patient makes voluntary saccades between two targets or reflexive saccades to alternately lit targets gives a qualitative measure of latency, speed, and accuracy of the saccades. This procedure should be done at least for lateral saccades in right and left gaze orientation. Each eye should be observed independently. The targets should be relatively close together, because most natural saccades are less than 15 degrees,[79] and large excursions encourage hypometric saccades or recruit head movement. Scoring systems for these observations are reviewed by Griffin.[81]

A more quantitative approach, which can provide additional data, is provided by the Developmental Eye Movement Test (DEM).* This is a timed test in which the patient must saccade to numbers that are arrayed on a page and name them as quickly as possible. The DEM is a substantial improvement over earlier saccadic tests of this genre in that timed baseline measurements are taken with the patient reading columns of evenly spaced vertical numbers so that difficulties with decoding or verbal expression can be differentiated from difficulty with the ocular–motor task. Next, a series of horizontal rows of digits are read. The number of errors and the time required to read all the digits are combined into separate scores for the vertical and horizontal tasks, with a higher score being slower or less accurate performance. A high ratio of horizontal score/vertical score indicates a saccadic problem. The DEM does not differentiate between difficulties in speed, latency, or accuracy, although error scores give some indication of the latter. Normative data by age are provided for times and error scores on both the vertical and horizontal tasks, as well as the ratio between them. Note, though, that this test concentrates on reading-type saccades, mostly left to right, and should be used in conjunction with other tests.

A variety of instruments has been designed to monitor and record eye movements objectively. These eye movement monitors give the most easily interpreted data but are less frequently used in the clinical setting because of issues of availability and expense.

Ordinarily, when training, saccades, latency, speed, and accuracy are lumped into the same scores; one trains for accuracy and then for speed, which improves as any one of the three parameters improves. Therapy may start with something as simple as "saccading" from one penlight to another as they are alternately lit in a dim room and may progress to complex search tasks, such as finding the next in a series of letters or numbers scrambled

---

* Developmental Eye Movement Test: Available from Bernell Corporation, Mishawaka, IN, www.bernell.com.

on a page. Instruments, such as the Wayne Saccadic Fixator[*] or the Dynavision2000,[†] with various programs for training saccades in combination with eye–hand coordination, are both useful and motivational. A number of computer-based programs has also been developed for orthoptic treatment of ocular–motor and binocular disorders. If difficulty inhibiting saccades or sustaining fixation is noted, one can apply therapies, such as making saccades only on a designated command to each in a series of targets. The ultimate goal of therapy is to develop fast, accurate saccades—both large and small—which can be sustained and performed with a high degree of automaticity. The latter is tested by adding a cognitive load, such as addition or spelling, while the patient does a saccadic task. This is an important concept in much of the visual therapy of eye movements. When a cognitive load is added, performance of the ocular–motor task will break down in patients *who are allocating excessive resources to what should be, for the most part, an automatic task.* Griffin[81] and Press[82] have written excellent texts for vision-care providers interested in learning about vision therapy programming and specific therapeutic techniques. Many of these therapy techniques may be prescribed by vision-care practitioners for application by occupational therapists in the rehabilitation setting.

9.7.1.1.2 Pursuits

Pursuits are the smooth eye movements used to follow a moving object and to hold a clear image of it stationary on the retina. They are complementary to the VOR in holding images stationary on the retina when we are moving. Pursuits are limited in speed to about 30 degrees per second. Attempts to track a faster target cause saccadic intrusions and "cogwheeling" of the movement. Pursuits are usually tested at the same time that the range of extraocular muscle motion in each eye is tested. Simple observation gives qualitative information about the ability to track a target to the full range of motion of each of the extraocular muscles monocularly, and then binocularly. The ability to track should be judged on smoothness, accuracy, and stamina, and the ability to track without head movement. As with saccades, a cognitive load should be applied to judge automaticity. Griffin[81] outlines systems for scoring pursuits.

Therapy for pursuits is often combined with extraocular stretching exercises relieving restrictions or contractures of the extraocular muscles by following targets to the farthest peripheral directions of gaze possible. These exercises are also important in the initial stages of therapy for binocular disorders. If there is any deficit on monocular testing, extraocular movements are trained monocularly prior to training binocularly so that equal facility is gained with each eye before adding a fusional load to the task.

For most vision therapy, one goal is to make the patient self-monitoring. Pursuit therapy is most effective when patients can be made aware of jerkiness or saccadic intrusions in their pursuits so that they can try to correct them. Many patients will be able to feel their eyes jump when their attention is directed to noticing interruptions in their smooth pursuit. However, in many TBI patients, proprioception from the extraocular muscles seems to be diminished or absent so that they are unable to feel when their eyes jump. In such cases, cues can be added to assist the patient. One technique is to use afterimages to tag the fovea by using a camera flash that has been masked off except for a small central target on which the patient fixates while the flash is triggered. The patient tries to maintain this afterimage on the pursuit target without interruption. A simpler technique that is

---

[*] Wayne Saccadic Fixator: Available from Wayne Engineering, Skokie, IL.
[†] Dynavision2000: Available from Dynavision2000, Markham, Ontario, Canada. www.info@dynavision2000.com.

sometimes effective is to have the therapist tell patients every time their eyes jump until the patients can begin to feel it for themselves.

Various instruments, from rotating disks with targets on them to computer-generated pursuit games, have been designed for facilitating pursuit therapy under both monocular and fused conditions. The ultimate goal of therapy is to be able to sustain smooth pursuits with either or both eyes in all fields of gaze with a high degree of automaticity, initially without moving one's head, and then adding head and, later, body movement.

9.7.1.1.3 Vestibular-Driven Eye Movements

Vestibular-driven eye movements—in particular, the VOR—help hold the visual world steady as we move within it. Patients who do not spontaneously adapt to damage affecting the VOR may complain of oscillopsia, or rhythmic movement of stationary objects. One way to test for a VOR problem is to have patients read a near point acuity card while shaking their head side to side and then up and down. In the case of a VOR dysfunction, the visual acuity will be severely degraded compared with an acuity taken with the stationary target.[83] Although therapy techniques have not been specifically developed for VOR dysfunction, applying the afterimage techniques discussed earlier with the patient attempting to stabilize the afterimage, initially, while sitting still, and later, with head movements, may give enough extra feedback to assist in recovery. Whether the patient recovers or learns to adjust to the movement, oscillopsia should be taken into consideration in driving rehabilitation.

The VOR must be coordinated with the cervical–ocular reflex (COR), a proprioceptive mechanism that also contributes to gaze stabilization. With the COR, eye movement is elicited by rotation of the neck. The VOR decreases with age, and the COR covaries in the opposite direction, increasing with age.[84] The COR is increased in whiplash, interfering with the synergy between COR and VOR, and may contribute to symptoms in these patients, including dizziness and vertigo.[85] In the differential diagnosis of dizziness and balance disorders, the COR must be considered along with the visual and vestibular contributions.

9.7.1.1.4 Fixation

Fixation, or the act of holding gaze steady on a target, was once thought to be a function of the pursuit system at zero velocity. This may be why fixation, itself, is seldom evaluated except in relation to strabismic amblyopia. However, recent evidence implicates an independent visual fixation system, perhaps located in the parietal lobe.[78] Disturbances in fixation may be considered in terms of inability to sustain fixation, as well as inability to fixate centrally and steadily. The former can be easily observed by having the patient hold fixation on a target for a minute. The ability to fixate steadily and centrically is only observable with special techniques. The easiest, most objective measure is with a visuoscope or, similarly, an ophthalmoscope with a central target. The examiner looks into the patient's eye with the scope, which projects a target onto the retina. The anatomy of the posterior pole of the eye and the projected target are viewed simultaneously. The patient is instructed to fixate the target while covering the other eye. The stability of the foveal reflex and centricity with regard to the target are easily observed in this manner. Other methods require reliable subjective feedback. For instance, the Haidinger brush, an entoptic phenomenon that marks the fovea, may be elicited with an instrument such as the Macular Integrity Tester* in which the patient fixates a target and reports the location and stability of the Haidinger brush in relation to the fixated target.

---

* Macula Integrity Tester: Available from Bernell Corporation, Mishawaka, IN, www.bernell.com.

In the case of inadequate ability to sustain fixation, the first step is to rule out refractive, binocular, accommodative, or other ocular–motor dysfunctions that may lead to asthenopia (i.e., eyestrain and/or headache) or discomfort. Such dysfunctions may make extended viewing aversive. They are also remediable, whereas a primary attention or fixation mechanism dysfunction might not be.

Unsteady or eccentric fixation is most typically encountered as a developmental phenomenon associated with strabismic amblyopia. In this manifestation, they cause decreased visual acuity but are seldom accompanied by asthenopic symptoms. There is an effective arsenal of therapeutic techniques to remediate developmental eccentric fixation routinely.[36,81] Unfortunately, unsteady fixation, which is acquired following TBI, may cause asthenopic symptoms because it may be bilateral rather than unilateral and it may be more resistant to treatment.

9.7.1.2 Binocular Dysfunction

9.7.1.2.1 Accommodation

Accommodative dysfunctions are common in the TBI population.[11] They can cause blur or asthenopic symptoms at near point, as well as slow focus change from distance to near and back. A *simple near point acuity test does not rule out an accommodative problem*, because it only indicates whether the patient can momentarily hold focus at near point. It does not indicate either that patients can sustain that focus or that they have any focusing flexibility. Objective techniques, such as near point retinoscopy performed while the patient processes visual information (e.g., reading or active involvement in viewing a picture), give an accurate assessment of the patient's lag of accommodation and ability to sustain accommodation on a near point task. Use of such tools as convex to concave lens flippers (i.e., devices with two pairs of lenses for viewing—one pair of convex lenses that requires accommodative relaxation to clear the target and one pair of concave lenses that requires accommodative effort to clear the target—set into a holder so that one can flip between the pairs of lenses) of various powers can give measurements of facility. These can be used as a subjective test with patients reading small print as they are able to clear it or as an objective test during retinoscopy. As discussed earlier, accommodative difficulties can cause convergence dysfunction, and convergence difficulties can cause accommodative dysfunction. In many cases, it is impossible to tell which problem is primary.

Typical treatments for accommodative dysfunctions are vision therapy or convex lenses worn either as single vision reading glasses or bifocals. In a prepresbyopic patient, vision therapy is an effective way to improve the amplitude and facility of accommodation, provided that the innervation subserving the function is sufficiently intact. Near-to-far focusing jumps and concave-to-convex lens jumps with near point targets may increase both amplitude and facility. Associated vergence difficulties must be treated in conjunction with the accommodative problem for effective remediation. If rehabilitation of accommodative function is not possible in the young patient, compensatory convex reading lenses should be prescribed, generally in a bifocal format. Some practitioners have suggested that bifocals should not be used for patients with brain injury or that only lined bifocals should be used. However, a bifocal, with the reading portion set low, so that it is not a safety hazard during mobility, is generally much easier to use than having the patient keep track of two pairs of glasses and figure out when to use which. In cases when lenses, but no active vision rehabilitation therapy, or only home vision rehabilitation therapy are being applied, the bifocal should be prescribed as a standard, lined bifocal. In cases when the bifocal add is less than +2.00 D, and the patient is undergoing in-office vision rehabilitation therapy, many patients do well with a "no-line" progressive bifocal because the therapy helps them adapt to the distortions in the progressive bifocal, and they receive the added advantage of clarity at intermediate distances, such as grocery store shelves, faces in conversation, and computer monitors. There are, of course, cases when the patient has limited downgaze or when the bifocal creates too much visual confusion to be applied. In this case, separate reading glasses are indicated. Often, when separate reading glasses are required, the patient requires a great deal of cuing and support to get the proper glasses on their nose for various tasks.

9.7.1.2.2 Nonstrabismic Binocular Disorders

Nonstrabismic binocular disorders are those eye-teaming difficulties that do not result in a frank strabismus (eye turn). Convergence insufficiency—difficulty pulling the eyes inward for near work—may be the most common nonstrabismic binocular finding in TBI patients. *Convergence insufficiency will often be missed by the simple pushup or near point of convergence test.* Krohel et al.[50] found that 6 of 23 TBI patients with convergence insufficiency had a normal near point of convergence but showed abnormal convergence reserves on prism testing. Prism vergence ranges should be mandatory in the visual evaluation of the TBI patient. Convergence insufficiency can lead to fatigue, headache, tearing, blurred vision, and eyestrain.[50] Often, it will cause skipping of words while reading, or transpositions when reading digits in numbers, as the eyes struggle to converge after each saccade. High exophoria (i.e., nonstrabismic outward resting posture of the eyes) is also a common finding in TBI patients. Padula et al.[11] hypothesizes that exodeviations of the eyes following TBI are caused by damage to the midbrain structures, which integrate ambient vision and spatial orientation.[71] This would be anatomically consistent with simultaneous damage to the mesencephalic structures involved in convergence control.[21] Padula et al. have described posttrauma vision syndrome,[25,26,86] a cluster of common posttraumatic visual deficits which may include high exophoria, convergence insufficiency, and accommodative dysfunction. Using brain response testing (VEPs), Padula et al.[26] demonstrated visual processing abnormalities in posttrauma vision syndrome, as well as improvement in the brain response to visual stimuli with application of low amounts of base-in prism and binasal patching. Their work also provides a clinical protocol for diagnosing posttrauma vision syndrome using the VEP. If posttrauma vision syndrome is diagnosed or suspected, early application of base-in prism and/or binasal patches may be profitable in treatment.

Prior to treating other binocular disorders, monocular eye movement and accommodative dysfunctions should be treated insofar as possible. Treatment of exobinocular disorders may include prism in reading or distance lenses, binasal patches, or therapy. One difficulty with putting base-in prism in lenses is that patients may "prism adapt" over a matter of days or weeks, developing the same phoria through the prisms as they had prior to introduction of the prisms. In such cases, the prescription of base-in prism increases the tonic error in binocular posture, leading some optometrists to argue that prism is poison. However, in a significant number of patients, base-in prisms provide an immediate reduction of symptoms and the patients do not prism adapt. The difficulty is in determining for which patients this will be the case. In-office, short-term trials may help in this decision. In any case, patients wearing base-in prism in their habitual spectacles should be monitored carefully. If they prism adapt, additional prism should not be prescribed.

Besides use of base-in prism, Padula and Shapiro[12] recommend use of bitemporal or binasal occluders (i.e., occluders covering only the temporal portion of both lenses or nasal portion of both lenses, respectively) applied to the patient's habitual spectacles for nonstrabismic visual dysfunctions. They suggest that bitemporal patches may reduce confusion by reducing input from the midbrain ambient vision system when the patient is attempting focal tasks such as reading. Binasal patches may be used in an effort to increase patients' awareness of their ambient vision while eliminating physiologic diplopia (i.e., the normal diplopia for objects in front of or behind the plane of fixation), which may initially cause confusion in the post-TBI patient. They also argue that this encourages reorganization of the midbrain-based ambient visual system, which is critical for visual–spatial organization and vision during movement.

Vision therapy for poorly compensated exophoria or convergence insufficiency should include fusional exercises to improve the amplitude of and the ability to sustain convergence as well as the speed of reflex fusion. Convex lenses may be used to work fusional convergence through the accommodative–convergence loop. Viewing through the convex lens relaxes accommodative–convergence so that the patient must exert more fusional convergence to avoid diplopia. Prisms can be used for manipulating images, causing the fusional vergence system to respond to the displaced image. Polarized or anaglyphic materials may be used to create second- or third-degree fusion targets (i.e., flat fusion or stereoscopic fusion, respectively) that can be manipulated to expand vergence ranges. At the same time, matches are developed between the ocular–motor feedback and position-in-space interpretation. Many specialized instruments have been developed for treatment of such binocular disorders. Some of these techniques may be prescribed for application by occupational therapists. Many of these techniques require more experience in vision therapy or more extensive instrumentation for effective application and therefore need to be performed in the vision-care setting.

Esophoric (i.e., nonstrabismic inward resting posture of the eyes) deviations of binocular vision are less common. This may be the result of anatomic considerations or because esophorias are more difficult to compensate for and are more likely to break down into a strabismus. Poorly compensated esophoria will often cause eyestrain or headache around the eyes or temples. Treatment may include use of convex lenses for near work, base-out prism, and vision therapy similar to that described for exodeviations. The same cautions regarding use of prisms apply here, perhaps even more so, because base-out prism is more difficult to remove once the patient has become dependent on it.

9.7.1.2.3 Strabismus

In strabismic deviations secondary to TBI, diplopia causes disorientation, as well as difficulty with spatial judgments, eye–hand coordination, mobility, and reading. Patients will often squint, close one eye, or assume head turns or tilts to try to block one eye or to keep objects in a field of gaze where they are able to fuse. In children, suppression and amblyopia may result. Patients who are diplopic should have a visual examination early during their rehabilitative program. Assessment of refractive status, binocularity, and ocular health do not require verbal communication from the patient. The same objective techniques that one would use to determine these conditions in a 4-month-old infant can be applied in the TBI population, when necessary. Prisms or partial patching (as discussed later) can be prescribed to eliminate diplopia so that other ongoing therapies can be more effective. Any time that prisms or patches are prescribed, frequent follow-up is required to keep pace with spontaneous and therapy-related recovery.

Fresnel (flat stick-on) prisms may be applied in an effort to reestablish fusion at the angle of the deviation. Lenses may also be applied in a therapeutic manner, using the accommodative–convergence relationship to mediate the angle of the deviation. For patients who are able, therapy is then applied, as described earlier for nonstrabismic errors, creating equal, efficient monocular skills, followed by vergence exercises combined with fusion, depth, and spatial localization training. Initial attempts at reestablishing fusion in adjustable instruments or with variable prisms may be met with horror fusionislike responses in which the images from the two eyes will approach each other and then jump to the other side, or may be superimposed, but not fuse into one object with the percept of depth.[87] The prognosis for recovery is best for patients with horizontal strabismus, uncomplicated by vertical deviations. However, vertical deviations will often resolve with therapy or as therapy is applied to the horizontal component of the strabismus. Residual vertical deviations can often be managed with prism ground into the patient's lenses. Patients who are not able to perform vision therapy for remediation of their strabismus are generally managed over the long term with patches and prism. They may also be managed surgically beyond the time period when spontaneous recovery might continue to lessen the angle of deviation.

Traditionally, TBI patients have been advised to use constant patching of one eye to resolve diplopia. However, this has undesirable consequences, such as loss of peripheral vision on the patched side while patched, and disuse of the patched eye, which may lead to suppression and/or diminish the chances of spontaneous recovery of fusion. *Partial* patching to eliminate diplopia or *patching for limited time periods* to facilitate other therapies is more desirable. If patients are unable to access rehabilitative vision care in a timely manner and diplopia is a major problem, patching the eyes on a daily alternating schedule may minimize the detrimental effects of patching until they can access such care.

Partial patches are tailored to the patient's particular deficit and should encourage recovery. As discussed earlier, binasal patches applied to the patient's spectacles allow for a full field of vision while eliminating diplopia. They are a particularly good patching method for treatment of esotropia and may enhance peripheral awareness while encouraging abduction. If the esotropia is unilateral, a single patch may be applied to the nasal portion of the patient's spectacles over the nondeviating eye. This technique encourages abduction of the esotropic eye because patients must either abduct that eye or turn their head to view in the visual field ipsilateral to the deviating eye. Exotropic deviations may sometimes be treated with translucent bitemporal patches. Thus, each eye must adduct to view in the contralateral field. However, bitemporal patches limit peripheral vision and are not recommended for long-term application or during ambulation. For patients who fuse in some fields of gaze but who have noncomitant strabismic deviations, partial patches may be applied to a portion of one spectacle lens to occlude only the diplopic field of gaze, allowing for fusion, most of the time. At the same time, vision therapy should be applied to expand the field of comfortable binocular vision.

Partial patches may be as inexpensive as a piece of translucent tape applied to the patient's spectacle lenses. Cling patches[*] are also available commercially. These patches, which stick to the lenses electrostatically, may be easily removed for therapy and reapplied. These also come in varying densities to degrade visual acuity to approximately 20/100, 20/200, or 20/400. The less dense patches enhance patient acceptance because they are, cosmetically, quite good and can hardly be discerned on the spectacle lenses by outside observers. Binasal, bitemporal, and partial patching may not work well for persons with various types of field defects.

Because most TBI patients with secondary strabismus had normal fusion prior to their injury, their prognosis is good for recovering fusion, even if one or more muscles are palsied.

---

[*] Cling Patch: Available from Bernell Corporation, Mishawaka, IN, www.bernell.com.

Even in apparent paresis of the muscle, recovery can occur, although the prognosis is more guarded. If a horror fusionislike response is elicited on initial testing, peripheral fusion techniques emphasizing depth and SILO (smaller in/larger out; described later) may be used until the patient is able to fuse more central targets. *Antisuppression therapy should not be used on these patients until there is evidence of their ability to attain central fusion because there is a strong possibility of creating intractable diplopia where there previously was none.*

9.7.1.2.4 Suppression

Suppression is the ability to diminish or eliminate the central vision originating from one eye to avoid diplopia. In children, it may lead to development of amblyopia in a unilaterally suppressed eye. Once suppression develops, antisuppression therapies must be applied to continue with fusional training.

Suppression may be considered either a blessing or a curse, depending on the goal of rehabilitation. If the goal is to restore central fusion with all the fine motor and stereoscopic advantages that come with it, then suppression is to be avoided through proper application of prisms, patching, or early application of vision therapy. If spontaneous resolution and 3 months of intensive vision therapy show no progress at all toward fusion, then perhaps encouraging suppression to develop may be the most effective way of avoiding diplopia.

If the patient cannot learn to fuse or suppress successfully, then a monovision refractive correction may be prescribed in which the spectacle or contact lens for one eye is set for near work and the other lens is set for distance clarity. This creates one clear image at each distance so that, with practice, the patient learns to attend easily to the clear image, giving a stable referent at each distance.

9.7.1.3 Decreased Visual Acuity

TBI patients with decreased visual acuity that cannot be improved by refractive means or by increased contrast will generally profit from standard low vision rehabilitation techniques. Unfortunately, the prospect of accepting their limitations and working hard to learn to use the remaining vision in the most efficient manner possible is not as motivating as the prospect of performing other types of therapy to recover lost visual function. This makes low vision rehabilitation a less positive experience for many patients.

Numerous small telescopes have been developed for magnification of distant objects. These may be hand-held for stationary viewing or for spotting and identification. Increased magnification results in reduced visual field. Therefore, telescopes used only for spotting and identification will generally have higher magnification than telescopes used for distance viewing. Telescopes may also be mounted in the top portion of a spectacle lens for frequent spot reference during such tasks as driving and note taking. A slight downward tilt of the head allows access to the telescope.

For near point tasks, aids range from high-powered convex lenses for near point work, allowing the patient to hold reading material closer, to video enhancement of images via closed circuit television. Bar magnifiers may assist low visual acuity patients in keeping their place during reading. Magnifiers that are hand-held or stand mounted for stability are also frequently used.

One of the difficulties in prescribing for the patient with moderately reduced acuity (20/60 to 20/120) is that many magnifying techniques will slow the process of reading. One must judge whether the patient can be rehabilitated with convex lenses and proper training or whether a magnifier will be of greater assistance. Trial and error to find the correction with which the patient is most comfortable will be a large part of the decision.

9.7.1.4 Decreased Contrast Sensitivity

Contrast sensitivity is the ability to discriminate differences in luminance between adjacent areas. Low contrast situations occur in fog and darkness, and when viewing through media opacities in the eye, such as cataracts. Reduced contrast sensitivity should be suspected when patients with good visual acuity complain of not seeing well. Neural damage in the visual system may also cause poor contrast sensitivity.[88] Damage to the magno system results in a reduction of contrast sensitivity for middle to low spatial frequency (larger contours). Damage to the parvo system results in loss of contrast sensitivity in detailed targets and may result in decreased visual acuity. Patients with diminished contrast sensitivity in the high-frequency range resulting in decreased visual acuity may find magnifying low vision aids helpful. Those with diminished contrast sensitivity for middle to low spatial frequencies are not helped by magnification. Printed material for these patients should be good quality and high contrast. In well-lit conditions, contrast enhancing tints (usually yellow to amber tints that screen out blue light) or overlays may be used. The selection of tint is usually based on the patient's subjective assessment of the quality of their vision. The Cerium Intuitive Colorimeter* is an instrument that allows presentation of colored wavelength filters that can be tested through the spectrum of hues, varying the saturation and brightness to find the lens tint that provides maximal comfort, efficiency, or contrast.

9.7.1.5 Visual Field Loss

Many patients with TBI have resultant visual field loss. Knowledge of visual field defects is important in helping patients adjust their behavior. It is also important for other rehabilitative therapists working with the patient to adjust their therapy, taking the field defect into account. Field defects may be either absolute, when there is no sensation of light or movement from within the scotoma; or relative, when brighter, larger, or moving stimuli may still be sensed within the scotoma. Assessment may range from simple confrontation testing, to tangent screen, to automated perimetry with a fixation monitor. Each has advantages and drawbacks. Confrontation testing can be done with no special equipment on patients who are unable to sit as required for the other tests. It gives a gross assessment of the extent of the visual field in each direction with each eye. However, it will not reveal scotomas within those boundaries. Tangent screen testing allows the examiner to map very closely small scotomas and islands of vision within the field that may not be mapped well on an automated perimeter that presents test points in a predetermined pattern. Automated perimeters with fixation monitoring give a relatively reliable measurement against which one may chart change in the visual field through repeated measures across time. However, the testing is often lengthy, taxing both posture and attention. Although for the general population, a 30-degree automated visual field has become standard of care, in patients with brain injury, a 60-degree field frequently gives a much better understanding of the patient's visual world. Furthermore, one should remember the peripheral crescents that may be spared fall outside even the 60-degree field, so if a patient presents with extremely constricted visual fields but navigates well, confrontation testing should be done to attempt to discover whether he or she is using blindsight, or whether they have a spared peripheral crescent.

---

* Cerium Intuitive Colorimeter: Available from Cerium Optical Products, Tenterden, Kent, England, www. ceriumoptical.com/vistech/colorimetry.aspx.

Probably the most common visual field defect necessitating rehabilitative services is homonymous hemianopia. Rehabilitation has mainly been concentrated on recognizing the field defect and working on compensatory scanning patterns, as well as prism devices to allow more peripheral areas of the scotoma to be viewed with smaller excursions of the head or eyes. Patients with hemianopia may also have mild balance difficulties (with their center of gravity shifted toward the blind field).[89] Yoked prism (discussed later) may be helpful in reestablishing balance.

Compensatory visual search into the scotomatous field is found to expand as a result of training, and these gains remain stable over time. Patients with hemianopic field defects who do not receive training do not tend to use adaptive search strategies.[90] Mirrors can be mounted on spectacle lenses,[91,92] but this technology is not much used anymore, because it is cumbersome. More commonly, Fresnel prisms with their apices toward the pupil are added in the peripheral portion of the lens in the scotomatous fields.[93] These devices move the images that fall in the periphery of the scotomatous field closer to the center of vision. These techniques enhance peripheral awareness because it is easier to view farther into the scotomatous field without head movement, and having the device applied to the spectacles serves as a reminder to do so. Considerable training and motivation are required for successful application of these devices because, when one scans into binocularly applied peripheral prism, the visual world jumps. If the prism is applied monocularly, then patients are diplopic while scanning into the prism and must turn their heads to fixate the object of interest singly after locating it. Rather than using Fresnel prisms, the prism may be ground with patients' spectacle prescription and mounted into their spectacle lens, reducing the optical blur induced by the Fresnel–type prism. Limited visual field recovery has been reported in some patients with this type of peripheral prism system applied monocularly,[52] perhaps from reallocation of cortical receptive fields. For patients with severe visual field constriction, the prism technique may be used in all affected fields.[94]

Peli[95] recommends application of horizontal strips of Fresnel prism (typically 40 pd) placed (base toward the visual field defect) superiorly and inferiorly across the lens on the side of the field defect; for a left hemianopia, one would place the prism strips on the left lens. Peli[95] argues that this creates peripheral diplopia, which is easier to adapt to than a peripheral prism that one scans into, and it cues attention to the unsighted visual field without regard to the lateral position of the eyes. In monocular patients, it may be beneficial to place Peli prisms superiorly only so that the prism does not interfere with vision for mobility. All the peripheral prism systems are useful tools. Each requires adaptation and training. Various patients will prefer one over the other. Peli prisms may also be useful in cases of visual–spatial neglect (discussed later) because there are no eye movements necessary to impose the neglected field on the attended field.

Field expanders or reverse telescopes may be helpful in occasional sighting for orientation, as when entering a room or locating objects on a table. Distortion and minification when viewing through field expanders make them difficult to use and, again, considerable training and motivation are required.[96]

Perceptual speed and perceptual span, often trained with tachistoscopic techniques, are also important. During mobility, the patient with visual field loss must make more fixations to cover the necessary visual expanse. Perceptual speed and span are also important for reading because any visual field loss that approaches the midline will tend to slow the reading process. Patients with left field loss may not see the beginnings of longer words and may misread them as similar words. They also have difficulty returning to the beginning of the next line. The simplest technique for remediating this problem is to keep a finger at the beginning of the next line down, or use an L-shaped marker that marks the line being read and has a bright flag at the beginning of the line to indicate the position of the beginning of the line. Typoscopes or rulers may also be helpful. A contrasting strip of ribbon placed vertically along the left margin is a simple, effective technique. Patients with right hemianopias lose the preview information that allows them to judge the placement of the next saccade and guess at the content of the next word. They also have difficulty judging where to return at the end of a line of print and will often return to the next line too early. A finger, hand, or strip of ribbon held at the end of the line serves as an easy marker. These patients may do better reading upside down or rotating the text 90 degrees and reading vertically so that they can preview the text coming up in their sound visual field.[97] Although this may be more cumbersome initially, vertical or upside down reading improves with time, whereas the left-to-right reading will always be impaired as a result of lack of peripheral vision guiding the saccade to the next word.

There have been reports in the literature of some partial resolution of hemianopia through training with lit targets moving from the scotoma toward the intact visual field and scanning into the scotoma.[51,98] These findings have been questioned by Balliet et al.[99] who were unable to replicate findings of recovery by training with lit targets. They bring up valid concerns regarding this controversial issue. However, Balliet et al. used smaller targets in their training than were used in the original studies because the smaller target led to less intrasubject variability. In therapy, variable responses may be the hallmark of recovery. In their desire for scientific reproducibility, Balliet et al. may have thrown away the therapeutic effect. Kerkhoff et al.,[51] in a study that had positive results, used a three-step training procedure that included (1) performing large saccades into the blind field, (2) improving visual search on projected slides, and (3) transfer of both to activities of daily living. With this procedure, they were training skills that the patient needed to acquire, and partial resolution of the scotoma seemed to be an additional gift for some of their patients. More recently, computerized systems that present stimuli in the blind field have been marketed for visual restitution of homonymous visual field deficits. The evidence demonstrates no more visual field recovery with these systems than with scanning prism systems.[100]

9.7.1.6 Blindsight

An interesting phenomenon that occurs in some patients with large areas of visual field loss from lesions to primary cortex is blindsight. Patients with blindsight are not consciously aware of vision in the "blind" field. However, they are able to report, at levels well above chance, such things as direction of movement and, on forced-choice "guessing," can discriminate such things as color, location, and sometimes shape. They consistently deny being able to "see" objects, but may navigate obstacle courses, avoiding objects in their path. Subcortical visual pathways have been implicated previously (reviewed by Stoerig and Cowey[101]), including those to the superior colliculus, inferior pulvinar, and the koniocellular layers of the dorsal lateral geniculate nucleus (dLGN). Furthermore, functional neuroimaging has shown that cortical areas in the ventral stream can respond to object stimuli presented to the blind field in blindsight-trained patients. Bridge et al.[102] recently demonstrated, using diffusion-weighted MRI tractography, a direct ipsilateral pathway between the lateral geniculate nucleus to the middle temporal area (MT/V5), without passing through the "primary" visual cortex. Such tracts were reported earlier in the macaque, by Sincich et al.[103] Both Bridge et al.[102] and Sincich et al.[103] hypothesize that this tract may provide for visual detection of moving stimuli following destruction of primary cortex. Furthermore, in a patient who had damage to primary visual cortex at age eight, Bridge et al.[102] demonstrated tracts between visual areas that did not exist in the control subjects. The implication is that using alternative brain areas for processing information following cortical damage (at least during childhood) may enhance other connections, or establish new connections. There have been multiple reports of training blindsight. For example, Chokron et al.[104] trained nine patients with unilateral occipital damage for 22 weeks, presenting forced-choice visual tasks such as pointing to visual targets, letter recognition and identification, visual comparison between the two hemifields, and target localization. All patients improved on blindsight tasks following training, and eight of the nine patients showed enlargement of their visual field on automated perimetry.

9.7.1.7 Photophobia

Photophobia (i.e., extreme light sensitivity) is a common aftereffect of head trauma.[105] Jackowski,[106] using dark adaptation studies, has demonstrated damage to rod-mediated visual mechanisms in brain injury patients with significant photophobia, even though they seldom complain of their night vision being reduced. The rods (i.e., dim light vision receptors) mainly feed into the magnovisual subsystem. Cone-mediated visual mechanisms were also damaged in these patients, but these deficits were small in comparison with the rod-mediated visual loss. The cones (i.e., daylight vision receptors) mainly feed into the parvo pathway. The magno and parvo pathways are mutually inhibitory. Jackowski[106] has hypothesized from her findings that damage to the rod system (or magno pathway) disinhibits the cone (or parvo pathway), causing this bright-light-sensing pathway to be overly responsive; this mechanism may be the cause of posttraumatic photophobia in many patients.

Patients who have posttraumatic binocular disorders or pupil dilation of one or both eyes may also complain of photophobia. Successful treatment of the binocular dysfunction will lessen the photophobia in cases when this is the primary cause. Otherwise, photophobia may be handled with any number of tints in the patient's spectacle lenses, the color and density of which are mainly prescribed for subjective comfort. Patients with extreme photophobia who also experience imbalance and/or visual confusion in visually busy spaces frequently benefit from indoor tints determined by Intuitive Colorimeter testing. These should not be prescribed with maximal brightness attenuation, even if the patient prefers this, because they will be too dark for indoor wear.

Photochromic lenses that darken in sunlight and lighten indoors may be helpful, although they do not darken well for driving applications. Although eye protection from ultraviolet radiation should be a consideration for everyone, it is even more important to incorporate ultraviolet protection into tinted lenses for patients with mydriatic pupils. In extreme cases of mydriasis, it is sometimes possible to prescribe an opaque custom contact lens with a small transparent pupil to decrease the light entering the eye. However, often, patients with mydriatic pupils have dry eyes, and contact lenses would be contraindicated.

9.7.2 Assessment and Rehabilitation of Perception/Integration

9.7.2.1 Localization and Spatial Vision

There is little information on effects of brain injury on the magno pathway until it reaches cortex. However, it is known that the large axon diameter of the magno cells makes them more vulnerable to various types of damage, as in glaucoma and Alzheimer's disease.[65] Disorders of motion perception are rare.[107] Indeed, studies in monkeys show that a lesion in the middle temporal area produces disorders of motion perception but that most of these disappear within a few days, presumably because the function is taken over by redundant pathways. Damage to the posterior cerebral cortex often results in spatial inattention to the contralateral visual field known as *unilateral spatial neglect* (USN) or *visual–spatial neglect* (VSN), both of which are discussed later.

A number of reception dysfunctions affect perception of spatial localization and orientation. For instance, we use the feedback from our vergence system to assist us in judging distance. If our eyes are more converged, then the target we are fixating is seen as closer. In persons with good binocularity, this effect, called *SILO*,[108] can be demonstrated by the use of prisms. If one fixates a target and places base-out prism in front of the eyes, the images of the target are moved in a convergent direction and the eyes must converge to avoid diplopia. The target will be perceived as having moved *in* toward the observer and will appear smaller than before. Size constancy dictates that objects get larger as they come closer, but because the target has not really moved, the image size on the retina remains unchanged. Therefore, because the vergence system says the object is closer but the image size remains unchanged, the interpretation must be that the object is now smaller. Base-in prism produces the opposite effect—the eyes diverge, the object appears to move out and away from the observer, and appears larger. As a result of the roles of accommodation and convergence in depth perception,[73] sudden onset of dysfunctions in accommodation or convergence secondary to TBI can make objects appear closer or farther away than they actually are, effectively collapsing or expanding visual space.

Conversely, feedback from the cortical and subcortical spatial processors affects the vergence system. For example, one type of convergence is driven strictly by proximity to an object; targets close to the face make us converge even though we may be viewing through an optical system set at infinity. The TBI patient with a primary visual–spatial disturbance will often have inaccurate eye pointing.

Feedback in visual–spatial processing runs both ways, from the binocular system to visual–spatial processors and from visual–spatial processors to the binocular system. Therefore, the most effective therapy for disorders of spatial perception in depth must take into account the binocular response. Similarly, the most effective treatment for eye teaming will often concentrate not only on achieving the correct motor response but also on creating correct spatial judgments, which can be used to guide the motor response.

Other difficulties in spatial organization may be reflected in inability to localize objects properly in relation to oneself. Egocentric "midline shifts" of varied etiologies have been noted in patients following brain injury. These shifts in midline perception can cause shifts in posture and weight distribution, which may cause difficulty with balance and gait. They may also affect eye–hand coordination. Tests used to detect egocentric visual midline shifts include line bisection tasks[109,110] and, more commonly, subjective judgment by the patient of when a wand or pencil, held in a vertical orientation and moved laterally, is directly on the horizontal midline (i.e., in front of nose).[12] Visual field defects, hemifield visual neglect, disruption of the midbrain ambient visual system, tonic ocular–motor imbalance, and imbalances in extraocular proprioception, or efferent copy commands to the extraocular muscles, are all possible causes of midline shift. As described by De Renzi,[111] tonic ocular–motor imbalance is an increased tone in the muscles turning the eyes to the side contralateral to the lesion. During routine testing, it is masked by the fixation mechanism, but it can be elicited by having the patient attempt to look straight ahead in darkness. During development, we learn to maintain position constancy of objects despite eye movements by comparing the efferent copy (commands going out to the eye muscles) and proprioceptive information received from the eye muscles, with the movement of the retinal image.[78] As the eyes, extraocular muscles, and separation between the eyes grow and change, slow adjustments in these systems take place. However, in TBI, a sudden change in any one of these systems may occur, changing the perceived location of objects in relation to ourselves.

Therapy for spatial distortions may include therapy for accommodative and convergence disorders as described earlier, with special emphasis on development of SILO and spatial localization. Lenses and prisms may be applied in either a compensatory manner or for therapy purposes. Spatial and postural effects of these optical devices are thoroughly reviewed by Press.[112] Padula et al.[11] advocate the use of small amounts of base-in prism to facilitate reorganization of the ambient system by reducing stress on the peripheral fusional system in cases of exophoria. Yoked prisms (i.e., equal amounts of prism in front of each eye with both bases in the same direction—up, down, right, or left) are an effective intervention for many cases of egocentric midline shift. These prisms move images of the surrounds in the direction of the apex of the prism for both eyes. Low amounts of yoked prism may be used in a compensatory manner[25,113] to shift images of objects that belong on the visual midline to the recently misplaced perceived visual center; this relieves the perceptual mismatch between what actually *is* and what is perceived, often restoring balance, normal gait, and the ability to move about easily in the world. More often, large amounts, such as 15 prism diopters, will be used in therapy to force problem solving and increase flexibility in the sensorimotor system. Activities, such as walking or tapping a swinging ball, while wearing these prisms involve recalibration and integration of vestibular, proprioceptive, kinesthetic, and extraocular efferent copy systems. This is an extremely effective technique for disrupting habitual patterns in patients who have been unresponsive to more instrument-based therapies so that, with guidance, they can reorganize their visual–motor system in a more adaptive manner. It is important to note that, in an observer with a normal visual system, prism adaptation would be expected to occur with long-term wear. Therapeutically, yoked prisms are only worn for periods extending from a few minutes to a few hours. Presumably, those individuals who experience a long-term compensatory effect wearing yoked prism full time have visual dysfunction that precludes prism adaptation to this prescription. This reasoning makes sense in that, if these patients had been able to do the sort of reorganization that prism adaptation requires, they would probably not have sustained an egocentric visual midline shift.

9.7.2.2 Visual Spatial Neglect

VSN, sometimes termed *visual hemi-inattention* when it affects an entire hemifield, is a phenomenon during which a portion of space is simply unattended, as if nothing existed there. On a visual field test, it may appear as a hemianopia. But, worse, patients are unaware of the defect. This makes them more prone to accident and more difficult to rehabilitate than the patient with hemianopia without neglect. When neglect affects only the visual system, it may easily be mistaken for hemianopia and, indeed, often coexists with true hemianopia. VSN is frequently concomitant with neglect of other senses, such as audition, as well as motor neglect, in which case the entire phenomenon is termed *unilateral spatial neglect* or *unilateral hemi-inattention*. Split-brain research[114] has provided evidence that the right hemisphere allocates attention to both visual fields, whereas the left hemisphere allocates attention to only the contralateral field (Figure 9.4). This finding in split-brain patients suggests that the right hemisphere allocation of attention to the right visual field is probably mediated through subcortical mechanisms. It may also help explain why most cases of overt neglect are secondary to right brain damage.

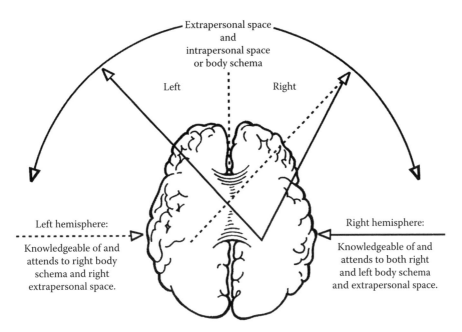

FIGURE 9.4
Allocation of spatial attention by the cortical hemispheres. The right hemisphere allocates spatial attention to both the right and left visual fields, whereas the left hemisphere allocates attention only to the right visual field. Thus, USN of the left visual field (following right brain damage) is considerably more common than USN of the right visual field. (Adapted from Moore, J. C. and Warren, M., *Effect of Visual Impairment on Postural and Motor Control following Adult Brain Injury*, Continuing education workbook by visABILITIES Rehab Services, Inc., www.visabilities.com. With permission.)

Although VSN of an entire hemispace is easily mistaken for hemianopia, the mechanisms and damaged brain substrates underlying VSN are quite different from hemianopia. Hemianopia is a sensory loss, in which the damaged neural substrates are in the postchiasmal visual pathway up to and including primary visual cortex. VSN is a perceptual deficit, in which the neural substrates necessary for sight are intact, but the visual substrates or pathways necessary to attend to or perceive the sensory input are not. VSN may best be thought of as a competitive process, where gradients of attention are distributed across the two halves of the visual field and, often, also in a superior–inferior direction. The more stimuli there are on the more attended side, the denser the neglect for the less attended side becomes. VSN may involve, separately or concurrently, the patient's own body (personal neglect), the space within arms reach (peripersonal neglect), or the space beyond arms reach (distant neglect). Object perception may be involved such that only half the object is perceived. VSN should be thought of as a syndrome that involves one or more multiple neural substrates, rather than a unitary disorder.[115]

The neural substrates for neglect lie in multiple centers of the brain. The posterior parietal cortex, temporoparietal junction, portions of the dorsolateral frontal lobes, as well as the parietofrontal pathways, the caudate portion of the superior temporal gyrus, the cingulated gyrus of the limbic system, and subcortical areas such as the pulvinar in the thalamus, and the putamen and caudate nucleus in the basal ganglia have all been implicated in neglect.[7,116–118]

Various tests, including drawing, line cancelation, pointing to objects scattered around the room, reading a newspaper article, and line bisection, have been developed to determine the presence of VSN. VSN may vary in degree and appear on some tests but not others.[119] Inattention may also be differentially distributed along the vertical meridian of the neglected field.[110,120] As reviewed by Kerkhoff et al.[51] during line bisection tasks, patients with neglect typically transect the line off to the side contralateral to the field defect. Patients with hemianopia generally do the opposite, deviating in the direction of the scotoma. Patients with both are more likely to bisect the line. Compared with patients with hemianopia without VSN, patients with VSN have even more abnormal scan paths when viewing simple figures and with fewer excursions into the blind field.[121]

Clinically, three considerations are important during therapy for VSN (N. W. Margolis, pers. comm.). First, the patient must be made aware of the condition. Second, compensatory strategies, such as scanning and reading strategies, should be taught. Last, these strategies must be generalized to both static, predictable stimuli (e.g., those encountered in reading or walking down a familiar corridor) and to dynamic, unpredictable stimuli (i.e., encountered in new environments). Margolis and Suter[122] review treatments for VSN. However, a singular therapy is worth mentioning here. Rosetti et al.[123] reported that large amounts of yoked prism (15–20 pd) with the bases oriented into the neglected field worn during visual–motor activities created immediate improvement in VSN that lasted hours or days following this therapy. Clinical experience shows that the results can be dramatic in some patients when used in conjunction with other standard VSN therapies. Gordon et al.[124] present a three-step program for remediation of perceptual deficits in patients with right brain damage. Step 1 is basic scanning training. Step 2 is somatosensory awareness and horizontal size estimation, and step 3 is complex visual perception training combined with left-to-right visual scanning within these tasks. They present evidence that, with extensive training, these functions generalize to daily living. Gianutsos and Mathesno[55] reviewed the literature on perceptual rehabilitation in USN and concluded that, overall, the efficacy of therapeutic intervention is supported. However, studies of solely microcomputer-based scanning therapy have not been shown to generalize.[125,126]

9.7.2.3 Object Perception

The visual percept we construct from sensory signals supersedes even the concrete sensation of touch. For instance, if an object (e.g., a square of plastic) is viewed through a minifying lens and is simultaneously manipulated by the hand (with the hand covered so that it cannot be used as a visual cue), the observer reports the square as being smaller than the real square. This is true whether the method of report is visual (e.g., picking a matching square out of a range of squares of various sizes), visual and tactile (e.g., drawing the square to size), or, surprisingly, tactile (e.g., picking a matching square by touch alone).[127]

It has been suggested that, visually, we construct perceptual objects via a two-step process.[128] First, preattentive data-driven filtering produces shapes and registers their features, as in reception. Then, focal attention is used to select a spatial location and integrate the features registered there into a perceptual object. This is analogous to figure–ground organization and should be concept-driven processing rather than data driven or sensation driven. Evidence arguing for this feature integration theory comes from the way that stabilized retinal images fade feature by feature rather than in small random parts. Principles at work during the second integration stage may be the Gestalt principles of proximity, good continuation, similarity, closure, and pragnanz (i.e., simplicity, regularity, or symmetry) or local versus global processing. In addition to integrating visual features, object perception includes cross-modality integration (i.e., integrating auditory, tactile, and olfactory sensations with visual information to complete the perceptual object). Spatial orientation, both the ability to process the orientation of external objects (extrapersonal orientation) and the ability to process the orientation of ourselves with regard to other objects (personal orientation), is discussed here because the treatment modalities are generally more similar to those used with object perception than other spatial dysfunctions. Personal orientation may be supported by the frontal lobe (particularly in the left hemisphere); extrapersonal orientation may be supported by the "where" pathway, particularly the right posterior parietal area.

Assessment and treatment of perceptual/integrative vision must take into account dysfunctions in reception. Multiple tests, with some redundancy, are necessary to diagnose differentially perceptual dysfunction of the visual system. For instance, copy-form tests are useful and may tell you something about spatial organization, but if the forms are poorly reproduced, you do not know whether this is a result of difficulties in reception, perception, visual–motor integration, or fine motor coordination. One must have a battery of tests that probe perceptual functions, such as figure–ground discrimination, closure, and spatial organization, as well as cross-modality and visual–motor integrative functions from different perspectives using different modalities. Gianutsos and Matheson[55] reviewed most of the available perceptual tests in the literature. For a sample test battery, see Aksionoff and Falk.[129] The perceptual workup will generally take 2 to 3 hours to administer and may need to be broken up into multiple sessions for TBI patients who fatigue easily.

During therapy, the patient and therapist must constantly keep in mind that it is the process, not the final answer, that is important. When possible, the strategies patients are using to solve a particular problem in therapy should be discussed. This creates awareness of the process and insight for the therapist, and provides the opportunity for the therapist to suggest modifications to the patient's problem-solving strategy. As reviewed by Groffman,[130] perceptual therapies may be considered as falling into a number of treatment modalities: (1) motor activities; (2) manipulatives; (3) instruments; (4) vision therapy; (5) lens therapy; (6) auditory therapy; (7) workbooks, toys, and games; and (8) computers. The modality is tailored to fit the level and perceptual deficit of the patient.

Although gross motor activities applied in vision therapy have often been criticized by those not involved in therapy, they are sometimes necessary to create more optimal support for the visual system. The eyes and visual system do not exist in isolation; the eyes are horizontally displaced from each other in the head and the biomechanics are such that they are intended to work with a horizontal disparity in relation to gravity. Tilting the head induces ocular torsion. Gross motor activities are also used for creating visual–proprioceptive and visual–kinesthetic matches in ambient space. Vision is dominant over touch in the normal visual system. However, in therapy, proprioceptive and kinesthetic feedback can help teach veridical visual perception. In the rehabilitation setting, many therapeutic activities with these two goals can be taken over by physical or occupational therapists.

Manipulatives are objects that can be used on the tabletop so that they can be handled, rotated, rearranged, and examined in a very concrete way. They allow for learning higher order visual concepts such as visual discrimination, form perception, and spatial orientation and organization with very concrete tools. These include blocks and puzzles specifically designed to teach perceptual skills. Other common examples of manipulatives are flannel boards (used with felt shapes of varied sizes and colors), geo boards (i.e., boards with evenly spaced pegs on which designs are made by stretching rubber bands between the pegs), or Peg-Boards, which can be used for reproducing patterns with or without rotations in orientation. Manipulatives also provide excellent eye–hand coordination activity.

A variety of instruments have been developed for visual perceptual training. Instrument techniques are varied and seem to provide additional motivation to many patients. An example would be adjustable-speed tachistoscopes, which are used to increase visual perceptual speed and span, as well as visual attention and short-term memory. Tachistoscope targets may vary from abstract geometric forms to be copied, to digit strings or words. They are also useful to demonstrate VSN or hemifield loss to the patient because, without time to scan, they will only see the portion of the word presented in the intact field.

Application of vision therapy to remediate receptive dysfunction often involves visual perception, both in spatial organization as discussed earlier and in that many fusion tasks require figure–ground discrimination. Lens and prism therapy were discussed earlier in terms of shifts in the localization and orientation of local surrounds.

Use of the auditory modality can enhance integration of visual and auditory senses. A number of tape and record programs are available for development of various perceptual and perceptual–motor skills including spatial relations, directionality, and visual–motor integration.[131]

Many workbooks, toys, and games are available in educational supply stores, including popular activities with hidden pictures or words for figure–ground discrimination, and form perception. Worksheets with simple, incomplete figures to be completed by the patient may be used for development of closure, as well as form perception. These tools also help develop eye–hand coordination. They are generally two-dimensional representations but have the advantage that, after patients understand the process, they may practice unsupervised with worksheets.

With most of these activities, the understanding of the visual goals, experience, and creativity of the therapist are key to the success of therapy. However, through development of computer programs, perceptual therapy has become more accessible and more easily administered by other rehabilitation disciplines, such as occupational therapy. A number of perceptual programs that combine the challenge and motivation of a video game with good perceptual therapy are commercially available. Such programs were reviewed by Press[132] in 1987. Although more programs have been marketed since then, many of the same companies are developing them, and Press' review[132] is a good resource for those interested in applying these techniques. Computer therapy generally requires the ability to manipulate a joystick or press a limited number of response keys. For patients with motor control problems, this may be easier than using workbooks or manipulatives.

9.7.2.3.1 Visual Agnosias

Agnosia is the inability to recognize objects visually. Object recognition may be apperceptive, where the perception of the object is faulty, or associative, where the object is perceived correctly but cannot be associated with prior memories or past experience.[133] In apperceptive agnosia, patients might not be able to match similar objects, draw or copy objects or shapes, or name objects by sight. However, if allowed to use tactile input, they could both name and match the object, as well as describe its function. Apperceptive agnosia is rare and is associated with diffuse cerebral damage of the occipital lobes and surrounding areas.

In associative agnosia, objects and shapes can be matched, but the patients are unable to associate them with past experience or function. For instance, they may be able to draw a key that is placed before them but be unable to name it or describe its function. When allowed to handle the key, they could both name it and relate that it is used to unlock a door. Associative agnosias can be surprisingly specific. The more common types of agnosia include object agnosia, prosopagnosia (i.e., inability to recognize familiar faces), and color agnosia.

Diagnosis of visual agnosias is important in deciding the proper course of treatment— therapy or compensation. Associative agnosias may be the result of lesions in the pathway that connect the visual "what" pathway with memory areas. De Haan et al.[134] have shown that covert recognition of objects and faces may exist in the absence of overt recognition. They suggest that this may provide a foundation for rehabilitation. Sergent and Poncet[135] report some restoration of overt face recognition under specific circumstances in one patient. Although, in some cases, restoration of function may be possible, therapy to address the agnosia directly is likely to be a long process, and success is not guaranteed. Compensatory strategies, as for low vision/blind patients, may be the best alternative for immediate management of agnosia.

9.7.2.3.2 Alexia

An important part of text recognition is the decoding of visual percepts into language. Interruption of visual pathways at the left angular gyrus[136] or splenium[137] prevent this decoding process from occurring, resulting in acquired alexia or inability to read. Most case reports of this dysfunction show some residual reading function. Treatment of alexia using integration strategies and based on the patient's residual reading skills has been successful. Often, a letter-by-letter reading strategy can be used by these patients, although it severely slows reading. Motor rehearsal, in terms of copying or tracing letters and words, as well as flash card techniques pairing the written with the spoken word have been applied with some success.

A successful strategy used with one patient is described by Daniel et al.[136] Initially, the patient spelled words aloud from flash cards and then said the word (as he recognized the word from auditory spelling). With practice, the patient was able to substitute covert spelling. Continued practice in this manner significantly increased his ability in reading and naming so that he was able to return to work within 4 months postinjury. At the 1 year follow-up, reading was still laborious, but the patient was able to read sufficiently to function in his job.

9.7.3 Assessment and Rehabilitation of Motor Output/Behavior

Visually directed motor output includes not only the planning and execution of eye–hand coordination and visually guided movement through space, but also the planning and execution of the next eye movement. As in the model presented in Figure 9.3, reception affects perception, which affects cognition, and both of the latter affect programming of the next eye movement, feeding back into reception (control of binocularity, eye movements, and fixation). This is a flexible, but closed, loop.

9.7.3.1 The Eyes

Most aspects of assessment and rehabilitation of motor output to the eyes have been discussed in Section 9.7.1 in this chapter. The rehabilitation already discussed is generally performed in the vision-care setting. Some specific exercises may be prescribed for application by occupational therapists in either inpatient or outpatient rehabilitation settings.

In addition to the aspects of ocular–motor and binocular control, which have already been discussed, ocular–motor planning and integration with the output controllers to the eyes are involved. Ocular–motor gaze apraxia is the inability to execute purposeful eye movements (reviewed by Roberts[133]). Patients with ocular–motor gaze apraxia may be differentially affected for various stimuli (e.g., unable to change fixation in response to verbal commands or peripheral visual, auditory, or touch stimuli). This may be exploitable in that one may be able to practice saccades to a multimodality stimulus and wean out the intact modality. An activity such as letter tracking,* during which one underlines rows of letters until a target letter is reached and then circles the target letter, may allow tactile–proprioceptive feedback to help guide eye movements. Treatment here falls into the realms of neuropsychology, occupational therapy, and vision therapy.

Compensatory strategies should be trained at the same time that remediation is attempted. Many compensatory strategies developed for low vision or the blind may be useful. Other strategies that lessen the necessity of looking in a particular location or reduce the need to scan can also be taught. For instance, moving the television away or using a small screen lessens the need to scan the scene in an organized fashion.

9.7.3.2 The Hands

Eye–hand coordination will be affected by receptive and perceptual problems, as well as by motor planning and integration of percepts with motor output controllers. Mild difficulties that occur developmentally in these areas will often result in clumsiness or difficulty with such tasks as producing clear handwriting. More severe dysfunction is described by two terms: *optic ataxia* and *constructional apraxia*.

Optic ataxia is an inability to guide the hand visually toward an object. Differentiating optic ataxia from primary dysfunctions in motor control can be achieved by having patients touch their index finger on one hand with the index finger on the other. Usually, in optic ataxia, the misreaching occurs for objects in the peripheral field. However, in more severe cases, misreaching will occur for visually fixated objects.[133] For milder cases, training the patient to visually fixate manipulated objects may be all that is required.

Constructional apraxia generally results from lesions of the posterior parietal lobe or the junction between the occipital, parietal, and temporal lobes. It may be the result of perceptual deficits, more frequently associated with right-hemisphere lesions, or motor function deficits, more frequently associated with left-hemisphere lesions. Walsh[138] lists differential effects on drawing that may be used to discriminate between perceptual and motor etiologies. For instance, right-hemisphere lesions will tend to result in energetic, scattered, or fragmented drawings with a loss of spatial relations and orientation; left-hemisphere involvement tends to result in drawings that are spatially intact and coherent, but are simplified and laborious, lacking in detail.

Again, treatment here falls into the realms of neuropsychology, occupational therapy, and vision therapy. A multitude of hand–eye coordination activities exists in the literature. For constructional apraxia, the differentiation should be made as to whether it is primarily perceptual or primarily motor, and treatment should emphasize that modality.

---

* Letter Tracking: Available from Academic Therapy Publications, Novato, CA.

9.7.3.3 The Body

As discussed earlier, receptive and perceptual dysfunctions can lead to adoption of head tilts or turns and shifts in posture, creating or complicating problems in balance during standing and walking. Patients are often unaware of these postural adjustments and, when asked, will deny any distortion in their percept and usually in their posture, even though something as easily noticed as a pronounced head tilt may be present. Testing for binocular dysfunctions and conditions that may contribute to egocentric midline shifts in the vertical and horizontal directions has been discussed. The vision practitioner must take a careful history and specifically ask about difficulty with balance, instability, mobility, and so forth, because most patients with these symptoms will often not bother to tell an eye doctor about these difficulties, because they assume the symptoms are unrelated to their eyes.

If a binocular dysfunction exists, the associated postural problems generally resolve as the binocular problem is remediated or when appropriate patching is applied. Treating the binocular difficulty not only relieves the diplopia or intermittent loss of fusion that can cause patients to adopt compensatory head and body postures, it may also involve teaching patients to reorganize their visual space in which the binocular problem has created distortions.

In the case of an egocentric midline shift, the specific etiology is often not diagnosed. Tests for midline shift or observing immediate responses to large amounts of yoked prism may be the extent of the diagnostic procedures. The effects of yoked prism on spatial organization and resultant shifts in posture with a normal visual system are well documented (reviewed by Press[112]). Yoked prisms move the images of the ambient surrounds in the direction of the apex of the prism for both eyes. In the normal visual system, this gives a fun house effect. It is, initially, rather disturbing during head movements and walking to have the world shifted to the right or left or, seemingly, stretched upward or squashed downward before you. Base-up prism will generally cause wearers to shift their weight backward onto their heels; base-down prism generally has the opposite effect, causing the wearer to shift weight forward onto the toes. Sometimes, these prisms may be prescribed to assist the physical therapist in rehabilitation of standing and walking. Often, with TBI patients, yoked prism applied in one lateral direction will create no noticeable difference and application in the opposite direction will make them unable to walk as they try to balance against the shift in surrounds. This type of behavior is a good indication that yoked prism therapy or compensatory yoked prism in patients' spectacle lenses can help normalize their posture and balance, either by reorienting their egocentric visual midline or by moving the image of the outside world to match their new internal visual midline. Patients who veer in one direction while walking may also benefit. Even without a visual midline shift, yoked prisms used for short therapy periods may be useful in breaking down maladaptive habitual postures that are resistant to treatment.

Similarly, visual interventions may be useful in patients with upper limb hemiparesis, although there is not a visual cause. Practicing visual imagery of movement of the paralyzed limb in conjunction with physical and occupational therapy can improve outcomes over therapy alone.[139]

9.7.4 Assessment and Rehabilitation of Visual Thinking/Memory

Visual images may be stored in either analogue or verbal storage. Therefore, when attempting to rehabilitate visual thinking and memory, it is important to be sure that the patient is not merely encoding the information verbally, but actually forming the mental image. Unlike visual perception, which is largely a bottom-up process, visual imagery is largely a top-down process. Visual imagery uses visual information that has been previously organized and stored; therefore, it is often possible to use visual imagery even though, after a TBI, visual input and perception may be disordered. Thus, sometimes, it may be trained in parallel with, or even in the absence of, organized visual perception.

Visualization, or use of visual imagery, has long been considered a useful high-end visual task by therapy-oriented optometrists. Visualization can be used for visual memory enhancement, such as visualizing the spelling of a word, or for spatial relations and spatial organization, such as visualizing object rotations or visualizing a map of how to get home from the grocery store. Numerous studies using various biologic indices (e.g., electrophysiology, cerebral blood flow, and other types of brain activity imaging) as well as studies of adults with brain damage show that, when internally constructing visual imagery, we may use many of the same visual representations as in constructing visual percepts from sensory input (reviewed by Farah[140] and Kosslyn and Thompson[141]). Techniques based on visual imagery may be used effectively for perceptual therapy for those patients who do not have manipulative abilities, provided that they are effective at using imagery. Problem solving with visual imagery occurs by using both visual imagery from memory and from imagination. These are separate skills and are used differently in problem solving.[142]

Visual memory, particularly visual sequential memory, is frequently impaired following TBI. Often, when there is post-TBI memory loss, verbal compensatory strategies are used, such as list making and writing in a calendar or log. These techniques rely heavily on left-hemisphere mechanisms. Rehabilitation of visual memory, which can be built on visual imagery, a heavily right-hemisphere function,[143] can provide supportive memory function and help organize incoming visual information, reducing general confusion.

There are many well-standardized tests that tap visual memory. One such test, which taps short-term visual memory and visual sequential memory, is the Test of Visual-Perceptual Skills.[144] An advantage of the Test of Visual-Perceptual Skills is that it allows the patient simply to point to the correct answer, minimizing the need to generate complex motor or verbal responses. It also provides separate assessments of visual memory for figures and visual sequential memory, the latter being critical in reading comprehension and in creating order from the visual information received.

One representative technique for practicing visual imagery from memory and improving visual memory is to use flannel boards. The therapist and patient have matching felt forms such as squares, circles, rectangles, and triangles of varying sizes and colors; each of them also has a flannel board on which to place the forms. The therapist places some of the forms on a flannel board in a spatial or sequential pattern. The patient is instructed to form a mental image of the pattern presented without using words to describe it. Then, the therapist's board is covered and the patient reproduces the pattern on his or her flannel board. As the performance improves, the number of forms is increased, the exposure time is reduced, and the delay between exposure and reproduction is increased to encourage transfer to long-term memory. Distracters may be interposed during the delay between exposure and reproduction. Flat, three-dimensional blocks, available commercially in foam or wood, can be used for patients who have difficulty manipulating felt forms.

Using visual imagery from imagination is a separate skill and is used in problem solving. Activities that emphasize this skill would include solving constructional or rotational problems.

9.8 Summary

The term *visual rehabilitation* is so broad that it often encompasses the services of neuro-psychologists, occupational therapists, and psychotherapists, in addition to ophthalmologists and optometrists, and specially trained orthoptists, vision therapists, or orientation and mobility specialists. Besides damage to the receptive structures, such as the eye and optic nerve, visual dysfunction may be caused by damage to any lobe of the brain, as well as midbrain structures and cranial nerves. Functional deficits include photophobia, decreased visual acuity or contrast sensitivity, ocular–motor disorders, binocular dysfunction (including strabismus), visual field loss, spatial disorientation, imbalance, unilateral spatial neglect, other visual perceptual disorders, integration disorders, and problems with visually guided motor planning and motor output.

Visual sequelae are quite commonplace in the TBI patient, but are often overlooked. Therefore, when the medical/surgical rehabilitation of the visual system is complete, the issue of functional recovery or compensation must be examined. Vision-care specialists who provide other patient populations with orthoptic or vision therapy or low vision services will generally be able to adapt many of their techniques to working with the TBI patient. Treatments often must be innovative and coordinated among the various professionals providing rehabilitative services. Visual sequelae to TBI can affect the patient's ability to perform such varied tasks as reading, walking, and driving. Unrehabilitated functional visual deficits can interfere with other therapies and with the patient's ability to perform activities of daily living, as well as return to work or school. They may also be a source of emotional turmoil, because the patient may experience unexplained feelings of imbalance, spatial distortion, or visual confusion, and may be unjustly suspected of malingering.

The neuroanatomy of the visual system is so complex that, to provide effective therapy, one must have a working model with which to organize rehabilitation. Such a model is presented in Figure 9.3. The major components of the model to be considered in diagnosis and therapy are (1) sensory input/reception, (2) perception/integration, (3) motor output/behavior, and (4) visual thinking/memory. In this model, each component affects the other. Our receptive functions affect perception and survival motor outputs. Our percepts affect our motor planning/output, as well as our thinking and memories. Our thinking and memories mediate our perceptions, as well as affect our motor planning/output; motor planning and output determine where our bodies are and how we are going to use our eyes next, mediating receptive function. Carefully planned vision therapy or use of lenses and prisms can intervene in any of these areas in a constructive way, or disruptively to break down bad adaptations.

The redundancy of the visual system as well as the flexibility of the visual system—demonstrated by experiments such as adaptation to inverting prisms, together with clinical experience such as therapeutic remediation of strabismus and amblyopia in adults—makes recovery of function a reasonable goal for many visual dysfunctions following TBI. Although one cannot always predict which patients will respond to such therapy, it seems inappropriate to offer less if there is a chance of recovery. When therapy is ineffective at restoring function within a reasonable time frame, there are many compensatory devices and strategies that can be applied, such as partial patching, prisms, or low vision devices and techniques. Even these should be prescribed with an eye toward maximizing function within the limits set by the patient's condition. The multiple deficits in sensation, speech and language, cognition, behavior, emotional state, and motor control encountered in TBI patients add to the challenge of providing effective vision care and make an interdisciplinary team approach most effective in returning the patient to optimal function.

9.9 Illustrative Visual Case Studies

9.9.1 Patient J.G.

J.G. was seen for vision evaluation 4 years after sustaining a mild TBI when she slipped and hit her head. Since then, she had been unable to read, sew, or do any near work for more than 10 minutes without getting a headache. She also complained of dizziness and photophobia. She had been through vision therapy previously, but on an intermittent basis as a result of geographic constraints. She was admitted to a postacute inpatient rehabilitation setting for treatment.

J.G. was diagnosed with accommodative and convergence insufficiencies, as well as a saccadic dysfunction. Based on her symptoms and these findings, a working diagnosis of posttrauma vision syndrome was indicated. Glasses were prescribed for full-time wear. Because J.G. was orthophoric at distance, base-in prism was not prescribed. However, she received a bifocal (to compensate for her accommodative insufficiency) with binasal patches (to help reduce her visual confusion and reorient her in space). J.G. reported immediate relief of many symptoms, with decreased photophobia and increased ability to do near work while wearing this prescription. Because her stay would be limited and her visual complaints were central to her rehabilitation, J.G. was seen weekly in the optometrist's office for vision therapy. Exercises were prescribed for convergence, accommodation, and saccadic dysfunction, which were administered by occupational therapists daily at the rehabilitation center. J.G. responded well to her prescription, binasal patching, and vision therapy. She simultaneously underwent vestibular therapy with the physical therapists. Within 3 months, the binasal patches were removed from her glasses, and she was able to read and sew as long as she liked (which turned out to be for hours at a time). She continued to wear the glasses full-time. The rehabilitation center arranged for her to spend an evening waitressing in a local restaurant (this was her former occupation), and she performed so well that the owner offered her a job. She returned to her home feeling fully rehabilitated and ready to return to her preinjury work and home life.

Two factors may have contributed to J.G.'s dramatic recovery in this case. She was in a rehabilitation setting where she was able to take advantage of coordinated rehabilitation services on a constant, rather than intermittent, basis. Also, placing her in a full-time prescription with binasal patches provided her with consistent, organized, visual input so that she could create a stable visual environment.

9.9.2 Patient J.R.

J.R. was seen for vision analysis 2 years post-TBI. He suffered a severe TBI in a motor vehicle accident. His chief complaint was double vision. He was referred by a local optometrist for treatment of large, constant exotropia. His case is notable because, although he had seen at least two ophthalmologists and an optometrist since his injury, no one had diagnosed him with a right hemianopia with visual neglect. He was unaware that he had a visual field defect. He and his family assumed that his spatial disorientation was simply part of his brain injury. When advised of the diagnosis, his mother asked if that was why he always veered to the left when driving. Fortunately, he had only been driving on their property. J. R. also suffered significant memory loss.

J.R. was seen on an outpatient basis, intermittently, for several years. Because he had no previous rehabilitation, working in a half day at the rehabilitation center several times a week and a vision therapy office visit once weekly proved to be a challenge for the family, and J.R. was inconsistent in his attendance and his homework. Nonetheless, over a period of approximately 18 months, the exotropia for which J.R. had been wearing a pirate patch for more than 2 years resolved with vision therapy. Therapeutic techniques included both orthoptic visual therapy and spatial organization. Scanning and visual memory therapy activities were prescribed and administered by occupational therapists and his parents. J.R. learned to scan effectively in familiar environments, but had residual difficulty in busy, unfamiliar environments, such as the shopping mall. Unfortunately, although his memory improved, it remained significantly impaired.

Although his rehabilitation was extended because of less than ideal compliance, J.R. was happy to be rid of his patch and to have better ability to move about in his space-world. He continued to live with his parents and young son. Although he required cueing for many tasks, he was able to help raise his son, participate in sports, and maintain a part-time job as a dishwasher in a restaurant.

9.9.3 Patient C.L.

C.L. was seen for visual evaluation 13 years after a TBI sustained in a motor vehicle accident. Her chief complaints at the time of the vision examination were that her eyes rolled back in her head during seizures and she experienced some eyestrain, although her occupational therapist had noted that C.L. complained of headaches and blurred vision after near work.

Examination revealed a convergence insufficiency exotropia (i.e., strabismus when viewing at near point resulting from the inability to converge her eyes). She was diplopic almost constantly when doing tasks within arm's length. When queried about the diplopia, she said that the doctor she saw just after her accident had told her it would go away in time, so she just waited.

Although her phorias were not large (9 prism diopters of exophoria at near), she had almost no elicitable base-out reflex fusion, and abnormal convergence ranges on prism vergence testing with a negative recovery (i.e., after fusion was broken with base-out prism, it required base-in prism to reestablish fusion). Her near point of convergence on pushup testing was 16 inches. Because she had so little fusion response, we were unable to prescribe any outpatient therapy.

C.L. was treated on a daily basis for 2 weeks, 45 minutes per day, using large fusion targets projected on a wall to attain peripheral fusion and SILO. Instrument (amblyoscope) convergence techniques were also applied. After 2 weeks, she was fusing well enough at near point that we were able to prescribe convergence exercises for practice with her occupational therapist at the rehabilitation facility. She continued in-office therapy once weekly and made continued progress with this regimen.

9.9.4 Patient L.R.

L.R. was seen 4 months postinjury with chief complaints of poor depth perception and difficulty keeping things level. Examination revealed a mild (approximately 10 prism diopters) right esotropia and a mild left superior rectus palsy that resulted in a noncomitant vertical component to the eye turn (6 prism diopters in primary gaze, increasing on left gaze). The superior rectus also intorts the eye. Her complaint of difficulty keeping things level probably resulted from a combination of extorsion of the eye and the noncomitancy of the vertical component. Pursuits were jerky. Ductions were full with the right eye and showed a superior temporal restriction with the left eye. Although she appeared to fixate with her left eye during the entire examination, she showed alternating suppression on her stereopsis testing. She also had reduced accommodative amplitude and facility.

Therapy progressed from monocular and biocular (i.e., two eyes open, without fusion) skills to antisuppression activities and in-instrument fusion with vertical and base-in vergences. After 12 weekly sessions in office with an hour of home therapy daily, her extraocular range of motion was full with each eye, with smooth pursuits. She showed no vertical or horizontal phoria, at distance or near, and she was comfortable with her vision. Therapy was continued for six additional sessions to improve fusional and accommodative flexibility. At her 1-year progress check, she had maintained all of her visual gains.

9.9.5 Patient B.B.

Patient B.B. was seen for examination 4 months postinjury. He had no light perception from his right eye as result of optic nerve atrophy following his injury. His left eye was healthy and intact. He presented with decreased acuity (20/80 when reading a vertical column and 20/30 when reading horizontally). He had reduced contrast sensitivity for medium spatial frequencies. He also had a left hemianopia with macular sparing. He had difficulty reading. He watched his feet when walking and tended to veer leftward. Saccades were slow and pursuits were jerky. He had a reduced amplitude of accommodation and was already wearing a bifocal correction, which he found useful. He read at approximately 8 inches from his eyes for the additional magnification.

B.B. was aware that he had a field defect but did little to compensate for it. The physical therapists had already taught him to use a walking stick on the blind side, both for physical support and to protect that side. However, like most patients with hemianopia, he did not scan toward the affected side. During tachistoscopic procedures, he generally missed the first few letters or digits and he, initially, had poor perceptual speed and span. On line bisection tasks, he transected the line at the center or contralateral to the blind field. This is the expected performance for a patient with hemianopia combined with VSN, rather than just a hemianopic defect. On some other tasks, his performance was consistent with a mild case of neglect. For instance, when instructed to scan a wall for target figures, he would scan from right (his intact field) to left. When asked to scan again from left to right, he would become argumentative, stating that he always scanned left to right and then would proceed to scan from right to left again. He showed few other indications of neglect. Copied forms were complete. On crossing-out tasks, he generally covered the entire page, always starting from right to left, but was careful to reach the left margin of the page.

Therapy began with monocular skills and tachistoscopic procedures for perceptual speed and span. These skills improved rapidly with therapy. Peripheral awareness techniques for expanding awareness within his intact field were applied with good success. B.B.'s overall reading speed improved along with his saccadic speed, perceptual span, and perceptual speed.

A number of techniques were applied for making B.B. more aware of space within his blind field. Some of these met with more success than others. He rejected application of Fresnel prism, saying he would rather move his eyes farther without the prism. He actively participated in both tabletop and wall-projected scanning activities, trying to adopt an efficient scanning pattern, moving from far left in his blind field, rightward. However, initially, these activities did not seem to generalize outside the therapy room. He was able to adopt a scanning pattern while walking. He looked left on every fourth step, which helped him walk without deviating leftward. His mobility and reading improved enough through his course of therapy that he was able to return to his life as a student at a junior college.

Acknowledgments

I thank my son, Andrew Suter, for his help, understanding, love, and support through the writing of this chapter. I am also grateful to the patients who have worked so hard in rehabilitation and have taught me so much and to many individual members of the Neuro-Optometric Rehabilitation Association who have contributed greatly to my understanding of the clinical issues herein.

References

1. Suter, P. S., A quick start in post-acute vision rehabilitation following brain injury, *Journal of Optometric Vision Development* 30, 73–82, 1999.
2. Van Essen, D. C., Functional organization of primate visual cortex, in A. Peters and E. G. Jones (Eds.), *Cerebral Cortex: Vol. 3, Visual Cortex*, Plenum Press, New York, 1985, Ch. 7, 259–329.
3. Felleman, D. J. and Van Essen, D. C., Distributed hierarchical processing in the primate cerebral cortex, *Cerebral Cortex*, 1(1), 1–47, 1991.
4. Kaas, J. H., Changing concepts of visual cortex organization in primates, in J. W. Brown (Ed.), *Neuropsychology of Visual Perception*, Lawrence Erlbaum Associates, Hillsdale, NJ, 1989, Ch. 1, 3–32.
5. Mishkin, M., Ungerleider, L. G., and Macko, K. A., Object vision and spatial vision: Two cortical pathways, *Trends in Neurosciences*, 6, 414–417, 1983.
6. Stuss, D. T. and Benson, D. F., Neuropsychological studies of the frontal lobes, *Psychological Bulletin*, 95(1), 3–28, 1984.
7. Mesulam, M. M., Spatial attention and neglect: Parietal, frontal, and cingulate contributions to the mental representation and attentional targeting of salient extrapersonal events, *Philosophical Transactions of the Royal Society of London, Series B, Biological Sciences*, 354(1387), 1325–1346, 1999.
8. Han, M. H., Craig, S. B., Rutner, D., Kapoor, N., Ciuffreda, K. J., and Suchoff, I. B., Medications prescribed to brain injury patients: A retrospective analysis, *Optometry*, 79(5), 252–248, 2008.
9. London, R., Wick, B., and Kirschen, D., Post-traumatic pseudomyopia, *Optometry*, 75(3), 143, 2004.
10. Chan, R. V. and Trobe, J. D., Spasm of accommodation associated with closed head trauma, *Journal of Neuroophthalmology*, 22(1), 15–17, 2002.
11. Padula, W. V., Shapiro, J. B., and Jasin, P., Head injury causing post trauma vision syndrome, *New England Journal of Optometry*, 41(2), 16–20, 1988.
12. Padula, W. V. and Shapiro, J., Post trauma vision syndrome caused by head injury, in W. V. Padula (Ed.), *A Behavioral Vision Approach for Persons with Physical Disabilities*, Optometric Extension Program Foundation, Inc., Santa Ana, CA, 1988, Ch. 14.
13. Goodrich, G. L., Kirby, J., Cockerham, G., Ingalla, S. P., and Lew, H. L., Visual function in patients of a polytrauma rehabilitation center: A descriptive study, *Journal of Rehabilitation Research and Development*, 44(7), 929–936, 2007.
14. Freeman, C. F. and Rudge, N. B., Cerebrovascular accident and the orthoptist, *British Orthoptic Journal*, 45, 8–18, 1988.
15. McKenna, K., Cooke, D. M., Fleming, J., Jefferson, A., and Ogden, S., The incidence of visual perceptual impairment in patients with severe traumatic brain injury, *Brain Injury*, 20(5), 507–518, 2006.

16. Roca, P. D., Ocular manifestations of whiplash injuries, *Annals of Ophthalmology*, 4(1), 63–73, 1972.
17. Gaetz, M. and Weinberg, H., Electrophysiological indices of persistent post-concussion symptoms, *Brain Injury*, 14(9), 815–832, 2000.
18. Lachapelle, J., Ouimet, C., Bach, M., Ptito, A., and McKerral, M., Texture segregation in traumatic brain injury: A VEP study, *Vision Research*, 44(24), 2835–2842, 2004.
19. Lachapelle, J., Bolduc-Teasdale, J., Ptito, A., and McKerral, M., Deficits in complex visual information processing after mild TBI: Electrophysiological markers and vocational outcome prognosis, *Brain Injury*, 22(3), 265–274, 2008.
20. Schlageter, K., Gray, B., Hall, K., Shaw, R., and Sammet, R., Incidence and treatment of visual dysfunction in traumatic brain injury, *Brain Injury*, 7(5), 439–448, 1993.
21. Cohen, M., Groswasser, Z., Barchadski, R., and Appel, A., Convergence insufficiency in brain-injured patients, *Brain Injury*, 3(2), 187–191, 1989.
22. Lepore, F. E., Disorders of ocular motility following head trauma, *Archives of Neurology*, 52(9), 924–926, 1995.
23. Fitzsimons, F. and Fells, P., Ocular motility problems following road traffic accidents, *British Orthoptic Journal*, 46, 40–48, 1989.
24. Ciuffreda, K. J., Kapoor, N., Rutner, D., Suchoff, I. B., Han, M. E., and Craig, S., Occurrence of oculomotor dysfunctions in acquired brain injury: A retrospective analysis, *Optometry*, 78(4), 155–161, 2007.
25. Padula, W. V. and Argyris, S., Post trauma vision syndrome and visual midline shift syndrome, *NeuroRehabilitation*, 6(3), 165–171, 1996.
26. Padula, W. V., Argyris, S., and Ray, J., Visual evoked potentials (VEP) evaluating treatment for post-trauma vision syndrome (PTVS) in patients with traumatic brain injuries (TBI), *Brain Injury*, 8(2), 125–133, 1994.
27. Groswasser, Z., Cohen, M., and Blankstein, E., Polytrauma associated with traumatic brain injury: Incidence, nature, and impact on rehabilitation outcome, *Brain Injury*, 4(2), 161–166, 1990.
28. Schwab, K., Grafman, J., Salazar, A. M., and Kraft, J., Residual impairments and work status 15 years after penetrating head injury: Report from the Vietnam Head Injury Study, *Neurology*, 43(1), 95–103, 1993.
29. Wehman, P., Kregel, J., Sherron, P., Nguyen, S., Kreutzer, J., Fry, R., and Zasler, N., Critical factors associated with the successful supported employment placement of patients with severe traumatic brain injury, *Brain Injury*, 7(1), 31–44, 1993.
30. Najenson, T., Groswasser, Z., Mendelson, L., and Hackett, P., Rehabilitation outcome of brain damaged patients after severe head injury, *International Rehabilitation Medicine*, 2(1), 17–22, 1980.
31. Murray, R., Shum, D., and McFarland, K., Attentional deficits in head-injured children: An information processing analysis, *Brain and Cognition*, 18(2), 99–115, 1992.
32. Shum, D. H., McFarland, K., Bain, J. D., and Humphreys, M. S., Effects of closed-head injury on attentional processes: An information-processing stage analysis, *Journal of Clinical and Experimental Neuropsychology*, 12(2), 247–264, 1990.
33. Stratton, G. M., Some preliminary experiments on vision without inversion of the retinal image, *Psychological Review*, 3(6), 611–617, 1896.
34. DeGutis, J. M., Bentin, S., Robertson, L.C., and D'Esposito, M., Functional plasticity in ventral temporal cortex following cognitive rehabilitation of a congenital prosopagnostic, *Journal of Cognitive Neuroscience*, 19(11), 1790–1802, 2007.
35. May, A., Hajak, G., Gänβbauer, S., Steffens, T., Langguth, B., Kleinjung, T., and Eichhammer, P., Structural brain alterations following 5 days of intervention: Dynamic aspects of neuroplasticity, *Cerebral Cortex*, 17(1), 205–210, 2007.
36. Etting, G. L., Strabismus therapy in private practice: Cure rates after three months of therapy, *Journal of the American Optometric Association*, 49(12), 1367–1373, 1978.
37. Selenow, A. and Ciuffreda, K. J., Vision function recovery during orthoptic therapy in an adult esotropic amblyope, *Journal of the American Optometric Association*, 57(2), 132–140, 1986.
38. Garzia, R. P., Efficacy of vision therapy in amblyopia: A literature review, *American Journal of Optometry and Physiological Optics*, 64(6), 393–404, 1987.

39. Freed, S. and Hellerstein, L. F., Visual electrodiagnostic findings in mild traumatic brain injury, *Brain Injury*, 11(1), 25–36, 1997, Jan.

40. Flax, N. and Duckman, R. H., Orthoptic treatment of strabismus, *Journal of the American Optometric Association*, 49(12), 1353–1361, 1978.

41. Suchoff, I. B. and Petito, G. T., The efficacy of visual therapy: Accommodative disorders and non-strabismic anomalies of binocular vision, *Journal of the American Optometric Association*, 57(2), 119–125, 1986.

42. The 1986/87 Future of Visual Development/Performance Task Force, The efficacy of optometric vision therapy, *Journal of the American Optometric Association*, 59(2), 95–105, 1988.

43. Cohen, A. H., Visual rehabilitation of a stroke patient, *Journal of the American Optometric Association*, 49(7), 831–832, 1978.

44. Cohen, A. H. and Soden, R., An optometric approach to the rehabilitation of the stroke patients, *Journal of the American Optometric Association*, 52(10), 795–800, 1981.

45. Gianutsos, R., Ramsey, G., and Perlin, R. R., Rehabilitative optometric services for survivors of acquired brain injury, *Archives of Physical Medicine and Rehabilitation*, 69(8), 573–578, 1988.

46. Berne, S. A., Visual therapy for the traumatic brain-injured, *Journal of Optometric Vision Development*, 21, 13–16, 1990.

47. Wagenaar, R. C., Van Wieringen, P. C. W., Netelenbos, J. B., Meijer, O. G., and Kuik, D. J., The transfer of scanning training effects in visual inattention after stroke: Five single-case studies, *Disability and Rehabilitation*, 14(1), 51–60, 1992.

48. Kerkhoff, G. and Stögerer, E., Recovery of fusional convergence after systematic practice, *Brain Injury*, 8(1), 15–22, 1994.

49. Ron, S., Plastic changes in eye movements of patients with traumatic brain injury, in A. F. Fuchs and W. Becker (Eds.), *Progress in Oculomotor Research*, Elsevier, New York, 1981, 233.

50. Krohel, G. B., Kristan, R. W., Simon, J. W., and Barrows, N. A., Posttraumatic convergence insufficiency, *Annals of Ophthalmology*, 18(3), 101–102, 104, 1986.

51. Kerkhoff, G., Münβinger, U., and Meier, E. K., Neurovisual rehabilitation in cerebral blindness, *Archives of Neurology*, 51(5), 474–481, 1994.

52. Gottlieb, D. D., Fuhr, A., Hatch, W. V., and Wright, K. D., Neuro-optometric facilitation of vision recovery after acquired brain injury, *NeuroRehabilitation*, 11(3), 175–199, 1998.

53. Weinberg, J., Diller, L., Gordon, W. A., Gerstman, L. J., Lieberman, A., Lakin, P., Hodges, G., and Ezrachi, O., Training sensory awareness and spatial organization in people with right brain damage, *Archives of Physical Medicine and Rehabilitation*, 60(11), 491–496, 1979.

54. McCabe, P., Nason, F., Demers Turco, P., Friedman, D., and Seddon, J. M., Evaluating the effectiveness of a vision rehabilitation intervention using an objective and subjective measure of functional performance, *Ophthalmic Epidemiology*, 7(4), 259–270, 2000.

55. Gianutsos, R. and Matheson, P., The rehabilitation of visual perceptual disorders attributable to brain injury, in M. J. Meier, A. L. Benton, and L. Diller (Eds.), *Neuropsychological Rehabilitation*, Guilford Press, New York, 1987, Ch. 10, 202–241.

56. Mazow, M. L. and Tang, R., Strabismus associated with head and facial trauma, *American Orthoptic Journal*, 32, 31–35, 1982.

57. Gianutsos, R., Cognitive rehabilitation: A neuropsychological specialty comes of age, *Brain Injury*, 5(4), 353–368, 1991.

58. Moore, J. C., Recovery potentials following CNS lesions: A brief historical perspective in relation to modern research data on neuroplasticity, *American Journal of Occupational Therapy*, 40(7), 459–463, 1986.

59. Cohen, A. H. and Rein, L. D., The effect of head trauma on the visual system: The doctor of optometry as a member of the rehabilitation team, *Journal of the American Optometric Association*, 63(8), 530–536, 1992.

60. Schor, C., Imbalanced adaptation of accommodation and vergence produces opposite extremes of the AC/A and CA/C ratios, *American Journal of Optometry and Physiological Optics*, 65(5), 341–348, 1988.

61. Ciuffreda, K. J., The scientific basis for and efficacy of optometric vision therapy in nonstrabismic accommodative and vergence disorders, *Optometry*, 73(12), 735–762, 2002.
62. Bullier, J., Feedback connections and conscious vision, *Trends in Cognitive Sciences*, 5(9), 369–370, 2001.
63. Lamme, V. A. F., Blindsight: The role of feedforward and feedback corticocortical connections, *Acta Psychologica*, 107(1–3), 209–228, 2001.
64. Finkel, L. H. and Sajda, P., Constructing visual perception, *American Scientist*, 82(3), 224–237, 1994.
65. Bassi, C. J. and Lehmkuhle, S., Clinical implications of parallel visual pathways, *Journal of the American Optometric Association*, 61(2), 98–110, 1990.
66. Shapley, R., Parallel neural pathways and visual function, in M. S. Gazzaniga (Ed.), *The Cognitive Neurosciences*, MIT Press, Cambridge, MA, 1995, Ch. 19.
67. Kessels, R. P., Postma, A., and de Haan, E. H., P and M channel-specific interference in the what and where pathway, *NeuroReport*, 10(18), 3765–3767, 1999.
68. De Russo, F. and Spinelli, D., Spatial attention has different effects on the magno- and parvocellular pathways, *NeuroReport*, 10(13), 2755–2762, 1999.
69. Milner, A. D. and Goodale, M. A., Two visual systems re-viewed, *Neuropsychologia*, 46(3), 774–785, 2008.
70. Van Essen, D. C., Anderson, C. H., and Felleman, D. J., Information processing in the primate visual system: An integrated systems perspective, *Science*, 255(5043), 419–423, 1992.
71. Trevarthen, C. and Sperry, R. W., Perceptual unity of the ambient visual field in human commissurotomy patients, *Brain*, 96(3), 547–570, 1973.
72. Lewald, J., Ehrenstein, W. H., and Guski, R., Spatio-temporal constraints for auditory–visual integration, *Behavioral Brain Research*, 121(1–2), 69–79, 2001.
73. Morrison, J. D. and Whiteside, T. C., Binocular cues in the perception of distance of a point source of light, *Perception*, 13(5), 555–566, 1984.
74. Glickstein, M., Cortical visual areas and the visual guidance of movement, in J. F. Stein (Ed.), *Vision and Visual Dysfunction, Vol. 13, Vision and Visual Dyslexia*, CRC Press, Ann Arbor, MI, 1991, Ch. 1, 1–11.
75. Tulving, E., Organization of memory: Quo vadis?, in M. S. Gazzaniga (Ed.), *The Cognitive Neurosciences*, MIT Press, Cambridge, MA, 1995, Ch. 54, 839–847.
76. Baddeley, A., Working memory, in M. S. Gazzaniga (Ed.), *The Cognitive Neurosciences*, MIT Press, Cambridge, MA, 1995, Ch. 47, 755–764.
77. Warren, M., Identification of visual scanning deficits in adults after cerebrovascular accident, *American Journal of Occupational Therapy*, 44(5), 391–399, 1990.
78. Leigh, R. J. and Zee, D. S., *The Neurology of Eye Movements*, 2nd ed., F. A. Davis, Philadelphia, PA, 1991, Ch. 1.
79. Ciuffreda, K. J. and Tannen, B., *Eye Movement Basics for the Clinician*, Mosby, St. Louis, MO, 1995.
80. Rayner, K. and Pollatsek, A., *The Psychology of Reading*, Prentice-Hall, Englewood Cliffs, NJ, 1989, Ch. 11, 393–435.
81. Griffin, J. R., *Binocular Anomalies: Procedures for Vision Therapy*, 2nd ed., Professional Press Books, Fairchild Publications, New York, 1982.
82. Press, L. J. (Ed.), *Applied Concepts in Vision Therapy*, Mosby-Year Book, St. Louis, MO, 1997.
83. Burde, R. M., Savino, P. J., and Trobe, J. D., *Clinical Decisions in Neuro-Ophthalmology*, 2nd ed., Mosby-Year Book, St. Louis, MO, 1992.
84. Kelders, W. P., Kleinrensink, G. J., van der Geest, J. N., Feenstra, L., de Zeeuw, C. I., and Frens, M. A., Compensatory increase of the cervico-ocular reflex with age in healthy humans, *The Journal of Physiology*, 553(Pt. 1), 311–317, 2003.
85. Montfoort, I., van der Geest, J. N., Slijper, H. P., de Zeeuw, C. I., and Frens, M. A., Adaptation of the cervico- and vestibulo-ocular reflex in whiplash injury patients, *Journal of Neurotrauma*, 25(6), 687–693, 2008.
86. O'Dell, M. W., Bell, K. R., and Sandel, M. E., 1998 Study guide: Brain injury rehabilitation, *Archives of Physical Medicine and Rehabilitation*, 79(Suppl. 1), S10, 1998.

87. London, R. and Scott, S. H., Sensory fusion disruption syndrome, *Journal of the American Optometric Association*, 58(7), 544–546, 1987.

88. Kupersmith, M. J., Siegel, I. M., and Carr, R. E., Subtle disturbances of vision with compressive lesions of the anterior visual pathway measured by contrast sensitivity, *Ophthalmology*, 89(1), 68–72, 1982.

89. Rondot, P., Odier, F., and Valade, D., Postural disturbances due to homonymous hemianopic visual ataxia, *Brain*, 115(Pt. 1), 179–188, 1992.

90. Kerkhoff, G., Münβinger, U., Haaf, E., Eberle-Strauss, G., and Stögerer, E., Rehabilitation of homonymous scotomata in patients with postgeniculate damage of the visual system: Saccadic compensation training, *Restorative Neurology and Neuroscience*, 4, 245–254, 1992.

91. Nooney, T. W., Jr., Partial visual rehabilitation of hemianopic patients, *American Journal of Optometry and Physiological Optics*, 63(5), 382–386, 1986.

92. Weiss, N. J., Remediation of peripheral visual field defects in low vision patients, in R. G. Cole and B. P. Rosenthal (Eds.), *Problems in Optometry: Vol. 4, Patient and Practice Management in Low Vision*, J. B. Lippincott, Philadelphia, 1992, Ch. 4.

93. Perlin, R. R. and Dziadul, J., Fresnel prisms for field enhancement of patients with constricted or hemianopic visual fields, *Journal of the American Optometric Association*, 62(1), 58–64, 1991.

94. Hoeft, W. W., The management of visual field defects through low vision aids, *Journal of the American Optometric Association*, 51(9), 863–864, 1980.

95. Peli, E., Vision multiplexing: An engineering approach to vision rehabilitation device development, *Optometry and Vision Science*, 78(5), 304–315, 2001.

96. Drasdo, N. and Murray, I. J., A pilot study on the use of visual field expanders, *British Journal of Physiological Optics*, 32, 22–29, 1978.

97. Prokopich, L. and Pace, R., Visual rehabilitation in homonymous hemianopia due to cerebral vascular accident, *Journal of Vision Rehabilitation*, 3, 29, 1989.

98. Zihl, J. and von Cramon, D., Restitution of visual field in patients with damage to the geniculo-striate visual pathway, *Human Neurobiology*, 1(1), 5–8, 1982.

99. Balliet, R., Blood, K. M., and Bach-y-Rita, P., Visual field rehabilitation in the cortically blind?, *Journal of Neurology, Neurosurgery, and Psychiatry*, 48(11), 1113–1124, 1985.

100. Reinhard, J., Schreiber, A., Schiefer, U., Kasten, E., Sabel, B. A., Kenkel, S., Vonthein, R., and Trauzettel-Klosinski, S., Does visual restitution training change homonymous visual field defects? A fundus controlled study, *British Journal of Ophthalmology*, 89(1), 30–35, 2005.

101. Stoerig, P. and Cowey, A., Blindsight, *Current Biology*, 17(19), R822–R824, 2007.

102. Bridge, H., Thomas, O., Jbabdi, S., and Cowey, A., Changes in connectivity after visual cortical brain damage underlie altered visual function, *Brain*, 131(Pt. 6), 1433–1444, 2008.

103. Sincich, L. C., Park, K. F., Wohlgemuth, M. J., and Horton, J. C., Bypassing V1: A direct geniculate input to area MT, *Nature Neuroscience*, 7(10), 1123–1128, 2004.

104. Chokron, S., Perez, C., Obadia, M., Gaudry, I., Laloum, L., and Gout, O., From blindsight to sight: Cognitive rehabilitation of visual field defects, *Restorative Neurology and Neuroscience*, 26(4–5), 305–320, 2008.

105. Bohnen, N., Twijnstra, A., Wijnen, G., and Jolles, J., Recovery from visual and acoustic hyper-aesthesia after mild head injury in relation to patterns of behavioural dysfunction, *Journal of Neurology, Neurosurgery, and Psychiatry*, 55(3), 222–224, 1992.

106. Jackowski, M. M., Altered visual adaptation in patients with traumatic brain injury, in K. J. Ciuffreda, I. B. Suchoff, and N. Kapoor (Eds.), *Visual and Vestibular Consequences of Acquired Brain Injury*, Optometric Extension Program, Santa Ana, CA, 2001, 145–173.

107. Husain, M., Visuospatial and visuomotor functions of the posterior parietal lobe, in J. F. Stein (Ed.), *Vision and Visual Dysfunction, Vol. 13, Vision and Visual Dyslexia*, CRC Press, Ann Arbor, MI, 1991, Ch. 2, 12–36.

108. Borish, I. M., *Clinical Refraction*, 3rd ed., Professional Press, Chicago, 1975, Ch. 30.

109. Halligan, P. W. and Marshall, J. C., Two techniques for the assessment of line bisection in visuo-spatial neglect: A single case study, *Journal of Neurology, Neurosurgery, and Psychiatry*, 52(11), 1300–1302, 1989.

110. Kerkhoff, G., Displacement of the egocentric visual midline in altitudinal postchiasmatic scotomata, *Neuropsychologia*, 31(3), 261–265, 1993.

111. De Renzi, E., Oculomotor disturbances in hemispheric disease, in C. W. Johnston and F. J. Pirozzolo (Eds.), *Neuropsychology of Eye Movements,* Lawrence Erlbaum Associates, Hillsdale, NJ, 1988, 177–199.

112. Press, L. J., Lenses and behavior, *Journal of Optometric Vision Development*, 21(2), 5–17, 1990.

113. Tilikete, C., Rode, G., Rossetti, Y., Pichon, J., Li, L., and Boisson, D., Prism adaptation to rightward optical deviation improves postural imbalance in left hemiparetic patients, *Current Biology*, 11(7), 524–528, 2001.

114. Mangun, G. R., Luck, S. J., Plager, R., Loftus, W., Hillyard, S. A., Handy, T., Clark, V. P., and Gazzaniga, M. S., Monitoring the visual world: Hemispheric asymmetries and subcortical processes in attention, *Journal of Cognitive Neuroscience*, 6(3), 267–275, 1994.

115. Bartolomeo, P. and Chokron, S., Levels of impairment in unilateral neglect, in M. Behrmann (Ed.), *Handbook of Neuropsychology*, 2nd ed., vol. 4, Amsterdam, Elsevier Science B V, 2001, 67–98.

116. Karnath, H. O., Ferber, S., and Himmelbach, M., Spatial awareness is a function of the temporal not the posterior parietal lobe, *Nature*, 411(6840), 950–953, 2001.

117. Karnath, H. O., Himmelbach, M., and Rorden, C., The subcortical anatomy of human spatial neglect: Putamen, caudate nucleus, and pulvinar, *Brain*, 125(Pt. 2), 350–360, 2002.

118. Thiebaut de Schotten, M., Urbanski, M., Duffau, H., Volle, E., Lévy, R., Dubois, B., and Bartolomeo, P., Direct evidence for a parietal–frontal pathway subserving spatial awareness in humans, *Science*, 309(5744), 2226–2228, 2005.

119. Stone, S. P., Halligan, P. W., and Greenwood, R. J., The incidence of neglect phenomena and related disorders in patients with an acute right or left hemisphere stroke, *Age and Ageing*, 22(1), 46–52, 1993.

120. Halligan, P. W. and Marshall, J. C., Is neglect (only) lateral? A quadrant analysis of line cancellation, *Journal of Clinical and Experimental Neuropsychology*, 11(6), 793–798, 1989.

121. Ishiai, S., Furukawa, T., and Tsukagoshi, H., Eye-fixation patterns in homonymous hemianopia and unilateral spatial neglect, *Neuropsychologia*, 25(4), 675–679, 1987.

122. Margolis, N. W., and Suter, P. S., Visual field defects and unilateral spatial inattention: Diagnosis and treatment, *Journal of Behavioral Optometry*, 17(2), 31, 2006.

123. Rosetti, Y., Rode, G., Pisella, L., Farne, A., Li, L., Boisson, D., and Perenin, M. T. Prism adaptation to a rightward optical deviation rehabilitates left hemispatial neglect, *Nature*, 395(6698), 166–169, 1998.

124. Gordon, W. A., Hibbard, M. R., Egelko, S., Diller, L., Shaver M. S., Lieberman, A., and Ragnarsson, K., Perceptual remediation in patients with right brain damage: A comprehensive program, *Archives of Physical Medicine and Rehabilitation*, 66(6), 353–359, 1985.

125. Robertson, I. H., Gray, J. M., Pentland, B., and Waite, L. J., Microcomputer-based rehabilitation for unilateral left visual neglect: A randomized controlled trial, *Archives of Physical Medicine and Rehabilitation*, 71(9) 663–668, 1990.

126. Ross, F. L., The use of computers in occupational therapy for visual-scanning training, *American Journal of Occupational Therapy*, 46(4), 314–322, 1992.

127. Rock, I. and Harris, C. S., Vision and touch, in *Perception: Mechanisms and Models*, Readings from Scientific American, San Francisco, 1972, 269–277.

128. Treisman, A. M., Features and objects in visual processing, *Scientific American*, 255(5), 114–125, 1986.

129. Aksionoff, E. B. and Falk, N. S., The differential diagnosis of perceptual deficits in traumatic brain injury patients, *Journal of the American Optometric Association*, 63(8), 554–558, 1992.

130. Groffman, S., Treatment of visual perceptual disorders, *Practical Optometry*, 4, 76, 1993.

131. Groffman, S. and Press, L. J., Computerized perceptual therapy programs: Part I, *Optometric Extension Program Curriculum II*, 61, 387, 1989.

132. Press, L. J., Computers and vision therapy programs, *Optometric Extension Program Curriculum II*, 60, 29, 1987.

133. Roberts, S. P., Visual disorders of higher cortical function, *Journal of the American Optometric Association*, 63(10), 723–732, 1992.

134. De Haan, E. H., Young, A. W., and Newcombe, F., Covert and overt recognition in prosopagnosia, *Brain*, 114(Pt. 6), 2575–2591, 1991.

135. Sergent, J. and Poncet, M., From covert to overt recognition of faces in a prosopagnostic patient, *Brain*, 113(Pt. 4), 989–1004, 1990.

136. Daniel, M. S., Bolter, J. F., and Long, C. J., Remediation of alexia without agraphia: A case study, *Brain Injury*, 6(6), 529–542, 1992.

137. Trobe, J. R. and Bauer, R. M., Seeing but not recognizing, *Survey of Ophthalmology*, 30(5), 328–336, 1986.

138. Walsh, K., *Neuropsychology: A Clinical Approach*, 2nd ed., Churchill Livingstone, New York, 1987.

139. Page, S. J., Levine, P., Sisto, S., and Johnston, M. V., A randomized efficacy and feasibility study of imagery in acute stroke, *Clinical Rehabilitation*, 15(3), 233–240, 2001.

140. Farah, M. J., Is visual imagery really visual? Overlooked evidence from neuropsychology, *Psychological Review*, 95(3), 307–317, 1988.

141. Kosslyn, S. M. and Thompson, W. L., Shared mechanisms in visual imagery and visual perception: Insights from cognitive neuroscience, in M. S. Gazzaniga (Ed.), *The New Cognitive Neurosciences*, MIT Press, Cambridge, MA, 2000, 975–985.

142. Adeyemo, S. A., Imagery in thinking and problem solving, *Perceptual and Motor Skills*, 92(2), 395–398, 2001.

143. Pegna, A. J., Khateb, A., Spinelli, L., Seeck, M., Landis, T., and Michel, C. M., Unraveling the cerebral dynamics of mental imagery, *Human Brain Mapping*, 5(6), 410–421, 1997.

144. Martin, N. A., *Test of Visual–Perceptual Skills (Non-motor)*, 3rd Ed., Academic Therapy Publications, Hydesville, CA, 2006.

Appendix

Organizations to contact for information regarding orthoptic or vision therapy, or referral to member doctors who may provide or prescribe therapy:

College of Optometrists in Vision Development

243 North Lindbergh Blvd., #310

St. Louis, MO 63141

(888) 268-3770

www.covd.org

Neuro-Optometric Rehabilitation Association

PO Box 1408

Guilford, CT 06437

(866) 222-3887

www.nora.cc

Optometric Extension Program Foundation, Inc.

1921 East Carnegie Ave. Ste. 3-L

Santa Ana, CA 92705

(949) 250-8070

www.oepf.org

10

Auditory Function Assessment in Posttraumatic Brain Injury Rehabilitation

Juan J. Bermejo

CONTENTS

10.1 Introduction

At its core, the profession of audiology is dedicated to the study of the human auditory system and its disorders, to the understanding of the impact that hearing loss has on human communication processes, and to the implementation of habilitation and rehabilitation strategies to assist persons identified as hearing impaired. Audiology has spread broadly beyond its initial focus on aural rehabilitation of military personnel returning from World War II. Currently, audiologists are involved in diagnostic assessment of auditory function in neonatal to geriatric subpopulations, in improving hearing sensitivity and communication effectiveness through the fitting of traditional and newer forms of amplification, and in the programming and maintenance of electronic implants impacting the auditory system. In addition, audiologists contribute expertise and guidance in clinical service areas such as industrial hearing conservation, vestibular assessment and rehabilitation, and tinnitus assessment and management.

In traumatic brain injury (TBI) rehabilitation, various clinical specialties seek to address effectively the educational, psychological, vocational, communication, medical, and other needs of those persons requiring such intervention. Knowledge of the patient's hearing ability is thus crucial to the effectiveness of these therapies because audition plays a key role in communication between patient and therapist. Jury and Flynn state that, at present, current TBI rehabilitation practices "can fail to adequately identify the possible neuro-otologic sequelae of TBI and to recognise the implications for expensive rehabilitation programmes."[1, p.288] As we shall see later, hearing loss is a common occurrence among persons with TBI. The various clinical therapies provided to them can be rendered more effectively by awareness of possible auditory dysfunction. Providing this awareness though diverse clinical assessment procedures is the role of audiologists.

The sections that follow describe the incidence of hearing loss among persons with TBI. Peripheral and central auditory anatomy and physiology are then discussed. The hope is that we can begin to appreciate how fragile and susceptible to injury the auditory system can be. Description of traditional tests and electrophysiologic examinations will help provide insight into the clinical tools available to audiologists in their quest to quantify peripheral and central auditory function in various clinical populations. Tinnitus evaluation and management have assumed an important role in clinical audiology because of the prevalence of tinnitus in the general hearing-impaired population and among TBI patients. The psychological impact tinnitus can have on the mental well-being of persons affected by it is well recognized.

10.1.1 Demographics

According to the Center for Disease Control, National Center for Injury Prevention and Control,[2] 1.4 million Americans sustain TBI annually, with 1.1 million discharged from hospital emergency rooms to deal with the sequelae associated with TBI. The National Institute of Neurological Disorders and Stroke[3] estimates that about 50% of all TBIs are caused by moving accidents (i.e., motorized vehicles and bicycles), 20% by violence, and 3% by sports-related injuries. There were approximately 313,700 head injuries related to sport activities in 2007, with cycling injuries occurring most frequently, followed by football injuries.[4] A frequently overlooked statistic is the incidence of TBI among the elderly. Falls among persons 65 years or older accounted for 56,000 hospitalizations for TBI in 2005.[5]

Combat in Iraq and Afghanistan has introduced the improvised explosive device with devastating consequences for American troops. Taber et al.[6] cited injury statistics that indicated in excess of 80% of treated personnel were injured by improvised explosive devices and a significant percentage sustained blast-related head injury. According to Eshel, blast-related head injuries have become "the signature wound of soldiers returning from Iraq."[7, p.2] Sayer et al.[8] found that, of 188 service members admitted to polytrauma rehabilitation centers, 56% had sustained blast-related injuries that included auditory and otologic impairments. Primary blasts cause more tympanic membrane perforations than other injuries, and high-frequency neurosensory hearing loss and tinnitus are the most frequently experienced sequelae.[9] Lew et al.[10] studied the occurrence of hearing loss among returning service personnel with TBI resulting from nonblast incidents and blast incidents. Neurosensory hearing loss was most frequently found in both groups, with 44% of nonblast-related injury patients reporting hearing loss and 62% of blast-related injury patients complaining of hearing difficulty. Tinnitus was reported by 38% of personnel with blast-related TBI versus 11% of those with nonblast-related TBI. A higher percentage of neurosensory hearing loss or mixed hearing loss was found in those injured by blasts.

These statistics indicate the great potential for auditory disorders resulting from blunt force or blast-related TBI, regardless of severity. Abd al-Hady et al.[11] found that 20% of their subjects with minor head injury had varying degrees of hearing loss. In a study of 130 individuals with minor head injury, five were found to have temporal bone fractures that caused greater high-frequency hearing loss than found in those with no temporal bone fracture.[12] Of 123 people with temporal bone fractures, Ghorayeb and Rafie[13] reported varying degrees of hearing loss in all of them. Zimmerman et al.[14] analyzed audiologic data from 50 children who sustained head trauma and noted the occurrence of hearing loss in 48% of them.

Vartiainen et al.[15] concluded that their head-injured patients with neurosensory hearing loss sustained cochlear lesions. They based this conclusion on their analysis of audiologic data from 199 Finnish children with blunt head injury. Dorman and Morton[16] studied 40 New Zealand children treated for minor head injury. Audiologic data from 25% of them revealed mild hearing loss. A more recent study by Jury and Flynn,[1] also conducted in New Zealand, found that, in 30 people affected by TBI for 19 months to 27 years, persistent hearing loss occurred in 33%. In 1989, Wennmo and Svensson[17] found that 75% of their 20 Swedish subjects with temporal bone fractures sustained hearing loss. Bergemalm and Borg[18] studied audiologic data from 25 TBI patients admitted to two Swedish hospitals. They concluded that changes in auditory function are common in TBI, vary in site of lesion, and can become progressively worse.

In their study involving 16 subjects seen for operative repair for conductive hearing loss, Basson and Van Lierop[19] found that blunt force head trauma or penetration wound to the head caused various ossicular chain or middle ear defects. Incudomalleolar joint disarticulations were more common, followed by stapedial fractures, with both injury types causing substantial conductive hearing loss that responded favorably to surgical repair.

From these studies, it is clear that even mild TBI can affect auditory function. For this reason, hearing loss should always be suspected in a person with TBI until clinically proved otherwise.

10.2 The Human Auditory System

The conventional approach to a discussion of human auditory anatomy, physiology, and neurophysiology is the division of the auditory system into external, middle ear, inner ear, and retrocochlear sections. This compartmentalization will aid in understanding pathophysiology as well as site-of-lesion testing.

A good starting point is a brief description of the skull. There are four sections of bone that comprise the skull: the frontal, temporal, parietal, and occipital. Of principal importance to this discussion is the temporal bone. The temporal bone has four sections, the most important of these being the petrous portion because it houses the sensory organs for audition and balance. Other bony sections (the tympanic, mastoid, and squamous) help form the ear canal and middle ear cavity.

10.2.1 External Ear

The external ear consists of the auricle or pinna and the osseous and cartilaginous portions of the ear canal (Figure 10.1). The auricle is cartilaginous, quite flexible, and helps to collect sound and direct it inward to the ear canal. The concha, the helix, the antihelix,

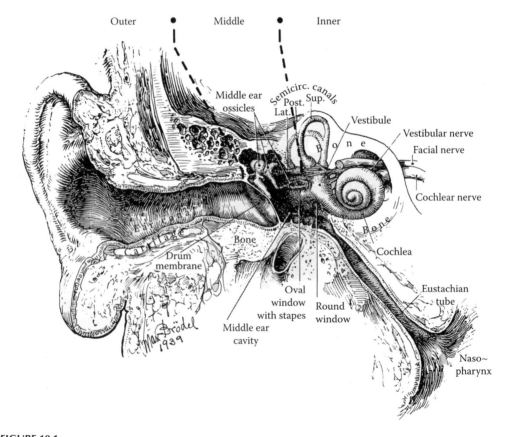

FIGURE 10.1
Drawing of the outer, middle, and inner ear. (From Durrant, J. and Lovrinic, J., *Bases of Hearing Science*, 2nd ed., Williams & Wilkins, Baltimore, 1984. With permission.)

the tragus, and the antitragus are principal features of the auricle. Of these, the concha, a large bowl-shaped depression near the middle of the auricle, is important because it helps funnel sound into the ear canal and is involved in providing slight amplification of high-frequency sounds. Yost and Nielsen[20] point to the auricle's role in helping to localize high-pitched sounds and to identify sound sources occurring behind or in front of the head. A more passive function is to protect the middle and inner ears by maintaining constant temperature and humidity, and to help in keeping out foreign bodies.

The human external auditory meatus (EAM) averages 28 mm in length and 7 mm in diameter.[21] The orifice of the EAM is generally oval in shape and is situated slightly lower than the medial portion near the eardrum; this may help keep water from lodging there.[22] The EAM is divided into cartilaginous and osseous portions. The cartilaginous portion occupies the lateral one third to one half, whereas the medial half to third thirds is osseous. Sebaceous and ceruminous glands located in the cartilaginous portion produce cerumen or earwax.

Functionally, the EAM appears to respond best (resonate) to sounds with frequencies that approximate 3800 Hz.[22] Together, the EAM and concha provide increased amplification in the 3000- to 5000-Hz range. This fact is important to consider in patients with EAM blockages caused by cerumen, dried or oozing blood, or foreign debris.

10.2.2 Middle Ear

The human tympanic membrane (TM) is the medial terminus for the ear canal, anchored fast to the annulus and measuring about 55 to 90 mm² in area.[20] The stiffness of the ear-drum is provided by the pars tens; a portion of the TM, the pars flaccida or Schrapnell's membrane, lacks stiff fibers and is, therefore, very flexible. As such, it may allow for some small degree of pressure equalization between external and middle parts of the ear.[22] On direct observation, the appearance of TMs may vary from translucent to opaque. In most individuals, the manubrium of the malleus in its attachment to the TM can be easily observed during otoscopic examination.

The role of the TM is to propagate sound energy from air to the inner ear. Sound transmission is accomplished by air conduction, by bone conduction, and through resonation of the air in the middle ear cavity.[20] Recently, Freeman et al.,[23] studying small mammals, described another mode of sound transmission. They were able to record auditory neural responses by directly applying a bone conduction stimulus to exposed brains. They postulated that cerebrospinal fluid may transmit sound pressure through to the inner ear fluids during bone conduction stimulation.

The air-filled middle ear space or tympanic cavity has a volume of approximately 2 cm³ and communicates anteriorly with the nasopharynx via the eustachian tube and posteriorly with the air cells of the mastoid bone. Suspended in the middle ear space are the ossicles or middle ear bones: the malleus, incus, and stapes. These are the smallest bones in the body. Also found in the middle ear space are the stapedius and tensor tympani muscles, the chorda tympani, and ligaments supporting the ossicles.

The malleus has its manubrium attached to the TM. A middle ear muscle, the tensor tympani, has its insertion on the manubrium and neck of the malleus. The incus and malleus articulate via a "saddle-type" joint. The incus attaches to the head of the stapes, forming the incudostapedial joint. Medially, the stapes footplate is fastened to the oval window. The malleus is supported by the anterior, lateral, and superior ligaments. Support for the incus is provided by the posterior ligament. The stapes is lodged in the oval window recess, held in place, but not fixated, by the annular ligament.

The stapedius and tensor tympani muscles are the auditory muscles and have an important role in stiffening the ossicular chain upon contraction through acoustic or nonacoustic stimulation. On the posterior wall of the middle ear cavity is the pyramidal eminence that houses the stapedius muscle. The tendon of the stapedius muscle emerges from the pyramidal eminence to attach to the head of the stapes. Innervation of the stapedius muscle is by the facial nerve. On the anterior wall of the middle ear is the semicanal of the tensor tympani muscle.[21] The tendon of the tensor tympani muscle inserts to the manubrium and neck of the malleus. The trigeminal nerve innervates the tensor tympani muscle. The chorda tympani, a branch of the facial nerve, also courses through the superior part of the middle ear cavity on its path to taste receptors on the tongue.

The role of the ossicles is to facilitate sound transmission. Sound energy in the air must be delivered efficiently to the cochlea, a fluid-filled chamber. Because of the difference in the densities of air and cochlear fluids, sound energy will be impeded by the greater density of the latter, resulting in some loss of this energy. Such impedance mismatch would be expected to decrease auditory sensitivity. The ossicles rotate in such a way that they perform a lever action, transferring a greater force to the stapes than that exerted on the tympanic membrane. This effectively increases the gain of the human auditory system by about 30 dB.[22]

The eustachian tube plays an important role in middle ear function. By opening and closing during chewing, swallowing, or yawning, the entry of air through the eustachian tube allows air pressure in the middle ear space to match that of ambient atmospheric pressure and, subsequently, effective sound transmission.

10.2.3 Bony Labyrinth

Within the petrous portion of the temporal bone are cavities that interconnect to form the osseous or bony labyrinth. Removal of surrounding bone permits a clear view of the complex system known as the *bony labyrinth:* the bony semicircular canals, the bony cochlea, and the vestibule between them. The orientation of the human osseous labyrinth is such that the semicircular canals lie posteriorly and to the side whereas the cochlea sits anteriorly and medially relative to the vestibule. Posterior and anterior semicircular canals are aligned almost 90 degrees to one another whereas the horizontal semicircular canal angles up 30 degrees from the horizontal plane. The semicircular canals have visible bulges or dilatations, known as *ampullae,* that open onto the vestibule.

The cochlea, an extension of the vestibule,[22] is a coiled structure measuring about 32 to 35 mm in length. It is wrapped around a bony structure called the *modiolus,* the base of which is the internal auditory meatus through which the cochleovestibular and facial nerves pass to reach auditory nuclei in the brainstem. There are two cochlear ducts—the scala tympani and the scala vestibuli—that are partially separated by the bony spiral lamina.

On the bony vestibule's lateral wall is the oval window that is covered by the stapedial footplate. The oval window connects the vestibule to the scala vestibuli. The round window is located in the inferior portion of the vestibule facing the middle ear cavity. It is the lateral terminus of the scala tympani.

Perilymph, one of two labyrinthine fluids and a filtrate of cerebrospinal fluid, fills the osseous labyrinth. The cochlear aqueduct, a small passage starting near the round window and continuing to the subarachnoid space, is believed to facilitate the transport of perilymph to the labyrinth.[24]

10.2.4 Membranous Labyrinth

Inside the bony labyrinth is a smaller, similarly shaped structure known as the *membranous labyrinth* (Figure 10.2). There are three divisions: the endolymphatic duct and sac, the membranous semicircular canals and the utricle, and the cochlear duct (or scala media) and saccule.[25] The saccule, utricle, and membranous semicircular canals contain the sensory organs for detecting angular and linear head motion. Auditory sensory epithelia (organ of Corti) reside in the scala media. The membranous labyrinth is filled with endolymph, a fluid different in chemical composition from perilymph. The endolymphatic duct and sac regulate the pressure of endolymphatic fluid.[26]

Because the focus of this discussion is the auditory system, only a brief discussion of the membranous semicircular canals follows. The utricle is a saclike structure inside the bony vestibule. The semicircular canals have five openings into the utricle. An enlarged bulb or ampulla at each opening contains the vestibular sensory epithelia—the crista ampullaris—supported by connective tissue. The crista contain hair cells with cilia that embed into a gelatinous structure called the *cupula*. Angular head movement causing endolymph to move in one direction across the crista will deflect the cupula and cilia and result in a receptor potential. This electrical event results in a discharge of the afferent vestibular nerve fibers. Deflection of the cupula in the opposite direction will fail to generate a receptor potential.

In the saccule and utricle are areas called *maculae* that consist of "fanlike" sensory structures with a covering called the *otolithic membrane.* This membranous structure is a gelatinous mass with a thin layer of calcium carbonate particles called *otoconia*. The sensory receptors are hair cells with stereocilia that project into the otolithic membrane. Movement

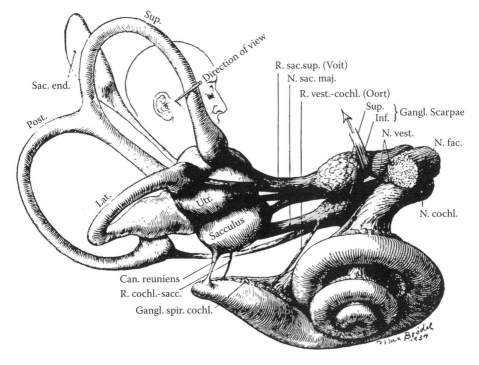

FIGURE 10.2
The membranous labyrinth. (From Hardy, M., *The Anatomical Record*, 59(4), 403–418, 1934. With permission.)

of this membrane in one direction will cause stereocilia to bend in the opposite direction, resulting in a physiologic response. The otolith organs thus respond to linear as well as angular head movements.[25]

10.2.5 The Cochlea

The spiral ligament, a crescent-shaped thickening of periosteum attached to the lateral wall of the cochlea, projects inward and anchors the basilar membrane laterally (Figure 10.3). On its medial side, the basilar membrane is attached to the spiral lamina, a bony shelf that partially divides the cochlear scalae. Thus, the basilar membrane is the roof of the scala tympani and the floor of the scala media. The roof of the scala media is formed by Reissner's membrane. The basilar membrane, about 32 mm long, is composed of transverse fibers lying perpendicular to its long axis. Unlike the scala media, the basilar membrane is wider toward its apex and narrower toward its basal end. This arrangement has had important implications for the development of the many theories of hearing.

The sensory epithelium for hearing, or the organ of Corti, rests on the basilar membrane. A single row of receptor cells, the inner hair cells (IHCs), and three rows of outer hair cells (OHCs) wind their way from base to apex. IHCs appear "flasklike" in shape and have two rows of stereocilia.[22] The shape of OHCs is more cylindrical, and each sensory cell has three to four rows of stereocilia arranged in a W shape. The tips of the tallest of the stereocilia are embedded in the tectorial membrane. The shorter of the OHC stereocilia are freestanding, whereas the IHC stereocilia are either freestanding or loosely attached to the tectorial membrane.[24] In simple terms, the hearing process is initiated by sound pressure acting on the TM. Through a pistonlike motion, the ossicles convey sound energy at a significantly higher gain to the oval window. A pressure gradient develops across the basilar membrane and organ of Corti creating a pressure wave that travels apically. Shearing forces act on the tectorial membrane, which in turn deflects the hair bundles toward their kinocilium, thereby depolarizing the hair cell and leading to a receptor potential. This physiologic excitation increases the number of spike discharges from afferent neurons, culminating in a whole nerve action potential. Only IHCs participate in the generation of an action potential. OHCs are the key elements in a cochlear amplifier that increases the sensitivity and frequency selectivity of the hearing organ.[27]

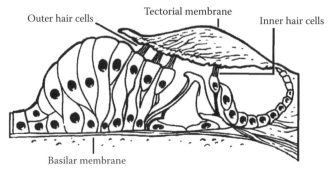

FIGURE 10.3
Structures of the organ of Corti.

10.2.6 The Auditory Nerve

As discussed previously, receptor cells depolarize when their stereocilia bend in response to shearing forces from the tectorial membrane during the traveling wave. Each IHC may be innervated by several afferent neurons, whereas many OHCs may be innervated, through multiple branching, by a single neuron. Approximately 30,000 nerve fibers comprise the auditory nerve; about 90% to 95% of these are type I radial neurons—thick, myelinated fibers that synapse with IHCs. Thin, scarcely myelinated type II, or outer spiral fibers, make up a smaller percentage (5% to 10%) of all afferent neurons, and these synapse with the OHCs.

An olivocochlear efferent system exists alongside the afferent neuronal pathway. Efferent fibers arise from either the lateral or medial superior olivary complex.[27] Lateral efferent axons tend to be unmyelinated, originate in the vicinity of the lateral superior olivary complex, and directly synapse with afferent dendrites at the base of the IHCs. From areas near the medial superior olivary complex are larger neurons with axons that are myelinated and synapse directly on OHCs. The role of the efferent system appears to involve the lowering of the sensitivity of the hearing organ in response to high-intensity sounds, reducing the effects of low-level background noise on moderate-intensity acoustic stimuli, and may serve to facilitate selective attention.[28]

10.2.7 Central Auditory Pathways

Primary auditory fibers are the central processes of bipolar neurons. The peripheral processes attach to the cochlear hair cells whereas the central fibers enter the brainstem to terminate on diverse cells in the dorsal and ventral cochlear nuclei (Figure 10.4). The latter are divided into anteroventral and posteroventral sections. A tonotopic arrangement is

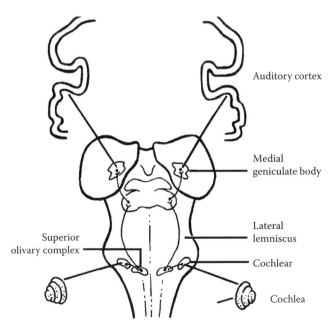

FIGURE 10.4
Central auditory pathways.

evident in the cochlear nuclei, whereby afferent nerve fibers responsive to high-frequency stimuli and, thus, originating from the basal end of the cochlea, terminate on cells of the dorsal side of the dorsal cochlear nuclei. The cochlear apex is sensitive to low-frequency sounds; nerve fibers from this cochlear area connect to cells on the ventral portion of the dorsal cochlear nuclei and to the ventral cochlear nuclei.

Secondary auditory nerve fibers are those that are arranged into three striae: the dorsal acoustic stria, the intermediate acoustic stria, and the ventral acoustic stria. Fibers from the dorsal acoustic stria project from the dorsal cochlear nuclei and cross the midline. Some nerve fibers terminate on the contralateral superior olivary complex with the majority entering the contralateral lateral lemniscus. From there, fibers project to the central nucleus of the inferior colliculus of the midbrain.

From cells in the posteroventral cochlear nucleus arise the intermediate acoustic striae to connect to cells in the periolivary and retro-olivary nuclei. From there, they cross the midline and terminate on the contralateral periolivary and retro-olivary nuclei. Afferent fibers continue contralaterally and join the lateral lemniscus and terminate in the inferior colliculus. Efferent auditory nerve fibers that attach to OHCs arise in these olivary nuclei to make up the olivocochlear bundle and, as described earlier, play a role in altering the sensitivity of auditory sensory receptors.

The ventral acoustic stria begins in the ventral cochlear nucleus and forms the trapezoid body. Many of its fibers course across the midline and form the lateral lemniscus. This nerve fiber bundle ascends to terminate on the central nucleus of the inferior colliculus within the midbrain.

The lateral lemniscus is comprised mainly of crossed secondary nerve fibers from the three acoustic striae. A few fibers from its nucleus will cross the midline and terminate at the contralateral inferior colliculus. From the inferior colliculus, ascending fibers continue on to the medial geniculate body of the thalamus. Fibers originating within the medial geniculate body form the geniculocortical fiber tract that connects to the transverse temporal gyrus in the temporal lobe.[29]

Typically, the presence of sound is perceived through air conduction, whereby the ear detects and processes sound carried through air. Sound transmission can also take place through the vibration of bones of the skull or teeth. Hearing sensitivity can become impaired as a result of defects occurring at the peripheral level (i.e., from the ear canal to the auditory nerve inclusive) or at the central level (i.e., from the brainstem to the auditory cortex). Four types of hearing losses are recognized clinically and are discussed later in the chapter. To assess an individual's hearing sensitivity, it is necessary to perform preliminary, yet essential, procedures.

10.3 Clinical Examination

10.3.1 Patient History

By careful questioning, a clinician should be able to gather enough information about a person's hearing status to help guide audiologic testing. Was hearing sensitivity normal or was hearing loss documented or suspected prior to injury? Was there exposure to excessively loud occupational or recreational noise, toxic industrial chemicals, or use of ototoxic medications? Did the person report tinnitus, or "ringing of the ears," prior to injury?

Did background noise appear to affect detrimentally the person's ability to comprehend speech? Were family members becoming sufficiently concerned with the person's hearing difficulty that hearing aid use was contemplated? During hospitalization, was there bleeding from either ear or was trauma to either pinna noted? Did radiologic studies discover fracture of temporal bone? Was the person found to exhibit hearing difficulty by hospital staff? Was hearing sensitivity assessed during hospitalization or shortly after discharge?

10.3.1.1 Standard Audiologic Procedures

Following the taking of a case history, the person is prepared for standard audiologic procedures. Many people with TBI who are seen as outpatients are capable of cooperating during testing and providing reliable responses. Standard pure tone and speech audiometric techniques are the basis for conventional audiologic studies of cooperative patients. By evaluating air conduction and bone conduction sensitivity, the audiologist can determine whether hearing sensitivity is within normal limits or whether hearing impairment is present unilaterally or bilaterally, and its severity can be established.

Speech audiometric data aid in determining the impact of hearing loss on the person's ability to perceive speech at normal intensity levels (sometimes referred to as *conversational speech levels*). Along with pure tone data, speech audiometric data can help ascertain communication problems likely to be experienced by the individual with hearing impairment.

It should be obvious that hearing testing is best performed in a quiet setting. Controlling the acoustical environment ensures that all persons receive hearing testing in optimal listening surroundings and that test data are reliable and accurately reflect hearing status at the time of examination. For these reasons, quantitative data obtained through standard audiologic procedures, rather than qualitative measures (e.g., "whisper test," watch test, single tuning fork test, etc.), are preferred.

A clinical audiometer is an electronic instrument used to generate pure tones and various types of noise stimuli. These, as well as recorded or live-voice speech stimuli, are presented to a listener through circumaural or insert earphones or a bone oscillator placed on the mastoid bone or forehead. When loudspeakers are used instead of earphones, hearing sensitivity is assessed in what is known as *soundfield testing*.

10.3.1.2 The Audiogram

With a person wearing earphones, pure tones ranging from 250 to 8000 Hz are presented at different sound intensity levels. Bone conduction thresholds can also be established in the frequency range of 250 to 4000 or 6000 Hz. Thresholds are determined at each specific frequency. Theoretically, a threshold represents the sound intensity level at which a listener is able to detect successfully a stimulus 50% of the time. Clinically, a pure tone threshold represents the faintest sound a person can hear. These test results can be depicted on a form known as an audiogram (Figure 10.5). In this graphical representation of hearing sensitivity, pure tone thresholds are plotted in terms of frequency versus intensity level, relative to normal hearing level.

Although pure tones are simple acoustic stimuli, speech is a complex stimulus. Conventional speech audiometric testing can be performed with single words, nonsense words or phrases, short sentences, or continuous discourse. Use of speech stimuli for evaluation of hearing sensitivity is essential because of the significant impact of hearing loss on one's ability to communicate orally.

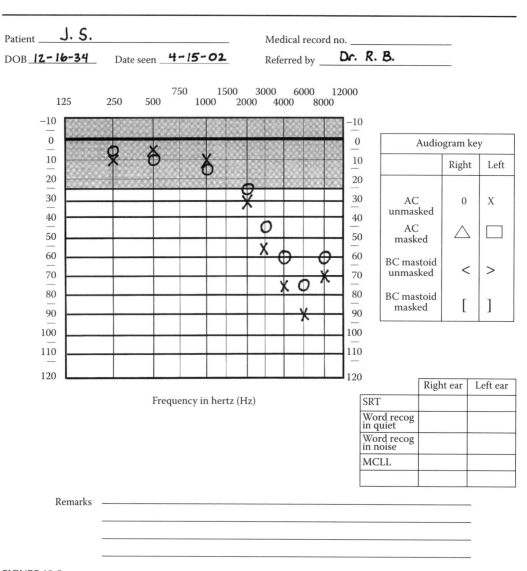

Patient _____J. S._____   Medical record no. _____

DOB _12-16-34_   Date seen _4-15-02_   Referred by _____Dr. R. B._____

	Right ear	Left ear
SRT		
Word recog in quiet		
Word recog in noise		
MCLL		

Remarks _____

FIGURE 10.5
Audiogram depicting loss of high-frequency hearing sensitivity.

Together, pure tone and speech stimuli help delineate the patient's hearing sensitivity. An individual with normal hearing sensitivity will typically have air conduction and bone conduction thresholds falling between –10 dBHL and 26 dBHL. Air conduction thresholds may differ from bone conduction thresholds by 5 to 15 dBHL. Because the normal hearing range is fairly wide, pure tone thresholds approximating 25 dBHL (and therefore technically within normal limits) may present mild auditory problems. Hearing sensitivity in the normal range facilitates, for most individuals in quiet surroundings, almost effortless reception of speech and nonspeech sounds. Of course, this may not hold true in geriatric patients because of aging effects on sensory and neural function.

10.3.1.3 Acoustic Immittance

Acoustic immittance encompasses tympanometry as well as measurements of middle ear compliance or impedance and eustachian tube function. In addition, testing for the presence of stapedial muscle contractions in response to loud acoustic stimuli is included. As described earlier, the middle ear serves to transfer effectively as much of the acoustical stimulus to the inner ear as possible through the action of the ossicular chain. Acoustic impedance refers to the amount of opposition to sound transmission posed by the middle ear. In ears with no otologic disease, acoustic impedance is minimal. Ears with TM or ossicular chain defects will demonstrate increased acoustic impedance, resulting in significant reflection of sound off a stiffened TM and out through the ear canal. This implies a reduction of sound energy flow to the inner ear.

By presenting a pure tone to the ear while varying air pressure in a closed ear canal, tympanometry quantifies the effect on transmission of that stimulus through the middle ear. A tympanometer measures how middle ear compliance varies as ear canal pressure changes to values above and below ambient atmospheric pressure. The data obtained permit assessment of the integrity of the TM, the stiffness of the middle ear, the operational function of the eustachian tube, and the status of the ossicular chain (Figure 10.6).

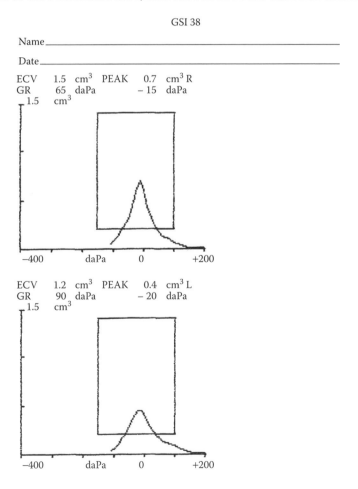

FIGURE 10.6
Tympanogram.

Patients with occluded ear canals will demonstrate abnormally low ear canal volume. Perforations of the TM will yield larger than normal ear canal volumes because the measurement is that of the combined volume values of both ear canal and middle ear space. Ossicular chain fixation will cause abnormally restricted movement of the TM and increased resistance to sound transmission as air pressure is varied. Discontinuity of the ossicular chain will do the opposite; because of increased flaccidity, the TM is hypermobile, and abnormal high middle compliance values are recorded by the tympanometer.

10.3.1.4 Acoustic Reflex Testing

The acoustic reflex is a contraction of the stapedius muscle when a sufficiently loud acoustic stimulus is presented to a healthy ear. This acoustic reflex arc consists of afferent auditory nerve fibers that terminate on the ventral cochlear nuclei, neurons arising from the ventral cochlear nucleus terminating near the ipsilateral facial motor nucleus as well as ipsilateral and contralateral medial superior olive (MSO), neurons from the MSO or peri-MSO that end ipsilaterally and contralaterally at the facial motor nucleus, and, finally, the facial motor nerve fibers that innervate the stapedius muscle.

In the normal ear, acoustic reflexes can be elicited by ipsilateral or contralateral stimulation. Pure tones, white noise, or bands of noise in the range of 70 to 100 dB above pure tone threshold are effective stimuli. The acoustic reflex is a stiffening of the TM that, in turn, increases the resistance to sound energy flow. Instrumentation is used to detect the sudden increase in acoustic impedance upon eliciting an acoustic reflex.

If conductive hearing loss (discussed later) is present, testing usually fails to elicit an acoustic reflex, often because of differing circumstances. For instance, persons with conductive hearing loss resulting from middle ear disease or trauma usually do not register the expected change in impedance because middle ear stiffness is already abnormally high. Thus, it is rare that these individuals would present with acoustic reflexes. On the other hand, a person with disarticulation of the ossicles has a middle ear with an abnormally high degree of flaccidity. In such a case, no acoustic reflex may be present because of the loss of continuity within the ossicular chain itself and between the ossicular chain and the TM.

Individuals with neurosensory hearing loss (discussed later) may or may not present with acoustic reflexes. If the neurosensory hearing loss (i.e., elevated pure tone thresholds) is mild, acoustic reflexes may be recorded, suggesting that recruitment is present. Recruitment is a clinical symptom in which the ear's ability to process loudness is impaired. A person with recruitment usually complains that certain sounds are annoying or even painful to hear. This is frequently the result of damage to the cochlea. In cases when the neurosensory hearing loss is moderate to severe, acoustic reflexes are generally absent.

10.3.1.5 Conductive Hearing Loss

When bone conduction pure tone thresholds are better than air conduction thresholds by more than 10 to 15 dBHL, a conductive hearing loss is said to be present. Common causes of conductive hearing loss include cerumen impactions, perforated TMs, middle ear disease, ossicular chain fixation or decoupling, and eustachian tube dysfunction. Less commonly encountered are atresia (i.e., absent ear canal), ear canal stenosis (i.e., narrowing of the ear canal orifice), active bleeding or dried blood occluding the ear canal, fracture across the osseous portion of the ear canal or across the middle ear, hemotympanum or blood occupying the middle ear space, vascular tumor in the middle ear space, and foreign debris in the ear canal or middle ear.

A patient with conductive hearing loss typically exhibits difficulty responding to verbal or nonverbal stimuli unless presented with louder than normal intensity levels. Most conductive hearing losses exist as long as the underlying medical condition persists. Medical and/or surgical treatment may help resolve most conductive hearing losses, and hearing sensitivity may return to normal in most cases.

10.3.1.6 Neurosensory Hearing Loss

Air conduction and bone conduction thresholds lying outside of normal and approximating one another indicate neurosensory hearing loss. Most individuals will acquire neurosensory hearing loss as a result of the aging process. Temporary or chronic exposure to dangerously loud sound without hearing protection is one of the leading causes of hearing loss. Autoimmune ear disease, endolymphatic hydrops, perilymphatic fistula, genetic or hereditary factors, viral infiltration into the cochlea, metabolic disease (such as hypothyroidism), and anemia are other bases for neurosensory hearing loss. Most individuals with typical neurosensory hearing losses are not medically treatable, except through amplification. Hearing aids, alternative listening devices, and the advent of middle ear, cochlear, and brainstem implants have made audition possible for many people with neurosensory hearing loss.

10.3.1.7 Mixed Hearing Loss

When low-frequency bone conduction thresholds are in the normal range but those in the mid- to high-frequency range approximate diminished air conduction pure tone thresholds, the hearing loss is referred to as *mixed*. Otosclerosis, a disease involving the growth of bone around the stapes footplate, commonly causes mixed hearing loss. The stapes footplate becomes increasingly fixated and unable to pivot freely within the oval window, resulting in diminished hearing sensitivity. Individuals with presbycusis (i.e., hearing loss secondary to the aging process) may also exhibit mixed hearing loss should an outer or middle ear lesion exist concomitantly. For instance, a person with earwax blockage of the ear canal, TM perforation, or middle ear disease will exhibit hearing loss resulting from conductive as well as neurosensory involvement. The conductive component of a mixed hearing loss may be resolved through medical or surgical treatment. The neurosensory portion of the hearing loss, however, may be permanent.

Fractures of the temporal bone can be longitudinal or transverse. Longitudinal fractures occur more frequently, usually spare cranial nerve VIII, and commonly cause conductive hearing loss as a result of damage to middle ear structures and the TM. Transverse fractures tend to produce total loss of auditory function because of the severe damage to the labyrinth.[25] Labyrinthine concussions can induce permanent change to hearing ability, especially to high-frequency hearing sensitivity.

10.3.1.8 Central Hearing Loss

People with central hearing loss generally have difficulty with cognitive processing of complex sounds while maintaining normal or neurosensory hearing loss. What is striking, from a clinical perspective, is the person's apparent ability to perceive sounds in a seemingly normal manner, but with obvious difficulty or failure to recognize specific sounds. It is not surprising that these individuals are mistakenly deemed to have functional or "nonorganic" hearing loss. For instance, a person may completely fail to attend to, recognize, or discriminate speech stimuli in light of apparently normal peripheral hearing sensitivity on audiometric testing. Central auditory processing and associated cortical or subcortical lesions that underlie central hearing loss are beyond the scope of this chapter. For this information, the reader is encouraged to review the work by Pinheiro and Musiek.[30]

10.4 Electrodiagnostic Procedures

10.4.1 Otoacoustic Emissions

The existence of "echoes" emanating from the cochlea and out the ear canal was first described by Kemp[31] in 1978. Briefly, acoustic stimuli presented to the ear at threshold were found to generate a return wave or echo detected within the ear canal. These echoes or emissions are the result of distortions in the traveling wave, and their presence reflects the health of OHCs. The ability to test for the presence of these otoacoustic emissions has provided clinicians with another tool for assessing the functional integrity of the human cochlea.

Testing is accomplished using a probe, having both a microphone and a stimulus generator, which is inserted into the ear canal. Clicks or pure tones are stimuli used to elicit responses that are then detected by the microphone inside the probe. These otoacoustic emissions (OAEs) are then analyzed to assess cochlear function in all patient age groups. Evoked OAEs are of two types: distortion and transient. The distinction is based on the type of stimulus used to elicit the cochlear response.

Transient OAEs are evoked using click or tone burst stimuli. Because such stimuli include a broad range of frequency components, their energy stimulates the basal as well as apical regions of the cochlea. Distortion-product OAEs are generated by using two pure tones (by convention, labeled F1 and F2). These stimuli are most effective when separated in frequency by an F2-to-F1 ratio of 1.22.[28] For instance, F2 may be a 1600-Hz pure tone whereas F1 may be 1311 Hz. Their ratio is thus 1600 Hz divided by 1311 Hz or 1.22. Distortion-product OAE findings are graphed, as in Figure 10.7.

Clinically, OAEs are used to assess the integrity of cochlear outer hair cells through an analysis of their amplitude. Most individuals with hearing loss exceeding 45 dBHL would be expected to have absent OAEs.[28] OAE testing thus serves to supplement other behavioral audiologic data to ascertain presence or absence of hearing loss and to distinguish sensory from neural hearing impairment.

10.4.2 Auditory Evoked Responses

There has always been a need to improve identification of hearing loss in difficult-to-test individuals. Individuals with TBI may be unable or unwilling to cooperate for standard behavioral audiometric testing. There may be a need to assess the neural integrity of cortical structures responsible for cognition, memory recall, speech recognition, language function, or attention. For these purposes, a battery of electrophysiologic techniques has

SmartOAE 4.24 USBezDP-OAE report

Juan J. Bermejo, Ph.D., FAAA
2201 Mount Vernon Ave., Ste. 109

661-872-7000

Name: D   H
SS#   :
DOB : 09/28/1965
Sex   : Female

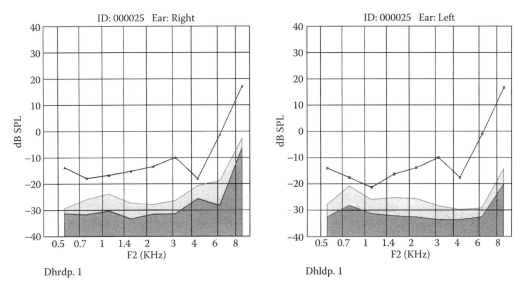

ID: 000025 Ear: Right

Dhrdp. 1

ID: 000025 Ear: Left

Dhldp. 1

FIGURE 10.7
Distortion-product otoacoustic emissions from a patient with normal hearing sensitivity.

been evolving since the 1930s. Known collectively as *auditory evoked responses,* these cortical responses to diverse acoustic stimuli have been used to delineate normal from abnormal cortical function, to identify neuroanatomic generators of these responses, and to evaluate their potential as clinical diagnostic measures. During the past 40 years, it has become clear that some of these techniques are more useful than other evoked potential methodologies in estimating hearing sensitivity.

The auditory evoked responses include electrocochleography (ECochG), brainstem auditory evoked response (BAER), auditory middle latency response (AMLR), auditory late response (ALR), and auditory P300 response (Figure 10.8). These electrophysiologic procedures utilize electrodes to measure tiny electrical voltages arising from various auditory neural substrates in response to clicks, tone pips, tone bursts, tones, or speech stimuli.

The utility of the tests is in the assessment of the neurophysiologic status of the cochlea (ECochG), the auditory nerve and auditory centers in the lower and middle brainstem (BAER), and higher level auditory processing centers (AMLR and ALR). These evoked responses are known as exogenous because their appearance is not dependent on any cognitive effort by the listener. That is, the evoked potentials from persons with normal hearing will appear regardless of whether the stimuli are attended to. On the other hand, the auditory P300 response is known as an endogenous or event-related evoked response. Its appearance requires considerable cognitive effort, such as attention to specific, randomly occurring auditory stimuli. These cognitive responses are believed to reflect the listener's capacity to attend or to ignore.

The ECochG and BAER techniques are used more frequently to complement or supplement standard behavioral audiologic findings. The sensory or neural events recorded via these two procedures represent very fast (i.e., in msec) processing of incoming auditory stimuli occurring at the periphery of the auditory system. The AMLR and ALR generally reflect auditory processing as it progresses through the brainstem and onto the auditory cortex. The auditory P300 response is a cumulative neural event arising from the involvement of cortical structures and sensory association areas.

10.4.3 Electrocochleography

ECochG testing is performed to evaluate the status of cochlear function. A transtympanic or extratympanic electrode is used to record electrical voltages in response to clicks presented to the ear. Responses arise within a 3- to 5-msec time window following stimulus onset and consist of the cochlear microphonic, the summating potential (SP), and the compound action potential (CAP) (see Figure 10.8). The cochlear microphonic reflects electrical voltages generated at the sensory hair cell level within the cochlea. The SP is also generated within the cochlea and is, most likely, a product of distortion occurring during in the processing of sound by sensory hair cells. The CAP is actually the collective response from hundreds of auditory nerve fibers departing the cochlea on their way to the brainstem.

ECochG components are analyzed with respect to amplitude and time of occurrence or latency. Although not a true hearing test, ECochG is useful for determining OHC function and the integrity of the auditory nerve. Because of its dependence on intact high-frequency hearing sensitivity, ECochG response parameters may be affected by different cochlear pathologies. For example, ECochG may be reduced in amplitude when sensory hearing loss more than 1000 Hz is present. The relationship between the SP and the CAP may be larger than normal in patients with endolymphatic hydrops.[32] Thus, ECochG may be an appropriate component in a test battery for establishing auditory function in a person with TBI, especially if standard audiometric testing is not deemed possible.

10.4.4 Brainstem Auditory Evoked Response

The BAER is perhaps the most commonly used neurophysiologic technique for evaluating the auditory nerve and nuclei in the lower brainstem, as well as auditory structures in the pontine and midbrain regions. Typically, clicks are used as stimuli, although tone

Electrocochleography (ECochG)

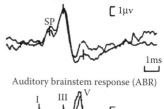

Auditory brainstem response (ABR)

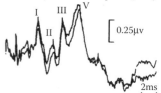

Auditory middle latency response (AMLR)

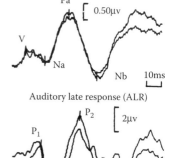

Auditory late response (ALR)

Auditory P300 response

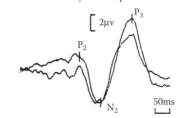

FIGURE 10.8
Waveforms representing the auditory evoked responses that are currently investigated clinically. (From James W. Hall, *Handbook of Auditory Evoked Responses*, published by Allyn and Bacon, Boston, MA. Copyright © 1992 by Pearson Education. Reprinted by permission of the publisher.)

bursts may be used to elicit frequency-specific auditory neural responses. Clicks are presented at a rate between 10 to 25 per second. Stimulus intensity is varied to elicit consistent neural responses at the lowest presentation level. Electrodes, placed on the scalp and on the earlobes or on the mastoid bones, are used to detect subcortical responses. These are submitted to signal averaging to generate five to seven waveforms (refer to Figure 10.8). These are patterns of negative and positive voltages occurring within a 10-msec time window (i.e., after the ECochG response). Auditory nerve conduction, interwave latencies, wave amplitudes, and the presence or absence of expected waveforms are analyzed for departure from data norms. Wave I and wave II are attributed to the auditory CAP. Wave III is thought to arise from the cochlear nuclei. The superior olivary complex is believed to generate wave IV, whereas wave V probably has its origins in the lateral lemniscus and inferior colliculus.[32]

BAER testing is usually performed on persons unable to cooperate during routine behavioral audiologic evaluation. Because BAER recordings are generally unaffected by sedation or sleep and require only that the patient rest quietly, clinicians have a reliable technique for estimating hearing sensitivity in this clinical population. Some individuals with suspected brainstem lesions secondary to head trauma will undergo BAER to help identify possible site of lesion, although the use of magnetic resonance imaging, computed tomographic scan, and other more advanced neuroradiologic studies have, in recent years, become the method of first choice. However, BAER recordings can provide information about the neural integrity of auditory structures in a compromised brainstem. In addition, serial BAER recordings can be used to assess improvement in the neural activity of auditory brainstem generators as a person progresses through TBI rehabilitation.

10.4.5 Middle Latency Response

Although auditory recordings such as the BAER and ECochG are known as fast electrophysiologic responses, the MLR occurs after the BAER but before the slow cortical responses such as the ALR and the P300 response (refer to Figure 10.8). Typically, clicks or tone bursts are presented at a stimulation rate of 7 to 10 per second. Stimulus intensity is generally held to less than 60 to 70 dB above threshold to minimize the large myogenic (i.e., postauricular muscle) response (discussed later). Electrodes are placed over the lateral temporal aspects of the scalp to record negative and positive voltage waves in response to auditory stimuli. Typically, four to five peaks and troughs with latency of 12 to 15 msec extend out to about 50 msec. A first prominent positive peak (Pa) occurs at about 25 to 30 msec, a large negative trough (Na) at about 40 to 45 msec, and a second large positive peak (Pb) at about 50 to 55 msec. The auditory structures responsible for generating the MLR are believed to be the auditory thalamus and primary auditory cortex.[32,33]

Of concern in recording the MLR is the ability to generate large muscle activity through the use of a high-intensity sound. This myogenic response can be recorded within the 15 to 50-msec MLR time window by an electrode placed near the ear. During ECochG and BAER testing, this myogenic response does not usually figure prominently in recordings because it typically appears after 10 msec (i.e., after the BAER time window). However, use of high-intensity stimulation can often cause the appearance of a robust triphasic myogenic response that is easily misinterpreted as the neurogenic MLR being sought.

Since its discovery in the 1960s, MLR testing has been performed in hopes of more easily identifying persons with hearing loss or brainstem and central nervous system disorders. Specific to TBI rehabilitation, using MLR has proved less useful than the BAER technique. The person's arousal state can influence the amplitude of the MLR, with natural or sedation-induced sleep reducing the amplitude of the waveform. Muscle artifact from body movement or from the presentation of the stimulus itself, if intense enough, will appear as a prominent triphasic response that mimics the MLR. MLR parameters are more easily affected by stimulus duration and latency than are BAER recordings.

10.4.6 Auditory Late Response

The origin of the ALR is debated among researchers because different studies have shown variability in response parameters that is contingent on cephalic versus noncephalic placement of the reference electrode. Most researchers concur that the origin of the ALR is the vicinity of the fissure of Sylvius and the primary auditory cortex in the temporal lobe.[21,22]

The ALR is evoked using tone bursts with long duration or plateaus exceeding 3 to 4 msec at very slow stimulus rates on the order of –0.5 or 1 per second. Evoked potential recordings are generally obtained within the range of 50 to 250 msec. The nomenclature used to identify the components of the ALR consists of P1, N1, P2, and N2 waves.

Clinical application of the ALR is very limited because of better, faster, more reliable electrophysiologic procedures that are used to estimate hearing sensitivity. As a measure of cortical function, the ALR has serious limitations because it is easily affected by arousal state, sleep, sedation, and medications that impact central nervous system function.

10.4.7 Auditory P300 Event-Related Potential

The ability to record the auditory P300 response depends very much on the participation of the listener. This endogenous or event-related potential, the P300, owes its appearance to attention to the presence, or in some cases, the absence, of a specific auditory stimulus. In a typical testing paradigm, a listener will have electrodes attached to the scalp. Clicks, tone bursts, speech stimuli, nonspeech stimuli, or practically any acoustic signal can be used as the "constant" or "frequent" stimulus. The listener may hear the constant stimulus 90% of the time. An auditory evoked response waveform is generated regardless of whether the listener attends to the constant stimulus (Figure 10.9). The technique calls for another acoustic stimulus, differing on some predetermined parameter, to be introduced, infrequently and at random, to the listener. The listener is instructed to attend (e.g., simply by counting) to the occurrence of the target stimulus. For instance, the letter "e" may serve as the "constant" stimulus and the letter "o" may serve as the "rare" stimulus. Completely at random, the letter "o" may be presented 10% of the time. Separate scalp recordings are then made in response to both the presentation of and attention to this rare stimulus. It is the listener's act of attending (a cognitive act) to the presence of the rare stimulus that generates the P300 waveform.

The P300 response is typically seen in the range of 250 to 700 msec. It is comprised of P1, N1, P2, N2, P3, and N3 peaks and troughs, with P3 generally occurring at about 300 msec. In general, the appearance of P300 depends on both the random occurrence of a rare stimulus and the ability of the listener to attend to the rare stimulus.

Efforts are less to identify neural generators of the P300 response than to identify those producing the auditory evoked responses described here because the P300 response itself is viewed as the product of a cognitive effort such as attention. Nevertheless, there is some speculation that the P300 response recorded intracranially may arise from the hippocampal region and the amygdala.[32]

Clinical application of P300 recordings have been performed on persons with mild to severe TBI. Again, it should be clear that estimating hearing sensitivity has not been the

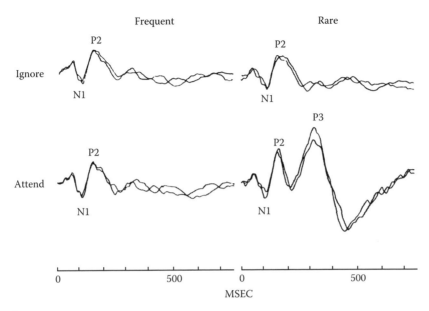

FIGURE 10.9
Auditory late response waveforms from a subject under attending or ignoring test conditions. (From Squires, K. C. and Hecox, K. E., *Seminars in Hearing*, 4(4), 422, 1983. With permission.)

focus of such use. Instead, interest is primarily on establishing the relationship between P300 latency and amplitude and various cognitive tasks. For instance, several recent studies of interest to TBI rehabilitation examined P300 recordings to investigate whether mild TBI caused deficits in attention,[34–37] increased distractibility during attending tasks,[38] or impaired information processing time.[39–42]

The role of auditory P300 in TBI rehabilitation continues to be of clinical interest because of efforts to uncover the relationship between neurophysiologic events at the cerebral level and a TBI individual's performance on behavioral scales.

10.5 Tinnitus Intervention

Tinnitus is the perception of sound when no external sounds are present to elicit the experience. Persons reporting tinnitus may describe tinnitus as "roaring," "ringing," "humming," "buzzing," or "pulsations" perceived in the ears or in the head. Tinnitus may be objective or, more commonly, subjective. According to Shulman,[43] objective tinnitus is audible to both patient and others. Subjective tinnitus is perceived only by the patient. Objective tinnitus may have its basis, among others, in eustachian tube dysfunction, cerebrovascular or cervicovascular lesion, or middle ear muscle myoclonus.[43] In their patients with pulsatile tinnitus, Sonmez et al.[44] found jugular vein defects and internal carotid artery lesions were the most common cause of objective tinnitus. Medical or surgical intervention for objective tinnitus is beyond the focus of this discussion. Therefore, the following sections will only address subjective tinnitus.

The mechanism or mechanisms underlying subjective tinnitus remain unknown, although injury to the auditory system, especially to sensory hair cells in the cochlea, is suspected as an underlying cause. Thus, subjective tinnitus may occur when the function of the auditory system is impaired (e.g., by noise, aging, otologic disease, drug side effects, and so forth). Noble[45] suggests, based on findings by Brozoski et al.[46] and Kaltenbach et al.,[47] that, in normal cochleae, inhibitory processes restrict the spread of spontaneous neural activity within the cochlea. When sensory hair cells are damaged, these inhibitory processes may become less effective in restraining the spread of spontaneous neural activity from other cochlear regions. This, in turn, may precipitate tinnitus awareness at the cortical level.[45]

In the general adult population, approximately 15% of individuals perceive tinnitus.[48] Welch and Dawes[49] found that, of 970 nonclinical subjects, almost 7% reported being aware of tinnitus 50% or more of the time. Forty-two percent of their subjects rated their tinnitus as "not at all annoying," 49% rated it as "slightly annoying," and almost 9% reported their tinnitus as "moderately or severely annoying." The personality of the tinnitus sufferer may have a significant bearing on how tinnitus is tolerated. Not surprisingly, Welch and Dawes[49] found that individuals more likely to react negatively to stress appeared to have heightened annoyance with tinnitus, with more men affected than women.

Treatment for tinnitus may involve the use of pharmacologic agents (e.g., anxiolytic medications such as alprazolam); personal or nonwearable electronic devices that generate masking noises (e.g., broadband, narrow band, or tonal music, or environmental sounds); hearing aids; psychological counseling/therapy; or combinations of sound therapy and counseling. Dobie,[50] in a review of 69 randomized clinical trials using either drug or non-drug therapies for tinnitus, concluded that drugs are not effective in long-term reduction of the frequency of occurrence of subjective tinnitus or in helping to improve the deleterious effects of tinnitus in most patients' everyday lives. However, the use of tricyclic antidepressants (e.g., nortriptyline and amitriptyline) showed effectiveness in helping tinnitus patients overcome sleep interference.

In addition, Dobie's[50] review of studies evaluating the efficacy of tinnitus maskers and hearing aids found these to provide somewhat limited relief. In contrast, Trotter and Donaldson[51] in the United Kingdom found that digitally programmable hearing aids fitted unilaterally or bilaterally provided significant relief from tinnitus awareness among their subjects with neurosensory hearing loss and tinnitus. Henry et al.[52] suggest that all tinnitus patients be given the option of using hearing aids to assist hearing sensitivity principally and, as a side benefit, to help reduce their perception of tinnitus.

Dobie[50] and Trotter and Donaldson[51] observed that the attention and reassurance given to patients by clinicians when discussing the nature of tinnitus and hearing loss may be therapeutic enough for many patients. In this light, various forms of cognitive–behavior therapy have been promoted for many years in tinnitus management for those individuals experiencing moderate or severe difficulty tolerating tinnitus. In essence, cognitive–behavior therapy attempts to change the way in which a tinnitus patient thinks about, reacts to, and acclimates to the presence of tinnitus. Noble[45] promotes the use of psychotherapy for those individuals with tinnitus experiencing emotional distress.

Audiologists frequently encounter TBI patients with complaint of tinnitus. Many audiologists have received little, if any, training in tinnitus intervention or are reluctant to undertake tinnitus management for various reasons. To aid audiologists wanting to implement tinnitus management, Henry et al.[52] proposed a five-tier progressive audiologic tinnitus management model. In essence, their program seeks to identify tinnitus sufferers requiring medical, audiologic, or mental health services. Patients with tinnitus usually contact their primary care providers first. These providers, in turn, can identify where to refer the patient: to an audiologist; to an ear, nose, and throat specialist; to emergency care; or to a mental health facility or provider. Audiologists undertake evaluation of hearing sensitivity, assess the impact of tinnitus on the patient's well-being through tinnitus questionnaires, fit hearing aids or tinnitus maskers, and provide group or individualized tinnitus management.

10.6 Summary

The person with TBI is typically confronted with a lengthy rehabilitation process. Skills once performed unconsciously may now require supreme conscious effort, often with the assistance of various TBI rehabilitation specialists. To ensure that therapeutic goals and objectives are met as efficiently as possible, effective communication between therapist and patient must take place. For this to occur, rehabilitation personnel must be cognizant of patients' ability to hear well enough to participate actively in their rehabilitation. Audiologists serve to provide the comprehensive audiologic assessments, using various and diverse audiologic techniques, needed to allow patient participation to be more effective.

References

1. Jury, M. A. and Flynn, M. C., Auditory and vestibular sequelae to traumatic brain injury: A pilot study, *The New Zealand Medical Journal*, 114(6), 286–288, 2001.
2. Center for Disease Control, National Center for Injury Prevention and Control, What is traumatic brain injury?, 2006, http://www.cdc.gov/ncipc/tbi/TBI.htm (accessed April 4, 2008).
3. National Institute of Neurological Disorders and Stroke, Traumatic brain injury: Hope through research, 2008, http://www.ninds.nih.gov/disorders/tbi/detail_tbi.htm (accessed April 4, 2008).
4. American Association of Neurological Surgeons, NeurosurgeryToday.org, What is neurosurgery?: Sports-related head injury, 2006, http://www.neurosurgerytoday.org/what/patient_e/sports.asp (accessed April 4, 2008).
5. Center for Disease Control and Prevention, Traumatic brain injuries can result from senior falls, 2008, http://www.cdc.gov/ncipc/tbi/elder_fall.htm (accessed June 30, 2008).
6. Taber, K. H., Warden, D. L., and Hurley, R. A., Blast-related traumatic brain injury: What is known?, *The Journal of Neuropsychiatry and Clinical Neurosciences*, 18(2), 141–145, 2006.
7. Eshel, D., IED blast related brain injuries: The silent killer, 2007, http://www.defense-update.com/analysis/analysis_270507_blast.htm (accessed June 30, 2008).
8. Sayer, N. A., Chiros, C. E., Sigford, B., Scott, S., Clothier, B., Pickett, T., and Lew, H. L., Characteristics and rehabilitation outcomes among patients with blast and other injuries sustained during the Global War on Terror, *Archives of Physical Medicine and Rehabilitation*, 89(1), 163–170, 2008.
9. Ritenour, A. E., Wickley, A., Ritenour, J. S., Kriete, B. R., Blackbourne, L. H., Holcomb, J. B., and Wade, C. E., Tympanic membrane perforation and hearing loss from blast overpressure in Operation Enduring Freedom and Operation Iraqi Freedom wounded, *Journal of Trauma*, 64(2 Suppl.), S174–S178, 2008.
10. Lew, H. L., Thomander, D., Chew, K. T., and Bleiberg, J., Review of sports-related concussion: Potential for application in military settings, *Journal of Rehabilitation Research and Development*, 44(7), 963–974, 2007.

11. Abd al-Hady, M. R., Shehata, O., el-Mously, M., and Sallam, F. S., Audiological findings following head trauma, *The Journal of Laryngology and Otology*, 104(12), 927–936, 1990.
12. Browning, G. G., Swain, I. R., and Gatehouse, S., Hearing loss in minor head injury, *Archives of Otolaryngology*, 108(8), 474–477, 1982.
13. Ghorayeb, B. Y. and Rafie, J. J., Fracture of the temporal bone: Evaluation of 123 cases, *Journal of Radiologie*, (Paris), 70(12), 703–710, 1989.
14. Zimmerman, W. D., Ganzel, T. M., Windmill, I. M., Nazar, G. B., and Phillips, M., Peripheral hearing loss following head trauma in children, *The Laryngoscope*, 103(1 pt 1), 87–91, 1993.
15. Vartiainen, E., Karjalainen, S., and Kärjä, J., Auditory disorders following head injury in children, *Acta Otolaryngologica*, 99(5–6), 529–536, 1985.
16. Dorman, E. B. and Morton, R. P., Hearing loss in minor head injury, *The New Zealand Medical Journal*, 95(711), 454–455, 1982.
17. Wennmo, C. and Svensson, C., Temporal bone fractures: Vestibular and other related ear sequela, *Acta Otolaryngologiva Supplementum*, 468, 379–383, 1989.
18. Bergemalm, P. O. and Borg, E., Long-term objective and subjective audiologic consequences of closed head injury, *Acta Otolaryngologica*, 121(6), 724–734, 2001.
19. Basson, O. J. and Van Lierop, A. C., Conductive hearing loss after head trauma: Review of ossicular pathology, management and outcomes, Paper presented at the Annual Academic Meeting of the South African Society of Otorhinolaryngology, Head and Neck Surgery, Port Elizabeth, South Africa, November 14–17, 2004.
20. Yost, W. A. and Nielsen, D. W., *Introduction to Hearing*, 2nd ed., Holt, Rinehart & Winston, New York, 1985.
21. Durrant, J. D. and Lovrinic, J. H., *Bases of Hearing Science*, 2nd ed., Williams & Wilkins, Baltimore, 1984.
22. Zemlin, W. R., *Speech and Hearing Science*, Prentice-Hall, Englewood Cliffs, NJ, 1968.
23. Freeman, S., Sichel, J. Y., and Sohmer, H., Bone conduction experiments in animals: Evidence for a non-osseous mechanism, *Hearing Research*, 146(1–2), 72–80, 2000.
24. Dallos, P., Overview: Cochlear neurobiology, in P. Dallos, A. N. Popper, and R. R. Fay (Eds.), *The Cochlea*, 1–43, Springer-Verlag, New York, 1996.
25. Baloh, R. W. and Honrubia, V., *Clinical Neurophysiology of the Vestibular System*, 2nd ed., F. A. Davis, Philadelphia, PA, 1990.
26. Wangemann, P. and Schact, J., Homeostatic mechanisms in the cochlea, in P. Dallos, A. N. Popper, and R. R. Fay (Eds.), *The Cochlea*, 130–185, Springer-Verlag, New York, 1996.
27. Guinan, J. J., Jr., Physiology of olivocochlear efferents, in P. Dallos, A. N. Popper, and R. R. Fay (Eds.), *The Cochlea*, 435–502, Springer-Verlag, New York, 1996.
28. Hall, J. W., *Handbook of Otoacoustic Emissions*, Singular Publishing, San Diego, CA, 2000.
29. Willis, W. D. and Grossman, R. G., *Medical Neurobiology*, 3rd ed., C. V. Mosby, St. Louis, MO, 1981.
30. Pinheiro, M. L. and Musiek, F. E., *Assessment of Central Auditory Dysfunction: Foundations and Clinical Correlates*, Williams & Wilkins, Baltimore, 1985.
31. Kemp, D. T., Stimulated acoustic emissions from within the human auditory system, *The Journal of the Acoustical Society of America*, 64(5), 1386–1391, 1978.
32. Hall, J. W., *Handbook of Auditory Evoked Responses*, Allyn & Bacon, Needham Heights, MA, 1992.
33. Chiappa, K. H., *Evoked Potentials in Clinical Medicine*, 2nd ed., Raven Press, New York, 1991.
34. Segalowitz, S. J., Dywan, J., and Unsal, A., Attentional factors in response time variability after traumatic brain injury: An ERP study, *Journal of the International Neuropsychological Society*, 3(2), 95–107, 1997.
35. Lew, H. L., Slimp, J., Price, R., Massagli, T. L., and Robinson, L. R., Comparison of speech-evoked *v* tone-evoked P300 response: Implications for predicting outcomes in patients with traumatic brain injury, *American Journal of Physical Medicine and Rehabilitation*, 78(4), 367–371, 1999.
36. Alberti, A., Sarchielli, P., Mazzotta, G., and Gallai, V., Event-related potentials in posttraumatic headache, *Headache*, 41(6), 579–585, 2001.

37. Potter, D. D., Bassett, M. R., Jory, S. H., and Barrett, K., Changes in event-related potentials in a three-stimulus auditory oddball task after mild head injury, *Neuropsychologia*, 39(13), 1464–1472, 2001.
38. Segalowitz, S. J., Bernstein, D. M., and Lawson, S., P300 event-related potential decrements in well-functioning university students with mild head injury, *Brain and Cognition*, 45(3), 342–356, 2001.
39. Kaipio, M. L., Cheour, M., Ceponiene, R., Ohman, J., Alku, P., and Näätänen, R., Increased distractibility in closed head injury as revealed by event-related potentials, *Neuroreport*, 11(7), 1463–1468, 2000.
40. Reinvang, I., Nordby, H., and Nielsen, C. S., Information processing deficits in head injury assessed with ERPs reflecting early and late processing stages, *Neuropsychologia*, 38(7), 995–1005, 2000.
41. Deacon, D. and Campbell, K. B., Effects of performance feedback on P300 and reaction time in closed head-injured outpatients, *Electroencephalography and Clinical Neurophysiology*, 78(2), 133–141, 1991.
42. Bernstein, D. M., Information processing difficulty long after self-reported concussion, *Journal of the International Neuropsychological Society*, 8(5), 673–682, 2002.
43. Shulman, A., Clinical types of tinnitus, in A. Shulman, J.- M. Aran, J. Tonndorf, H. Feldmann, and J. A. Vernon (Eds.), *Tinnitus: Diagnosis/Treatment*, 323–341, Lea & Febiger, Philadelphia, 1991.
44. Sonmez, G., Basekim, C. C., Ozturk, E., Gungor, A., and Kizilkaya, E., Imaging of pulsatile tinnitus: A review of 74 patients, *Clinical Imaging*, 31(2), 102–108, 2007.
45. Noble, W., Treatments for tinnitus, *Trends in Amplification*, 12, 236–241, 2008, http://tia.sagepub.com (accessed November 11, 2008).
46. Brozoski, T. J., Spires, T. J., and Bauer, C. A., Vigabatrin, a GABA transaminase inhibitor, reversibly eliminates tinnitus in an animal model, *Journal of the Association for Research in Otolaryngology*, 8(1), 105–118, 2007.
47. Kaltenbach, J. A., Rachel, J. D., Mathog, T. A., Zhang, J., Falzarano, P. R., and Lewandowski, M., Cisplatin-induced hyperactivity in the dorsal cochlear nucleus and its relation to outer hair cell loss: Relevance to tinnitus, *Journal of Neurophysiology*, 88(2), 699–714, 2002.
48. Henry, J. A., *Using Sound to Manage Tinnitus*, Featured Session, Presented at the American Academy of Audiology Convention, Charlotte, NC, April 3, 2008.
49. Welch, D. and Dawes, P. J., Personality and perception of tinnitus, *Ear and Hearing*, 29(5), 1–9, 2008.
50. Dobie, R. A., A review of randomized clinical trials in tinnitus, *Laryngoscope*, 109(8), 1202–1211, 1999.
51. Trotter, M. I. and Donaldson, I., Hearing aids and tinnitus therapy: A 25-year experience, Paper presented at the British Academic Conference in Otolaryngology, Birmingham, UK, July 5–7, 2006
52. Henry, J. A., Zaugg, T. L., Myers, P. J., and Schechter, M. A., The role of audiologic evaluation in progressive audiologic tinnitus management, *Trends in Amplification*, 12, 170–187, 2008, http://tia.sagepub.com (accessed November 11, 2008).

11

Issues in Aging Following Traumatic Brain Injury

Alan Weintraub and Mark J. Ashley

CONTENTS

11.1 Introduction

Neuromedical issues are faced by a rapidly growing population of more than 3.1 million persons living with traumatic brain injury (TBI) in the United States.[1] As the TBI population ages, survivors, practitioners, caregivers, and financially responsible parties alike must consider the neuromedical issues associated with aging and the complex sequelae of TBI. These parties must attempt to anticipate the issues to be faced by this population and further attempt to put in place mechanisms that might address those problems.

There is an average of at least 1.4 million TBIs that occur in the United States each year.[2] This includes 1.1 million emergency department visits, 235,000 to 288,000 hospitalizations, and 50,000 deaths.[2,3] This number is thought to be an underestimate because it accounts only for cases that present for medical treatment. Another 200,000 individuals are treated in hospital outpatient settings or physicians' offices.[4] These figures do not account for injuries in the military or unrecognized TBI.[2] Concussion arising from sporting or recreational activities are estimated to be around 300,000 injuries,[5] although a much higher estimate of between 1.6 million and 3.8 million sports-related TBIs is suggested as a result of inclusion of concussion associated both with, and without, a loss of consciousness.[2]

Approximately 475,000 children age 0 to 14 years sustain TBI each year.[2] The number is comprised of 2685 TBI-related deaths, 37,000 estimated hospitalizations, and 435,000 emergency department visits. In general, nearly 90% of all TBI cases are considered to be mild TBIs. (However, it is known that deficits may persist with some children.) Given the large number of such cases, much more consideration of this group is needed, including attention to recurrent, cumulative brain injuries and their sequela.

The highest incidence of TBI is bimodal in nature. Individuals 15 to 24 years of age constitute the first grouping, whereas the second is comprised of those people age 75 years and older. Prevalence is estimated at around 3.1 million individuals in the United States,[1] with incidence reported at 90 per 100,000.[6] Thurman et al.[7] estimates that between 80,000 and 90,000 persons per year become disabled as a result of TBI. Another study of TBI hospitalizations in South Carolina extrapolated lifelong disability prevalence to be approximately 125,000 people per year.[3] It has been estimated that 20% of hospitalized survivors of TBI do not return to work as a result of injury-related disability. The total lifetime productivity costs have been estimated at $51.2 billion in 2000 dollars.[4] As such, TBI presents a major public health concern, both as a diagnosis in itself and, in particular, as the effects of aging are applied.[3,8]

Age has been identified as contributory to outcome for persons who sustain TBI, although in a nonlinear way. It seems logical to assume that TBI inflicted upon a chronologically older brain would yield more devastating sequelae, and perhaps a more disabling outcome, when compared with a similar injury sustained by a younger brain.[9–12] Although this seems to hold true for cases of severe injury,[13,14] there is less support for injuries of lesser severity. This may be the result of the neurobiology of injury and the potential for greater neuroplasticity in the younger brain.[15] A prospective study by Rapoport and Feinstein[16] found an inverse relationship associated with age and mild TBI. Older subjects (60+ years) fared better than their younger counterparts (18–59 years) with higher Glasgow outcome scores, less physical symptomatology, less psychosocial impairment, and less psychological distress. A reason for these surprisingly better outcomes in an elderly mild TBI population raises relevant theoretical considerations. Although the younger brain has clear biologic advantages for recovery of function, the older person usually will have well-established "real-life" knowledge, structures, and routines in their day-to-day experience that may give them compensatory advantage to facilitate a better functional outcome. In addition, environmental demands associated with older adult lifestyles are often diminished in comparison with the demands placed upon younger adults.

Consequently, it is difficult, at best, to attempt to make definitive statements about likely long-term neuromedical issues following TBI based "solely" upon the age of the individual and even the level of severity of a given injury. Clearly, additional factors play into the long-term neuromedical outlook.

It seems logical to consider these factors together with other pertinent information that may bear on the long-term scenario. Insight may also be gleaned from review of known, frequently encountered acute medical complications associated with TBI, rehospitalization experiences for individuals with TBI, the pathophysiology of TBI, neurologic conditions associated with aging and/or TBI, and morbidity and mortality statistics. This chapter reviews various neuromedical issues associated with TBI, along with the interplay that exists between TBI and other conditions/diseases associated with advancing age.

11.2 Acute Medical Complications and Rehospitalization Rates in TBI

TBI impacts the central nervous system (CNS) and numerous other organ systems as a result of the traumatic mechanistic nature of injury, such as motor vehicle accidents, falls, and so on. An early review of medical complications and associated injuries provides valuable insight into different types of intracerebral, extracerebral, and systemic complications in TBI.[17] The study reported differences in outcome as measured by Disability Rating Scale scores[18] and length of stay for both acute and rehabilitation hospitalization as they related to severity of intracerebral and extracerebral injury and observed complications. Intracranial hemorrhages and other cerebral complications included subdural, epidural, subarachnoid, intraparenchymal, and other hemorrhages. Of individuals studied, 68% had one or more intracerebral hemorrhages. Other cerebral complications included intracranial hypertension, cerebrospinal fluid (CSF) leak, hydrocephalus, and seizures. Extracerebral complications included respiratory failure, pneumonitis, urinary tract infection, soft tissue infection, coagulopathy, renal failure, and septic shock. Associated injuries included fractures, cranial nerve injuries, hemothorax/pneumothorax, intra-abdominal injury, spinal cord injury (SCI), peripheral nerve injury, brachial plexus injury, and amputation. The frequency of these complications is shown in Table 11.1 through Table 11.3.

Englander et al.[19] also reported that respiratory complications were seen in 39% of 637 individuals during acute hospitalization. Twenty-one percent of individuals required gastrostomies and 23% required jejunostomies. More detailed information was available from this study pertaining to upper extremity fractures (humerus, radius, or ulna), which occurred in 11% of the study population, and pelvis or lower extremity fractures, which occurred in 21% of persons studied.

Of the four reported intracerebral acute medical complications, only hydrocephalus and seizures appear to impact the long-term neuromedical status of people with TBI. Of the seven reported extracerebral complications, it could be argued that respiratory and coagulopathic complications might reasonably bear some long-term neuromedical importance for persons with TBI.[20] It is less clear that early infectious complications, once resolved, impact long-term neuromedical status. Finally, of the eight associated injuries reported, cranial nerve injuries, SCI, peripheral nerve, and brachial plexus injuries might bear some significance from a strict neuromedical perspective, but only cranial nerve injury and SCI[21] seem to bear on likely neuromedical conditions impacting the CNS.

A second source of insight into the nature of long-term neuromedical issues associated with aging in TBI is found in literature that reviews rehospitalization rates and reasons in the TBI population. People with disabilities, in general, are more likely to be rehospitalized than the nondisabled population.[22,23] Several studies have examined medical

TABLE 11.1

Intracerebral Complications

Complication	%
Intracranial hypertension	20
Seizure	17
CSF leak	8
Hydrocephalus	5

TABLE 11.2

Extracerebral Complications

Complication	%
Respiratory failure	39
Pneumonitis	26
Urinary tract infection	21
Soft tissue infection	16
Coagulopathy	5
Septic shock	3

TABLE 11.3

Associated Injuries

Injury	%
Fractures	62
Cranial nerve	19
Hemo-/pneumothorax	11
Intra-abdominal injury	7
SCI	2
Peripheral nerve injury	2
Brachial plexus injury	<1
Amputation	<1

complications resulting in rehospitalization a number of years postinjury in TBI. Cifu et al.[24] found that rehospitalization rates were relatively stable over the first 3 years postinjury when all reasons for rehospitalization were grouped together. An increase in rehospitalizations resulting from behavioral/psychiatric problems, seizures, and general health maintenance from years 1 to 3 was observed. Rehospitalization for infectious processes peaked in year 2 and decreased somewhat in year 3 (Table 11.4).

A report of rehospitalizations was conducted 1 and 5 years after TBI for 1547 consecutive patients[25] enrolled in the National Institute of Disability and Rehabilitation Research (NIDRR) Model Systems for Traumatic Brain Injury. Of these, 799 were eligible for 5-year follow-up. The authors reported findings that were similar to those of Cifu et al.[24] in that rehospitalization for seizures and psychiatric problems increased from year 1 to year 5 (Table 11.4). It is interesting to note that, between the two studies by Cifu et al.[24] and Marwitz et al.,[25] rehospitalization rates for general health maintenance increased over the time periods studied. Clearly, disabled persons are less able to participate in their own health maintenance at the level seen in the general population, and general health may be an issue of concern in the discussion of aging. In persons who have sustained TBI, cognitive, social, financial, and physical disabilities may serve as barriers to self-initiated health maintenance activities and practices.

Psychiatric issues also pose a substantial concern for the aging TBI population. Rehospitalization rates for psychiatric issues remained relatively stable between the two studies from year 2 (15.3%) to year 3 (15%)[24] and year 5 (16%).[25] Burg et al.[26] reported finding an incidence of self-reported TBI of one or more injuries in psychiatrically hospitalized individuals of 66%. This increase in psychiatric rehospitalization correlated with substantially more aggression toward family members and caregivers between years 1 and 5 postinjury.[27] Specifically, Brooks et al.[27] reported the incidence of threats of violence at a rate of 15% at year 1. By year 5, these incidents were reported by 54% of caregivers. Physical assault of a family member was reported by 10% of caregivers in year 1 and 20% in year 5.

Rehospitalization rates for seizures increased steadily over years 1, 2, and 3 in the study by Cifu et al.,[24] peaking at 15% in year 3. The study by Marwitz et al.[25] found seizure rehospitalization rates at 18.7% at year 5.

Rehospitalization rates for orthopedic/reconstructive procedures remained surprisingly high during the first 3 years postinjury, ranging from 44.3% in year 1 to a relatively stable 23.7% to 25% in years 2 and 3, respectively. By year 5, the rate dropped to 13.3%, still fairly

TABLE 11.4

Etiology of Rehospitalizations by Year Postinjury

Reason	Year 1[a] (*n* = 79) [22.5%])	Year 2[a] (*n* = 59) [21.0%])	Year 3[a] (*n* = 40) [20.0%])	Year 5[b] (*n* = 75) [17.0%])
Rehabilitation	3 (3.8%)	0 (0%)	0 (0%)	1 (1.3%)
Seizures	8 (10.1%)	8 (13.6%)	6 (15.0%)	14 (18.7%)
Neurologic disorder	4 (5.1%)	8 (13.6%)	2 (5.0%)	2 (2.7%)
Psychiatric	5 (6.3%)	9 (15.3%)	6 (15.0%)	12 (16.0%)
Infectious	9 (11.4%)	10 (16.9%)	3 (7.5%)	6 (8.0%)
Orthopedic/reconstructive	35 (44.3%)	14 (23.7%)	10 (25.0%)	10 (13.3%)
General health maintenance	11 (13.9%)	10 (16.9%)	9 (22.5%)	27 (36.0%)
Unknown	4 (5.1%)	0 (0%)	4 (10.0%)	3 (4.0%)

Source: [a]Cifu et al., *Archives of Physical Medicine and Rehabilitation*, 80(1), 85–90, 1990. [b]Marwitz et al., *Journal of Head Trauma Rehabilitation*, 16(4), 307–317, 2001.

high for 5 years postinjury. Rehospitalization rates of 8% at 5 years postinjury for infectious disease are also high and may be a reflection of antibiotic-resistant organisms that have increased in recent years.

In summary, the rehospitalization data up to 5 years postinjury suggests that seizures, neurologic disorders, psychiatric/behavioral disorders, and maintenance of general health are issues of concern. Acute hospitalization complications and relatively short-term rehospitalization rates out to 5 years provide limited insight into likely neuromedical concerns for a population that can be reasonably expected to live from 10 to 55 years postinjury, depending upon age at injury, injury type, injury severity, and functional status.[28]

11.3 Cognitive Decline

The relationship among a history of TBI, age or aging, and cognitive decline must be examined from two perspectives. The first considers whether cognitive decline associated with normal aging is, in some manner, impacted or accelerated by interaction with some neurologic mechanism associated with the abnormal brain following TBI. The second considers whether the cognitive impairment often seen following TBI persists throughout life or worsens over time in comparison to the cognitive performance of persons without TBI. The clinician considering cognitive decline must be able to differentiate normal age-related cognitive decline from early signs of dementia, especially in attempting to prognosticate and make recommendations to individuals and their families. Several studies have attempted to examine the reality, persistence, and perception of TBI-related progressive cognitive impairments with aging.

Subjects with mild to moderate TBI were evaluated several years postinjury for cognitive performance and were compared with two groups of age-matched normals.[29] Middle-age persons and older persons with, and without, TBI were also matched and compared. The TBI subjects reported the belief that they sustained no long-term sequela associated with the TBI, although test results demonstrated cognitive performance to be impaired. The authors reported TBI sustained early in life, which results in permanent sequelae in specific domains of cognitive functioning, did not interact with changes in cognitive function arising from normal aging. In fact, middle-age persons with TBI actually performed at the level of older, non-TBI subjects.[29]

Goldstein and Shelly[30] reported that deficits in cognitive performance persisted over time for persons with TBI when compared with a normal population. In addition, these authors found that the magnitude of the difference in cognitive performance between persons with, and without, TBI remained stable over time. These findings suggest that the effect of TBI on cognitive performance is additive to declines in cognitive performance associated with normal aging.

Ashman et al.[31] evaluated the degree of cognitive decline seen within 2 to 5 years of injury for a group of individuals with TBI age 55 years and older compared with a noninjured, age-matched group. Neither group demonstrated any significant decline in cognitive performance over the period of study, although there were clear differences in overall cognitive performance between the two groups. Further analysis of a subgroup of individuals in both groups with the apolipoprotein-epsilon 4 (APOE-4) allele also did not demonstrate any significant differences in performance or decline.

Thus, it appears that individuals with TBI may accommodate to some level of decrement in cognitive performance over time. Without reference to potentially escalating neurobehavioral sequelae with aging, these studies show that differences exist between individuals with TBI and those without. These differences persist but seem to remain stable in magnitude.

The literature of cognitive decline in normal aging suggests that there may be a high level of predictive accuracy of general intelligence over time or with advancing age.[32] Duncan and others[33-35] have shown, with functional magnetic resonance imaging (MRI) and positron emission tomography (PET) studies, that general intelligence may recruit essentially the same neural structures as frontal function. Therefore, investigation of cognitive decline after TBI may need, then, to account for differences in preinjury general intelligence function as a probable cofounder, as well. Clearly, frontal structures and neural networks are frequently anatomically disrupted during TBI. Even though this will result in correlative clinical impairments of both intelligence and frontal executive functions, there still does not appear to be strong conclusive support for "accelerated" cognitive decline for the general TBI population.

11.3.1 Dementia and Alzheimer's Disease

Along the seeming continuum of cognitive decline associated with normal aging comes a point at which the level of cognitive decline interferes with normal function and becomes dementia. The prevalence of the "dementia syndrome," in and of itself, increases with advancing age.[36] There is also some degree of intellectual and cognitive dysfunction affecting about 15% of the population older than the age of 65.[37] This makes it difficult to investigate whether TBI directly causes dementia and/or Alzheimer's disease (AD). The research issue is further clouded by difficulty in proper characterization of normal cognitive decline and early-onset dementia.

The contribution of TBI to the development of AD and other dementias has been a topic of considerable focus in the literature. The literature has revealed an intriguing relationship between a history of TBI and AD, in particular. The linkage of TBI to AD will be examined but it is important to consider the scientific limitations in research design and methodology. Much of the literature provides retrospective reviews of coincidental diagnoses such as stroke or TBI and the development of AD or other dementia.[38] Correlational studies are useful in pointing to potential causal relationships; however, attribution of causality resulting from the finding of correlation is inappropriate. Care must be taken to avoid this common error in the application of statistical analysis.[39]

The presence of neurofibrillary tangles has been identified in the brains of boxers who suffered from the syndrome of pugilistica dementia. AD-like pathology appeared to arise from a protracted history of repeated blows to the head.[40] Beta-amyloid protein deposition was not found, however, in these subjects. Conversely, in a study by Roberts et al.,[41] immunocytochemical methodology further clarified the neuropathology of pugilistica dementia. The use of immunocytochemical methodology allowed identification of both substantial beta-amyloid protein deposition and development of neurofibrillary tangles in pugilistica dementia similar to that found in AD. Increased expression of beta-amyloid precursor protein is found as an acute-phase response to traumatic neuronal injury. In addition, such increased expression is a marker of immunoreactivity. The authors suggested that the extensive overexpression of this response may lead to the deposition of beta-amyloid protein, thereby initiating an AD-type process within days postinjury.[41]

Several retrospective and case-controlled studies demonstrated a higher incidence of AD in individuals with a history of TBI.[42–45] Salib and Hillier[46] examined the relationship among TBI and AD and other dementias, looking at relative risk/odds ratios. Although there was an association found between a history of TBI and the development of AD (only in males) and other dementias, greater risk ratios were observed for other dementias rather than AD. In this study, head trauma was not identified to be a significant risk for AD. The interval observed between TBI and the development of AD was several decades.

Later research added still further information in determining the relationship between a history of TBI and the development of AD. Mayeux et al.[47] determined that it was the presence of APOE-4 that materially increased the risk of AD. TBI, in the absence of the APOE-4 allele, did not increase the risk of AD and only the presence of the APOE-4 allele in persons with a TBI did so.[48] Although the presence of the APOE-4 allele increased the risk of AD, cerebral deposition of beta-amyloid with age, a genetic mutation, or brain injury were felt to contribute further to the pathogenesis of AD.[49,50] The effects of brain injury and APOE genotype on AD risk was studied by Guo et al.,[48] who evaluated 2233 subjects who met criteria for probable or definitive AD. The study continued to demonstrate a relationship between TBI injury severity and genetic subtype.

A population-based study conducted by Nemetz et al.[51] investigated the incidence of persons with TBI who later developed AD. It was concluded that the incidence of AD was no different than that of the normal population. The onset of AD for persons with a history of TBI, however, was observed to occur an average of 10 years earlier than for those without a history of TBI. In a prospective, population-based study of 6645 participants who were free of dementia at baseline, Mehta et al.[52] compared them with a cohort of individuals diagnosed with dementia. Their findings included no increased risk of AD or dementia associated with a history of trauma with a loss of consciousness. Multiple head traumas, time since head trauma, and duration of unconsciousness also did not significantly influence the risk of dementia. Finally, the presence of the APOE-4 allele was not found to interact with the time to onset of dementia.

The production of beta-amyloid plaques has been found to occur within hours of injury to the brain.[53,54] Postmortem studies have shown the presence of diffusely distributed beta-amyloid plaques in 30% to 50% of cases of severe TBI.[53,55] Surgically resected temporal cortex from survivors of severe TBI shows similar presence of beta-amyloid plaques,[56] suggesting that plaque formation is initiated quite soon following injury and in relation to the rapid upregulation of amyloid precursor protein (APP). Perhaps more important, the production of amyloid precursor protein is upregulated after TBI[57] along with microglia-derived interleukin 1 (IL-1; a potent anti-inflammatory cytokine) resulting in increased expression[58,59] and processing of APP.[60] IL-1 activates astrocytes[61] and promotes increased expression of astrocyte-derived APOE-4.[62] Traumatic axonal injury results in a local accumulation of APP and may represent a source for intraneuronal processing of APP with the production of beta-amyloid peptides.[41,63] APP is produced by endothelium, glia, and neurons[64] and seems to play a role in intra- and interneuronal signaling, synaptic transmission, neuronal growth, plasticity, learning, and memory.[65,66]

Certain mechanisms of injury have been shown to result in a surge of APP messenger RNA or its translation in ischemia,[67–70] axotomy,[71] and in chemical injury to cholinergic structures.[72] The precise role of APP and IL-1 in AD and brain injury of various types has to be further elucidated.

AD is a heterogeneous disorder that may be caused by genetic or environmental factors or a combination of both.[73] Chromosomal abnormalities on 1, 14, and 21 have been implicated in the pathogenesis of the early-onset form of AD. The epsilon-4 allele of the apolipoprotein E gene on chromosome 19 is a risk factor for early- and late-onset sporadic and familial AD. As detailed earlier, TBI is an environmental trigger for the upregulation of beta-amyloid protein, which is found to be present in approximately 30% of patients who die after a single episode of brain injury. For those individuals who develop AD after a TBI, there is an overrepresentation of the APOE-4 allele;[74] however, it is clear that not all who possess the APOE-4 allele go on to develop AD.

Still other factors may bear on the earlier manifestation of AD and the association of TBI with other dementias. Brain trauma damages the blood–brain barrier, permitting extravasation of serum proteins into the surrounding parenchyma.[75,76] The introduction of serum proteins into the surrounding parenchyma may portend an activation of an immunologic response later in life in instances when the blood–brain barrier is again compromised. Because permeability of the blood–brain barrier is not well understood in normal aging, the issue of potential leakage as a trigger for a secondary immunologic response needs further exploration.[77]

Study of regional cerebral blood flow in AD reveals diminution of regional cerebral blood flow in the posterior temporal and inferior frontal/parietal areas in subjects who developed AD.[78] Therefore, the nature of the TBI itself may yield predictive insight into whether AD will more likely manifest. For example, focal and multifocal injuries to the brain tend to predominate in the frontal poles and anterior temporal structures of the brain.

Utilizing PET, regional brain metabolism for individuals with cognitive symptoms of dementia was found to be a sensitive indicator of both AD and neurodegenerative disease by Silverman et al.[79] A negative PET scan indicated that cognitive impairments were unlikely to progress over at least a 3-year period.

A salient neuroimaging feature of AD and the frontotemporal dementias is progressive brain atrophy, also a characteristic of chronic TBI. Chan et al.[80] obtained serial magnetic resonance images to quantify rates of cerebral atrophy in individuals with AD, frontotemporal dementia, and control subjects. They found the annual rate of atrophy was significantly greater in individuals with dementia (2.7%) than in control subjects (0.5%). Although the results of this study were able to distinguish normals from individuals with dementia, it could not differentiate between the types of dementia, such as AD or frontotemporal dementia. These atrophy measurement techniques are currently confined to the research environment. In the future, brain atrophy measurement techniques may provide a means of assessing the differential characteristics of post-TBI cerebral atrophy resulting from aging contrasted with an index of a more specific separate dementia entity, such as AD or frontotemporal dementia. The implications of this regional volumetry technology may help in the development of treatments with the goal of delaying a progressive neurodegenerative process.

The loss of neural structures associated with TBI earlier in life does reduce overall neuronal availability and thereby diminishes the redundancy of neural structures. As such, a diminished reserve may contribute to an earlier manifestation of dementias. To the extent that AD and other dementias may have a genetic basis, persons with TBI may experience the development of these dementias in concurrence with the TBI sequelae, just as they might other diseases, such as cancer or heart disease.

As one attempts to draw conclusions regarding TBI and its relationship to the development of AD or other dementias, multidimensional factors need to be considered. The clinician must evaluate the potential interrelationships between age, various neuropathologies associated with different injury types, idiopathic neuronal atrophy, the potential contribution of repetitive trauma, genetic predisposition, and immunosusceptibility. These relationships may all play a role in the timing of the onset of dementia, the rapidity of progression of dementia, and/or the development of other neurodegenerative disorders.

11.3.2 Other Neurologic Disorders

The majority of studies investigating the relationship of TBI and neurologic disease have focused on brain injury as either a precipitating risk factor for the *de novo* development or exacerbation of the progression of AD, Parkinson's disease, amyotrophic lateral sclerosis, and multiple sclerosis (MS).[81–86] Given case reports relating post-TBI syndromes that resemble Parkinson's disease,[87,88] the theoretical consideration of trauma as an etiology of parkinsonism is necessary.[89] Goetz and Stebbins[90] found that TBI seemed to modify the course of Parkinson's disease in a small series of 10 individuals. Following TBI, they found a transient increase in disability status lasting a few weeks, but after 1 year, there was no difference in disability compared with age-matched control subjects.

Williams et al.[86] examined the medical records of 821 people with TBI, between 1935 and 1974, who were more than 40 years old. These people were followed for the development of dementia and other degenerative neurologic diseases. Utilizing a standardized morbidity ratio, there was no evidence that brain trauma was a significant risk factor for the development of Parkinsonism, Parkinson's disease, or amyotrophic lateral sclerosis.

Over the many years, the issue of injuries precipitating MS or promoting new relapses of MS has also been passionately debated in the literature. Well-designed studies have concluded that TBI and other types of injuries do not precipitate MS, nor do they lead to relapses of MS. Sibley et al.[82] reported a large number of prospectively studied individuals with MS and identified a subgroup of 67 individuals who incurred a total of 140 episodes of "closed head injury." It should be noted that only nine of these episodes were associated with a period of definite or probable loss of consciousness, with none lasting more than a few minutes. Siva et al.[84] examined individuals with significant TBI to determine whether any of these individuals subsequently developed MS. The study did not consider individuals with MS who incurred TBI.

However, to our knowledge, there are no other studies describing the interaction of "significant TBI" with underlying MS. Many clinicians have wrestled with the issue of a coincidental MS relapse versus the consequences from the TBI. It has been postulated that the pathobiologic interaction of TBI with damage to axons in previously demyelinated pathways may explain these unexpected clinical scenarios.[91,92]

The majority of studies addressing trauma and MS concern the issue of trauma as an environmental etiologic trigger of MS or relapses of MS. In 1987, Poser[93] suggested that TBI may exacerbate the underlying disease process of MS. Bamford et al.,[81] Sibley et al.,[82,83] Siva et al.,[84] and Kurland,[85] on the basis of longitudinal studies of cohorts, found no indication that either the onset or exacerbation of MS was the result of physical trauma. A major limitation of these studies was that their design did not evaluate the consequences of "significant TBI" in people with MS.

In general, the effect of preexisting neurologic disorders and their attendant neuropathology interacting with the pathobiology caused by TBI appear significant, but how this modifies outcome is unknown. Conversely, how the pathobiology of TBI modifies the subsequent course of the underlying neurologic disease is also unknown. In this regard, demyelinating diseases, such as MS, may interact differently than neuronal diseases, such as Parkinson's disease, in the setting of TBI and with the consequences of aging. This, again, may be an additive effect related to neuronal loss with increasing brain age, thus magnifying the pathobiologic effects of the TBI and the neuropathology of other neuronal diseases, such as Parkinson's disease, and demyelinating diseases, such as MS.

Recently, studies examining the history of recurrent concussions and even repetitive subconcussive contacts to the head have been evaluated regarding the risk factors in developing later life cognitive impairment and/or AD. In a study of retired professional football players who had a previous head injury exposure, the risk of developing late-life cognitive impairments was examined by Guskiewicz et al.[94] This study demonstrated a dose–response relationship among concussions, frequencies, and the increased lifetime burden of cognitive impairment. More specifically, retired players who had sustained three or more reported concussions had a fivefold prevalence of mild cognitive impairments as a diagnosis[95,96] and a threefold prevalence of reported significant memory problems when compared with other retired players who did not have a history of concussion. As it relates to mild TBI and concussion, future prospective studies were recommended. Specifically, these studies need to document more clearly the history related to type and severity of concussion, correlative rigorous diagnostic criteria, genetic evaluation, and serial clinical evaluations, including neurocognitive testing and functional neuroimaging.

11.4 Seizures

Seizures are considered to be the clinical manifestation of an abnormal and excessive discharge of a set of neurons within the brain, including cortical cells. Although seizure phenomena can be associated with an acute insult to the CNS or a generalized systemic metabolic disturbance, this does not necessarily constitute a condition of "epilepsy."[74] Epilepsy is defined as a condition characterized by recurrent, unprovoked seizures.[76]

Epilepsy occurs within the general population with varying incidence depending upon age. This topic must consider, independently, seizures associated with "normal aging," aging-related diseases, TBI, and their potential interactions.

11.4.1 Normal Aging

Seizure incidence appears to be highest in children, although incidence increases substantially in people older than 70 years of age.[97,98] Hauser et al.,[97] in a prospective epidemiologic population-based study, followed the incidence of epilepsy and unprovoked seizures in Rochester, Minnesota, over a 50-year period. Incidence in people older than age 70 was found to be two to three times greater than in children. Incidence at age 40 was 30/100,000 and, by age 80, increased to 140/100,000. No gender difference observed. Generalized seizures occurred most frequently in children, whereas the elderly had a higher incidence of partial-onset seizures. In people older than age 75, partial epilepsy was five times more frequent than at earlier ages. Approximately two thirds of seizures in people younger than age 40 were tonic–clonic seizures. The rate of tonic–clonic seizures decreased to 54% for the age group 40 to 65 years and to 40% in people 65 years and older.[97] Overall, the cumulative incidence of epilepsy ranged from 1.2% from 0 to 24 years, 3% from 25 to 74 years, and 4.4% from 75 to 85 years. Age-specific incidence is highest in the first year of life. Incidence decreases during childhood and remains stable up to age 54, when incidence begins to increase again.[97]

Hauser et al.[97] determined the three most common etiologies for seizure disorders in people older than age 65 were cerebrovascular disease, degenerative diseases of the CNS, and CNS tumors. Approximately two thirds of all cases had a cerebrovascular etiology. Included in this category are cerebrovascular accident (embolic stroke and intracerebral hemorrhage), hypertension, vasculitis, and arteriovenous malformation.[99–104] Seizures are fairly common within the first 2 weeks of cerebral infarction and are considered to be an acute effect of the infarction.[105,106] Cerebral cortex involvement, the presence of multiple lesions, hemorrhage, and embolic infarcts have been identified as risk factors for recurrent seizures following stroke.[107]

Degenerative diseases are associated with an incidence of seizures that ranges from 10% to 22%.[108–111] McAreavey et al.[108] found that people with dementia who had seizures were younger and more cognitively impaired than a control group of people with dementia only. There did not appear to be any dementia etiologic differences between the two groups.

Hauser et al.[97] found CNS infections, tumors, and neurologic defects arising from birth or trauma to be of equal frequency as antecedents to seizure disorders in people age 15 to 34 years. Neoplasms and trauma were equally frequent antecedents in people age 35 to 64 years, and cerebrovascular disease emerged as the most frequent. Cerebrovascular insults preceded the diagnosis of epilepsy in 15% of this age group. In the group of individuals older than 65 years of age, 28% of all newly identified seizure cases were preceded by cerebrovascular disease and 20% of seizures had associated degenerative disease.

Management of seizures is impacted by physiologic changes in aging.[112] Pharmacokinetics, routes of administration, drug interactions, pharmacodynamic interactions, and even drug cost must all be considered because they influence treatment selection.[98] Aging is associated with decreases in serum concentration of plasma proteins and albumin necessary for pharmacologic binding, absorption, and bioavailability.[113,114] Inefficiencies in hepatic and renal function with advancing age also impact metabolism and excretion.[113,114] Swallowing and cognitive decline may contribute to difficulty with an oral route of administration. Nasogastric, intramuscular, and rectal options for drug delivery must be made available.[115] Finally, in people older than 60 years of age, the average number of drugs taken at one time is seven, with up to 13 taken over a year.[116] The risk of pharmacokinetic and pharmacodynamic polypharmacy interactions is quite high.

11.4.2 Traumatic Brain Injury

Seizures play a relatively prominent role in a discussion of either aging or TBI. Seizures represent the second most frequent intracerebral complication, occurring at a rate of 17%. Only intracranial hypertension, as an intracerebral complication, is higher and, then, by only 3%.[17] Seizures increase in frequency from year 1 to year 5 as a reason for rehospitalization and become the second most common reason for rehospitalization, following general health maintenance.[24,25]

Studies of seizure incidence and prevalence in the general population logically have individuals with TBI as a subgroup. Consequently, direct comparison of data sets between the two groups should be cautiously interpreted. The causes of epilepsy that are germane to the discussion of "aging-related" posttraumatic seizures can be idiopathic, tumor, trauma, and vascular, which may include hypoxic/ischemic cerebral insult.[117] A thorough review of the subject can be found in Chapter 2 (this volume). Also, Dalmady-Israel and Zasler[118] published a critical review of the literature related to current concepts of definition, incidence, and risk factors pertaining to posttraumatic seizures. This review, together with an overview of the topic by Yablon,[119] offers a good literature review of posttraumatic seizures over the past 50 years, including incidence, natural history, and predictive characteristics. These articles discuss rehabilitation management topics, such as anticonvulsant prophylaxis, symptom management, and other problems encountered in the rehabilitation setting.

Posttraumatic epilepsy (PTE), to some degree, is the result of neuronal biochemical changes related to the injury process and may play a role in seizures or recurrent ictal episodes.[120] In addition, differences in types of force, mechanical factors, and anatomic injury may help determine one's predilection for developing posttraumatic seizures.[120] A positive correlation between brain injury severity and the development of one or more seizures has been identified. When brain trauma results in cortical injury and neurologic deficits without interruption of the dura matter, PTE incidence ranges between 7% and 39%. When dural disruption and neurologic abnormalities coexist, the incidence increases dramatically to between 20% and 57%. Interestingly, however, injury severity and the persistence of ictal episodes do not appear to have a correlation.[121]

In practical terms, rehabilitation professionals have considered missile penetrating injuries, depressed skull fractures, intracerebral/intracranial hematomas, and early epilepsy, defined as seizures within the first week after brain trauma, as the highest at-risk group for developing PTE.[122–125] Feeney and Walker[126] developed a mathematical model to estimate the probability of posttraumatic seizures. This classic study found individuals with central parietal injury, dural penetration, hemiplegia, missile wounds, and intracerebral hematomas to be at greatest risk for development of PTE.

Clinicians' experience and Feeney and Walker's[126] work suggesting dural penetration to be a key risk factor has also been substantiated in the literature. Although the risk of seizures is, in fact, very high following penetrating missile injury and has been estimated at 35% to 53%,[127] the risk in diffuse closed head injury, without contusion or laceration of the cortex, is much lower, at approximately 5%.[128]

PTE can occur during the early period following TBI. The early period is defined as occurring within the first 7 days of injury.[129] PTE can also have its first manifestation many months or years postinjury, thereby defining late seizures. The risk of PTE after cerebral parenchyma-penetrating injury remains for up to 15 years. Approximately 95% of individuals who remain free of seizures during the first 3 years after injury remain seizure free in the long term.[130–132] Approximately 56% of individuals with TBI, without missile injuries, who develop late seizures do so within the first year of injury.[133]

Age at the time of injury appears to figure into the risk of developing PTE.[122] In a study by Kennedy and Freeman,[134] risk of early posttraumatic seizures was found to be higher in children, although fewer developed late seizures, defined as after the first week posttrauma. When late seizures occurred, approximately 40% were noted to have focal features, 70% became unconscious, and 20% had disturbed consciousness, with or without focality, defined as partial–complex seizures.

In a study of 490 consecutive people with TBI, Asikainen et al.[135] studied factors active in the development of early and late seizures and their subsequent influence on long-term outcome. They determined that young children were more prone to early seizures than adolescents and adults, who were more prone to late seizures. The main risk factors for late posttraumatic seizures were the known presence of early seizures and depressed skull fracture. Brain injury severity, as measured by a low Glasgow Coma Scale (GCS) score, prolonged unconsciousness, and posttraumatic amnesia, without localized brain pathology, was not found to be a risk factor for the development of late PTE. It was recommended that people with TBI who developed seizure disorders have appropriate anticonvulsant therapy and thorough follow-up. Individuals receiving this level of care were able to attain higher rehabilitation goals and functional outcomes, such as employment.[135]

To explore further the risks of developing PTE with advancing age, the coexistence of genetic predisposition must be considered. Investigation of the influence of apolipoprotein alleles in nonlesional temporal lobe epilepsy (TLE) saw no relationship between APOE polymorphisms and TLE.[136] However, a later investigation found that, although the distribution of APOE genotype was similar between temporal lobe lesional and nonlesional patients and control subjects, higher levels of plasma APOE were observed in TLE patients 4.9 times more than control subjects,[137] suggesting that APOE may play a role in TLE.

It is always of great interest to be able to discern whether a seizure will be an isolated event or whether recurrence is likely or inevitable. This is of concern for operation of automobiles and mechanized equipment, independence and safety in the community or living environment, and return to school or work. Haltiner et al.[138] studied the incidence and risk factors for seizure recurrence after the onset of late PTE. This longitudinal, cohort design showed that when late seizures developed following severe TBI, the probability of recurrence was high. The importance of aggressive anticonvulsant medication management following a first, unprovoked late seizure was emphasized.

Although the importance of treating defined seizures and epilepsy is clear, the issue of suppressive treatment versus prevention is somewhat controversial. *Suppressive treatment* is defined as medication intervention to decrease the occurrence of seizures during the time in which the individual is at greatest risk. *Prevention* refers to an approach of ongoing treatment following the epileptogenic-at-risk phase. Several older retrospective studies suggested antiepileptic prophylaxis may prevent the genesis of epileptic foci.[139–141]

However, most clinicians now practice in a manner consistent with a study conducted by Temkin et al.[129] This randomized, double-blind study of phenytoin coverage for the prevention of posttraumatic seizures was designed on the assumption that seizure prophylaxis following brain injuries (i.e., medicating to attempt to prevent the first seizure) would prevent the development of eventual posttraumatic epilepsy. Convincing evidence was demonstrated regarding the effectiveness of phenytoin seizure prophylaxis when treating during the first week following severe TBI. When compared with placebo, treatment with phenytoin was associated with a 73% decrease in the risk of seizures during the first week. However, no significant protective effect was detected between day 8 and the end of the second year of study. Therefore, the early, but not late, effect of phenytoin appears to have an early suppressive effect (i.e., during the vulnerable epileptogenic phase), but not necessarily a true long-term prophylactic or preventative effect. This hallmark study concluded that phenytoin reduces the incidence of seizures during the first week after injury, but not thereafter.

Hepatic metabolism, when considering seizure issues, has implications with advancing age. More specifically, hepatic metabolism been shown to be altered following acute neurotrauma.[142,143] This altered metabolism following neurotrauma[142] may persist for at least 2 to 4 weeks in some patients. The degree of metabolic alteration appears to be associated with older age, ethanol on admission, increased severity of neurologic injury, tube feeding, total parenteral nutrition, and postinjury neurosurgical intervention. Time to normalization of unbound clearance is longer for patients with TBI and may be the result of activation of proinflammatory cytokines, tumor necrosis factor alpha, and IL-1 and -6.[143] This study demonstrated that metabolism of valproic acid is increased following TBI. Animal studies suggest that valproic acid may have neuroprotective properties counteracting neuronal damage in the hippocampal formation, including the dentate gyrus, seen after status epilepticus.[144]

Therapies for epilepsy are largely focused on symptom management (i.e., reducing or eliminating seizures). However, these interventions also affect the underlying mechanisms of disease progression of epileptogenesis.[145] There is some suggestion that antioxidant therapies may be of interest in preventing PTE, specifically those cases arising from the increased presence of reactive oxygen species.[146,147]

PTE represents an opportunity for repeated brain injury both from falls associated with seizures as well as from the direct effects of seizures.[148] It may be appropriate to consider status epilepticus as even a separate brain injury when it occurs.[149]

While managing people with TBI throughout their entire life, the clinician must be cognizant of the unique presentations of the types of seizures that present with aging and the elderly, appropriate methods of diagnosis, and the complexity of different treatment paradigms.[115,150,151] Care should be taken to avoid overattribution of seizures to a history of TBI alone in the elderly.

11.5 Cerebral Atrophy, Ventricular Size, and Hydrocephalus

Posttraumatic ventriculomegaly is a frequent neuroimaging finding following moderate to severe TBI.[152,153] Ventriculomegaly following TBI remains a controversial condition regarding what it signifies. Chronic neuroimaging findings of cerebral or subcortical atrophy do not necessarily have clinical implications.

Chronically aging TBI reveals a relationship between cortical atrophy and ventricular volume in neuroimaging studies. Volumetric measures of brain morphology show that the generalized effects of most traumatic diffuse axonal injuries are more evident via ventricular dilatation, whereas the effects of focal and multifocal injury appear to be more evident in cortical atrophy measures.[154]

Computed tomographic (CT) volumetric studies of the cortical/subcortical mass-to-ventricular size ratio[155] have shown that marked encephalomalacia occurs over many years postinjury.[154,156] As the processes of neurodegeneration and gliosis associated with injury advance over time, cortical/subcortical volume decreases, and there is an associated compensatory increase in ventricular size. Over time, the CT pattern in TBI is one of mild to moderate ventricular enlargement and normal sulcal prominence, except in cases of focal injury. This process is far greater than that seen in normal aging, although a similar, less pronounced change in cortical volume and ventricular size is seen in normal aging. MRI of elderly persons with a history of diffuse axonal injury demonstrates progressive atrophy within the corpus callosum over many years.[157–159]

Normally, CSF is produced by the choroid plexus in the ventricular system. CSF is extruded into the ventricles and flows from the ventricle of origin to the sequential ventricles via the aqueduct of Sylvius, ultimately exiting the ventricular system to be reabsorbed by the arachnoid villi in the superior sagittal sinus. Noncommunicating or obstructive hydrocephalus develops when an obstruction blocks the flow of CSF and a buildup of CSF occurs behind the obstruction, causing the ventricles behind the obstruction to enlarge. Obstructive hydrocephalus can occur as a result of hematoma, subarachnoid hemorrhage, or meningitis.[160] Communicating hydrocephalus occurs when CSF production continues at a normal rate, but reabsorption in the subarachnoid space is slowed, causing a buildup of CSF within the ventricular system. Ventricular enlargement stretches fibers in the surrounding regions, thereby impairing function. Clinically significant hydrocephalus, whether obstructive or communicating, may be of a high- or normal-pressure variant.[161]

Differentiation of ventriculomegaly, in which the underlying process is the result of subcortical atrophy, and "hydrocephalus," which implies an active obstruction of CSF or diminished reabsorption, is quite difficult at times. The progression of ventricular enlargement, which results from cerebral atrophy associated with diffuse axonal injury and normal aging, can further complicate this clinical differentiation. The importance of differentiation of the typical symptoms of normal-pressure hydrocephalus[162] from symptoms related to brain trauma, itself, is reviewed by Beyerl and Black.[163] The imaging criteria of Kishore et al.[152] are still widely accepted for progressive ventriculomegaly with the distended appearance of the anterior horns of the lateral ventricles, enlargement of the temporal horns of the third ventricle, with normal or absent sulci, and, if present, enlargement of the basilar cisterns and fourth ventricle. Periventricular decreased density on CT scanning was also felt to be a diagnostic indicator of communicating hydrocephalus, as well as enhanced transependymal and periventricular flow patterns on MRI.

The classic triad of normal-pressure hydrocephalus is impaired gait, incontinence, and dementia.[162,164,165] During the early stages of this phenomenon, gait may be unsteady or apraxic and cognitive decline can be noted, as opposed to an absolute loss of consciousness in more severe cases.[166]

Even though ventricular shunting is frequently regarded as a routine procedure, clinicians must be cognizant of the possibilities of mechanical, biologic, or technical complications.[167] Complications of ventricular shunting for hydrocephalus can include shunt failure, hemorrhage, delayed wound closure, infection, and seizures.[168] Dan and Wade[167] reviewed the incidence of seizures after ventricular shunting in 180 of 207 consecutive cases for hydrocephalus arising from various causes. A total of 9.4% developed seizures. Incidence appeared to be age related, with a 15.2% occurrence in children younger than 1 year, 10% occurrence in people age 1 to 49 years, and 6.9% incidence in people older than 49 years. Risk of postshunt seizures decreased with time after surgery, from 5% during the first year to 1.1% after the third year. The incidence of seizures rose with multiple shunt revisions. Cortical puncture site for ventricular catheterization significantly affected rates of seizures. In 168 individuals with a posterior parietal insertion, incidence of seizures was 6.6%. In 11 individuals with frontal catheter placement, 54.5% experienced seizures.

Shunt implantation outcomes were also reviewed in 48 individuals following severe TBI in whom implantation was performed a mean of 27 months postinjury.[168] Improvement in clinical status occurred in 52.1% of patients, whereas 47.9% showed no improvement. Immediate seizures occurred within 1 hour of surgery in five patients. Seizures occurred within the first week of surgery in one patient and after the first week in 29 patients. Prior to shunt implantation, 14 individuals had seizures, whereas 17 developed seizures after shunt implantation. Postoperative complications that required shunt revision were shown by 15 individuals. Three individuals had postoperative complications that did not require shunt revision, one of whom developed marked cerebral edema.

In summary, clinical differentiation between cerebral atrophy resulting from aging, and subcortical atrophy resulting from trauma, must be made. The clinical and imaging differentiation is furthered by determination of the degree to which the observed recovery pattern is, or is not, consistent with an expected recovery pattern related to the underlying pathophysiologic correlates of injury. When incongruence between the observed and expected recovery patterns exists, the interaction of communicating hydrocephalus, with or without pressure, should be considered. Careful selection for shunt placement should be based on a realistic appraisal of the risk/benefit ratio for surgical complications versus better outcomes. Favorable outcomes from CSF shunting in appropriately selected individuals are reported, and technical considerations include timing, the type of shunt valve used, seizure prophylaxis, and methods of long-term follow-up.[169] A recent technologic advance is found in the development of programmable shunt valves. An improved understanding of intracranial pressure dynamics and their clinical correlates, before and after CSF shunting, may lead to a more scientific rationale for the application of these valves and their safe use.

11.6 Neuroendocrine Dysfunction

TBI has been associated with neuroendocrine dysfunction in both the acute and chronic states.[170–174] Endocrine abnormalities following brain trauma vary with the comparative degree of injury to the hypothalamus, the anterior or posterior pituitary, the upper or lower portion of the pituitary stalk, and the connections of these structures to other subcortical and brainstem structures.[175] These traumatic neurohypophyseal system injuries acutely may lead to abnormalities in salt and water metabolism, including syndrome of insufficient antidiuretic hormone (SIADH), temporary or permanent diabetes insipidus, thyroid function, control of body temperature, abnormalities in adrenocorticotropic hormone (ACTH)–cortisol levels, and glucose metabolism, to name a few. Yuan and Wade[175] felt it was unusual to find "classic" features of hypothalamic or pituitary dysfunction in the TBI population. Koiv et al.[170] found serum catecholamine and ACTH levels were reduced in people with severe brain injury who had CT evidence of severe alterations in mesencephalic/diencephalic regions. In these patients, cortisol levels were elevated.

Early reports of neuroendocrine dysfunction following head trauma appeared in 1942[176]; however, reports of hypopituitarism following head trauma were scarce enough that its prevalence was thought to be quite low.[177] The condition of posttraumatic hypopituitarism can become clinically significant at any time postinjury, with 15% of patients diagnosed 5 or more years after trauma.[177] Hypopituitarism in its most severe form can be life threatening, and in lesser manifestations can impair adaptation to stressful events.[177]

Neuroendocrine dysfunction following chronic TBI has recently been systematically evaluated as a potential contributor to outcome. Lieberman et al.[172] studied 70 adults with TBI on average who were 4 years postinjury. Serum thyrotropin stimulation hormone (TSH), free T_4, insulinlike growth factor 1, prolactin, testosterone (males), and cosyntropin stimulation were evaluated. Abnormal results were followed by dynamic tests of gonadotropin, TSH, and growth hormone (GH) secretion. The authors reported that 31.4% of subjects had no abnormalities. A single abnormal axis was found in 51.4% of the subjects (26 adrenal, 8 thyroid, and 2 GH), and 12 subjects had dual-axis abnormalities (5 adrenal and thyroid, 4 adrenal and GH, 1 GH and thyroid, 1 gonadal and thyroid, and 1 adrenal and prolactin). There was no correlation with initial GCS score. GH deficiency was found in 15% of subjects and low morning cortisol levels in 46% of these patients. Hypogonadism and diabetes insipidus were not observed.

Kelly et al.[171] reported some degree of hypopituitarism in nearly 40% of persons who had sustained moderate to severe head injury. Long-term anterior pituitary dysfunction was most common, whereas thyrotroph and corticotroph deficiencies were less common. The authors suggest that pituitary–hypothalamic axis testing is warranted for people with moderate to severe brain injury or subarachnoid hemorrhage, particularly those who experienced hypotensive or hypoxic events, evidence of diffuse brain swelling, and/or basilar skull fractures that involve the sella turcica. Although direct trauma to the pituitary gland may account for dysfunction, the authors feel that vascular causes may be more prominent.

Bushnik et al.[178] found an inordinately high prevalence of endocrine abnormalities associated with brain injury in evaluation of a group of 64 individuals averaging 42 years of age and 10 years postinjury. Utilizing definitions of severe growth hormone deficiency (GHD) of peak GH of less than 3 ng/mL and moderate GHD of peak GH of 3 to 9.9 ng/mL, more than 90% of individuals showed moderate or severe GHD following glucagon provocation. Utilizing the more conservative GHD definition of peak GH of less than 3 ng/mL, the study still found a high incidence of a single-axis abnormality of 79%. Cortisol deficiency was defined as a fasting serum cortisol less than 15 µg/dL, and a prevalence of 19% was found. Central hypothyroidism, defined as low serum free T4 in the presence of low normal serum TSH, was found in 19% of individuals as well.

Leon-Carrion et al.[179] compared individuals with TBI with GHD to those without GHD and found greater deficits in attention, executive function, memory, and emotion in those with GHD. GH replacement has been identified to improve many of these deficits.[180–182] Kelly et al.[183] showed elevated levels of depression and reduced quality of life associated with GHD in TBI. Furthermore, mitochondrial damage arising as part of the degenerative cascade in widespread/diffuse cortical traumatic axonal injury (TAI)[184] likely impacts overall neurologic function and may be particularly evident in higher executive skills. GH impacts both mitochondrial function and myelin repair and production.[185–187] GH increases insulinlike growth factor 1, which in turn impacts a host of functions, including oligodendrocyte production of myelin,[187] cell proliferation, myogenesis, exercise tolerance, and energy metabolism.

Neuroendocrine function may be important for rehabilitative success, neuromedical function, and overall health. It is illustrative to consider examples of how specific endocrine abnormalities may correlate and further contribute to an individual's functional life challenges over time.

GH is involved in myelin formation and repair, oligodendrocyte development, energy metabolism, and mitochondrial function. GH has implications for attention, working memory, and long-term memory. GH deficiency manifests in exercise intolerance, reduced strength, dyslipidemia, impaired psychological well-being, fatigue, osteoporosis, and abnormal body composition as decreased lean body mass and increased abdominal adiposity.[188,189]

Neuronal growth is regulated by cytoskeletal proteins and depends on thyroid hormone equilibrium.[190] The highest concentration of thyroid hormone receptors has been found in the adult rat hippocampus, amygdala, and cerebral cortex.[191] Both thyroid and estrogen have been demonstrated to impact dendritic tree density in the cerebral cortex.[146,192–195] Thyroid is involved in gene regulation for encoding proteins of myelin, mitochondria, neurotrophins, neurotrophic receptors, transcription factors, cellular matrix proteins, adhesion molecules, and intracellular signaling. It plays an integral role in mitochondrial energy transduction. Thyroid deficiency can result in cerebellar ataxia, leading to instability and a predisposition to falling and reinjury. Thyroid deficiency can also further contribute to cognitive and emotional difficulties in the domains of memory and new learning. Symptoms of thyroid deficiency include fatigue, myopathy, weakness, decreased cognitive function, decreased libido, depression, irritability, and menstrual irregularity.[188,189]

Glucocorticoid receptors, like thyroid receptors, are found in concentration in the hippocampus.[196] Cortisol impacts memory and mood disorders via the limbic/medial temporal lobe. The subsequent paralimbic neurobehavioral consequences of glucocorticoid insufficiency include apathy, depression, irritability, and psychosis. Increased cortisol decreases the expression of brain-derived neurotrophic factor expression and downregulates hippocampal synaptic connectivity.

The direct result of endocrine dysfunction as it relates to TBI and aging may lead to an array of chronic physical, neurobehavioral, and functional disabilities. This comorbidity should be further explored in individuals who display chronic symptoms of fatigue, loss of muscle strength, decreased energy, cognitive dysfunction, inability to regulate body temperature, emotional lability, decreased aerobic capacity, and decreased bone mineral density. Combined with the direct effects of TBI, an endocrinopathy may further result in a diminished sense of well-being, social isolation, and overall reduced quality of life.[197,198]

Endocrine function should be monitored in brain-injured individuals who may be particularly susceptible beyond the postacute phase of management. Ghigo et al.[189] provide specific guidelines for endocrine surveillance following TBI. TBI individuals at particular risk with aging to this comorbidity are those with known basilar skull fracture, history of severe diffuse axonal injury with dysautonomia, protracted posttraumatic amnesia, or those with a history of syndrome of insufficient antidiuretic hormone or diabetes insipidus.

11.7 Sleep

Sleep is beneficial for the rejuvenation of human functioning, and animal studies have shown it necessary for survival. Deprivation and disturbance of this rejuvenating process can have many adverse effects. With aging, these effects include excessive daytime sleepiness, fatigue, frustration, depression, poor quality of life, impaired performance, decreased productivity, and increased health care costs.[199] Sleep disturbance is a relatively common complication following TBI. Sleep dysfunction and its relationship to TBI-related fatigue merits consideration.

Beetar et al.[200] reported that subjects with brain injury had significantly more insomnia (56%) and pain complaints (59%) than nonbrain-injured subjects. Fatigue has been reported to be as high as 68% at 2 years and 73% at 5 years postinjury.[201] Sleep–wake disturbances consisting of excessive daytime sleepiness and fatigue have been found in 55% of patients, and posttraumatic hypersomnia in 22%, although insomnia and circadian rhythm disturbances were not found.[202] This study did report on a group of patients with overall better outcomes than reported in large clinical outcome studies, suggesting the possibility of a biased population.

Clinchot et al.[203] reported 50% of brain-injured individuals had difficulty sleeping during inpatient rehabilitation. Another study reported 30% of individuals with brain injury were found to experience insomnia.[204] Interestingly, they reported that the more severe brain injury was associated with less likelihood of sleep disturbance. A single-night study of 14 patients with mild to severe TBI averaging approximately 20 months postinjury showed that these individuals had more awakenings lasting longer than 5 minutes and shorter rapid eye movement (REM) latency when compared with a group of healthy sleepers.[205] Stage 1 sleep was statistically greater than control subjects, whereas there were no statistical differences in stage 2, stage 3–4, or REM sleep. A two-consecutive-night study of 16 individuals with severe TBI comparing postinjury intervals at 1 month, 6 months, and 12 months showed increased number of awakenings, increased percentage of wakefulness, and decreased percentage of REM sleep.[206] Improvement was noted at 6 months; however, at 12 months, sleep disturbances increased again, particularly in those between 35 to 45 years of age.

Many of the sequelae of sleep disturbance may be particularly disruptive to the neurobehavioral functioning of individuals with TBI. This includes agitation, poor performance, decreased attention, memory, confusion, somatic complaints, and decreased seizure threshold. One study revealed self-reported sleep disturbance in 73% of rehabilitation inpatients and 52% of outpatients with brain injury, and two other studies reported a correlation between sleep pattern abnormalities and cognitive deficits following brain injury.[207–209]

The particular sleep disorders individuals with TBI are at risk for include posttraumatic hypersomnia, narcolepsy, central sleep apnea, obstructive sleep apnea (OSA), nocturnal seizures, periodic limb movement disorder, and insomnia.[210] In a study of 20 individuals 1 and 9 months after brain injury who complained of excessive daytime sleepiness, eight subjects had sleep apnea/hypopnea syndrome.[211] Sleep apnea was found in 47% of individuals with brain injury in acute inpatient rehabilitation.[212] In 71 brain-injured individuals in a residential/day rehabilitation program, excessive daytime sleepiness was reported in 65% of subjects. Eleven percent had sleep apnea/hypopnea, 25% had periodic limb movement disorders, and one subject had narcolepsy.[213] Finally, Castriotta and Lai[214] found 7 of 10 individuals with brain injury had complaints of excessive daytime sleepiness, sleep-disordered breathing, and narcolepsy. They reported that all subjects were treated with either continuous positive airway pressure (for sleep-disordered breathing) or Provigil (for narcolepsy and posttraumatic hypersomnia), which resulted in subjectively improved quality of life and substantial improvement in daytime function.[214]

It is important to note that some studies point out discrepancies between self-reports of fatigue/sleep and objective findings.[178,215] Individuals with brain injury appear to be less accurate in reporting. Inaccuracy may be related to impaired self-perception (anosognosia), memory deficits, or other factors such as accommodation to fatigue at prolonged postinjury intervals. The inaccuracy of reporting, however, points to the need for objective diagnostic studies of sleep in all patients.

Lankford et al.[216] reported on nine cases of narcolepsy following TBI. They concluded that narcolepsy may become manifest following even a minor brain injury in six of the nine cases where human leucocyte antigen testing showed a genetic predisposition to narcolepsy. Ebrahim et al.[217] relate two cases of narcolepsy following TBI to potential hypocretin deficiency and related hypothalamic damage. They suggest that posttraumatic narcolepsy may vary by clinical presentation, nature and severity of injury, time from injury to onset of narcolepsy, and human leucocyte antigen type.

The incidence of sleep disorders for persons with TBI is much higher than that in the general population. Sleep apnea/hypopnea is estimated to occur in 2% to 4% of the general populace. Periodic limb movement disorder occurrence is about 5% and hypersomnolence occurs in 0.3% to 13% of the general population.[213] Sleep disorders clearly contribute to a number of other neuromedical conditions, including reduced seizure threshold, psychiatric and behavioral disorders, cognitive dysfunction, and overall feeling of reduced psychological well-being.[164,218–220] From a social perspective, sleep disorders have been associated with increased incidence of motor vehicle collisions[221,222] and unintentional injuries.[223]

OSA also represents a potential area of concern. The incidence of OSA is an extreme contributor as well to sleep–wake disturbances following TBI. Cognitive impairment consisting of impaired sustained attention and memory has been found in patients with

OSA following TBI.[224] Reduced mammillary body volume in patients with OSA supports impaired memory associated with OSA as well.[137] Anterograde memory disorders have also been associated with OSA.[225] Such memory deficits do not seem to be completely reversible following treatment with continuous positive airway pressure, suggesting permanent neurologic damage.

Cerebral damage is not routinely observed via standard MRI in OSA in a non-TBI population; however, more sophisticated imaging techniques show structural changes involving the anterior cingulate, hippocampus, frontal cortical regions, cerebellar, and brainstem areas.[226–231] Multiple regions of lower fractional anisotropy within white matter of the anterior corpus callosum; anterior and posterior cingulate cortex and cingulum bundle; right column of the fornix; portions of the frontal, ventral prefrontal, parietal, and insular cortices; bilateral internal capsule, left cerebral peduncle and corticospinal tract; and deep cerebellar nuclei were found in diffusion tensor imaging of nonbrain-injured patients with OSA.[232] Metabolite levels indicative of axonal loss or injury have been reported in nonbrain-injured patients with OSA.[229,231] Axonal changes may include reduction in diameter and/or myelin without axonal death, however, with potential functional modification of axons. Animal studies show exposure to intermittent hypoxia accompanying apneic incidents to simulate OSA results in damage to corpus callosal fibers[233] and cellular injury in the hippocampus, basal forebrain, brainstem, frontal cortex, and cerebellum.[233–235] Oxidative processes are increased following apneic episodes found in animals,[236,237] and inflammatory markers are increased in both animals and humans following apneic episodes.[236,238] Neurodegenerative processes are associated with increased inflammatory markers.[239] The potential for an interaction between depression as both arising from damage to brain structures and furthering damage to brain structures has been raised.[240] A finding of more damage to anterior insulae and anterior cingulate was associated with depressive symptoms in OSA in nonbrain-injured patients.

Sleep disturbances can be assessed using subjective measures such as self-rating scales.[241,242] However, sleep disturbance can also be measured using more objective techniques that range from monitoring changes in select physiologic processes (heart rate, temperature, cortisol levels, blood/oxygen levels, and so forth) to full polysomnography and sleep lab studies.[243,244]

The role of hypocretins (orexins) in sleep regulation has been raised recently.[245] Hypocretins are produced by a group of neurons in the posterolateral hypothalamus. They provide excitatory input to a number of regions of the CNS, including the serotonergic cells of the dorsal raphe nucleus, norepinephrinergic neurons of the locus ceruleus, cholinergic cells of the basal forebrain and the laterodorsal/pedunculopontine tegmental area of the brainstem, histaminergic cells of the tuberomammillary nucleus, dopaminergic cells of the substantia nigra, and the ventral tegmental area. These neurotransmitter systems inhibit sleep-active neurons in the ventrolateral preoptic area via excitatory signals sent via the forebrain and thalamus.[245] Hypocretin was first implicated in the onset of narcolepsy; however, recent studies have found depletion of hypocretin 1 levels in acute moderate to severe TBI.[246] The role of hypocretin in brain injury will require further investigation as the increasingly important role of damage to the hypothalamus and the hypothalamic–pituitary axis is better understood.

A combination of subjective and objective measures, combined with serial clinical evaluation throughout the aging process, will assist clinicians in appropriate management strategies.[247,248] Depending on etiology, management strategies include extension of time in bed, naps, surgery, various medical devices (e.g., oral appliances, continuous positive airway pressure), and pharmacotherapy.[248,249]

11.8 Mortality and Life Expectancy

One of the most frequently asked questions concerns what impact TBI has on life expectancy. This issue presents a number of pragmatic concerns for families of people with TBI and bears on the development of suitable support systems that will be able to address lifelong issues effectively.[250] Logistical and financial planning for the individual, and public health planning on a larger scale, require the most accurate appraisal possible of what will need to be provided for an individual living with TBI and for how long.

There is a significant amount of literature describing the risk factors, shortened life expectancies, and causes of death in persons with chronic, disabling CNS conditions that may be illustrative in the discussion of such issues in TBI.[251–254] In certain subgroups of persons with severe mental and physical disabilities, several studies have shown abbreviated life expectancies. In a study examining life expectancy of profoundly handicapped persons with mental retardation, Eyman et al.[255] collected data on mortality and other factors for 99,543 persons with developmental disabilities. This comprehensive review between 1984 and 1987 examined subgroups with functional disability related to mobility, personal activity of daily living abilities (e.g., self-feeding), and incontinence. People with severe mental retardation were found to have decreased life expectancy, either as children or adults, if they had severe limitations in mobility, were dependent on nutritional tube feeds, and were incontinent. This subgroup represented the most medically fragile group and had an average life expectancy of less than 5 years. However, as mobility, nutritional, and bowel and bladder independence improved, so did life expectancy, adding a range of up to an additional 23 years. This study did not, however, account for differences in environmental factors, such as the level and intensity of care and the enrichment of the environment in which the person was being cared for, thus allowing them to thrive. Roboz[256] found that people with mental retardation had the highest mortality when there was extensive brain damage and a completely bedridden condition was present. This study in a non-TBI-disabled population with mental retardation demonstrated the influence of functional predictors of long-term morbidity and mortality, and the contribution of comorbid neurologic factors.

Much of the literature on mortality after TBI in adults has focused on predictors of early mortality (i.e., less than 1 year after injury). Mortality studies involving hospitalized individuals have found that approximately 90% of those individuals admitted to a hospital with TBI are discharged alive.[257,258] Risk factors such as age, admission GCS score, associated injuries, hypotension, hypoxia, and intracranial hemorrhage are associated with survival. A study by Marshall et al.[259] reported 6-month mortality at 36% among those with an admission GCS score of less than 8 points, by itself, or associated with the presence of subdural hematoma and elevated intracranial pressure. In another study, 1-year mortality was found to be associated with factors such as age, GCS score, injury severity, and presence of intracranial hemorrhage. Although neither of these studies focused on individuals who received inpatient rehabilitation, Fiedler et al.[260] examined first rehabilitation admissions for TBI in 1998 using data from the Uniform Data System for Medical Rehabilitation. They found mortality within this population was 1% to 2% 3 months postdischarge. This study was focused on functional independence as a correlate of mortality. It did not attempt to determine survival status in those persons lost to follow-up, nor was any analysis done to identify predictors of mortality.

Most relevant to issues of aging are studies reporting on mortality and life expectancy beyond 1 year after TBI. In a study of Vietnam veterans with penetrating cerebral injuries, the cause of death after TBI appeared to have similar patterns to those seen in the general population as soon as 2 years postinjury.[261] However, earlier studies implicated seizures as a cause of death unique to the TBI population.[262,263] More recently, seizures appeared as the third leading cause of death in reviewing a California database analyzing post-TBI mortality.[20] However, in that study, both circulatory and respiratory causes of death were more common than seizures and both of these causes appeared consistently over time and across populations.

A preliminary study utilizing the NIDRR-funded TBI Model Systems National Data Base has identified a range of possible predictors of future mortality.[264] These include age, previous TBI, having an injury that was caused by a fall, blood alcohol level, posttraumatic amnesia, and discharge disposition. However, only age at the time of injury and blood alcohol level were significant predictors of mortality in this study's multivariate analysis. Alcohol was not shown to be a significant risk factor in a similar study conducted in Australia.[265]

Overall, a few studies do suggest that life expectancy for individuals with TBI is shorter than for those in the general population.[28,262,263] However, the evidence explaining why life expectancy is shorter is very mixed.[20,28,261,264–267] In persons who have sustained severe TBI and are considered "low functioning" or dependent, life expectancies seem to be much shorter. Ashwal et al.,[268] in a study reporting on the most severely injured of TBI survivors, found that those who remained in a persistent vegetative state had a mortality rate of 82% at 3 years postinjury and 95% at 5 years postinjury.

People with TBI who remain in a persistent vegetative state represent a subgroup of TBI with the least functional status and mobility. There is some suggestion that a distinction might be made even between life expectancy for persons with the "minimally conscious state" versus "persistent vegetative state" (PVS). In this vain, Jennett and Plum[269] differentiated PVS from other types of chronic unconsciousness and suggested that life expectancy for PVS differed when compared with other types of unconsciousness. The Multi-Society Task Force on PVS,[270] in a literature review of the medical aspects of the persistent vegetative state, examined data available on survival. The review concluded that a reduction of life expectancy to approximately 2 to 5 years for both children and adults resulted when neurologic injury was severe enough to produce PVS. Examination of the records of 251 individuals diagnosed with PVS resulted in the conclusion that survival beyond 15 years was rare.

Morbidity and mortality show differences between those people in coma immediately after a nontraumatic versus a traumatic injury, with the nontraumatic group having a poorer prognosis.[270] Rates of death and PVS combined are higher at 1 year postinjury for the nontraumatic group than for the traumatic group. By 1 year, 85% of nontraumatically injured people who immediately entered coma remained in PVS or died contrasted with 48% for the traumatically injured group. A shortened life expectancy in PVS was noted to be the result of several factors. Reported causes of death include infection (usually of the pulmonary or urinary tract), generalized systemic failure, sudden death, respiratory failure, and other disease-related causes, such as recurrent strokes or tumors. It was stated that age was an important factor both in young infants and children, and that the elderly have a shorter life expectancy than young or middle-age adults. It was not well delineated whether the cause of the vegetative state or the subsequent medical complications were the etiologies of death.

In contrast, two studies of "highly functioning," ambulatory adults suggested that life expectancy was reduced by 3 to 5 years.[262,263] Roberts[271] followed approximately 500 individuals with severe disabilities up to 25 years. An estimated reduction in life expectancy of 4 to 5 years was found among individuals who became mobile enough to walk unaided. Strauss et al.[28] reviewed life expectancies across all severity levels of TBI. They also found diminution of life expectancy to be dependent upon level of mobility. That is, life expectancy for people with no mobility ranged from 10 to approximately 15 years depending upon age at the time of injury. The shortest life expectancies were associated with older age at injury. This trend remained stable for people with poor mobility and fair to good mobility. Those with poor mobility ranged from 17.9 to 34.2 years' life expectancy and those with fair to good mobility ranged from 26.5 to 54.8 years' life expectancy, again depending upon age at injury. The youngest people at injury had the greatest decrease in life expectancy.

There appears to be some reduction in life expectancy related to TBI associated with other comorbidities. Weiss et al.,[267] in a study examining post World War I head-injured veterans, found that the occurrence of posttraumatic seizures was a prognostic factor for a higher death rate after the age of 50 years. Although other indicators of injury severity did not lead to differences in death rates, there were significantly more deaths resulting from cerebrovascular causes in the head-injured group compared with control subjects. In post-World War II studies, Corkin et al.[266] found that penetrating head injury, coupled with posttraumatic epilepsy, shortened life expectancy in persons who survived the initial postinjury period when compared with head injury alone. Educational level was found to be independent of the influence of seizures on life expectancy, meaning people with more education survived longer than those with less. Walker and Blumer[272] also found the death rate of World War II veterans with posttraumatic epilepsy to be higher than that of normal men. In addition, wounds involving the right cerebral hemisphere seemed to shorten life span more than similar injuries of the left hemisphere.

Strauss et al.[28] reviewed the records of 946 persons who sustained TBI, age 5 to 21 years, who were receiving disability services in California between 1987 and 1995. The study explored risk factors associated with mortality after TBI: male gender, no mobility, poor mobility, tube fed, fed completely by others, attempts to finger feed, and assistance with activities of daily living. Cognitive skills did not contribute to prediction of mortality. Age at injury was not found to relate systematically to mortality risk, either. Time since injury was found to impact relative risk of mortality. After the initial acute period, time since injury during the first 1 to 2 years showed less than half the risk of mortality when compared with children with cerebral palsy. However, in the longer run, mortality rates between the two groups seemed to converge. The greatest predictor of mortality appeared to be mobility. Known causes of death were listed as late effect of accidental history (n = 19), subsequent vehicle and other accidents (*n* = 3), infections (n = 3), pulmonary (*n* = 2), epilepsy (*n* = 2), cerebrovascular (*n* = 1), suffocation (*n* = 1), burning (n = 1), suicide (*n* = 1), unspecified (*n* = 2), and missing (*n* = 3).[28]

The findings of causes of death reported by Strauss et al.[28] are similar to those reported by Roberts.[271] Although Roberts[271] reported that causes of death for people with TBI were not very different from the general population for many causes, some stood out as being different. These included meningitis, epilepsy, accidents, suicides, and respiratory disease. The causes of death reported by Roberts[271] and Strauss et al.[28] closely follow the causes for rehospitalization reported by Cifu et al.[24] and Marwitz et al.[25]

The mortality risk factor of "functional status" has also been explored in the literature related to TBI mortality. In particular, feeding and mobility are reported to be major determinants of life expectancy in both children and adults.[28] One study found that mobility was a stronger predictor of mortality than consciousness in "poorly" responsive individuals.[273] Shavelle et al.[20] reported standardized mortality ratios for those with TBI that range from a low of 180% in ambulatory individuals to 196% in those who are partially ambulatory and as high as 660% in nonambulatory individuals. These studies are beginning to lend credence to the concept of function as a predictor of mortality. In future prospective, longitudinal studies, knowledge of objective functional measures at rehabilitation admission, discharge, and in selected time frames postinjury may, themselves, be predictive of survival, life expectancy, neuromedical complications, and other relevant comorbidities.[254]

Finally, medical–legal issues encompassing life expectancy and the need for long-term planning seem relevant.[274] The logistics and costs of these long-term planning considerations are immense.[250] The anticipated progression of communicative, physical, and neurobehavioral changes over a lifetime is not yet an exact science. Planning for later life events and end of life can be furthered to a degree by not only the knowledge of neuromedical complications and long-term issues, but also recognition of associated functional changes arising from either the neurologic injury or associated nonneurologic injuries.[250] It is not possible, at this time, to enumerate fully the exhaustive implications of aging on such functional skills and limitations because investigation into these arenas has only just begun for the TBI population. The work done thus far in SCI should serve as an excellent model for this endeavor.[21,251–253] This will only help to further the understanding of the efficacy of specific medical rehabilitative interventions and allow better understanding of society's duty in resource allocation.[275]

Estimating life expectancy in a "specific" person with TBI is a complex and challenging endeavor. Statistical methods are often valuable in making life expectancy estimates for persons with SCI and other neurologic disabilities when grouped by particular characteristics. However, in a heterogeneous TBI population characterized by different injury types and severity with discrepant medical, neurologic, and functional disabilities, a statistical methodology may be inaccurate. Furthermore, the impact of pre- and comorbid variables and different rehabilitative and long-term supportive care paradigms may also have a differential impact on long-term morbidity and mortality. In an article by Kraus[276] reviewing accuracy of life expectancy estimates in life care plans, it was felt important to consider nonbiographic and noninjury factors, as well as the injury itself. That article emphasized a host of important variables that may impact life expectancy, such as income, access to health care, health behaviors, and psychosocial adaptations.

11.9 Successful Aging

Successful aging is a wonderful goal for an individual with the disabling physical, cognitive, neurobehavioral, and emotional disabilities associated with TBI. Successful aging is defined as an optimal state of overall functioning and well-being. Successful aging can be difficult to achieve, even in the general population. In a cross-sectional aging study that obtained information from 599 participants in Leiden, Netherlands, successful aging, from a public health perspective, was defined as a state of being.[277] All participants were classified as "successful" or "not successful" based on optimal scores for physical, social, and psychocognitive functioning, and feelings of well-being using validated quantitative instruments. Although 45% of the participants had optimal scores for well-being, only 13% had optimal scores for overall functioning. In total, 10% of the participants satisfied all the criteria and could be classified as "successfully aged." The qualitative interviews showed that most elderly people viewed success as a process of adaptation rather than a state of being. The participants recognized the various domains of successful aging, but valued well-being and social functioning more than physical and psychocognitive functioning. Therefore, aging people with TBI are not unlike the elderly population and should view successful aging as a process of adaptation.

A study conducted by Harrison-Felix et al.[278] investigated mortality in a cohort of 2178 individuals with TBI completing inpatient rehabilitation. It was found that individuals with TBI were twice as likely to die compared with individuals in the general population of similar age, gender, and race. This resulted in an estimated average life expectancy reduction of 7 years for individuals with TBI. The strongest risk factors for death 1 year postinjury were older age, greater disability at rehabilitation discharge, and, interestingly, unemployment at the time of injury.

As a follow-up to this retrospective cohort study, "causes of death" in individuals with TBI were further investigated.[278] Databases utilized to investigate causes of death included the TBI Model Systems National Database, Social Security Death Indices, Death Certificates and the U.S. Population Age–Race–Gender Cause specific mortality rates from 1994 in comparison. Outcome measurement tools were the International Classification of Diseases-9 (ICD-9) revision clinical modification-coded death certificates. Individuals with TBI were 37 times more likely to die of seizures when compared with other causes. Individuals with TBI were 12 times more likely to die of septicemia, four times more likely to die of pneumonia, and approximately three times more likely to die of other respiratory conditions (excluding pneumonia), digestive conditions, and other external causes of injury.

In summary, the relative known risk of morbidity and mortality following TBI with increasing age makes it important for individuals to have vigilant follow-up and monitoring. Specifically, the prevention, diagnosis, and optimal management of frequent comorbidities that are most frequently involved in death (circulatory disorders) and other relatively high-risk factors for death (seizures, septicemia, respiratory, and digestive conditions) and other external causes of injury need to be monitored and managed over a lifetime.

Further studies need to evaluate more specifically the effects of different severities and subtypes of TBI and comorbidities, and to explore different avenues toward improved care, enhancement of long-term survival, and maintenance of quality of life.[278]

References

1. Zaloshnja, E., Miller, T., Langlois, J. A., and Selassie, A. W., Prevalence of long-term disability from traumatic brain injury in the civilian population of the United States, 2005, *Journal of Head Trauma Rehabilitation*, 23(6), 394–400, 2008.
2. Langlois, J. A., Rutland-Brown, W., and Thomas, K. E., *Traumatic Brain Injury in the United States: Emergency Department Visits, Hospitalizations, and Deaths*, Centers for Disease Control and Prevention, National Center for Injury Prevention and Control, Atlanta, GA, 2006.
3. Selassie, A. W., Zaloshnja, E., Langlois, J. A., Miller, T., Jones, P., and Steiner, C., Incidence of long-term disability following traumatic brain injury hospitalization, United States, *The Journal of Head Trauma Rehabilitation*, 23(2), 123–131, 2008.
4. Finkelstein, E., Corso, P., and Miller, T., *The Incidence and Economic Burden of Injury in the United States*, Oxford University Press, New York, 2006.
5. Thurman, D. J., Branche, C. M., and Sniezek, J. E., The epidemiology of sports-related traumatic brain injuries in the United States: Recent developments, *Journal of Head Trauma Rehabilitation*, 13(2), 1–8, 1998.

6. Gabella, B., Hoffman, R. E., Marine, W. W., and Stallones, L., Urban and rural traumatic brain injuries in Colorado, *Annals of Epidemiology*, 7(3), 207–212, 1997.

7. Thurman, D. J., Alverson, C., Dunn, K. A., Guerrero, J., and Sniezek, J. E., Traumatic brain injury in the United States: A public health perspective, *Journal of Head Trauma Rehabilitation*, 14(6), 602–615, 1999.

8. National Institutes of Health, Rehabilitation of persons with traumatic brain injury, *NIH Consensus Statement*, 16(1), 1–41, 1998.

9. Fields, R. B. and Coffey, C. E., Traumatic brain injury, in C. E. Coffey and J. L. Cummings (Eds.), *Textbook of Geriatric Neuropsychiatry*, American Psychiatric Press, Washington, DC, 479–508, 1994.

10. Pennings, J. L., Bachulis, B. L., Simons, C. T., and Slazinski, T., Survival after severe brain injury in the aged, *Archives of Surgery*, 128(7), 787–794, 1993.

11. Vollmer, D. G., Torner, J. C., Jane, J. A., Sadovnic, B., Charlebois, D., Eisenberg, H. M. et al., Age and outcome following traumatic coma: Why do older patients fare worse?, *Journal of Neurosurgery*, 75(Suppl.), S37–S49, 1991.

12. Rothweiler, B., Temkin, N. R., and Dikmen, S. S., Aging effect on psychosocial outcome in traumatic brain injury, *Archives of Physical Medicine and Rehabilitation*, 79(8), 881–887, 1998.

13. Mazzucchi, A., Cattelani, R., Missale, G., Gugliotta, M., Brianti, R., and Parma, M., Head-injured subjects aged over 50 years: Correlations between variables of trauma and neuropsychological follow-up, *Journal of Neurology*, 239(5), 256–260, 1992.

14. Rapoport, M. J. and Feinstein, A., Outcome following traumatic brain injury in the elderly: A critical review, *Brain Injury*, 14(8), 749–761, 2000.

15. Bach y Rita, P., Central nervous system lesions: Sprouting and unmasking in rehabilitation, *Archives of Physical Medicine and Rehabilitation*, 62(9), 413–417, 1981.

16. Rapoport, M. J. and Feinstein, A., Age and functioning after mild traumatic brain injury: The acute picture, *Brain Injury*, 15(10), 857–864, 2001.

17. Bontke, C. F., Lehmkuhl, L. D., Englander, J., Mann, N., Ragnarsson, K. T., Zasler, N. D., et al., Medical complications and associated injuries of persons treated in the traumatic brain injury model systems programs, *Journal of Head Trauma Rehabilitation*, 8(2), 34–46, 1993.

18. Rappaport, M., Hall, K. M., Hopkins, K., Belleza, T., and Cope, D. N., Disability rating scale for severe head trauma: Coma to community, *Archives of Physical Medicine and Rehabilitation*, 63(3), 118–123, 1982.

19. Englander, J. S., Cifu, D. X., Wright, J., Zafonte, R., Mann, N., Yablon, S., et al., The impact of acute complications, fractures, and motor deficits on functional outcome and length of stay after traumatic brain injury: A multi-center analysis, *Journal of Head Trauma Rehabilitation*, 11(5), 15–26, 1996.

20. Shavelle, R. M., Strauss, D., Whyte, J., Day, S. M., and Yu, Y. L., Long-term causes of death after traumatic brain injury, *American Journal of Physical Medicine and Rehabilitation*, 80(7), 510–516, 2001.

21. Charlifue, S. W. and Lammertse, D. P., Aging in spinal cord injury, in S. Kirshblum, D. I. Campagnolo, and J. A. DeLisa (Eds.), *Spinal Cord Medicine*, Williams & Wilkins, Philadelphia, PA, 409–423, 2001.

22. Burns, T. J., Batavia, A. I., Smith, Q. W., and DeJong, G., Primary health care needs of persons with physical disabilities: What are the research and service priorities?, *Archives of Physical Medicine and Rehabilitation*, 71(2), 138–143, 1990.

23. Davidoff, G., Schultz, J. S., Lieb, T., Andrews, K., Wardner, J., Hayes, C., et al., Rehospitalization after initial rehabilitation for acute spinal cord injury: Incidence and risk factors, *Archives of Physical Medicine and Rehabilitation*, 71(2), 121–124, 1990.

24. Cifu, D. X., Kreutzer, J. S., Marwitz, J. H., Miller, M., Hsu, G. M., Seel, R. T., et al., Etiology and incidence of rehospitalization after traumatic brain injury: A multicenter analysis, *Archives of Physical Medicine and Rehabilitation*, 80(1), 85–90, 1999.

25. Marwitz, J. H., Cifu, D. X., Englander, J., and High, W. M., A multi-center analysis of rehospitalizations five years after brain injury, *Journal of Head Trauma Rehabilitation*, 16(4), 307–317, 2001.

26. Burg, J. S., Williams, R., Burright, R. G., and Donovick, P. J., Psychiatric treatment outcome following traumatic brain injury, *Brain Injury*, 14(6), 513–533, 2000.

27. Brooks, N., Campsie, L., Symington, C., Beattie, A., and McKinlay, W., The five year outcome of severe blunt head injury: A relative's view, *Journal of Neurology, Neurosurgery, and Psychiatry*, 49(7), 764–770, 1986.

28. Strauss, D. J., Shavelle, R. M., and Anderson, T. W., Long term survival of children and adolescents after traumatic brain injury, *Archives of Physical Medicine and Rehabilitation*, 79(9), 1095–1100, 1998.

29. Klein, M., Houx, P. J., and Jolles, J., Long-term persisting cognitive sequelae of traumatic brain injury and the effect of age, *Journal of Nervous and Mental Disease*, 184(8), 459–467, 1996.

30. Goldstein, G. and Shelly, C. H., Similarities and differences between psychological deficit in aging and brain damage, *Journal of Gerontology*, 30(4), 438–455, 1975.

31. Ashman, T. A., Cantor, J. B., Gordon, W. A., Sacks, A., Spielman, L., Egan, M., et al., A comparison of cognitive functioning in older adults with and without traumatic brain injury, *Journal of Head Trauma Rehabilitation*, 23(3), 139–148, 2008.

32. Rabbitt, P., Frontal brain changes and cognitive performance in old age, *Cortex*, 41(2), 238–240, 2005.

33. Duncan, J., Burgess, P., and Emslie, H., Fluid intelligence after frontal lobe lesions, *Neuropsychologia*, 33(3), 261–268, 1995.

34. Duncan, J. and Owen, A. M., Common regions of the human frontal lobe recruited by diverse cognitive demands, *Trends in Neurosciences*, 23(10), 475–483, 2000.

35. Duncan, J., Seitz, R. J., Kolodny, J., Bor, D., Herzog, H., Ahmed, A., et al., A neural basis for general intelligence, *Science*, 289(5478), 457, 2000.

36. Rocca, W. A., Amaducci, L. A., and Schoenberg, B. S., Epidemiology of clinically diagnosed Alzheimer's disease, *Annals of Neurology*, 19(5), 415–424, 1986.

37. Katzman, R., Editorial: The prevalence and malignancy of Alzheimer's disease: A major killer, *Archives of Neurology*, 33(4), 217–218, 1976.

38. Tatemichi, T. K., How acute brain failure becomes chronic: A view of the mechanisms of dementia related to stroke, *Neurology*, 40(11), 1652–1659, 1990.

39. Susser, M., *Causal Thinking in the Health Sciences: Concepts and Strategies in Epidemiology*, Oxford University Press, New York, 1973.

40. Corsellis, J. A., Bruton, C. J., and Freeman-Browne, D., The aftermath of boxing, *Psychological Medicine*, 3(3), 270–303, 1973.

41. Roberts, G. W., Gentleman, S. M., Lynch, A., Murray, L., Landon, M., and Graham, D. I., Beta amyloid protein deposition in the brain after severe head injury: Implications for the pathogenesis of Alzheimer's disease, *Journal of Neurology, Neurosurgery, and Psychiatry*, 57(4), 419–425, 1994.

42. Mortimer, J. A., French, L. R., Hutton, J. T., and Schuman, L. M., Head injury as a risk factor for Alzheimer's disease, *Neurology*, 35(2), 264–267, 1985.

43. Mortimer, J. A., van Duijn, C. M., Chandra, V., Fratiglioni, L., Graves, A. B., Heyman, A., et al., Head trauma as a risk factor for Alzheimer's disease: A collaborative re-analysis of case–control studies, EURODEM Risk Factors Research Group, *International Journal of Epidemiology*, 20(Suppl. 2), S28–S35, 1991.

44. Rasmusson, D. X., Brandt, J., Martin, D. B., and Folstein, M. F., Head injury as a risk factor in Alzheimer's disease, *Brain Injury*, 9(3), 213–219, 1995.

45. Heyman, A., Wilkinson, W. E., Stafford, J. A., Helms, M. J., Sigmon, A. H., and Weinberg, T., Alzheimer's disease: A study of epidemiological aspects, *Annals of Neurology*, 15(4), 335–341, 1984.

46. Salib, E. and Hillier, V., Head injury and the risk of Alzheimer's disease: A case control study, *International Journal of Geriatric Psychiatry*, 12(3), 363–368, 1997.

47. Mayeux, R., Ottman, R., Maestre, G., et al., Synergistic effects of traumatic head injury and apolipoprotein-epsilon 4 in patients with Alzheimer's disease, *Neurology*, 46(3), 889–891, 1996.

48. Guo, Z., Cupples, L. A., Kurz, A., Auerbach, S. H., Volicer, L., Chui, H., et al., Head injury and the risk of AD in the MIRAGE study, *Neurology*, 54(6), 1316–1323, 2000.
49. Jordan, B. D., Chronic traumatic brain injury associated with boxing, *Seminars in Neurology*, 20(2), 179–185, 2000.
50. Roberts, G. W., Allsop, D., and Bruton, C., The occult aftermath of boxing, *Journal of Neurology, Neurosurgery, and Psychiatry*, 53(5), 373–378, 1990.
51. Nemetz, P. N., Leibson, C., Naessens, J. M., Beard, M., Kokmen, E., Annegers, J. F., et al., Traumatic brain injury and time to onset of Alzheimer's disease: A population-based study, *American Journal of Epidemiology*, 149(1), 32–40, 1999.
52. Mehta, K. M., Ott, A., Kalmijn, S., Slooter, A. J., van Duijn, C. M., and Hofman, A., Head trauma and risk of dementia and Alzheimer's disease: The Rotterdam study, *Neurology*, 53(9), 1959–1962, 1999.
53. Roberts, G. W., Gentleman, S. M., Lynch, A., and Graham, D. I., Beta A4 amyloid protein deposition in brain after head trauma, *Lancet*, 338(8780), 1422–1423, 1991.
54. Van Den Heuvel, C., Lewis, S., Wong, M., Manavis, J., Finnie, J., Blumbergs, P., et al., Diffuse neuronal perikaryon amyloid precursor protein immunoreactivity in a focal head impact model, *Acta Neurochirurgica*, 71(Suppl.), 209–211, 1998.
55. Huber, A., Gabbert, K., Kelemen, J., and Cervos-Navarro, J., Density of amyloid plaques in brain after head injury, *Journal of Neurotrauma*, 10(Suppl. 1), S180, 1993.
56. Ikonomovic, M. D., Uryu, K., Abrahamson, E. E., Ciallella, J. R., Trojanowski, J. Q., Lee, V. M. Y., et al., Alzheimer's pathology in human temporal cortex surgically excised after severe brain injury, *Experimental Neurology*, 190(1), 192–203, 2004.
57. McKenzie, J. E., Gentleman, S. M., Roberts, G. W., Graham, D. I., and Royston, M. C., Increased numbers of beta APP-immunoreactive neurones in the entorhinal cortex after head injury, *Neuroreport*, 6(1), 161–164, 1994.
58. Goldgaber, D., Harris, H. W., Hla, T., Maciag, T., Donnelly, R. J., Jacobsen, J. S., Vitek, M. P., and Gajdusek, D. C., Interleukin 1 regulates synthesis of amyloid beta-protein precursor mRNA in human endothelial cells, *Proceedings of the National Academy of Sciences of the United States of America*, 86(19), 7606–7610, 1989.
59. Forloni, G., Demicheli, F., Giorgi, S., Bendotti, C., and Angeretti, N., Expression of amyloid precursor protein mRNAs in endothelial, neuronal and glial cells: Modulation by interleukin-1, *Brain Research, Molecular Brain Research*, 16(1–2), 128–134, 1992.
60. Buxbaum, J. D., Oishi, M., Chen, H. I., Pinkas-Kramarski, R., Jaffe, E. A., Gandy, S. E., et al., Cholinergic agonists and interleukin 1 regulate processing and secretion of the Alzheimer beta/A4 amyloid protein precursor, *Proceedings of the National Academy of Sciences of the United States of America*, 89(21), 10075–10078, 1992.
61. Giulian, D., Young, D. G., Woodward, J., Brown, D. C., and Lachman, L. B., Interleukin-1 is an astroglial growth factor in the developing brain, *Neuroscience*, 8(2), 709–714, 1988.
62. Das, S. and Potter, H., Expression of the Alzheimer amyloid-promoting factor antichymotrypsin is induced in human astrocytes by IL-1, *Neuron*, 14(2), 447–456, 1995.
63. Smith, D. H., Chen, X. H., Iwata, A., and Graham, D. I., Amyloid beta accumulation in axons after traumatic brain injury in humans, *Journal of Neurosurgery*, 98(5), 1072–1077, 2003.
64. Schmechel, D. E., Goldgaber, D., Burkhart, D. S., Gilbert, J. R., Gajdusek, D. C., and Roses, A. D., Cellular localization of messenger RNA encoding amyloid-beta-protein in normal tissue and in Alzheimer disease, *Alzheimer Disease and Associated Disorders*, 2(2), 96–111, 1988.
65. Bayer, T. A., Wirths, O., Majtenyi, K., Hartmann, T., Multhaup, G., Beyreuther, K., et al., Key factors in Alzheimer's disease: Beta-amyloid precursor protein processing, metabolism and intraneuronal transport, *Brain Pathology*, 11(1), 1–11, 2001.
66. Turner, P. R., O'Connor, K., Tate, W. P., and Abraham, W. C., Roles of amyloid precursor protein and its fragments in regulating neural activity, plasticity and memory, *Progress in Neurobiology*, 70(1), 1–32, 2003.
67. Abe, K., Tanzi, R. E., and Kogure, K., Selective induction of Kunitz-type protease inhibitor domain-containing amyloid precursor protein mRNA after persistent focal ischemia in rat cerebral cortex, *Neuroscience Letters*, 125(2), 172–174, 1991.

68. Heurteaux, C., Bertaina, V., Widmann, C., and Lazdunski, M., K+ channel openers prevent global ischemia-induced expression of c-fos, c-jun, heat shock protein, and amyloid beta-protein precursor genes and neuronal death in rat hippocampus, *Proceedings of the National Academy of Sciences of the United States of America*, 90(20), 9431–9435, 1993.

69. Koistinaho, J., Pyykonen, I., Keinanen, R., and Hokfelt, T., Expression of beta-amyloid precursor protein mRNAs following transient focal ischaemia, *Neuroreport*, 7(15–17), 2727–2731, 1996.

70. Kim, H. S., Lee, S. H., Kim, S. S., Kim, Y. K., Jeong, S. J., Ma J., et al., Post-ischemic changes in the expression of Alzheimer's APP isoforms in rat cerebral cortex, *Neuroreport*, 9(3), 533–537, 1998.

71. Scott, J. N., Parhad, I. M., and Clark, A. W., Beta-amyloid precursor protein gene is differentially expressed in axotomized sensory and motor systems, *Brain Research, Molecular Brain Research*, 10(4), 315–325, 1991.

72. Wallace, W. C., Bragin, V., Robakis, N. K., Sambamurti, K., VanderPutten, D., Merril, C. R., et al., Increased biosynthesis of Alzheimer amyloid precursor protein in the cerebral cortex of rats with lesions of the nucleus basalis of Meynert, *Brain Research, Molecular Brain Research*, 10(2), 173–178, 1991.

73. Van Broeckhoven, C. L., Molecular genetics of Alzheimer disease: Identification of genes and gene mutations, *European Neurology (Basel)*, 35(1), 8–19, 1995.

74. Graham, D. I., Horsburgh, K., Nicoll, J. A., and Teasdale, G. M., Apolipoprotein E and the response of the brain to injury, *Acta Neurochirurgica*, 73(Suppl.), 89–92, 1999.

75. Rinder, L. and Olsson, Y., Studies on vascular permeability changes in experimental brain concussion. I. Distribution of circulating fluorescent indicators in brain and cervical cord after sudden mechanical loading of the brain, *Acta Neuropathologica*, 11(3), 183–200, 1968.

76. Rapoport, S. I., *Blood Brain Barrier in Physiology and Medicine*, Raven Press, New York, 1976.

77. Rapoport, S. I., Ohno, K., and Pettigrew, K. D., Blood–brain barrier permeability in senescent rats, *Journal of Gerontology*, 34(2), 162–169, 1979.

78. Nobili, F., Copello, F., Buffoni, F., Vitali, P., Girtler, N., Bordoni, C., et al., Regional cerebral blood flow and prognostic evaluation in Alzheimer's disease, *Dementia and Geriatric Cognitive Disorders*, 12(2), 89–97, 2001.

79. Silverman, D. H., Small, G. W., Chang, C. Y., Lu, C. S., Kund De Aburtto, M. A., Chen, W., et al., Positron emission tomography in evaluation of dementia: Regional brain metabolism and long-term outcome, *Journal of the American Medical Association*, 286(17), 2120–2127, 2001.

80. Chan, D., Fox, N. C., Jenkins, R., Scahill, R. I., Crum, W. R., and Rossor, M. N., Rates of global and regional cerebral atrophy in AD and frontotemporal dementia, *Neurology*, 57(10), 1756–1763, 2001.

81. Bamford, C. R., Sibley, W. A., Thies, C., Laguna, J. F., Smith, M. S., and Clark, K., Trauma as an etiologic and aggravating factor in multiple sclerosis, *Neurology*, 32(10), 1229–1234, 1981.

82. Sibley, W. A., Bamford, C. R., Clark, K., Smith, M. S., and Laguna, J. F., A prospective study of physical trauma and multiple sclerosis, *Journal of Neurology, Neurosurgery, and Psychiatry*, 54(7), 584–589, 1991.

83. Sibley, W. A., Physical trauma and multiple sclerosis, *Neurology*, 43(10), 1871–1874, 1993.

84. Siva, A., Radhakrishnan, K., Kurland, L. T., O'Brien, P. C., Swanson, J. W., and Rodriguez, M., Trauma and multiple sclerosis: A population-based cohort study from Olmsted County, Minnesota, *Neurology*, 43(10), 1878–1882, 1993.

85. Kurland, L. T., Trauma and multiple sclerosis, *Annals of Neurology*, 36(Suppl.), S33–S37, 1994.

86. Williams, D. B., Annegers, J. F., Kokmen, E., O'Brien, P. C., and Kurland, L. T., Brain injury and neurologic sequelae: A cohort study of dementia, parkinsonism, and amyotrophic lateral sclerosis, *Neurology*, 41(10), 1554–1557, 1991.

87. Bhatt, M., Desai, J., Mankodi, A., Elias, M., and Wadia, N., Posttraumatic akinetic-rigid syndrome resembling Parkinson's disease: A report on three patients, *Movement Disorders*, 15(2), 313–317, 2000.

88. Doder, M., Jahanshahi, M., Turjanski, N., Moseley, I. F., and Lees, A. J., Parkinson's syndrome after closed head injury: A single case report, *Journal of Neurology, Neurosurgery, and Psychiatry*, 66(3), 380–385, 1999.

89. Factor, S. A., Sanchez-Ramos, J., and Weiner, W. J., Trauma as an etiology of parkinsonism: A historical review of the concept, *Movement Disorders*, 3(1), 30–36, 1988.

90. Goetz, C. G. and Stebbins, G. T., Effects of head trauma from motor vehicle accidents on Parkinson's disease, *Annals of Neurology*, 29(2), 191–193, 1991.

91. Povlishock, J. T. and Jenkins, L. W., Are the pathobiological changes evoked by traumatic brain injury immediate and irreversible?, *Brain Pathology*, 5(4), 415–426, 1995.

92. Povlishock, J. T., Erb, D. E., and Astruc, J., Axonal response to traumatic brain injury: Reactive axonal change, deafferentation, and neuroplasticity, *Journal of Neurotrauma*, 9(Suppl. 1), S189–S200, 1992.

93. Poser, C. M., Trauma and multiple sclerosis: An hypothesis, *Journal of Neurology*, 234(3), 155–159, 1987.

94. Guskiewicz, K., Marshall, S., Bailes, J., McCrea, M., Cantu, R. C., Randolph, C., et al., Association between recurrent concussion and late-life cognitive impairment in retired professional football players, *Neurosurgery*, 57(4), 719–724, 2005.

95. Petersen, R. C., Doody, R., Kurz, A., Mohs, R. C., Morris, J. C., Rabins, P. V., et al., Current concepts in mild cognitive impairment, *Archives of Neurology*, 58(12), 1985–1992, 2001.

96. Meyer, J., Xu, G., Thornby, J., Chowdhury, M., and Quach, M., Longitudinal analysis of abnormal domains comprising mild cognitive impairment (MCI) during aging, *Journal of Neurological Sciences*, 201(1–2), 19–25, 2002.

97. Hauser, W. A., Annegers, J. F., and Kurland, L. T., Incidence of epilepsy and unprovoked seizures in Rochester, Minnesota: 1935–1984, *Epilepsia*, 34(3), 453–468, 1993.

98. Ramsay, R. E. and Pryor, F., Epilepsy in the elderly, *Neurology*, 55(5 Suppl. 1), S9–S14, discussion, S54–S58, 2000.

99. Louis, S. and McDowell, F., Epileptic seizures in non-embolic cerebral infarction, *Archives of Neurology*, 17(4), 414–418, 1967.

100. Cocito, L., Favale, E., and Reni, L., Epileptic seizures in cerebral arterial occlusive disease, *Stroke*, 13(2), 189–195, 1982.

101. Holmes, G. L., The electroencephalogram as a predictor of seizures following cerebral infarction, *Clinical Electroencephalography*, 11(2), 83–86, 1980.

102. Meyer, J. S., Charney, J. Z., Rivera, V. M., and Mathew, N. T., Cerebral embolization: Prospective clinical analysis of 42 cases, *Stroke*, 2(6), 541–554, 1971.

103. Richardson, Jr., E. P. and Dodge, P. R., Epilepsy in cerebral vascular disease: A study of the incidence and nature of seizures in 104 consecutive autopsy-proven cases of cerebral infarction and hemorrhage, *Epilepsia*, C 3(1), 49–74, 1954.

104. Shinton, R. A., Gill, J. S., Zezulka, A. V., and Beevers, D. G., The frequency of epilepsy preceding stroke: Case–control study in 230 patients, *Lancet*, 1(8523), 11–13, 1987.

105. Viitanen, M., Eriksson, S., and Asplund, K., Risk of recurrent stroke, myocardial infarction and epilepsy during long-term follow-up after stroke, *European Neurology*, 28(4), 227–231, 1988.

106. Munoz, M., Boutros-Toni, F., Preux, P. M., Chartier, J. P., Ndzanga, E., Boa, F., et al., Prevalence of neurological disorders in Haute-Vienne department (Limousin region—France), *Neuroepidemiology*, 14(4), 193–198, 1995.

107. Faught, E., Peters, D., Bartolucci, A., Moore, L., and Miller, P. C., Seizures after primary intracerebral hemorrhage, *Neurology*, 39(8), 1089–1093, 1989.

108. McAreavey, M. J., Ballenger, B. R., and Fenton, G. W., Epileptic seizures in elderly patients with dementia, *Epilepsia*, 33(4), 657–660, 1992.

109. Hauser, W. A., Seizures disorders: The changes with age, *Epilepsia*, 33(Suppl. 4), S6–S14, 1992.

110. Sjogren, T., Sjogren, H., and Lindgren, A. G., Morbus Alzheimer and morbus Pick: A genetic, clinical and patho-anatomical study, *Acta Psychiatrica et Neurologica Scandinavica*, 82(Suppl.), 1–152, 1952.

111. Pearce, J. and Miller, E., *Clinical Aspects of Dementia*, Bailliere Tindall, London, 1973.

112. Boggs, J. G., Elderly patients with systemic disease, *Epilepsia*, 42(Suppl. 8), 18–23, 2001.

113. Faught, E., Pharmacokinetic considerations in prescribing antiepileptic drugs, *Epilepsia*, 42(Suppl. 4), 19–23, 2001.

114. Kramer, G., Epilepsy in the elderly: Some clinical and pharmacotherapeutic aspects, *Epilepsia*, 42(Suppl. 3), 55–59, 2001.
115. Faught, E. and Pellock, J. M., The challenge of treatment selection for epilepsy, *Epilepsia*, 42(Suppl. 8), 4–5, 2001.
116. White, P., Polypharmacy and the older adult, *Journal of the American Academy of Nurse Practitioners*, 7(11), 545–548, 1995.
117. Browne, T. R. and Holmes, G. L., Epilepsy, *New England Journal of Medicine*, 344(15), 1145–1151, 2001.
118. Dalmady-Israel, C. and Zasler, N. D., Post-traumatic seizures: A critical review, *Brain Injury*, 7(3), 263–273, 1993.
119. Yablon, S. A., Posttraumatic seizures, *Archives of Physical Medicine and Rehabilitation*, 74(9), 983–1001, 1993.
120. Dugan, E. M. and Howell, J. M., Posttraumatic seizures, *Emergency Medicine Clinics of North America*, 12(4), 1081–1087, 1994.
121. Caveness, W. F., Epilepsy, a product of trauma in our time, *Epilepsia*, 17(2), 207–215, 1976.
122. Jennett, B., *Posttraumatic Epilepsy: Advances in Neurology*, Raven Press, New York, 1979.
123. Annegers, J. F., Grabow, J. D., Groover, R. V., Laws, Jr., E. R., Elveback, L. R., and Kurland, L. T., Seizures after head trauma: A population study, *Neurology*, 30(7 Pt. 1), 683–689, 1980.
124. Jennett, B., Early traumatic epilepsy: Incidence and significance after non-missile injuries, *Archives of Neurology*, 30(5), 394–398, 1974.
125. Jennett, B. and Teasdale, G., *Management of Head Injuries*, F. A. Davis, Philadelphia, 1981.
126. Feeney, D. M. and Walker, A. E., The prediction of posttraumatic epilepsy. A mathematical approach, *Archives of Neurology*, 36(1), 8–12, 1979.
127. Salazar, A. M., Jabbari, B., Vance, S. C., Grafman, J., Amin, D., and Dillon, J. D., Epilepsy after penetrating head injury. I. Clinical correlates: A report of the Vietnam Head Injury Study, *Neurology*, 35(10), 1406–1414, 1985.
128. McQueen, J. K., Blackwood, D. H., Harris, P., Kalbag, R. M., and Johnson, A. L., Low risk of late post-traumatic seizures following severe head injury: Implications for clinical trials of prophylaxis, *Journal of Neurology, Neurosurgery, and Psychiatry*, 46(10), 899–904, 1983.
129. Temkin, N. R., Dikmen, S. S., Wilensky, A. J., Keihm, J., Chabal, S., and Winn, H. R., A randomized, double-blind study of phenytoin for the prevention of post-traumatic seizures, *New England Journal of Medicine*, 323(8), 497–502, 1990.
130. Hauser, W. A., Anderson, V. E., Loewenson, R. B., and McRoberts, S. M., Seizure recurrence after a first unprovoked seizure, *New England Journal of Medicine*, 307(9), 522–528, 1982.
131. Weiss, G. H., Feeney, D. M., Caveness, W. F., Dillon, D., Kistler, J. P., Mohr, J. P., et al., Prognostic factors for the occurrence of posttraumatic epilepsy, *Archives of Neurology*, 40(1), 7–10, 1983.
132. Weiss, G. H., Salazar, A. M., Vance, S. C., Grafman, J. H., and Jabbari, B., Predicting posttraumatic epilepsy in penetrating head injury, *Archives of Neurology*, 43(8), 771–773, 1986.
133. Jennett, B., *Epilepsy after Non-Missile Head Injuries*, 2nd ed., Heinemann, London, 1975.
134. Kennedy, C. R. and Freeman, J. M., Posttraumatic seizures and posttraumatic epilepsy in children, *Journal of Head Trauma Rehabilitation*, 1(4), 66–73, 1986.
135. Asikainen, I., Kaste, M., and Sarna, S., Early and late posttraumatic seizures in traumatic brain injury rehabilitation patients: Brain injury factors causing late seizures and influence of seizures on long-term outcome, *Epilepsia*, 40(5), 584–589, 1999.
136. Cambardella, A., Aguglia, U., Cittadella, R., Romeo, N., Sibilia, G., LePiane, E., et al., Apolipoprotein E polymorphisms and the risk of non-lesional temporal lobe epilepsy, *Epilepsia*, 40(12), 1804–1807, 1999.
137. Kumar, A., Tripathi, M., Pandey, R. M., Ramakrishnan, L., Srinivas, M., and Luthra, K., Apolipoprotein E in temporal lobe epilepsy: A case–control study, *Disease Markers*, 22(5/6), 335–342, 2006.
138. Haltiner, A. M., Temkin, N. R., and Dikmen, S. S., Risk of seizure recurrence after the first late posttraumatic seizure, *Archives of Physical Medicine and Rehabilitation*, 78(8), 835–840, 1997.

139. Young, B., Rapp, R. P., Norton, J. A., Haack, D., Tibbs, P. A., and Bean, J. R., Failure of prophylactically administered phenytoin to prevent early posttraumatic seizures, *Journal of Neurosurgery*, 58(2), 231–235, 1983.

140. Wohns, R. N. and Wyler, A. R., Prophylactic phenytoin in severe head injuries, *Journal of Neurosurgery*, 51(4), 507–509, 1979.

141. Rish, B. L. and Caveness, W. F., Relation of prophylactic medication to the occurrence of early seizures following craniocerebral trauma, *Journal of Neurosurgery*, 38(2), 155–158, 1973.

142. Boucher, B. A. and Hanes, S. D., Pharmacokinetic alterations after severe head injury: Clinical relevance, *Clinical Pharmacokinetics*, 35(3), 209–221, 1998.

143. Anderson, G. D., Temkin, N. R., Awan, A. B., and Winn, R. H., Effect of time, injury, age, and ethanol on interpatient variability in valproic acid pharmacokinetics after traumatic brain injury, *Clinical Pharmacokinetics*, 46(4), 307–318, 2007.

144. Brandt, C., Gastens, A. M., Sun, M., Hausknecht, M., and Löscher, W., Treatment with valproate after status epilepticus: Effect on neuronal damage, epileptogenesis, and behavioral alterations in rats, *Neuropharmacology*, 51(4), 789–804, 2006.

145. Boison, D., The adenosine kinase hypothesis of epileptogenesis, *Progress in Neurobiology*, 84(3), 249–262, 2008.

146. Pagni, C. A. and Zenga, F., Posttraumatic epilepsy with special emphasis on prophylaxis and prevention, *Acta Neurochirurgica*, 93(Suppl.), 27–34, 2005.

147. Gupta, Y. K. and Gupta, M., Posttraumatic epilepsy: A review of scientific evidence, *Indian Journal of Physiology and Pharmacology*, 50(1), 7–16, 2006.

148. Brown, S., Deterioration, *Epilepsia* 47, 19–23, 2006.

149. DeLorenzo, R. J., Sun, D. A., and Deshpande, L. S., Cellular mechanisms underlying acquired epilepsy: The calcium hypothesis of the induction and maintenance of epilepsy, *Pharmacology and Therapeutics*, 105(3), 229–266, 2005.

150. Anonymous, *Pharmacological Management of Insomnia*, 2001, http://www.sleepfoundation.org. publications/execusum.html (accessed March 26, 2001).

151. Loring, D. W. and Meador, K. J., Cognitive and behavioral effects of epilepsy treatment, *Epilepsia*, 42(Suppl. 8), 24–32, 2001.

152. Kishore, P. R., Lipper, M. H., Miller, J. D., Girevendulis, A. K., Becker, D. P., and Vines, F. S., Posttraumatic hydrocephalus in patients with severe head injury, *Neuroradiology*, 16(1), 261–265, 1978.

153. Levin, H. S., Meyers, C. A., Grossman, R. G., and Sarwar, M., Ventricular enlargement after closed head injury, *Archives of Neurology*, 38(10), 623–629, 1981.

154. Massman, P. J., Bigler, E. D., Cullum, C. M., and Naugle, R. I., The relationship between cortical atrophy and ventricular volume, *International Journal of Neuroscience*, 30(1–2), 87–99, 1986.

155. Turkheimer, E., Cullum, C. M., Hubler, D. W., Paver, S. W., Yeo, R. A., and Bigler, E. D., Quantifying cortical atrophy, *Journal of Neurology, Neurosurgery, and Psychiatry*, 47(12), 1314–1318, 1984.

156. Yamaura, A., Ono, J., Watanabe, Y., and Saeki, N., CT findings and outcome in head injuries: Effects of aging, *Neurosurgical Review*, 12(Suppl. 1), 178–183, 1989.

157. Levin, H. S., Williams, D. H., Valastro, M., Eisenberg, H. M., Crofford, M. J., and Handel, S. F., Corpus callosal atrophy following closed head injury: Detection with magnetic resonance imaging, *Journal of Neurosurgery*, 73(1), 77–81, 1990.

158. Gentry, L. R., Imaging of closed head injury, *Radiology*, 191(1), 1–17, 1994.

159. Levin, H. S., Mendelsohn, D., Lilly, M. A., Yeakley, J., Song, J., Scheibel, R. S., et al., Magnetic resonance imaging in relation to functional outcome of pediatric closed head injury: A test of the Ommaya-Gennarelli model, *Neurosurgery*, 40(3), 432–440, 1997.

160. Katz, R. T., Brander, V., and Sahgal, V., Updates on the diagnosis and management of posttraumatic hydrocephalus, *American Journal of Physical Medicine and Rehabilitation*, 68(2), 91–96, 1989.

161. Zasler, N. D. and Marmarou, A., Posttraumatic hydrocephalus: Special topic report, *TBI Transmit*, 3(3), 5–8, 1992.

162. Fisher, C. M., The clinical picture in occult hydrocephalus, *Clinical Neurosurgery*, 24, 270–284, 1977.
163. Beyerl, B. and Black, P. M., Posttraumatic hydrocephalus, *Neurosurgery*, 15(2), 257–261, 1984.
164. Hakin, S. and Adams, R. D., The special clinical problem of symptomatic hydrocephalus with normal cerebrospinal fluid pressure: Observations on cerebrospinal fluid hydrodynamics, *Journal of Neurological Sciences*, 2(4), 307–327, 1965.
165. Adams, R. D., Fisher, C. M., Hakim, S., Ojemann, R. G., and Sweet, W. H., Symptomatic occult hydrocephalus with "normal" cerebrospinal-fluid pressure: A treatable syndrome, *New England Journal of Medicine*, 273(3), 117–126, 1965.
166. Graff-Radford, N. R. and Godersky, J. C., Normal-pressure hydrocephalus: Onset of gait abnormality before dementia predicts good surgical outcome, *Archives of Neurology*, 43(9), 940–942, 1986.
167. Dan, N. G. and Wade, M. J., The incidence of epilepsy after ventricular shunting procedures, *Journal of Neurosurgery*, 65(1), 19–21, 1986.
168. Tribl, G. and Oder, W., Outcome after shunt implantation in severe head injury with posttraumatic hydrocephalus, *Brain Injury*, 14(4), 345–354, 2000.
169. Phuenpathom, N., Ratanalert, S., Saeheng, S., and Sripairojkul, B., Post-traumatic hydrocephalus: Experience in 17 consecutive cases, *Journal of the Medical Association of Thailand*, 82(1), 46–53, 1999.
170. Koiv, L., Merisalu, E., Zilmer, K., Tomberg, T., and Kaasik, A. E., Changes of sympatho-adrenal and hypothalamo-pituitary–adrenocortical system in patients with head injury, *Acta Neurologica Scandinavica*, 96(1), 52–58, 1997.
171. Kelly, D. F., Gonzalo, I. T., Cohan, P., Berman, N., Swerdloff, R., and Wang, C., Hypopituitarism following traumatic brain injury and aneurysmal subarachnoid hemorrhage: A preliminary report, *Journal of Neurosurgery*, 93(5), 743–752, 2000.
172. Lieberman, S. A., Oberoi, A. L., Gilkison, C. R., Masel, B. E., and Urban, R. J., Prevalence of neuroendocrine dysfunction in patients recovering from traumatic brain injury, *Journal of Clinical Endocrinology and Metabolism*, 86(6), 2752–2756, 2001.
173. Cernak, I., Savic, V. J., Lazarov, A., Joksimovic, M., and Markovic, S., Neuroendocrine responses following graded traumatic brain injury in male adults, *Brain Injury*, 13(12), 1005–1015, 1999.
174. Childers, M. K., Rupright, J., Jones, P. S., and Merveille, O., Assessment of neuroendocrine dysfunction following traumatic brain injury, *Brain Injury*, 12(6), 517–523, 1998.
175. Yuan, X. Q. and Wade, C. E., Neuroendocrine abnormalities in patients with traumatic brain injury, *Frontiers in Neuroendocrinology*, 12(3), 209–230, 1991.
176. Escamilla, R. F. and Lisser, H., Simmonds disease, *Journal of Clinical Endocrinology and Metabolism*, 2(2), 65–96, 1942.
177. Benvenga, S., Campenni, A., Ruggeri, R. M., and Trimarchi, F., Hypopituitarism secondary to head trauma, *Journal of Clinical Endocrinology and Metabolism*, 85(4), 1353–1361, 2000.
178. Bushnik, T., Englander, J., and Katznelson, L., Fatigue after TBI: Association with neuroendocrine abnormalities, *Brain Injury*, 21(6), 559–566, 2007.
179. Leon-Carrion, J., Leal-Cerro, A., Cabezas, F. M., Atutxa, A. M., Gomez, S. G., Cordero, J. M. F., et al., Cognitive deterioration due to GH deficiency in patients with traumatic brain injury: A preliminary report, *Brain Injury*, 21(8), 871–875, 2007.
180. Arwert, L. I., Veltman, D. J., Deijen, J. B., Sytze van Dam, P., and Drent, M. L., Effects of growth hormone substitution therapy on cognitive functioning in growth hormone deficient patient: A functional MRI study, *Neuroendocrinology*, 83(1), 12–19, 2006.
181. Oertel, H., Schneider, H. J., Stalla, G. K., Holsboer, F., and Zihl, J., The effect of growth hormone substitution on cognitive performance in adult patients with hypopituitarism, *Psychoneuroendocrinology*, 29(7), 839–850, 2004.
182. Deijen, J. B., de Boer, H., and van der Veen, E. A., Cognitive changes during growth hormone replacement in adult men, *Psychoneuroendocrinology*, 23(1), 45–55, 1998.

183. Kelly, D. F., McArthur, D. L., Levin, H., Swimmer, S., Dusick, J. R., Cohan, P., et al., Neurobehavioral and quality of life changes associated with growth hormone insufficiency after complicated mild, moderate, or severe traumatic brain injury, *Journal of Neurotrauma,* 23(6), 928–942, 2006.

184. Povlishock, J. T. and Katz, D. I., Update of neuropathology and neurological recovery after traumatic brain injury, *Journal of Head Trauma Rehabilitation,* 20(1), 76–94, 2005.

185. Strobl, J. and Thomas, M. J., Human growth hormone, *Pharmacological Reviews,* 46(1), 1–34, 1994.

186. Kulinskiĭ, V. I. and Kolesnichenko, L. S., [Regulation of metabolic and energetic mitochondrial functions by hormones and signal transduction systems], *Biomeditsinskaya Khimiya,* 52(5), 425–427, 2006. [In Russian.]

187. Yao, K. L., Liu, X., Hudson, L. D., and Webster, H. D., Insulin-like growth factor I treatment reduces demyelination and up-regulates gene expression of myelin-related proteins in experimental autoimmune encephalomyelitis, *Proceedings of the National Academy of Sciences of the United States of America,* 92(13), 6190–6194, 1995.

188. Elovic, E., Anterior pituitary dysfunction after traumatic brain injury: Part I, *Journal of Head Trauma Rehabilitation,* 18(6), 541–543, 2003.

189. Ghigo, E., Masel, B., Aimaretti, G., Leon-Carrion, J., Casaneuva, F. F., Dominguez-Morales, M. R., Elovic, E., et al., Consensus guidelines on screening for hypopituitarism following traumatic brain injury, *Brain Injury,* 19(9), 711–724, 2005.

190. Nunez, J., Effects of thyroid hormones during brain differentiation, *Molecular and Cellular Endocrinology,* 37(2), 125–132, 1984.

191. Dussault, J. H. and Ruel, J., Thyroid hormones and brain development, *Annual Review of Physiology,* 49, 321–334, 1987.

192. Ruiz-Marcos, A., Cartagena Abella, P., Garcia Garcia, A., Escobar del Rey, F., and Morreale de Escobar, G., Rapid effects of adult-onset hypothyroidism on dendritic spines of pyramidal cells of the rat cerebral cortex, *Experimental Brain Research,* 73(3), 583–588, 1988.

193. Ruiz-Marcos, A., Sanchez-Toscano, F., Obregon, M. J., Escobar del Rey, F., and Morreale de Escobar, G., Thyroxine treatment and recovery of hypothyroidism-induced pyramidal cell damage, *Brain Research* (*Netherlands*), 239(2), 559–574, 1982.

194. Wooley, C. S. and McEwen, B. S., Estradiol regulates synapse density in the CA1 region of the hippocampus in the adult female rat, *Society of Neuroscience Abstracts,* 16(12), 144, 1990.

195. Luine, V. N., Estradiol increases choline acetyltransferase activity in specific basal forebrain nuclei and projection areas of female rats, *Experimental Neurology,* 89(2), 484–490, 1985.

196. McEwen, B. S., Weiss, J. M., and Schwartz, L. S., Selective retention of corticosterone by limbic structures in rat brain, *Nature,* 220(5170), 9111–9112, 1968.

197. Lieberman, S. A. and Hoffman, A. R., Growth hormone deficiency in adults: Characteristics and response to growth hormone replacement, *Journal of Pediatrics,* 128(5 Pt. 2), S58–S60, 1996.

198. Carroll, P. V., Christ, E. R., Bengtsson, B. A., Carlsson, L., Christiansen, J. S., Clemmons, D., et al., Growth hormone deficiency in adulthood and the effects of growth hormone replacement: A review, Growth Hormone Research Society Scientific Committee, *Journal of Clinical Endocrinology and Metabolism,* 83(2), 382–395, 1998.

199. National Institutes of Health, *Brain Basics: Understanding Sleep,* 2007, http://www.ninds.nih.gov/healthandmedical/pubs/understandingsleepbrainbasic.html (accessed April 24, 2009).

200. Beetar, J. T., Guilmette, T. J., and Sparadeo, F. R., Sleep and pain complaints in symptomatic traumatic brain injury and neurologic populations, *Archives of Physical Medicine and Rehabilitation,* 77(12), 1298–1302, 1996.

201. Olver, J. H., Ponsford, J. L., and Curran, C. A., Outcome following traumatic brain injury: A comparison between 2 and 5 years after injury, *Brain Injury,* 10(11), 841–848, 1996.

202. Baumann, C. R., Werth, E., Stocker, R., Ludwig, S., and Bassetti, C. L., Sleep–wake disturbances 6 months after traumatic brain injury: A prospective study, *Brain,* 130(7), 1873–1883, 2007.

203. Clinchot, D. M., Bogner, J., Mysiw, W. J., Fugate, L., and Corrigan, J., Defining sleep disturbance after brain injury, *American Journal of Physical Medicine and Rehabilitation*, 77(4), 291–295, 1998.

204. Fichtenberg, N. L., Zafonte, R. D., Putnam, S., Mann, N. R., and Millard, A. E., Insomnia in a post-acute brain injury sample, *Brain Injury*, 16(3), 197–206, 2002.

205. Ouellet, M. C. and Morin, C. M., Subjective and objective measures of insomnia in the context of traumatic brain injury: A preliminary study, *Sleep Medicine*, 7(6), 485–497, 2006.

206. George, B. and Landau-Ferey, J., Twelve months' follow-up by night sleep EEG after recovery from severe head trauma, *Neurochirurgie*, 29(2), 45–47, 1986.

207. Hammond, F. M. and Zafonte, R. D., Drugs for management of sleep disorders, *Physical Medicine and Rehabilitation Clinics of North America*, 8(4), 801–825, 1997.

208. Alexandre, A., Rubini, L., Nertempi, P., and Farinello, C., Sleep alterations during post-traumatic coma as a possible predictor of cognitive defects, *Acta Neurochirurgica Supplementum*, 28(1), 188–192, 1979.

209. Ron, S., Algom, D., Hary, D., and Cohen, M., Time-related changes in the distribution of sleep stages in brain injured patients, *Electroencephalography and Clinical Neurophysiology*, 48(4), 432–441, 1980.

210. Young, T., Palta, M., Dempsey, J., Skatrud, J., Weber, S., and Badr, S., The occurrence of sleep-disordered breathing among middle-aged adults, *New England Journal of Medicine*, 328(17), 1230–1235, 1993.

211. Guilleminault, C., Faull, K. F., Miles, L., and van den Hoed, J., Posttraumatic excessive daytime sleepiness: A review of 20 patients, *Neurology*, 33(12), 1584–1589, 1983.

212. Webster, J. B., Bell, K. R., Hussey, J. D., Natale, T. K., and Lakshminarayan, S., Sleep apnea in adults with traumatic brain injury: A preliminary investigation, *Archives of Physical Medicine and Rehabilitation*, 82(3), 316–321, 2001.

213. Masel, B. E., Scheibel, R. S., Kimbark, T., and Kuna, S. T., Excessive daytime sleepiness in adults with brain injuries, *Archives of Physical Medicine and Rehabilitation*, 82(11), 1526–1532, 2001.

214. Castriotta, R. J. and Lai, J. M., Sleep disorders associated with traumatic brain injury, *Archives of Physical Medicine and Rehabilitation*, 82(10), 1403–1406, 2001.

215. Castriotta, R. J., Wilde, M. C., Lai, J. M., Atanasov, S., Masel, B. E., and Kuna, S. T., Prevalence and consequences of sleep disorders in traumatic brain injury, *Journal of Clinical Sleep Medicine*, 3(4), 349–356, 2007.

216. Lankford, D. A., Wellman, J. J., and O'Hara, C., Posttraumatic narcolepsy in mild to moderate closed head injury, *Sleep*, 17(8 Suppl.), S25–S28, 1994.

217. Ebrahim, I. O., Peacock, K. W., and Williams, A. J., Posttraumatic narcolepsy: Two case reports and a mini review, *Journal of Clinical Sleep Medicine*, 1(2), 153–156, 2005.

218. Findley, L. J., Barth, J. T., Powers, D. C., Wilhoit, S. C., Boyd, D. G., and Suratt, P. M., Cognitive impairment in patients with obstructive sleep apnea and associated hypoxemia, *Chest*, 90(5), 686–690, 1986.

219. Greenberg, G. D., Watson, R. K., and Deptula, D., Neuropsychological dysfunction in sleep apnea, *Sleep*, 10(3), 254–262, 1987.

220. Montplaisir, J., Bedard, M. A., Richer, F., and Rouleau, I., Neurobehavioral manifestations in obstructive sleep apnea syndrome before and after treatment with continuous positive airway pressure, *Sleep*, 16(6 Suppl.), S17–S19, 1992.

221. Young, T., Blustein, J., Finn, L., and Palta, M., Sleep-disordered breathing and motor vehicle accidents in a population-based sample of employed adults, *Sleep*, 20(8), 608–613, 1997.

222. Teran-Santos, J., Jimenez-Gomez, A., and Cordero-Guevara, J., The association between sleep apnea and the risk of traffic accidents, Cooperative Group Burgos-Santander, *New England Journal of Medicine*, 340(11), 847–851, 1999.

223. Horstmann, S., Hess, C. W., Bassetti, C., Gugger, M., and Mathis, J., Sleepiness-related accidents in sleep apnea patients, *Sleep*, 23(3), 383–389, 2000.

224. Wilde, M. C., Castriotta, R. J., Lai, J. M., Atanasov, S., Masel, B. E., and Kuna, S. T., Cognitive impairment in patients with traumatic brain injury and obstructive sleep apnea, *Archives of Physical Medicine and Rehabilitation*, 88(10), 1284–1288, 2007.

225. Ferini-Strambi, L., Baietto, C., Di Gioia, M. R., Castaldi, P., Castronovo, C., Zucconi, M., et al., Cognitive dysfunction in patients with obstructive sleep apnea (OSA): Partial reversibility after continuous positive airway pressure (CPAP), *Brain Research Bulletin*, 61(1), 87–92, 2003.

226. Macey, P. M., Henderson, L. A., Macey, K. E., Alger, J. R., Frysinger, R. C., Woo, M. A., Harper, R. K., Yan-Go, F. L., and Harper, R. M., Brain morphology associated with obstructive sleep apnea, *American Journal of Respiratory and Critical Care Medicine*, 166(10), 1382–1387, 2002.

227. Morrell, M. J., McRobbie, D. W., Quest, R. A., Cummin, A. R., Chiassi, R., and Corfield, D. R., Changes in brain morphology associated with obstructive sleep apnea, *Sleep Medicine*, 4(5), 451–454, 2003.

228. Bartlett, D. J., Rae, C., Thompson, C. H., Byth, K., Joffee, D. A., Enright, T., et al., Hippocampal area metabolites relate to severity and cognitive function in obstructive sleep apnea, *Sleep Medicine*, 5(6), 593–596, 2004.

229. Kamba, M., Inoue, Y., Higami, S., Suto, Y., Ogawa, T., and Chen, W., Cerebral metabolic impairment in patients with obstructive sleep apnoea: An independent association of obstructive sleep apnoea with white matter change, *Journal of Neurology, Neurosurgery, and Psychiatry*, 71(3), 334–339, 2001.

230. Halbower, A. C., Ishman, S. L., and McGinley, B. M., Childhood obstructive sleep-disordered breathing: A clinical update and discussion of technological innovations and challenges, *Chest*, 132(6), 2030–2041, 2007.

231. Tonon, C., Vetrugno, R., Lodi, R., Gallassi, R., Provini, F., Lotti, S., et al., Proton magnetic resonance spectroscopy study of brain metabolism in obstructive sleep apnoea syndrome before and after continuous positive airway pressure treatment, *Sleep*, 30(3), 305–311, 2007.

232. Macey, P. M., Kumar, R., Woo, M. A., Valladares, E. M., Yan-Go, F. L., and Harper, R. M., Brain structural changes in obstructive sleep apnea, *Sleep*, 31(7), 967–977, 2008.

233. Veasey, S. C., Davis, C. W., Fenik, P., Zhan, G., Hsu, Y. J., Pratico, D., et al., Long-term intermittent hypoxia in mice: Protracted hypersomnolence with oxidative injury to sleep–wake brain regions, *Sleep*, 27(2), 194–201, 2004.

234. Pae, E.-K., Chien, P., and Harper, R. M., Intermittent hypoxia damages cerebellar cortex and deep nuclei, *Neuroscience Letters*, 375(2), 123–128, 2005.

235. Gozal, D., Daniel, J. M., and Dohanich, G. P., Behavioral and anatomical correlates of chronic episodic hypoxia during sleep in the rat, *Journal of Neuroscience*, 21(7), 2442–2450, 2001.

236. Zhan, G., Fenik, P., Pratico, D., and Veasey, S. C., Inducible nitric oxide synthase in long-term intermittent hypoxia: Hypersomnolence and brain injury, *American Journal of Respiratory and Critical Care Medicine*, 171(12), 1414–1420, 2005.

237. Zhu, Y., Fenik, P., Zhan, G., Mazza, E., Kelz, M., Aston-Jones, G., and Veasey, S. C., Selective loss of catecholaminergic wake active neurons in a murine sleep apnea model, *Journal of Neuroscience*, 27(37), 10060–10071, 2007.

238. Shamsuzzaman, A. S., Winnicki, M., Lanfranchi, P., Wolk, R., Kara, T., Accurso, V., and Somers, V. K., Elevated C-reactive protein in patients with obstructive sleep apnea, *Circulation*, 105(21), 2462–2464, 2002.

239. McLaurin, J., D'Souza, S., Stewart, J., Blain, M., Beaudet, A., Nalbantoglu, J., et al., Effect of tumor necrosis factor [alpha] and [beta] on human oligodendrocytes and neurons in culture, *International Journal of Developmental Neuroscience*, 13(3–4), 369–381, 1995.

240. Cross, R. L., Kumar, R., Macey, P. M., Doering, L. V., Alger, J. R., Yan-Go, F. L., et al., Neural alterations and depressive symptoms in obstructive sleep apnea patients, *Sleep*, 31(8), 1103–1109, 2008.

241. Lee, K. A., Hicks, G., and Nino-Murcia, G., Validity and reliability of a scale to assess fatigue, *Psychiatry Research*, 36(3), 291–298, 1991.

242. Krupp, L. B., LaRocca, N. G., Muir-Nash, J., and Steinberg, A. D., The Fatigue Severity Scale: Application to patients with multiple sclerosis and systemic lupus erythematosus, *Archives of Neurology*, 46(10), 1121–1123, 1989.

243. Closs, S. J., Assessment of sleep in hospital patients: A review of methods, *Journal of Advanced Nursing*, 13(4), 501–510, 1988.

244. Closs, S. J., Patient's sleep–wake rhythms in hospital: Part 2, *Nursing Times*, 84(2), 54–55, 1988.
245. Baumann, C. R., and Bassetti, C. L., Hypocretins (orexins) and sleep–wake disorders, *The Lancet Neurology*, 4(10), 673–682, 2005.
246. Baumann, C. R., Stocker, R., Imhof, H. G., Trentz, O., Hersberger, M., Mignot, E., and Bassetti, C. L., Hypocretin-1 (orexin A) deficiency in acute traumatic brain injury, *Neurology*, 65(1), 147–149, 2005.
247. Johns, M. W., A new method for measuring daytime sleepiness: The Epworth Sleepiness Scale, *Sleep*, 14(6), 540–545, 1991.
248. Zafonte, R. D., Mann, N. R., and Fichtenberg, N. L., Sleep disturbance in traumatic brain injury: Pharmacological options, *Neurorehabilitation*, 7(3), 189–195, 1996.
249. Morin, C. M., Colecchi, C., Stone, J., Sood, R., and Brink, D., Behavioral and pharmacological therapies for late-life insomnia: A randomized controlled trial, *Journal of the American Medical Association*, 281(11), 991–999, 1999.
250. Bush, G. W., Calculating the cost of long-term living: A four-step process, *Journal of Head Trauma Rehabilitation*, 5(1), 47–56, 1990.
251. DeVivo, M. J. and Ivie, 3rd, C. S., Life expectancy of ventilator-dependent persons with spinal cord injuries, *Chest*, 108(1), 226–232, 1995.
252. Geisler, W. O., Jousse, A. T., Wynne-Jones, M., and Breithaupt, D., Survival in traumatic spinal cord injury, *Paraplegia*, 21(6), 364–373, 1983.
253. Whiteneck, G. G., Charlifue, S. W., Frankel, H. L., Fraser, M. H., Gardner, B. P., Gerhart, K. A., et al., Mortality, morbidity, and psychosocial outcomes of persons spinal cord injured more than 20 years ago, *Paraplegia*, 30(9), 617–630, 1992.
254. Signorini, D. F., Andrews, P. J., Jones, P. A., Wardlaw, J. M., and Miller, J. D., Predicting survival using simple clinical variables: A case study in traumatic brain injury, *Journal of Neurology, Neurosurgery, and Psychiatry*, 66(1), 20–25, 1999.
255. Eyman, R. K., Grossman, H. J., Chaney, R. H., and Call, T. L., The life expectancy of profoundly handicapped people with mental retardation, *New England Journal of Medicine*, 323(9), 584–589, 1990.
256. Roboz, P., Mortality rate in institutionalized mentally retarded children, *The Medical Journal of Australia*, 1(5), 218–221, 1972.
257. Luerssen, T. G., Klauber, M. R., and Marshall, L. F., Outcome from head injury related to patient's age: A longitudinal prospective study of adult and pediatric head injury, *Journal of Neurosurgery*, 68(3), 409–416, 1988.
258. Conroy, C. and Kraus, J. F., Survival after brain injury: Cause of death, length of survival, and prognostic variables in a cohort of brain-injured people, *Neuroepidemiology*, 7(1), 13–22, 1988.
259. Marshall, L. F., Gautille, T., Klauber, M. R., Eisenberg, H. M., Jane, J. A., Luerssen, T. G., et al., The outcome of severe closed head injury, *Journal of Neurosurgery*, 75(Suppl. 1), S28–S36, 1991.
260. Fiedler, R. C., Granger, C. V., and Post, L. A., The Uniform Data System for Medical Rehabilitation: Report of first admissions for 1998, *American Journal of Physical Medicine and Rehabilitation*, 79(1), 87–92, 2000.
261. Rish, B. L., Dillon, J. D., and Weiss, G. H., Mortality following penetrating craniocerebral injuries: An analysis of the deaths in the Vietnam Head Injury Registry population, *Journal of Neurosurgery*, 59(5), 775–780, 1983.
262. Lewin, W., Marshall, T. F., and Roberts, A. H., Long-term outcome after severe head injury, *British Medical Journal*, 2(6204), 1533–1538, 1979.
263. Walker, A. E., Leuchs, H. K., Lechtape-Gruter, H., Caveness, W. F., and Kretschman, C., Life expectancy of head injured men with and without epilepsy, *Archives of Neurology*, 24(2), 95–100, 1971.
264. Hammond, F. M., Wiercisiewski, D. R., Grattan, K. D., Norton, J. A., and Yablon, S., Mortality following traumatic brain injury: Who dies and when, *Archives of Physical Medicine and Rehabilitation*, 81(9), 1260, 2000. [Abstract.]
265. Baguley, I., Slewa-Younan, S., Lazarus, R., and Green, A., Long-term mortality trends in patients with traumatic brain injury, *Brain Injury*, 14(6), 505–512, 2000.

266. Corkin, S., Sullivan, E. V., and Carr, F. A., Prognostic factors for life expectancy after penetrating head injury, *Archives of Neurology*, 41(9), 975–977, 1984.

267. Weiss, G. H., Caveness, W. F., Einsiedel-Lechtape, H., and McNeel, M. L., Life expectancy and causes of death in a group of head-injured veterans of World War I, *Archives of Neurology*, 39(12), 741–743, 1982.

268. Ashwal, S., Eyman, R. K., and Call, T. L., Life expectancy of children in a persistent vegetative state, *Pediatric Neurology*, 10(1), 27–33, 1994.

269. Jennett, B. and Plum, F., Persistent vegetative state after brain damage: A syndrome in search of a name, *Lancet*, 1(7753), 734–737, 1972.

270. Multi-Society Task Force on PVS, Medical aspects of the persistent vegetative state (second of two parts), *New England Journal of Medicine*, 330(22), 1572–1579, 1994.

271. Roberts, A. H., *Severe Accidental Head Injury: An Assessment of Long-Term Prognosis*, The MacMillan Press, London, 1979.

272. Walker, A. E. and Blumer, D., The fate of World War II veterans with posttraumatic seizures, *Archives of Neurology*, 46(1), 23–26, 1989.

273. Strauss, D. J., Ashwal, S., Day, S. M., and Shavelle, R. M., Life expectancy of children in vegetative and minimally conscious states, *Pediatric Neurology*, 23(4), 312–319, 2000.

274. Kolpan, K. I., Medicolegal issues regarding lifelong care, *Journal of Head Trauma Rehabilitation*, 5(1), 100–101, 1990.

275. DeJong, G. and Betavia, A. I., Societal duty and resource allocation for persons with severe traumatic brain injury, *Journal of Head Trauma Rehabilitation*, 4(1), 1–12, 1989.

276. Kraus, J. S., Accuracy of life expectancy estimates in life care plans: Consideration of non-biographical and non-injury factors, *Topics in Spinal Cord Rehabilitation*, 7(4), 59–68, 2002.

277. von Faber, M., Bootsma-van der Siel, A., van Exel, E., Gussekloo, J., Lagaay, A. M., van Dongen, E., et al., Successful aging in the oldest old: Who can be characterized as successfully aged?, *Archives of Internal Medicine*, 161(22), 2694–2700, 2001.

278. Harrison-Felix, C., Whiteneck, G., DeVivo, M. J., Hammond, F. M., and Jha, A., Causes of death following 1 year postinjury among individuals with traumatic brain injury, *The Journal of Head Trauma Rehabilitation*, 21(1), 22–33, 2006.

12

Bioscience Frontiers in Neuromedical Interventions Following Brain Injury

Mark J. Ashley, Alan Weintraub, and David L. Ripley

CONTENTS

12.1 Introduction

The purpose of this chapter is to consider whether clinical interventions might evolve toward restitution of normalized metabolic and neurophysiologic activity following traumatic insult to the brain. To accomplish this, bioscience research and clinical trials will have to focus on complex cellular neural networks under tremendous physiologic strain and consider the recovery demands that this system must achieve. Can we treat cellular metabolic challenges, prevent or reverse early structural senescence, or promote neurogenesis, synaptogenesis, angiogenesis, and gliogenesis needed for neurologic remodeling after brain injury? The following discussion may provide some clues or potential pathways to optimization of function in the injured or recovering central nervous system (CNS).

The common response following brain injury can be characterized as slow and inconsistent. It is clear that there is tremendous metabolic disruption following traumatic brain injury (TBI) in all levels of severity postinjury.[1] It seems to be assumed that residual neurologic structures return to a normal metabolic and functional state after a period of time. However, there may be reason to question whether this is, in fact, the case. Interventions that may be considered to encourage healing within the brain must take this into consideration.

The brain has evolved into an organ supremely efficient at data acquisition, reduction, and storage. Novel information arriving into the CNS requires the greatest recruitment of structures and resources. As the brain processes information, it is stored in a fashion that is hierarchically built upon previously stored information via continuous synaptic remodeling. Familiarity with information results in increasing efficiency of neural structures, with fewer neural resources required for representation of information. In fact, it appears that a primary function of some neurons in the prefrontal cortex is to control neural networks that pertain to specific information.[2] The ability of single neurons to take on complex function has also been demonstrated in temporal regions.[2,3] Because recruitment of large networks on a continual basis would require tremendous energy utilization, the CNS adaptation appears to be reduction of neural representation of lesser numbers of structures, thus requiring less energy expenditure.

Continuous remodeling of neural ensembles and networks logically requires energy and connectivity to achieve efficiency. Energy utilization includes energy for normal cellular function, repair, protein synthesis, organelle synthesis and transport, membrane permeability maintenance, neuromodulator production and reuptake, myelin repair, synaptic remodeling, and synaptic transmission.

Not only must energy be supplied for these activities, but the neuron must deal with the metabolic consequences of respiration, glycolysis, oxidative phosphorylation, and lipid peroxidation. Generation of reactive oxygen species (ROS) increases as metabolic demand increases. The presence of ROS triggers a host of reactions and cellular defense mechanisms, the activation of which is dependent upon ready availability of a wide variety of substrates. Adenosine triphosphate (ATP) production and calcium buffering are reduced or impaired with dysfunction of mitochondrial energy metabolism, resulting in increased generation of ROS.[4] The increase in the generation of ROS damages cell membranes via lipid peroxidation, resulting in acceleration of the rate of mitochondrial DNA mutation and damage. The brain consumes about 20% of the body's oxygen and, thus, is highly vulnerable to excessive oxidative stress. Excessive oxidative stress and excessive calcium loading result in a loss of the impermeability of the inner mitochondrial membrane. Ultimately, mitochondrial swelling and the release of cytochrome C and Apaf-1 induce caspase-mediated apoptosis.[5,6] These underlying neuronal concepts play a large role in cellular homeostasis and may be clearly affected not only initially post-TBI, but also during recovery and rehabilitation.

12.2 Pathophysiology of Traumatic Brain Injury

It is important to appreciate the pathophysiologic complexity and heterogeneity of TBI. Structural changes associated with acute and chronic TBI logically serve as a basis for recovery. As such, consideration of the nature and type of injury to neural structures may be important to consider as well. TBI can result in focal or diffuse metabolic, hypoxic, ischemic, or traumatic axonal damage.[7] Focal damage can be expected to impact certain motor, sensory, or cognitive functions, depending upon the neural structures or systems involved.

Diffuse axonal injury (DAI) is recognized as a primary component of neurophysiologic dysfunction in 40% to 50% of all brain injury of traumatic etiology.[8] DAI tends to affect, predictably, specific regions of the human brain, such as the parasagittal white matter of the cerebral cortex, the corpus callosum, and the pontine–mesencephalic junction adjacent to the superior cerebellar peduncles.[9] At the cellular level, direct forces of sufficient magnitude breach the neuronal/axonal cytoplasmic cellular membrane, initiating a cytotoxic biochemical cascade of events that impacts neuronal health and function in the immediate vicinity of the primary damage.[10] The damage inflicted by this cytotoxic biochemical cascade, however, is not restricted to the locality of the primary site of damage and can reach far distant cellular structures within the CNS.[11]

More specifically, axolemmal permeability is induced by trauma resulting in a local influx of Ca^{2+}. Cysteine proteases, calpain, and caspases promote proteolytic digestion of spectrin, which is a major constituent of the cytoskeletal membrane. Calpain activation causes mitochondrial injury that results in release of cytochrome C and caspase activation. Caspases and calpain participate in the cytoskeletal membrane degradation that occurs over time.[12]

Neurofilamentary changes also occur in a subset of severe TBI. These changes may result in mechanical failure of the axonal cytoskeleton,[13] which may impact mitochondrial migration from their site of biosynthesis in the cell body to positions along the axon or terminal.[14–17] Neurofilamentary changes associated with Wallerian degeneration, however, are not immediate. Wallerian-type axonal degeneration progresses from axonal swelling to swelling of the axonal bulbs, leading to the development of small clusters of microglia.[18] At a cellular level, this includes residual endogenous brain peptides and small proteins,[19] immunoreactive astrocytes in injured areas,[20,21] beta-amyloid protein deposition,[22] and neurofibrillary tangles.[23] These changes occur from days to months to years after injury. Active myelin degeneration occurs as the final stage in the neurodegenerative process during the first 2 years after DAI.[24]

Some evidence also exists for the presence of chronic perivascular iron deposition (siderosis) associated with previous perivascular hemorrhage in cortical, subcortical, brainstem, and cerebellar structures.[25] Primary areas of involvement include the parasagittal white matter, the corpus callosum, the internal capsule, and the deep gray matter.

12.3 Mitochondrial Function

Mitochondrial function is crucial for energy transduction and is crucial to CNS function. Cell survival and death are regulated by mitochondria. What may have begun as a symbiotic relationship between a primitive bacteria and a single-cell anaerobic organism more than 1 billion years ago has evolved into mitochondrial structures that provide energy for cellular function, regulate Ca^{2+}, and determine the life cycle of the cell.[26–28]

Although the brain accounts for only 2% of the body's weight, it receives 15% of total cardiac output and uses 20% of the total body oxygen consumption.[29] This is, in part, a result of the proliferation of mitochondria in neural cellular structures. Mitochondria provide for aerobic respiration, calcium regulation, and apoptosis. Damage to mitochondria results in bioenergetic crisis or failure and leads to both necrosis when profound and apoptosis when less complete.[5,29,30] Energy is continuously required to maintain ion gradients across neuronal plasma membranes that are critical to the ability to generate action potentials. Mitochondria are the primary intracellular source of cytotoxic free radicals because they produce 90% of cellular ATP, the principal energy source for energy-requiring actions in plants and animals.[31,32] Lesser amounts of ATP are also produced by glycolysis. They are organelles of varying size that fuse, divide, and branch in a dynamic reticular network.[27,28] Perinuclear mitochondria replicate more actively than those elsewhere in the cell, and many are distributed to synapses.[29] They can move within the cytoplasm, which allows them to distribute themselves within cells and to partition between dividing cells.[28] Failure to resculpt mitochondria dynamically compromises organelle localization and neuronal function. Mitochondria are found in axons and, to a lesser degree, in dendrites.[33–35] Mitochondrial energy transduction appears to be compartmentalized at synapses.

Neurofilaments impact axon caliber, cell shape, and organelle transport as integral components of the cytoskeleton. Cytoskeletal defects may impact synaptic mitochondrial localization and defects in molecular motors that drive both anterograde and retrograde axonal transport of organelles and proteins. The breakdown of microtubules is thought to be the result of hyperphosphorylation of tau protein.[36,37]

Neurotransmission is dependent upon energy supply. Therefore, the role of ATP is highlighted in maintaining synaptic membrane potential and fueling numerous steps in the synaptic neurotransmitter vesicle cycle such as scission, uncoating, and refilling of vesicles with neurotransmitters.[38] Movement and sequestration of mitochondria appear to impact regulation of synaptic strength.

Mitochondria are found in higher concentrations in cellular regions with high metabolic demand, accumulating in the vicinity of active growth cones of developing neurons.[39] Mitochondria redistribute into dendritic protrusion in response to synaptic excitation and correlated with synaptic spine formation and synaptogenesis.[17] Figure 12.1 depicts mitochondrial location, migration, and concentration.

The dynamics of mitochondrial motility are important in consideration of bioenergetic demand and capacity. Extension into dendritic protrusions is induced by local synaptic stimulation. Increased activity of mitochondria correlates with the ability of a neuron to form new excitatory synapses in response to stimulation. There appears to be reciprocity between regulation of synapses and mitochondria. Neuronal activity can affect the motility, fusion/fission balance, and distribution within the cell of mitochondria in dendrites. Repetitive excitatory depolarization of a synapse causes mitochondrial redistribution in dendritic protrusions. As a result of the length and compartmentalization of neurons, to meet the spatial and temporal metabolic demands of neurons, mitochondria must be adequately and properly distributed within subcellular compartments. In comparison with axons, mitochondria within dendrites are less motile overall and move shorter distances.[40] Excitotoxic doses of glutamate have been shown to inhibit mitochondrial movement and to alter mitochondrial shape from elongated to round.[41] Depolarization suppresses mitochondrial motility, whereas neuronal inactivity speeds up mitochondrial movement. Mitochondrial distribution appears to be affected by dendritic activity in that mitochondria become concentrated in the region of synaptic activity as opposed to more widely distributed.

Mitochondriopathies usually follow a slow progression involving multiple organ systems.[42] Most are associated with increased free oxygen radical production arising from deficits in electron transport and resulting in reduced energy production. Damage to mitochondria causes disruption of ATP production and increases in ROS production that are capable of overwhelming the cell's normal antioxidant defenses.[31,43] The brain is particularly susceptible because of its high energy consumption rate and its normally high ROS production.[29,44] These arise, in turn, from the brain's high content of "peroxidizable"

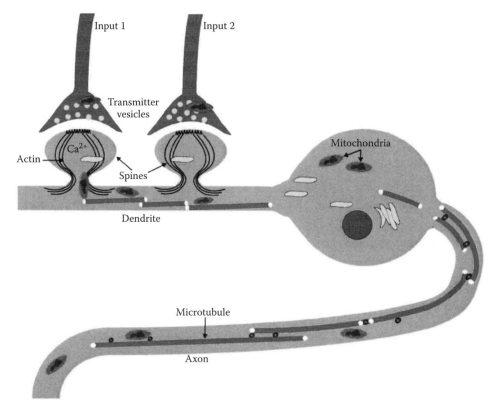

FIGURE 12.1

Involvement of mitochondrial motility in synaptic plasticity. Mitochondria migrate along microtubules in dendrites and axons. Mitochondria migrate to areas of greater energy demand as needed, such as dendritic spines and transmitter vesicles. (From Mattson, M. P., Gleichmann, M., and Cheng, A., *Neuron*, 60(5), 752, 2008. With permission.)

unsaturated fatty acids, its high oxygen consumption, and a comparative paucity of anti-oxidant enzymes when compared with other organ systems.

Frequent consequences of mitochondrial dysfunction include dementias, epilepsy, and ataxias.[45] Oxidative stress that results in energy inhibition has been shown to alter amyloid precursor protein (APP) processing, thereby potentially contributing to amyloidosis.[46,47] β-amyloid decreases the stability of mitochondria, in turn, and can induce oxidative stress and subsequent bioenergetic crisis or failure.[48–50] Mitochondrial impairment enhances β-amyloid production.[51] Further complication arises from difficulties in mitochondrial migration that disallows mitochondrial distribution to high-energy-requiring cellular targets, such as synapses, where continual remodeling may be required or needed for function or learning, respectively.

12.4 Neuroendocrine Function

Neuroendocrine dysfunction following TBI has been recently documented and has become the topic of numerous reviews.[52–56] The presence of posterior pituitary dysfunction and its resultant disorders of salt and fluid balance has long been recognized by clinicians as a result of the ready availability of laboratory evidence routinely collected during the acute stages of recovery following TBI, as well as the potentially life-threatening consequences of posterior pituitary dysfunction. Recently, however, a greater awareness has grown of the presence of anterior pituitary dysfunction following TBI, as well. This is becoming an important area for clinical interventions to promote recovery following TBI. Prevalence of deficiency along the four primary hormone axes is as follows: somatotroph, 6% to 25%; gonadotroph, 8% to 12%; thyrotroph, 4% to 6%; and corticotroph, 4% to 6%.[52,54,57–62]

Guidelines exist specific to screening for hypopituitarism following TBI.[63] However, the premise behind the timing of current guidelines is that most individuals will recover endocrine function following TBI, as well as the uncertainty about the implications for endocrine supplementation during the recovery after TBI. It is possible that as more information is collected regarding the impact of endocrine dysfunction following TBI, the clinical guidelines for screening and provocative testing will change accordingly. The clinician must realize that hypopituitarism may not manifest immediately after injury and may take months or years to do so.[64] Diagnosis of a hormone deficiency often does not take on the importance that it perhaps should. In addition, some controversy exists over definition of hormone insufficiency versus deficiency and, to be sure, neither the field of endocrinology itself nor the payer sector have become current with the most recent information from the literature.

An area where this is very clear is with respect to growth hormone deficiency (GHD) following TBI. Agreement about what constitutes GHD versus growth hormone (GH) insufficiency has not been universal, and as a result, payer practices vary considerably with regard to coverage for GH therapy. Because growth hormone is secreted in a pulsatile fashion, serum levels of GH are unreliable as a measure of GH secretory production, and stimulation testing is necessary to determine whether GHD is present. Insulinlike growth factor 1 (IGF-1) is frequently used to reflect an averaging of GH production, because circulating IGF-1 derives from GH-stimulated biosynthesis, primarily in the liver. However, clinical studies of the impact of IGF-1, both as an indicator and a correlate of GH function, have been mixed. IGF-1 levels following TBI should be monitored, and provocative testing should be strongly considered for any IGF-1 levels less than 200 µg/dL.

Hormone replacement therapy (HRT) is not yet routinely performed following TBI. There are several questions regarding HRT:

1. Does the patient improve by returning hormone levels to within a normal range?
2. Is reacquisition of cortical function by residual neurologic structures dependent upon or enhanced by HRT?
3. Does HRT impact the return of normal neuroendocrine function following TBI?
4. What are the potential complications of HRT and does it worsen risk of the development of complications following TBI, such as agitation or deep venous thrombosis?
5. To what extent, if any, does neuroendocrine function impact the bioenergetics of brain function?

Crucial to determination of efficacy of such interventions is whether assessment of the effects of treatment is properly defined. Independent variables such as rate and extent of recovery versus recovery of function alone may be more pertinent. As one considers these questions, recovery of function may be more or less immediate. Expectations pertaining to recovery of function may be tempered by the knowledge that the intent of HRT is for both an immediate and a long-term effect. HRT may play both a restorative and a neuroprotective role, improving and preserving function, as discussed later in the chapter.

Research is revealing that some hormones appear to be synthesized on a local basis by neurons and glia within the CNS. It is not clear whether responsible mechanisms for endogenous localized production function normally or in an altered fashion following injury to the brain.

In general, we shall review the impact a few major hormones have on cellular function, regeneration, and repair.

12.4.1 Somatotrophic Axis

GH and IGF-1 are increasingly implicated in neural protection, regeneration, and functional plasticity.[65,66] The effects of GH and IGF-1 are exerted at structural and metabolic levels. They impact myelination, somatic growth, oligodendrocyte function and production, levels of neurotransmitters and neurotransmitter receptors, glucose metabolism, cerebral blood flow, neuronal dendritic arborization, and intercellular communication in astrocytes.[65] Impacted neurotransmitters include serotonin, norepinephrine, dopamine, glutamate, and acetylcholine.

GH levels in the blood derive primarily from pituitary function, whereas IGF-1 derives primarily from the liver. However, within the CNS there is evidence to suggest that levels of both GH and IGF-1 may be related to levels that cross the blood–brain barrier as well as related to levels that may be produced in various parts of the brain. It is well established that IGF-1 from the body reaches the brain parenchyma and cerebrospinal fluid.[65]

The trophic effects of GH within the CNS have been demonstrated for neurons and astrocytes.[67] GH affects both neuron and astrocyte proliferation in development, and conversely, decreased dendritic branching and smaller neuronal somas have been associated with lower GH levels.[68] GH appears to affect neuronal dendritic branching in the cerebral cortex[68] whereas IGF-1 affects arborization within the developing cerebellum[69,70] and the developing adult cerebral cortex.[71–73] Peripheral IGF-1 has been shown to increase both cellular proliferation within the dentate subgranular zone and the subsequent migration and differentiation of progenitor cells within the dentate gyrus.[74,75]

Exercise increases peripheral and intracerebral GH and IGF-1 in adult animals and results in similar hippocampal neurogenesis.[76] Exercise has been shown preferentially to impact learning and memory, functional recovery after brain injury, and mental decline associated with senescence.[77–80] Underlying this improvement appears to be increases in brain-derived neurotrophic factor within the hippocampus.[81] IGF-1 appears to mediate the impact of exercise on cognitive function.[82] GH stimulates cellular protein synthesis.[83] Cellular enzymatic homeostasis supporting normal cellular function including maintenance, repair, and normal metabolic function is altered, in turn, by impaired protein synthesis.[84]

GH and IGF-1 appear to impact both angiogenesis and cerebral blood flow. Arteriolar density in the cerebral cortex in older animals increases with GH treatment, and increased density has been correlated with increased serum IGF-1 levels.[85] In addition, brain vessel density in the hippocampus and cerebellum increases with IGF-1.[75] Elderly humans demonstrate an association of greater cerebral blood flow in the left premotor and left dorsolateral prefrontal cortices with higher IGF-1 levels.[86]

IGF-1 has been shown to be successful in reducing damage following ischemic lesions in experimental animals; however, human studies have yet to be performed.[87] IGF-1 appears to enhance glucose uptake in neurons exposed to glucose deprivation,[88] and this may be one of the mechanisms exercised by estradiol as a neuroprotectant.[89] Glucose utilization was observed to increase 11% to 14% in the anterior cingulate of the cortex, the CA1 region of the hippocampus, and the arcuate nucleus of the hypothalamus following IGF-1 administration in older animals.[90]

IGF-1 was found to correlate positively with cognitive functioning and overall degree of improvement following rehabilitation for individuals with ischemic stroke.[91] Outcomes were significantly better for those with IGF-1 levels more than 161.8 μg/dL. Administration of IGF-1 in animals reduces infarct volume and improves neurologic function after ischemia.[92,93]

GH and IGF-1 have been the subject of a number of research articles regarding various aspects of functioning following TBI. The most studied area has involved the association of GHD or low IGF-1 with fatigue. Most of these studies have had mixed results.[62,94–98]

In summary, GH and/or IGF-1 interact with oligodendrocytes, neurons, astrocytes, blood vessels, and erythrocytes within the CNS, impacting along with neurogenesis, gliogenesis, glucose metabolism and cellular survival, protein synthesis, cerebral blood flow, neurotransmitter synthesis and reception, gap junction formation, myelin sheath formation, and arborization.[65,83] As such, attention paid to these substances during the postinjury phases following TBI or other brain injury may well provide for enhanced neuroprotection, metabolic and physiologic functioning of residual structures, enhanced synaptic remodeling during learning and skill acquisition, better neuromodulatory availability and function, and, perhaps, more complete and rapid recovery of CNS capacity.

12.4.2 Gonadotroph Axis

12.4.2.1 Testosterone

It is clear that androgens alter the morphology, survival, and axonal regeneration of motor neurons. Androgen receptors are found throughout the brain; however, their distribution shows a sexual dimorphism.[99–101] Testosterone, in the free form, can cross the blood–brain barrier and influence neuronal cells.[102] Increases in neurite outgrowth in cultured neural cells have been observed.[103–105] Interestingly, neuronal steroids that are synthesized within the nervous system by neurons and glial cells appear to exert neurotrophic action, with some showing an anticonvulsant effect.[106–108]

Testosterone may exert protection against neurodegeneration by prevention of tau protein hyperphosphorylation. Tau proteins are predominantly axonal microtubule or binding proteins that stabilize the neuronal skeleton.[109] Amyloid-β formation may be prevented by decreases in amyloid-β peptides after treatment with testosterone.[110] Increased plasma amyloid-β levels have been reported with androgen deprivation,[111] and reduced amyloid-β-mediated apoptosis has been reported.[112] Testosterone increases expression of nerve growth factor, and mediates neurite growth and interneural communication via branching and arborization.[113,114] Testosterone is acted upon by the estrogen-synthesizing enzyme aromatase and is converted to estradiol. Aromatase itself plays an important role in neuroprotection,[115] and the neuroprotective benefits of androgens appear to be mediated by their conversion to estrogens.[116,117]

Testosterone increases the rate of axonal regeneration via selective alterations of the neuronal cytoskeleton in peripheral nerves.[118] Testosterone affects a synergistic stimulation of protein synthesis with the cytokine IGF-1 and others.[119]

On a more functional level, androgen precursors have been demonstrated to affect functional outcome in rats following experimental brain injury. In one study, dehydroepi-androsterone (DHEA) administered 1 week postinjury in rodents resulted in a significant improvement in tests of both physical and cognitive function in rats following experimental TBI.[120] Studies in humans have also suggested a correlation between functional status and T levels.[96,121]

There are a number of mechanisms by which this may occur, both physically and cognitively. Testosterone has been shown to enhance spatial cognition in healthy men age 60 to 75 years when testosterone levels were increased for 3 months to a level commonly found in young men.[122] Testosterone enanthate supplementation for 6 weeks improved spatial and verbal memory in healthy older men age 50 to 80 years.[123] Another study showed improved working memory following testosterone enanthate.[122] Alleviation of depression after testosterone supplementation in individuals with low testosterone levels and selective serotonin reuptake inhibitor-refractory depression has been observed, as well as improvement in verbal and spatial memory in aging men.[124–126] Interestingly, testosterone levels are significantly lower in both men and women with amyotrophic lateral sclerosis (ALS).[127]

12.4.2.2 Estrogen

Gender differences in outcomes following TBI has led to a number of studies investigating the impact of female steroid hormones on neuroprotection and neurogenesis following TBI.[128] Initial efforts focused on estrogen as the potential source for these differences. Estrogen has a number of properties that makes it a unique candidate for investigation into potential sources for clinical intervention following TBI. The role of estrogen in protection from oxidative stress is considerable and includes protection from serum deprivation, amyloid-β peptide-induced toxicity, glutamate-induced excitotoxicity, hydrogen peroxide, oxygen–glucose deprivation, iron, hemoglobin, and mitochondria toxins.[129–151] Estrogen's neuroprotective effects have also been demonstrated in a number of models of acute cerebral ischemia and subarachnoid hemorrhage.[152–159] Although controversial, it appears that the neuroprotective mechanisms exhibited by estrogen do not directly affect neuronal structures, but rather other cell types, such as astrocytes.[160]

Estrogens have a multitude of effects on mitochondrial function that are most notable when the cell is placed under stress. They are active in preservation of ATP production, prevention of production of ROS, moderating excessive cellular and mitochondrial Ca^{2+} loading, and preservation of mitochondrial membrane stability during stress.[29] Nonfeminizing estrogens have been found to be as effective as the potent feminizing hormone, 17 β-estradiol (E2), in prevention of mitochondrial Ca^{2+} influx,[161] and more selective neuroprotective synthetic estrogenlike compounds have been developed in response to the potential benefits of their use in treatment of neurodegenerative conditions.[32,162–165]

Ischemia-induced learning disability and neuronal loss is prevented in both sexes by estradiol.[155,166,167] At the same time, when levels of estradiol are reduced, both the function and survivability of neurons are compromised.[168,169] Early onset and increased deposition of β-amyloid peptide are associated with estrogen depletion in the brain.[170]

There are some reports that raise concern that estrogen may not be neuroprotective in all circumstances. Administration of estrogen prior to TBI was protective for males, but worsened mortality in female rats in one study.[171] Transient forebrain ischemia has been shown to worsen hippocampal neuronal loss with estrogen.[172] Overall, there is some evidence that estrogen increases neuronal excitability whereas progesterone has anticonvulsant properties.[173]

A potential area for clinical impact of estrogen may be in its apparent neuroregenerative properties. Estrogen receptors have been found to be selectively upregulated in certain areas of the brain following injury. Estrogen has important roles in modulating brain homeostasis, synaptic plasticity, cognition, and neuroprotection[174] through traditional and nontraditional cell-signaling mechanisms. Some of the receptors code for specific genetic intracellular signals responsible for neurogenesis. In particular, some of these messengers, such as c-Fos and PELP1, appear to demonstrate properties responsible for activation of genetic mechanisms responsible for cellular repair. In addition, some receptor-mediated responses may be responsible for causing stem cells to differentiate into neuroprogenitor cells.

12.4.2.3 Progesterone

Progesterone, another female steroid hormone, has been implicated in a number of mechanisms that are important for neuroprotection following CNS insult. The role of progesterone, as with others mentioned earlier, is considered here primarily for its effects on neurophysiologic function. The discussion of progesterone to follow refers to the natural hormone and its natural metabolites. Natural progestogens are metabolized in very different ways from synthetic progestogens, sometimes termed *progestins*. Technical issues pertaining to rationale for avoidance of specific progestins are reviewed by Schumacher et al.[175] Progesterone and its metabolites are effective in maintenance of neuronal viability and in regeneration of neurons. They also act on oligodendrocytes, promoting myelination in the CNS and the peripheral nervous system.[175–178] Progesterone impacts remyelination[178] despite age-related declines in capacity for myelin regeneration.[179] A sexual dimorphism exists in remyelination with middle-age female animals better able to remyelinate than male animals whereas no differences are found in younger animals.[180]

Progesterone is similar to estradiol in its protection of neurons against glucose deprivation,[181] glutamate toxicity,[182] β-amyloid peptides,[183] upregulation of brain-derived neurotrophic factor,[184] reduction of inflammation by suppression of activation of microglia,[185,186] and inhibition of cytokine production.[187] Progesterone is involved in the modulation of a number of neurotransmitter receptors, including nicotinic acetylcholine receptors,[188] and acts as a potent positive modulator of γ-aminobutyric acid A (GABA$_A$). Anesthetic, analgesic, and anxiolytic effects of progestogens may be explained by modulation of GABA$_A$.[189]

Progesterone, like several other steroids, is produced locally in the brain and is part of a group of neurosteroids, so termed because they are produced by neurons and glia *de novo* from cholesterol. The effect of progesterone varies, like GH, with the compartment of the CNS in which it is found. Its effects are mediated by estrogen priming within the hypothalamus and in some limbic structures; however, not so in the cerebral cortex, septum, caudate putamen, midbrain, or cerebellum.[190,191] In structures where estrogen priming is involved, progesterone receptors are downregulated by progesterone treatment, whereas they are unaffected in brain regions where estrogen priming is ineffective.[192,193]

Progesterone has been found to restore retrograde axonal transport,[194] which has been proposed as active in the development of Alzheimer's disease (AD).[195] Also active in the development of AD are the untoward effects of lipid peroxidation of neuronal lipids.[196]

Reduction of lipid peroxidation is achieved after TBI with progesterone treatment,[197] along with increased activity of antioxidant superoxide dismutases.[198] Mitochondrial protection by increased expression of antiapoptotic proteins in the outer mitochondrial membrane has been demonstrated associated with both progesterone and estrogen,[181,199] and complete reversal of alterations in mitochondrial respiration has been attributed to progesterone in a low physiologic range in female animals.[200]

Animal studies show progesterone reduces edema and secondary neuronal losses after TBI and promotes more complete recovery of function after TBI.[201,202] Neurons that are particularly susceptible to injury during cerebral ischemia benefit from progesterone,[203,204] and infarct size has been shown to be smaller in middle cerebral artery occlusion after pre-treatment with progesterone.[205,206] When hormone administration is prolonged, behavioral recovery is more complete.[207] The timing of intervention, ranging from preinjury treatment to up to 24 hours postinjury, has been shown to be effective.[208]

Benefits have been demonstrated in one human trial. Patients treated with intravenous infusion of natural progesterone for 3 days showed a 50% reduction in mortality compared with patients treated with conventional state-of the-art treatment in the same facility.[209] Moderately injured patients treated with progesterone had better functional outcomes than nontreated patients. There was no difference observed in functional outcomes for those with severe injury, but this may have been the result, in part, of the survival of more severely injured individuals in the treatment group.[209]

12.5 Thyrotroph Axis

Thyroid hormones are the primary endocrine influence for regulation of metabolic rate. Thyrotrophic dysfunction following TBI is less common than the somatotrophic or gonad-otrophic axes in terms of frank deficiency. Subclinical hypothyroidism, however, is common in adults without brain injury, and decreased resting energy expenditure has been found in those who have abnormally high TSH levels.[210] The risk for metabolic syndrome is raised in the presence of subclinical hypothyroidism.[211] Thyroid hormones have a substantial impact upon mitochondrial function,[212] are involved in mitochondrial biogenesis, and enhance ATP generation.[213] The effect of thyroid hormones on mitochondrial function is both nongenomic and genomic.[212]

Thyroid hormones are readily transported from the blood to the brain. It crosses into the brain via the chord plexus and cerebrospinal fluid.[214] The active thyroid hormone 3,5,3'-triiodothyronine (T3) is locally synthesized from thyroxine (T4) by glial cells, tanycytes, and astrocytes via the action of type II deiodinase.[215] T3 is regulated by type III deiodinase to degrade both T4 and T3. Type III deiodinase is expressed by neurons.[215] Thyroid regulates gene-encoding proteins for a host of structures and substances: myelin, mitochondria, neurotrophins, cellular matrix proteins, cellular adhesion molecules, and proteins involved in intracellular signaling.[215,216]

The role of thyroid in brain development may be instructive to its potential role in the recovering brain. Thyroid deficiency during development impairs cytoarchitecture in the neocortex and cerebellum.[217] Changes in cortical patterns of lamination occur together with changes in dendritic morphology and axonal projections.[218,219] Cell migration, outgrowth of neuronal polarity, synaptogenesis, and myelin formation are slowed.[216] Glial cell proliferation and neuronal cell death are both increased.[216] Lastly, thyroid is also involved in microtubule assembly and polarization differences in axons and dendrites.[216]

12.6 Neuroendocrinimmunology

TBI clearly leads to increased risk for other health conditions such as psychiatric illness[220] and depression,[221] alcohol misuse,[222] chronic hypopituitarism,[52,53,56,223,224] chronic pain,[225] AD,[226–234] myocardial disease,[235] posttraumatic epilepsy,[236–240] heterotopic ossification,[241] hydrocephalus,[242] hypoadrenalism,[243,244] hypothyroidism,[245] hypogonadism,[246] impotence,[247] osteoporosis,[246] hyponatremia,[248] sleep disorders,[249] obesity,[62] substance abuse,[250] and a host of other conditions.

Between 1975 and 1986, Besedovsky et al.[251–253] began to investigate the interactions between nervous, endocrine, and immunologic systems, including the relationship among immune system evocation of noradrenergic neuronal changes, mediation of immunoregulation by the sympathetic nervous system, and immunoregulatory feedback between interleukin 1 (IL-1) and glucocorticoid hormones. Since then, the sciences of neuroendocrinimmunology, neuroimmunomodulation, and psychoneuroimmunology have emerged, focusing on the investigation and study of bidirectional intercommunication links between the nervous, endocrine, and immunologic systems.[254,255] Interaction between the CNS, endocrine, and immune systems and TBI can all result in perturbations of cytokine production. These perturbations may result, in turn, in many health conditions promoted by proinflammatory cytokine expressions. Examples include cardiovascular disease, type 2 diabetes, and inflammatory bowel disease.

The immune and endocrine systems have been more recently conceptualized partly as "sensory" systems that are exquisitely interrelated and interdependent to the extent that changes in one system result in changes in the other.[256] These systems continuously interact to regulate a number of other diverse physiologic processes in a bidirectional fashion also mediated by the secretion and action of cytokines and hormones.[257–259] The CNS modulates immune system function via the autonomic nervous system and neuroendocrine pathways. Immune function is altered by neurotransmitters and hormones produced and released along these pathways. Interaction between the CNS and the immune system is necessary to maintain homeostasis, ensuring the proper turning on and off of the immune system.

Neurotransmitters involved in immune system modulation include acetylcholine, norepinephrine, vasoactive intestinal peptide, substance P, and histamine.[260] Hormones include corticotrophin-releasing hormone, leptin, and alpha-melanocyte-stimulating hormone[260]; prolactin, growth hormone, IGF-1, thyroid-stimulating hormone, and glucocorticoids[256,261]; and other steroid hormones such as androgens, estrogens, mineralocorticoids, and progestins.[262] Lymphocytes are also known to synthesize multiple hormones, including adrenocorticotropic hormone (ACTH), prolactin, and growth hormone.[255]

Cytokines can be anti-inflammatory or proinflammatory. Proinflammatory cytokines can act as a negative regulatory feedback tempering the action of hormones and growth factors within the CNS. Dysregulation of this homeostatic process can result in comorbid conditions associated with chronic inflammatory disease such as type 2 diabetes, cardiovascular disease, inflammatory bowel disease, rheumatoid arthritis, and major depression.[256] IGF-1 regulation can be achieved also by the actions of proinflammatory cytokines such as tumor necrosis factor (TNF) and IL-1.[256] TNF regulates immune cells, can induce apoptosis and inflammation, and can inhibit tumorigenesis and viral replication. IL-1 actually is a group of cytokines: IL-1α, IL-1β, and IL-1RA.[263] IL-1α and IL-1β are proinflammatory and are involved in immune system activation against infection. They are produced by macrophages, monocytes, and dendritic cells. Although IL-1 is involved in the pathogenesis of many diseases, in smaller amounts it assists in healing and infection.

Cytokines are produced along autonomic and endocrine pathways. The cytokine IL-1 influences the release of corticotrophin-releasing hormone by the hypothalamus, increasing stress hormone levels and suppressing immune function.[264] IL-1 and TNF-α signal neuroendocrine, autonomic, and limbic and cortical regions of the CNS impacting neural activity and modifying behaviors. These behaviors include sleep and directly impact social behavior, mood, activity, cognition, and pain.[265] Disordered sleep following TBI also has the potential to complicate neuroendocrine dysfunction even more.

To complicate matters further, many neuroendocrine anomalies result in sleep disturbances, creating a cyclical problem with vast neuroimmunomodulatory implications. Hormones regulate a wide variety of immune functions, and cytokines arising from immune system response in turn affect the neuroendocrine system. These hormones include prolactin, GH, IGF-1, and thyroid-stimulating hormone, at the very minimum.

Microglia in the CNS play an important role in neural inflammation following brain injury.[266] Microglia are distributed around and migrate within the CNS, analyzing for damaged neurons, plaques, and infectious agents.[267] Microglia are derived from monocytes that are produced in the bone marrow during hematopoiesis. Microglial proliferation increases in response to brain injury.[268] Streit[269,270] suggests that microglia may play an important role in neuronal function, providing endogenous CNS immune function when microglial cells themselves are viable and fully functional. Increased microglial apoptosis and dystrophy are seen in aged brain and in AD. Microglial cells appear to become senescent with age and therefore unable to provide endogenous CNS immune support.[266,271]

The use of embryonic stem cell transplants has provided an opportunity to understand some additional dynamics of neurocellular repair. Embryonic stem cells of hematopoietic origin, specifically human umbilical cord blood cells (HUCB), have been used extensively to treat various nonmalignant, malignant, and hematopoietic diseases in children.[272,273] There is some suggestion that the actual cell replacement itself is not the responsible mechanism for functional improvements.[274–277] Instead, HUCB cells release certain chemokines, trophic factors, or possibly, cytokines that aid in repair and recovery. Newman et al.[278] found elevations of IL-8, monocyte chemoattractant protein 1 (MCP-1), and IL-1α in cultured HUCB. IL-8, a chemokine, is a strong chemoattractant for neutrophils and lymphocytes, causing activation of motile apparatus, directional migration, increases in surface adhesion molecules, lysosomal enzyme release, and production of reactive oxygen intermediates.[161] IL-8 is elevated in the sera of humans following multiple sclerosis, TBI, and ischemic stroke.[279–281] In addition, TNF-α and IL-1 have been implicated in stimulating release of IL-8 and MCP-1.[282–284] MCP-1, a beta-chemokine, is a strong chemoattractant for monocytes in the brain, especially after disease onset or injury as part of the inflammatory response.[285]

IL-1 is derived from microglia, is involved in activation of astrocytes, and promotes increased expression of astrocyte-derived apolipoprotein E 4 allele (APOE-4).[286,287] Both APP and IL-1 expression are upregulated following TBI, likely contributing to the increased production of β-amyloid plaques within hours of injury[288–291] and resulting in increased processing of APP.[292] A main hypothesis of the etiology of AD is based upon "the neurotoxic effects of amyloid β leading to disruption of calcium homeostasis, energy failure, induction of oxidative stress, mitochondrial and, consequently, synaptic dysfunction, and hyperphosphorylation of tau protein."[293, p. 669] Mitochondrial dysfunction may also contribute to the pathogenesis of AD as a result of impairment of mitochondrial oxidative phosphorylation.[293,294]

The brain accounts for nearly 20% of the total body cholesterol.[295] Repair and maintenance of myelin by oligodendrocytes within the brain represents the highest use of energy in the uninjured brain, and most of the cholesterol in the brain is found within myelin, with the balance found in neurons, glial cells, or extracellular lipoproteins.[296] The brain synthesizes the majority of the cholesterol in the brain *de novo*,[297] with very little of the cholesterol present outside the brain passing the blood–brain barrier. Cholesterol is important for lipid organization and for neurosteroid biosynthesis.[298] Cholesterol may affect APP processing and function, thereby impacting APOE expression.[299] APOE participates in the redistribution of cholesterol within the brain, which usually occurs as a result of axonal/synaptic remodeling, although this can also occur as a result of insult or disease.[299] APOE is involved in the redistribution of cholesterol from cells during membrane synthesis, neuritic growth extension, and branching.[300–302] APOE is also involved in maintenance of vascular integrity.

IGF-1 is produced primarily by the liver as an endocrine hormone. Its production is stimulated by GH. More important, GHD is one of the more frequently occurring posttraumatic endocrine disorders.[54,246,303] Malnutrition, GH insensitivity, lack of GH receptors, or underproduction of GH can result in lowered IGF-1. IGF-1 levels are also affected by exercise status, stress levels, body mass index, nutritional status, estrogen status, and xenobiotic intake. IGF-1 is crucial for a number of vital physiologic processes, including myogenesis, cell proliferation, cholesterol production within the CNS, and mitochondrial function, at least. IGFs also promote cellular proliferation, differentiation and nutrient transport, energy storage, gene transcription, and protein synthesis.[304]

Proinflammatory cytokine-induced hormone resistance has been recently implicated in a number of hormone systems including glucocorticoids, GH, and IGF-1.[305–308] Proinflammatory cytokines are known to suppress apoptosis in a variety of cancer cells,[309,310] induce skeletal muscle wasting,[311] and induce CNS changes resulting in behavioral and motivational problems, such as sickness and depression.[312,313] Common to all is IGF-1 resistance induced by proinflammatory cytokines.

Increasingly, as we consider interventions in acute, postacute, and chronic phases of the disease of brain injury, the interface between immune, endocrine, and neurologic functions will be important. The characterization of disease processes following TBI and the approaches taken to prevent, ameliorate, or cure this disease will need to consider carefully the interactions of these systems.

Of course, these issues point to the need for continued health surveillance for people with acquired brain injury. It is apparent that a number of processes are altered that, in turn, place the body's immune response at jeopardy or put processes into play that may, in some individuals, place the individual at greater risk for certain health conditions. Potentially, these include diseases arising from proinflammatory cytokine upregulation such as diabetes, cardiovascular disease, inflammatory bowel disease, and major depression.

Alterations of the endocrine system, apart from the interrelated imposition on immune function, may result in a host of neuroendocrine-related disease states arising from posttraumatic hypopituitarism that require identification and treatment. Clearly, the TBI population is not a homogenous one, and clinical and research investigations need to elucidate further the differences within the population that culminate in greater or lesser likelihood of the development of specific disease states. Add genetic predisposition such as APOE-4 expression or other familial disease connections to this mix and it may be possible to create better predictive models for the development and/or mitigation of certain diseases following TBI.

12.7 Treatment Implications

12.7.1 Theoretical Antioxidant Options

The body's natural defenses provide clues to potential augmentative measures. Substances identified as neuroprotective include estrogen, progesterone, alpha-tocopherol (vitamin E), antioxidants, and free radical scavengers.

Beneficial effects of antioxidants as neuroprotective for hypoxia–ischemia have been demonstrated in studies in which animals were fed diets rich in polyphenols.[314–318] Anthocyanins—dietary polyphenols found in blueberries, strawberries, raspberries, and cranberries—decrease platelet aggregation,[316,319–321] reduce the release of inflammatory mediators, and inhibit oxidation of low-density lipoprotein and normal blood lipid profiles in humans. Another polyphenol, commonly known as *resveratrol*, inhibits platelet aggregation, promotes vasodilation, exerts antiatherosclerotic effects,[322] and has been shown to have neuroprotective effects against ischemia/reperfusion.[323–325] Polyphenols like resveratrol have been observed in rats to attenuate age-related cognitive and motor decline, reduce cognitive deficits in a mouse model of AD, protect against β-amyloid in oxidative stress in neurons, and preserve cellular energy associated with formation of *de novo* mitochondria.[326–328]

Two potential mechanisms for the beneficial effects of antioxidants are upregulation of endogenous antioxidant systems and induction of heme oxidase in the brain. Resveratrol, curcumin, caffeic acid, phenethyl ester, and ethyl ferulate[329,330] induce heme oxidase, thus exerting a direct effect on neuronal genes, preconditioning those neurons to withstand hypoxia better.

Slemmer et al.[331] articulate a number of strategies directed at reducing age-related increases in brain oxidative damage. These strategies include utilization of vitamin E, curcumin, and nonsteroidal anti-inflammatory drugs including indomethacin and ibuprofen. These authors also include resveratrol-rich diets.

Vitamin E has been demonstrated to preserve learning and memory with chronic administration and to enhance long-term potentiation in rats.[332,333] Cognitive function in humans is also positively correlated with plasma levels of vitamin E,[334] and improvements in cognitive function have been associated with diets rich in vitamin E.[335] Vitamin E increases rapid, nonsustained proliferation of microglia in rat cultures.[336] Pharmacokinetics of vitamin E are altered significantly by cigarette smoking whereas absorption is enhanced with a high-fat versus low-fat diet.[337–339]

Nonsteroidal anti-inflammatory drugs have been suggested to improve AD.[340] Microglial activation is reduced in correlation with nonsteroidal anti-inflammatory treatment.[341,342] Reduced chronic microglial activation may result in a decrease in oxidative damage.[343] Oxidized proteins and β-amyloid plaques have been observed to be reduced in association with curcumin along with enhanced antioxidant activity in rats.[342,344]

Diets rich in omega-3 polyunsaturated fatty acids are associated with less age-related cognitive decline, perhaps because these diets are less susceptible to oxidative damage.[345,346]

It has been difficult to demonstrate the beneficial effects of antioxidant treatment of ischemic stroke in humans despite very promising results in animals. This may result, in part, from high levels of endogenous antioxidants in humans compared with other mammalian species,[347] making it difficult for researchers to reach substantially higher levels of antioxidant presence. Another explanation may be antioxidants are prone to oxidation, diminished shelf life, and degradation.[331] Some disappointing results have been encountered with application of antioxidant therapy for TBI. Additional explanations offered include that perhaps the mechanical damage is so substantial following TBI, that it becomes difficult to elucidate the subtle, but perhaps very relevant, neuropsychological and cognitive improvements that may be achieved.

What remains to be seen is whether antioxidants can exert a beneficial impact effectively mitigating damage caused by oxidative stress in an altered CNS following brain injury from other etiologies. It is also interesting to consider whether long-term antioxidant therapies that extend neuroprotection are effective in minimizing antioxidant change in residual neurologic structures that are recruited to assume new suprahysiologic functional states required by new demands for synaptic remodeling necessary for cortical reorganization. Perhaps antioxidant therapies, in combination with other bioenergetic strategies, may be found to be beneficial in recovery after brain injury.

12.7.2 Theoretical Combination Therapies

The array of neurophysiologic complications encountered by residual neurologic structures following brain injury is impressive. At the very least, changes occur in myelination and remyelination; synaptic remodeling; synaptic transmission; neurotransmitter synthesis, release, reuptake, and deactivation; axonal transport; neurotransmitter receptor function; glial support; immune system actions; and bioenergetic function.

Figure 12.2 depicts a summary of events reviewed in the preceding text that represents challenges in the bioenergetic cycle and may result in bioenergetic failure. Many may constitute potential therapeutic targets. Although perhaps all of these could be addressed in

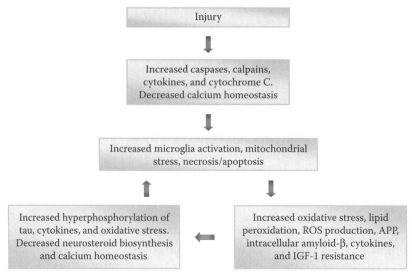

FIGURE 12.2
Summary of neurodegenerative events.

time, many are accessible today with tools and interventions that can be designed and implemented.

Available long-term interventions for TBI, thus far, have been exceptionally limited. Perhaps a paradigmatic shift in how brain function after injury is viewed is in order. Is it possible that the upregulation of trophic factor expression and immune system activation immediately following injury is intended to assist with preservation and/or recovery of function? What can be done to extend the period of time during which upregulation of trophic factors occurs? As the brain accommodates to injury over time, does the metabolic milieu of the brain change in favor of support for active neural networks and away from inactive or less active networks? Does the brain simply respond to environmental demand in its newly kindled state of synaptic remodeling immediately following injury, and then settle into a new normative state in which synaptic remodeling continues to occur but at a slower pace? Do the bioenergetic dysfunctions result in an earlier senescence of neurologic structures and, if so, can early cellular senescence be reversed? Do the bioenergetic changes that occur following injury slowly stabilize, or do they remain jeopardized or marginalized by the tension between bioenergetic demands, and the resultant consequences of toxic metabolic oxidative physiologies and immune system activation?

The clinical opportunity is to attempt to influence these substrates with available interventions. Obvious opportunities can be found addressing oxidative stress; ROS production; inflammatory response; hormonal insufficiencies, deficiencies, and imbalances; and neurotransmitter bioavailability and receptor function. We have numerous examples in medical management of TBI with success that likely stems from their impact at this level. Careful evaluation of the extent to which medical and therapeutic interventions likely impact one or more of these areas (i.e., oxidative stress; ROS production; inflammatory response; hormonal insufficiencies, deficiencies, and imbalances; and neurotransmitter bioavailability and receptor function) may lead to better bioenergetic function and support for organelle biogenesis, neurogenesis, synaptogenesis, angiogenesis and gliogenesis, and ultimately, support for protracted and more complete recovery of function.

Care must always be taken as one considers manipulation or titration of these functions. Although few would argue with the likely beneficial effects of antioxidant support to address oxidative stress and ROS production, there is evidence that a minimal ROS production is necessary to promote adequate thyroid hormone function.[348] Concern is ever present, although often exaggerated (particularly in the context of risk/benefit ratios in these patients) about tumorigenesis associated with GH treatment or estrogen replacement therapies. Progesterone, in its natural form, is quite safe and very effective in many of the desired targeted areas.[175] Application of dopaminergic, serotonergic, and cholinergic medications is fairly common in TBI; however, can we use these with a different mindset as we consider targeting facets of the bioenergetic cycle? Will we advocate the continuation of enriched and hierarchically organized environmental demand such as that found in intense rehabilitation therapies for longer durations? Will we view this as an integral method for sustaining trophic factor upregulation? Will we target, and successfully improve, the bioenergetic processes of residual neurologic structures as they recover from the initial and secondary anatomic and physiologic disruptions of injury? Can we slow or stop the metabolic neurodegenerative cascade and normalize bioenergetic production? Will or should interventions be limited by consequences of increasing metabolic rate and associated oxidative processes by regimens designed to impose a maximal rate of reacquisition of function? How will we safely promote support for new epigenetic, morphologic, and functional changes in surviving neurons and glia? From everything that neuroscience has learned about plasticity in the CNS, we should combine environmental demand with these metabolically targeted interventions, and we should expect enhanced rate and extent of recovery as a result.

So what does the cure look like? Perhaps the cure includes titration of neuroendocrine levels, paying particular attention to GH, neurosteroids, IGF-1, and thyroid hormones.[349,350] Perhaps it includes dietary management of nutriceuticals such as antioxidants, vitamin E, curcumin, polyphenols, and flavonoids.[331] Perhaps it looks like provision of supports like vitamin B complex, alpha lipoic acid, and acetyl-L-carnitine.[351,352] Perhaps it involves discriminant application or manipulation of levels of neurotransmitters such as dopamine, serotonin, acetylcholine, or GABA. It may include incorporation of physical exercise as a means of enriching IGF-1 availability and improving neurotrophic factor expression in the hippocampus. It may involve looking at fatigue, sleep disorders, depression, hypercholesteremia, and others as symptoms of bioenergetic and/or neuroendocrine failure rather than as the diagnosis. It may be steeped in lessons gleaned from these same factors in the maturing brain. It may be that the individuality of brain injury suggests an individualized assessment of the previously mentioned options and a tailored combination applied to each patient and monitored for requisite modification as the residual neurophysiology adopts and provides for new functional response and ultimately returns to a truly normal bioenergetic state.

But whatever it looks like, it likely should embrace neuroendocrinimmunology, and it should be very different from the approach currently underway that is steeped in ever-shortening rehabilitation treatment and reactive medical and sociologic management of overt complications of the disease of brain injury.

This chapter is intended to provoke thinking that will, at some point, bridge the gap between the worlds of basic neuroscience laboratory research and clinical rehabilitation. The hope is that, ultimately, success in doing so will effectuate significant differences in the treatment paradigm for TBI and, subsequently, make enormous differences in the lives of people with TBI and their families.

Acknowledgment

The authors thank the Centre for Neuro Skills Clinical Research and Education Foundation (CNS-CREF) team (Jessica Ashley, PhD; Richard Helvie, MD; Lisa Kreber, PhD; Robert Lehr, PhD; and Craig Persel, BA) for their assistance in review and refinement of this manuscript.

References

1. Bergsneider, M., Hovda, D. A., Lee, S. M., Kelly, D. F., McArthur, D. L., Vespa, P. M., et al., Dissociation of cerebral glucose metabolism and level of consciousness during the period of metabolic depression following human traumatic brain injury, *Journal of Neurotrauma*, 17(5), 389–401, 2000.
2. Thomas, E., Van Hulle, M. M., and Vogels, R., Encoding of categories by noncategory-specific neurons in the inferior temporal cortex, *Journal of Cognitive Neuroscience*, 13(2), 190, 2001.

3. Sigala, N. and Logothetis, N. K., Visual categorization shapes feature selectivity in the primate temporal cortex, *Nature*, 415(6869), 318–320, 2002.

4. Beal, M. F., Bioenergetic approaches for neuroprotection in Parkinson's disease, *Annals of Neurology*, 53(S3), S39–S48, 2003.

5. Zou, H., Henzel, W. J., Liu, X., Lutschg, A., and Wang, X., Apaf-1, a human protein homologous to *C. elegans* CED-4, participates in cytochrome c-dependent activation of caspase-3, *Cell*, 90(3), 405–413, 1997.

6. Stavrovskaya, I. G. and Kristal, B. S., The powerhouse takes control of the cell: Is the mitochondrial permeability transition a viable therapeutic target against neuronal dysfunction and death?, *Free Radical Biology and Medicine*, 38(6), 687–697, 2005.

7. Katz, D. I. and Alexander, M. P., Traumatic brain injury: Predicting course of recovery and outcome for patients admitted to rehabilitation, *Archives of Neurology*, 51(7), 661–670, 1994.

8. Meythaler, J. M., Peduzzi, J. D., Eleftheriou, E., and Novack, T. A., Current concepts: Diffuse axonal injury-associated traumatic brain injury, *Archives of Physical Medicine and Rehabilitation*, 82(10), 1461–1471, 2001.

9. Graham, D. I., Adams, J. H., and Genneralli, T. A., Pathology of brain damage in head injury, in P. Cooper (Ed.), *Head Injury*, 2nd ed., Williams and Wilkins, Baltimore, MD, 72–88, 1987.

10. Povlishock, J. T. and Jenkins, L. W., Are the pathobiological changes evoked by traumatic brain injury immediate and irreversible?, *Brain Pathology*, 5(4), 415–426, 1995.

11. Povlishock, J. T., Erb, D. E., and Astruc, J., Axonal response to traumatic brain injury: Reactive axonal change, deafferentation, and neuroplasticity, *Journal of Neurotrauma*, 9(Suppl. 1), S189–S200, 1992.

12. Büki, A. and Povlishock, J. T., All roads lead to disconnection? Traumatic axonal injury revisited, *Acta Neurochirurgica*, 148(2), 181–194, 2006.

13. Povlishock, J. T., Pathobiology of traumatically induced axonal injury in animals and man, *Annals of Emergency Medicine*, 22(6), 980–986, 1993.

14. Hollenbeck, P. J. The pattern and mechanism of mitochondrial transport in axons, *Frontiers in Bioscience*, 1(1), 91–102, 1996.

15. Miller, K. E. and Sheetz, M. P., Axonal mitochondrial transport and potential are correlated, *Journal of Cell Science*, 117(Pt 13), 2791–2804, 2004.

16. Ly, C. V. and Verstreken, P., Mitochondria at the synapse (Neuroscience Update), *The Neuroscientist*, 12(4), 291–299, 2006.

17. Li, Z., Okamoto, K.- I., Hayashi, Y., and Sheng, M., The importance of dendritic mitochondria in the morphogenesis and plasticity of spines and synapses, *Cell*, 119(6), 873–887, 2004.

18. Maxwell, W. L., Povlishock, J. T., and Graham, D. L., A mechanistic analysis of nondisruptive axonal injury: A review, *Journal of Neurotrauma*, 14(7), 419–440, 1997.

19. Slemmon, J. R. and Flood, D. G., Profiling of endogenous brain peptides and small proteins: Methodology, computer-assisted analysis, and application to aging and lesion models, *Neurobiology of Aging*, 13(6), 649–660, 1992.

20. Jiang, M. H., Hoog, A., Ma, K. C., Nie, X. J., Olsson, Y., and Zhang, W. W., Endothelin-1-like immunoreactivity is expressed in human reactive astrocytes, *Neuroreport*, 4(7), 935–937, 1993.

21. Zhang, P., Hirsch, E. C., Damier, P., Duyckaerts, C., and Javoy-Agid, F., C-fos protein-like immunoreactivity: Distribution in the human brain and over-expression in the hippocampus of patients with Alzheimer's disease, *Neuroscience*, 46(1), 9–21, 1992.

22. Roberts, G. W., Gentleman, S. M., Lynch, A., Murray, L., Landon, M., and Graham, D. I., Beta amyloid protein deposition in the brain after severe head injury: Implications for the pathogenesis of Alzheimer's disease, *Journal of Neurology, Neurosurgery, and Psychiatry*, 57(4), 419–425, 1994.

23. Dale, G. E., Leigh, P. N., Luthert, P., Anderton, B. H., and Roberts, G. W., Neurofibrillary tangles in dementia pugilistica are ubiquitinated, *Journal of Neurology, Neurosurgery, and Psychiatry*, 54(2), 116–118, 1991.

24. McLellan, D. R., The structural bases of coma and recovery: Insights from brain injury in humans and experimental animals, in M. E. Sandel and D. W. Ellis (Eds.), *The Coma-Emerging Patient*, Hanley & Belfus, Philadelphia, 389–407, 1990.

25. Adams, C. W. and Bruton, C. J., The cerebral vasculature in dementia pugilistica, *Journal of Neurology, Neurosurgery, and Psychiatry*, 52(5), 600–604, 1989.
26. Dyall, S. D., Brown, M. T., and Johnson, P. J., Ancient invasions: From endosymbionts to organelles, *Science*, 304(5668), 253–257, 2004.
27. Karbowki, M. and Youle, R. J., Dynamics of mitochondrial morphology in healthy cells and during apoptosis, *Cellular Death and Differentiation*, 10(8), 870–878, 2003.
28. Yaffe, M. P., The machinery of mitochondrial inheritance and behavior (cover story), *Science*, 283(5407), 1493, 1999.
29. Simpkins, J. W. and Dykens, J. A., Mitochondrial mechanisms of estrogen neuroprotection, *Brain Research Reviews*, 57(2), 421–430, 2008.
30. Kroemer, G. and Reed, J. C., Mitochondrial control of cell death, *Nature Medicine*, 6(5), 513–519, 2000.
31. Dykens, J. A., Mitochondrial free radical production and the etiology of neurodegenerative disease, in M. F. Beal, I. Bodis-Wollner, and N. Howell (Eds.), *Neurodegenerative Diseases: Mitochondria and Free Radicals in Pathogenesis*, Wiley, Hoboken, NJ, 29–55, 1997.
32. Green, D. R. and Kroemer, G., The pathophysiology of mitochondrial cell death, *Science*, 305(5684), 626–629, 2004.
33. Adams, I. and Jones, D. G., Quantitative ultrastructural changes in rat cortical synapses during early-, mid- and late-adulthood, *Brain Research*, 239, 349–363, 1982.
34. Cameron, H. A., Kaliszewski, C. K., and Greer, C. A., Organization of mitochondria in olfactory bulb granule cell dendritic spines, *Synapse*, 8(2), 107–118, 1991.
35. Chicurel, M. E. and Harris, K. M., Three-dimensional analysis of the structure and composition of CA3 branched dendritic spines and their synaptic relationships with mossy fiber boutons in the rat hippocampus, *The Journal of Comparative Neurology*, 325(2), 169–182, 1992.
36. Cash, A. D., Perry, G., Ogawa, O., Raina, A. K., Zhu, X., and Smith, M. A., Is Alzheimer's disease a mitochondrial disorder?, *Neuroscientist*, 8(5), 489–496, 2002.
37. Swerdlow, R. H., Mitochondrial DNA-related mitochondrial dysfunction in neurodegenerative diseases, *Archives of Pathology and Laboratory Medicine*, 126(3), 271–280, 2002.
38. Murphy, V. N. and De Camilli, P., Cell biology of the presynaptic terminal, *Annual Review of Neuroscience*, 26, 701–728, 2003.
39. Morris, R. L. and Hollenbeck, P. J., The regulation of bidirectional mitochondrial transport is coordinated with axonal outgrowth, *The Journal of Cell Science*, 104(Pt 3), 917–927, 1993.
40. Overly, C. C., Rieff, H. I., and Hollenbeck, P. J., Organelle motility and metabolism in axons vs. dendrites of cultured hippocampal neurons, *Journal of Cell Science (Cambridge)*, 109(5), 971–980, 1996.
41. Rintoul, G. L., Filiano, A. J., Brocard, J. B., Kress, G. J., and Reynolds, I. J., Glutamate decreases mitochondrial size and movement in primary forebrain neurons, *Journal of Neuroscience*, 23(21), 7881–7888, 2003.
42. Finsterer, J., Mitochondriopathies, *European Journal of Neurology*, 11(3), 163–186, 2004.
43. Lemasters, J. J., Qian, T., Bradham, C. A., Brenner, D. A., Cascio, W. E., Trost, L. C., et al., Mitochondrial dysfunction in the pathogenesis of necrotic and apoptotic cell death, *Journal of Bioenergetics and Biomembranes*, 31(4), 305–319, 1999.
44. Finsterer, J., Central nervous system manifestations of mitochondrial disorders, *Acta Neurologica Scandinavica*, 114(4), 217–238, 2006.
45. Betts, J., Lightowlers, R. N., and Turnbull, D. M., Neuropathological aspects of mitochondrial DNA disease, *Neurochemical Research*, 29(3), 505–511, 2004.
46. Gabuzda, D., Busciglio, J., Chen, L. B., Matsudaira, P., and Yankner, B. A., Inhibition of energy metabolism alters the processing of amyloid precursor protein and induces a potentially amyloidogenic derivative, *Journal of Biological Chemistry*, 269(18), 13623–13628, 1994.
47. Drake, J., Link, C. D., and Butterfield, D. A., Oxidative stress precedes fibrillar deposition of Alzheimer's disease amyloid [beta]-peptide (1-42) in a transgenic *Caenorhabditis elegans* model, *Neurobiology of Aging*, 24(3), 415–420, 2003.
48. Muller, W. E., Kirsch, C., and Eckert, G. P., Membrane-disordering effects of beta-amyloid peptides, *Biochemical Society Transactions*, 29(Pt 4), 617–623, 2001.

49. Casley, C. S., Canevari, L., Land, J. M., Clark, J. B., and Sharpe, M. A., Beta-amyloid inhibits integrated mitochondrial respiration and key enzyme activities, *Journal of Neurochemistry*, 80(1), 91–100, 2002.
50. Canevari, L., Abramov, A. Y., and Duchen, M. R., Toxicity of amyloid beta peptide: Tales of calcium, mitochondria and oxidative stress, *Neurochemical Research*, 29(3), 637–650, 2004.
51. Busciglio, J., Pelsman, A., Wong, C., Pigino, G., Yuan, M., Mori, H., et al., Altered metabolism of the amyloid beta precursor protein is associated with mitochondrial dysfunction in Down's syndrome, *Neuron*, 33(5), 677–688, 2002.
52. Kelly, D. F. G., Cohan, P., Berman, N., Swerdloff, R., and Wang, C., Hypopituitarism following traumatic brain injury and aneurysmal subarachnoid hemorrhage: A preliminary report, *Journal of Neurosurgery*, 93(5), 743–752, 2000.
53. Lieberman, S. A., Oberoi, A. L., Gilkison, C. R., Masel, B. E., and Urban, R. J., Prevalence of neuroendocrine dysfunction in patients recovering from traumatic brain injury, *Journal of Clinical Endocrinology and Metabolism*, 86(6), 2752–2756, 2001.
54. Bondanelli, M., De Marinis, L., Ambrosio, M. R., Monesi, M., Valle, D., Zatelli, M. C., Fusco, A., Bianchi, A., Farneti, M., and Degli Uberti, E. C., Occurrence of pituitary dysfunction following traumatic brain injury, *Journal of Neurotrauma*, 21(6), 685–696, 2004.
55. Elovic, E., Anterior pituitary dysfunction after traumatic brain injury: Part I, *Journal of Head Trauma Rehabilitation*, 18(6), 541–543, 2003.
56. Schneider, H. J., Kreitschmann-Andermahr, I., Ghigo, E., Stalla, G. K., and Agha, A., Hypothalamopituitary dysfunction following traumatic brain injury and aneurysmal subarachnoid hemorrhage: A systematic review, *Journal of the American Medical Association*, 298(12), 1429–1438, 2007.
57. Agha, A., Rogers, B., Mylotte, D., Taleb, F., Tormey, W., Phillips, J., et al., Neuroendocrine dysfunction in the acute phase of traumatic brain injury, *Clinical Endocrinology*, 60(5), 584–591, 2004.
58. Agha, A., Phillips, J., O'Kelly, P., Tormey, W., and Thompson, C. J., The natural history of posttraumatic hypopituitarism: Implications for assessment and treatment, *The American Journal of Medicine*, 118(12), 1416.e1–1416.e7, 2005.
59. Aimaretti, G., Ambrosio, M. R., Di Somma, C., Gasperi, M., Cannavo, S., Scaroni, C., et al., Residual pituitary function after brain injury-induced hypopituitarism: A prospective 12-month study, *Journal of Clinical Endocrinology and Metabolism*, 90(11), 6085–6092, 2005.
60. Aimaretti, G., Ambrosio, M. R., Benvenga, S., Borretta, G., De Marinis, L., De Menis, E., et al., Hypopituitarism and growth hormone deficiency (GHD) after traumatic brain injury (TBI), *Growth Hormone & IGF Research*, 14(Suppl. 1), 114–117, 2004.
61. Leal-Cerro, A., Flores, J. M., Rincon, M., Murillo, F., Pujol, M., Garcia-Pesquera, F., et al., Prevalence of hypopituitarism and growth hormone deficiency in adults long-term after severe traumatic brain injury, *Clinical Endocrinology*, 62(5), 525–532, 2005.
62. Popovic, V., GH deficiency as the most common pituitary defect after TBI: Clinical implications, *Pituitary*, 8(3–4), 239–243, 2005.
63. Ghigo, E., Masel, B., Aimaretti, G., Leon-Carrion, J., Casaneuva, F. F., Dominquez-Morlaes, M. R. R., Elovic, E., et al., Consensus guidelines on screening for hypopituitarism following traumatic brain injury, *Brain Injury*, 19(9), 711–724, 2005.
64. Benvenga, S., Campenni, A., Ruggeri, R. M., and Trimarchi, F., Hypopituitarism secondary to head trauma, *Journal of Clinical Endocrinology and Metabolism*, 85(4), 1353–1361, 2000.
65. Aberg, N. D., Brywe, K. G., and Isgaard, J., Aspects of growth hormone and insulin-like growth factor-I related to neuroprotection, regeneration, and functional plasticity in the adult brain, *The Scientific World Journal*, 6(1), 53–80, 2006.
66. Aberg, N. D., Aberg, M. A. I., and Eriksson, P. S., Growth hormone and insulin-like growth factor I and cellular regeneration in the adult brain, in F. Nyberg (Ed.), *The Somatotrophic Axis in Brain Function*, Elsevier, San Diego, CA, 121–141, 2005.
67. Diamond, M. C., The effects of early hypophysectomy and hormone therapy on brain development, *Brain Research*, 7(3), 407–418, 1968.

68. Ransome, M. I., Goldshmit, Y., Bartlett, P. F., Waters, M. J., and Turnley, A. M., Comparative analysis of CNS populations in knockout mice with altered growth hormone responsiveness, *European Journal of Neuroscience*, 19(8), 2069–2079, 2004.

69. Kakizawa, S., Yamada, K., Iino, M., Watanabe, M., and Kano, M., Effects of insulin-like growth factor I on climbing fibre synapse elimination during cerebellar development, *European Journal of Neuroscience*, 17(3), 545–554, 2003.

70. Nieto-Bona, M. P., Garcia Segura, L. M., and Torres Aleman, I., Transsynaptic modulation by insulin-like growth factor I of dendritic spines in Purkinje cells, *International Journal of Developmental Neuroscience*, 15(6), 749–754, 1997.

71. Noguchi, T. and Sugisaki, T., Abnormal neuronal growth in the little (lit) cerebrum, *Experimental Neurology*, 89(1), 274–278, 1985.

72. Niblock, M. M., Brunso-Bechtold, J. K., and Riddle, D. R., Insulin-like growth factor I stimulates dendritic growth in primary somatosensory cortex, *Journal of Neuroscience*, 20(11), 4165–4176, 2000.

73. Cheng, C. M., Mervis, R. F., Niu, S. L., Salem, Jr., N., Witters, L. A., Tseng, V., et al., Insulin-like growth factor I is essential for normal dendritic growth, *Journal of Neuroscience Research*, 73(1), 1–9, 2003.

74. Aberg, M. A. I., Aberg, N. D., Hedbacker, H., Oscarsson, J., and Eriksson, P. S., Peripheral infusion of IGF-I selectively induces neurogenesis in the adult rat hippocampus, *Journal of Neuroscience*, 20(8), 2896–2903, 2000.

75. Lopez-Lopez, C., LeRoith, D., and Torres-Aleman, I., Insulin-like growth factor I is required for vessel remodeling in the adult brain, *Proceedings of the National Academy of Sciences of the United States of America*, 101(26), 9833–9838, 2004.

76. Trejo, J. L., Carro, E., and Torres-Aleman, I., Circulating insulin-like growth factor I mediates exercise-induced increases in the number of new neurons in the adult hippocampus, *Journal of Neuroscience*, 21(5), 1628–1634, 2001.

77. Fordyce, D. E. and Wehner, J. M., Physical activity enhances spatial learning performance with an associated alteration in hippocampal protein kinase C activity in C57BL/6 and DBA/2 mice, *Brain Research*, 619(1–2), 111–119, 1993.

78. Kramer, A. F., Hahn, S., Cohen, N. J., Banich, M. T., McAuley, E., Harrison, C. R., et al., Ageing, fitness and neurocognitive function, *Nature*, 400(6743), 418–419, 1999.

79. Grealy, M. A., Johnson, D. A., and Rushton, S. K., Improving cognitive function after brain injury: The use of exercise and virtual reality, *Archives of Physical Medicine and Rehabilitation*, 80(6), 661–667, 1999.

80. Laurin, D., Verreault, R., Lindsay, J., MacPherson, K., and Rockwood, K., Physical activity and risk of cognitive impairment and dementia in elderly persons, *Archives of Neurology*, 58(3), 498–504, 2001.

81. Gomez-Pinilla, F., Ying, Z., Roy, R. R., Molteni, R., and Edgerton, V. R., Voluntary exercise induces a BDNF-mediated mechanism that promotes neuroplasticity, *Journal of Neurophysiology*, 88(5), 2187–2195, 2002.

82. Ding, Q., Vaynman, S., Akhavan, M., Ying, Z., and Gomez-Pinilla, F., Insulin-like growth factor I interfaces with brain-derived neurotrophic factor-mediated synaptic plasticity to modulate aspects of exercise-induced cognitive function, *Neuroscience*, 140(3), 823–833, 2006.

83. Nørrelund, H., Riis, A. L., and Møller, N., Effects of GH on protein metabolism during dietary restriction in man, *Growth Hormone & IGF Research*, 12(4), 198–207, 2002.

84. Rattan, S. I. S., Synthesis, modifications, and turnover of proteins during aging, *Experimental Gerontology*, 31(1–2), 33–47, 1996.

85. Sonntag, W. E., Lynch, C. D., Cooney, P. T., and Hutchins, P. M., Decreases in cerebral microvasculature with age are associated with the decline in growth hormone and insulin-like-growth factor 1, *Endocrinology*, 138, 3515–3520, 1997.

86. Arwert, L. I., Veltman, D. J., Deijen, J. B., Lammertsma, A. A., Jonker, C., and Drent, M. L., Memory performance and the growth hormone/insulin-like growth factor axis in elderly: A positron emission tomography study, *Neuroendocrinology*, 81(1), 31–40, 2005.

87. Carro, E., Trejo, J. L., Busiguina, S., and Torres Aleman, I., Circulating insulin-like growth factor I mediates the protective effects of physical exercise against brain insults of different etiology and anatomy, *Journal of Neuroscience*, 21(15), 5678–5688, 2001.

88. Russo, V. C., Kobayashi, K., Najdovska, S., Baker, N. L., and Werther, G. A., Neuronal protection from glucose deprivation via modulation of glucose transport and inhibition of apoptosis: A role for the insulin-like growth factor system, *Brain Research*, 1009(1–2), 40–53, 2004.

89. Cheng, C. M., Cohen, M., Wang, J., and Bondy, C. A., Estrogen augments glucose transporter and IGF1 expression in primate cerebral cortex, *Federation of American Societies for Experimental Biology Journal*, 15(5), 907–915, 2001.

90. Lynch, C. D., Lyons, D., Khan, A., Bennett, S. A., and Sonntag, W. E., Insulin-like growth factor-1 selectively increases glucose utilization in brains of aged animals, *Endocrinology*, 142, 506–509, 2001.

91. Bondanelli, M., Ambrosio, M. R., Onofri, A., Bergonzoni, A., Lavezzi, S., Zatelli, M. C., et al., Predictive value of circulating insulin-like growth factor I levels in ischemic stroke outcome, *Journal of Clinical Endocrinology and Metabolism*, 91(10), 3928–3934, 2006.

92. Liu, X., Fawcett, J. R., Thorne, R. G., and Frey I. W. H., Non-invasive intranasal insulin-like growth factor-I reduces infarct volume and improves neurologic function in rats following middle cerebral artery occlusion, *Neuroscience Letters*, 308(2), 91–94, 2001.

93. Guan, J., Miller, O. T., Waugh, K. M., McCarthy, D. C., and Gluckman, P. D., Insulin-like growth factor-1 improves somatosensory function and reduces the extent of cortical infarction and ongoing neuronal loss after hypoxia–ischemia in rats, *Neuroscience*, 105(2), 299–306, 2001.

94. Bushnik, T., Englander, J., and Katznelson, L., Fatigue after TBI: Association with neuroendocrine abnormalities, *Brain Injury*, 21(6), 559–566, 2007.

95. Bondanelli, M., Ambrosio, M. R., Cavazzini, L., Bertocchi, A., Zatelli, M. C., Carli, A., et al., Anterior pituitary function may predict functional and cognitive outcome in patients with traumatic brain injury undergoing rehabilitation, *Journal of Neurotrauma*, 24(11), 1687–1698, 2007.

96. Carlson, N. E., Brenner, L. A., Wierman, M. E., Harrison-Felix, C., Morey, C., Gallagher, S., et al., Hypogonadism on admission to acute rehabilitation is correlated with lower functional status at admission and discharge, *Brain Injury*, 23(4), 336–344, 2009.

97. Hatton, J., Kryscio, R., Ryan, M., Ott, L., and Young, B., Systemic metabolic effects of combined insulin-like growth factor-I and growth hormone therapy in patients who have sustained acute traumatic brain injury, *Journal of Neurosurgery*, 23(6), 928–942, 2006.

98. Kelly, D. F., McArthur, D. L., Levin, H., Swimmer, S., Dusick, J. R., Cohan, P., et al., Neurobehavioral and quality of life changes associated with growth hormone insufficiency after complicated mild, moderate, or severe traumatic brain injury, *Journal of Neurotrauma*, 23(6), 928–942, 2006.

99. Belle, M. D. C. and Lea, R. W., Androgen receptor immunolocalization in brains of courting and brooding male and female ring doves (*Streptopelia risoria*), *General and Comparative Endocrinology*, 124(2), 173–187, 2001.

100. Larsson, D. G. J., Sperry, T. S., and Thomas, P., Regulation of androgen receptors in Atlantic croaker brains by testosterone and estradiol, *General and Comparative Endocrinology*, 128(3), 224–230, 2002.

101. Lu, S.- F., McKenna, S. E., Cologer-Clifford, A., Nau, E. A., and Simon, N. G., Androgen receptor in mouse brain: Sex differences and similarities in autoregulation, *Endocrinology*, 139(4), 1594–1601, 1998.

102. Iqbal, M. J., Dalton, M., and Sawers, R. S., Binding of testosterone and oestradiol to sex hormone binding globulin, human serum albumin and other plasma proteins: Evidence for nonspecific binding of oestradiol to sex hormone binding globulin, *Clinical Science* (*London*), 64(3), 307–314, 1983.

103. Lustig, R. H., Sex hormone modulation of neural development in vitro, *Hormones and Behavior*, 28(4), 383–395, 1994.

104. Beyer, C., Green, S. J., and Hutchison, J. B., Androgens influence sexual differentiation of embryonic mouse hypothalamic aromatase neurons in vitro, *Endocrinology*, 135(3), 1220–1226, 1994.

105. Beyer, C. and Hutchison, J. B., Androgens stimulate the morphological maturation of embryonic hypothalamic aromatase-immunoreactive neurons in the mouse, *Developmental Brain Research*, 98(1), 74–81, 1997.

106. Baulieu, E. E., Robel, P., and Schumacher, M., Neurosteroids: Beginning of the story, *International Review of Neurobiology*, 46, 1–32, 2001.

107. Budziszewska, B., Siwanowicz, J., Lekiewicz, M., Jaworska-Feil, L., and Laso, W., Protective effects of neurosteroids against NMDA-induced seizures and lethality in mice, *European Neuropsychopharmacology*, 8(1), 7–12, 1998.

108. Frye, C. A. and Reed, T. A.W., Androgenic neurosteroids: Anti-seizure effects in an animal model of epilepsy, *Psychoneuroendocrinology*, 23(4), 385–399, 1998.

109. Lim, D., Flicker, L., Dharamarajan, A., and Martins, R. N., Can testosterone replacement decrease the memory problem of old age? *Medical Hypotheses*, 60(6), 893–896, 2003.

110. Gouras, G. K., Xu, H., Gross, R. S., Greenfield, J. P., Hai, B., Wang, R., et al., Testosterone reduces neuronal secretion of Alzheimer's β-amyloid peptides, *Proceedings of the National Academy of Sciences of the United States of America*, 97(3), 1202–1205, 2000.

111. Almeida, O. P., Waterreus, A., Spry, N., Corica, T., Martins, G., Martins, R. N., et al., Effect of testosterone deprivation on the cognitive performance of a patient with Alzheimer's disease, *International Journal of Geriatric Psychiatry*, 16(8), 823–825, 2001.

112. Pike, C. J., Testosterone attenuates [beta]-amyloid toxicity in cultured hippocampal neurons, *Brain Research*, 919(1), 160–165, 2001.

113. Kujawa, K. A., Tanzer, L., and Jones, K. J., Inhibition of the accelerative effects of testosterone on hamster facial nerve regeneration by the antiandrogen flutamide, *Experimental Neurology*, 133(2), 138–143, 1995.

114. Tirassa, P., Thiblin, I., Ågren, G., Vigneti, E., Aloe, L., and Stenfors, C., High-dose anabolic androgenic steroids modulate concentrations of nerve growth factor and expression of its low affinity receptor (p75-NGFr) in male rat brain, *Journal of Neuroscience Research*, 47(2), 198–207, 1997.

115. Schumacher, M., Guennoun, R., Stein, D. G., and De Nicola, A. F., Progesterone: Therapeutic opportunities for neuroprotection and myelin repair, *Pharmacology & Therapeutics*, 116(1), 77–106, 2007.

116. Wozniak, A., Hutchison, R. E., Morris, C. M., and Hutchison, J. B., Neuroblastoma and Alzheimer's disease brain cells contain aromatase activity, *Steroids*, 63(5–6), 263–267, 1998.

117. Veiga, S., Garcia-Segura, L. M., and Azcoitia, I., Neuroprotection by the steroids pregnenolone and dehydroepiandrosterone is mediated by the enzyme aromatase, *Journal of Neurobiology*, 56(4), 398–406, 2003.

118. Jones, K. J., Sotrer, P. D., Drengler, S. M., and Oblinger, M. M., Differential regulation of cytoskeletal gene expression in hamster facial motoneurons: Effects of axotomy and testosterone treatment, *Journal of Neuroscience Research*, 57(6), 817–823, 1999.

119. Yoshizawa, A., Clemmons, D. R., Testosterone and insulin-like growth factor (IGF) I interact in controlling IGF-binding protein production in androgen-responsive foreskin fibroblasts, *Journal of Clinical Endocrinology and Metabolism*, 85(4), 1627–1633, 2000.

120. Hoffman, S. W., Virmani, S., Simkins, R. M., and Stein, D. G., The delayed administration of dehydroepiandrosterone sulfate improves recovery of function after traumatic brain injury in rats, *Journal of Neurotrauma*, 20(9), 859–870, 2003.

121. Young, T. P., Hoaglin, H. M., and Burke, D. T., The role of serum testosterone and TBI in the in-patient rehabilitation setting, *Brain Injury*, 21(6), 645–649, 2007.

122. Janowsky, J. S., Chavez, B., and Orwoll, E., Sex steroids modify working memory, *Journal of Cognitive Neuroscience*, 12(3), 407–414, 2000.

123. Cherrier, M. M. P., Asthana, S. M., Plymate, S. M., Baker, L. P., Matsumoto, A. M. M., Peskind, E. M., et al., Testosterone supplementation improves spatial and verbal memory in healthy older men, *Neurology*, 57(1), 80–88, 2001.

124. Seidman, S. N. and Rabkin, J. G., Testosterone replacement therapy for hypogonadal men with SSRI-refractory depression, *Journal of Affective Disorders*, 48(2–3), 157–161, 1998.

125. Sternbach H. Age-associated testosterone decline in men: Clinical issues for psychiatry, *American Journal of Psychiatry,* 155(10), 1310–1318, 1998.

126. Zitzmann, M., Testosterone and the brain, *Aging Male*, 9(4), 195–199, 2006.

127. Militello, A., Vitello, G., Lunetta, C., Toscano, A., Maiorana, G., Piccoli, T., et al., The serum level of free testosterone is reduced in amyotrophic lateral sclerosis, *Journal of the Neurological Sciences*, 195(1), 67–70, 2002.

128. Stein, D. G., Sex differences in brain damage and recovery of function: Experimental and clinical findings, *Progress in Brain Research*, 161, 339–351, 2007.

129. Bae, Y. H., Hwang, J. Y., Kim, Y. H., and Koh, J. Y., Anti-oxidative neuroprotection by estrogens in mouse cortical cultures, *Journal of Korean Medical Science*, 15(3), 327–336, 2000.

130. Bishop, J. and Simpkins, J. W., Estradiol treatment increases viability of glioma and neuroblastoma cells in vitro, *Molecular and Cellular Neuroscience*, 5(4), 303–308, 1994.

131. Green, P. S., Bishop, J., and Simpkins, J. W., 17Alpha-estradiol exerts neuroprotective effects on SK-N-SH cells, *Journal of Neuroscience*, 17(2), 511–515, 1997.

132. Behl, C., Widmann, M., Trapp, T., and Holsboer, F., 17-[Beta] estradiol protects neurons from oxidative stress-induced cell death in vitro, *Biochemical and Biophysical Research Communications*, 216(2), 473–482, 1995.

133. Goodman, Y., Bruce, A. J., Cheng, B., Estrogens attenuate and corticosterone exacerbates excitotoxicity, oxidative injury, and amyloid beta-peptide toxicity in hippocampal neurons, *Journal of Neurochemistry*, 66(5), 1836–1844, 1996.

134. Green, P. S. and Simpkins, J. W., Neuroprotective effects of estrogens: Potential mechanisms of action, *International Journal of Developmental Neuroscience*, 18(4–5), 347–358, 2000.

135. Green, P. S., Gridley, K. E., and Simpkins, J. W., Estradiol protects against [beta]-amyloid (25-35)-induced toxicity in SK-N-SH human neuroblastoma cells, *Neuroscience Letters*, 218(3), 165–168, 1996.

136. Gridley, K. E., Green, P. S., and Simpkins, J. W., Low concentrations of estradiol reduce [beta]-amyloid (25-35)-induced toxicity, lipid peroxidation and glucose utilization in human SK-N-SH neuroblastoma cells, *Brain Research*, 778(1), 158–165, 1997.

137. Gridley, K. E., Green, P. S., and Simpkins, J. W., A novel, synergistic interaction between 17 beta-estradiol and glutathione in the protection of neurons against beta-amyloid 25-35-induced toxicity in vitro, *Molecular Pharmacology*, 54(5), 874–880, 1998.

138. Mattson, M. P., Robinson, N., and Guo, Q., Estrogens stabilize mitochondrial function and protect neural cells against the pro-apoptotic action of mutant presenilin-1, *Neuroreport*, 8(17), 3817–3821, 1997.

139. Mook-Jung, I., Joo, I., Sohn, S., Jae Kwon, H., Huh, K., and Whan Jung, M., Estrogen blocks neurotoxic effects of [beta]-amyloid (1-42) and induces neurite extension on B103 cells, *Neuroscience Letters*, 235(3), 101–104, 1997.

140. Pike, C. J., Estrogen modulates neuronal Bcl-x$_l$ expression and beta-amyloid-induced apoptosis, *Journal of Neurochemistry*, 72(4), 1552–1563, 1999.

141. Singer, C. A., Rogers, K. L., Strickland, T. M., and Dorsa, D. M., Estrogen protects primary cortical neurons from glutamate toxicity, *Neuroscience Letters*, 212(1), 13–16, 1996.

142. Singer, C. A., Rogers, K. L., and Dorsa, D. M., Modulation of Bcl-2 expression: A potential component of estrogen protection in NT2 neurons, *Neuroreport*, 9(11), 2565–2568, 1998.

143. Weaver, C. E., Park-Chung, M., Gibbs, T. T., and Farb, D. H., 17[Beta]-estradiol protects against NMDA-induced excitotoxicity by direct inhibition of NMDA receptors, *Brain Research*, 761(2), 338–341, 1997.

144. Zaulyanov, L. L., Green, P. S., and Simpkins, J. W., Glutamate receptor requirement for neuronal death from anoxia–reoxygenation: An in vitro model for assessment of the neuroprotective effects of estrogens, *Cellular and Molecular Neurobiology*, 19(6), 705–718, 1999.

145. Moosmann, B. and Behl, C., The antioxidant neuroprotective effects of estrogens and phenolic compounds are independent from their estrogenic properties, *Proceedings of the National Academy of Sciences of the United States of America*, 96(16), 8867–8872, 1999.

146. Sawada, H., Ibi, M., Kihara, T., Urushitani, M., Akaike, A., and Shimohama, S., Estradiol protects mesencephalic dopaminergic neurons from oxidative stress-induced neuronal death, *Journal of Neuroscience Research*, 54(5), 707–719, 1998.

147. Regan, R. F. and Guo, Y., Estrogens attenuate neuronal injury due to hemoglobin, chemical hypoxia, and excitatory amino acids in murine cortical cultures, *Brain Research*, 764(1-2), 133–140, 1997.

148. Wilson, M. E., Dubal, D. B., and Wise, P. M., Estradiol protects against injury-induced cell death in cortical explant cultures: A role for estrogen receptors, *Brain Research*, 873(2), 235–242, 2000.

149. Blum-Degen, D., Haas, M., Pohli, S., Harth, R., Römer, W., Oettel, M., et al., Scavestrogens protect IMR 32 cells from oxidative stress-induced cell death, *Toxicology and Applied Pharmacology*, 152(1), 49–55, 1998.

150. Wang, J., Green, P. S., and Simpkins, J. W., Estradiol protects against ATP depletion, mitochondrial membrane potential decline and the generation of reactive oxygen species induced by 3-nitroproprionic acid in SK-N-SH human neuroblastoma cells, *Journal of Neurochemistry*, 77(3), 804–911, 2001.

151. De Girolamo, L. A., Hargreaves, A. J., and Billett, E. E., Protection from MPTP-induced neurotoxicity in differentiating mouse N2a neuroblastoma cells, *Journal of Neurochemistry*, 76(3), 650–660, 2001.

152. Simpkins, J.W., Rajakumar, G., Zhang, Y. Q., Simpkins, C. E., Greenwald, D., Yu, C. J., et al., Estrogens may reduce mortality and ischemic damage caused by middle cerebral artery occlusion in the female rat, *Journal of Neurosurgery*, 87(5), 724–730, 1997.

153. Alkayed, N. J. M. D. P., Harukuni, I. M. D., Kimes, A. S. P, London, E. D. P., Traystman, R. J. P., and Hurn, P. D. P., Gender-linked brain injury in experimental stroke, *Stroke*, 29(1), 159–165, 1998.

154. Dubal, D. B., Kashon, M. L., Pettigrew, L. C., Ren, J. M., Finklestein, S. P., Rau, S. W., et al., Estradiol protects against ischemic injury, *Journal of Cerebral Blood Flow and Metabolism*, 18(11), 1253–1258, 1998.

155. Sudo, S., Wen, T.- C., Desaki, J., Matsuda, S., Tanaka, J., Arai, T., et al., [Beta]-Estradiol protects hippocampal CA1 neurons against transient forebrain ischemia in gerbil, *Neuroscience Research*, 29(4), 345–354, 1997.

156. He, Z., He, Y.- J., Day, A. L., and Simpkins, J. W., Proestrus levels of estradiol during transient global cerebral ischemia improves the histological outcome of the hippocampal CA1 region: Perfusion-dependent and -independent mechanisms, *Journal of the Neurological Sciences*, 193(2), 79–87, 2002.

157. Fukuda, K., Yao, H., Ibayashi, S., Nakahara, T., Uchimura, H., and Fujishima, M., Ovariectomy exacerbates and estrogen replacement attenuates photothrombotic focal ischemic brain injury in rats, *Stroke*, 31(1), 155–160, 2000.

158. Mendelowitsch, A., Ritz, M.- F., Ros, J., Langemann, H., and Gratzl, O., 17[Beta]-estradiol reduces cortical lesion size in the glutamate excitotoxicity model by enhancing extracellular lactate: A new neuroprotective pathway, *Brain Research*, 901(1–2), 230–236, 2001.

159. Yang, S.- H., He, Z., Wu, S. S., He, Y.- J., Cutright, J., Millard, W. J., et al., 17-[bgr] Estradiol can reduce secondary ischemic damage and mortality of subarachnoid hemorrhage, *Journal of Cerebral Blood Flow and Metabolism*, 21(2), 174–181, 2001.

160. Dhandapani, K. M. and Brann, D. W., Role of astrocytes in estrogen-mediated neuroprotection, *Experimental Gerontology*, 42(1–2), 70–75, 2007.

161. Wang, J. M., Xu, L., Murphy, W. J., Taub, D. D., and Chertov, O., IL-8 induced T-lymphocyte migration: Direct as well as indirect mechanisms, *Methods*, 10(1), 191–200, 1996.

162. Brinton, R. D., Requirements of a brain selective estrogen: Advances and remaining challenges for developing a NeuroSERM, *Journal of Alzheimer's Disease*, 6(6 Suppl.), S27–S35, 2004.

163. Zhao, L., O'Neill, K., Diaz Brinton, R., Selective estrogen receptor modulators (SERMs) for the brain: Current status and remaining challenges for developing NeuroSERMs, *Brain Research Reviews*, 49(3), 472–493, 2005.

164. Manthey, D. and Behl, C., From structural biochemistry to expression profiling: Neuroprotective activities of estrogen, *Neuroscience*, 138(3), 845–850, 2006.

165. Simpkins, J. W., Yang, S.- H., Liu, R., Perez, E., Cai, Z. Y., Covey, D. F., et al., Estrogen-like compounds for ischemic neuroprotection, *Stroke*, 35(11 Suppl. 1), 2648–2651, 2004.

166. Wise, P. M., Estrogens and neuroprotection, *Trends in Endocrinology and Metabolism*, 13(6), 229–230, 2002.

167. Wise, P. M., Dubal, D. B., Rau, S. W., Brown, C. M., and Suzuki, S., Are estrogens protective or risk factors in brain injury and neurodegeneration? Reevaluation after the Women's Health Initiative, *Endocrine Reviews*, 26(3), 308–312, 2005.

168. McEwen, B, S., The molecular and neuroanatomical basis for estrogen effects in the central nervous system, *Journal of Clinical Endocrinology and Metabolism*, 84(6), 1790–1797, 1999.

169. Garcia-Segura, L. M., Azcoitia, I., and Don Carlos, L. L., Neuroprotection by estradiol, *Progress in Neurobiology*, 63(1), 29–60, 2001.

170. Yue, X., Lu, M., Lancaster, T., Cao, P., Honda, S.- I., Staufenbiel, M., et al., Brain estrogen deficiency accelerates Aβ plaque formation in an Alzheimer's disease animal model, *Proceedings of the National Academy of Sciences of the United States of America*, 102(52), 19198–19203, 2005.

171. Emerson, C. S., Headrick, J. P., and Vink, R., Estrogen improves biochemical and neurologic outcome following traumatic brain injury in male rats, but not in females, *Brain Research*, 608(1), 95–100, 1993.

172. Harukuni, I., Hurn, P. D., and Crain, B. J., Deleterious effect of [beta]-estradiol in a rat model of transient forebrain ischemia, *Brain Research*, 900(1), 137–142, 2001.

173. Smith, S. S. and Woolley, C. S., Cellular and molecular effects of steroid hormones on CNS excitability, *Cleveland Clinic Journal of Medicine*, 71(Suppl. 2), S4–S10, 2004.

174. Raz, L., Khan, M. M., Mahesh, V. B., Vadlamudi, R. K., and Brann, D. W., Rapid estrogen signaling in the brain, *Neurosignals*, 16(2–3), 140–153, 2008.

175. Schumacher, M., Guennoun, R., Mercier, G., Désarnaud, F., Lacor, P., Bénavides, J., et al., Progesterone synthesis and myelin formation in peripheral nerves, *Brain Research Reviews*, 37(1–3), 343–359, 2001.

176. Ghoumari, A. M., Ibanez, C., El-Etr, M., Leclerc, P., Eychenne, B., O'Malley, B. W., et al., Progesterone and its metabolites increase myelin basic protein expression in organotypic slice cultures of rat cerebellum, *Journal of Neurochemistry*, 86(4), 848–859, 2003.

177. Magnaghi, V., Cavarretta, I., Galbiati, M., Martini, L., and Melcangi, R. C., Neuroactive steroids and peripheral myelin proteins, *Brain Research Reviews*, 37(1–3), 360–371, 2001.

178. Ibanez, C., Shields, S. A., El-Etr, M., Baulieu, E. E., Schumacher, M., and Franklin, R. J. M., Systemic progesterone administration results in a partial reversal of the age-associated decline in CNS remyelination following toxin-induced demyelination in male rats, *Neuropathology & Applied Neurobiology*, 30(1), 80–89, 2004.

179. Gilson, J. and Blakemore, W. F., Failure of remyelination in areas of demyelination produced in the spinal cord of old rats, *Neuropathology and Applied Neurobiology*, 19(2), 173–181, 1993.

180. Li, W.- W., Penderis, J., Zhao, C., Schumacher, M., and Franklin, R. J. M., Females remyelinate more efficiently than males following demyelination in the aged but not young adult CNS, *Experimental Neurology*, 202(1), 250–254, 2006.

181. Nilsen, J. and Brinton, R. D., Impact of progestins on estrogen-induced neuroprotection: Synergy by progesterone and 19-norprogesterone and antagonism by medroxyprogesterone acetate, *Endocrinology*, 143(1), 205–212, 2002.

182. Ogata, T., Nakamura, Y., Tsuji, K., Shibata, T., and Kataoka, K., Steroid hormones protect spinal cord neurons from glutamate toxicity, *Neuroscience*, 55(2), 445–459, 1993.

183. Ogata, T., Nakamura, Y., Tsuji, K., Shibata, T., and Kataoka, K., Steroid hormones protect spinal cord neurons from glutamate toxicity, *Neuroscience*, 55(2), 445–459, 1993.

184. González, S. L., Labombarda, F., González Deniselle, M. C., Guennoun, R., Schumacher, M., and De Nicola, A. F., Progesterone up-regulates neuronal brain-derived neurotrophic factor expression in the injured spinal cord, *Neuroscience*, 125(3), 605–614, 2004.

185. Drew, P. D. and Chavis, J. A., Female sex steroids: Effects upon microglial cell activation, *Journal of Neuroimmunology*, 111(1–2), 77–85, 2000.

186. He, J., Evans, C.-O., Hoffman, S. W., Oyesiku, N. M., and Stein, D. G., Progesterone and allopregnanolone reduce inflammatory cytokines after traumatic brain injury, *Experimental Neurology*, 189(2), 404–412, 2004.

187. Miller, L. and Hunt, J. S., Regulation of TNF-{alpha} production in activated mouse macrophages by progesterone, *Journal of Immunology*, 160(10), 5098–5104, 1998.

188. Valera, S., Ballivet, M., and Bertrand, D., Progesterone modulates a neuronal nicotinic acetylcholine receptor, *Proceedings of the National Academy of Sciences of the United States of America*, 89(20), 9949–9953, 1992.

189. Rupprecht, R. and Holsboer, F., Neuroactive steroids: Mechanisms of action and neuropsychopharmacological perspectives, *Trends in Neurosciences*, 22(9), 410–416, 1999.

190. Maclusky, N. J. and McEwen, B. S., Oestrogen modulates progestin receptor concentrations in some rat brain regions but not in others, *Nature*, 274(5668), 276–278, 1978.

191. Parsons, B., Rainbow, T. C., MacLusky, N. J., and McEwen, B. S., Progestin receptor levels in rat hypothalamic and limbic nuclei, *Journal of Neuroscience*, 2(10), 1446–1452, 1982.

192. Camacho-Arroyo, I., Pérez-Palacios, G., Pasapera, A. M., and Cerbón, M. A., Intracellular progesterone receptors are differentially regulated by sex steroid hormones in the hypothalamus and the cerebral cortex of the rabbit, *The Journal of Steroid Biochemistry and Molecular Biology*, 50(5–6), 299–303, 1994.

193. Guerra-Araiza, C., Villamar-Cruz, O., González-Arenas, A., Chavira, R., and Camacho-Arroyo, I., Changes in progesterone receptor isoforms content in the rat brain during the oestrous cycle and after oestradiol and progesterone treatments, *Journal of Neuroendocrinology*, 15(10), 984–990, 2003.

194. Gonzalez Deniselle, M. C., Garay, L., Gonzalez, S., Guennoun, R., Schumacher, M., and De Nicola, A.F., Progesterone restores retrograde labeling of cervical motoneurons in Wobbler mouse motoneuron disease, *Experimental Neurology*, 195(2), 518–523, 2005.

195. Stokin, G. B., Lillo, C., Falzone, T. L., Brusch, R. G., Rockenstein, E., Mount, S. L., et al., Axonopathy and transport deficits early in the pathogenesis of Alzheimer's disease, *Science*, 307(5713), 1282–1288, 2005.

196. Praticò, D. and Sung, S., Lipid peroxidation and oxidative imbalance: Early functional events in Alzheimer's disease, *Journal of Alzheimer's Disease*, 6(2), 171–175, 2004.

197. Roof, R. L., Hoffman, S. W., and Stein, D. G., Progesterone protects against lipid peroxidation following traumatic brain injury in rats, *Molecular and Chemical Neuropathology*, 31(1), 1–11, 1997.

198. Moorthy, K., Yadav, U., Siddiqui, M., Mantha, A., Basir, S., Sharma, D., et al., Effect of hormone replacement therapy in normalizing age related neuronal markers in different age groups of naturally menopausal rats, *Biogerontology*, 6(5), 345–356, 2005.

199. Garcia-Segura, L. M., Cardona-Gomez, P., Naftolin, F., and Chowen, J. A., Estradiol upregulates Bcl-2 expression in adult brain neurons, *Neuroreport*, 9(4), 593–597, 1998.

200. Robertson, C. L., Puskar, A., Hoffman, G. E., Murphy, A. Z., Saraswati, M., and Fiskum, G., Physiologic progesterone reduces mitochondrial dysfunction and hippocampal cell loss after traumatic brain injury in female rats, *Experimental Neurology*, 197(1), 235–243, 2006.

201. Cutler, S. M., VanLandingham, J. W., Murphy, A. Z., and Stein, D. G., Slow-release and injected progesterone treatments enhance acute recovery after traumatic brain injury, *Pharmacology Biochemistry and Behavior*, 84(3), 420–428, 2006.

202. Rodrigue, G., Stuart, W. H., and Donald, G. S., Effects of the duration of progesterone treatment on the resolution of cerebral edema induced by cortical contusions in rats, *Restorative Neurology and Neuroscience*, 18(4), 161–166, 2001.

203. González-Vidal, M. D., Cervera-Gaviria, M., Ruelas, R., Escobar, A., Moralí, G., and Cervantes, M., Progesterone: Protective effects on the cat hippocampal neuronal damage due to acute global cerebral ischemia, *Archives of Medical Research*, 29(2), 117–124, 1998.

204. Cervantes, M., González-Vidal, M. D., Ruelas, R., Escobar, A., and Moralí, G., Neuroprotective effects of progesterone on damage elicited by acute global cerebral ischemia in neurons of the caudate nucleus, *Archives of Medical Research*, 33(1), 6–14, 2002.

205. Jiang, N., Chopp, M., Stein, D., and Feit, H., Progesterone is neuroprotective after transient middle cerebral artery occlusion in male rats, *Brain Research*, 735(1), 101–107, 1996.
206. Kumon, Y., Kim, S. C., Tompkins, P., Stevens, A., Sakaki, S., and Loftus, C. M., Neuroprotective effect of postischemic administration of progesterone in spontaneously hypertensive rats with focal cerebral ischemia, *Journal of Neurosurgery*, 92(5), 848–852, 2000.
207. Galani, R., Hoffman, S. W., and Stein, D. G., Effects of the duration of progesterone treatment on the resolution of cerebral edema induced by cortical contusions in rats, *Restorative Neurology and Neuroscience*, 18(4), 161–166, 2001.
208. Roof, R. L., Duvdevani, R., Heyburn, J. W., and Stein, D. G., Progesterone rapidly decreases brain edema: Treatment delayed up to 24 hours is still effective, *Experimental Neurology*, 138(2), 246–251, 1996.
209. Wright, D. W., Kellermann, A. L., Hertzberg, V. S., Clark, P. L., Frankel, M., Goldstein, F. C., Salomone, J. P., et al., ProTECT: A randomized clinical trial of progesterone for acute traumatic brain injury, *Annals of Emergency Medicine*, 49(4), 391–402, 2007.
210. Tagliaferri, M., Berselli, M. E., Calo, G., Minocci, A., Savia, G., Petroni, M. L., et al., Subclinical hypothyroidism in obese patients: Relation to resting energy expenditure, serum leptin, body composition, and lipid profile, *Obesity*, 9(3), 196–201, 2001.
211. Uzunlulu, M., Yorulmaz, E., and Oguz, A., Prevalence of subclinical hypothyroidism in patients with metabolic syndrome, *Endocrine Journal*, 54(1), 71–76, 2007.
212. Harper, M.- E. and Seifert, E. L., Thyroid hormone effects on mitochondrial energetics, *Thyroid*, 18(2), 145–156, 2008.
213. Menzies, K. J., Robinson, B. H., and Hood, D. A., Effect of thyroid hormone on mitochondrial properties and oxidative stress in cells from patients with mtDNA defects, *American Journal of Physiology–Cell Physiology*, 296(2), C355–C362, 2009.
214. Chanoine, J. P., Alex, S., Fang, S. L., Stone, S., Leonard, J. L., Korhle, J., et al., Role of transthyretin in the transport of thyroxine from the blood to the choroid plexus, the cerebrospinal fluid, and the brain, *Endocrinology*, 130(2), 933–938, 1992.
215. Bernal, J., Action of thyroid hormone in brain, *Journal of Endocrinological Investigation*, 25(3), 268–288, 2002.
216. Bernal, J. and Nunez, J., Thyroid hormones and brain development, *European Journal of Endocrinology*, 133(4), 390–398, 1995.
217. Balázs, R., Kovács, S., Cocks, W. A., Johnson, A. L., and Eayrs, J. T., Effect of thyroid hormone on the biochemical maturation of rat brain: Postnatal cell formation, *Brain Research*, 25(3), 555–570, 1971.
218. Berbel, P., Guadaño-Ferraz, A., Martínez, M., Quiles, J. A., Balboa, R., and Innocenti, G. M., Organization of auditory callosal connections in hypothyroid adult rats, *European Journal of Neuroscience*, 5(11), 1465–1478, 1993.
219. Gravel, C., Sasseville, R., and Hawkes, R., Maturation of the corpus callosum of the rat: II. Influence of thyroid hormones on the number and maturation of axons, *Journal of Comparative Neurology*, 291(1), 147–161, 1990.
220. Fann, J. R., Burington, B., Leonetti, A., Jaffe, K., Katon, W. J., and Thompson, R. S., Psychiatric illness following traumatic brain injury in an adult health maintenance organization population, *Archives of General Psychiatry*, 61(1), 53–61, 2004.
221. Jorge, R. E., Robinson, R. G., Moser, D., Tateno, A., Crespo-Facorro, B., and Arndt, S., Major depression following traumatic brain injury, *Archives of General Psychiatry*, 61(1), 42–50, 2004.
222. Jorge, R. E., Starkstein, S. E., Arndt, S., Moser, D., Crespo-Facorro, B., and Robinson, R. G., Alcohol misuse and mood disorders following traumatic brain injury, *Archives of General Psychiatry*, 62(7), 742–749, 2005.
223. Behan, L. A., Phillips, J., Thompson, C. J., and Agha, A., Neuroendocrine disorders after traumatic brain injury, *Journal of Neurology, Neurosurgery, and Psychiatry*, 79(7), 753–759, 2008.
224. Bavisetty, S. B. S., McArthur, D. L. P. D. M. P. H., Dusick, J. R. M. D., Wang, C. M.D., Cohan, P. M. D., Boscardin, W. J. P. D., et al., Chronic hypopituitarism after traumatic brain injury: Risk assessment and relationship to outcome, *Neurosurgery*, 62(5), 1080–1094, 2008.

225. Nampiaparampil, D. E., Prevalence of chronic pain after traumatic brain injury: A systematic review, *Journal of the American Medical Association*, 300(6), 711–719, 2008.
226. Mortimer J. A., French, L. R., Hutton, J. T., and Schuman, L. M., Head injury as a risk factor for Alzheimer's disease, *Neurology*, 35(2), 264–267, 1985.
227. Amaducci, L. A., Fratiglioni, L., Rocca, W. A., Fieschi, C., Livrea, P., Pedone, D., et al., Risk factors for clinically diagnosed Alzheimer's disease: A case–control study of an Italian population, *Neurology*, 36(7), 922–931, 1986.
228. O'Meara, E. S., Kukull, W. A., Sheppard, L., Bowen, J. D., McCormick, W. C., Teri, L., et al., Head injury and risk of Alzheimer's disease by apolipoprotein E genotype, *American Journal of Epidemiology*, 146(5), 373–384, 1997.
229. Gottlieb, S., Head injury doubles the risk for Alzheimer's disease, *British Medical Journal*, 321(7269), 1100, 2000.
230. Lye, T. C. and Shores, E. A., Traumatic brain injury as a risk factor for Alzheimer's disease: A review, *Neuropsychology Review*, 10(2), 115–129, 2000.
231. Jellinger, K. A., Paulus, W., Wrocklage, C., and Litvan, I., Effects of closed traumatic brain injury and genetic factors on the development of Alzheimer's disease, *European Journal of Neurology*, 8(6), 707–710, 2001.
232. Nemetz, P. N., Leibson, C., Naessens, J. M., Beard, M., Kokmen, E., Annegers, J. F., et al., Traumatic brain injury and time to onset of Alzheimer's disease: A population-based study, *American Journal of Epidemiology*, 149(1), 32–40, 1999.
233. Fleminger, S., Oliver, D. L., Lovestone, S., Rabe-Hesketh, S., and Giora, A., Head injury as a risk factor for Alzheimer's disease: The evidence 10 years on: A partial replication, *Journal of Neurology, Neurosurgery, and Psychiatry*, 74(7), 857–862, 2003.
234. Plassman, B. L., Havlik, R. J., Steffens, D. C., Helms, M. J., Newman, T. N., Drosdick, D., et al., Documented head injury in early adulthood and risk of Alzheimer's disease and other dementias, *Neurology*, 55(8), 1158–1166, 2000.
235. Mashaly, H. A. and Provencio, J. J., Inflammation as a link between brain injury and heart damage: The model of subarachnoid hemorrhage, *Cleveland Clinic Journal of Medicine*, 75(Suppl. 2), S26–S30, 2008.
236. Caveness, W. F., Epilepsy, a product of trauma in our time, *Epilepsia*, 17(2), 207–215, 1976.
237. Feeney, D. M. and Walker, A. E., The prediction of posttraumatic epilepsy: A mathematical approach, *Archives of Neurology*, 36(1), 8–12, 1979.
238. Jennett, B., Early traumatic epilepsy: Incidence and significance after nonmissile injuries, *Archives of Neurology*, 30(5), 394–398, 1974.
239. Annegers, J. F., Grabow, J. D., Groover, R. V., Laws, Jr., E. R., Elveback, L. R., and Kurland, L. T., Seizures after head trauma: A population study, *Neurology*, 30(7 Pt. 1), 683–689, 1980.
240. Jennett, B. and Teasdale, G., *Management of Head Injuries*, F. A. Davis, Philadelphia, 1981.
241. Garland, D. E. and Keenan, M. A. E., Orthopedic strategies in the management of the adult head-injured patient, *Physical Therapy*, 63(12), 2004–2009, 1983.
242. Poca, M. A., Sahuquillo, J., Mataro, M., Benejam, B., Arikan, F., and Baquena, M., Ventricular enlargement after moderate or severe head injury: A frequent and neglected problem, *Journal of Neurotrauma*, 22(11), 1303–1310, 2005.
243. Bernard, F., Outtrim, J., Menon, D. K., and Matta, B. F., Incidence of adrenal insufficiency after severe traumatic brain injury varies according to definition used: Clinical implications, *British Journal of Anaesthesia*, 96(1), 72–76, 2006.
244. Tsagarakis, S., Tzanela, M., and Dimopoulou, I., Diabetes insipidus, secondary hypoadrenalism and hypothyroidism after traumatic brain injury: Clinical implications, *Pituitary*, 8(3), 251–254, 2005.
245. Klose, M., Juul, A., Poulsgaard, L., Kosteljanetz, M., Brennum, J., and Feldt-Rasmussen, U., Prevalence and predictive factors of post-traumatic hypopituitarism, *Clinical Endocrinology*, 67(2), 193–201, 2007.
246. Agha, A. and Thompson, C. J., Anterior pituitary dysfunction following traumatic brain injury (TBI), *Clinical Endocrinology*, 64, 481–488, 2006.

247. Ascoli, P. and Cavagnini, F., Hypopituitarism, *Pituitary* 9(4), 335–342, 2006.

248. Chang, C.- H., Liao, J.- J., Chuang, C.- H., and Lee, C.- T. E., Recurrent hyponatremia after traumatic brain injury, *American Journal of the Medical Sciences*, 335(5), 390–393, 2008.

249. Castriotta, R. J., Wilde, M. C., Lai, J. M., Atanasov, S., Masel, B. E., and Kuna, S. T., Prevalence and consequences of sleep disorders in traumatic brain injury, *Journal of Clinical Sleep Medicine*, 3(4), 349–356, 2007.

250. Corrigan, J. D. and Cole, T. B., Substance use disorders and clinical management of traumatic brain injury and posttraumatic stress disorder, *Journal of the American Medical Association*, 300(6), 720–721, 2008.

251. Besedovsky, H. O., del Rey, A. E., Sorkin, E., DaPrada, M., Burri, R., and Honegger, C., The immune response evokes changes in brain noradrenergic neurons, *Science*, 221(4610), 564–566, 1983.

252. Besedovsky, H. O., Del Rey, A. E., Sorkin, E., and Dinarello, C. A., Immunoregulatory feedback between interleukin-1 and glucocorticoid hormones, *Science*, 233(4764), 652–654, 1986.

253. Besedovsky, H. O., Rey, A. D., Sorkin, E., Da Prada, M., and Keller, H. H., Immunoregulation mediated by the sympathetic nervous system, *Cellular Immunology*, 48(2), 346–355, 1979.

254. Ziemssen, T. and Kern, S., Psychoneuroimmunology: Cross-talk between the immune and nervous systems, *Journal of Neurology*, 254(Suppl. 2), II8–II11, 2007.

255. Wilder, R. L., Neuroendocrine-immune system interactions and autoimmunity, *Annual Review of Immunology*, 13, 307–338, 1995.

256. O'Connor, J. C., McCusker, R. H., Strle, K., Johnson, R. W., Dantzer, R., and Kelley, K. W., Regulation of IGF-I function by proinflammatory cytokines: At the interface of immunology and endocrinology, *Cellular Immunology*, 252(1–2), 91–110, 2008.

257. Hehlgans, T. and Pfeffer, K., The intriguing biology of the tumour necrosis factor/tumour necrosis factor receptor superfamily: Players, rules and the games, *Immunology*, 115(1), 1–20, 2005.

258. Valverde, A. M., Benito, M., and Lorenzo, M., The brown adipose cell: A model for understanding the molecular mechanisms of insulin resistance, *Acta Physiologica Scandinavica*, 183(1), 59–73, 2005.

259. Frystyk, J., Free insulin-like growth factors: Measurements and relationships to growth hormone secretion and glucose homeostasis, *Growth Hormone & IGF Research*, 14(5), 337–375, 2004.

260. Steinman, L., Elaborate interactions between the immune and nervous systems, *Nature Immunology*, 5(6), 575–581, 2004.

261. Arkins, S., Johnson, R. W., Minshall, R., Dantzer, R., and Kelley, K. W., Immunophysiology: The interaction of hormone lymphohemopoietic cytokines and the neuroimmune axis, in B. S. McEwen (Ed.), *Coping with the Environment: Neural and Endocrine Mechanisms, Handbook of Physiology*, Oxford, New York, 469–495, 2001.

262. Butts, C. L. and Sternberg, E. M., Neuroendocrine factors alter host defense by modulating immune function, *Cellular Immunology*, 252(1–2), 7–15, 2008.

263. Dinarello, C. A., The interleukin-1 family: 10 Years of discovery, *Federation of American Societies for Experimental Biology Journal*, 8(15), 1314–1325, 1994.

264. McEwen, B. S., Biron, C. A., Brunson, K. W., Bulloch, K., Chambers, W. H., Dhabhar, F. S., et al., The role of adrenocorticoids as modulators of immune function in health and disease: Neural, endocrine and immune interactions, *Brain Research Reviews*, 23(1–2), 79–133, 1997.

265. Lorton, D., Lubahn, C. L., Estus, C., Millar, B. A., Carter, J. L., Wood, C. A., et al., Bidirectional communication between the brain and the immune system: Implications for physiological sleep and disorders with disrupted sleep, *Neuroimmunomodulation*, 13(5–6), 357–374, 2006.

266. Miller, K. R. and Streit, W. J., The effects of aging, injury and disease on microglial function: A case for cellular senescence, *Neuron Glia Biology*, 3(3), 245–253, 2007.

267. Gehrmann, J., Matsumoto, Y., and Kreutzberg, G. W., Microglia: Intrinsic immuneffector cell of the brain, *Brain Research Reviews*, 20(3), 269–287, 1995.

268. Streit, W. J., Hurley, S. D., McGraw, T. S., and Semple-Rowland, S. L., Comparative evaluation of cytokine profiles and reactive gliosis supports a critical role for interleukin-6 in neuron–glia signaling during regeneration, *Journal of Neuroscience Research*, 61(1), 10–20, 2000.

269. Streit, W. J., Microglia as neuroprotective, immunocompetent cells of the CNS, *Glia*, 40(2), 133–139, 2002.

270. Streit, W. J., Microglia and neuroprotection: Implications for Alzheimer's disease, *Brain Research Reviews*, 48(2), 234–239, 2005.

271. Conde, J. R. P. and Streit, W. J. P., Microglia in the aging brain, *Journal of Neuropathology & Experimental Neurology*, 65(3), 199–203, 2006.

272. Cohen, S. B., Gluckman, E., Rubinstein, P., and Madrigal, J. A. (Eds.), *Cord Blood Characteristics: Role in Stem Cell Transplantation*, Martin Dunitz, London, 2000.

273. Lu, L., Shen, R. N., and Broxmeyer, H. E., Stem cells from bone marrow, umbilical cord blood and peripheral blood for clinical application: Current status and future application, *Critical Reviews in Oncology/Hematology*, 22(2), 61–78, 1996.

274. Chen, S. H., Chang, F. M., Tsai, Y. C., Huang, K. F., Lin, C. L., and Lin, M. T., Infusion of human umbilical cord blood cells protect against cerebral ischemia and damage after heatstroke in the rat, *Experimental Neurology*, 199(1), 2682–2688, 2006.

275. Vendrame, M., Cassady, C. J., Newcomb, J., Bulter, T., Pennypacker, K. R., Zigova, T., et al., Infusion of human umbilical cord blood cells in rat model of stroke dose-dependently rescues behavioral deficits and reduces infarct volume, *Stroke*, 35(10), 1–6, 2004.

276. Willing, A. E., Lixian, A., Milliken, M., Poulos, S., Zigova, T., Song, S., et al., Intravenous versus intrastriatal cord blood administration in a rodent model of stroke, *Journal of Neuroscience Research*, 73(3), 296–307, 2003.

277. Willing, A. E., Vendrame, M., Mallery, J., Cassady, C. J., Davis, C. D., and Sanchez-Ramos, J., et al., Mobilized peripheral blood cells administered intravenously produce functional recovery and stroke, *Cell Transplant*, 12(4), 449–454, 2003.

278. Newman, M. B., Willing, A. E., Manresa, J. J., Sanberg, C. D., and Sanberg, P. R., Cytokines produced by cultured human umbilical cord blood (HUCB) cells: Implications for brain repair, *Experimental Neurology*, 199(1), 201–208, 2006.

279. Lund, B. T., Ashikian, N., Ta, H. Q., Chakryan, Y., Manoukian, K., Goroshen, S., et al., Increased CXCL8 (IL-8) expression in multiple sclerosis, *Journal of Neuroimmunology*, 155(1–2), 161–171, 2004.

280. Kushi, H., Saito, T., Majkino, K., and Hayashi, N., IL-8 is a key mediator of neuroinflammation in severe traumatic brain injuries, *Acta Neurochirurgica*, 86(Suppl.), 347–350, 2003.

281. Kostulas, N., Pelidou, S. H., Kivisakk, P., Kostulas, V., and Link, H., Increased IL-8 beta, IL-8, and IL-17 mRNA expression in blood mononuclear cells observed in a prospective ischemic stroke study, *Stroke*, 30(10), 2174–2179, 1999.

282. Kasahara, T., Mukaida, N., Yamashita, K., Yagisawa, H., Akahoshi, T., and Matsushima, K., IL-1 and TNF-alpha induction of IL-8 and monocyte chemotactic and activating factor (MCAF) mRNA expression in a human astrocytoma cell line, *Immunology*, 74(1), 60–67, 1991.

283. Kim, J. S., Cytokines and adhesion molecules in stroke and related diseases, *Journal of Neurological Science*, 137(2), 69–78, 1996.

284. Yang, Y. Y., Hu, C. J., Chang, S. M., Tai, T. Y., and Leu, S. J., Aspirin inhibits monocyte chemoattractant protein-one and interleukin-eight expression in TNF-alpha stimulated human umbilical vein endothelial cells, *Atherosclerosis*, 174(2), 207–213, 2004.

285. Yoshimura, T. and Ueda, A., Monocyte chemoattractant protein-one, in B. B. Aggarwal, J. U. Gutterman (Eds.), *Human Cytokines: Handbook for Basic and Clinical Research*, 2nd ed., Blackwell Science, Cambridge, 198–221, 1996.

286. Giulian, D., Woodward, J., Young, D. G., Krebs, J. F., and Lachman, L. B., Interleukin-1 injected into mammalian brain stimulates astrogliosis and neovascularization, *Journal of Neuroscience*, 8(7), 2485–2490, 1988.

287. Das, S. and Potter, H., Expression of the Alzheimer amyloid-promoting factor antichymotrypsin is induced in human astrocytes by IL-1, *Neuron*, 14(2), 447–456, 1995.

288. McKenzie, J. E., Gentleman, S. M., Roberts, G. W., Graham, D. I., and Royston, M. C., Increased numbers of beta APP-immunoreactive neurones in the entorhinal cortex after head injury, *Neuroreport*, 6(1), 161–164, 1994.

289. Goldgaber, D., Harris, H. W., Hla, T., Maciag, T., Donnelly, R. J., Jacobsen, J. S., et al., Interleukin 1 regulates synthesis of amyloid beta-protein precursor mRNA in human endothelial cells, *Proceedings of the National Academy of Sciences of the United States of America*, 86(19), 7606–7610, 1989.

290. Forloni, G., Demicheli, F., Giorgi, S., Bendotti, C., and Angeretti, N., Expression of amyloid precursor protein mRNAs in endothelial, neuronal and glial cells: Modulation by interleukin-1, *Brain Research, Molecular Brain Research*, 16(1–2), 128–134, 1992.

291. Van Den Heuvel, C., Lewis, S., Wong, M., Manavis, J., Finnie, J., Blumbergs, P., et al., Diffuse neuronal perikaryon amyloid precursor protein immunoreactivity in a focal head impact model, *Acta Neurochirurgica*, 71(Suppl.), 209–211, 1998.

292. Buxbaum, J. D., Oishi, M., Chen, H. I., Pinkas-Kramarski, R., Jaffe, E. A., Gandy, S. E., et al., Cholinergic agonists and interleukin 1 regulate processing and secretion of the Alzheimer beta/A4 amyloid protein precursor, *Proceedings of the National Academy of Sciences of the United States of America*, 89(21), 10075–10078, 1992.

293. Hauptmann, S., Keil, U., Scherping, I., Bonert, A., Eckert, A., and Müller, W. E., Mitochondrial dysfunction in sporadic and genetic Alzheimer's disease, *Experimental Gerontology*, 41(7), 668–673, 2006.

294. Chagnon, P., Betard, C., Robitaille, Y., Cholette, A., and Gauvrea, D., Distribution of brain cytochrome oxidase activity in various neurodegenerative diseases, *Neuroreport*, 6(5), 711–715, 1995.

295. Dietschy, J. M. and Turley, S. D., Thematic review series: Brain lipids, cholesterol metabolism in the central nervous system during early development and in the mature animal, *Journal of Lipid Research*, 45(8), 1375–1397, 2004.

296. Snipes, G. J. and Suter, U., Cholesterol and myelin, *Subcellular Biochemistry*, 28, 173–204, 1997.

297. Simons, M. M. D., Keller, P. P., Dichgans, J. M. D., and Schulz, J. B. M. D., Cholesterol and Alzheimer's disease: Is there a link?, *Neurology*, 57(6), 1089–1093, 2001.

298. Adibhatla, R. M. and Hatcher, J. F., Altered lipid metabolism in brain injury and disorders, *Subcellular Biochemistry*, 49, 241–268, 2008.

299. Fenili, D. and McLaurin, J., Cholesterol and APOE: A target for Alzheimer's disease therapeutics, current drug targets, *CNS & Neurological Disorders*, 4(5), 553–567, 2005.

300. Mauch, D. H., Nagler, K., Schumacher, S., Goritz, C., Muller, E.- C., Otto, A., et al., CNS synaptogenesis promoted by glia-derived cholesterol, *Science*, 294(5545), 1354, 2001.

301. Göritz, C., Mauch, D. H., Nägler, K., and Pfrieger F. W., Role of glia-derived cholesterol in synaptogenesis: New revelations in the synapse–glia affair, *Journal of Physiology* (*Paris*), 96(3–4), 257–263, 2002.

302. Graham, D. I., Horsburgh, K., Nicoll, J. A., and Teasdale, G. M., Apolipoprotein E and the response of the brain to injury, *Acta Neurochirurgica*, 73(Suppl.), 89–92, 1999.

303. Urban, R., Harris, P., and Masel, B. Anterior hypopituitarism following traumatic brain injury, *Brain Injury*, 19(5), 349–358, 2005.

304. McCuster, R. H., Strle, K., Broussard, S. R., Dantzer, R., Bluthe, R. M., and Kelley, K. W., Crosstalk between insulin-like growth factors and proinflammatory cytokines, in R. Ader, R. Dantzer, C. Glaser, C. Heijnen, M. Irwin, and D. Padgett et al., (Eds.), *Psychoneuroimmunology*, 171–192, Academic Press, New York, 2006.

305. Avitsur, R., Kavelaars, A., Heijnen, C., and Sheridan, J. F., Social stress and the regulation of tumor necrosis factor-[alpha] secretion, *Brain, Behavior, and Immunity*, 19(4), 311–317, 2005.

306. Silverman, M. N., Pearce, B. D., Biron, C. A., and Miller, A. H., Immune modulation of the hypothalamic–pituitary–adrenal (HPA) axis during viral infection, *Viral Immunology*, 18(1), 41–78, 2005.

307. Lang, C. H., Hong-Brown, L., and Frost, R. A., Cytokine inhibition of JAK-STAT signaling: A new mechanism of growth hormone resistance, *Pediatric Nephrology*, 20(3), 306–312, 2005.

308. Shen, W.- H., Zhou, J.- H., Broussard, S. R., Freund, G. G., Dantzer, R., and Kelley, K. W., Proinflammatory cytokines block growth of breast cancer cells by impairing signals from a growth factor receptor, *Cancer Research*, 62(16), 4746–4756, 2002.

309. Mocellin, S., Rossi, C. R., Pilati, P., and Nitti, D., Tumor necrosis factor, cancer and anticancer therapy, *Cytokine & Growth Factor Reviews*, 16(1), 35–53, 2005.

310. Wajant, H., Gerspach, J., and Pfizenmaier, K., Tumor therapeutics by design: Targeting and activation of death receptors, *Cytokine & Growth Factor Reviews*, 16(1), 55–76, 2005.

311. Spate, U. and Schulze, P. C., Proinflammatory cytokines and skeletal muscle, *Current Opinion in Clinical Nutrition and Metabolic Care*, 7(3), 265–269, 2004.

312. Kelley, K. W., Bluthé, R.- M., Dantzer, R., Zhou, J.- H., Shen, W.- H., Johnson, R. W., et al., Cytokine-induced sickness behavior, *Brain, Behavior, and Immunity*, 17(1, Suppl. 1), 112–118, 2003.

313. Schiepers, O. J. G., Wichers, M. C., and Maes, M., Cytokines and major depression, *Progress in Neuro-Psychopharmacology and Biological Psychiatry*, 29(2), 201–217, 2005.

314. Sweeney, M. I., Kalt, W., MacKinnon, S. L., Ashby, J., and Gottschall-Pass, K. T., Feeding rats diets enriched in low-bush blueberries for six weeks decreases ischemia-induced brain damage, *Nutritional Neuroscience*, 5(6), 427–431, 2002.

315. Wang, Y., Chang, C.- F., Chou, J., Chen, H.- L., Deng, X., Harvey, B. K., et al., Dietary supplementation with blueberries, spinach, or spirulina reduces ischemic brain damage, *Experimental Neurology*, 193(1), 75–84, 2005.

316. Kalt, W., Forney, C. F., Martin, A., and Prior, R. L., Antioxidant capacity, vitamin C, phenolics, and anthocyanins after fresh storage of small fruits, *Journal of Agricultural and Food Chemistry*, 47(11), 4638–4644, 1999.

317. Sellappan, S. and Akoh, C. C., Flavonoids and antioxidant capacity of Georgia-grown Vidalia onions, *Journal of Agricultural and Food Chemistry*, 50(19), 5338–5342, 2002.

318. Neto, C. C., Cranberry and blueberry: Evidence for protective effects against cancer and vascular diseases, *Molecular Nutrition & Food Research*, 51(6), 652–664, 2007.

319. Morazzoni, P. and Magistretti, M. J., Activity of myrtocyan, an anthocyanoside complex from *Vaccinium myrtillus* (VMA), on platelet aggregation and adhesiveness, *Fitoterapia*, 61(13), 13–21, 1990.

320. Youdim, K. A., McDonald, J., Kalt, W., and Joseph, J. A., Potential role of dietary flavonoids in reducing microvascular endothelium vulnerability to oxidative and inflammatory insults, *The Journal of Nutritional Biochemistry*, 13(5), 282–288, 2002.

321. Heinonen, I. M., Meyer, A. S., and Frankel, E. N. Antioxidant activity of berry phenolics on human low-density lipoprotein and liposome oxidation, *Journal of Agricultural and Food Chemistry*, 46(10), 4107–4112, 1998.

322. Frémont, L., Biological effects of resveratrol, *Life Sciences*, 66(8), 663–673, 2000.

323. Huang, S. S., Tsai, M. C., Chih, C. L., Hung, L. M., and Tsai, S. K., Resveratrol reduction of infarct size in Long-Evans rats subjected to focal cerebral ischemia, *Life Sciences*, 69(9), 1057–1065, 2001.

324. Sinha, K., Chaudhary, G., and Kumar Gupta, Y., Protective effect of resveratrol against oxidative stress in middle cerebral artery occlusion model of stroke in rats, *Life Sciences* 71(6), 655–665, 2002.

325. Inoue, H., Jiang, X.- F., Katayama, T., Osada, S., Umesono, K., and Namura, S., Brain protection by resveratrol and fenofibrate against stroke requires peroxisome proliferator-activated receptor [alpha] in mice, *Neuroscience Letters*, 352(3), 203–206, 2003.

326. Joseph, J. A., Denisova, N. A., Arendash, G., Gordon, M., Diamond, D., Shukitt-Hale, B., et al., Blueberry supplementation enhances signaling and prevents behavioral deficits in an Alzheimer disease model, *Nutritional Neuroscience*, 6(3), 153, 2003.

327. Bastianetto, S. and Quirion, R., Natural extracts as possible protective agents of brain aging, *Neurobiology of Aging*, 23(5), 891–897, 2002.

328. Dasgupta, B. and Milbrandt, J., Resveratrol stimulates AMP kinase activity in neurons, *Proceedings of the National Academy of Sciences of the United States of America*, 104(17), 7217–7222, 2007.

329. Hean, Z., Potential mechanism by which resveratrol, a red wine constituent, protects neurons, *Annals of the New York Academy of Sciences*, 993, 276–286, 2003.

330. Scapagnini, G., Butterfield, D. A., Colombrita, C., Sultana, R., Pascale, A., and Calabrese, V., Ethyl ferulate, a lipophilic polyphenol, induces HO-1 and protects rat neurons against oxidative stress, *Antioxidants & Redox Signaling*, 6(5), 811–818, 2004.

331. Slemmer, J. E., Shacka, J. J., Sweeney, M. I., and Weber, J. T., Antioxidants and free radical scavengers for the treatment of stroke, traumatic brain injury and aging, *Current Medicinal Chemistry*, 15(4), 404–414, 2008.

332. Socci, D. J., Crandall, B. M., and Arendash, G. W., Chronic antioxidant treatment improves the cognitive performance of aged rats, *Brain Research*, 693(1–2), 88–94, 1995.

333. Xie, Z. and Sastry, B. R., Induction of hippocampal long-term potentiation by [alpha]-tocopherol, *Brain Research*, 604(1–2), 173–179, 1993.

334. Haller, J., Weggemans, R. M., and Ferry, M. G., Mental health: Mini-Mental State Examination and Geriatric Depression Score of elderly Europeans in the SENECA study of 1993, *European Journal of Clinical Nutrition*, 50(Suppl. 2), S112–S116, 1996.

335. Ortega, R. M., Requejo, A. M., Andres, P., Lopez-Sobaler, A. M., Quintas, M. E., Redondo, M. R., et al., Dietary intake and cognitive function in a group of elderly people, *American Journal of Clinical Nutrition*, 66(4), 803–809, 1997.

336. Flanary, B. E., and Streit, W. J., Alpha-tocopherol (vitamin E) induces rapid, nonsustained proliferation in cultured rat microglia, *Glia*, 53(6), 669–674, 2006.

337. Lodge, J. K., Hall, W. L., Jeanes, Y. M., and Proteggente, A. R., Physiological factors influencing vitamin E biokinetics, *Annals of the New York Academy of Sciences*, 1031, 60–73, 2004.

338. Lodge, J. K., Vitamin E bioavailability in humans, *Journal of Plant Physiology*, 162(7), 790–796, 2005.

339. Bruno, R. S. and Traber, M. G., Vitamin E biokinetics, oxidative stress and cigarette smoking, *Pathophysiology*, 13(3), 143–149, 2006.

340. Veld, B. A., Ruitenberg, A., Hofman, A., Launer, L. J., van Duijn, C. M., Stijnen, T., et al., Nonsteroidal anti-inflammatory drugs and the risk of Alzheimer's disease, *New England Journal of Medicine*, 345(21), 1515–1521, 2001.

341. Mackenzie, I. and Munoz D. G., Nonsteroidal anti-inflammatory drug use and Alzheimer-type pathology in aging, *Neurology*, 50(4), 986–990, 1998.

342. Yan, Q., Zhang, J., Liu, H., Babu-Khan, S., Vassar, R., and Biere, A. L., et al., Anti-inflammatory drug therapy alters {beta}-amyloid processing and deposition in an animal model of Alzheimer's disease, *Journal of Neuroscience*, 23(20), 7504–7509, 2003.

343. Lim, G. P., Chu, T., Yang, F., Beech, W., Frautschy, S. A., and Cole, G. M., The curry spice curcumin reduces oxidative damage and amyloid pathology in an Alzheimer transgenic mouse, *Journal of Neuroscience*, 21(21), 8370–8377, 2001.

344. Bala, K., Tripathy, B., and Sharma, D., Neuroprotective and anti-ageing effects of curcumin in aged rat brain regions, *Biogerontology*, 7(2), 81–89, 2006.

345. Kalmijn, S., Feskens, E. J. M., Launer, L. J., and Kromhout, D., Polyunsaturated fatty acids, antioxidants, and cognitive function in very old men, *American Journal of Epidemiology*, 145(1), 33–41, 1997.

346. Kalmijn, S., Launer, L. J., Ott, A., Witteman, J. C., Hofman, A., and Breteler, M. M., Dietary fat intake and the risk of incident dementia in the Rotterdam Study, *Annals of Neurology*, 42, 776–782, 1997.

347. Choi, S. W., Benzie, I. F. F., Collins, A. R., Hannigan, B. M., and Strain, J. J., Vitamins C and E: Acute interactive effects on biomarkers of antioxidant defence and oxidative stress, *Mutation Research/Fundamental and Molecular Mechanisms of Mutagenesis*, 551(1–2), 109–117, 2004.

348. Poncin, S., Colin, I., and Gerard, A. C., Minimal oxidative load: A prerequisite for thyroid cell function, *Journal of Endocrinology*, 201(1), 161–167, 2009.

349. Oertel, H., Schneider, H. J., Stalla, G. K., Holsboer, F., and Zihl, J., The effect of growth hormone substitution on cognitive performance in adult patients with hypopituitarism, *Psychoneuroendocrinology*, 29(7), 839–850, 2004.

350. Gibney, J., Wolthers, T., Johannsson, G., Umpleby, A. M., and Ho, K. K. Y., Growth hormone and testosterone interact positively to enhance protein and energy metabolism in hypopituitary men, *American Journal of Physiology, Endocrinology, and Metabolism*, 289(2), E266–E271, 2005.
351. Long, J., Gao, F., Tong, L., Cotman, C., Ames, B., and Liu, J., Mitochondrial decay in the brains of old rats: Ameliorating effect of alpha-lipoic acid and acetyl-ʟ-carnitine, *Neurochemical Research*, 34(4), 755–763, 2009.
352. Kidd, P. M., Neurodegeneration from mitochondrial insufficiency: Nutrients, stem cells, growth factors, and prospects for brain rebuilding using integrative management, *Alternative Medicine Review*, 10(4), 268–293, 2005.

13

Neuroplasticity and Rehabilitation Therapy

Robert P. Lehr, Jr.

CONTENTS

13.1 Introduction

The skilled therapist of the brain-injured person requires an understanding of the underlying anatomy and physiology, its relationship to the injury, the mechanisms of learning, and the creative array of multimodal therapeutic skills that they have at their disposal. The 21st century brings an ever-increasing understanding of the mechanisms involved in how the brain accomplishes learning and how these mechanisms are impacted by the traumatic event. We are at a point where we must view more than just the injury to the neurons but must consider the damage to the environment in which the neurons exist. This chapter reviews some of these issues and provides some insight into the therapeutic process.

Therapies are what have been described as being *activity dependent*.[1] Being activity dependent means the therapy is focused to the point that the recipient of the therapy is actively engaged in the therapeutic process. Therapies are designed by the therapist to elicit a key response from the client, and this leads to one part of a successful rehabilitative program. Learned skills have their foundation in the nervous system, and we now know that there are physical changes that take place at the synaptic level to produce the rehabilitative results. It is the synaptic environment that is the ultimate target of the therapeutic process. The purpose of this chapter is to provide therapists with a better understanding of neuronal changes and how the human brain is altered by their therapies.

Neuroplasticity refers to the ability of the brain to change its structure and organization as the organism encounters its environment.[2] The human brain is composed of a collection of neurons that have been shown to be pliable and subject to changes in structure, individually as well as collectively, if the interaction between them is initiated with purposeful intent. Just because the brain is active does not mean it is learning. Learning comes from purposeful activity in which the learner is fully participating. As you will recall, just sitting in the classroom did not guarantee the acquisition of the material of the lecture. It was not until you actively studied the material, committed it to memory, or put it to use that you learned the material. In a like manner, the traumatic brain-injured client must be committed and actively engaged in the therapeutic process.

Now let us look at some of the learning processes therapists initiate and see them on the cellular level. It is hoped that this insight will provide you with a better appreciation of the processes involved and perhaps lead to some innovative therapies.

The early prediction by Hebb[3] that there would be observable changes in the neurons or their synapses was further elaborated by neuroscientists to suggest that the behavioral changes an organism makes in response to the influences of the environment would be reflected in changes in synapses in the central nervous system.[4] Neurobiologists (Bailey and Chen,[5] Kandel,[6] and others) followed with elegant experiments that demonstrated the importance of this synaptic organization and the interactions that occur between the neurons and, as we see later in the chapter, the supporting glia. Using very simple animals, such as marine snails and moving on to rodents and mammals, these investigators were able to clarify the role of the synapse in learning.

Learning is a complex process that has several levels. We will look at learning in terms of habituation, sensitization, classical conditioning, and operant conditioning. These are by no means the only concepts involved in learning, but they will allow us to illustrate some changes that take place at the cellular organization of the brain and to place them in the context of therapy.

13.2 Habituation

Kandel,[6] using the California marine snail *Aplysia,* has demonstrated the simple form of learning known as *habituation*. This form of learning is characterized by the reduced response to a presentation of a novel stimulus. The experimental setup is demonstrated in Figure 13.1. When a stimulus is applied to the siphon, the snail responds by reflex withdrawal of its gill, mantle, and tail. With repeated stimulation to the siphon, there

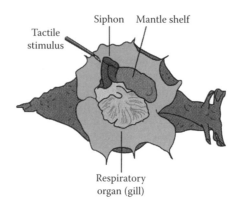

FIGURE 13.1

Marine snail *Aplysia*: experimental setup. (From E. R. Kandel, J. H. Schwartz, and T. M. Jessell, Eds., *Principles of Neural Science*, 4th ed., McGraw-Hill, New York, 2000, chap. 63, p. 1248. With permission.)

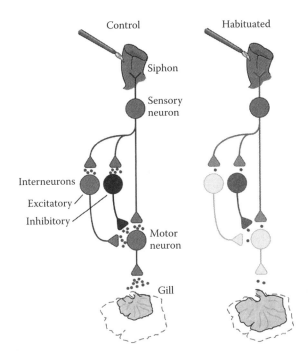

FIGURE 13.2

Marine snail *Aplysia*: gill-withdrawal reflex circuit. (From E. R. Kandel, J. H. Schwartz, and T. M. Jessell, Eds., *Principles of Neural Science*, 4th ed., McGraw-Hill, New York, 2000, chap. 63, p. 1248. With permission.)

is a depression of the reflex response. The decreased response is characterized by a decrease in the synaptic transmission from the presynaptic sensory neurons to the interneurons and motor neurons in the reflex circuit (Figure 13.2). There is a decrease, over time, of the amount of transmitter released. These changes are internal to the presynaptic neuron and can last for a few minutes or a few hours. This is known as *short-term habituation*.

When stimulation occurs over several training sessions, there has been demonstrated an actual reduction in the number of synapses present to the postsynaptic neuron, and this process is known as *long-term habituation*. Although this has not been demonstrated in humans, it can be speculated that this is what occurs when we condition a client who has symptoms of dizziness by constant exposure to a revolving swing. The constant presentation of a stimulus that produces the dizziness will, in time, habituate. First, there is a reduction of neurotransmitter, and then, eventually, a reduction of synaptic connections so that a stable equilibrium may be obtained, without nausea.

13.3 Sensitization

In *sensitization*, the process involves an additional neuron and is more complex. The additional neuron is one that "facilitates" the signal by reinforcement (Figure 13.3). It is an enhancement of the reflex response after the presentation of a strong stimulus. After a strong stimulus, the organism is more attentive to all stimulations to itself, and the

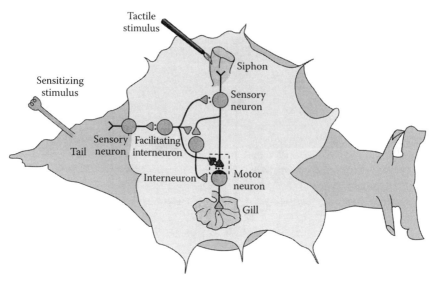

FIGURE 13.3
Marine snail *Aplysia*: gill sensitization. (From E. R. Kandel, J. H. Schwartz, and T. M. Jessell, Eds., *Principles of Neural Science*, 4th ed., McGraw-Hill, New York, 2000, chap. 63, p. 1251. With permission.)

nature of the synapse physically changes.[7] There is an increase in the size of the synaptic zone[7] (Figure 13.4) and in the number of vesicles containing neurotransmitter in the active zone.[8] These changes in the circuit demonstrate that there is a "memory" of what has happened to them. These changes last several minutes and are known as *short-term sensitization*.

Long-term sensitization also occurs following several training sessions. (Figure 13.4) This process produces proteins that enhance the short-term mechanisms and also promotes the growth of axons with new synapses. These newly produced proteins have been shown to be persistently active for up to 24 hours without requiring a continuous signal of any sort. This is an exciting opportunity for the therapy regimen. These new synapses cause the postsynaptic neuron to increase its dendritic branches to accommodate the new synapses from the axons of the presynaptic neurons.[8]

Recent research by Fellin et al.[9] has demonstrated the active role of the glial astrocyte in the coordination of the synaptic processes. Although the details of the exact role of this interaction have not been clarified, there is evidence of a feed forward as well as a feedback modulation of the activity at the "tripartite" synapse (Figure 13.5).

This synaptic plasticity is "activity dependent," and with the increased axonal sproutings, increased neurotransmitters, and corresponding dendritic field expansion, there are changes in the surrounding tissue. There are increases in the glial cell components and an increase in the vascular supply to the region. These changes are rapid and have been identified to take place within 10 to 15 minutes.[10] The therapist must move quickly to reinforce the target behavior when the client demonstrates the acquisition of the sought behavior.

In addition, exercise has been demonstrated to increase the number of synapses in the cerebellum of experimental animals that undergo complex motor skill learning, but not mere motor activity.[11] These demonstrations of the plasticity of the brain at the cellular level show that a new foundation for the behavior has been formed, and the repetition of the behavior will reinforce the newly formed synaptic connection. As we repeat the

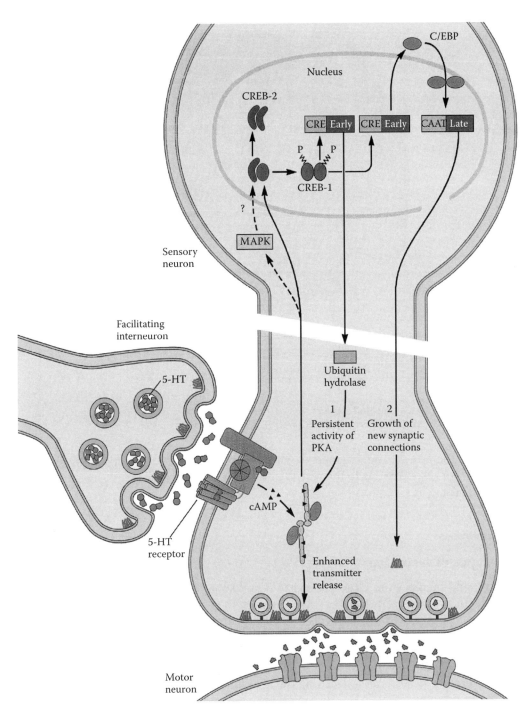

FIGURE 13.4

Schematic model for short-term enhancement and persistent synaptic enhancement with long-term sensitization. 5-HT, serotonin; CAAT, cytidine-adenosine-adenosine-thymidine; cAMP, cyclic adenosine monophosphate; C/EBP, CCAAT-enhancer-binding-proteins; CRE, cyclic AMP response element; CREB-1, cyclic AMP response element-binding proteins-1; CREB-2, cyclic AMP response element-binding proteins-2; MAPK, mitogen-activated protein kinase; PKA, protein kinase A. (From E. R. Kandel, J. H. Schwartz, and T. M. Jessell, Eds., *Principles of Neural Science*, 4th ed., McGraw-Hill, New York, 2000, chap. 63, p. 1255. With permission.)

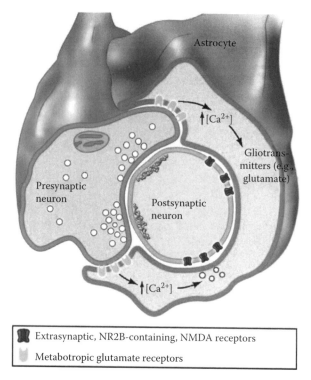

FIGURE 13.5
Schematic representation of the glial astrocyte in the coordination of the synaptic processes. (From Fellin, T., Pascual, O., and Haydon, P. G., *Physiology*, 21(3), 208–215, 2006. With permission.)

activity in a therapy setting, we increase the effectiveness of the corresponding synapses and this, in turn, contributes to the reacquisition of the skills.

13.4 Types of Learning

Learning and memory are closely associated and sometimes difficult to separate except for academic purposes. For the therapist, however, they are intertwined in a more specific way. The rehabilitation process involves the returning to wholeness of the entire person and, as such, makes demands on many systems, from the locomotor to the cognitive. The cellular mechanisms involved in the learning and memory processes we are discussing are the same. The two types of learning we discussed earlier, habituation and sensitization, are forms of *nonassociative* learning during which the organism learns the properties of a single stimulus.

In another form of learning, *associative*, the organism learns about the relationship between two stimuli or between a stimulus and a behavior.[12] For the therapist, it might be more productive to view the learning/memory process as being based on the classification of *explicit* and *implicit* memory. It is not our purpose to engage in an extensive discussion of memory, but to set the stage for the learning process within the therapeutic setting.

Explicit memory deals with facts and events. This form of memory is recalled by a deliberate conscious effort. Facts and remembering events are the purview of the entire rehabilitative team. It is also the area where the cognitive functions of the skills of daily living are rehabilitated. The skills to plan the day, to shop for groceries, and to make change for a dollar are some of the items of concern, and these require the reestablishment of the explicit memory.

Explicit memory has been shown to involve *long-term potentiation* (LTP) in the hippocampus. In fact, the presence of LTP in the hippocampus was the first confirmation of Hebb's rule[3] that learning would be based in the physical changes in the synapse. LTP represents the receptiveness and increased facilitation of the excitatory synaptic potentials in the postsynaptic neurons that can last for hours, weeks, or months.[8] The relationship, in time, of two presenting stimuli increases the efficacy of the two synaptically related cells and is a reminder to the cells of that relationship.

This synaptic enhancement can take different forms in different parts of the hippocampus. Recent research has shown that the hippocampus is a key component in early memory and in the final distribution of information to the multimodal association areas of the cerebral cortex. The left hippocampus seems to be involved with verbal memory, whereas the right hippocampus seems to be more involved with the representation of the environment and the ability to find our way in it.[8] Suffice it to say that the association of the hippocampal and multimodal association cortical neurons and their associated astrocyte cell support is established in the synapses of their respective neurons.[9] The reinforcement with repeated practice is what produces a successful therapeutic regimen.

Implicit memory, on the other hand, refers to how to perform an act. These memories of a specific task do not require conscious effort to recall or to reestablish. They require concentration and a focus on the task at hand, but not the conscious effort of recall. Implicit memory is seen in the training of skilled movements and perceptual skills. These are the skills of walking, driving a car, or performing other motor tasks.[8]

Implicit memories involve habituation and sensitization, but they also include two other processes: *classical conditioning* and *operant conditioning*. These processes involve the concept of association. In classical conditioning, there are two stimuli presented that, after a series of associations with each other, begin to produce a new response. These associations are established in the synapses of the cooperating neurons. This new response then enables the organism to predict the environment.

In operant conditioning, the associative relationship is between the organism and a subsequent behavior produced. The organism learns that, for a specific action, there is a related reward. Thus, if behavior is controlled, then the individual receives an appropriate reward for that action. This is the foundation for the wide use of behavioral modification programs (see Chapter 20, this volume).

Classical conditioning relies on an association in which a stimulus that had been previously incapable of producing a response is paired with a strong stimulus that does produce the response, and the association between the two will eventually produce the response from the weaker stimulus. Classical conditioning results in a greater and longer lasting enhancement. This process is one in which there is a presynaptic facilitation of the synaptic transmission. It is the pairing, in time, of a meaningful relationship that produces the result. The internal mechanisms of the process are solidly established and involve several enzymes and genes.[8] The combinations of enzymes and genes are the same that we saw in the process of long-term sensitization. The production of the cellular proteins by this process forms the foundation for the results seen in the therapeutic program.

13.5 Hierarchical Learning

Rehabilitation, as a process, requires the work of several respective professions. Among these, the professions of physical and occupational therapy hold, as a major tenet, the developmental concepts in neurodevelopmental therapy.[13,14] Neurodevelopmental theory says that there is a basic developmental sequence in the individual from the time of conception to adulthood. The function that is expressed is built on previously learned foundations. We must crawl before we walk. Therefore, it is important that the process of restoration of function should follow the same sequences that occurred in development.

Kandel[6] has shown that the stages of learning mentioned earlier are sequential. The infant *Aplysia* is first capable of only habituation; then, with maturity, dishabituation occurs and finally, sensitization. These sequential stages of learning confirm that learning is a process that builds on previously developed mechanisms and is not complete at birth. This understanding seen in the simple snail lends support to the foundation of some long-standing therapies of rehabilitation[3,4] that suggest a hierarchy exists in the development of the individual, and successful therapy must be carried out in the same order.

It is clear that learning is a hierarchical process and has a neuronal basis. It is not so clear in the cognitive area where we have only begun to investigate the cognitive functions with modern imaging techniques and cellular neurophysiologic experiments. The literature on cognition is rich, indeed, and has provided a foundation of strategies that has been successfully incorporated into the rehabilitation environment (Chapter 18, this volume).

Cognitive scientists will tell us that we are first able to describe objects using very simple descriptions of color, size, and shape. From this base, we can move to the descriptions of their usefulness and, eventually, to the features of the object, allowing use of the object for other extended purposes.[15]

Current concepts in the neural sciences are beginning to reveal a neural concreteness to constructing the visual image from the features of the object. The neural pathway for vision is known to have two parallel pathways that convey different types of information.[16] One pathway, the P pathway, is concerned with form, size, and shape, or *what* the object is. The P pathway projects to the temporal multimodal association cortex. The other pathway, the M pathway, is concerned with movement and depth perception, or *where* the object is located. This M pathway projects to the parietal multimodal association cortex.

As these two pathways project to separate areas of the cerebral cortex, this helps explain the selective loss of some features of an object. As an example, object agnosia, the ability to name an object, is associated with Brodmann areas 18, 20, and 21 on the left temporal cortex, whereas color anomia, the ability to name a color, is associated with the speech zones or connections for Brodmann areas 18 and 37. The mechanism of the complete visual construct is pulled together by a yet-unknown *binding mechanism*.

The binding mechanism takes the properties of form (rectangle), color (yellow), and dimensions in depth (box) and says, "We have a long yellow box!" Thus, the binding mechanism pulls together a single representation of an object from several multimodal association cortices. Treisman et al.[17] and Julesz[18] have suggested that such associations require focused *attention*. They further divide the process into two steps. One is the *preattentive* stage, during which the object is scanned for the size, shape, color, and movement by the parallel processing P and M pathways. A serial processing that is responsible for identifying how to categorize the visually constructed object follows. This categorization is dependent on the hippocampus and the eventual storage of the information about the object in the various association cortices.[10]

Attention is a function of working memory. Baddeley[19] proposed a model in which verbal working memory has two components: a subvocal rehearsal system of a phonologic log accessed by reading words or numbers, and a short-term memory store activated by speech. This "articulatory loop" allows us to retain phone numbers or addresses for short periods of time. He also demonstrated a nonverbal working memory that he called a *visuospatial scratchpad*. Both of these components are greatly dependent on the multimodal association areas of the frontal lobe and its executive function.

Until recently, we have assigned the basal ganglia to a simple role in motor behaviors. Recent work has demonstrated that they also play a key role in cognition, mood, and behavior.[20] Three circuits have been described that originate in the prefrontal association and limbic regions of the cortex and interact with specific areas of the basal ganglia. These areas of the frontal cortex are frequently the ones implicated in the deficits and behaviors seen in the traumatically brain-injured individual in the rehabilitation setting.

The first circuit is the *dorsolateral prefrontal* circuit (Figure 13.6), and this is the one frequently characterized by the term *director of executive functions*. It is the one most closely corresponding to the "articulatory loop" described by Baddeley[19] that is important for working memory. The circuit begins in the prefrontal cortex, projects to the basal ganglia, then to the thalamus, and back to the prefrontal cortex. This circuit undertakes cognitive tasks such as organizing behavioral responses and using verbal responses in problem solving.

The second circuit is the *lateral orbitofrontal* circuit (Figure 13.7). This circuit begins in the lateral orbitofrontal cortex, projects to the basal ganglia and to the thalamus, and returns to the orbitofrontal cortex. This circuit seems to be involved in mediating empathetic and socially appropriate responses. Injury to this area results in the individual being irritable and failing to respond to social cues.

The third circuit is the *anterior cingulate* (Figure 13.8). This circuit is distinguished by its role in motivated behavior, and it may play a role in conveying reinforcing stimuli to diffuse areas of cortical and subcortical regions.[21] This circuit begins in the anterior

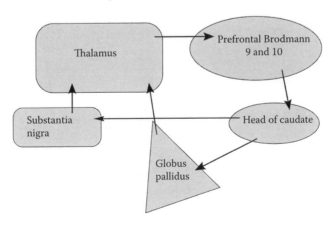

FIGURE 13.6
Dorsolateral prefrontal circuit.

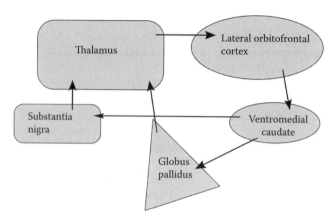

FIGURE 13.7
Lateral orbitofrontal circuit.

cingulate gyrus on the medial surface of the cerebral cortex and projects to the ventral striatum, which in turn receives inputs from the hippocampus, amygdala, and entorhinal cortices. From the ventral striatum, the projection goes to other parts of the basal ganglia, then to the thalamus, and back to the anterior cingulate gyrus. This particular circuit includes dopamine-containing neurons in the midbrain that have inputs to the basal ganglia. It has been suggested that these neurons may deliver reward predictive signals. This circuit may be deeply involved in procedural learning and, as such, this circuit may be important in the behavior modification programs in which reinforcement and reward are utilized.

13.6 Multimodal Rehabilitation

Multimodal rehabilitation refers to a therapeutic approach that attempts to address the individual as a whole person. This places a responsibility on the rehabilitative team to take into

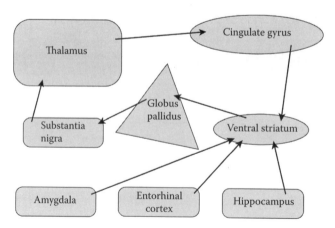

FIGURE 13.8
Anterior cingulate circuit.

account all the rehabilitative possibilities. The process must address the physical aspects of movement and awareness of the environment as well as the cognitive, behavioral, social, and psychological aspects of the individual.

We have just discussed the role of the multimodal association cortices and their role in learning and memory. It was shown that the long-term storage of memories was a function of the hippocampus distributing the component parts of the memory to the parietal, frontal, and temporal lobes. In a similar manner, we noted the distribution of the visual pathways to the multimodal, parietal, and temporal cortices. And the three circuits of the basal ganglia were related to the limbic and frontal association cortices. Saper et al.[22] provided an excellent overview of the association areas of the cerebral cortex and how these structures form the foundations for the cognitive capabilities of the brain.

In each of these descriptions of the related pathway, we mentioned the route through the thalamus. The thalamus is a central structure of ancient origin. Before the development of the cerebral cortex, there was a thalamus that performed the functions of integrating the sensory and motor functions of the organism. It acts as a gatekeeper for information that is conveyed to the cerebral cortex.[23] In this role, it is central to the integration of all the sensory modalities, except olfaction. In addition, it plays a role in the extrapyramidal motor output from the basal ganglia, as well as the three mentioned basal ganglia–cortical circuits concerned with cognition, mood, and behavior.

The thalamus is composed of several nuclei that have different roles (Figure 13.9). Some of the nuclei function for specific sensory modalities such as vision and auditory functions. Others have a motor integrative function, such as pathways to the extrapyramidal tract. Yet others are of a diffuse nature to serve the organism's arousal system. In any case, it is important for the therapist to remember that the thalamus holds the potential to be involved in many of the observed deficits of the head-injured person.

13.7 Neurogenesis in Adult Humans

The old concept that we are born with all the neurons we will ever have and that some neurons die off over our lifetime was recently found to be false. This long-held belief was overturned in an elegant experiment. P. S. Eriksson of Goteborg University, Sweden, and F. H. Gage of the Salk Institute, San Diego, California, demonstrated that new neurons, as defined by biologic markers, are generated from dividing progenitor cells in the dentate gyrus of adult humans.[24] Furthermore, they and their colleagues indicated that the human hippocampus retains its ability to generate neurons throughout life. Exciting prospects and intensive investigations are underway. Their work was built upon that of Gould et al.,[25] who had demonstrated this phenomenon in macaque monkeys. She has subsequently shown that some of these new neurons have an apparent transient existence of only 9 weeks.

This transient existence perhaps holds some promise for utilization for future therapies. Arsenijevic et al.[2] have demonstrated that there are multipotent precursor cells able to generate neurons, astrocytes, and oligodendrocytes in the human brain. Furthermore, they noted that these precursor cells are widely distributed, having been found in many brain regions studied, including the temporal and the frontal cortices, the amygdala, the

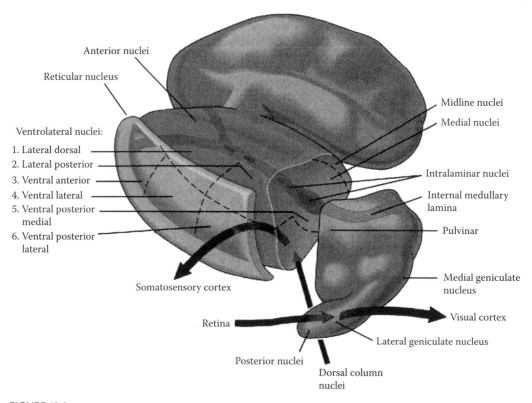

Anterior nuclei

Reticular nucleus

Ventrolateral nuclei:

1. Lateral dorsal
2. Lateral posterior
3. Ventral anterior
4. Ventral lateral
5. Ventral posterior
   medial
6. Ventral posterior
   lateral

Somatosensory cortex

Retina

Posterior nuclei

Dorsal column
nuclei

Midline nuclei

Medial nuclei

Intralaminar nuclei

Internal medullary
lamina

Pulvinar

Medial geniculate
nucleus

Visual cortex

Lateral geniculate nucleus

FIGURE 13.9
The major subdivisions of the thalamus. (From E. R. Kandel, J. H. Schwartz, and T. M. Jessell, Eds., *Principles of Neural Science*, 4th ed., McGraw-Hill, New York, 2000, chap. 18, p. 343. With permission.)

hippocampus, and the periventricular zone. This work demonstrates a possible new platform to study adult human neurogenesis.

A summary of recent work that reflects on the restoration of function indicates that it requires synaptic regeneration even with precursor cells for regions of the injured brain. The injured environment is altered so that the previously permissive nurturing one is altered to make synaptogenesis difficult. In order for the synapses to be regenerated, the proper target must be found by the seeking axon. The postsynaptic membrane must be responsive to the particular neurotransmitter that is released. The proper supporting cells must be viable. The milieu of the surrounding environment must be one of balance of the proper ions and nutrients. Lastly, several key factors that limit regeneration of central axons have been identified and the hope is that, through manipulation, regeneration of synapses may be enhanced.[26]

The discovery of the multipotent precursor cells and the work on manipulating the factors that limit regeneration of central axons suggest that the possibility of transplantation and the rehabilitation of the individual in an enriched environment hold promise for development and recovery of lost functions. The synaptogenesis stimulated by the activity-dependent therapeutic setting should give the cellular basis of learning we have been discussing a strong chance to bring about the rehabilitative results we want. However, these prospects remain speculative, but tantalizing, and will require much further experimental effort to develop to their potential for rehabilitation.

13.8 Constraint-Induced Therapy

More recent has been the discovery of *constraint-induced* therapy for stroke victims.[27] This therapy restricts the movements of the undamaged limb to make maximum use of the appendage that has been impaired. This therapy is not limited to limb movement, but has been seen to be useful in therapy for language disorders, such as aphasia.[28] Such restriction of movement to the impaired structure causes changes in the brain, altering the synapses and enhancing the neuronal connections. These changes can take several forms, such as the assumption of the function by the same region in the other hemisphere, a change in the type of sensory processing from one modality to a new one, or an enlargement of a functional brain region resulting from its expanded use.[29]

In a like manner, it has been demonstrated that exercise, and not just motor activity, can produce physical changes in the brain structure.[30] Gómez-Pinilla et al.[30] have demonstrated in experimental animals that an increase in challenging exercise activity potentiates the effects of physical activity on trophic factor induction in the cerebellum, and that the trophic factor involvement in behavior may provide a molecular basis for the enhanced cognitive function associated with active lifestyles and may guide development of strategies to improve rehabilitation. In addition to the experimental animals, changes that take place in the human motor cortex have been demonstrated with neuroimaging.[31]

This change wrought by the action of the therapist on the impaired person brings about the positive result of rehabilitation. It is the active interaction of the therapist, client, and the environment that causes physical changes in the structure of the brain that have formed the basis of all the therapies ever used. It is only during the past decade or so that we have been able to demonstrate that these changes are taking place at the level of the neurons. These changes in the brain tissue have been demonstrated conclusively by new neuroimaging technology.[32]

13.9 Summary

These are exciting times for researchers and rehabilitation specialists alike. The prospect of new possibilities is incentive to press the frontiers of knowledge. However, it should be remembered that therapies have worked for years without a clear understanding of the underlying foundations of the changes wrought on the brain itself. The constant repetition of the target activity has brought about restoration of function. It is with the deeper knowledge of the changes in the brain that do occur that insights into new therapies may develop.

References

1. Kandel, E. R., Sensory experience and the fine-tuning of synaptic connections, in E. R. Kandel, J. H. Schwartz, and T. M. Jessell (Eds.), *Principles of Neural Science*, 4th ed., McGraw-Hill, New York, 2000, 1114–1130.

2. Arsenijevic, Y., Villemure, J. G., Brunet, J. F., Bloch, J. J., Déglon, N., Kostic, C., Zurn, A., and Aebischer, P., Isolation of multipotent neural precursors residing in the cortex of the adult human brain, *Experimental Neurology*, 170(1), 48–62, 2001.

3. Hebb, D. O., *The Organization of Behavior*, Wiley, New York, 1949.

4. Sejnowski, T. J. and Tesauro, G., The Hebb rule for synaptic plasticity: Algorithms and implementations, in J. H. Burn and W. O. Berry (Eds.), *Neural Models of Plasticity*, Academic Press, San Diego, 1989, 94–101.

5. Bailey, C. H. and Chen, M., Morphological basis of long-term habituation and sensitization, *Science*, 220(4592), 91–93, 1983.

6. Kandel, E. R., Cellular mechanisms of learning and the biological basis of individuality, in E. R. Kandel, J. H. Schwartz, and T. M. Jessell (Eds.) *Principles of Neural Science*, 4th ed., McGraw-Hill, New York, 2000, 1247–1279.

7. Kandel, E. R., Cellular mechanisms of learning and the biological basis of individuality, in E. R. Kandel, J. H. Schwartz, and T. M. Jessell (Eds.) *Principles of Neural Science*, 4th ed., McGraw-Hill, New York, 2000, Ch. 63, Fig. 63-5 B, p. 1255.

8. Kandel, E. R., The molecular biology of memory storage: A dialogue between genes and synapses, *Science*, 294(5544), 1030–1038, 2001.

9. Fellin, T., Pascual, O., and Haydon, P. G., Astrocytes coordinate synaptic networks: Balanced excitation and inhibition, *Physiology*, 21(3), 208–215, 2006.

10. Chang, F. L. F. and Greenough, W. T., Transient and enduring morphological correlates of synaptic activity and efficacy changes in the rat hippocampal slice, *Brain Research*, 309(1), 35–46, 1984.

11. Kleim, J. A., Swaim, R. A., Armstrong, K. A., Napper, R. M., Jones, T. A., and Greenough, W. T., Selective synaptic plasticity within the cerebellar cortex following complex motor skill learning, *Neurobiology of Learning and Memory*, 69(3), 274–289, 1998.

12. Kandel, E. R., Kupfermann, I., and Iversen, S., Learning and memory, in E. R. Kandel, J. H. Schwartz, and T. M. Jessell (Eds.), *Principles of Neural Science*, 4th ed., McGraw-Hill, New York, 2000, 1227–1246.

13. Bobath, B., Treatment of neuromuscular disorders by imposing patterns of coordination, *Physiotherapy*, 55(1), 18–22, 1969.

14. Ayers, A. J., *Sensory Integration and Learning Disorders*, Western Psychological Services, Los Angeles, CA, 1972.

15. Ashley, M. J. and Krych, D. K., Cognitive disorders: Diagnosis and treatment in the TBI Patient, in M. J. Ashley and D. K. Krych (Eds.), *Traumatic Brain Injury Rehabilitation*, CRC Press, Boca Raton, FL, 1995, 289–318.

16. Kandel, E. R. and Wurtz, R. H., Constructing the visual image, in E. R. Kandel, J. H. Schwartz, and T. M. Jessell (Eds.), *Principles of Neural Science*, 4th ed., McGraw-Hill, New York, 2000, 492–506.

17. Treisman, A., Sykes, M., and Glade, G., Selective attention stimulus integration, in S. Dornie (Ed.), *Attention and Performance VI*, Lawrence Erlbaum Associates, Hilldale, NJ, 1977, 333–361.

18. Julesz, B., Toward an axiomatic theory of preattentive vision, in G. M. Edelman, W. E. Gall, and W. M. Cowan (Eds.), *Dynamic Aspects of Neocortical Function*, Wiley, New York, 1984, 585–612.

19. Baddeley, A., Cognitive psychology and human memory, *Trends in Neuroscience*, 11(4), 176–181, 1988.

20. DeLong, M. R., The basal ganglia, in E. R. Kandel, J. H. Schwartz, and T. M. Jessell (Eds.), *Principles of Neural Science*, 4th ed., McGraw-Hill, New York, 2000, 853–867.

21. Graybiel, A. M., The basal ganglia, 2001, R509–R511, http://cogsci.ucsd.edu/~imerzlya/107C/BasalGanglia.pdf.

22. Saper, C. B., Iversen, S., and Frackowiak, R., Integration of sensory and motor function, in E. R. Kandel, J. H. Schwartz, and T. M. Jessell (Eds.), *Principles of Neural Science*, 4th ed., McGraw-Hill, New York, 2000, 349–380.

23. Amaral, D. G., The functional organization of perception and movement, in E. R. Kandel, J. H. Schwartz, and T. M. Jessell (Eds.), *Principles of Neural Science*, 4th ed., McGraw-Hill, New York, 2000, 337–348.

24. Eriksson, P. S., Perfilieva, E., Björk-Eriksson, T., Alborn, A. M., Nordborg, C., Peterson, D. A., and Gage, F. H., Neurogenesis in the adult human hippocampus, *Nature Medicine*, 4(11), 1313–1317, 1998.

25. Gould, E., Vail, N., Wagers, M., and Gross, C. G., Inaugural article: Adult-generated hippocampal and neocortical neurons in macaques have a transient existence, *Proceedings of the National Academy of Sciences of the United States of America*, 98(19), 10910–10917, 2001.

26. Sanes, J. R., and Jessell, T. M., The formation and regeneration of synapses, in E. R. Kandel, J. H. Schwartz, and T. M. Jessell (Eds.), *Principles of Neural Science*, 4th ed., McGraw-Hill, New York, 2000, 1108–1114.

27. Taub, E. and Morris, D. M., Constraint-induced movement therapy to enhance recovery after stroke, *Current Atherosclerosis Report*, 3(4), 279–286, 2001.

28. Pulvermüller, F., Neininger, B., Elbert, T., Mohr, B., Rockstroh, B., Koebbel, P., and Taub, E., Constraint-induced therapy of chronic aphasia after stroke, *Stroke*, 32(7), 1621–1626, 2001.

29. Grafman, J., Conceptualizing functional neuroplasticity, *Journal of Communication Disorders*, 33(4), 345–355, 2000.

30. Gómez-Pinilla, F., So, V., and Kesslak, J. P., Spatial learning and physical activity contribute to the induction of fibroblast growth factor: Neural substrates for increased cognition associated with exercise, *Neuroscience*, 85(1), 53–61, 1998.

31. Levy, C. E., Nichols, D. S., Schmalbrock, P. M., Keller, P., and Chakeres, D. W., Functional MRI evidence of cortical reorganization in upper-limb stroke hemiplegia treated with constraint-induced movement therapy, *American Journal of Physical Medicine and Rehabilitation*, 80(1), 4–12, 2001.

32. Nudo, R. J., Plautz, E. J., and Frost, S. B., Role of adaptive plasticity in recovery of function after damage to motor cortex, *Muscle*, 24(8), 1000–1019, 2001.

14

Pituitary Dysfunction after Traumatic Brain Injury

Sorin G. Beca, Brent Masel, and Randall J. Urban

CONTENTS

14.1 Pathophysiology of the TBI-Induced Pituitary Dysfunction

It has been suspected for almost a century that traumatic brain injury (TBI) can produce pituitary dysfunction, but only during the past decade have we completed prospective studies that document that hypothalamic–pituitary axis damage occurs after TBI. Previously, there were only case reports associating pituitary dysfunction with brain injury. In 2000, Benvenga et al.,[1] reviewed these case reports, raising the possibility of an association between TBI and pituitary dysfunction. They further noted that endocrine dysfunction can occur more than 10 years after the initial injury, and that the injury may not have been substantial enough to require hospitalization, or even be remembered by the patient. Similarly, it is only recently that a clear association has emerged between post-TBI neuroendocrine dysfunction and neurobehavioral and quality of life impairments.

An important aspect of TBI-induced hypopituitarism is the potential impact on brain recovery. It is accepted in the literature[2–6] that the most common neurobehavioral and quality-of-life complaints affecting TBI survivors are memory and concentration deficits, anxiety, depression, fatigue, and loss of emotional well-being. The fact that receptors for pituitary hormones, especially growth hormone (GH) and insulinlike growth factor 1 (IGF-1), are widely present in the brain supports the assumption that they are integral to effective brain repair and recovery.[2–6] It is yet unproved in any study that acute hormonal deficiencies have a deleterious impact on the neuroprotective and early repair processes that follow a TBI. Future studies will address this important possibility.

The exact mechanisms of injury to the pituitary after TBI are not completely understood. To discuss the pathophysiology of pituitary damage, we must first briefly point out the functional anatomy of the gland. The pituitary gland is seated at the base of the skull within the sella turcica and is tethered to the hypothalamus by the infundibulum.

The diaphragma sella separates it from the suprasellar cistern. Both the anterior and the posterior pituitary receive blood supply from the internal carotids. The blood supplied by the long hypophyseal portal veins is fed from the superior hypophyseal arteries and other small branches of the circle of Willis, and it provides the anterior pituitary gland with 70% to 90% of its blood supply. Moreover, hypothalamic releasing hormones are carried by this vascular system to the anterior pituitary. The cellular distribution in the pituitary gland supplied by the long hypophyseal veins includes the somatotrophs (located in the lateral wings of the gland) and the gonadotrophs (mostly located in the peripheral parts of the gland). The short hypophyseal portal veins arise from branches of the intracavernous internal carotid artery, the inferior hypophyseal arteries that enter the sella from below the diaphragma sella, and together provide less than 30% of its vascular supply, predominantly in the medial portion of the gland. The posterior lobe receives its blood supply through the inferior hypophyseal arterial branches.

The most possible mechanisms of injury are direct brain injury event, indirect injuries such as hypoxia and hypotension, and the transient effects of critical illness and medication. Direct mechanisms refer to fractures through the skull base and sella turcica, as well as the shearing injuries of the pituitary, infundibulum, and/or hypothalamus. Although the risk or injury to the anterior lobe is greatest from a basilar skull fracture, the anterior lobe can be injured by any skull fracture or even by severe brain trauma in the absence of fracture.[7] Fractures of the sella turcica after fatal brain injury are found on autopsy in as many as 20% of cases, depending on whether the petrous temporal bone is included in the statistics.[8] Transection or rupture of the pituitary stalk results in anterior lobe infarction because of disruption of the portal blood supply from the hypothalamus to the anterior pituitary. Therefore, it can be inferred that shearing forces delivered from different angles and with varying forces could impair blood flow through the long hypophyseal portal veins to the peripheral pituitary and cause isolated, multiple, or partial deficiencies of anterior pituitary hormone secretion. Currently, there are no adequate animal models to confirm this inference, and imaging techniques have not been developed to assess blood flow to the pituitary through the hypophyseal portal veins after TBI.

Indirectly, functional damage at the hypothalamic–pituitary region can be the result of a secondary hypoxic insult. Another possibility is diffuse axonal injury (DAI) caused by acceleration–deceleration along with rotational forces in motor vehicle crashes. DAI is the principal pathology in 40% to 50% of TBI hospital admissions and is the predominant cause of loss of consciousness (LOC). Secondary to shearing injury, DAI is seen in the midline structures.[9]

Head trauma presents a substantial risk to pituitary function because of that gland's encasement within the sella turcica, its delicate infundibular hypothalamic structures, and its vulnerable vascular supply (Figure 14.1).[10] Therefore, mechanical compression from injury or pituitary gland swelling may play a part in diffuse vascular injury DVI.[11] The long hypophyseal portal vessels and the pituitary stalk are thought to be particularly vulnerable to mechanical trauma, low cerebral blood flow, brain swelling, and intracranial hypertension. The first study that showed traumatic infarction of the anterior pituitary gland was conducted by Daniel et al. half a century ago in a report on fatal head injuries,[12] and one decade later in larger studies proved by Ceballos[13] and Kornblum and Fisher.[14]

Benvenga et al.[1] commented on the peculiar vascularization of the pituitary, noting that the peripheral layer of anterior pituitary cells under the capsule receives arterial blood from the capsule, and not from the two systems of portal veins. Therefore, these cells and those in a small area close to the posterior lobe are the only surviving cells in cases

Arteries and veins of hypothalamus and hypophysis

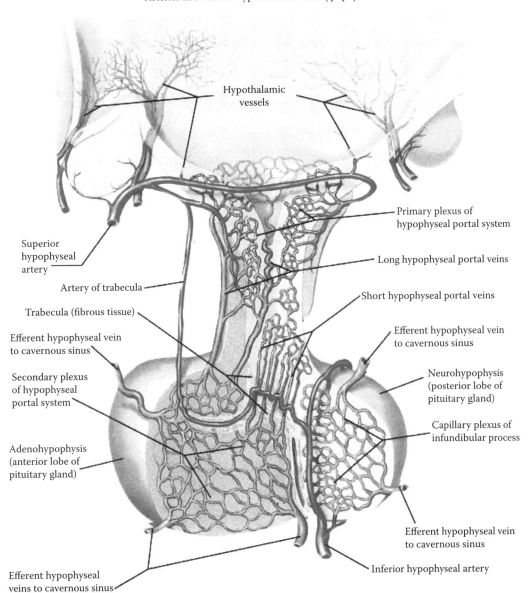

Hypothalamic vessels

Primary plexus of hypophyseal portal system

Long hypophyseal portal veins

Superior hypophyseal artery

Artery of trabecula

Trabecula (fibrous tissue)

Short hypophyseal portal veins

Efferent hypophyseal vein to cavernous sinus

Efferent hypophyseal vein to cavernous sinus

Secondary plexus of hypophyseal portal system

Neurohypophysis (posterior lobe of pituitary gland)

Capillary plexus of infundibular process

Adenohypophysis (anterior lobe of pituitary gland)

Efferent hypophyseal vein to cavernous sinus

Efferent hypophyseal veins to cavernous sinus

Inferior hypophyseal artery

FIGURE 14.1
Blood supply of the hypothalamus and pituitary. (Reproduced from Netter Images, 2006. Used with permission of Elsevier. All rights reserved.)

of pure anterior lobe necrosis. Interestingly, severed portal vessels can regenerate, which may explain the occasional report of recovery from anterior pituitary insufficiency that is a complication of head trauma.[15]

Pathophysiology of acute hypopituitarism after TBI is even less studied because of the complicated nature of a severely ill patient. Recently, Cohan et al.[16] demonstrated that acute central (pituitary) adrenal insufficiency was present in a majority of patients with moderate to severe TBI, measured by acute cortisol and adrenocorticotropic hormone (ACTH) levels. Factors that correlated with adrenal insufficiency were younger age, lower Glasgow Coma Scale (GCS) score (trauma severity), early ischemic insults, as well as etomidate use. Metabolic suppressive agents (such as propofol and pentobarbital) or etomidate had a transient and reversible effect on the corticotrophic function of the pituitary.

The stress of critical illness has serious effects on the acute functioning of all anterior pituitary hormonal axes. Euthyroid syndrome (low thyroid-stimulating hormone [TSH], low T3 and high reverse T3) occurs commonly in critically ill patients. The gonadotropic axis is also suppressed, with acute lowering of gonadal hormones.

14.2 Clinical Symptoms of Hypopituitarism

For those who survive a (severe) TBI, the clinical manifestations vary widely depending on the type, site, and severity of the injury, including direct or indirect injury to the hypothalamus and pituitary. Any of the hormones produced by the anterior or posterior pituitary can be affected by TBI. Release of the anterior pituitary hormones (GH, TSH, luteinizing hormone [LH], follicle-stimulating hormone [FSH], and ACTH) is stimulated by the neuropeptide-releasing hormones from the hypothalamus. The posterior pituitary hormones (vasopressin, oxytocin) are produced by the hypothalamus and are carried by long axonal projections into the posterior pituitary, from which they are later released. Pituitary hormones regulate many processes that are critical for normal metabolic function and normal life expectancy. As a result, deficiency of one or more of these hormones will produce diverse symptoms and signs, with consequent severe morbidity and possibly reduced life expectancy. Failure to identify hypopituitarism could adversely affect a patient's ability to adapt physically and mentally after TBI. Reductions in muscle mass, exercise capacity, and energy are associated with GH deficiency.[17] Thyroid hormone deficiency and testosterone deficiency[18] are a significant concern in patients attempting to maximize their recovery from a TBI. The patient's history and physical examination may help determine whether hypopituitarism is present. For example, decreased ACTH may lead to complaints of weakness or fatigue or to symptoms of hypoglycemia. Patients with decreased TSH may experience cold intolerance or fatigue. Decreased LH or FSH may result in sexual dysfunction, menstrual abnormalities, and infertility. In GH deficiency, lean body mass decreases and body fat increases. Exercise tolerance is decreased and the patient will complain of a loss of well-being and overall quality of life. The GH–IGF-1 axis plays an important role in executive function and memory function. GH deficiency is associated with poor cognition, and GH replacement in severe GH deficiency results in improved cognition in patients without TBI.[19] Leon-Carrion et al.[20] demonstrated cognitive impairments in GH-deficient patients after TBI and suggested that treatment with GH could improve cognition. The anterior pituitary deficiencies with corresponding clinical symptoms are summarized in Table 14.1. Posterior pituitary deficiencies after TBI are common in the acute phase, but they usually are not permanent and are easily detectable in acute settings by assessment of urine osmolality.

Because the clinical manifestations of these anterior pituitary hormone deficiencies may be nonspecific and are often attributed to the physical and psychological sequelae of the brain trauma itself,[1] the clinical diagnosis of hypopituitarism is challenging and the diagnosis may be delayed for months or years. Education regarding TBI and pituitary dysfunction is an important next step for endocrinologists, neurologists, neurosurgeons, and rehabilitation health care providers.

TABLE 14.1

Clinical Signs and Symptoms of Hypopituitarism

Signs and Symptoms	Associated Hormones
Weakness, fatigue, decreased exercise tolerance	ACTH, GH, LH, FSH, TSH
Increased body fat	GH, LH, FSH
Decreased muscle mass	GH, LH, FSH
Loss of libido, erectile dysfunction, oligo-/amenorrhea, infertility	LH, FSH
Ischemic heart disease	GH
Shortened life span	GH
Weight loss, weight gain	ACTH, TSH
Cognition, psychomotor speed	GH, TSH
Attention, learning	GH, TSH
Memory	GH, TSH, LH, FSH

ACTH, adrenocorticotropic hormone; FSH, follicle stimulating hormone; GH, growth hormone; LH, luteinizing hormone; TSH, thyroid-stimulating hormone.

14.3 Guidelines for Screening for Hypopituitarism

The probability of developing hypopituitarism has been based on the severity of the TBI,[1,10] especially when associated with cranial fractures, cerebral damage, and a prolonged period of LOC (Figure 14.2).[21] Therefore, a major distinction for consideration of who to treat is based on moderate to severe versus mild head injury. There is a lack of studies on mild TBI, whereas moderate to severe TBI has been extensively studied. The most widely used clinical classification of TBI severity is the GCS. It defines the severity of TBI within the past 48 hours and is based on the patient's eye opening and verbal and motor response to stimuli. A score of 13 to 15 points is considered mild; 9 to 12 points, moderate, and ≤8 points, severe.[22] Other factors that define clinical severity of TBI include duration of LOC, posttraumatic amnesia, and radiologically identified intracranial lesion.[11,21] The radiologic findings on computed tomography (CT) are based on Marshall Classification. Kelly et al.[10] identified GCS scores of <10 points, diffuse brain swelling on initial CT, and hypotensive or hypoxic insults as significant predictors of developing hypopituitarism. By contrast, Lieberman et al.[23] found no correlation between severity of head injury and pituitary dysfunction as assessed by GCS score. Although mild TBI was not included in the study by Agha et al.,[24] patients with severe or moderate TBI did not display a relationship between hypopituitarism and TBI severity, as measured by either GCS score or CT scan findings. In addition, in two prominent studies by Aimaretti et al.,[25,26] the degree of hypopituitarism was not related to the GCS or the Fisher scale.

Many questions remain regarding which patients are at greatest risk for TBI-induced hypopituitarism.[27] Techniques used to identify and assess TBI have yielded conflicting results. Low serum IGF-I levels are indicative of GH deficiency, but they also may be caused by other diseases or result from advancing age.[28] Continuous monitoring of electroencephalograms can be a useful prognostic tool for patients with moderate to severe TBI during the first 3 days after injury,[29] but routine use of electroencephalograms for very slight head injury is discouraged.[30] Confounding the issue even further is the lack of consensus on the criteria for defining TBI as mild, moderate, or severe.[18,31] The patients with TBI are first seen by the trauma surgeons and neurosurgeons, neurologists and physiatrists. Subsequent

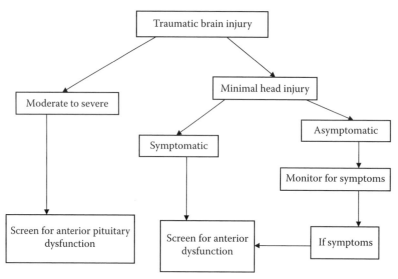

FIGURE 14.2
Screening for hypopituitarism based on the severity of brain injury.

therapy is provided by the rehabilitation physicians. Because the pituitary deficiency may not be diagnosed for many years after TBI, rehabilitation physicians must continuously monitor their patient for signs and symptoms indicative of hypothalamic–pituitary impairment. There is a body of evidence that patients with severe TBI need to be screened. Several studies show the importance to screen patients with moderate to severe TBI for anterior and posterior dysfunction. In conclusion, all patients with moderate to severe TBI and symptoms should be studied. However, physicians should also be aware of clinical symptoms of anterior or posterior pituitary dysfunction in patients with mild TBI.

At this time, we can outline a time frame for the evolution of TBI-induced pituitary dysfunction, allowing us to suggest recommendations for testing and treatment (Table 14.2). Hypopituitarism identified immediately after TBI may not always persist or may require long-term treatment. We will briefly discuss three prominent studies with specific phases: acute[24] (7–21 days), recovery[25,26] (3 months–1 year), and chronic (>1 year).[32] These studies display specific phases of TBI (and subarachnoid hemorrhage) to assist with the guidelines of when to treat. Agha et al.[24] examined the prevalence of anterior and posterior pituitary dysfunction during the acute (7–21 days) phase following TBI. This series identified deficiencies in need of immediate replacement such as ACTH deficiency and posterior pituitary dysfunction. Aimaretti et al.[25,26] examined head injury (TBI and subarachnoid hemorrhage) during the recovery phase (3 months–1 year). Panhypopituitarism

TABLE 14.2

Phases of Pituitary Deficiencies after Traumatic Brain Injury

Phase	Pituitary Axis Dysfunction
Acute, 7–21 days	ACTH, antidiuretic hormone (ADH) (evaluate and treat)
Recovery, 3–12 months	Panhypopituitarism: definitive Multiple deficiencies: variable (can recover partially/completely) Isolated deficiency: good chance of recovery
Chronic, >1 year	Usually remain permanent

at 3 months showed no recovery at 1 year. Isolated hormonal deficits could change between 3 months and 1 year. In the study by Bondanelli et al.,[32] there were patients who developed anterior pituitary deficiencies more than 1 year after their TBI.

In conclusion, we recommend screening the moderate to severe TBI subject acutely for diabetes insipidus (DI) and ACTH deficiency. Anterior hormone screening should be considered at 3 months to make certain that a patient does not have panhypopituitarism. For most TBI patients, endocrine screening at 1 year will detect treatable deficiencies that are permanent. In TBI patients who show normal pituitary function after 1 year, the clinician should be alert to pituitary dysfunction in the years following TBI.

14.4 Endocrine Testing

The hospital record at the time of admission should be reviewed for low GCS score and other indicators of moderate to severe brain injury, hypoxic and hypotensive episodes, brain swelling, and diabetes insipidus, all of which may increase the probability of hypopituitarism. Although diabetes insipidus is routinely attributed to pituitary insult, it only occurs in approximately 30% of patients with both TBI and hypopituitarism, and it is usually transient. Endocrine evaluation should therefore be considered despite the absence of DI. A full endocrinologic evaluation should be considered in all patients with the aforementioned conditions. In addition, patients with mild trauma should be considered for evaluation if they develop symptoms without the confounding physical disabilities.

For TBI patients, pituitary gland function should be tested prospectively or retrospectively.[27] Routine basal hormonal testing should be performed for any patient hospitalized with a TBI who has symptoms such as polyuria, hyponatremia, or hypotension. Acutely, the adrenal axis should be treated. Prospectively, moderate to severe TBI patients should undergo a baseline hormonal evaluation at 3 and 12 months after the primary brain insult. Retrospectively, all patients with any signs or symptoms of hypopituitarism with a history of moderate or severe TBI more than 12 months earlier should undergo hormonal testing.

In terms of testing, each individual axis needs to be evaluated.[27] Basal free T4 and TSH levels should be measured to evaluate the thyroid axis. To evaluate gonadal function, baseline LH and FSH levels, together with a morning testosterone level should be obtained in men and an estradiol level should be obtained in premenopausal women who are not menstruating regularly. Prolactin levels should be measured in all patients. A basal morning (9 am) cortisol level should be measured initially to screen for severe adrenal insufficiency. If cortisol levels are less than 500 nmol/L (18 µg/dL), the patient should be referred to an endocrinologist for further assessment. This involves a dynamic stimulatory test for adrenal reserve using the insulin tolerance test (ITT), glucagon stimulation test, or short ACTH (Cosyntropin) test. Patients should have normal thyroid function, or be on appropriate thyroid hormone replacement, before stimulation testing. The ITT is contraindicated in patients with a history of ischemic heart disease or epilepsy. For this reason, some clinicians prefer to avoid the ITT in head trauma patients.[23,33,34] One stimulation test is sufficient for the diagnosis of adult growth hormone deficiency (GHD). For adult GHD, the gold standard for diagnosis is the ITT, but ITT is contraindicated in many trauma patients because of risk of seizures. Among the classic provocative tests, a good alternative for both GH and ACTH is the glucagon stimulation test. The other provocative tests to consider are growth hormone-releasing hormone in combination with arginine, as well with

TABLE 14.3

Routine Basal Hormonal Screening Tests for TBI-Induced Hypopituitarism

Basal Hormone Test	Test Time
Serum cortisol (morning)	9 AM
Free T4, TSH, free T3	9 AM
Insulinlike growth factor 1	9 AM
Follicle-stimulating hormone, luteinizing hormone, testosterone (in men) or 17βE2 (in women)	9 AM
Prolactin	9 AM
Patients with polyuria: diuresis, urine density, Na^{++}, and plasma osmolality	Any time
Dynamic Testing	
Cosyntropin (ACTH) stimulation test: 250 μg ACTH intramuscularly/intravenously and measure serum cortisol 30 minutes and 60 minutes later (normal, >500 nmol/L or 18 μg/dL)	Any time

Source: Ghigo, E., Masel, B., Aimaretti, G., Leon-Carrion, J., Casanueva, F. F., Dominguez-Morales, M. R., Elovic, E., et al., *Brain Injury*, 19(9), 711–724, 2005.

GH secretagogues.[35] Not all patients suspected of having GHD, however, require a GH stimulation test for diagnosis. Patients with three or more pituitary hormone deficiencies and an IGF-1 less than the reference range have a greater than 97% chance of being GH deficient, and therefore, do not need a GH stimulation test. A normal serum IGF-1 level does not exclude the diagnosis. Dynamic stimulatory testing for GH reserve will usually be required. Hypoglycemia is the most potent stimulus for both somatotropic and corticotropic functions. The ITT or glucagon tests enable adrenal and GH reserves to be assessed simultaneously. Table 14.3 provides an algorithm for routine basal hormonal testing for TBI-induced hypopituitarism and Table 14.4 provides the main provocation/dynamic tests required for diagnosis of the pituitary deficiencies.

Cranial magnetic resonance imaging provides the most specific cross-sectional views of the hypothalamus and pituitary. Although radiographic assessment of the pituitary is often not useful in diagnosis, imaging studies may reveal the nature of the pituitary injury and may help localize the insult.[36] Visualization of a pituitary stalk interruption

TABLE 14.4

Summary of Typical Provocation Tests Performed by Endocrinologists for Hypopituitarism

Provocative Agent and Dosage	Assay Times (min)	Response
Insulin-induced hypoglycemia[a]: 0.05–0.15 regular insulin IU/kg intravenously at 0 min	0, 30, 45, 60, 75, 90	Cortisol, >500 mmol/L (18 mg/dL)
		Normal GH, peak >5 mg/L
		Severe GHD, peak GH <3 mg/L
Glucagon stimulation test: 1 mg intramuscularly at 0 min	0, 90, 120, 150, 180	Cortisol, >500 mmol/L (18 mg/dL)
		Normal GH, peak >5 mg/L
		Severe GHD, peak GH <3 mg/L
Cosyntropin ACTH stimulation test: 250 μg intravenously/intramuscularly	0, 30, 60	Cortisol, >500 mmol/L (18 mg/dL)
GHRH–arginine: GHRH, 1 mg/kg intravenously at 0 min; arginine, 0.5 g/kg (maximum dose, 30 g)	0, 30, 45, 60	Normal GH, peak >16.5 mg/L
		Severe GHD, peak GH <9 mg/L

[a] The insulin tolerance test is contraindicated in patients with central nervous system pathologies.
GHD, growth hormone deficiency; GHRH, growth hormone-releasing hormone.

confirms the diagnosis and is predictive of multiple anterior pituitary hormone deficiencies. However, the absence of visual damage on imaging studies does not exclude hormonal abnormalities.

14.5 Replacement Therapy Rationale

Most endocrinopathies following TBI are the result of failure at the anterior pituitary level. Studies investigating the benefits of hormone replacement in TBI patients are ongoing, but there are published studies of the benefits of hormone replacement in deficient patients from causes other than TBI. Treatment involves replacement of individual hormones, depending on the specific deficiencies, to control signs and symptoms and to enable patients to perform normal daily activities. After hormone dosages are determined, they generally remain unchanged except during periods of illness or other unusual stress, and there is a need for life-long treatment.[7] Therapy should follow the general progression of the pituitary dysfunction after TBI: acute phase (1–3 weeks), recovery phase (3–12 months), and chronic (>1 year; Table 14.4). It is well known that pituitary hormone secretions are affected immediately after TBI, but these may not always persist or require long-term treatment. During the acute phase, Agha et al.[28] demonstrated deficiencies in need of immediate replacement: ACTH deficiency (secondary adrenal insufficiency) and posterior pituitary dysfunction (DI and syndrome of inappropriate antidiuretic hormone [SIADH]).

TBI can cause central adrenal deficiency, which can be life threatening, and hydrocortisone therapy should begin as soon as the diagnosis is confirmed by an ACTH stimulation test or other appropriate test. If TSH deficiency is identified, thyroid replacement therapy can start only after serum cortisol levels are normalized (the thyroid hormone enhances the metabolism for cortisol; therefore, it could unmask/worsen a compensated adrenal insufficiency/deficiency). Sex hormone replacement therapy may be initiated in men and in premenopausal women with LH and FSH deficiencies. Replacement of sex hormones improves body composition, energy levels, and general well-being. Replacement can also normalize sexual function and reduce the risk of osteoporosis.

There is a consensus among the endocrinologists that patients with panhypopituitarism or multiple pituitary deficits should undergo immediate replacement therapy for all pituitary deficiencies, with the notable exception of GHD. It is demonstrated that the other hormonal deficits, once replaced, can restore the normal GH response to the provocative tests. For isolated pituitary deficit of GH, provocative testing should be postponed until 12 months after trauma to prove that GHD is persistent. Similarly, the gonadotropic deficit is recommended to be replaced only after retesting, because it is known that gonadal function is transiently impaired as a result of concurrent stressful conditions and can recover over time. In addition, secondary hypogonadism is not a clinical emergency.

The neuropsychological benefits for the replacement of anterior pituitary hormones in patients with TBI have not been studied, but they represent a promising possibility for improved mental function. Such studies are currently being initiated in patients with TBI. There are suggestions in the literature that the efficacy of hormonal replacement should include neuropsychiatric evaluation tests for fatigue (Fatigue Severity Scale, [Multidimensional Fatigue Inventory 20]), emotion (visual analogue mood scale and neurologic changes of personality inventory), cognition (digit vigilance task), and quality of life (assessment of GHD in adults).

14.6 Summary

TBI is one of the important causes of disability and pituitary dysfunction after moderate to severe TBI occurs in a significant proportion of these patients. The exact mechanism of pituitary damage is not completely understood. Symptoms of hypopituitarism in TBI survivors are difficult to differentiate from other posttraumatic sequelae. Hormone replacement is helping patients to recover on physical and psychological levels. With this chapter we hope to increase the awareness of the medical community for the need to screen and treat pituitary dysfunction actively, even many years after TBI.

References

1. Benvenga, S., Campenni, A., Ruggeri, R. M., and Trimarchi, F., Clinical review 113: Hypopituitarism secondary to head trauma, *Journal of Clinical Endocrinology and Metabolism,* 85(4), 1353–1361, 2000.
2. D'Ercole, A. J., Ye, P., Calikoglu, A. S., and Gutierrez-Ospina, G., The role of the insulin-like growth factors in the central nervous system, *Mol. Neurobiol.,* 13(3), 227–255, 1996.
3. Dusick, J. R., Wang, C., Cohan, P., Swerdloff, R., and Kelly, D. F., Pathophysiology of hypopituitarism in the setting of brain injury, in *Pituitary,* (Epub ahead of print), 2008.
4. Hellawell, D. J., Taylor, R. T., and Pentland, B., Cognitive and psychosocial outcome following moderate or severe traumatic brain injury, *Brain Injury,* 13(7), 489–504, 1999.
5. Kelly, D. F., McArthur, D. L., Levin, H., Swimmer, S., Dusick, J. R., Cohan, P., Wang, C., and Swerdloff, R., Neurobehavioral and quality of life changes associated with growth hormone insufficiency after complicated mild, moderate, or severe traumatic brain injury, *Journal of Neurotrauma,* 23(6), 928–942, 2006.
6. Scheepens, A., Sirimanne, E. S., Breier, B. H., Clark, R. G., Gluckman, P. D., and Williams, C. E., Growth hormone as a neuronal rescue factor during recovery from CNS injury, *Neuroscience,* 104(3), 677–687, 2001.
7. Mitchell, A., Steffenson, N., and Davenport, K., Hypopituitarism due to traumatic brain injury: A case study, *Critical Care Nurse,* 17(4), 34–37, 40–42, 46–51, 1997.
8. Samadani, U., Reyes-Moreno, I., and Buchfelder, M., Endocrine dysfunction following traumatic brain injury: Mechanisms, pathophysiology, and clinical correlations, *Acta Neurochirurgica,* 93(Suppl.), 121–125, 2005.
9. Estes, S. M. and Urban, R. J., Hormonal replacement in patients with brain injury-induced hypopituitarism: Who, when, and how to treat?, *Pituitary,* 8(3–4), 267–270, 2005.
10. Kelly, D. F., Gonzalo, I. T., Cohan, P., Berman, N., Swerdloff, R., and Wang, C., Hypopituitarism following traumatic brain injury and aneurysmal subarachnoid hemorrhage: A preliminary report, *Journal of Neurosurgery,* 93(5), 743–752, 2000.
11. Greenwald, B. D., Burnett, D. M., and Miller, M. A., Congenital and acquired brain injury, 1. Brain injury: Epidemiology and pathophysiology, *Archives of Physical Medicine and Rehabilitation,* 84(3 Suppl. 1), S3–S7, 2003.
12. Daniel, P. M., Prichard, M. M., and Treip, C. S., Traumatic infarction of the anterior lobe of the pituitary gland, *Lancet,* 2(7109), 927–931, 1959.
13. Ceballos, R., Pituitary changes in head trauma (analysis of 102 consecutive cases of head injury), *Alabama Journal of Medical Sciences,* 3(2), 185–198, 1966.
14. Kornblum, R. N. and Fisher, R. S., Pituitary lesions in craniocerebral injuries, *Archives of Pathology,* 88(3), 242–248, 1969.

15. Iglesias, P., Gomez-Pan, A., and Diez, J. J., Spontaneous recovery from post-traumatic hypopituitarism, *Journal of Endocrinological Investigation*, 19(5), 320–323, 1996.

16. Cohan, P., Wang, C., McArthur, D. L., Cook, S. W., Dusick, J. R., Armin, B., Swerdloff, et al., Acute secondary adrenal insufficiency after traumatic brain injury: A prospective study, *Critical Care Medicine*, 33(10), 2358–2366, 2005.

17. Beca, S. G., High, Jr., W. M., Masel, B. E., Mossberg, K. A., and Urban, R. J., What are critical outcome measures for patients receiving pituitary replacement following brain injury?, *Pituitary*, (Epub ahead of print), 2008.

18. Carroll, L. J., Cassidy, J. D., Holm, L., Kraus, J., and Coronado, V. G., Methodological issues and research recommendations for mild traumatic brain injury: The WHO Collaborating Centre Task Force on Mild Traumatic Brain Injury, *Journal of Rehabilitation Medicine*, 43(Suppl.), 113–125, 2004.

19. Aleman, A., Verhaar, H. J., de Haan, E. H., de Vries, W. R., Samson, M. M., Drent, M. L., Van der Veen, E. A., and Kippeschaar, H. P., Insulin-like growth factor-I and cognitive function in healthy older men, *Journal of Clinical Endocrinology and Metabolism*, 84(2), 471–475, 1999.

20. Leon-Carrion, J., Leal-Cerro, A., Cabezas, F. M., Atutxa, A. M., Gomez, S. G., Cordero, J. M., Moreno, A. S., Ferrari, M. D., and Dominguez-Morales, M. R., Cognitive deterioration due to GH deficiency in patients with traumatic brain injury: A preliminary report, *Brain Injury*, 21(8), 871–875, 2007.

21. Marshall, L. F., Marshall, S. B., Klauber, M. R., Van Berkum, C. M., Eisenberg, H., Jane, J. A., Luerssen, T. G., Marmarou, A., and Foulkes, M. A., The diagnosis of head injury requires a classification based on computed axial tomography, *Journal of Neurotrauma*, 9(Suppl. 1), S287–S292, 1992.

22. Teasdale, G. and Jennett, B., Assessment of coma and impaired consciousness: A practical scale, *Lancet*, 2(7872), 81–84, 1974.

23. Lieberman, S. A., Oberoi, A. L., Gilkison, C. R., Masel, B. E., and Urban, R. J., Prevalence of neuroendocrine dysfunction in patients recovering from traumatic brain injury, *Journal of Clinical Endocrinology and Metabolism*, 86(6), 2752–2756, 2001.

24. Agha, A., Rogers, B., Mylotte, D., Taleb, F., Tormey, W., Phillips, J., and Thompson, C. J., Neuroendocrine dysfunction in the acute phase of traumatic brain injury, *Clinical Endocrinology*, 60(5), 584–591, 2004.

25. Aimaretti, G., Ambrosio, M. R., Di Somma, C., Fusco, A., Cannavo, S., Gasperi, M., Scaroni, C., et al., Traumatic brain injury and subarachnoid haemorrhage are conditions at high risk for hypopituitarism: Screening study at 3 months after the brain injury, *Clinical Endocrinology*, 61(3), 320–326, 2004.

26. Aimaretti, G., Ambrosio, M. R., Di Somma, C., Gasperi, M., Cannavo, S., Scaroni, C., Fusco, A., et al., Residual pituitary function after brain injury-induced hypopituitarism: A prospective 12-month study, *Journal of Clinical Endocrinology and Metabolism*, 90(11), 6085–6092, 2005.

27. Ghigo, E., Masel, B., Aimaretti, G., Leon-Carrion, J., Casanueva, F. F., Dominguez-Morales, M. R., Elovic, E., et al., Consensus guidelines on screening for hypopituitarism following traumatic brain injury, *Brain Injury*, 19(9), 711–724, 2005.

28. Urban, R. J., Harris, P., and Masel, B., Anterior hypopituitarism following traumatic brain injury, *Brain Injury*, 19(5), 349–358, 2005.

29. Vespa, P. M., Boscardin, W. J., Hovda, D. A., McArthur, D. L., Nuwer, M. R., Martin, N. A., Nenov, V., et al., Early and persistent impaired percent alpha variability on continuous electroencephalography monitoring as predictive of poor outcome after traumatic brain injury, *Journal of Neurosurgery*, 97(1), 84–92, 2002.

30. Korinthenberg, R., Schreck, J., Weser, J., and Lehmkuhl, G., Post-traumatic syndrome after minor head injury cannot be predicted by neurological investigations, *Brain and Development*, 26(2), 113–117, 2004.

31. de Kruijk, J. R., Twijnstra, A., Meerhoff, S., and Leffers, P., Management of mild traumatic brain injury: Lack of consensus in Europe, *Brain Injury*, 15(2), 117–123, 2001.

32. Bondanelli, M., De Marinis, L., Ambrosio, M. R., Monesi, M., Valle, D., Zatelli, M. C., Fusco, A., Bianchi, A., Farneti, M., and Degli Uberti, E. C., Occurrence of pituitary dysfunction following traumatic brain injury, *Journal of Neurotrauma*, 21(6), 685–696, 2004.
33. Biller, B. M., Samuels, M. H., Zagar, A., Cook, D. M., Arafah, B. M., Bonert, V., Stavrou, S., Kleinberg, D. L., Chipman, J. J., and Hartman, M. L., Sensitivity and specificity of six tests for the diagnosis of adult GH deficiency, *Journal of Clinical Endocrinology and Metabolism*, 87(5), 2067–2079, 2002.
34. Ho, K. K. and 2007 GH Deficiency Consensus Workshop Participants, Consensus guidelines for the diagnosis and treatment of adults with GH deficiency II: A statement of the GH Research Society in association with the European Society for Pediatric Endocrinology, Lawson Wilkins Society, European Society of Endocrinology, Japan Endocrine Society, and Endocrine Society of Australia, *European Journal of Endoerinology*, 157(6), 695–700, 2007.
35. Ghigo, E., Aimaretti, G., Arvat, E., and Camanni, F., Growth hormone-releasing hormone combined with arginine or growth hormone secretagogues for the diagnosis of growth hormone deficiency in adults, *Endocrine*, 15(1), 29–38, 2001.
36. Argyropoulou, M., Perignon, F., Brauner, R., and Brunelle, F., Magnetic resonance imaging in the diagnosis of growth hormone deficiency, *Journal of Pediatrics*, 120(6), 886–891, 1992.

Part II

Allied Health Themes

15

The Therapeutic Potential of Diet and Exercise on Brain Repair

Fernando Gomez-Pinilla and Sandeep Sharma

CONTENTS

15.1   Introduction

The brain has a remarkable capacity for plasticity, an aptitude that ironically contrasts with the limited efficacy of current therapeutic approaches to reduce the consequences of brain injury. Despite the large number of clinical trials to test the action of many pharmacologic compounds in minimizing the burden of neurologic disorders, the results of many of these trials have been unsuccessful. Another concern frequently encountered in neurosurgery is that the patient outcome after brain surgery does not match the prognosis. These facts create many questions about what unaccounted variables as part of the history of the patient can be determinant for the final expression of brain plasticity and repair. An increasing number of studies indicate that environmental conditions and experiences encountered in the daily routine of individuals can dramatically affect the capacity of the brain to react to challenges. In particular, certain types of dietary factors (e.g., omega-3 fatty acids) can increase production of molecular systems that serve synaptic function, whereas diets rich in saturated fats do the opposite. In turn, exercise similarly displays healing effects on the human brain by counteracting the mental decline associated with age[1] and facilitating function recovery resulting from brain injury and disease.[2]

The overall evidence indicates that diet and exercise are two noninvasive approaches that can be used to improve molecular mechanisms of neural repair, most likely by modulating synaptic transmission.[3] As discussed here, studies have been conducted that indicate that select diets and exercise modulate levels of molecules important for synaptic plasticity, such as brain-derived neurotrophic factor (BDNF), thus affecting normal brain function and recovery events following brain insults.

15.2 BDNF Supports Cognitive Function

BDNF is a neurotrophin with a status as a regulator of the survival, growth, and differentiation of neurons during development[4,5] that has matured to include the adult nervous system. Indeed, it is now known that BDNF functions to translate activity into synaptic and cognitive plasticity in the adult animal. BDNF is able to modulate the efficacy of neurotransmitter release,[6] to stimulate the synthesis of vesicle-associated proteins,[7,8] and to regulate transcriptional factors.[9,10] In the hippocampus, BDNF is capable of inducing a rapid potentiation of glutamate-mediated synaptic transmission[11] and long-lasting potentiation of perforant path–dentate gyrus connections in vivo.[12]

Long-term potentiation (LTP), considered an electrophysiologic correlate of learning and memory,[13] selectively increases BDNF messenger RNA levels in the hippocampus. Transgenic animals with diminished BDNF expression are impaired in learning a spatial memory task.[14] Functional blocking of BDNF has been demonstrated to impair learning and memory in rats on the water maze and on an avoidance task.[15,16] Similarly, blocking endogenous BDNF was able to significantly reduce LTP.[15] Moreover, replenishing the depleted hippocampus with exogenous BDNF seems to ameliorate these deficits. Exogenous BDNF application[17] or transfection of hippocampal slices with a BDNF-expressing adenovirus[18] has been shown to restore the ability to induce LTP. BDNF, but not nerve-growth factor (NGF) or neurotrophin-3 (NT-3), seems to play a role in consolidating long-term memories.[19] Clinical studies support the importance of BDNF in learning and memory in humans.[20,21] A study conducted by Egan et al.[20] has found that individuals expressing a specific polymorphism in the BDNF gene exhibit learning impairments.

15.3 Role of Nutritional Factors in Normal Brain Health and after Brain Trauma

15.3.1 Omega-3

A number of studies point to the health effects of dietary factors on the brain. For example, fish-derived omega-3 fatty acids have been shown to counteract the deterioration in cognition and synaptic plasticity after traumatic brain injury. One of the most important forms of omega-3 fatty acids, docosahexaenoic acid (DHA), has been found to be a key component of neuronal membranes at sites of signal transduction at the synapse, suggesting that its action is vital to brain structure and function.[22] Evidence suggests that DHA serves to improve neuronal function by supporting synaptic membrane fluidity and function, and regulating gene expression and cell signaling.[23] Because the human body is not efficient in producing its own DHA, supplementation of diet with foods rich in DHA is important in ensuring proper function of neurons and in facilitating neuronal recovery after injury.[24] An additional benefit of omega-3 fatty acids that we observed in our studies is that they appear to reduce oxidative stress damage that results from trauma, indicating the possibility of their application in assisting the recovery process.[24,25] Recently, DHA dietary supplementation along with exercise has been shown to have beneficial effects on synaptic plasticity and cognition in rodents under normal conditions.[26]

Another dietary supplement that has shown promise in protecting neurons is vitamin E, found in certain oils, nuts, and spinach. Vitamin E functions as an antioxidant, reducing free radicals in the brain that would otherwise impede optimal function of neurons. Vitamin E has shown positive effects on memory performance in older people,[27] indicating its ability to maintain neuronal health. A different study in aging mice revealed the benefits of vitamin E by showing a correlation between the amount of ingested vitamin E and improved neurologic performance, survival, and brain mitochondrial function.[28]

15.3.2 Dietary Polyphenols

Polyphenols can be broadly divided into two categories: flavonoids and nonflavonoids. Although numerous studies have reported flavonoid-mediated neuroprotection, there is little information about the interaction of flavonoids or their metabolites with the blood–brain barrier (BBB). The flavonoid epigallocatechin gallate, a polar polyphenol, has been reported to enter the brain after a gastric administration of [3H] epigallocatechin gallate.[29] The citrus flavonoids naringin and hesperetin readily cross the BBB, whereas the less lipophilic glucuronide or glycoside conjugates have greater difficulty.[30] It also appears that methylated flavonoids cross the BBB more readily than their phenolic counterparts.[31]

15.3.3 Curcumin

Curcumin is a major chemical component of turmeric (*Curcuma longa*) and is used as a spice to give a specific flavor and yellow color to Indian curries and is used in food preservation. Interestingly, the prevalence of Alzheimer's disease (AD) in people age 70 to 79 years in India is 4.4-fold less than in the United States.[32] Turmeric is derived from the rhizome, or root, of the plant. There is substantial *in vitro* evidence indicating that curcumin has antioxidant, anti-inflammatory, and antiamyloid activities.[33] For instance, curcumin could inhibit lipid peroxidation,[34] activate glutathione *S*-transferase,[34] or induce heme oxygenase-1.[35] When fed to older Tg2576 mice with advanced amyloid accumulation, curcumin reduced amyloid beta (Aβ) levels and plaques.[36] In this study, low (160 ppm) and high (5000 ppm) doses of curcumin significantly lowered oxidized proteins and interleukin, 1β, whereas low doses reduced plaque burden. Subsequent *in vivo* studies using multiphoton microscopy demonstrated that curcumin could cross the BBB, targeting senile plaques in Tg2576 mice and disrupting existing plaques.[37] In accordance with these observations, our own studies have shown that the supplementation of curcumin into the diets of rats reduced the effects of experimental concussive injury on cognitive function tasks.[38]

15.3.4 Green Tea

Green tea is rich in flavonoids (30% of dry weight of a leaf),[39] with the main compounds being epigallocatechin-gallate, (–)-epigallocatechin, (–)-epicatechin, and (–)-epicatechin-3-gallate. Catechin intake has been associated with a wide variety of beneficial health effects.[40] The prevention of cerebrovascular diseases or stroke by green tea has been evidenced during a 4-year follow-up study with 5910 individuals. The incidence of cerebral hemorrhage and stroke was 2-fold higher in those who consumed less than five cups than in those who consumed five cups or more daily.[41] An inverse correlation between black tea consumption and the incidence of stroke was also replicated in a cohort of 552 men age 50 to 69 years and followed up for 15 years.[42] Although there is no significant outcome relative to tea consumption in AD case control, there are several *in vitro* studies showing that green tea extract may protect neurons from Aβ-induced damages.[43–46]

15.3.5 Resveratrol

Resveratrol is a nonflavonoid polyphenolic found in grapes, red wine, and berries. There are two isomeric forms of resveratrol, the biologically inactive *cis*-resveratrol and the most biologically active *trans*resveratrol (*trans*-3,4,5-trihydroxystilbene). This compound has been the focus of a number of studies demonstrating its antioxidant, anti-inflammatory, antimutagenic, and anticarcinogenic effects.[47–49] Interestingly, several epidemiologic studies indicate an inverse correlation of wine consumption and incidence of AD.[50–52] It is well-known that reducing food intake or caloric restriction extends life span in a wide range of species. Recently, it has been found that resveratrol can mimic dietary restriction and trigger sirtuin proteins.[53] The sirtuin enzymes are a phylogenetically conserved family of enzymes that catalyze nicotinamide adenine dinucleotide (NAD)-dependent protein deacetylation. In yeast, sir2 is essential for life span extension by caloric restriction and a variety of other stresses, including increased temperature, amino acid restriction, and osmotic shock.[54,55]

15.3.6 Effects of Polyphenols on Cognitive Performance

Berries are rich sources of phenolic compounds, such as phenolic acids, as well as anthocyanins, proanthocyanidins, and other flavonoids. Interestingly, a significant positive correlation between serum anthocyanin content and postprandial antioxidant status has been observed.[56] This absorption could have some positive effects in the brain through several processes, as has been demonstrated in various animal studies. Dietary supplementation for 8 weeks with blueberry extracts reversed cognitive deficits in the Morris water maze performance test in 19-month-old rats.[57] Additional evidence was seen in a recent study with the double-transgenic mice model of AD overexpressing amyloid precursor protein (APP) and presenilin 1, in which genetic mutations promote the production of the Aβ peptide and the hallmark of AD-like senile plaques in several regions. When these mice were supplemented with blueberry extract (2% of diet) at 4 months and continued until 12 months of age, their performance in a Y-maze cognitive performance test was similar to that of nontransgenic mice and significantly better than that of nonsupplemented transgenic mice.[58] In the mice supplemented with blueberry extract, the concentrations of hippocampal extracellular signal-regulated kinase (ERK), as well as striatal and hippocampal protein kinase C receptor (PKCR), were higher than in transgenic mice supplemented with control diet. Both protein kinase C and ERK have been shown to be involved in early and late stages of memory formation.[59] These results indicate that blueberry extract supplementation might prevent cognitive and motor deficits through various neuronal signaling pathways.

15.3.7 Caloric Intake

Cognition and plasticity of the brain have also been shown to be affected by caloric intake and the frequency of food consumption. Restriction of calories seems to increase levels of BDNF, resulting in improved neuronal function. Fasting every other day has been shown to protect neurons in the hippocampus against excitotoxicity-induced death.[60] In the study, rats put on an every-other-day fasting diet for 2 to 4 months had hippocampus neurons that were much more resistant to degeneration induced by kainic acid, and greater preserved memory than rats fed *ad lib*. The effects of caloric restriction have also been described in animal models of spinal cord injury, in which every-other-day fasting improves functional recovery after a partial cervical spinal cord injury.[61]

Although certain foods seem to contribute positively to neuronal health, diets that are rich in saturated fats and sugar decrease levels of BDNF in the brain and lead to poorer neuronal performance. Molteni et al.[62] have shown that rats fed a diet high in saturated fats and refined sugars (similar in content to the "junk food" that has become popular today) for a period of 1 to 2 months performed significantly worse on the spatial learning water maze test than rats fed a healthier diet that was low in fat and contained complex carbohydrates. The effects of this high-caloric diet seem to be related to elevated levels of oxidative stress, which may be reversed by antioxidant treatment[63] or exercise.[64]

15.4 From Nutrition to Nutrigenomics

There is increasing support for the possibility that the physiologic effects of dietary factors can be inheritable in the form of epigenetic regulation. Genetic variation in selected single nucleotide polymorphism, haplotypes, and copy number variants can have A remarkable effect, not only in our response to dietary components, but also on our food preferences and their optimal utilization.[65] Recent evidence suggests that nutrients/phytochemicals can alter the degree of histone acetylation. Administration of the sulforaphane present in *Brassica* (broccoli) to human embryonic kidney cells and to human colorectal tumor cells inhibited histone deacetylase.[66] Sulforaphane has also been shown to have histone deacetylase activity in human subjects, albeit transiently.[67] This type of modulation of gene expression is termed *epigenetics* (changing expression without altering the DNA nucleotide sequence) and may be crucial in terms of the benefit of the diet in preventing chronic disease.

15.5 Effect of Exercise on Brain Health

Given that most of our current genome remains unchanged from the times of our ancestors,[68] who had to perform abundant exercise for survival, the prevalence of inactivity in U.S. society is abnormal. The lack of physical activity and our genetics may therefore contribute to the prevalence of obesity in modern industrialized societies[69,70] and derived metabolic dysfunctions, such as type 2 diabetes, hypertension, and cardiovascular disease.[69,71,72] A sedentary lifestyle or the lack of physical activity seems to be the primary causal factor responsible for about one third of deaths resulting from coronary heart disease, colon cancer, and type 2 diabetes.[73]

During the past two decades, the benefits of exercise on cognitive function have been commended by many studies conducted on both humans and animals. These studies have shown that exercise has the capacity to enhance learning and memory[74–76] under a variety of conditions, from counteracting the mental decline that comes with age to facilitating functional recovery after brain injury and disease.[2,77,78] A meta-analysis of the human literature conducted by Colcombe and Kramer[79] has provided reproducible findings that exercise has a positive effect on cognitive function in humans. An analysis of 18 longitudinal fitness-training studies revealed that cardiovascular fitness training improved overall cognitive function regardless of task type. In addition, the effects that exercise seems to have on ameliorating the cognitive decline in aging animals also extend to human senescence.[1,80,81]

15.6 Exercise and Neural Repair

Much like a healthy diet, physical activity is thought to benefit neuronal function by increasing BDNF levels and reducing oxidative stress. More specifically, exercise has been found to play an important role in the regulation of neurite development,[82] maintenance of the synaptic structure,[83] axonal elongation,[64] and neurogenesis in the adult brain.[76] Studies have indicated that physical activity displays long-lasting changes in morphology and function of the nervous system, suggesting that a lifestyle that implements regular exercise can lead to a brain more resistant to insults. Preinjury exercise has been shown to have benefits in animal models of Parkinson's disease.[84] Postinjury application of exercise also seems promising in facilitating recovery, but more studies are needed to determine when, and to what extent, it should be integrated into a patient's lifestyle. When physical therapy was implemented to treat Parkinson's disease, patients showed signs of increased motor ability.[85] Exercise applied after experimental traumatic brain injury has also been shown to have beneficial effects, but these effects seem to depend on the postinjury resting period and the severity of the injury.[86]

15.7 Mechanisms of Action for the Effects of Exercise on the Brain

Exercise seems to exert its action on brain and body physiology using molecular systems that have an intrinsic dependence on activity, principally impacting the neurotrophin BDNF, a recognized arbitrator of metabolic efficiency, eating behavior, synaptic plasticity, and learning and memory. The use of a novel microbead injection method for drug-mediated blocking experiments has elucidated the contribution of different pathways that may be responsible for mediating the exercise-induced changes in hippocampal synaptic plasticity.[87] Accordingly, it was determined that exercise uses several different conduits of signal transduction, such as mitogen-activated protein kinase (MAPK), calcium/calmodulin protein kinase II (CAMKII), and the *N*-methyl-D-aspartate receptor (NMDA-R), to mediate its effects on hippocampal synaptic plasticity. More important, MAPK, CAMKII, and the NMDA-R were found to impact downstream effectors of BDNF action on gene expression and synaptic transmission (i.e., cyclic adenosine monophosphate [cAMP] response element binding protein (CREB) and synapsin I, respectively.[87]

CREB is critical for activity-dependent long-term neuronal plasticity and is believed to be an evolutionarily conserved molecule requisite for the formation of long-term memory; specifically, CREB has been described as a molecular switch for the activation of transcription necessary for long-term memory.[88–90] CREB seems to be an important piece in the BDNF-mediated machinery responsible for the potentiating effects of exercise on learning and memory. Blocking BDNF action during exercise was sufficient to abrogate the exercise-induced enhancement in learning and memory, and to prevent exercise-induced increase in CREB messenger RNA levels and the active form of CREB.[91] An additional player determined to promote the effects of exercise on hippocampal synaptic plasticity is NMDA-R. BDNF can potentiate synaptic transmission through NMDA-R,[92] providing an alternative path to CAMKII and MAPK-mediated changes. NMDA-R activation[93] can initiate CAMKII[94] to converge on the MAPK cascade.[95] Like the forerunners described before it, NMDA-R is critical for modulating LTP, and mediating learning and memory processes.[96] Other ways that exercise may benefit brain function is by modulating the transmission properties of synapse. Studies have shown that BDNF regulates synapsin I, a phosphoprotein localized to the presynaptic membrane, and synaptophysin, a major integral protein on synaptic vesicles.[97]

15.8 Energy Expenditure, Metabolism, and BDNF

The discovery that BDNF is intimately connected with energy metabolism has opened new avenues to understanding the action of BDNF on the brain. Mice that either lack one copy of the BDNF gene or have a conditioned deletion of BDNF in the postnatal brain are hyperphagic and develop obesity.[98] Moreover, mice with reduced BDNF levels are both obese and hyperglycemic.[99,100] Peripheral or central infusion of BDNF has been found to reduce body weight, normalize glucose levels,[101] ameliorate lipid metabolism in diabetic rodents,[102] and increase insulin sensitivity.[102] Hypoglycemia and intermittent fasting both increase BDNF levels whereas hyperphagia and high oxidative stress levels, the harmful by-products of energy metabolism, decrease BDNF levels.[63,78,103] It is also notable that, in the mature central nervous system, the BDNF protein is most abundant in brain areas foremost associated with cognitive and neuroendocrine regulation: the hippocampus and hypothalamus, respectively.[104] TrkB-mediated signaling is coupled with the melanocortin-4 receptor, a critical receptor involved in energy balance, such that melanocortin-4 receptor has been shown to regulate the expression of BDNF in the ventral medial hypothalamus.[105] Recent evidence from our own lab demonstrated that, during exercise, cellular energy metabolism can modulate BDNF-mediated synaptic plasticity in the hippocampus.[106] By infusing 1,25-dihydroxyvitamin D3, a modulator of energy metabolism, directly into the hippocampus during 3 days of voluntary wheel running, we found that BDNF, synapsin I, and CREB where significantly reduced.[3] Moreover, disrupting energy metabolism in the hippocampus reduced the expression p-CAMKII, the signal transduction cascade downstream to

BDNF action. Other findings from the study showed that exercise increases the expression of the uncoupling protein 2, a mitochondrial protein that uncouples substrate oxidation from adenosine triphosphate synthesis.[107–110] The overall evidence seems to suggest that exercise uses various elements intrinsic to cell energy metabolism to modulate synaptic plasticity and cognition.

15.9 Summary

Lifestyle conditions, such as diet and exercise, can contribute to the ability of the brain to counteract neurologic disorders. Specific diets and exercise routines have been shown to impact select factors that can make the brain more resistant to damage, facilitate synaptic transmission, and improve cognitive abilities. Accordingly, managed dietary manipulations and exercise have strong therapeutic potential. The overall evidence in the neural repair field indicates that this capacity could be implemented as a precondition to improve the outcome of brain surgery. Because diet and exercise are an integral part of human life, applying them to facilitate regeneration of neurons after injury or surgery would be a noninvasive and practical approach for enhancing recovery. The findings presented in this chapter stress that lifestyle implementations, such as exercise, seem to activate inherently systems concerned with whole body metabolism and brain plasticity. In a modern world where the ills of the body and brain can be delineated to sedentary lifestyle and bad diet choices, it is ever more so important to realize the connection that the body holds with the brain. Behaviors, such as exercise, that are concerned with activity and metabolism may have developed simultaneously and interdependently during evolution to determine ultimately how lifestyle influences cognitive function.

Given the ability of exercise to augment BDNF levels, exercise may be an effective life style implementation that can abate, if not combat, the effects of stress-related lifestyle choices. In particular, it has been found that exercise can counteract the decrease in hippocampal BDNF levels resulting from the consumption of a high-fat diet.[64] It should be emphasized that other complementary lifestyle alterations, such as changes in the nutrient content of one's diet,[24,62] can also be implemented to increase both body and brain health. When diet and exercise are combined, the success of regeneration and healing seems more pronounced than when either option is implemented by itself. Emerging studies indicate that exercise is capable of boosting the health effects of certain diets, such as omega-3 fatty acids.[26] It has also been observed that exercise can counteract some of the deleterious effects of a saturated-fat diet on synaptic plasticity and cognitive function of rats.[64]

References

1. Kramer, A. F., Hahn, S., Cohen, N. J., Banich, M. T., McAuley, E., Harrison, C. R., Chason, J., et al., Ageing, fitness, and neurocognitive function, *Nature*, 400(6743), 418–419, 1999.
2. Grealy, M. A., Johnson, D. A., and Rushton, S. K., Improving cognitive function after brain injury: The use of exercise and virtual reality, *Archives of Physical Medicine and Rehabilitation*, 80(6), 661–667, 1999.

3. Vaynman, S. and Gomez-Pinilla, F., Revenge of the "sit": How lifestyle impacts neuronal and cognitive health through molecular systems that interface energy metabolism with neuronal plasticity, *Journal of Neuroscience Research,* 84(4), 699–715, 2006.

4. Barde, Y. A., Neurotrophins: A family of proteins supporting the survival of neurons, *Progress in Clinical and Biological Research,* 390, 45–56, 1994.

5. Wang, T., Xie, K., and Lu, B., Neurotrophins promote maturation of developing neuromuscular synapses, *Journal of Neuroscience,* 15(7 pt. 1), 4796–4805, 1995.

6. Bolton, M. M., Pittman, A. J., and Lo, D. C., Brain-derived neurotrophic factor differentially regulates excitatory and inhibitory synaptic transmission in hippocampal cultures, *Journal of Neuroscience,* 20(9), 3221–3232, 2000.

7. Lu, B. and Chow, A., Neurotrophins and hippocampal synaptic transmission and plasticity, *Journal of Neuroscience,* 58(1), 76–87, 1999.

8. Schinder, A. F. and Poo, M., The neurotrophin hypothesis for synaptic plasticity, *Trends in Neuroscience,* 23(12), 639–645, 2000.

9. Finkbeiner, S., Tavazoie, S. F., Maloratsky, A., Jacobs, K. M., Harris, K. M., and Greenberg, M. E., CREB: A major mediator of neuronal neurotrophin responses, *Neuron,* 19(5), 1031–1047, 1997.

10. Tully, T., Regulation of gene expression and its role in long-term memory and synaptic plasticity, *Proceedings of the National Academy of Sciences of the United States of America,* 94(9), 4239–4241, 1997.

11. Lessmann, V. and Heumann, R., Modulation of unitary glutamatergic synapses by neurotrophin-4/5 or brain-derived neurotrophic factor in hippocampal microcultures: Presynaptic enhancement depends on pre-established paired-pulse facilitation, *Neuroscience,* 86(2), 399–413, 1998.

12. Messaoudi, E., Bardsen, K., Srebro, B., and Bramham, C. R., Acute intrahippocampal infusion of BDNF induces lasting potentiation of synaptic transmission in the rat dentate gyrus, *Journal of Neurophysiology,* 79(1), 496–499, 1998.

13. Patterson, S. L., Grover, L. M., Schwartzkroin, P. A., and Bothwell, M., Neurotrophin expression in rat hippocampal slices: A stimulus paradigm inducing LTP in CA1 evokes increases in BDNF and NT-3 mRNAs, *Neuron,* 9(6), 1081–1088, 1992.

14. Linnarsson, S., Bjorklund, A., and Ernfors, P., Learning deficit in BDNF mutant mice, *European Journal of Neuroscience,* 9(12), 2581–2587, 1997.

15. Ma, Y. L, Wang, H. L., Wu, H. C., Wei, C. L., and Lee, E. H., Brain-derived neurotrophic factor antisense oligonucleotide impairs memory retention and inhibits long-term potentiation in rats, *Neuroscience,* 82(4), 957–967, 1998.

16. Mu, J. S., Li, W. P., Yao, Z. B., and Zhou, X. F., Deprivation of endogenous brain-derived neurotrophic factor results in impairment of spatial learning and memory in adult rats, *Brain Research,* 835(2), 259–265, 1999.

17. Patterson, S. L., Abel, T., Deuel, T. A. S., Martin, K. C., Rose, J. C., and Kandel, E. R., Recombinant BDNF rescues deficits in basal synaptic transmission and hippocampal LTP in BDNF knockout mice, *Neuron,* 16(6), 1137–1145, 1996.

18. Korte, M., Carroll, P., Wolf, E., Brem, G., Thoenen, H., and Bonhoeffer, T., Hippocampal long-term potentiation is impaired in mice lacking brain-derived neurotrophic factor, *Proceedings of the National Academy of Sciences of the United Sates of America,* 92(19), 8856–8860, 1995.

19. Johnston, A. N. and Rose, S. P., Memory consolidation in day-old chicks requires BDNF but not NGF or NT-3: An antisense study, *Molecular Brain Research,* 88(1–2), 26–36, 2001.

20. Egan, M. F., Kojima, M., Callicott, J. H., Goldberg, T. E., Kolachana, B. S., Bertolino, A., Zaitsev, E., et al., The BDNF val66met polymorphism affects activity-dependent secretion of BDNF and human memory and hippocampal function, *Cell,* 122(2), 257–269, 2003.

21. Hariri, A. R., Goldberg, T. E., Mattay, V. S., Kolachana, B. S., Callicott, J. H., Egan, M. F., and Weinberger, D. R., Brain-derived neurotrophic factor val66met polymorphism affects human memory-related hippocampal activity and predicts memory performance, *Journal of Neuroscience,* 23(45), 6690–6694, 2003.

22. Jones, C. R., Arai, T., and Rapoport, S. I., Evidence for the involvement of docosahexaenoic acid in cholinergic stimulated signal transduction at the synapse, *Neurochemical Research*, 22(6), 663–670, 1997.

23. Salem, N., Litman, B., Kim, H. Y., and Gawrisch, K., Mechanisms of action of docosahexaenoic acid in the nervous system, *Lipids*, 36(9), 945–959, 2001.

24. Wu, A., Ying, Z., and Gomez-Pinilla, F., Dietary omega-3 fatty acids normalize BDNF levels, reduce oxidative damage, and counteract learning disability after traumatic brain injury in rats, *Journal of Neurotrauma*, 21(11), 1457–1467, 2004.

25. Wu, A., Ying, Z., and Gomez-Pinilla, F., Omega-3 fatty acids supplementation restores mechanisms that maintain brain homeostasis in traumatic brain injury, *Journal of Neurotrauma*, 24(10), 1587–1595, 2007.

26. Wu, A., Ying, Z., and Gomez-Pinilla, F., Docosahexaenoic acid dietary supplementation enhances the effects of exercise on synaptic plasticity and cognition, *Neuroscience*, 155(3), 751–759, 2008.

27. Perkins, A. J., Hendrie, H. C., Callahan, C. M., Gao, S., Unverzagt, F. W., Xu, Y., Hall, K. S., and Hui, S. L., Association of antioxidants with memory in a multiethnic elderly sample using the Third National Health and Nutrition Examination Survey, *American Journal of Epidemiology*, 150(1), 37–44, 1999.

28. Navarro, A., Gomez, C., Sanchez-Pino, M. J., Gonzalez, H., Bandez, M. J., Boveris, A. D., and Boveris, A., Vitamin E at high doses improves survival, neurological performance, and brain mitochondrial function in aging male mice, *American Journal Physiology, Regulatory, Integrative and Comparative Physiology*, 289(5), 1392R–1399R, 2005.

29. Suganuma, M., Okabe, S., Oniyama, M., Tada, Y., Ito, H., and Fujiki, H., Wide distribution of [3H] (–)-epigallocatechin gallate, a cancer preventive tea polyphenol, in mouse tissue, *Carcinogenesis*, 19(10), 1771–1776, 1998.

30. Youdim, K. A., Dobbie, M. S., Kuhnle, G., Proteggente, A. R., Abbott, N. J., and Rice-Evans, C., Interaction between flavonoids and the blood–brain barrier: In vitro studies, *Journal of Neurochemistry*, 85(1), 180–192, 2003.

31. Youdim, K. A., Shukitt-Hale, B., and Joseph, J. A., Flavonoids and the brain: Interactions at the blood–brain barrier and their physiological effects on the central nervous system, *Free Radical Biology and Medicine*, 37(11), 1683–1693, 2004.

32. Ganguli, M., Chandra, V., Kamboh, M. I., Johnston, J. M., Dodge, H. H., Thelma, B. K., Juyal, R. C., Pandav, R., Belle, S. H., and DeKosky, S. T., Apolipoprotein E polymorphism and Alzheimer disease: The Indo–US Cross-National Dementia Study, *Archives of Neurology*, 57(6), 824–830, 2000.

33. Menon, V. P. and Sudheer, A. R., Antioxidant and anti-inflammatory properties of curcumin, *Advances in Experimental Medicine and Biology*, 595, 105–125, 2007.

34. Wei, Q. Y., Chen, W. F., Zhou, B., Yang, L., and Liu, Z. L., Inhibition of lipid peroxidation and protein oxidation in rat liver mitochondria by curcumin and its analogues, *Biochimica et Biophysica Acta*, 1760(1), 70–77, 2006.

35. Motterlini, R., Foresti, R., Bassi, R., and Green, C. J., Curcumin, an antioxidant and anti-inflammatory agent, induces heme oxygenase-1 and protects endothelial cells against oxidative stress, *Free Radical Biology and Medicine*, 28(8), 1303–1312, 2000.

36. Lim, G. P., Chu, T., Yang, F., Beech, W., Frautschy, S. A., and Cole, G. M., The curry spice curcumin reduces oxidative damage and amyloid pathology in an Alzheimer transgenic mouse, *Journal of Neuroscience*, 21(21), 8370–8377, 2001.

37. Garcia-Alloza, M., Borrelli, L. A., Rozkalne, A., Hyman, B. T., and Bacskai, B. J., Curcumin labels amyloid pathology in vivo, disrupts existing plaques, and partially restores distorted neuritis in an Alzheimer mouse model, *Journal of Neurochemistry*, 102(4), 1095–1104, 2007.

38. Wu, A., Ying, Z., and Gomez-Pinilla, F., Dietary curcumin counteracts the outcome of traumatic brain injury on oxidative stress, synaptic plasticity, and cognition, *Experimental Neurology*, 197(2), 309–317, 2006.

39. Graham, H. N., Green tea composition, consumption, and polyphenol chemistry, *Preventative Medicine*, 21(3), 334–350, 1992.

40. Sutherland, B. A., Rahman, R. M., and Appleton, I., Mechanisms of action of green tea catechins, with a focus on ischemia-induced neurodegeneration, *Journal of Nutritional Biochemistry*, 17(5), 291–306, 2006.
41. Sato, Y., Nakatsuka, H., Watanabe, T., Hisamichi, S., Shimizu, H., Fujisaku, S., Ichinowatari, Y., et al., Possible contribution of green tea drinking habits to the prevention of stroke, *Tohoku Journal of Experimental Medicine*, 157(4), 337–343, 1989.
42. Keli, S. O., Hertog, M. G., Feskens, E. J., and Kromhout, D., Dietary flavonoids, antioxidant vitamins, and incidence of stroke: The Zutphen study, *Archives of Internal Medicine*, 156(6), 637–642, 1996.
43. Bastianetto, S., Yao, Z. X., Papadopoulos, V., and Quirion, R., Neuroprotective effects of green and black teas and their catechin gallate esters against beta-amyloid-induced toxicity, *European Journal of Neuroscience*, 23(1), 55–64, 2006.
44. Choi, Y. T., Jung, C. H., Lee, S. R., Bae, J. H., Baek, W. K., Suh, M. H., Park, J., Park, C. W., and Suh, S. I., The green tea polyphenol (–)-epigallocatechin gallate attenuates beta-amyloid-induced neurotoxicity in cultured hippocampal neurons, *Life Sciences*, 70(5), 603–614, 2001.
45. Levites, Y., Amit, T., Mandel, S., and Youdim, M. B., Neuroprotection and neurorescue against Abeta toxicity and PKC-dependent release of nonamloidogenic soluble precursor protein by green tea polyphenol (–)-epigallocatechin-3-gallate, *Federation of American Societies for Experimental Biology Journal*, 17(8), 952–954, 2003.
46. Levites, Y., Amit, T., Youdim, M. B., and Mandel, S., Involvement of protein kinase C activation and cell survival/cell cycle genes in green tea polyphenol (–)epigallocatechin 3-gallate neuroprotective action, *Journal of Biological Chemistry*, 277(34), 30574–30580, 2002.
47. de la Lastra, C. A. and Villegas, I., Resveratrol as an anti-inflammatory and anti-aging agent: Mechanisms and clinical implications, *Molecular Nutrition and Food Research*, 49(5), 405–430, 2005.
48. Jang, M., Cai, L., Udeani, G. O., Slowing, K. V., Thomas, C. F., Beecher, C. W., Fong, H. H., et al., Cancer chemopreventive activity of resveratrol, a natural product derived from grapes, *Science*, 275(5297), 218–220, 1997.
49. Soleas, G. J., Diamandis, E. P., and Goldbert, D. M., Resveratrol: A molecule whose time has come? And gone?, *Clinical Biochemistry*, 30(2), 91–113, 1997.
50. Lindsay, J., Laurin, D., Verreault, R., Hebert, R., Helliwell, B., Hill, G. B., and McDowell, I., Risk factors of Alzheimer's disease: A prospective analysis from the Canadian Study of Health and Aging, *American Journal of Epidemiology*, 156(5), 445–453, 2002.
51. Orgogozo, J. M., Dartigues, J. F., Lafont, S., Letenneur, L., Commenges, D., Salamon, R., Renaud, S., and Breteler, M. B., Wine consumption and dementia in the elderly: A prospective community study in the Bordeaux area, *Revue Neuroloque (Paris)*, 153(3), 185–192, 1997.
52. Truelsen, T., Thudium, D., and Gronbaek, M., Amount and type of alcohol and risk of dementia: The Copenhagen City Heart Study, *Neurology*, 59(9), 1313–1319, 2002.
53. Baur, J. A. and Sinclair, D. A., Therapeutic potential of resveratrol: The in vivo evidence, *Nature Reviews Drug Discovery*, 5(6), 493–506, 2006.
54. Anderson, R. M., Latore-Esteves, M., Neves, A. R., Lavu, S., Medvedik, O., Taylor, C., Howitz, K. T., Santos, H., and Sinclair, D. A., Yeast life-span extension by calorie restriction is independent of NAD fluctuation, *Science*, 302(5653), 2124–2126, 2003.
55. Swiecilo, A., Krawiec, Z., Wawryn, J., Bartosz, G., and Bilinski, T., Effect of stress of the life span of the yeast Saccharomyces cerevisiae, *Acta Biochimica Polonica*, 47(2), 355–365, 2000.
56. Mazza, G., Kay, C. D., Cottrell, T., Holub, B. J., Absorption of anthocyanins from blueberries and serum antioxidant status in human subjects, *Journal of Agricultural and Food Chemistry*, 50(26), 7731–7737, 2002.
57. Andres-Lacueva, C., Shukitt-Hale, B., Galli, R. L., Jauregui, O., Lamuela-Raventos, R. M., and Joseph, J. A., Anthocyanins in aged blueberry-fed rats are found centrally and may enhance memory, *Nutritional Neuroscience*, 8(2), 111–120, 2005.
58. Joseph, J. A., Denisova, N. A., Arendash, G., Gordon, M., Diamond, D., Shukitt-Hale, B., and Morgan, D., Blueberry supplementation enhances signaling and prevents behavioral deficits in an Alzheimer disease model, *Nutritional Neuroscience*, 6(3), 153–162, 2003.

59. Micheau, J. and Riedel, G., Protein kinases: Which one is the memory molecule?, *Cellular and Molecular Life Sciences*, 55(3), 534–548, 1999.

60. Bruce-Keller, A. J., Umberger, G., McFall, R., and Mattson, M. P., Food restriction reduces brain damage and improves behavioral outcome following excitotoxic and metabolic insults, *Annals of Neurology*, 45(1), 8–15, 1999.

61. Plunet, W. T., Streijger, F., Lam, C. K., Lee, J. H. T., Liu, J., and Tetzlaff, W., Dietary restriction started after spinal cord injury improves functional recovery, *Experimental Neurology*, 213(1), 28–35, 2008.

62. Molteni, R., Ying, Z., and Gomez-Pinilla, F., Differential effects of acute and chronic exercise on plasticity-related genes in the rat hippocampus revealed by microarray, *European Journal of Neuroscience*, 16(6), 1107–1116, 2002.

63. Wu, A., Ying, Z., and Gomez-Pinilla, F., The interplay between oxidative stress and brain-derived neurotrophic factor modulates the outcome of a saturated fat diet on synaptic plasticity and cognition, *European Journal of Neuroscience*, 19(4), 1699–1707, 2004.

64. Molteni, R., Wu, A., Vaynman, S., Ying, Z., Barnard, R. J., and Gomez-Pinilla, F., Exercise reverses the harmful effects of consumption of a high-fat diet on synaptic and behavioral plasticity associated to the action of brain-derived neurotrophic factor, *Neuroscience*, 123(2), 429–440, 2004.

65. Ferguson, L. R., Nutrigenomics: Integrating genomic approaches into nutrition research, *Molecular Diagnosis and Therapy*, 10(2), 101–108, 2006.

66. Myzak, M. C., Karplus, P. A., Chung, F. L., and Dashwood, R. H., A novel mechanism of chemo-protection by sulforaphane: Inhibition of histone deacetylase, *Cancer Research*, 64(16), 5767–5774, 2004.

67. Dashwood, R. H. and Ho, E., Dietary histone deacetylase inhibitors: From cells to mice to man, *Seminars in Cancer Biology*, 17(5), 363–369, 2007.

68. Cordain, L., Gotshall, R. W., Eaton, S. B., and Eaton, S. B., 3rd, Physical activity, energy expenditure and fitness: An evolutionary perspective, *International Journal of Sports Medicine*, 19(5), 328–335, 1998.

69. Booth, F. W., Chakravarthy, M. V., Gordon, S. E., and Spangenburg, E. E., Waging war on physical inactivity: Using modern molecular ammunition against an ancient enemy, *Journal of Applied Physiology*, 93(1), 3–30, 2002.

70. Wendorf, M. and Goldfine, I. D., Archaeology of NIDDM: Excavation of the "thrifty" genotype, *Diabetes*, 40(2), 161–165, 1991.

71. Jung, R. T., Obesity as a disease, *British Medical Bulletin*, 53(2), 307–321, 1997.

72. Must, A., Spadano, J., Coakley, E. H., Field, A. E., Colditz, G., and Dietz, W. H., The disease burden associated with overweight and obesity, *Journal of the American Medical Association*, 282(16), 1523–1529, 1999.

73. Powell, K. E. and Blair, S. N., The public health burdens of sedentary living habits: Theoretical but realistic estimates, *Medicine and Science in Sports and Medicine*, 26(7), 851–856, 1994.

74. Rogers, R. L., Meyer, J. S., and Mortel, K. F., After reaching retirement age physical activity sustains cerebral perfusion and cognition, *Journal of the American Geriatrics Society*, 38(2), 123–128, 1990.

75. Suominen-Troyer, S., Davis, K. J., Ismail, A. H., and Salvendy, G., Impact of physical fitness on strategy development in decision-making tasks, *Perceptual and Motor Skills*, 62(1), 71–77, 1986.

76. van Praag, H., Kempermann, G., and Gage, F. H., Running increases cell proliferation and neurogenesis in the adult mouse dentate gyrus, *Nature Neuroscience*, 2(3), 266–270, 1999.

77. Bohannon, R. W., Physical rehabilitation in neurologic diseases, *Current Opinion in Neurology*, 6(5), 765–772, 1993.

78. Lindvall, O., Kokaia, Z., Bengzon, J., Elmer, E., and Kokaia, M., Neurotrophins and brain insults, *Trends in Neuroscience*, 17(11), 479–496, 1994.

79. Colcombe, S. and Kramer, A. F., Fitness effects on the cognitive function of older adults: A meta-analytic study, *Psychological Science*, 14(2), 125–130, 2003.

80. Colcombe, S. J., Kramer, A. F., McAuley, E., Erickson, K. I., and Schalf, P., Neurocognitive aging and cardiovascular fitness: Recent findings and future directions, *Journal of Molecular Neuroscience*, 24(1), 9–14, 2004.

81. Hillman, C. H., Erickson, K. I., and Kramer, A. F., Be smart, exercise your heart: Exercise effects on brain and cognition, *Nature Reviews Neuroscience*, 9(1), 58–65, 2008.

82. Zurmohle, U., Herms, J., Schlingensiepen, R., Brysch, W., Schlingensiepen, K. H., Changes in the expression of synapsin I and II messenger RNA during postnatal rat brain development, *Experimental Brain Research*, 108(3), 441–449, 1996.

83. Vaynman, S., Ying, Z., and Gomez-Pinilla, F., Exercises induces BDNF and synapsin I to specific hippocampal subfields, *Journal of Neuroscience Research*, 76(3), 356–362, 2004.

84. Crizzle, A. M. and Newhouse, I. J. P., Is physical exercise beneficial for persons with Parkinson's disease?, *Clinical Journal of Sports Medicine*, 16(5), 422–425, 2006.

85. Hirsch, M. A., Toole, T., Maitland, C. G., and Rider, R. A., The effects of balance training and high-intensity resistance training on persons with idiopathic Parkinson's disease, *Archives of Physical Medicine and Rehabilitation*, 84(8), 1109–1117, 2003.

86. Griesbach, G. S., Gómez-Pinilla, F., and Hovda, D. A., Time window for voluntary exercise-induced increases in hippocampal neuroplasticity molecules after traumatic brain injury is severely dependent, *Journal of Neurotrauma*, 24(7), 1161–1171, 2007.

87. Vaynman, S., Ying, Z., and Gomez-Pinilla, F., Interplay between brain-derived neurotrophic factor and signal transduction modulators in the regulation of the effects of exercise on synaptic-plasticity, *Neuroscience*, 122(3), 647–657, 2003.

88. Bourtchuladze, R., Frenguelli, B., Blendy, J., Cioffi, D., Schutz, G., and Silva, A. J., Deficient long-term memory in mice with a targeted mutation of the cAMP-responsive element-binding protein, *Cell*, 79(1), 59–68, 1994.

89. Dash, P. K., Hochner, B., and Kandel, E. R., Injection of the cAMP-responsive element into the nucleus of aplysia sensory neurons blocks long-term facilitation, *Nature*, 345(6277), 718–721, 1990.

90. Yin, J. C., Del Vecchio, M., Zhou, H., and Tully, T., CREB as a memory modulator: Induced expression of a dCREB2 activator isoform enhances long-term memory in Drosophila, *Cell*, 81(1), 107–115, 1995.

91. Vaynman, S., Ying, Z., and Gomez-Pinilla, F., Hippocampal BDNF mediates the efficacy of exercise on synaptic plasticity and cognition, *European Journal of Neuroscience*, 20(10), 2580–2590, 2004.

92. Song, D. K., Choe, B., Bae, J. H., Park, W. K., Han, I. S., Ho, W. K., and Earm, Y. E., Brain-derived neurotrophic factor rapidly potentiates synaptic transmission through NMDA, but suppresses it through non-NMDA receptors in rat hippocampal neuron, *Brain Research*, 799(1), 176–179, 1998.

93. Chosh, A., Carnahan, J., and Greenberg, M. E., Requirement for BDNF in activity-dependent survival of cortical neurons, *Science*, 263(5153), 1618–1623, 1994.

94. Bading, H. and Greenberg, M. E., Stimulation of protein tyrosine phosphorylation by NMDA receptor activation, *Science*, 253(5022), 912–914, 1991.

95. Platenik, J., Kuramoto, N., and Yoneda, Y., Molecular mechanisms associated with long-term consolidation of NMDA signals, *Life Sciences*, 67(4), 335–364, 2000.

96. Cammarota, M., Bevilaqua, L. R., Ardenghi, P., Paratcha, G., Levi de Stein, M., Izquierdo, I., and Medina, J. H., Learning-associated activation of nuclear MAPK, CREB and Elk-1, along with Fos production, in the rat hippocampus after a one-trial avoidance learning: Abolition by NMDA receptor blockade, *Molecular Brain Research*, 76(1), 36–46, 2000.

97. Vaynman, S., Ying, Z., Wu, A., and Gomez-Pinilla, F., Coupling energy metabolism with a mechanism to support brain-derived neurotrophic factor-mediated synaptic plasticity, *Neuroscience*, 139(4), 1221–1234, 2006.

98. Rios, M., Fan, G., Fekete, C., Kelly, J., Bates, B., Kuehn, R., Lechan, R. M., and Jaenisch, R., Conditional deletion of brain-derived neurotrophic factor in the postnatal brain leads to obesity and hyperactivity, *Molecular Endocrinology*, 15(10), 1748–1758, 2001.

99. Kernie, S. G., Liebl, D. J., and Parada, L. F., BDNF regulates eating behavior and locomotor activity in mice, *EMBO Journal*, 19(6), 1290–1300, 2000.

100. Lyons, W. E., Mammounas, L. A., Ricaurte, G. A., Coppola, V., Reid, S. W., Bora, S. H., Wihler, C., Koliatsos, V. E., and Tessarollo, L., Brain-derived neurotrophic factor-deficient mice develop aggressiveness hyperphagia in conjunction with brain serotonergic abnormalities, *Proceedings of the National Academy of Sciences of the United States of America*, 96(26), 15239–15244, 1999.

101. Tonra, J. R., Ono, M., Liu, X., Garcia, K., Jackson, C., Yancopoulos, G. D., Wiegland, S. J., and Wong, V., Brain-derived neurotrophic factor improves blood glucose control and alleviates fasting hyperglycemia in C57BLKS-Lepr(db)/lepr(db) mice, *Diabetes*, 48(3), 588–594, 1999.

102. Tsuchida, A., Nonomura, T., Nakagawa, T., Itakura, Y., Ono-Kishino, M., Yamanaka, M., Sugaru, E., Taiji, M., and Noguchi, H., Brain-derived neurotrophic factor ameliorates lipid metabolism in diabetic mice, *Diabetes, Obesity and Metabolism*, 4(4), 262–269, 2002.

103. Lee, J., Duan, W., and Mattson, M. P., Evidence that brain-derived neurotrophic factor is required for basal neurogenesis and mediates, in part, the enhancement of neurogenesis by dietary restriction in the hippocampus of adult mice, *Journal of Neurochemisty*, 82(6), 1367–1375, 2002.

104. Nawa, H., Carnahan, J., and Gall, C., BDNF protein measured by a novel enzyme immunoassay in normal brain and after seizure: Partial disagreement with mRNA levels, *European Journal of Neuroscience*, 7(7), 1527–1535, 1995.

105. Xu, B., Goulding, E. H., Zang, K., Cepoi, D., Cone, R. D., Jones, K. R., Tecott, L. H., and Reichardt, L. F., Brain-derived neurotrophic factor regulates energy balance downstream of melanocortin-4 receptor, *Nature Neuroscience*, 6(7), 736–742, 2003.

106. Gomez-Pinilla, F., Vaynman, S., and Ying, Z., Brain-derived neurotrophic factor functions as a metabotrophin to mediate the effects of exercise on cognition, *European Journal of Neuroscience*, 28(1), 2278–2287, 2008.

107. Bouillaud, F., Ricquier, D., Thibault, J., and Weissenbach, J., Molecular approach to thermogenesis in brown adipose tissue: cDNA cloning of the mitochondrial uncoupling protein, *Proceedings of the National Academy of Sciences of the United States of America*, 82(2), 445–458, 1985.

108. Mao, W., Yu, X. X., Zhong, A., Li, W., Brush, J., Sherwood, S. W., Adams, S. H., and Pan, G., UCP4, a novel brain-specific mitochondrial protein that reduces membrane potential in mammalian cells, *FEBS Letters*, 443(3), 326–330, 1999.

109. Sanchis, D., Fleury, C., Chomiki, N., Goubern, M., Huang, Q., Neverova, M., Gregoire, F., et al., BMCP1, a novel mitochondrial carrier with high expression in the central nervous system of humans and rodents, and respiration uncoupling activity in recombinant yeast, *Journal of Biological Chemistry*, 273(51), 34611–34615, 1998.

110. Vidal-Puig, A., Solanes, G., Grujic, D., Flier, J. A., and Lowell, B. B., UCP3: An uncoupling protein homologue expressed preferentially and abundantly in skeletal muscle and brown adipose tissue, *Biochemical and Biophysical Research Communications*, 235(1), 79–82, 1997.

16

The Traumatic Brain Injury Literature: Scholarship

John R. Muma, Steven J. Cloud, and Brett E. Kemker

CONTENTS

16.1 Introduction

Referring to the fact that the field of rehabilitation for traumatic brain injury (TBI) is in its infancy, Gonzalez-Rothi[1] commented: "There is much to be achieved before we are ready to meet the responsibility of our role effectively."[(p.195)] She outlined research phases toward establishing treatment efficacy, and then treatment effectiveness.

Although her outline is desirable, there are other substantive issues that need consideration, as well. The purposes of this chapter are the following:

1. To outline six levels of scholarship
2. To discuss rational evidence
3. To discuss the nominalist fallacy that is an obstacle for the field
4. To discuss alternatives for adducing effective rehabilitation strategies and procedures
5. To stress the importance of addressing the heterogeneous TBI population

16.2 Levels of Scholarship

Kaplan[2] outlined six levels of scholarship as a field strives to become scientific. These levels were modified slightly by Muma.[3] Table 16.1 outlines these levels of scholarship.

TABLE 16.1

An Abridged Version of Scholarly Levels as a Field Becomes Scientific

Levels	Characteristics
Formal	Coherence. Coherent views and perspectives derived from bona fide philosophical views and theoretical perspectives that underwrite empirical evidence.
Postulational	Formal logic. Reliance on the assumptions and propositions underlying the substantive aspects of a field.
Symbolic	Symbolism. Reliance on advanced experimental and statistical evidence.
Eristic	Empiricism. Reliance on statistical and experimental evidence.
Academic	Rationalism. Identification of parameters of populations with ad hoc speculations about their relationships. Loose or convenient logic including reductionism and impressionism.
Literary	Authoritarianism. Essays that delimit a field of study. Possible reliance on capriciousness, intuition, authoritarianism, dogma, elitism, popularity, currency, personalization, hype, and impressionism.

Sources: Kaplan, A., *The Conduct of Inquiry: Methodology for Behavioral Science*, Chandler Publishing, San Francisco, CA, 1964; Muma, J., *Scholarship in Communication Disorders: Raising the Bar*, Natural Child Publisher, Hattiesburg, MS, 2008.

In the *literary level*, which is the lowest level of scholarship, the focus is on essays that effectively delimit the scopes of practice. This level relies, to some extent, on capriciousness, intuition, authoritarianism, dogma, elitism, popularity, currency, personalization, hype, and impressionism.

Regarding capriciousness, Bruner[4] used the phrase "shooting from the hip," in which individuals are willing to ignore scholarly requirements for evidence, and they merely make arbitrary assertions. Such activities are detrimental to a field's credibility. The literary level holds considerable potential for launching a field appropriately and also for misleading a field by undermining scholarship. It becomes necessary to appreciate which literary activities contribute to a field and which do not.

As for *intuition*, perhaps one should be reminded that it is often wrong. Wanner,[5] the chief executive officer of the Russell Sage Corporation, made the following comment regarding understanding some formal aspects of grammar: "[P]erhaps we should not trust our intuitions."[(p.82)] His statement has a larger implication; although intuition may be right in some instances, it often is wrong in many others.

Authoritarianism refers to reliance on pronouncements that lack appropriate evidence. For example, the TBI literature has much to say about intervention guidelines, but little, if anything, to say concerning underlying philosophical views and theoretical perspectives that underwrite clinical services. Such authoritarian edicts undermine the credibility of a profession simply because the primary function of philosophical views and theoretical perspectives is to provide disciplined understandings. Such understandings warrant particular clinical services.

Dogma is unsubstantiated views and perspectives. Dogma is another form of authoritarianism.

Elitism is a social-based notion whereby those of "the elite" have special privileges that are presumably valued by the "less elite." Thus, elitism is a special case of authoritarianism in which elitist views are provided regardless of the evidence.

Popularity merely means the most popular views and practices. For example, reinforcement-based intervention, both traditional and the newer ecologically oriented versions, have become popular. Popularity does not ensure quality. Indeed, there is a major concern that reinforcement-based intervention is incompatible with language acquisition.[6,7]

Currency refers to the most current views, perspectives, and practices. On its face, currency appears to be desirable. However, appearances are deceptive. Currency does not ensure the most *appropriate or effective* services. For example, many current practices are in need of supporting evidence. Thus, currency perpetuates views, perspectives, and practices, but it provides no assurances of appropriateness or effectiveness.

Personalization occurs when individuals choose to focus on individuals rather than issues. Such activity is detrimental to scholarship because it is issues, not personalities, that count in scholarship.

Hype is an abbreviation for *hyperbole,* which means to exaggerate. To exaggerate is, in effect, to misrepresent. This is a form of dishonesty and it undermines scholarship.

Impressionism is a set of conclusions that reflect an individual's views regardless of the evidence. Said differently, when individuals choose to ignore the literature and operate as they want, such individuals are operating with impressionism. Furthermore, some views and perspectives may attain a life of their own by virtue of long-standing use. Reinforcement for intervention has a long-standing history, although the major language acquisition scholars have long since dismissed reinforcement as a viable account of language acquisition.[6,8–11] The more recent version of reinforcement has shifted to a more ecologic orientation, but it maintains the essential premises of reinforcement theory.

The *academic level* addresses characteristics of a population based on loose notions such as reductionism and impressionism rather than formal theories. Ad hoc speculation occurs, but it is questionable when it is unsupported by replication. The fundamental problem with *reductionism* is that when behavior is reduced, it is often changed, and it may not pertain to the original behavior.[4,11] *Impressionism* is not governed by the "rules of science." Consequently, any views and interpretations are permitted in impressionism.

The *eristic level* is based on canons of proof in the tradition of empiricism. Reliance is placed on inference based on experimental designs and statistical evidence. This level of science deals with clinical trials and the phases of development outlined by Gonzalez-Rothi.[1] In addition to within-subject designs and between-subjects designs, this level pertains to sampling, power, curtailment, programs of research, replication, and meta-analysis.

The *symbolic level*, as a more advanced version of the eristic level, relies on the progress of knowledge via symbolic means. It uses rather advanced statistical and mathematical mechanisms, but it is vulnerable to misinterpretation of those mechanisms that rely on complex inference.

The *postulational level* is vested on formal logic whereby reliance is placed on examining the underlying assumptions and propositions for the substantive and operational aspects of a field. This level establishes logical underpinnings issuing from philosophical views and theoretical perspectives.

The substantive bridge from the postulational level to the formal level is ascertained through the creation of *models.* As these models achieve measures of descriptive and explanatory adequacies,[12,13] they become bona fide theories. For example, Brown's[14] five early stages of language acquisition, with the attendant mean length of utterance values, comprise a possible model for understanding early language acquisition.

In language, *descriptive adequacy* is achieved by the following criteria: formal, complete, simple, and noncontradictory.[15] A theory is formal if it can be expressed in rules. A theory cannot address selected aspects of a domain. Rather, it should address the complete domain. A theory becomes simple when it is posited in the most parsimonious manner. A theory is noncontradictory when one aspect of the theory does not contradict another aspect.

Explanatory adequacy is achieved through either developmental evidence or evidence of mental processing. Such evidence *explains* how the mind functions in learning and using language.[11,16]

The *formal level* is concerned with the degree to which there is *coherence* among underlying assumptions, philosophical views, and theoretical perspectives. Moreover, this level ensures that theoretical perspectives are derived from philosophical views and that there is continuity between real-world applications and underlying views and perspectives.

Given these levels of scholarship, it is apparent that the field of intervention for TBI is very much oriented on the literary and academic levels, and it is struggling with the eristic level. Clearly, this field is not committed to intervention practices oriented on philosophical views and theoretical perspectives, save behaviorism. However, as indicated earlier, the behaviorist orientation is suspect because it is incompatible with the literature (theoretical perspectives) for both cognition and language. Accordingly, it is desirable for the TBI field to conceptualize and implement intervention practices based on rational evidence.

16.3 Rational Evidence

Rational evidence encompasses widely accepted philosophical views and theoretical perspectives. Inasmuch as the field of TBI rehabilitation is interested in cognition and language, it should be based on rational evidence for cognition and language. Searle[11] provided the most eloquent review of the major philosophical views of cognition and language. He considered monism, dualism, materialism, behaviorism, functionalism, and constructionism.

Monism is the view that only the mind or the brain needs to be considered, but not both. The TBI literature is monistic in this sense. TBI scholars focus primarily on the brain. As such, their primary interests pertain to the localization of mental skills in the cortices and to physiologic recovery.

Dualism is the view that both mind and brain are important. At first glance, a dualistic view appears to be the appropriate perspective for understanding TBI. Searle,[11] however, posited that dualism is deficient because it misses consciousness and intentions as specific instances of consciousness.

Materialism is the view that mental skills ultimately can be accounted for through the neurochemistry of synapses and the myelin coverings of neurons. That is, mental material at the microlevel accounts for the brain, thus the mind, and dysfunctions as the consequence of trauma or disease operate on mental material. Searle,[11] however, indicated that materialism does not account for consciousness because it does not address intent.

Behaviorism is the view that behavior can be explained in terms of positive or negative reinforcement and cueing. Searle[11] identified one of the fundamental flaws of behaviorism. He stated: "The absurdity of behaviorism lies in the fact that it denies the existence of any mental states."[(p.35)]

Functionalism holds that the functions of cognition and language have priority over structure. There are three major proponents of functionalism: behavioral, simulation, and cognitive socialization. The behavioral advocates contend that positive and negative reinforcement and cueing function to alter behavior. The simulation perspective pertains to computer simulations that presumably function *as if* they were cognitive processes. Brown[14] cautioned that as-if simulations are vulnerable to misrepresentation because a simulation is really not what is purported to be. A simulation is a likeness rather than an actual entity.

The cognitive socialization view of functionalism is that the primary *cognitive functions* of language are representation[9] and mediation,[16] and the primary *communicative functions* of language are intent,[4,11,16] implicit content or possible worlds,[4] and explicit content.[17–20] Adherents to these views maintain that language structures function to make intentions recognizable.[18,20]

Searle[11] showed that the most coherent philosophical view for both cognition and language is *constructionism*. Advocates of this view contend that individuals actively construct their perspectives of the world[21] or what has come to be known as *possible worlds*.[4] Thus, what is possible for one individual does not necessarily hold the same possibilities for another. Yet mutual social and cultural influences operate as leveling effects so that although individuals have different possibilities, their possibilities are essentially the same. The clinical implications are to ascertain each individual's available repertoire (pre- and/or posttrauma) for cognitive and grammatical systems. Furthermore, it is advisable to maintain social and cultural affiliations.

In addition to philosophical views, rational evidence deals with theoretical perspectives. These perspectives are important because theories offer disciplined understandings and explanations.[2,22] Such understandings and explanations provide a scholarly field with a substantive and operational base.

There is rather solid evidence that the TBI field is atheoretical. The various dependent and independent variables are not derived from bona fide theories. Furthermore, the TBI literature is remarkably myopic by considering the brain but not recognizing major mind–brain distinctions and other related issues that ultimately establish constructionism as the most coherent view.

The mind–brain issue was raised by 19th century scholars (Descartes, de Saussure, von-Helmbolt, and so forth). These considerations came to a climax with the debate between Frege and Russell at the beginning of the 20th century. Frege[23] held that the name of a referent is understood when it makes "sense" in context. However, Russell[24] contended that the name of a referent is understood logically. The perspective of making sense in context pertains to the mind. Reliance on logic also depends on the mind, but individuals rarely contemplate the underlying assumptions and propositions of a message. The most thorough and comprehensive understandings regarding mind–brain distinctions issue from the works of Bruner,[4] Lakoff,[21] Nelson,[16] and Searle.[11]

Considerations about the *mind* are oriented on the *cognitive functions* of the mind centering on consciousness in general, and intent as specific instances of consciousness.[11] In this arena, *intent* becomes the "irreducible nucleus" of both cognition and language.[4,11,16] Furthermore, both cognition and language operate in terms of narratives, or story lines, that make sense in one's own world.

From the mind perspective, it is necessary to address the following issues when treating individuals with TBI: intentionality, possible worlds or implicit content, explicit content, narratives, repertoires, active language learning loci, and executive functions.[25]

Regarding the latter, Ylvisaker and Feeney[26] outlined aspects of cognition.[(p.59)] Their outline cited some aspects of cognition, but it missed others—notably, the centrality of intent[27] discrepancy learning theory for orienting and establishing attention,[28–30] memory that cannot be separated from its applications,[31] and mental processing that is essentially not modality specific.[32,33]

Intentionality is the "irreducible nucleus" of language and cognition.[4,11,16] This means that accounts of language and cognition for individuals with brain injury should be centered on intention rather than elicitation. That is, spontaneous language and thinking in ecologically relevant contexts[25,34–37] provide the best evidence of what an individual can do with language and cognition rather than performances on contrived tasks (testing) or reinforcement schedules.[8]

Narratives are story lines of thought and communication. It is necessary to ascertain the nature of narratives used by individuals with brain injury to determine which aspects of narratives should be the focus of intervention.

Ylvisaker and Feeney[26] promoted "positive everyday routines" as an intervention strategy. However, they did not address different kinds of repertoires. Yet Ninio et al.[38] indicated that describing a speaker's repertoires is crucial for understanding that individual's language capacity. They wrote: "Describing speakers' repertoires of communicative intents and rules for expressing those intents is crucial to any complete description of the language capacity."[(p.157)]

There are several different kinds of repertoires that should be assessed with individuals with TBI. These include the following:

1. Repertoires for basic grammatical systems (subject–noun–phrase system repertoire, object–noun–phrase system repertoire, auxiliary system repertoire, verb–phrase system repertoire)

2. Repertoires for phonologic systems (phonologic processes, phonetic inventory, homonymy, phonologic avoidance)

3. Repertoires for pragmatic systems (openings, topic initiation, topic development, topic sharing, deictic reference, three types of anaphora, preclosings, and closings)

Repertoires are not discussed in the TBI literature. Yet a fundamental inquiry for these individuals is their available cognitive and communicative repertoires. The intervention implication is to expand an individual's repertoires. For example, some individuals may rely on a relatively small set of highly rehearsed utterances. The intervention ramification is to introduce lexical variation (new words that express ecologically relevant issues) into such utterances to expand a person's communicative skills.

Active language learning also is a fundamental principle of language acquisition. However, individuals with cerebral injury may have difficulty dealing with the vicissitudes of daily life. Consequently, they may rely on a constant set of utterances and even unvaried surroundings. It is not unusual for individuals with cerebral injury to become upset when their surroundings are varied. Yet variation enables an individual to deal with the vicissitudes of daily life.

There are many theories of cognition and language that have continuity with construc-tionism. Perera,[39] the editor of the *Journal of Child Language*, identified the five most influen-tial theories of language acquisition. The theories are as follows:

1. Relevance theory,[20] which is the newest rendition of speech act theory[18,19,31]
2. Bootstrapping theories[40–42]
3. Government and binding theory,[43–45] with the sister theories of learnability and parameter setting[10,46–48]
4. Modularity theory[49]
5. Parallel distributed processing theory[50]

Given Perera's[37] identification of the five most influential theoretical perspectives, conscientious professionals should consider the rehabilitation implications of these theories.

There are two very important observations to be made regarding this list. First, because reinforcement theory lacks descriptive and explanatory adequacies, reinforcement theory did not make the list. Second, the modality theory[51] also did not make this list on similar grounds.

Consequently, the most highly qualified scholars dismissed both reinforcement and modality theories in the 1970s and 1980s. Regarding reinforcement theory, Nelson[7] wrote: "Models of language acquisition built explicitly on assumptions of positive and negative reinforcement are no longer acceptable."[(p.33)]

This circumstance raises a paradox for the clinical fields. On the one hand, brain injury professionals are willing to rely on reinforcement theory[52] when rendering clinical ser-vices to individuals with TBI. On the other hand, scholars have indicated that reinforce-ment theory does not measure up to scholarly rigor.[11,53]

Clark and Clark[33] provided the most thorough account of information processing. They showed that the modality of a message becomes "purged" very early in information pro-cessing, before the essential cognitive processing takes place. Nelson[7,16] affirmed that cognitive processing of messages is not modality specific. Tallal,[54] who has done more research on auditory processing than anyone else, summarized her research by saying: "These deficits [language impairments] are neither specific to speech stimuli nor confined to the auditory modality."[(p.616)]

Another paradox concerning the field of TBI intervention pertains to language modali-ties. This field, like several other clinical fields, is willing to rely on the modality the-ory[51] by virtue of addressing *expressive language, receptive language, auditory processing*, and *visual processing*. Although there are differences in modality processing, these differences are marginal, and the core issues (cognition, codification, communication, and emotion) of language are missed.[3,36,37,55] Perhaps it should be noted that the most highly qualified scholars dismissed the modality theory several decades ago. Strangely, the clinical fields remain undaunted by their reliance on this theory.

There are many theories that could be beneficial to the field of TBI. The following is a partial list: the theory of natural categories,[56] the situated mind,[16] learnability theory,[10] bootstrapping theory,[41] discrepancy learning theory,[28–30] cognitive distancing theory,[57,58] and relevance theory.[20] These theories offer many potentials for providing appropriate clinical services to individuals with TBI.

Regarding relevance theory, the two main tenets are the centrality of intent for both cognition and language, and the distinctions between explicit and implicit content for messages. Sperber and Wilson[20] indicated that, when an individual wants (intent) to think or communicate, that is the most opportune time to learn. Furthermore, the purpose of messages is to make intentions recognizable. Thus, intervention for individuals with TBI should be vested on intent.

It is because of relevance theory that the communicative payoff principle has become clinically useful.[25,36,55] When an individual wants to communicate by whatever means (pointing, gesture, utterances), the clinician stays on the topic. Typically, that individual becomes progressively more confident and strives to communicate more and, more important, that individual attempts new means of communication.

Explicit content is the basic ideas entailed in a message. For example, the sentence "I want a Coke" has the following basic ideas: someone/desires/something. The particulars for these basic ideas reside in an individual's knowledge of the world or possible worlds. Thus, if an individual does not know the meaning of Coke, then this message does not work as intended. The clinical ramification is that intervention should always encompass topics within an individual's world. Following Bronfenbrenner,[34,35] such intervention would be ecologically valid.

16.4 The Nominalist Fallacy

Bohannon and Bonvillian[12] made the following comment concerning the nominalist fallacy: "Researchers fall into this fallacy when they think that giving a phenomenon a special name sufficiently explains the phenomenon."[(p.270)]

The intervention literature for TBI contains numerous instances of the nominalist fallacy, especially pertaining to cognition and language. There are many claims concerning memory, problem solving, executive functions, and language that relate to this fallacy.

This fallacy is evidenced when the dependent variables are only marginally relevant, or tangential, to a domain but the conclusions are domain conclusions. Bruner[59] used the phrase *going beyond the information given* to refer to an individual's cognitive ability to infer. Bruner's observation can be applied to researchers who generalize beyond the data given to draw conclusions about a domain.

For example, Butler and Copeland[60] used a cognitive remediation program that dealt with the digit span test, sentence memory, and the continuous performance test. They drew conclusions about memory based on digit memory and sentence memory. Yet these notions of memory were shown to lack validity many years ago.[61,62] Furthermore, Fivush and Hudson[31] showed that memory cannot be isolated from its applications. Under this circumstance, it is impossible to measure memory as an entity by itself. Rather, it becomes necessary to ascertain each individual's repertoire of skills for a particular aspect of a domain.

A study by van't Hooft et al.[63] utilized the Amsterdam Memory and Training Program. The participants were randomly assigned to experimental and control groups. The authors reported significant gains for the experimental group regarding sustained and short-term attention tests and a delayed word memory test. Inasmuch as significant gains were obtained, the question arises as to whether these results are generalizable to the TBI population.

There are three reasons to give pause about such generalizations:

1. Given the current literature on attention and memory, the dependent variables are questionable.
2. Theories on attention and memory were not used to derive these measures—notably, the theory for eliciting and maintaining attention.[28–30]
3. The number of participants ($n = 20$) in each group is likely to be insufficient to represent a heterogeneous population.

The TBI literature makes many claims concerning cognition (notably, attention, memory, problem solving, and various executive functions) and the language literature (notably, semantics, syntax, phonology, and pragmatics). Rather than the nominalist fallacy, it is more appropriate to tie specific claims to relevant theoretical perspectives. By doing so, the intervention literature becomes elevated to a higher level of scholarship—namely, at the postulational and formal levels. Accordingly, these higher levels offer more potential for providing appropriate and effective intervention.

The literature on theory of mind (TOM) also should be incorporated into the TBI literature.[64–71] In contrast to the Piagetian perspectives about the physical world, TOM pertains to the social–emotional world. Three substantive aspects of TOM are especially relevant to TBI. One substantive dimension is an individual's expressions concerning one's own emotions. (I am afraid.) Another substantive dimension is the perception of others. (He is silly.) A third dimension is the recognition of shared perspectives. (We want hot dogs.) The TOM literature, including the research paradigms, has much to offer the TBI rehabilitation literature.

16.5 Adducing Effective Rehabilitation Services: Alternatives

Some contend that the most appropriate evidence for ascertaining treatment efficacy and effectiveness is the result of randomized clinical trials. The research phases posited by Gonzalez-Rothi[1] reflected this view. Perhaps some additional comments should be made about within-subject and between-subject designs and some other related issues—notably, programs of research, replications, and meta-analyses.

One problem with some research designs, both multivariate and multiple baseline, is that the more variables that are included, the greater the likelihood of false findings. With these designs, it is essential to replicate treatments to weed out spurious findings.

Similarly, studies with small participant sample sizes and/or small cognitive or language sample sizes are likely to yield skewed results. Such results are highly vulnerable to type I and type II research errors. A type I error is rejecting the null hypothesis when, in fact, it should be accepted. A type II error occurs when the null hypothesis is accepted, but, in fact, it should have been rejected.

Another problem that is specific to within-subject designs is the reliance on interpretations of graphical evidence rather than statistical significance. Such interpretations result in impressionism rather than statistical rigor. Replication is necessary to clean up impressionism.

Reliance on control groups is desirable from the perspective of scholarly rigor. However, the use of control groups means that promising interventions may be withheld from those participants in the control groups. This is a very serious ethical dilemma. On the one hand, it is desirable to substantiate the effectiveness of a particular intervention approach. On the other hand, however, an approach that is withheld for research purposes from those in the control group raises the problem of unethical conduct. A watered-down solution for this dilemma is to provide an alternative intervention. However, this creates another issue with its confounded effects.

Programs of research that include replications offer another way to ascertain the effectiveness of various intervention approaches. Such programs provide opportunities to appreciate each intervention approach from different perspectives. Coupled with repertoire evidence rather than test scores, programs of research could become the most effective ways to substantiate the effectiveness of intervention approaches for heterogeneous populations.

Another promising way to establish effective intervention is the use of meta-analyses. Such analyses may be conducted by focusing attention on either the independent variables or the dependent variables for a group of studies. Such studies have both positive and negative dimensions. They are positive because they can be used to summarize a body of literature toward a firmer understanding of an issue. They are negative because they rely on selected aspects of the literature, and this may lead to impressionism.

Recognizing that the intervention literature is in its infancy, the best evidence for substantiating appropriate intervention policies and practices is not empirical evidence but rational evidence. As indicated earlier, rational evidence is the composite of philosophical views and theoretical perspectives that warrant particular clinical services. Here again, rational evidence underscores the need for the TBI literature to be derived from recognized philosophical views and theoretical perspectives.

16.6 Heterogeneity

Individuals with TBI comprise a heterogeneous population. Although a particular intervention approach may be effective for one individual, it does not necessarily mean that it will be effective for another. Indeed, a particular treatment may not be effective in one instance, but it may work surprisingly well under different circumstances.

Heterogeneity undermines those research designs that are implicitly based on the homogeneity assumption. Specifically, between-group designs are threatened by heterogeneous populations. There are two kinds of threats: loss of power and inadequate participant sample sizes. When between-group designs are used with heterogeneous populations, the resulting analyses become increasingly vulnerable to type I and type II errors, thereby losing power.

With homogeneous populations, the participant sample sizes should be about 40 for each variable. However, with heterogeneous populations, the participant sample sizes should be much larger, perhaps double. Yet the research with TBI participants is typically inordinately small. The results of such studies should only be regarded as suggestive of what one or a few individuals can do, rather than a population. The within-group designs are even more vulnerable to spurious findings that are only attributed to one or a few individuals.

16.7 Summary

In summary, this chapter raises some concerns about the current literature on TBI. There is reason to be cautious and introspective regarding some of the conclusions in this literature. The reasons for circumspection pertain to the following:

- Research samples that are exceedingly small and may not be representative of the population of individuals with TBI
- Research designs such as the within-subject designs that result in impressionism rather than statistical significance
- Cognitive terms that do not measure up to the substantive issues in the cognitive literature
- Willingness of some authors "to go beyond the information given" in a study when drawing conclusions

The absence of bona fide theories in conceptualizing, implementing, and drawing conclusions raises questions about the presumed effectiveness of some TBI interventions. Perhaps the following quote by Gonzalez-Rothi[1] will suffice as a summary: "We have an emerging literature involving 'exploratory' studies designed to begin the process of creating treatment options and honing these innovations toward effectiveness and application."[(p.196)]

References

1. Gonzalez-Rothi, L., Cognitive rehabilitation: The role of theoretical rationales and respect for the maturational process needed for our evidence, *Journal of Head Trauma Rehabilitation*, 21(2), 194–197, 2006.
2. Kaplan, A., *The Conduct of Inquiry: Methodology for Behavioral Science*, Chandler Publishing, San Francisco, CA, 1964.
3. Muma, J., *Scholarship in Communication Disorders: Raising the Bar*, Natural Child Publisher, Hattiesburg, MS, 2008.
4. Bruner, J., *Actual Minds, Possible Worlds*, Harvard University Press, Cambridge, MA, 1986.
5. Wanner, E., The parser's architecture, in F. Kessel (Ed.), *The Development of Language and Language Researchers*, Erlbaum, Hillsdale, NJ, 79–96, 1988.
6. Chomsky, N., *Language and Mind*, Harcourt, Brace, & Jovanovich, New York, 1968.
7. Nelson, K., *Making Sense: The Acquisition of Shared Meaning*, Academic Press, New York, 1985.
8. Macken, M., Representation, rules, and overgeneralization in phonology, in B. MacWhinney (Ed.), *Mechanisms of Language Acquisition*, Erlbaum, Hillsdale, NJ, 367–397, 1987.
9. Mandler, J., Representation, in P. H. Mussen (Series Ed.), J. H. Flavell, and E. M. Markman (Eds.), *Handbook of Child Psychology: Vol. 3, Cognitive Development*, 4th ed., Wiley, New York, 420–494, 1983.
10. Pinker, S., Learnability theory and the acquisition of a first language, in F. Kessel (Ed.), *The Development of Language and Language Researchers*, Erlbaum, Hillsdale, NJ, 97–120, 1988.
11. Searle, J., *The Rediscovery of the Mind*, MIT Press, Cambridge, MA, 1992.
12. Bohannon, J. N. and Bonvillian, J. D., Theoretical approaches to language acquisition, in J. Berko Gleason (Ed.), *The Development of Language*, 5th ed., Allyn & Bacon, Boston, 254–314, 2001.
13. Chomsky, N., *Syntactic Structures*, Mouton, The Hague, 1957.

14. Brown, R., *A First Language: The Early Stages*, Harvard University Press, Cambridge, MA, 1973.
15. Tuniks, G., Linguistic theory in the transformationalist approach, *Lingua*, 16, 364–376, 1966.
16. Nelson, K., *Language in Cognitive Development*, Cambridge University Press, New York, 1996.
17. Greenfield, P. M. and Smith, J. H., *Communication and the Beginnings of Language*, Academic Press, New York, 1976.
18. Grice, H. P., Logic and conversation, in P. Cole and J. L. Morgan (Eds.), *Syntax and Semantics: Vol. 3, Speech Acts*, Seminar Press, New York, 41–58, 1975.
19. Searle, J., *Speech Acts: An Essay in the Philosophy of Language*, Cambridge University Press, Cambridge, UK, 1969.
20. Sperber, D. and Wilson, D., *Relevance: Communication and Cognition*, Harvard University Press, Cambridge, MA, 1986.
21. Lakoff, G., *Women, Fire, and Dangerous Things: What Categories Reveal about the Mind*, University of Chicago Press, Chicago, IL, 1987.
22. Kerlinger, F., *Foundations of Behavioral Research*, 2nd ed., Holt, Rinehart, & Winston, New York, 1973.
23. Frege, G., On sense and reference, in P. Greach and M. Block (Eds.), *Translations from the Philosophical Writings of Gottleb Frege*, Blackwell, Oxford, UK, 1952 [1892].
24. Russell, B., On denoting, *Mind*, 14(56), 479–493, 1905.
25. Muma, J. and Cloud, S., *Advancing Communication Disorders: 60 Basic Issues*, Natural Child Publisher, Hattiesburg, MS, 2008.
26. Ylvisaker, M. and Feeney, T., *Collaborative Brain Injury Intervention: Positive Everyday Routines*, Singular, San Diego, CA, 1998.
27. Searle, J., *The Rediscovery of the Mind*, MIT Press, Cambridge, MA, 1992.
28. Kagan, J., Continuity in cognitive development during the first year, *Merrill-Palmer Quarterly*, 15(1), 101–119, 1969.
29. Kagan, J., *Change and Continuity in Infancy*, Wiley, New York, 1971.
30. Kagan, J., The determinants of attention in the infant, *American Scientist*, 58(3), 298–306, 1970.
31. Fivush, R. and Hudson, J., *Knowing and Remembering in Young Children*, Cambridge University Press, New York, 1990.
32. Baddeley, A., Working memory: The interface between memory and cognition, in D. Schacter and E. Tulving (Eds.), *Memory Systems: 1994*, MIT Press, Cambridge, MA, 351–368, 1994.
33. Clark, H. and Clark, E., *Psychology and Language*, Harcourt, Brace, & Jovanovich, New York, 1977.
34. Bronfenbrenner, U., Developmental research, public policy, and the ecology of childhood, *Child Development*, 45(1), 1–5, 1974.
35. Bronfenbrenner, U., *The Ecology of Human Development*, Harvard University Press, Cambridge, MA, 1979.
36. Muma, J., *Language Acquisition: A Functionalistic Approach*, Pro-Ed, Austin, TX, 1986.
37. Muma, J., *Effective Speech–Language Pathology: A Cognitive Socialization Approach*, Erlbaum, Mahwah, NJ, 1998.
38. Ninio, A., Snow, C. E., Pan, B. A., and Rollins, P. R., Classifying communicative acts in children's interactions, *Journal of Communicative Disorders*, 27(2), 157–187, 1994.
39. Perera, K., Editorial: Child language research: Building on the past, looking to the future, *Journal of Child Language*, 21(1), 1–7, 1994.
40. Bruner, J., The social context of language acquisition, *Language and Communication*, 1(2/3), 155–178, 1981.
41. Gleitman, L., The structural sources of verb meanings, in P. Bloom (Ed.), *Language Acquisition: Core Readings*, MIT Press, Cambridge, MA, 174–221, 1994.
42. Pinker, S., The bootstrapping problem in language acquisition, in B. MacWhinney (Ed.), *Mechanisms of Language Acquisition*, Erlbaum, Hillsdale, NJ, 399–442, 1987.
43. Chomsky, N., *Lectures on Government and Binding*, Foris, New York, 1982.
44. Chomsky, N., *Barriers*, MIT Press, Cambridge, MA. 1986.
45. Chomsky, N., A minimalist program for linguistic theory, in K. Hale and S. Keyser (Eds.), *The View from Building 20: Essays in Linguistics in Honor of Sylvain Bromberger*, MIT Press, Cambridge, MA, 1–52, 1993.

46. Hyams, N., *Language Acquisition and the Theory of Parameters*, Reidel, Dordrecht, Holland, 1986.

47. Lightfoot, D., The child's trigger experience: Degree-O learnability, *Behavioral and Brain Sciences*, 12(2), 321–375, 1989

48. Pinker, S., *Learnability and Cognition*, MIT Press, Cambridge, MA, 1989.

49. Fodor, J., *The Modularity of the Mind: An Essay on Faculty Psychology*, MIT Press, Cambridge, MA. 1983.

50. McClelland, J. and Rummelhart, D., *Parallel Distributed Processing*, vol. 2, Bradford, Cambridge, MA, 1986.

51. Osgood, C., Motivational dynamics of language behavior, *Nebraska Symposium on Motivation*, University of Nebraska Press, Lincoln, NE, 1957.

52. Skinner, B., *Verbal Behavior*, Appleton-Century-Crofts, New York, 1957.

53. Kohn, A., *Punished by Rewards*, Houghton & Mifflin, Boston, 1993.

54. Tallal, P., Fine-grained discrimination deficits in language-learning impaired children are specific neither to the auditory modality nor to speech perception, *Journal of Speech and Hearing Research*, 33(3), 616–619, 1990.

55. Muma, J., *Language Handbook*, Prentice-Hall, Englewood Cliffs, NJ, 1978.

56. Rosch, E., Natural categories, *Cognitive Psychology*, 4(3), 328–350, 1973.

57. Sigel, I., Language of the disadvantaged: The distancing hypothesis, in C. Lavatelli (Ed.), *Language Training in Early Childhood Education*, University of Illinois Press, Urbana, IL, 60–78, 1971.

58. Sigel, I. and Cocking, R., Cognition and communication: A dialectic paradigm for development, in M. Lewis and L. Rosenblum (Eds.), *Interaction, Conversation, and the Development of Language*, Wiley, New York, 207–226, 1977.

59. Bruner, J. and Olver, R. Development of equivalence transformation in children. In J. Bruner (Ed.), *Beyond the information given*, Norton, New York, 1973.

60. Butler, R. W. and Copeland, D. R., Attentional processes and their remediation in children treated for cancer: A literature review and the development of a therapeutic approach, *Journal of the International Neuropsychological Society*, 8(1), 115–124, 2002.

61. Blankenship, A., Memory span: A review of the literature, *Psychological Bulletin*, 35(1), 1–25, 1938.

62. Jenkins, J., Remember that old theory of memory? Well, forget it!, *American Psychologist*, 29(11), 785–795, 1974.

63. van't Hooft, I., Andersson, K., Bergman, B., Sejersen, T., Von Wendt, L., and Bartfai, A., Beneficial effect from a cognitive training programme on children with acquired brain injuries demonstrated in a controlled study, *Brain Injury*, 19(7), 511–518, 2005.

64. Astington, J. W. and Jenkins, J. M., A longitudinal study of the relation between language and theory-of-mind development, *Developmental Psychology*, 35(5), 1311–1320, 1999.

65. Bretherton, I. and Beeghly, M., Talking about internal states: The acquisition of an explicit theory of mind, *Developmental Psychology*, 18(6), 906–921, 1982.

66. Dunn, J., Brown, J, Slomkowski, C., Tesla, C., and Youngblade, L., Young children's understanding of other people's feelings and beliefs: Individual differences and their antecedents, *Child Development*, 62(6), 1352–1366, 1991.

67. Farrar, M. and Maag, L., Early language development and the emergence of a theory of mind, *First Language*, 22(65), 197–213, 2002.

68. Flavell, J. H., Flavell, E. R., Green, F. L., and Moses, L. J., Young children's understanding of fact beliefs versus value beliefs, *Child Development*, 61(4), 915–928, 1990.

69. Leslie, A., Some implications of pretence for mechanisms underlying the child's theory of mind, in J. Astington, P. Harris, and D. Olson (Eds.), *Developing Theories of Mind*, Cambridge University Press, Cambridge, 19–46, 1988.

70. Perner, J., Ruffman, T., and Leekam, S., Theory of mind is contagious: You catch it from your sibs, *Child Development*, 65(4), 1228–1238. 1994.

71. Wellman, H. M., Cross, D., and Watson, J., Meta-analysis of theory-of-mind development: The truth about false belief, *Child Development*, 72(3), 655–684, 2001.

17

Neuroanatomic Review of Cognitive Function: Anatomy and Plasticity

Mark J. Ashley

CONTENTS

17.1 Introduction

Traumatic brain injury (TBI) involves an unpredictable and wide array of neurologic structures. The clinician is faced with a tremendous variety of clinical presentations as a result. Advances in neuroscience have been considerable during the past two decades, and knowledge of neurologic anatomy and physiology has improved tremendously. Knowledge of the basic anatomy and physiology of the brain is important for understanding behavioral manifestations following injury at a minimum. That same knowledge should be integral to theoretical constructs and rationales for the development of treatment approaches for cognitive dysfunction following TBI.

The most basic levels of cognition relate to how information enters the central nervous system (CNS), is gathered, moved, reduced, used, and stored. This chapter provides a review of the anatomy that underlies information processing and a review of some aspects of the physiology of learning and memory.

17.1.1 Sensory Systems

Information flow throughout the CNS is a primary concern for cognitive function. Tactile sensory pathways include those responsible for pain and temperature (lateral spinothalamic tract), those responsible for conscious proprioception and discriminative touch (dorsal column–medial lemniscal pathway), and those responsible for unconscious proprioception (ventral and dorsal spinocerebellar tracts) (Figure 17.1). The lateral spinothalamic tract synapses in the ventral posterior thalamic nucleus and projects via thalamocortical fibers of the posterior limb of the internal capsule to sensory cortex in the postcentral gyrus of the frontal lobe. Collateral projections from the spinothalamic tract synapse in the

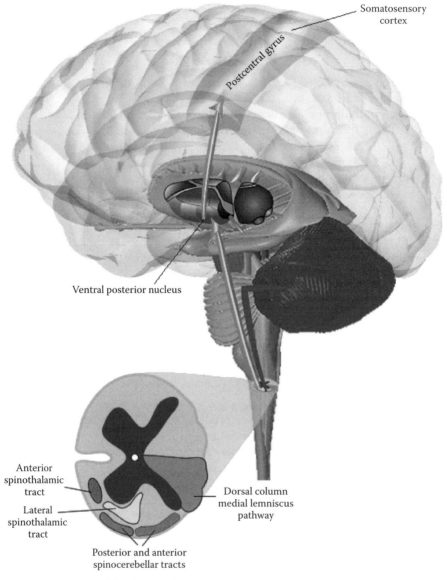

FIGURE 17.1 (See color insert following page 528.)
Diagram of the spinothalamic tract at the level of the spinal cord, brainstem, thalamus, and parietal cortex. Colors correspond to specific portions of the pathway.

brainstem within the reticular formation. The dorsal column–medial lemniscal pathway follows the same course as the lateral spinothalamic tract via the ventral posterior nucleus of the thalamus and posterior limb of the internal capsule on its way to the postcentral gyrus. The anterior spinothalamic tract, which is responsible for perceptions of simple touch, comprises a portion of the dorsal column. The ventral and dorsal spinocerebellar tracts terminate at the level of the cerebellum.

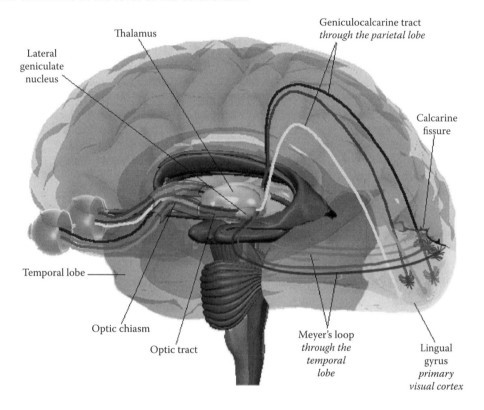

Left visual field

- Left upper quadrant crosses through the optic chiasm to the right geniculocalcarine tract and on to the calcarine fissure
- Left lower quadrant crosses via the optic chiasm to the right side Meyer's loop to the visual cortex
- Right upper quadrant passes along the optic tract via the left side Meyer's loop to the visual cortex
- Right lower quadrant passes along the optic tract via the left geniculocalcarine tract to the calcarine fissure

Right visual field

- Right lower quadrant crosses through the optic chiasm to the right geniculocalcarine tract and on to the calcarine fissure
- Right upper quadrant crosses via the optic chiasm to the left Meyer's loop to the visual cortex
- Left upper quadrant passes along the optic tract via the right side Meyer's loop to the visual cortex
- Left lower quadrant passes through the optic tract via the right geniculocalcarine tract to the calcarine fissure

FIGURE 17.2
Visual pathways from retinas, thalamus, geniculocalcarine tract, Meyer's loop, and occipital cortex.

Visual stimuli enter the system at a supratentorial level, coursing from the retina via the optic nerve to the lateral geniculate nucleus of the thalamus (Figure 17.2). The stimulus progresses from the lateral geniculate nuclei via Meyer's loop and the geniculocalcarine tract before terminating in the calcarine fissure and lingual gyrus of the occipital lobe, respectively. Visual stimuli travel to the occipital primary sensory regions via both temporal (Meyer's loop) and parietal lobe (geniculocalcarine tract) structures, depending upon the quadrant of the visual field represented. More detail is presented in Chapter 7 (this volume).

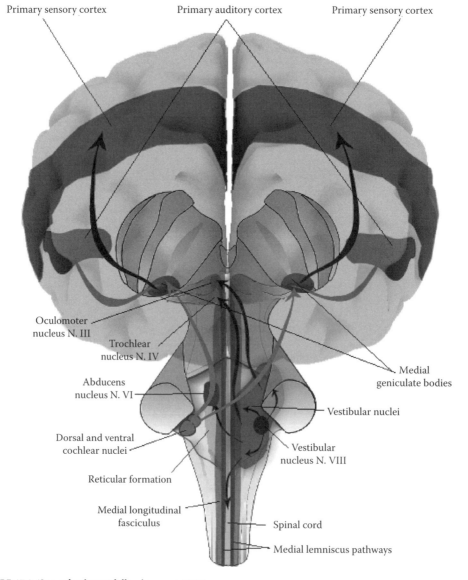

FIGURE 17.3 (See color insert following page 528.)
Auditory and vestibular sensory pathways depicting brainstem nuclei and thalamic relays via the medial geniculate bodies, progressing to parietal and temporal cortices.

Auditory stimuli first registers at the dorsal and ventral cochlear nuclei located in the pons (Figure 17.3). Auditory stimuli travel from these nuclei to the medial geniculate bodies of the thalamus before continuing to the auditory cortex of the temporal lobes. Vestibular stimuli also course through cranial nerve VIII, which synapses in the brainstem on the superior, medial, lateral, and inferior vestibular nuclei located in the upper medulla and lower pons (Figure 17.3). Stimuli project from these nuclei to the spinal cord, cerebellum, reticular formation, and to the nuclei of the oculomotor (III), trochlear (IV), and abducens (VI) cranial nerves via the medial longitudinal fasciculus. Vestibular signals terminate in the primary sensory area of the parietal lobe and auditory signals terminate in the superior temporal gyrus.

Olfactory stimuli travel from the olfactory bulb to the rhinencephalon and project to the piriform area of the medial temporal lobe (MTL), the anterior perforated substance and the terminal gyri of the medial basal frontal lobe, and the anterior uncus located in the medial surface of the temporal lobe (Figures 17.4 and 17.5). Olfactory stimuli also project to the amygdala and hippocampal gyrus. Like visual stimuli, olfactory stimuli enter the CNS at a supratentorial level. Olfactory stimuli reach the thalamus via projections from the piriform cortex and the amygdala. Odorant stimuli can reach the neocortex directly or indirectly via the thalamus.[1] The influence of olfactory stimuli on emotive state is supported by projections to the amygdala and hypothalamus. Pheromones signal via these same pathways. The orbitofrontal and frontal cortices are involved in conscious odor discrimination.

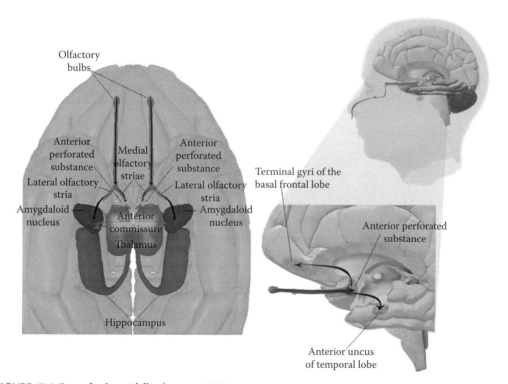

FIGURE 17.4 (See color insert following page 528.)
Olfactory system: olfactory bulb to anterior perforated substance to anterior and frontal lobe. Inferior and medial views.

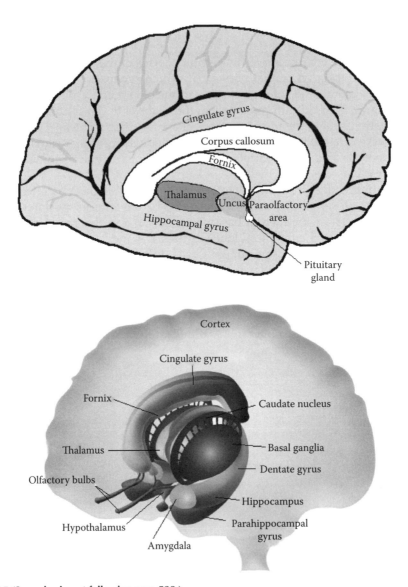

FIGURE 17.5 (See color insert following page 528.)
Medial and three-dimensional views of olfactory bulb, amygdala, thalamus, uncus, and paraolfactory area.

17.2 Reticular Formation

The pathways reviewed thus far are systems that relay to specific thalamic nuclei and act more directly upon the primary sensory cortices via various thalamic nuclei. The reticular formation acts indirectly to provide sensory input to the cortex, but does so via the nonspecific thalamic nuclei (Figure 17.6). Projections from the nonspecific thalamic nuclei connect to all areas of the cortex. Afferent input to the reticular formation is provided from collateral branches of the spinothalamic and lemniscal pathways, and information descending from the cortex through the corticoreticular pathways. The corticoreticular fibers include

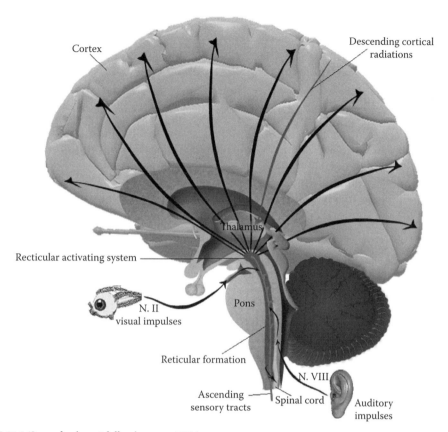

FIGURE 17.6 (See color insert following page 528.)
Reticular activating system with sensory input, ascending and descending pathways.

collateral branches of the corticospinal and corticobulbar tracts deriving from cortical areas that are widespread. The cerebellum, basal ganglia, hypothalamus, cranial nerve nuclei, and colliculi also provide afferent input to the reticular formation. The superior colliculus is implicated in the covert orientation of attention to visual space,[2] and the midbrain has been implicated in the orientation of attention and maintenance of arousal level.[3,4]

Reticular efferents deliver information from the reticular formation to the hypothalamus, the nonspecific nuclei of the thalamus,[5] and the descending reticulospinal pathway.[6] Pathways projecting from the reticular formation are part of the ascending projectional system.

17.2.1 Hypothalamus, Pituitary, Thalamus, and Basal Ganglia

17.2.1.1 Hypothalamus and Pituitary

A primary function of the hypothalamus is regulation of the autonomic nervous system. The hypothalamus integrates autonomic response and endocrine function with behavior to maintain homeostasis of certain systems. Blood pressure and electrolyte composition are maintained by control of drinking and salt appetite. Body temperature is regulated by control of metabolic thermogenesis and behaviors that seek to warm or cool the individual. Energy metabolism is regulated by feeding, digestion, and metabolic rate. Reproduction is regulated through hormonal control. Finally, emergency responses to stress are controlled by regulating blood flow to muscle and other tissues, and by the release of adrenal stress hormones. The hypothalamus receives inputs of sensory information from all over the body, compares this information with biologic set points and, upon detection of deviation from the set points, adjusts autonomic, endocrine, and behavioral responses to return to homeostasis.[7]

Hypothalamic influence is exerted directly upon the pituitary. The pituitary controls hormone production by serving as a feedback mechanism rather than by direct production of hormones. The anterior pituitary regulates the sex hormones, prolactin, growth hormone (GH), and cortisol. The posterior pituitary regulates antidiuretic hormone and insulin production (Figure 17.7).

Pituitary function following brain injury is frequently disrupted.[8,9] The anterior pituitary is most vulnerable to injury and this injury is often precipitated by elevated intracranial pressure, sustained hypotension, anoxia, and subarachnoid hemorrhage.[10] GH deficiency,

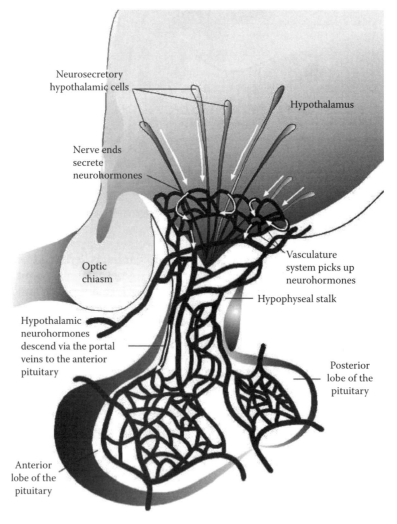

FIGURE 17.7

Hypothalamus, hypophyseal stalk, and pituitary showing anterior and posterior pituitary division and blood supply.

hypogonadism, and hypothyroidism are the most common sequelae of pituitary injury following TBI.[10] One review of 71 people with TBI found that, although not all met criteria for clinical deficiency, an overall trend was observed toward low normal ranges of hormone levels for the group as a whole (Brent Masel, pers. comm.).

GH deficiencies are implicated in cognitive dysfunction (attention, executive functioning, memory, and emotion); mitochondrial function; fatigue; dyslipidemia; reduced strength and exercise capacity; and osteoporosis. Correction of growth hormone has been suggested to benefit cognitive function postinjury.[11] Insulinlike growth factor 1 treatment has been shown to reduce demyelination and upregulate gene expression of myelin-related proteins in other populations[12] and may well play a role in recovery and/or preservation of function following brain injury. Six months of GH substitution in GH-deficient individuals was found to improve long-term and working memory.[13] Functional magnetic resonance imaging studies revealed activations in prefrontal, parietal, motor, and occipital cortices during a working memory task, and less recruitment compared with placebo in the ventrolateral prefrontal cortex (PFC), suggesting overall less effort required and more efficiency in neural recruitment.[13] Others have reported improvements in attentional performance at 3 months and 6 months of GH treatment.[14] GH impacts mitochondrial function, and decreased levels may directly impact energy production in the cell body as well as along the axon and in axonal and dendritic endplates, where mitochondrial function is necessary to meet energy demands throughout the cell.[15,16]

GH is also implicated in myelin production in the CNS. In the presence of axonal injury in spinal cord injury models designed to simulate demyelinating disease, administration of insulinlike growth factor 1 increases myelin generation through increased myelin protein synthesis and myelin regeneration via oligodendrocytes.[12]

Thyroid function is crucial for normal brain development and for proper production of oligodendrocytes.[17–21] Furthermore, thyroid administration early in a demyelinating inflammatory disease model enhances and accelerates remyelination, increasing expression of platelet-derived growth factor-α receptor, restoring normal levels of myelin basic protein messenger RNA and protein, and allows early and morphologically competent reassembly of myelin sheaths.[22] Thyroid is also clearly implicated in the regulation of mitochondrial function.[23]

Similarly, thyroid is implicated in enhancing remyelination in chronic inflammatory disease.[22] The impact of thyroid and steroid hormones on neural structures should be considered. Thyroid hormones regulates availability of cytoskeletal proteins necessary for neuronal growth.[24] Concentrations of thyroid hormone receptors have been found to be highest in the hippocampus, amygdala, and cerebral cortex of rats.[25] Depletion of thyroid in adult rats results in a significant reduction in dendritic density in the cerebral cortex.[26,27] Thyroid function is crucial in normal brain development and impacts gene regulation for encoding proteins of myelin, mitochondria, neurotrophins and neurotrophic receptors, cytoskeleton, transcription factors, splicing regulators, cell matrix proteins, adhesion molecules, and proteins involved in intracellular signaling.[20] Many of these, if not all, play a role in recovery of neuronal and astrocytic function following brain injury. Excess and deficient levels of thyroid hormones can impact neurodevelopment.[17] Two iodothyronines (T3 and T2) have been shown to be effectors of the actions of thyroid hormones on energy metabolism and the regulation of energy transduction performed by cellular mitochondria.[23]

Androgen deficiencies have clear implications for both cognition and mood. Sex steroid administration has been shown to be beneficial in improving working memory, particularly in men.[28] Estrogen has been shown to increase the number of synapses in the hippocampus in animals[29–31] and has been shown to improve verbal memory in women.[32,33] Estrogen has also been demonstrated to impact dendritic density as well as acetylcholine synthesis.[34,35] In fact, estrogen therapy has been shown to be effective in Alzheimer's disease.[36]

Glucocorticoid receptors are prominent in the limbic system.[26] As a significant portion of the information processing circuitry (in particular, as it relates to the MTL complex), the role of the limbic system is substantial in memory consolidation. The amygdala is important in mediating the influences of epinephrine, norepinephrine, and glucocorticoids on memory.[37] Additional information about neuroendocrine function can be found in Chapters 11 and 14 in this volume.

17.2.1.2 Thalamus

The thalamus is comprised of four groups of nuclei: the *anterior, medial, ventral,* and *posterior*.[38] The *anterior* nucleus is a single nucleus that receives its major input from the mammillary nuclei of the hypothalamus and the presubiculum of the hippocampal formation. It is interconnected with the cingulate and frontal cortices and may be involved in memory. The *medial* nucleus is comprised of the mediodorsal nucleus, which has three subdivisions. Each of these projects to a particular region of frontal cortex, and input is received from the basal ganglia, amygdala, and midbrain. The medial nucleus is also implicated in memory. The *ventral* nucleus is comprised of the ventral anterior and ventral lateral nuclei. These are involved in motor control. Input to these nuclei comes from the cerebellum and basal ganglia, and output is to the motor cortex. The ventral posterior nucleus, also part of the ventral nucleus, sends somatosensory information to the neocortex. Lastly, the *posterior* nucleus is made up of the medial geniculate, lateral geniculate, and lateral posterior nuclei and the pulvinar. The medial geniculate nucleus receives tonotopic auditory stimulus and projects it to the superior temporal gyrus. The lateral geniculate receives information from the retina and projects it to the primary visual cortex.[38]

The nuclei discussed thus far are referred to as *specific thalamic nuclei.* Figure 17.8 provides a detailed depiction of thalamic nuclei, their connections, and functions. They project to specific primary sensory areas of the cortex. Nonspecific nuclei, on the other hand, project diffusely to several cortical and subcortical regions. The thalamus receives a great deal of input from the cortex. In fact, cortical input to the lateral geniculate nucleus, for example, is greater in number of synapses than input from the retina. Most thalamic nuclei are similar. A single thalamic nucleus sends information to multiple cortical areas, which return information back to the thalamus but to different thalamic nuclei. Irrelevant information is suppressed whereas so-called "correct input" is facilitated by positive feedback via corticofugal projections.[39]

The thalamus is surrounded by the reticular thalamic nucleus, which forms an outer layer to the thalamus. The reticular nucleus uses the inhibitory neurotransmitter γ-aminobutyric acid, whereas most other thalamic nuclei utilize glutamate, an excitatory neurotransmitter. Neurons of the reticular nucleus do not interconnect with cortical neurons, but terminate, instead, on other thalamic nuclei as they exit the thalamus. The reticular nucleus exerts a modulatory effect on the actions of other thalamic nuclei in this manner. As a result, a degree of information processing occurs at the thalamus as a result of the monitoring of the thalamocortical stream of information made possible by the collaterals of other thalamic nuclei synapsing on reticular neurons as they pass through the outer layer of the reticular nucleus.[38]

Anterior nucleus—Receives input from the mammillary nuclei of the hypothalamus and the presubiculum of the hippocampal formation. Connected with the cingulate gyrus and frontal cortices. Involved in memory.

Lateral dorsal nucleus—Inputs from the hippocampal formation and mammillary bodies and projects to the cingulate cortex. Relays signals to the cingulate gyrus. May contribute to visceral–sensory integration.

Lateral posterior nucleus—Inputs from adjacent thalamic nuclei. Interconnected with superior parietal lobe. Aids in integrating and transcoding multiple sensory modalities underling higher mental functions.

Medial nucleus—Input from the basal ganglia, amygdala, and midbrain. Comprised of the mediodorsal nucleus which has three subdivisions. Each projects to a particular region of the frontal cortex. Implicated in memory.

Ventral anterior nucleus—Inputs from the basal ganglia and cerebellum. Outputs to the supplementary motor cortex. It initiates wanted movement and inhibits unwanted movement.

Ventral lateral nucleus—Input from the cerebellum and basal ganglia. Outputs to the primary motor cortex and premotor cortex. Aids coordination and planning of movement. Plays a role in learning movement.

Ventral posterior nucleus—Input from the medial and spinal lemniscus, and spinothalamic and trigeminothalamic tract. Ouputs to the somato sensory cortex and ascending reticuloactivation system. Functions in touch, body position, pain, temperature, itch, taste, and arousal.

Medial geniculate nucleus—Receives tonotopic auditory stimulus and projects it to the superior temporal gyrus.

Lateral geniculate nucleus—Receives information from the retina and projects it to the primary visual cortex.

Pulvinar—Connection with visual cortical, somatosensory cortical association areas, and with cingulate, posterior parietal, and prefrontal cortical areas. Aids in language formation and processing and reading and writing.

Reticular thalamic nucleus—Forms an outer layer of the thalamus. Neurons terminate on other thalamic nuclei as they exit the thalamus. Exerts a modulator effect on the actions of other thalamic nuclei.

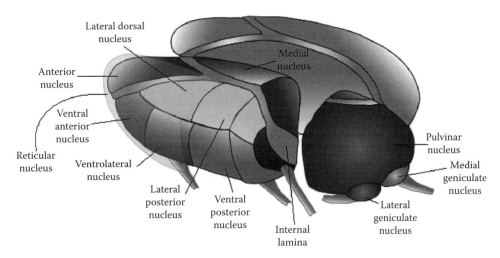

FIGURE 17.8 (See color insert following page 528.)
Thalamic nuclei locations, pathways, and functions.

17.2.1.3 Basal Ganglia

The basal ganglia are comprised of four major nuclei: the *striatum*, the *globus pallidus*, the *substantia nigra*, and the *subthalamic nucleus*. The *striatum* receives input from the cerebral cortex, thalamus, and brainstem and projects to the globus pallidus and the substantia nigra. The *globus pallidus* and *substantia nigra*, in turn, form the major output projections from the basal ganglia. The basal ganglia are involved in a variety of behaviors, including voluntary movement and skeletomotor, oculomotor, cognitive, and emotional functions.[40,41] Basal ganglia output is back to the cortex, via the thalamus, or to the brainstem. The basal ganglia serve as an important system linking the thalamus and cerebral cortex. Information that originates from a specific cortical area may be returned from the thalamus to other cortical areas.

17.3 Medial Temporal Lobe and Hippocampal Complex

The MTL includes the hippocampal region (CA fields, dentate gyrus, and subicular complex) and the entorhinal, perirhinal, and parahippocampal cortices (Figure 17.9). The

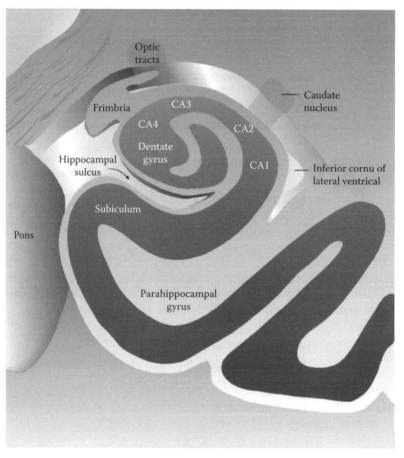

FIGURE 17.9
Coronal view of the hippocampal complex.

hippocampus has been widely studied because of its role in memory. The hippocampal gyri are located in the inferior medial temporal lobes.

Damage to the hippocampus, or any of the association areas in the temporal lobe with which it connects, will result in deficits in explicit memory.[29–31] Explicit memory is sometimes referred to as *declarative memory* and includes episodic and semantic memory. Declarative memory formation is impaired following MTL damage. Semantic memory is the capacity for acquisition and recollection of facts and other general knowledge about the world.[42–44] Episodic memory involves memory for events and experiences whereas semantic memory involves memory for factual information abstracted from specific incidents or episodes.[45,46] Characteristics of declarative memory include that it is flexible, consciously accessible, and integrated into a broad fund of stored knowledge.[47–50]

As damage in the MTL extends laterally, semantic knowledge becomes increasingly impaired. Formation of declarative knowledge may not be possible in complete MTL damage, even with the support of structures outside the MTL.[51] Processing of novel versus familiar auditory stimuli appears to activate the anterior and posterior hippocampal complex respectively, whereas processing of novel versus familiar visual information appears to be reversed.[52] Likewise, there appears to be a differential response for encoding and retrieval activity, with the anterior structures responding more to encoding whereas the posterior structures respond more to retrieval.[53,54]

Information appears to be processed first in the association areas of the prefrontal, limbic, and parieto-occipitotemporal cortices.[45,55] Information is then passed to the parahippocampal and perirhinal cortices and, from these, on to the entorhinal cortex. From the entorhinal cortex, information passes to the dentate gyrus, the subiculum, and the CA3 and CA1 regions of the hippocampus. The dentate gyrus passes information to the CA3 hippocampal region, which then passes information to the CA1 region and on to the subiculum. From there, information is sent back to the entorhinal cortex,[56] on to the parahippocampal and perirhinal cortices, and back to the cortices. Hippocampal projections to cortical areas are widely distributed.[56] The circuitous nature of these connections provides support for a role in detection of novel stimuli,[57,58] associative memory,[59,60] encoding of explicit memory,[58] retrieval of explicit memory,[61] attentional control of behavior,[62] spatial memory,[63,64] and, possibly, a role in the development of long-term memory.[45] The CA3 region of the hippocampus appears to deal primarily with previously stored information. The CA1 region, in contrast, seems to deal primarily with novel information. The CA3 region is hypothesized to provide sparsely encoded information arising from highly processed information received from the dentate gyrus.[65–67] CA3 is also thought to be an autoassociator and comparator.[65–67] It appears that CA3 may be able to retrieve entire patterns from partial or degraded input, comparing it with data arriving from entorhinal cortex and thereby acting to filter information sent to CA1.[68] Processing of spatial scenes appears to involve the parahippocampus, whereas spatial memory involves the right hippocampus. Context-dependent explicit memory is more dependent upon the left hippocampus.[64]

The connection of the association cortices and hippocampal structures is quite important for overall cognitive function. Information from several, widely distributed cortical regions must be integrated to perform complex mental functions. The association areas receive information from higher order sensory areas and, ultimately, convey the consolidated information to higher order motor areas.[69] The motor areas organize planned actions. The hippocampal role, together with involvement of other medial temporal and limbic lobe structures, is found in the manner in which hippocampal input is received from and output is projected to the associative cortices. These circuits appear to be active in processes whereas previously stored information is modified by new experience.[45]

Hippocampal efferents project to the amygdala, the septum, the fornix, the thalamus, the mammillary bodies, the medial preoptic area, and the perifornical nucleus of the hypothalamus.[70] The anterior hippocampus appears to exert an excitatory modulatory effect on the amygdala.[71] It exerts inhibitory effects on the fornix and both excitatory and inhibitory effects on the ventromedial nucleus of the hypothalamus. The amygdala is implicated in self-preservation activities, such as the search for food, feeding, fighting, and self-protection,[72] and the association of sensory information with emotional states. McGaugh[73] cites evidence that the basolateral region of the amygdala is crucial in memory consolidation arising from emotionally intense experiences. Stress hormone production and other neuromodulatory systems activated by such experiences are made possible via the anterior hippocampal projections to the amygdala, which progress to the hypothalamus and the basal forebrain. The posterior hippocampus also sends projections to the hypothalamus via the fornix. Motivational significance of incoming stimuli is determined by the amygdala, with subsequent coordination of multiple systems to enable an appropriate response.

Long-term potentiation (LTP) occurring in the hippocampus serves as a component of synaptic consolidation. LTP in the hippocampus is largely dependent upon dopaminergic availability.[74] Some authors suggest dopamine receptor (D1/D5) activation serves to initiate intracellular second messenger accumulation, functioning more in a modulatory role.[75] There actually may be a synergistic role between D1/D5 receptor activation and *N*-methyl-d-aspartate (NMDA) receptor activation for LTP induction.[76]

17.4 Inferior Temporal Lobe

The inferior temporal cortex includes the inferior and middle temporal gyri and is bounded posteriorly just anterior to the lateral occipital sulcus and bounded anteriorly just a couple of millimeters posterior to the temporal pole. It extends laterally to the occipitotemporal sulcus (Figure 17.10).

The inferior temporal lobe (ITL) interconnects with the visual peristriate cortex (V2, V3, and V4) and the polysensory areas of the superior temporal sulcus, the temporopolar prosiocortex, the PFC, and the limbic system (comprised of the limbic lobe, hippocampus, and amygdala). (For a detailed review of ITL anatomy in the primate, see Logothetis.[77])

The ITL appears to be important for object recognition and categorization. Category-specific impairments have been tied to temporal lobe-specific injuries.[78] Visual features that are important in category membership determination are instantiated in single neuron activity in primate ITL,[79] and neuronal selectivity for shape and color have been demonstrated.[80] It appears that short-term memory for the categorized visual[65] percept of pictures is represented in the ITL.[81]

The ITL in primates has been shown to be involved in visual discrimination,[82–85] visual attention,[86,87] and visual short-term memory.[86,88,89] Selective reactivity to stimulus dimensions of shape, orientation, and color has been demonstrated in single unit recordings in the ITL.[90–92] In addition, evidence has demonstrated modulation of ITL unit response by attention and situational variables.[93–95] The ITL does not appear to be directly involved in association memory in that neurons have not been found to discriminate on the basis of reward.[93] Acquisition of serial recognition tasks (when intervening stimuli occur between novel and familiar presentations) is associated with the ITL.[96]

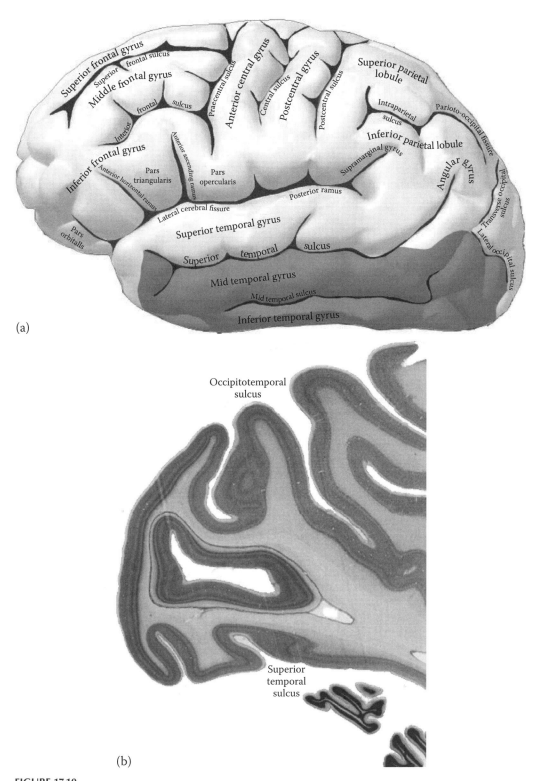

FIGURE 17.10

(a) Lateral view of the inferotemporal cortex. (b) Coronal view of the occipitotemporal and superior temporal sulci.

Thomas et al.[80] found that approximately 25% of sampled ITL neurons responded only to specific category exemplars during a visual categorization task. The exemplar specificity of ITL neurons may point to a larger role to be played by the PFC in categoric boundary determination. The majority of sampled neurons in the ITL were not category specific and appeared to be "broadly tuned," instead, for categorization activity. Unlike individual neurons in the PFC that are able to encode rules, neurons in the ITL do not appear able to respond individually to derive categorization, but rather function collectively.

Stimulation of the ITL in humans results in recall of visual imagery.[97] Because of its interconnections, it is structurally predisposed to integrate multiple aspects of vision, relay information to multisensory convergence areas, and interact with structures that play an important role in decision making, in short- and long-term memory, and in emotions.[77] ITL involvement includes sensitivity to the level of categorization and the level of expertise of the observer.

17.5 Frontal Lobe

The frontal lobe is organized to provide motor function in the primary motor cortex (Brodmann area 4) anterior to the central fissure. The primary motor cortex receives its input from the premotor cortex (areas 6 and 8) and from the somatosensory cortex. Fibers from areas 4, 6, and 8 of the frontal lobe and 3, 2, and 1 of the parietal lobe contribute to the corticospinal tract. Horizontal gaze is controlled by area 8. The motor component of speech is managed by areas 44 and 45 in the left hemisphere (Figure 17.11). The balance of the frontal lobe, comprising nearly two thirds of the entire frontal lobe, provides support for executive cognitive functions. Information flow in the postcentral fissure cortex progresses from primary to secondary to tertiary association cortices. However, that information flow is reversed in the frontal lobe, with flow progressing from tertiary to secondary to primary motor cortices. In fact, the frontal lobe is largely informed by postcentral fissure and subcortical structures.

Executive functions are managed by the PFC. The PFC can be subdivided into three major regions: orbital, medial, and lateral. The orbitofrontal cortex provides inhibitory control via its efferents to the hypothalamus, the basal ganglia, and other neocortical areas, some of which are within the PFC itself. Damage to the orbitofrontal cortex results in behaviors described as impulsive, disinhibited, irritable, contentious, tending toward coarse humor, and showing a disregard for social and moral principles.[98]

The medial PFC includes the most anterior portion of the cingulate gyrus. It is involved in attention and emotion. Damage to the medial frontal cortex can result in difficulty in initiating movement or speech[99,100] and akinetic mutism in larger lesions. Apathy, abulia, or a loss of spontaneity can be seen together with difficulty in concentration on behavioral or cognitive tasks.[98]

The lateral PFC is important to organization and execution of behavior, speech, and reasoning. Luria[101] found damage to this area to be associated with inability to formulate and carry out plans and sequences of actions, and conscious representation and construction of sequences of spoken and written language.[102] Damage in the lateral PFC is often accompanied by severe attention disorder.

Afferent connections to the PFC include the brainstem, thalamus, basal ganglia, limbic system, amygdala, hypothalamus, hippocampal association cortices, and each of the other

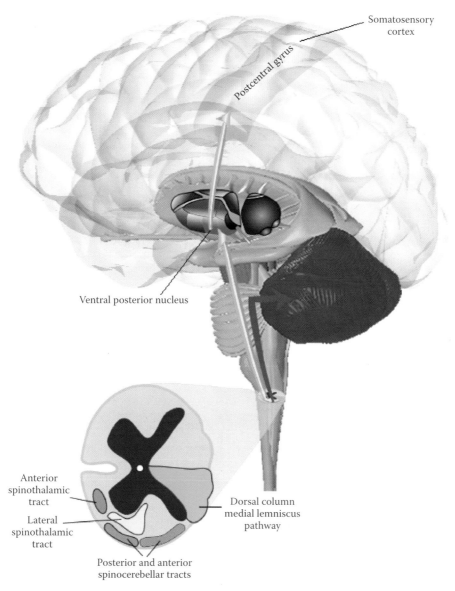

FIGURE 17.1

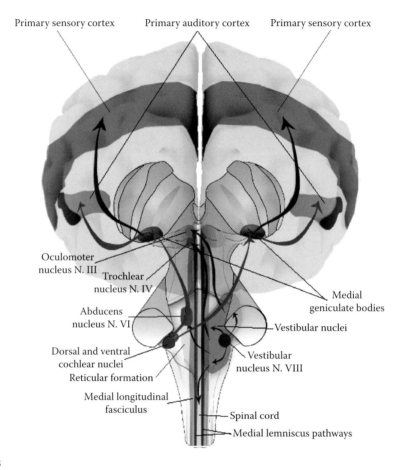

FIGURE 17.3

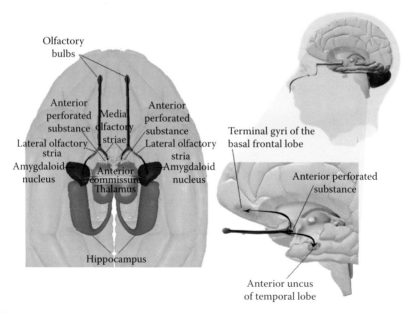

FIGURE 17.4

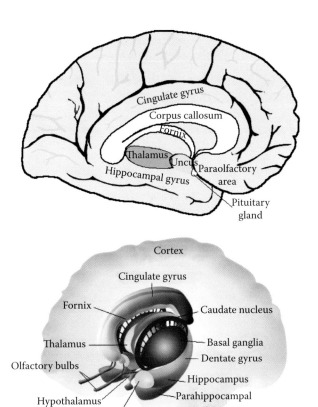

FIGURE 17.5

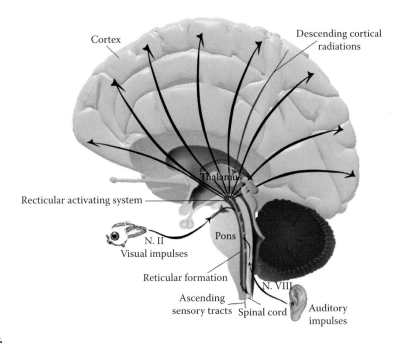

FIGURE 17.6

Anterior nucleus—Receives input from the mammillary nuclei of the hypothalamus and the presubiculum of the hippocampal formation. Connected with the cingulate gyrus and frontal cortices. Involved in memory.

Lateral dorsal nucleus—Inputs from the hippocampal formation and mammillary bodies and projects to the cingulate cortex. Relays signals to the cingulate gyrus. May contribute to visceral–sensory integration.

Lateral posterior nucleus—Inputs from adjacent thalamic nuclei. Interconnected with superior parietal lobe. Aids in integrating and transcoding multiple sensory modalities underling higher mental functions.

Medial nucleus—Input from the basal ganglia, amygdala, and midbrain. Comprised of the mediodorsal nucleus which has three subdivisions. Each projects to a particular region of the frontal cortex. Implicated in memory.

Ventral anterior nucleus—Inputs from the basal ganglia and cerebellum. Outputs to the supplementary motor cortex. It initiates wanted movement and inhibits unwanted movement.

Ventral lateral nucleus—Input from the cerebellum and basal ganglia. Outputs to the primary motor cortex and premotor cortex. Aids coordination and planning of movement. Plays a role in learning movement.

Ventral posterior nucleus—Input from the medial and spinal lemniscus, and spinothalamic and trigeminothalamic tract. Ouputs to the somato sensory cortex and ascending reticuloactivation system. Functions in touch, body position, pain, temperature, itch, taste, and arousal.

Medial geniculate nucleus—Receives tonotopic auditory stimulus and projects it to the superior temporal gyrus.

Lateral geniculate nucleus—Receives information from the retina and projects it to the primary visual cortex.

Pulvinar—Connection with visual cortical, somatosensory cortical association areas, and with cingulate, posterior parietal, and prefrontal cortical areas. Aids in language formation and processing and reading and writing.

Reticular thalamic nucleus—Forms an outer layer of the thalamus. Neurons terminate on other thalamic nuclei as they exit the thalamus. Exerts a modulator effect on the actions of other thalamic nuclei.

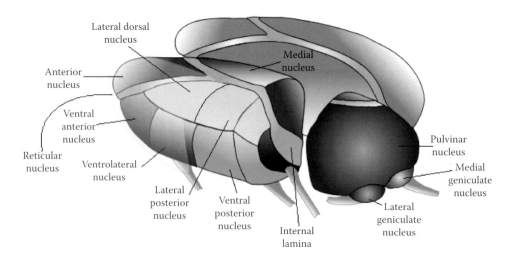

FIGURE 17.8

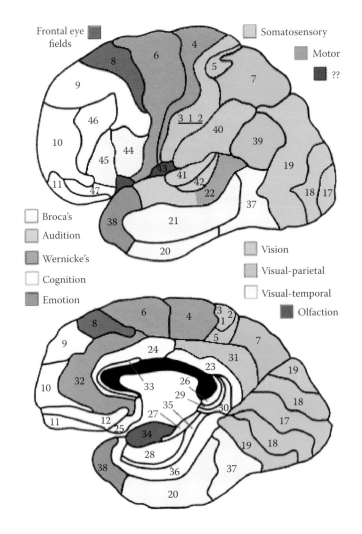

FIGURE 17.11

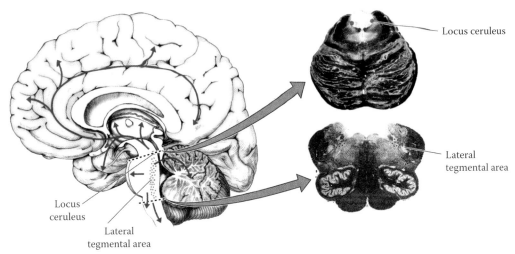

Locus ceruleus

Lateral tegmental area

FIGURE 17.12

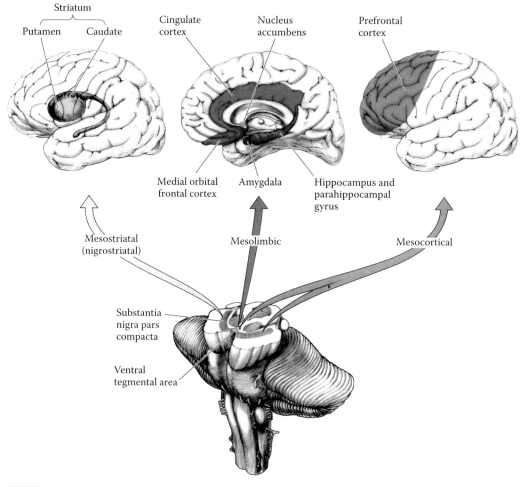

Striatum

Putamen   Caudate

Cingulate cortex

Nucleus accumbens

Prefrontal cortex

Medial orbital frontal cortex

Amygdala

Hippocampus and parahippocampal gyrus

Mesostriatal (nigrostriatal)

Mesolimbic

Mesocortical

Substantia nigra pars compacta

Ventral tegmental area

FIGURE 17.13

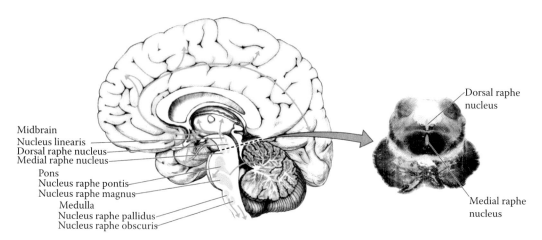

Midbrain
Nucleus linearis
Dorsal raphe nucleus
Medial raphe nucleus
Pons
Nucleus raphe pontis
Nucleus raphe magnus
Medulla
Nucleus raphe pallidus
Nucleus raphe obscuris

Dorsal raphe nucleus

Medial raphe nucleus

FIGURE 17.14

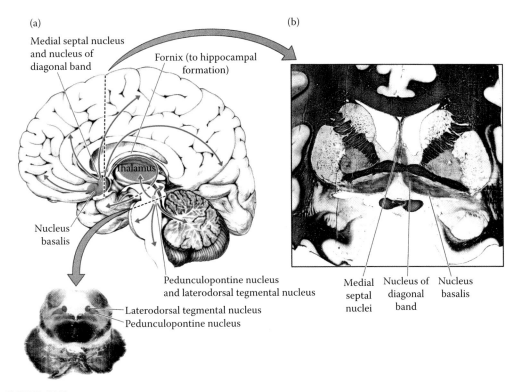

(a)

Medial septal nucleus
and nucleus of
diagonal band

Fornix (to hippocampal
formation)

Thalamus

Nucleus
basalis

Pedunculopontine nucleus
and laterodorsal tegmental nucleus

Laterodorsal tegmental nucleus
Pedunculopontine nucleus

(b)

Medial   Nucleus of   Nucleus
septal   diagonal   basalis
nuclei   band

FIGURE 17.15

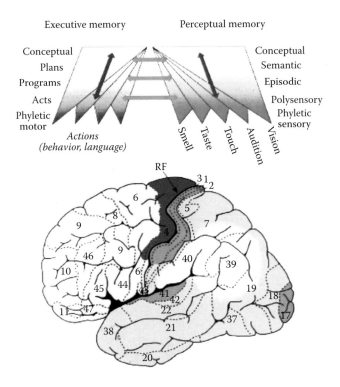

Executive memory   Perceptual memory

Conceptual   Conceptual
Plans   Semantic
Programs   Episodic
Acts   Polysensory
Phyletic   Phyletic
motor   sensory

Actions
(behavior, language)   Smell Taste Touch Audition Vision

RF

3 1
  2
6
    5
8
9   7
    4
46   9
10   40
             39
45 44
11 47   41
         42   19 18
       22
38   21   37   17
     20

FIGURE 19.1

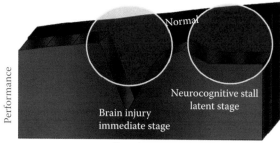

Pediatric TBI: Two stages of recovery

FIGURE 25.3

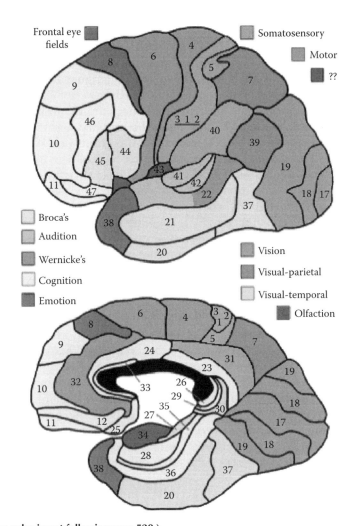

FIGURE 17.11 (See color insert following page 528.)
Brodmann areas color coded for primary functional significance. (From Prof. Mark W. Dubin, University of Colorado–Boulder, MCD Biology, http://spot.colorado.edu/~dubin/talks/brodmann/brodmann.html. With permission.)

prefrontal regions, but not primary sensory or motor cortices. The prefrontal regions are connected both to themselves and to each other with some cortical connectivity being interhemispheric. The memory networks of the posterior cortex acquire information and associations with action and forward that information to the PFC to influence the formation of networks of executive memory.[98] It is reasonable to compartmentalize information collection and retention as primarily a posterior cortical function, whereas formulation and execution of actionable concepts and events or refinement of previous knowledge is the purview of the anterior cortical structures. Clearly, however, the neurons of the PFC can also substantially modify previously acquired information.

The PFC serves as the substrate for executive memory whereas the postcentral fissure area of the parietal lobe serves as the substrate for perceptual memory. The PFC is the highest order of neocortex in both phylogenetic and ontogenetic terms and represents about one third of the neocortex. It is the latest maturing in myelogenic and synaptogenic terms[103–105] and does not reach full maturity until adolescence in humans.[106–108] The

PFC is crucial for propositional speech, reasoning, motor and executive memory, temporal organization of behavior, mediation of contingencies of action across time, retrospective (short and sensory memory) and prospective memory, active adaptation to the environment, skeletal and ocular movement, reasoning, spoken language, modulation of visceral actions, and emotional behavior.[109,110]

The neuronal networks that serve perceptual memory are found in the postcentral fissure area and are organized hierarchically upon the primary sensory cortices. Similarly, the precentral fissure region of the PFC provides an organization system of movement, behavior, speech, and reasoning based upon a similar hierarchy of inputs from disparate cortical and subcortical structures. The PFC utilizes these structures as efferent sources of information in addition to afferent networks to achieve the desired behavioral, speech, or reasoning outcome.[98,111] Higher cortical areas accommodate higher levels of memory, including episodic and semantic memory, together constituting declarative memory. Individual items of memory or knowledge are less hierarchically arranged and are better thought of as "heterarchical," relying upon mixtures of information from mixed memory types. Memory of a specific event relies upon a network of structures serving each of the mixed memory types.

Information flow in the CNS appears to utilize either primary or associative cortices, depending upon the degree of familiarity or novelty of the information. As novel information arrives and is compared with previously acquired information, comparative assessment appears to be conducted by the hippocampus and associative cortices acting in harmony. Previously acquired information is both impacted by and impacts the utilization of novel information. The posterior cortices appear to function as increasingly effective information processing and storage centers, providing information necessary for anterior cortical processing, such as executive function. Novel information requires the largest utilization of cortical resource resulting from heavy recruitment of multiple primary sensory areas. After the information is learned, much less cortical resource is utilized and the information appears to be more efficiently represented in smaller cortical areas of associative cortex. As new information arrives that bears upon previously acquired information, these networks are activated and modified to represent and assimilate the newly acquired information. This resource utilization pattern, from more to less cortical resource, can be seen also in studies examining cortical activation patterns during phases of skill acquisition.[112,113]

The prefrontal networks appear to function by prefrontal neuronal control exerted over existent networks. Neuromodulatory biasing of the network connections to address requisite needs in problem solving, reasoning, and other executive functions has been proposed. Neurons within the PFC provide biasing signals that guide the flow of neural activity along pathways to establish the proper interaction between inputs, internal states, and needed outputs for a given task.[114] The PFC appears to function to exert cognitive control in a top-down fashion upon existing networks, biasing them into controlled activity and disallowing their activity outside of the constraints of the current situation. The PFC marshals the same information and action networks that function to provide automaticity of response, however, through the neuromodulatory biasing of the network, disallows reflexive or automatic responses, and promotes the creation of event-specific responses that may be partially or entirely new. At the level of the cortex, neurotransmitters are better conceptualized therefore as neuromodulators.

Neurons in the PFC have been found to be individually capable of encoding abstract rules.[115] The PFC appears to be involved in guidance of behavior according to previously learned rules and in utilization of working memory.[116] Because the PFC receives highly processed information from other parts of the brain, its role appears to be to synthesize that information into learned task contingencies, concepts, and task rules.[117] PFC neurons are able to maintain task-relevant information and have a strong ability to resist interference from distraction.[111,118–120]

17.6 Commissural and Association Tract Fibers

Information must be moved from one cerebral area to another. Transport between subcortical and cortical areas is accomplished by projectional fibers that comprise the internal capsule. Fibers of the internal capsule carry information both toward and away from the cortex. Axons of the internal capsule spreading out to all areas of the cortex are known as the *corona radiata*. Fibers from the thalamus projecting to the cortex travel in the internal capsule. Projections from the anterior and medial thalamic nuclei carry visceral and other information and project to the frontal lobe via the anterior limb of the internal capsule. Projections from the ventral anterior and ventral lateral nuclei of the thalamus travel in the genu and posterior limb of the internal capsule and reach the motor and premotor areas of the frontal lobes. The ventral posterior and medial thalamic nuclei project to the sensory cortex of the parietal lobe via the fibers of the posterior limb of the internal capsule. The posterior limb of the internal capsule also contains optic and auditory fibers. Corticobulbar (head and face muscles) and corticospinal (neck and trunk muscles) motor pathways travel via the posterior limb of the internal capsule to the brainstem (corticobulbar) and spinal cord (corticospinal).

Interhemispheric connections are accomplished by the corpus callosum and two smaller commissural bundles. The anterior commissure interconnects the anterior temporal areas. The hippocampal gyri are connected to each other via the hippocampal commissure.

Intrahemispheric interconnection is accomplished by association fibers. The temporal and frontal lobes are joined by the uncinate fasciculus. The medial surfaces of the frontal, temporal, and parietal lobes are connected by the cingulum, which also connects the cingulate gyrus to the orbitofrontal cortex and the hippocampal cortex. Projectional fibers from the thalamus to these regions are contained in the cingulum. The anterior cingulate gyrus is implicated in executive attention[121] through the detection of conflicts occurring during information processing that signal the need to engage top-down attentional processes.[122] The anterior cingulate cortex is active in conscious attention during auditory processing.[123] It may provide an important connection between widely disparate aspects of attention, such as the mental operations of visual target detection and semantic content by integration of information arising from the various multimodal association cortices. The anterior cingulate gyrus has been implicated in episodic memory retrieval as well.[124] Finally, *arcuate fibers* connect adjacent gyri in neocortical areas. An excellent review of commissures, long tracts, and pathways connecting cortical and subcortical areas is provided by Taber and Hurley.[125]

Widespread/diffuse traumatic axonal injury (TAI) is a common characteristic of nearly all traumatically induced brain injury.[126] TAI impacts cortical and subcortical pathways, which serve the distributed network of discrete cortical regions where features that define an object or experience are stored. Both storage and recall of information are necessarily impacted by TAI and made less efficient. TAI is most frequently seen in the long tracts of the midline structures of the brain.[127] The cingulum is thought to be an important structure in the transfer of information from distributed regions of the brain to association cortices for integration. As such, the prevalence of TAI in the regions of the brain surrounding the cingulum will necessarily impact information transfer.

17.7 Principles of Neurophysiology and Cognition

The study of cognition has long been the realm of experimental psychology. Carefully designed research and detailed behavioral observation allowed insight into phenomena such as sensitization and habituation. The limitations of psychological investigation, however, rarely allowed for much beyond conjecture regarding the nature of the physiologic underpinnings of such behaviors. Cognitive processes, such as memory, have long been investigated, and early information regarding neurophysiologic issues arose from observation of persons with known injuries who may have been later studied at autopsy in an attempt to correlate, in gross anatomic terms, sites of lesion and observed premorbid behavioral changes.

Advances in neuroscience continue to expand the information available regarding neurophysiologic function and the cognitive processes that arise from that function. It is now possible to discuss neuronal function and neurotransmission at the level of the cell, gene, ion, and neurotransmitter. Neuroanatomic organization has advanced considerably from the early days, when primary debate consisted of whether nerve cells interconnected via a protoplasmic continuity or whether nerve cells existed individually and were contiguous rather than continuous.[56]

As neuroscience continues to expand available information, conceptions about neurocognitive function likewise will be necessarily advanced and refined. It is important to utilize available information, however incomplete it may still be, to develop rational theoretical constructs from which diagnosis and treatment of cognitive function are approached.

17.8 Information Processing, Neurotransmission, and Learning

Information processing has long been conceived as dependent upon the existence of three levels of storage: sensory stores, short-term memory, and long-term memory. Baddeley's[128] early conceptualization of these mechanisms led to the question of how information was transferred from short-term storage to long-term storage. Others have more recently suggested a need to revisit these concepts to consider frontal lobe structure, which may enable (1) the updating and maintenance of information; (2) the selection, manipulation, or monitoring of information; and (3) the selection of processes, subgoals, or planning.[129]

Memory consolidation implies a progression of staging of memory with variations in strength and reliability of memories across time. Consolidation occurs at the synaptic level and the systemic level. Much has been done recently to investigate the biologic mechanisms of memory consolidation. Synaptic tagging was identified as a factor in the synaptic consolidation process whereby requisite proteins for protein synthesis necessary for LTP accumulate in confined regions within the dendrite until LTP is instituted.[130,131] Genetic networks have been identified that, through upregulation or downregulation, are active in memory consolidation and memory retrieval, and are necessary constituents in both.[132] Memory is most recently viewed as a complex biologic process in which networks of neurons and genes function as the neurophysiologic basis for memory.[132] Genetic alteration in response to memory formation may be considered at both the synaptic and systemic levels of consolidation. At the systemic level of consolidation, information is stored in places other than the originally implicated synapses. Information is also altered once stored in systemic consolidation, seemingly comprised of a more synapse-efficient process.

At a cellular level, it has been demonstrated that different types of memory formation place different demands on the cellular mechanisms for protein synthesis. Protein synthesis occurs within the nucleus of the neuron in direct response to learning. Protein synthesis does not occur, though, for all types of memory. Short-term storage does not require protein synthesis. "All of the proteins, including receptors, ion channels, enzymes, and transporters, required for short-term memory formation and temporary storage are already present in sufficient abundance. In sharp contrast, however, long-term memory absolutely depends on the synthesis of new proteins or the increased synthesis of already existing proteins."[133, p. 235]

Synaptic activation and transmission lead to changes throughout the neuron. The nucleus, axon, dendrite, and synapse undergo structural changes that support information processing, learning, and memory. Changes at the synapse are such that they support the immediate, short-term, or long-term demands of the information processing process and either encourage or discourage further synaptic transmission. When transmission occurs across a synapse, the synapse becomes "potentiated," thereby making the synapse more responsive to the next transmission.[134] Potentiation of the synapse can be of varying durations, lasting seconds to years. Posttetanic potentiation lasts for a minute or less, whereas short-term potentiation lasts somewhat longer. Posttetanic potentiation and short-term potentiation result from increases in the number of quanta released and/or the strength of their postsynaptic effects.[135] LTP lasts weeks to years. LTP requires several simultaneous signals to be received by the neuron, and effectively "strengthens" the synapse. However, LTP alone does not provide adequate support for learning that is preserved over a lifetime. Declarative memory formation is highly dependent upon MTL structures including the hippocampus and entorhinal, perirhinal, and parahippocampal cortices. These structures are crucial for information acquisition and short-term storage; however, their role dissipates over time as information is transferred from recent to long-term storage.[136] In the latter instance, information appears to be distributed to other neocortical areas where it is stored.

LTP has an inhibitory counterpart known as *long-term depression* (LTD). LTD, a decrease in synaptic responsivity that is activity dependent, has been found to be induced postsynaptically, and it is possible that LTD may also require the production of a retrograde messenger.[137] Both LTP and LTD are viewed as cellular mechanisms involved in learning and memory. Habituation and sensitization are nonassociative types of learning and can be both short and long term in nature. Habituation and sensitization may be subserved by short- and long-term potentiation and depression.[138]

In studies with *Aplysia*, Frost et al.[138] demonstrated that short- and long-term potentiation were dependent upon the presentation of serotonin (5-hydroxytryptamine [5-HT]). A single presentation of 5-HT resulted in an increase in the excitatory postsynaptic potential between the sensory and motor neuron that lasted minutes. Presentation of five applications of 5-HT resulted in an increase in the excitatory postsynaptic potential that lasted 24 hours, required new RNA and protein synthesis, and involved the growth of new synaptic connections between the sensory and motor neuron. It is important to note that 5-HT is the modulatory neurotransmitter for the studied sensorimotor synapse in *Aplysia*. A number of studies have demonstrated, with differing species, similar mechanisms underlying learning and the development of nondeclarative motor skills and explicit (hippocampus-based) memory.[139–141]

In instances when LTP occurs, changes occur within the cell body and in gene expression. These changes may impact the function of all synapses or may be restricted to specific synapses. In instances when only select synapses undergo LTP, other synapses of the same neuron are more readily able to undergo LTP as a result of changes in the genetic expression at the cell body. Castelluci et al.[142] noted that both genetic expression and protein synthesis, not necessary for formation of short-term memory, likely were required for acquisition of long-term memory. In addition, it has been determined that neurotransmitters not only serve transmission of a signal across a synapse, but also function in the regulation of local protein synthesis, independent of the cell body used to establish synapse-specific changes in synaptic strength.[143] Frost et al.[144] found underlying circuit modification could be accomplished by at least four neuronal sites for short-term memory formation in *Aplysia*. Martin et al.[143] later demonstrated that local protein synthesis occurred at the synapse independent of the soma and its nucleus, thereby allowing for long-term, branch-specific facilitation.

LTP has been shown to last for varying periods of time throughout the brain. Within the dentate gyrus, LTP can last for months and up to a year.[145] LTP within the hippocampal area of CA1 and in the neocortex can last weeks.[146,147] LTP has at least two phases: a protein synthesis-independent phase and a protein synthesis-dependent phase. The protein synthesis-independent phase can last a few hours, whereas the protein synthesis-dependent phase lasts longer. Information that has passed into the protein synthesis-dependent phase is more resistant to loss. LTP can be more easily reversed early after its induction and becomes much less so 1 to 2 hours postinduction.[148] The development of resistance to reversal of LTP can be blocked by protein synthesis inhibitors.[149]

Reversal of LTP can be induced by transient anoxia,[150] low-frequency stimulation,[151,152] heterosynaptic high-frequency stimulation,[153] and seizure activity.[154] Brief exposure to novelty can result in a time-dependent reversal of LTP[155] and longer periods of exposure to novel enriched environments have been shown to reverse LTP gradually.[145] Abraham and Williams[148] suggest that protein synthesis-dependent LTP may not permanently "lock in" a memory but may simply act to raise the threshold for future change.

Immediate early genes (IEGs) have been identified that function in activity-dependent plasticity of dendrites.[156] The existence of IEGs (1) may account for rapid LTP formation that could not be accounted for by protein synthesis dependence alone, (2) may contribute to the protein synthesis-independent phase of LTP formation, and (3) are experience dependent. IEG expression has been demonstrated within both hippocampal and neocortical neurons. IEGs do not require *de novo* protein synthesis or previous activation of any other responsive genes. IEG transcription initiates following patterned synaptic activity that induces long-term synaptic plasticity.[157,158] Limitations of protein synthesis inhibitors used to study LTP and protein synthesis led one group to investigate IEGs as potential participants in memory formation.[132]

One of these IEGs, *Arc* (activity-regulated cytoskeleton-associated protein), has been implicated in the encoding process.[159] *Arc* was initially investigated as a growth factor that, when stimulated, induced rapid and transient expression of a set of genes, IEGs, which encoded transcription factors, cytokines, and other molecules that are believed to regulate long-term cellular responses.[160] Others have found that similarly rapid genomic responses are induced in neurons by neurotransmitter stimulation.[161,162] The IEG *Arc* is induced in response to neuronal activity. It is involved in synaptic and proteomic responses of memory formation.[132] Interestingly, *Arc* transcription is induced by NMDA receptor activation, which causes excitatory synaptic activity.[156,163] It should be recalled that a synergistic effect has been identified between dopamine and NMDA activation during LTP.[76] *Arc* is of interest because it was first found to be induced within 1 to 2 minutes of maximal electroconvulsive seizures and was found as intranuclear foci within most neurons. It disappears within about 15 minutes and subsequently becomes prominent in cytoplasmic and dendritic regions from 15 to 45 minutes poststimulus. Later, *Arc* can only be found in dendritic regions. Studies show that *Arc* can be behaviorally induced in the hippocampus following the same time patterns observed following maximal electroconvulsive seizures.[159] Finally, *Arc* is expressed after exploration of an environment and in learning tasks *in vivo*.[68,159,164]

Gene expression is just one factor active in determining a neuron's range of responses in recruitment or in stabilization of a neural circuit.[132] Memory formation depends then, at least, upon neural circuits and patterns of gene expression within individual neurons at any given time.

Although these studies are exciting in their implications, LTP and IEGs are not the only substrates of memory.[165] LTP, by itself, cannot account for all aspects of potentiation. The role of adhesion chemistry has been proposed by Lynch[165] as responsible for the explanation of the time constraints observed for LTP and memory function. Three transmembrane cell adhesion receptors have been identified: *integrin, cell adhesion molecules*, and *cadherins*. "Integrin activation/engagement thus emerges as that process whose temporal requirements dictate the particular time courses recently discovered for LTP and repeatedly described for memory."[165, pp. 143–144]

Other morphologic changes are known that may subserve LTP. Schubert[166] found that synaptic cleft modifications occur following synaptic transmission. Following repeated transmission across a synapse, the size of the synaptic cleft is reduced, and glycoproteins released into the cleft act to bind the synaptic endplates closer together. In addition, the synaptic endplates themselves broaden, resulting in greater exposure of neurotransmitter vesicles. The result is more rapid release of neurotransmitter into the synapse and less distance for the neurotransmitter to travel. As more rapid release and uptake of neurotransmitter occurs, more rapid transmission occurs.

Neurons are organized in adjacent columns of cells within the CNS. Cells within columns serve separate but similar functions, and greater numbers of computational columns are correlated with area size of the cortex dedicated to specific function.[8] Activation of a single neuron can cause increased electrical activity in adjacent cells and may cause a focal neuronal LTP response.[167] Aggregate groups of neurons are thought to function most probably together.[168] Activation of adjacent cells within columns may facilitate a desired level of processing or compound information processing. Both nitric oxide and carbon dioxide have been identified as retrograde messengers in neurotransmission, and they may play a role in widespread LTP.[169] Nitric oxide is a relatively short-acting neurotransmitter. Its release has been demonstrated to be experienced by closely adjacent synapses,[167] and it has been implicated in reference memory in studies of working versus reference memory in rats.[170,171]

Simple neural activation is not sufficient to bring about certain morphologic changes. *Reactive synaptogenesis* has been demonstrated to occur only when the neural activation is associated with learning.[172,173] During this process, new dendritic spine formation occurs at the synaptic level following repeated neurotransmission. This process is fairly rapid, with studies showing it to occur within 10 to 15 minutes.[174] Synaptogenesis must be supported by both glial cells[175] and adequate blood supply.[172] The time frame required for synaptogenesis to occur may be more than coincidental to the time required to allow for the transport of requisite proteins, which must transpire to allow for information to be transferred to long-term storage.

17.8.1 Neuromodulatory Neurotransmitters

Modulatory neurotransmitters play a major role in information processing. These substances most probably allow for a biasing of cortical and subcortical responsivity that is situationally determined.[114] The six primary modulatory neurotransmitter systems consist of the *noradrenergic* (norepinephrine), *adrenergic* (epinephrine), *dopaminergic, serotonergic, cholinergic*, and *histaminergic* cell groups. In addition, there are more than 50 neuroactive peptides that act as neurotransmitters, although not all are active, of course, within the brain.

A nucleus of interest in the noradrenergic system is the locus ceruleus (blue spot) located dorsally and lateral of midline in the periaqueductal and periventricular gray matter of the pons, near the fourth ventricle in the rostral pons. Noradrenergic neurons (Figure 17.12) are also located within the lateral tegmental area of the pons and medulla. Ascending projections from both regions reach the entire forebrain, the brainstem, cerebellum, and spinal cord, thereby impacting the entire CNS. Noradrenergic neurons of the medulla project to the hypothalamus, controlling endocrine and cardiovascular function. Those in the caudal regions of the pons and medulla are involved in sympathetic functions such as blood pressure control.[176] The locus ceruleus is implicated in maintenance of vigilance and responsiveness to unexpected stimuli. The norepinephrine system is involved in modulation of attention, sleep–wake states, and mood. Although firing of the locus ceruleus increases during waking and decreases during sleep, lesions of the locus ceruleus do not cause somnolence. Norepinephrine is implicated in depression, manic–depressive disorders, obsessive–compulsive disorders,

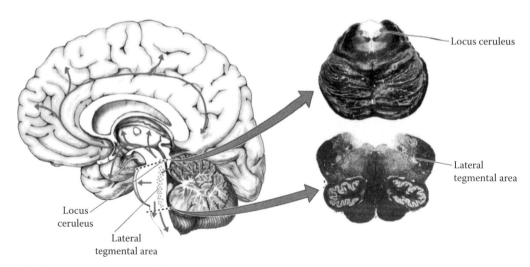

FIGURE 17.12 (See color insert following page 528.)
Noradrenergic projection systems. (Line drawing from Blumenfeld, H., *Neuroanatomy Through Clinical Cases*, Sinauer Associates, Inc., Sunderland, MA, 2002, pg. 596. With permission. Photograph reprinted from Martin, J. H., *Neuroanatomy: Text and Atlas*, 2nd ed., Appleton & Lange, Stamford, CT, 1996, pp. 512, 520. With permission from McGraw-Hill.)

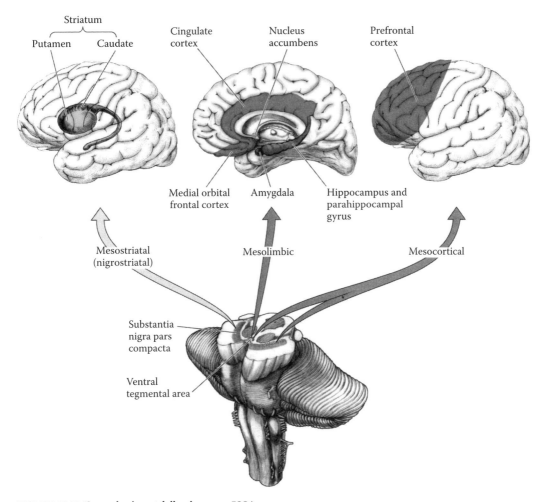

FIGURE 17.13 (See color insert following page 528.)
Dopaminergic projection systems. (From Blumenfeld, H., *Neuroanatomy Through Clinical Cases*, Sinauer Associates, Inc., Sunderland, MD, 2002, p. 595. With permission.)

and anxiety disorders, together with serotonin.[176] These cell groups constitute the long projection system of the reticular formation.[177]

Dopaminergic projections (Figure 17.13) arise from the substantia nigra pars compacta and the ventral tegmental area of the brainstem, and traverse many systems. Dopaminergic neurons project to the telencephalon. Neurons project to the frontal and temporal cortices as well as to the striatum, the limbic cortex, the amygdala, and the nucleus accumbens. These structures are involved in emotion; memory storage (encoding, retrieval, and working memory); movement; initiation/initiative; and thought.

Dopaminergic projections travel via the tuberoinfundibular, mesostriatal, mesocortical, and mesolimbic dopaminergic pathways. The tuberoinfundibular pathway projects from the hypothalamus to the pituitary. The mesostriatal pathway arises from the substantia nigra and serves the striatum—specifically, the caudate and putamen. Lesions of the mesostriatal pathway result in movement disorders, such as parkinsonism, and are often treated with dopaminergic agonists.[176] The mesolimbic pathway serves the medial temporal cortex, amygdala, cingulate gyrus, and the nucleus accumbens. As such, lesions

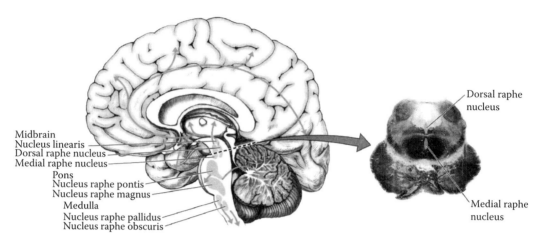

Midbrain
Nucleus linearis
Dorsal raphe nucleus
Medial raphe nucleus
Pons
Nucleus raphe pontis
Nucleus raphe magnus
Medulla
Nucleus raphe pallidus
Nucleus raphe obscuris

Dorsal raphe nucleus

Medial raphe nucleus

FIGURE 17.14 (See color insert following page 528.)
Serotonergic projection systems. (Line drawing from Blumenfeld, H., *Neuroanatomy Through Clinical Cases*, Sinauer Associates, Inc., Sunderland, MD, 2002, p. 597. With permission. Photograph from Martin, J. H., *Neuroanatomy: Text and Atlas*, 2nd ed., Appleton & Lange, Stamford, CT, 1996, pg. 522. With permission from McGraw-Hill.)

of this pathway may result in (1) difficulty encoding and retrieving information (medial temporal cortex); (2) information conflict resolution (cingulate gyrus); and (3) "positive" symptoms of schizophrenia, such as hallucination. Dopaminergic antagonists are used to treat symptoms of schizophrenia. The mesocortical pathway arises largely from the ventral tegmental area and projects to the PFC. Lesions of this pathway may result in deficits of working memory, attention, abulia, hypokinesis, and the "negative" symptoms of schizophrenia.

Most of the serotonergic neurons (Figure 17.14) of the brainstem are located in the raphe nuclei. These neurons project to essentially the whole of the telencephalon. Some pathways project to the hypothalamus and are involved in cardiovascular function, whereas those projecting to the forebrain act to modulate the responsiveness of cortical neurons. Serotonergic neurons are involved in regulating attention and complex cognitive function.[178] Serotonin also impacts sexual function via a pathway from the raphe nucleus down the spinal cord, eating behaviors and appetite through a pathway to the hypothalamus, emotions (including anxiety and panic) and memory through a pathway to the limbic system, obsessive–compulsive disorder through a pathway to the basal ganglia, and cognition via a pathway to the PFC.

Cholinergic neurons (Figure 17.15) project from the mesopontine tegmentum and the basal forebrain. The neurons of the pontine region provide a descending projectional pathway to the nuclei of the pontine and medullary reticular formation. They also project in a major ascending pathway to the thalamus. The ascending pathway to the thalamus exerts an arousal effect that is mediated indirectly by excitatory projections from the thalamus to the cortex.[176] Projections arising in the basal forebrain provide indirect cholinergic input to the cortex. By contrast, cholinergic projections arising from the nucleus basalis neurons project entirely to nearly all the cerebral cortex. The hippocampal formation is fed by projections from the medial septal nuclei and the nucleus of the diagonal band of Broca, and cholinergic neurons of the descending pathway are thought to impact the sleep–wake cycle via these projections. Cholinergic blockade of central cholinergic transmission results in delirium, whereas blockade of the striatal neurons results in movement disorders.[176] The primary function of acetylcholine is found in attention, memory, and learning.

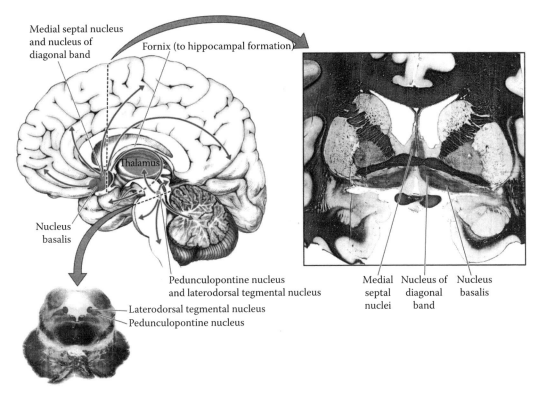

FIGURE 17.15 (See color insert following page 528.)
Cholinergic projection systems. (Line drawing from Blumenfeld, H., *Neuroanatomy Through Clinical Cases*, Sinauer Associates, Inc., Sunderland, MA, 2002, p. 594. With permission. Photograph from Martin, J. H., *Neuroanatomy: Text and Atlas*, 2nd ed., Appleton & Lange, Stamford, CT, 1996, pp. 522, 542. With permission from McGraw-Hill.)

Histaminergic neurons (Figure 17.16) are located in the posterior lateral hypothalamus and the tuberomamillary nucleus.[177] These neurons project to the spinal cord and to the entire cortex. These projections are thought to contribute to cortical arousal and to an arousal response at the level of the brainstem.

After neurotransmitters are released into a synapse, they must be removed from the cleft via one of three mechanisms to preserve responsivity of the synapse. Neurotransmitters can be removed by diffusion, enzymatic degradation, and reuptake. Reuptake is the most common mechanism used for inactivation. Enzymatic degradation and reuptake offer two important means of pharmacologic intervention in neurotransmission.

17.9 Summary

Injury to the body's most intricate and exquisite organ precipitates a combination of predictable and, as yet, unpredictable consequences that manifest in a wide variety of behavioral manifestations. The clinical reality is that most interventions today are geared toward reacting to the behavioral manifestations and applying treatments that remain

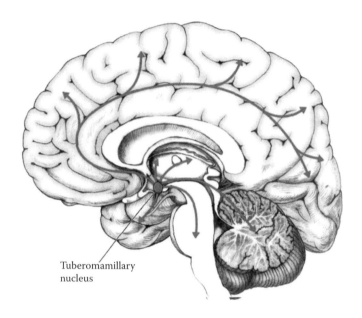

Tuberomamillary
nucleus

FIGURE 17.16
Histaminergic projection systems. (From Blumenfeld, H., *Neuroanatomy Through Clinical Cases*, Sinauer Associates, Inc., Sunderland, MD, 2002, p. 598. With permission.)

largely focused on compensation for lost or altered function. We hope this chapter provides you with information that may enable alternative approaches to brain injury that seek to take advantage of residual plasticity or enhance the plastic response of the brain as structures are encouraged to take on additional function. Cognitive recovery after brain injury occurs to varying degrees, with ample evidence of improvements in areas such as attention, perception, learning, memory, planning, and problem solving. The clinical question should be focused on what can be done to further cognitive recovery of function, in keeping with recovery usually demonstrated in physical function. Discovery of methods of securing true recovery of cognitive function will best derive from knowledge of neurologic anatomy and physiology associated with plasticity and targeted cognitive skill sets. We encourage you to consider how this information integrates with Chapters 12 and 19 in this volume on potential neuromedical interventions and cognitive rehabilitation.

References

1. Buck, L. B., Smell and taste: The chemical senses, in E. R. Kandel, J. H. Schwartz, and T. M. Jessell (Eds.), *Principles of Neural Science*, 4th edition, McGraw-Hill, New York, 627–647, 2000.
2. Posner, M. I., Psychobiology of attention, in M. S. Gazzinaga and C. Blakemore, (Eds.), *Handbook of Psychobiology*, Academic Press, New York, 441–480, 1975.
3. Goff, W. R., Evoked potential correlates of perceptual organization in man, in C. R. Evans and T. B. Mulholland, (Eds.), *Attention in Neurophysiology*, Appleton, New York, 1969.
4. Gummow, L., Miller, P., and Dustman, R. E., Attention and brain injury: A case for cognitive rehabilitation of attentional deficits, *Clinical Psychology Review*, 3(3), 255–274, 1983.
5. Scheibel, M. E. and Scheibel, A. B., Structural organization of nonspecific thalamic nuclei and their projection toward cortex, *Brain Research*, 6(1), 60–94, 1967.

6. Daube, J. R., Sandok, B. A., Reagon, T. J., and Westmoreland, B. F., *Medical Neurosciences: An Approach to Anatomy, Pathology, and Physiology by System and Levels*, Little, Brown, Boston, 1978.

7. Iversen, S., Iversen, L., and Saper, C. B., The autonomic nervous system and the hypothalamus, in E. R. Kandel, J. H. Schwartz, and T. M. Jessell, (Eds.), *Principles of Neural Science*, 4th ed., McGraw-Hill, New York, 960–981, 2000.

8. Bondanelli, M. D. E., Marinis, L., Ambrosio, M. R., Monesi, M., Valle, D., Zatelli, M. C., et al., Occurrence of pituitary dysfunction following traumatic brain injury, *Journal of Neurotrauma*, 21(6), 685–696, 2004.

9. Urban, R. J., Harris, P., and Masel, B., Anterior hypopituitarism following traumatic brain injury, *Brain Injury*, 19(5), 349–358, 2005.

10. Agha, A. and Thompson, C. J., Anterior pituitary dysfunction following traumatic brain injury, *Clinical Endocrinology*, 64(5), 481–488, 2006.

11. Leon-Carrion, J., Leal-Cerro, A., Murillo Cabezas, F., Madrazo Atutxa, A., Garcia Gomex, S., Flores Cordero, J. M., et al., Cognitive deterioration due to GH deficiency in patients with traumatic brain injury: A preliminary report, *Brain Injury*, 21(8), 871–875, 2007.

12. Yao, D. L., Liu, H., Hudson, L. D., and Webster, H. D., Insulin-like growth factor I treatment reduces demyelination and up-regulates gene expression of myelin-related proteins in experimental autoimmune encephalomyelitis, *Proceedings of the National Academy of Sciences of the United States of America*, 92(13), 6190–6194, 1995.

13. Artwert, L. I., Veltman, D. J., Deijen, J. B., van Dam, P. S., Delemarre-van de Wall, H. A., and Drent, M. L., Growth hormone deficiency and memory functioning in adults visualized by functional magnetic resonance imaging, *Neuroendocrinology*, 82(1), 32–40, 2005.

14. Oertel, H., Schneider, H. J., Stalla, G. K., Holsboer, F., and Zihl, J., The effect of growth hormone substitution on cognitive performance in adult patients with hypopituitarism, *Psychoneuroendocrinology*, 29(7), 839–850, 2004.

15. Strobl, J. S. and Thomas, M. J., Human growth hormone, *Pharmacological Reviews*, 46(1), 1–34, 1994.

16. Kulinskǐ, V. I. and Kilesnichenko, L. S., Regulation of metabolic and energetic mitochondrial functions by hormones and signal transduction systems, *Biomeditsinskaya Khimiya*, 52(5), 425–427.

17. Mussa, G. C., Mussa, F., Bretto, R., Zambelli, M. C., and Silvestro, L., Influence of thyroid in nervous system growth, *Minerva Pediatrica*, 53(4) 325–353, 2001.

18. Rodriguez-Pena, A., Oligodendrocyte development and thyroid hormone, *Journal of Neurobiology*, 40(4), 497–512, 1999.

19. Bernal, J., Thyroid hormones and brain development, *Vitamins and Hormones*, 71, 95–122, 2005.

20. Bernal, J., Action of thyroid hormone in brain, *Journal of Endocrinological Investigation*, 25(3), 268–288, 2002.

21. Bernal, J. and Nunez, J., Thyroid hormones and brain development, *European Journal of Endocrinology*, 133(4), 390–398, 1995.

22. Fernandez, M., Giuliani, A., Pirondi, S., D'Intino, G., Giardino, L., Aloe, L., et al., Thyroid hormone administration enhances remyelination in chronic demyelinating inflammatory disease, *Proceedings of the National Academy of Sciences of the United States of America*, 101(46), 16363–16368, 2004.

23. Goglia, F., Silvestri, E., and Lanni, A., Thyroid hormones and mitochondria, *Bioscience Reports*, 22(1), 17–32, 2002.

24. Nunez, J., Effects of thyroid hormones during brain differentiation, *Molecular and Cellular Endocrinology*, 37(2), 125–132, 1984.

25. Dussault, J. H. and Ruel, J., Thyroid hormones and brain development, *Annual Reviews of Physiology*, 49, 321–334, 1987.

26. Ruiz-Marcos, A., Cartagena Albella P., Garcia Garcia, A., Escobar del Rey, F., and Morreale de Escobar, G., Rapid effects of adult-onset hypothyroidism on dendritic spines of pyramidal cells of the rat cerebral cortex, *Experimental Brain Research*, 73(3), 583–588, 1988.

27. Ruiz-Marcos, A., Sanchez-Toscano, F., Obregon, M. J., Escobar del Rey, F., and Morreale de Escobar, G., Thyroxine treatment and recovery of hypothyroidism-induced pyramidal cell damage, *Brain Research*, 239(2), 559–574, 1982.

28. Janowsky, J. S., Chavez, B., and Orwoll, E., Sex steroids modify working memory, *Journal of Cognitive Neuroscience*, 12(3), 407–414, 2000.

29. Woolley, C. S. and McEwen, B. S., Estradiol mediates fluctuation in hippocampal synapse density during the estrous cycle in the adult rat, *Journal of Neuroscience*, 12(7), 2549–2554, 1992.

30. Woolley, C. S. and McEwen, B. S., Roles of estradiol and progesterone in regulation of hippocampal dendritic spine density during the estrous cycle in the rat, *The Journal of Comparative Neurology*, 336(2), 293–306, 1993.

31. Woolley, C. S. , Weiland, N. G., McEwen, B. S., and Schwartzkroin, P. A., Estradiol increases the sensitivity of hippocampal CA1 pyramidal cells to NMDA receptor-mediated synaptic input, correlation with dendritic spine density, *The Journal of Neuroscience*, 17(5), 1848–1859, 1997.

32. Kampen, D. L. and Sherwin, B. B., Estrogen use and verbal memory in healthy postmenopausal women, *Obstetrics and Gynecology*, 83(6), 979–983, 1994.

33. Sherwin, B. B., Estrogen and/or androgen replacement therapy and cognitive functioning in surgically menopausal women, *Psychoneuroendocrinology*, 13(4) 345–357, 1988.

34. Wooley, C. S. and McEwen B. S., Estradiol regulates synapse density in CA1 region of the hippocampus in the adult female rat, *Society of Neurosciences Abstracts*, 16, 144, 1990.

35. Luine, V. N., Estradiol increases choline acetyltransferase activity in specific basal forebrain nuclei and projection areas of female rats, *Experimental Neurology*, 89(2), 484–490, 1985.

36. Fillit, H., Weinreb, H. Cholst, I., Luine, V., McEwen, B., Amador, R., et al., Observations in a preliminary open trial of estradiol therapy for senile dementia–Alzheimer's type, *Psychoneuroendocrinology*, 11(3), 337–345, 1996.

37. McGaugh, J. L., Memory: A century of consolidation, *Science*, 287(5451), 248–251, 2000.

38. Amaral, D. G., A functional organization of perception and movement, in E. R. Kandel, J. H. Schwartz, and T. M. Jessell, (Eds.), *Principles of Neural Science*, 4th ed., McGraw-Hill, New York, 337–348, 2000.

39. Herrero, M. T., Barcia, C., and Navarro, M., Functional anatomy of thalamus and basal ganglia, *Childs Nervous System*, 18(8), 386–404, 2002.

40. Nauta, W. J. H., Circuitous connections linking cerebral cortex, limbic system, and corpus striatum, in B. K. Doane and K. R. Livingston, (Eds.), *The Limbic System: Functional Organization and Clinical Disorders*, Raven Press, New York, 43, 1986.

41. DeLong, M. R., The basal ganglia, in E. R. Kandel, J. H. Schwartz, and T. M. Jessell, (Eds.), *Principles of Neural Science*, 4th ed., McGraw-Hill, New York, 853–867, 2000.

42. Eichenbaum, H. and Cohen, N. J., *From Conditioning to Conscious Recollection: Memory Systems of the Brain*, Oxford University Press, New York, 2001.

43. Tulving, E., *Elements of Episodic Memory*, Oxford University Press, Cambridge, 1983.

44. Squire, L. R. and Zola-Morgan, S., The medial temporal lobe memory system, *Science*, 253(5026), 1380–1386, 1991.

45. Kandel, E. R., Kupferman, I., and Iversen, S., Learning and memory, in E. R. Kandel, J. H. Schwartz, and T. M. Jessell, (Eds.), *Principles of Neuroscience*, 4th ed., McGraw-Hill, New York, 1227–1246, 2000.

46. Tulving, E., Episodic memory: From mind to brain, *Annual Review of Psychology*, 53, 1–25, 2002.

47. Tulving, E., Hayman, C. A., and Macdonald, C. A., Long-lasting perceptual priming and semantic learning in amnesia: A case experiment, *Journal of Experimental Psychology: Learning and Cognition*, 17(4), 595–617, 1991.

48. Hamann, S. B. and Squire, L. R., On the acquisition of new declarative knowledge in amnesia, *Behavioral Neuroscience*, 109(6), 1027–1044, 1995.

49. Westmacott, R. and Moscovitch, M., Names and words without meaning: Incidental postmorbid semantic learning is a person with extensive bilateral medial temporal damage, *Neuropsychology*, 15(4), 586–596, 2001.

50. Shimamura, A. P. and Squire, L. R., Long-term memory in amnesia: Cued recall, recognition memory, and confidence ratings, *Journal of Experimental Psychology Learning, Memory, and Cognition*, 14(4), 763–770, 1988.

51. Bayley, P. J. and Squire, L. R., Failure to acquire new semantic knowledge in patients with large medial temporal lobe lesions, *Hippocampus*, 15(2), 273–280, 2005.

52. Saykin, A. J., Johnson, S. C., Flashman, L. A., McAllister, T. W., Sparling, M., Darcey, T. M., et al., Functional differentiation of medial temporal and frontal regions involved in processing novel and familiar words: An fMRI study, *Brain*, 122(Pt. 10), 1963–1971, 1999.

53. Schacter, D. L. and Wagner, A. D., Medial temporal lobe activations in fMRI and PET studies of episodic encoding and retrieval, *Hippocampus*, 9(1), 7–24, 1999.

54. Lepage, M., Habib, R., and Tulving, E., Hippocampal PET activations of memory encoding and retrieval: The HIPER model, *Hippocampus*, 8(4), 313–322, 1998.

55. Rolls, E. G., Neurophysiological and neuronal network analysis of how the primate hippocampus functions in memory, in J. Delacour (Ed.), *The Memory System of the Brain*, World Scientific, Singapore, 1994.

56. Willis, Jr., W. D. and Grossman, R. G., *Medical Neurobiology: Neuroanatomical and Neurophysiological Principles Basic to Clinical Neuroscience*, C. V. Mosby, St. Louis, MO, 1977.

57. Ranck, Jr., J. B., Studies on single neurons in dorsal hippocampal formation and septum in unrestrained rats, *Experimental Neurology*, 41(2), 462–531, 1974.

58. Tulving, E., Markowitsch, H. J., Kapur, S., Habib, R., and Houle, S., Novelty encoding networks in the human brain: Positron emission tomography data, *Neuroreport*, 5(18), 2525–2528, 1994.

59. Stark, C. E., Bayley, P. J., and Squire, L. R., Recognition memory for single items and for associations in similarly impaired damage to the hippocampal region, *Learning and Memory*, 9(5), 238–242, 2002.

60. Davachi, L. and Wagner, A. D., Hippocampal contributions to episodic encoding: Insights from relational and item-based learning, *Journal of Neurophysiology*, 88(2), 982–990, 2002.

61. Eichenbaum, H., The hippocampus and declarative memory: Cognitive mechanisms of neural codes, *Behavioural Brain Research*, 127(1–2), 199–207, 2001.

62. Wall, P. M. and Messier, C., The hippocampal formation: Orbitomedial prefrontal cortex circuit in the attentional control of active memory, *Behavioural Brain Research*, 127(1–2), 99–117, 2001.

63. Ramos, J. M. J., The perirhinal cortex and long-term spatial memory in rats, *Brain Research*, 947(2), 294–298, 2002.

64. Burgess, N., Maguire, E. A., and O'Keefe, J., The human hippocampus and spatial and episodic memory, *Neuron*, 35(4), 625–641, 2002.

65. McNaughton, B. L. and Nadel, L., Hebb-Marr networks and the neurobiological representations of action in space, in M. A. Gluck and D. E. Rumelhart, (Eds.), *Neuroscience and Connectionist Theory*, Erlbaum, Hillsdale, NJ, 1–64, 1990.

66. Treves, A. and Rolls, E. T., Computational analysis of the role of the hippocampus in memory, *Hippocampus*, 4(3), 374–391, 1994.

67. Vinogradova, O. S., Hippocampus as comparator: Role of the two input and two output systems of the hippocampus in selection and registration of information, *Hippocampus*, 11(5), 578–598, 2001.

68. Vazdarjanova, A. and Guzowski, J. F., Differences in hippocampal neuronal population responses to modifications of an environmental context: Evidence for distinct, yet complementary functions of CA3 and CA1 ensembles, *Journal of Neuroscience*, 24(29), 6489–6496, 2004.

69. Saper, C. B., Iversen, S., and Frackowiak, R., Integration of sensory and motor function, in E. R. Kandel, J. H. Schwartz, and T. M. Jessell, (Eds.), *Principles of Neural Science*, 4th ed., McGraw-Hill, New York, 349–380, 2000.

70. Poletti, C. E., Kinnary, M. A., and MacLean, P. D., Hippocampal influence on unit activity of hypothalamus, preoptic region, and basal forebrain in awake, sitting squirrel monkeys, *Journal of Neurophysiology*, 26(2), 308–324, 1973.

71. Poletti, C. E., Is the limbic system a limbic system? Studies of hippocampal efferents: Their functional and clinical implications, in B. K. Doane and K. F. Livingston, (Eds.), *The Limbic System: Functional Organization and Clinical Disorders*, Raven Press, New York, 1986.

72. MacLean, P. D., Culminating developments in the evolution of the limbic system: The thalamocingulate division, in B. K. Doane and K. F. Livingston, (Eds.), *The Limbic System: Functional Organization and Clinical Disorders*, Raven Press, New York, 1986.

73. McGaugh, J. L., Memory consolidation and the amygdala: A systems perspective, *Trends in Neuroscience*, 25(9), 456, 2002.

74. Wise, R. A., Dopamine, learning and motivation, *Nature Reviews Neuroscience*, 5(6), 483–494, 2004.

75. Mockett, B. G., Brooks, W. M., Tate, W. P., and Abraham, W. C., Dopamine D1/D5 receptor activation fails to initiate an activity-independent late-phase LTP in rat hippocampus, *Brain Research*, 1021(1), 92–100.

76. Navakkode, S., Sajikumar, S., and Frey, J. U., Synergistic requirements for the induction of dopaminergic D1/D5-receptor-mediated LTP in hippocampal slides of rat CA1 in vitro, *Neuropharmacology*, 52(7), 1547–1554, 2007.

77. Logothetis, N. K., Object vision and visual awareness, *Current Opinion in Neurobiology*, 8(4), 536–544, 1998.

78. Damasio, H., Grabowski, T. J., Tranel, D., Hichwa, R. D., and Damasio, A. R., A neural basis for lexical retrieval, *Nature*, 380(6574), 499–505, 1996.

79. Sigala, N. and Logothetis, N. K., Visual categorization shapes feature selectivity in the primate temporal cortex, *Nature*, 415(6869), 318–320, 2002.

80. Thomas, E., Van Hulle, M. M., and Vogel, R., Encoding of categories by noncategory-specific neurons in the inferior temporal cortex, *Journal of Cognitive Neuroscience*, 13(2), 190–200, 2001.

81. Miyashita, Y. and Chang, H. S., Neural correlate of pictorial short-term memory in the primate temporal cortex, *Nature*, 331(615), 68–70, 1988.

82. Wilson, M., Wilson, W. A., and Sunenshine, H. S., Perception, learning, and retention of visual stimuli by monkeys with inferotemporal lesions, *Journal of Comparative and Physiological Psychology*, 65(3), 404–412, 1968.

83. Iwai, E. and Mishkin, M., Further evidence on the locus of the visual area in the temporal lobe of the monkey, *Experimental Neurology*, 25(4), 585–594, 1969.

84. Cowey, A. and Gross, C. G., Effects of foveal prestriate and inferotemporal lesions on visual discrimination by rhesus monkeys, *Experimental Brain Research*, 11(2), 128–144, 1970.

85. Dean, P., Effects of inferotemporal lesions on the behavior of monkeys, *Psychological Bulletin*, 83(1), 41–71, 1976.

86. Fuster, J. M., Bauer, R. H., and Jervey, J. P., Effects of cooling inferotemporal cortex on performance of visual memory tasks, *Experimental Neurology*, 71(2), 398–409, 1981.

87. Wilson, M., Kaufman, H. M., Zieler, R. E., and Lieb, J. P., Visual identification and memory in monkeys with circumscribed inferotemporal lesions, *Journal of Comparative and Physiological Psychology*, 78(2), 178–183, 1972.

88. Kovner, R. and Stamm, J. S., Disruption of short-term visual memory by electrical stimulation of inferotemporal cortex in the monkey, *Journal of Comparative and Physiological Psychology*, 81(1), 163–172, 1972.

89. Delacour, J., Inferotemporal cortex and short term visual memory in monkeys: New data, *Experimental Brain Research*, 28(3–4), 301–310, 1977.

90. Gross, C. G., Rocha-Miranda, C. E., and Bender, D. B., Visual properties of neurons in inferotemporal cortex of the macaque, *Journal of Neurophysiology*, 35(1), 96–111, 1972.

91. Desimone, R. and Gross, C. G., Visual areas in the temporal cortex of the macaque, *Brain Research*, 178(2), 363–380, 1979.

92. Sato, T., Kawamura, E., and Iwai, E., Responsiveness of inferotemporal single units to visual pattern stimuli in monkeys performing discrimination, *Experimental Brain Research*, 38(3), 313–319, 1980.

93. Rolls, E. T., Judge, M. K., and Sanghera, M. K., Activity of neurons in the inferotemporal cortex of the alert monkey, *Brain Research*, 130(2), 229–238, 1977.

94. Gross, C. G., Bender, D. B., and Gerstein, G. L., Activity of inferior temporal neurons in behaving monkeys, *Neuropsychologica*, 17(2), 215–229, 1979.

95. Mikami, A. and Kubota, K., Inferotemporal neuron activities and color discrimination with delay, *Brain Research*, 182(1), 65–78, 1980.

96. Gaffan, D. and Weiskrantz, L., Recency effects and lesion effects in delayed non-matching to randomly baited samples by monkeys, *Brain Research*, 196(2), 373–386, 1980.

97. Penfield, W. and Perot, P., The brain's record of auditory and visual experience: A final summary and discussion, *Brain*, 86(pt. 4), 595–696, 1963.

98. Fuster, J. M., The prefrontal cortex: An update: Time is of the essence, *Neuron*, 30(2), 319–333, 2001.

99. Verfaellie, M. and Heilman, K. M., Response preparation and response inhibition after lesions of the medial frontal lobe, *Archives of Neurology*, 44(12), 1265–1271, 1987.

100. Cummings, J. L., Frontal–subcortical circuits and human behavior, *Journal of Psychosomatic Research*, 44(6), 627–628, 1998.

101. Luria, A. R., *Higher Cortical Functions in Man*, Basic Books, New York, 1966.

102. Luria, A. R., *Traumatic Aphasia*, Mouton, The Hague, 1970.

103. Flechsig, P., *Anatomie des menschichen Gehirns und Ruckenmarks auf Myelogenetischer Grundlage*, Thieme, Leipzig, 1920.

104. Huttenlocher, P. R. and Dabholkar, A. S., Regional differences in synaptogenesis in human cerebral cortex, *The Journal of Comparative Neurology*, 287(2), 167–178, 1997.

105. Conel, J., *The Postnatal Development of the Human Cerebral Cortex*, 6 vols., Harvard University Press, Cambridge, 1939–1963.

106. Chugani, H. T., Positron emission tomography: Principles and applications in pediatrics, *Mead Johnson Symposium on Perinatal and Development Medicine*, 25, 15–18, 1987.

107. Paus, T., Zijdenbos, A., Worsley, K., Collins, D. L., Blumenthal, J., Giedd, J. N., et al., Structural maturation of neural pathways in children and adolescents: In vivo study, *Science*, 283(5409), 1908–1911, 1999.

108. Sowell, E. R., Thompson, P. M., Holmes, C. J., Jernigan, T. L., and Toga, A. W., In vivo evidence for post-adolescent brain maturation in frontal and striatal regions, *Nature Neuroscience*, 2(10), 859–861, 1999.

109. Thomas, C. L., *Ed Taber's Cyclopedic Medical Dictionary*, 17th ed., F. A. Davis, Philadelphia, 1993.

110. Fuster, J. M., Executive frontal functions, *Experimental Brain Research*, 133(1), 66–70, 2000.

111. Fuster, J. M., *Memory in the Cerebral Cortex*, MIT Press, Cambridge, MA, 1995.

112. Little, D. M., Klein, R., Shobat, D. M., McClure, E. D., and Thulborn, K. R., Changing patterns of brain activation during category learning revealed by functional MRI, *Cognitive Brain Research*, 22(1), 84–93, 2004.

113. Little, D. M. and Thulborn, K. R., Correlations of cortical activation and behavior during the application of newly learned categories, *Cognitive Brain Research*, 25(1), 33–47, 2005.

114. Miller, E. K. and Cohen, J. D., An integrative theory of prefrontal cortex function, *Annual Review of Neuroscience*, 24(1), 167–202, 2001.

115. Wallis, J. D., Anderson, K. C., and Miller, E. K., Single neurons in prefrontal cortex encode abstract rules, *Nature*, 411(6840) 953–956, 2001.

116. White, I. M. and Wise, S. P., Rule-dependent neuronal activity in the prefrontal cortex, *Experimental Brain Research*, 126(3), 315–335, 1999.

117. Miller, E. K., Freedman, D. J., and Wallis, J. D., The prefrontal cortex: Categories, concepts and cognition, *Philosophical Transactions: Biological Sciences*, 357(1424), 1123–1136, 2002.

118. Fuster, J. M., Unit activity in prefrontal cortex during delayed-response performance: Neuronal correlates of transient memory, *Journal of Neurophysiology*, 36(1), 61–78, 1973.

119. Goldman-Rakic, P. S., Circuitry of primate prefrontal cortex and regulation of behavior by representational memory, in F. Plum (Ed.), *Handbook of Physiology: The Nervous System*, American Physiological Society, Bethesda, MD, 373–417, 1987.

120. Goldman-Rakic, P. S., The prefrontal landscape: Implications of functional architecture for understanding human mentation and the central executive, *Philosophical Transactions of the Royal Society of London*, Series B, 351(1346), 1445–1453, 1996.

121. Turak, B., Louvel, J., Buser, P., and Lamarche, M., Event-related potentials recorded from the cingulated gyrus during attentional tasks: A study in patients with implanted electrodes, *Neuropsychologia*, 40(1), 99–107, 2002.

122. VanVeen, V., Cohen, J. D., Botvinick, M. M., Stenger, V. A., and Carter, C. S., Anterior cingulated cortex, conflict monitoring, and levels of processing, *Neuroimage*, 14(6), 1302–1308, 2001.

123. Benedict, R. H., Shucard, D. W., Santa Maria, M. P., Schucard, J. L., Abara, J. P., Coad, M. L., et al., Covert auditory attention generates activation in the rostral/dorsal anterior cingulated cortex, *Journal of Cognitive Neuroscience*, 14(4), 637–645, 2002.

124. Lepage, M., Ghaffar, O., Nyberg, L., and Tulving, E., Prefrontal cortex and episodic memory retrieval mode, *Proceedings of the National Academy of Sciences of the United States of America*, 997(1), 506–511, 2000.

125. Taber, K. H. and Hurley, R. A., Traumatic axonal injury: Atlas of major pathways, *Journal of Neuropsychiatry and Clinical Neuroscience*, 19(2), iv–104, 2007.

126. Buki, A. and Povlishock, J. T., All roads lead to disconnection? Traumatic axonal injury revisited, *Acta Neurochirurgica*, 148(2), 181–193, 2006.

127. Meythaler, J. M., Peduzzi, J. D., Eleftheriou, E., and Novack, T. A., Current concepts: Diffuse axonal injury-associated traumatic brain injury, *Archives of Physical Medicine and Rehabilitation*, 82(10), 1461–1471, 2001.

128. Baddeley, A. D., Estimating the short-term component in free recall, *Quarterly Journal of Experimental Psychology*, 61(1), 13–15, 1970.

129. Fletcher, P. C. and Henson, R. N., Frontal lobes and human memory: Insights from functional neuroimaging, *Brain*, 124 (Pt. 5), 849–881, 2001.

130. Frey, U. and Morris, R. G. M., Weak before strong: Dissociating synaptic tagging and plasticity: Factor accounts of late-LTP, *Neuropharmacology*, 37(4–5), 545–552, 1998.

131. Frey, U. and Morris, R. G. M., Synaptic tagging: Implications for late maintenance of hippocampal long-term potentiation, *Trends in Neurosciences*, 21(5), 181–188, 1998.

132. Miyashita, T., Kubik, S., Lewandowski, G., and Guzowski, J. F., Networks of neurons, networks of genes: An integrated view of memory consolidation, *Neurobiology of Learning and Memory*, 89(3), 269–284, 2008.

133. Brinton, R. E., Biochemical correlates of learning and memory, in J. L. Martinez and R. P. Kesner, (Eds.), *Learning and Memory: A Biological View*, Academic Press, San Diego, 1991.

134. Kandel, E. R., Cellular mechanisms of learning and biological basis of individuality, in E. R. Kandel, J. H. Schwartz, and T. M. Jessell, (Eds.), *Principles of Neuroscience*, Elsevier, New York, 1991.

135. Hannay, T., Larkman, A., Stratford, K., and Jack, J. A., A common rule governs the synaptic locus of both short-term and long-term potentiation, *Current Biology*, 3(12), 832–841, 1993.

136. Bayley, P. J., Gold, J. J., Hopkins, R. O., and Squire, L. R., The neuroanatomy of remote memory, *Neuron*, 46(5), 799–810, 2005.

137. Bolshakov, V. Y. and Siegelbaum, S. A., Postsynaptic induction and presynaptic expression of hippocampal long-term depression, *Science*, 264(5162), 1148–1152, 1994.

138. Frost, W. N., Castellucci, V. F., Hawkins, R. D., and Kandel, E. R., Monosynaptic connections made by the sensory neurons of the gill- and siphon-withdrawal reflex in *Aplysia* participate in the storage of long-term memory for sensitization, *Proceedings of the National Academy of Sciences of the United States of America*, 82(23), 8266–8269, 1985.

139. Davis, R. L., Physiology and biochemistry of *Drosophila* learning mutants, *Physiological Reviews*, 76(2), 299–317, 1996.

140. Bliss, T. V. and Collingridge, G. L., A synaptic model of memory: Long-term potentiation in the hippocampus, *Nature*, 361(640), 31–39, 1993.

141. Squire, L. R., Memory and the hippocampus: A synthesis from findings with rats, monkeys, and humans, *Psychological Reviews*, 99(2), 195–231, 1992. [Published erratum appears in *Psychological Reviews*, 99(3), 582, 1992.]

142. Castellucci, V. F., Frost, W. N., Goelet, P., Montarolo, P. G., Schacher, S., Morgan, J. A., et al., Cell and molecular analysis of long-term sensitization in *Aplysia*, *Journal of Physiologie* (Paris), 81(4), 349–357, 1986.

143. Martin, K. C., Casadio, A., Zhu, H., Yaping, E., Rose, J. C., Chen, M. B., et al., Synapse-specific, long-term facilitation of *Aplysia* sensory to motor synapses: A function for local protein synthesis in memory storage, *Cell*, 91(7), 927–938, 1997.

144. Frost, W. N., Clark, G. A., and Kandel, E. R., Parallel processing of short-term memory for sensitization in *Aplysia, Journal of Neurobiology*, 19(4), 297–334, 1988.

145. Abraham, W. C., Logan, B., Greenwood, J. M., and Dragunow, M., Induction and experience-dependent consolidation of stable long-term potentiation lasting months in the hippocampus, *Journal of Neuroscience*, 22(21), 9626–9634, 2002.

146. Staubli, U. and Lynch, G., Stable long-term potentiation elicited by "theta" pattern stimulation, *Brain Research*, 435(1), 227–234, 1987.

147. Trepel, C. and Racine, R. J., Long-term potentiation in the neocortex of the adult, freely moving rat, *Cerebral Cortex*, 8(8), 719–729, 1998.

148. Abraham, W. C. and Williams, J. M., LTP maintenance and its protein synthesis-dependence, *Neurobiology of Learning and Memory*, 89(3), 260–268, 2008.

149. Woo, N. H. and Nguyen, P. V., Protein synthesis is required for synaptic immunity to depotentiation, *Journal of Neuroscience*, 23(4), 1125–1132, 2003.

150. Arai, A., Larson, J., and Lynch, G., Anoxia reveals a vulnerable period in the development of long-term potentiation, *Brain Research*, 511(1), 353–357, 1990.

151. Fujii, S., Saito, Y., Mayakawa, H., Ito, K., and Kato, H., Reversal of long-term potentiation (depotentiation) induced by tetanus stimulation of the input to CA1 neurons of guinea pig hippocampal slices, *Brain Research*, 555(1), 112–122, 1991.

152. Larson, J., Xiao, P., and Lynch, G., Reversal of LTP by theta frequency stimulation, *Brain Research*, 600(1), 97–102, 1993.

153. Abraham, W. C. and Huggett, A., Induction and reversal on long-term potentiation by repeated high-frequency stimulation in rat hippocampal slices, *Hippocampus*, 7(2), 137–145, 1997.

154. Hesse, G. W. and Teyler, T. J., Reversible loss of hippocampal LTP following electroconvulsive seizures, *Nature*, 264, 562–564, 1976.

155. Xu, L., Anwyl, R., and Rowan, M. J., Spatial exploration induces a persistent reversal of long-term potentiation in rat hippocampus, *Nature*, 394, 891–894, 1998.

156. Lyford, G. L., Yamagata, K., Kaufmann, W. E., Barnes, C. A., Sanders, L. K., Copeland, N. G., et al., *Arc*, a growth factor and activity-regulated gene, encodes a novel cytoskeleton-associated protein that is enriched in neuronal dendrites, *Neuron*, 14(2), 433–445, 1995.

157. Abraham, W. C., Mason, S. E., Demmer, J., Williams, J. M., Richardson, C. L., Tate, W. P., et al., Correlations between immediate early gene induction and the persistence of long-term potentiation, *Neuroscience*, 56(3), 717–727, 1993.

158. Worley, P. F., Bhat, R. V., Baraban, J. M., Erickson, C. A., McNaughton, B. L., and Barnes, C. A., Thresholds for synaptic activation of transcription factors in hippocampus: Correlation with long-term enhancement, *Journal of Neuroscience*, 13(11), 4776–4786, 1993.

159. Guzowski, J. F., McNaughton, B. L., Barnes, C. A., and Worley, P. F., Environment-specific expression of the immediate-early gene *Arc* in hippocampal neuronal ensembles, *Nature Neuroscience*, 2(12), 1120–1124, 1999.

160. Lau, L. F. and Nathans, D., Genes induced by serum growth factors, *The Hormonal Control of Gene Transcription*, Elsevier Science, Amsterdam, 257–293, 1991.

161. Greenberg, M. E., Ziff, E. B., and Green, L. A., Stimulation of neuronal acetylcholine receptors induces rapid gene transcription, *Science*, 234(4772), 80–83, 1986.

162. Sheng, M. and Greenberg, M. E., The regulation and function of c-fos and other immediate early genes in the nervous system, *Neuron*, 4(4), 477–485, 1990.

163. Link, W., Koneitzko, U., Kauselmann, G., Krug, M., Schwanke, B., Frey, U., et al., Somatodendritic expression of an immediate early gene is regulated by synaptic activity, *Proceedings of the National Academy of Sciences of the United States of America*, 92(12), 5734–5738, 1995.

164. Guzowski, J. F., Miyashita, T., Chawla, M. K., Sanderson, J., Maes, L. I., Houston, F. P., et al., Recent behavioral history modifies coupling between cell activity and *Arc* gene transcription in hippocampal CA1 neurons, *Proceedings of the National Academy of Sciences of the United States of America*, 103(4), 1077–1082, 2006.

165. Lynch, G., Memory consolidation and long-term potentiation, in M. S. Gazzaniga (Ed.), *The New Cognitive Neurosciences*, 2nd ed., MIT Press, Cambridge, MA, 43–44, 139–157, 2000.

166. Schubert, D., The possible role of adhesion in synaptic modification, *Trends in Neuroscience*, 14(4), 127–130, 1991.

167. Schuman, E. M. and Madison, D. V., Locally distributed synaptic potentiation in the hippocampus, *Science*, 263(5146), 532–536, 1994.

168. Barinaga, M., Learning by diffusion: Nitric oxide may spread memories, *Science*, 263(5146), 466, 1994.

169. Hawkins, R. D., Zhuo, M., and Arancio, O., Nitric oxide and carbon monoxide as possible retrograde messengers in hippocampal long-term potentiation, *Journal of Neurobiology*, 25(6), 652–665, 1994.

170. Ohno, M., Yamamoto, T., and Watanabe, S., Intrahippocampal administration of the NO synthase inhibitor L-NAME prevents working memory deficits in rats exposed to transient cerebral ischemia, *Brain Research*, 634(1), 173–177, 1994.

171. Ohno, M., Yamamoto, T., and Watanabe, S., Deficits in working memory following inhibition of hippocampal nitric oxide synthesis in the rat, *Brain Research*, 632(1–2), 36–40, 1993.

172. Black, J. E., Sirevaag, A. M., and Greenough, W. T., Complex experience promotes capillary formation in young rat visual cortex, *Neuroscience Letters*, 83(3), 351–355, 1987.

173. Anderson, B. J., Isaacs, K. R., Black, J. E., Vinci, L. M., Alcantara, A. A., and Greenough, W. T., Synaptogenesis in cerebellar cortex of adult rats after less than 15 hours of visuomotor training over 10 days, *Society of Neurosciences Abstracts*, 14, 1239, 1988.

174. Chang, F. L. and Greenough, W. T., Transient and enduring morphological correlates of synaptic activity and efficacy change in the rat hippocampal slice, *Brain Research*, 309(1), 35–46, 1984.

175. Sirevaag, A. M., Smith, S., and Greenough, W. T., Rats reared in a complex environment have larger astrocytes with more processes than rats raised socially or individually, *Society of Neurosciences Abstracts*, 14, 1135, 1988.

176. Blumenfeld, H., *Neuroanatomy Through Clinical Cases*, Sinauer Associates, Inc., Sunderland, MA, 2002.

177. Saper, C. B., Brain stem modulation of sensation, movement, and consciousness, in E. R. Kandel, J. H. Schwartz, and T. M. Jessell, (Eds.), *Principles of Neural Science*, 4th ed., McGraw-Hill, New York, 889–909, 2000.

178. Schwartz, J. H., Neurotransmitters, in E. R. Kandel, J. H. Schwartz, and T. M. Jessell, (Eds.), *Principles of Neural Science*, 4th ed., McGraw-Hill, New York, 280–297, 2000.

18

Principles of Cognitive Rehabilitation in Traumatic Brain Injury: An Integrative Neuroscience Approach

Fofi Constantinidou and Robin D. Thomas

CONTENTS

18.1 Introduction

The survivor of moderate to severe traumatic brain injury (TBI) is typically faced with an array of neuropsychological challenges. These include cognitive changes in attention, memory and learning difficulties, information processing impairments, and executive functioning deficits, and psychosocial issues such as emotional/anger management, anxiety, and depression. Neuropsychological deficits often hamper the individual's ability to function independently and return to productive living. Subsequently, cognitive rehabilitation (CR) is an integral component of TBI rehabilitation efforts.

18.1.1 Models of Cognitive Rehabilitation

Cognitive retraining falls under two primary categories: restorative and compensatory. Restorative rehabilitation is based on neuroanatomic and neurophysiologic models of learning. These models suggest that neuronal growth and synaptogenesis result directly from repeated exposure and repetition of stimulation through experience.[1] Consequently, cognitive training could potentially lead to the development of new neuronal circuits, which could cause reorganization of partially damaged systems, reduce cognitive impairment, and improve functional ability. It is possible that, if rehabilitation is withdrawn too early, the functional reorganization would not have an opportunity to occur; thus, treatment effects will not be permanent.

The compensatory rehabilitation approach operates under the assumption that certain functions cannot be recovered or restored completely. Therefore, the patient needs to use certain strategies to improve functional performance without relying on the restoration of the damaged neurocognitive systems.[2] The restorative and compensatory approaches could be used together in rehabilitation to maximize performance. For instance, assisting patients to develop self-awareness regarding their cognitive needs by the use of systematic strategies could have a restorative effect on planning and deliberate cognitive processing abilities.[2] There are several comprehensive approaches to CR, including works by Ben-Yishay, Prigatano, and others that focus on holistic rehabilitation,[3–7] and other approaches[8–12] that involve developing hierarchical strategies for the treatment of basic and complex cognitive systems and also helping the patient develop self-awareness and acceptance of changed abilities. Chapter 21 provides more in-depth information regarding the scope and objectives of neuropsychological rehabilitation. This chapter focuses on principles of cognitive organization. The integrative theoretical model presented in this chapter can form the basis for the development of therapy procedures to address cognitive deficits associated with TBI.

18.1.2 Cognitive Theory and Rehabilitation

Cognitive theory organizes human cognition into a hierarchy of basic and complex processes/systems. Basic processes, such as sensory perception, attention, and memory, underlie more complex systems, including categorization, problem solving, reasoning, and abstract thought processes.

Neurobiologic research in humans and animals provides support for the cognitive systems generated by cognitive theory. When these networks are disrupted, the observable outcomes include predictable cognitive deficits. The neuropathology of TBI is complex because it consists of both focal and diffuse cortical and subcortical lesions along with a cascade of neurobiologic changes. Therefore, unlike unilateral focal brain damage (e.g., resulting from a stroke or a neoplastic lesion), the cognitive disruption observed in TBI can be bilateral and extensive. The challenge of CR is to implement effective and efficient treatment modalities that will enable survivors to maximize their level of functioning in the face of this diffuse systemic disruption.

The purpose of this chapter is to apply cognitive theory, current findings in cognitive neuroscience, and brain research to develop principles of CR following moderate to severe brain injury. The following questions will be addressed:

1. What are the neuropathologic mechanisms that affect basic and complex cognitive systems following injury?

2. How does the brain recover from injury?

3. What are the general principles of basic and complex human cognitive systems and how does TBI interfere with these systems?

4. How can principles of cognitive theory be applied to treat cognitive deficits associated with TBI?

18.2 Effects of Brain Injury on Neuronal Function

The most common form of TBI is a closed head injury (CHI). The primary neuropathologies identified in CHI are the result of mechanical forces associated with movement of the brain within the skull. In addition to focal lesions, the inertial loading (resulting from acceleration or deceleration forces) causes linear and rotational acceleration that typically coexist or follow each other in CHI[13,14] and may cause greater impairment than focal injuries at the site of impact. Rotational acceleration forces may have more devastating effects than linear forces, because rotational forces lead to greater strain on the axons. The type of strain depends on the direction of the forces applied to the brain tissue. Specifically, tensile forces pull axons apart, compressive forces push axons together, and parallel deforming forces lead to shear strains.[13] Rotational forces may result in focal lesions of midline structures like the corpus callosum and the dorsolateral quadrants of the midbrain. However, it appears that the displacement of the brain tissue relative to the skull leads to more devastating results than the acceleration, per se.[13,15] The strain rate, according to Viano,[15] is a critical variable. That is, a particular group of axons will suffer more damage if strained (or displaced) with more intensity and longer duration than if the same axons were strained at a lower rate of intensity and shorter amount of time. The straining of the axon fibers is one mechanism leading to microscopic damage affecting the soma and the axon, and subsequently leading to diffuse axonal injury (DAI).

18.2.1 Cell Function/Cell Death

Upon contact, the individual may sustain a focal injury (coup or contrecoup) and inertial loading as a result of acceleration/deceleration forces resulting in multifocal and diffuse lesions.[13,16] The higher the velocity at the time of impact (as in the case of high-speed motor vehicle accidents), the stronger the inertia forces applied to the skull. The frontal and temporal lobes of the brain, which include systems critical for attention, categorization, strategy building, memory, and learning, are often compromised as a result of coup or contrecoup lesions in CHI. These lesions include contusions resulting from hemorrhagic lesions that can lead to cell death. The mechanism of diffuse neuronal cell loss involves both necrotic and apoptotic neurocascades. Necrotic death is attributed to ischemia (secondary to cell membrane failure), whereas apoptotic cell death evolves more slowly and is not clearly understood.[16]

18.2.2 Diffuse Axonal Injury

There is a gradient of injury that occurs both at the axonal level and grossly at the distribution of DAI. The distribution of DAI follows a gradient from peripheral hemispheres to deeper parts of the cerebrum in more severe injuries. In more severe injuries, the corpus callosum and dorsolateral midbrain tend to also be involved, often associated with macroscopic petechial hemorrhages seen on magnetic resonance images.

Studies with animal models and human autopsy findings have been used to study the pathophysiology of diffuse axonal injury.[17] Although the discussion on DAI has focused traditionally on myelinated axons, more recently there is evidence supporting the involvement of fine-fiber unmyelinated axons (like the cells found in the splenium of the corpus callosum).[16] Hence, focusing only on myelinated axons may underestimate the full effect of axonal damage. Animal models simulated severe injuries resulting in stretching or compressing of long tract axons, with maximal stretching or compression at focal points on the axons' length. At 12 to 24 hours postinjury, swollen axoplasmic masses, called *retraction balls*, formed and detached from more distal axonal segments. In less severe injuries, focal alterations of axolemma can lead to progressive changes and a cascade of electrochemical events interfering with axonal transport (anterograde and retrograde), focal axonal swelling, and detachment from the distal axonal segment.

The exact nature of the reactive axonal changes is unknown, but because the effects are delayed, future research might determine how to prevent certain axonal changes. The delayed autodestructive cellular phenomena have been linked to surges of the excitatory neurotransmitter glutamate, especially at *N*-methyl-D-aspartate receptors. These intracellular surges impede neuronal function. Areas of the brain with large numbers of *N*-methyl-D-aspartate receptors, such as the hippocampus, are very vulnerable to the aforementioned autotoxic changes.[13] Not all axonal swellings result in retraction balls. In an experimental mild/moderate brain injury with cats, some of the swellings showed numerous reactive neuritic sprouts in the brainstem area.[18] By the end of the first month, some of these swellings degenerated and some continued to mature. Some of these neuritic outgrowths were reorganized to course into the parenchyma (where myelin was absent) or course parallel to distended myelin sheath.

During the second and third month postinjury, there is great variability in the regenerative responses of animals. Some new sprouting originates from reactive axonal swellings. The more mature sprouting shows further maturation and seems to gain easy access to the rest of the brain.[18] It remains unclear, however, whether these neuroplastic changes will yield adaptive or maladaptive changes.[16]

A large array of processes can occur following damage to the brain, which may be extensive, and result in dramatic changes in behavior and cognition (Section 18.2.4). Some of these processes occur also during normal development, and some are evident in healthy individuals following experiences that produce learning and memory.[19] When dramatic changes in behavior or cognition occur following head trauma, it is normally assumed that some neurons in the brain have been damaged, and/or some axons have been severed. Other cells in the "penumbra" have also been damaged. Immediately following the injury, phagocytes infiltrate the area and dispose of the nonfunctioning tissue. Frequently, glial cells will then infiltrate the area vacated by the dead neurons. They either provide nutrients for regenerating axons, or form scar tissue that will retard functional reconnection between remaining cells. Areas of gliosis are observable in magnetic resonance images of severe TBI survivors taken several months or years after the trauma.

Future research needs to investigate the long-term outcomes of regenerative processes in relationship to neurobehavioral outcomes. The identification of targeted growth factors that enhance desirable regenerative processes would provide significant benefits to survivors of brain injury.

18.2.3 Metabolic Dysfunction

The mechanical and cellular changes described in the previous sections can lead to a wide array of metabolic changes. Similar to the aforementioned changes, the metabolic cascade can also be focal, multifocal, and/or diffuse. Even persons with mild brain injury are extremely sensitive to slight changes in cerebral blood flow (CBF), increases in intracranial pressure, and apnea. Although advances in technology, such as positron emission tomography, diffusion tensor imaging, nuclear magnetic resonance spectroscopy, and microdialysis studies, have been extremely helpful in understanding the metabolic effects of TBI, the exact mechanism of this injury-induced vulnerability is not fully understood. It appears that this metabolic imbalance is heterogeneous and affects brain areas differently. The metabolic cascade has become a major concern in brain injury management because it can lead to further tissue damage and contribute more extensively to the neurobehavioral outcomes following TBI than the initial mechanical damage.[20–22]

This vulnerable state following injury is thought to be a result of interactive neurochemical and metabolic cascades following injury, consisting of several mechanisms that are described in experimental and human brain injury:

1. A massive release of the excitatory neurotransmitter glutamate leading to excitotoxicity and also to an increase in glucose metabolism (hyperglycolysis). The temporal lobe and hippocampal areas are particularly vulnerable to the glutamate surges.[16,18,23]

2. Ionic fluctuations such as increased levels of extracellular potassium (K+). The increase in K+ activates the adenosine triphosphate-dependent sodium–potassium pumps and results in considerable metabolic stress and, possibly, hyperglycolysis.

3. Elevation in extracellular calcium (Ca++) has been shown to increase vasoconstriction, which may account for the reduction in CBF and may also activate destructive lipases and proteases.[23,24]

4. Production of reactive forms of oxygen species that cause damage via the induction of lipid and oxygen oxidation.

5. Loss of autoregulation, as evidenced by increased demand for glucose (hyperglycolysis) lasting from immediately after to up to 1 week following the injury,[23,25] and a reduction in CBF.

6. The acute period of hyperglycolysis is followed by a period of metabolic depression and reduction in glucose utilization (i.e., hypoglycolysis) that lasts for up to 10 days in experimental TBI.[25] During this period of time, there is a decrease in protein synthesis and oxidative metabolism, which suggests that the glycolysis is not the only metabolic pathway affected in brain injury.[16]

18.2.4 Brain Reorganization and Sprouting Following Injury

In the central nervous system, when neurons are killed or when axons are damaged, the axon terminals of those cells will degenerate, thus vacating synaptic contacts on postsynaptic neurons. The postsynaptic cell will die if enough of its presynaptic contacts are vacated. If the postsynaptic cell survives, its soma and/or dendrites will have vacant locations where presynaptic degeneration has occurred. At this point, a number of possible events can occur that can result in recovery of function. The damaged axons can regenerate and form new terminals on the cells they previously innervated, or axons from other neurons can sprout new terminals that form synapses at the vacant locations on the postsynaptic neuron. This sprouting constitutes a reorganization of the connections among the surviving brain structures and can serve as a major impetus for recovery of function. All sprouting is not, however, necessarily adaptive. As mentioned previously in this chapter, it is possible for the newly sprouted connections to result in maladaptive behaviors.[26]

The reorganization of the brain by axon terminal sprouting is not unique to the aftermath of neuron death in the brain. It occurs naturally in the healthy brain continually during development and later in life. During development, axon terminals compete for positions on various somata or dendrites of neurons. Similarly, when an otherwise healthy neuron looses synaptic contacts on its soma or dendrites, a variety of different afferent cells will compete for the vacant areas on its surface. The nature of the connectivity of the "recovered" brain should be very dependent upon the particular pattern of new synapses that form.

During development, it is clear that the patterns of connections that form and prevail are severely impacted by the nature of the organism's experience. For years, it has been known that there are gross differences in brain structure as a result of different experiences. Later studies have shown that the structure of individual neurons in the neocortex is dramatically affected by experience. A good example is shown in the studies of the brains of animals raised in enriched versus impoverished environments. Animals raised in an enriched environment have neurons with richer dendrite trees, containing a larger number of higher order dendritic branches and more synaptic contacts. These observations were first made in young animals, but have been shown to occur in adult animals as well. In fact, the richness of the connections of various neocortical cells will rise and fall in very short intervals with changes in inputs to those cells.[27] The particular pattern of new connections following brain damage should also be dramatically affected by the experience of the individual during recovery following the lesion. And some patterns may prove to be detrimental to the organism. The issue for rehabilitative therapy is to determine the patterns of experience that best optimize posttraumatic performance.

One of the most frequently used procedures to study synaptic plasticity examines the effects of repeated stimulation of the presynaptic cell on the excitability of the postsynaptic neuron. Depending on the parameters of the repeated stimulation, such stimulation frequently results in "potentiation" or "depression" of synaptic efficacy. Earlier studies revealed changes in the excitability of the postsynaptic neuron last for minutes, called *short-term potentiation* or *short-term depression*. However, later studies revealed that, at certain synapses, such changes could persist for longer periods of time—in some cases, for many days. Changes in synaptic efficacy that are seen following long-term potentiation and depression can result from an increase or decrease in the amount of neurotransmitter released from the presynaptic terminal, an increase or decrease in the number of active postsynaptic receptors, the sprouting of new synapses, the pairing down of existing synapses, or changes in the structure of existing synapses, such as changes in the size or shape of dendritic spines or modification of the synaptic cleft.

Currently, theories of the changes in cell interaction induced by experience or recovery following brain damage focus on modification in the properties of existing synapses or the sprouting of new synapses between cells that already have direct synaptic contact. However, during development, transformations in brain function and organization are attributed to the formation of new synapses between cells that did not previously interact. Clearly, before Purkinje cells exist in the cerebellum, there can be no synapses between climbing fibers or granule cell parallel fibers onto Purkinje cells. Obviously, the birth of new neurons that form functional synapses with other neurons requires one to address the issue that synapses must be forming between cells that previously had not interacted.

Despite the remarkable degree of behavioral and cognitive adjustments that accompany adult learning and memory, or recovery of function, most cellular models of neural plasticity do not consider these changes to be accompanied by synaptogenesis between previously noncommunicating neurons. The theories generally assume that the new synapses that are formed during learning or recovery only strengthen (or weaken) communication between already communicating neurons. This position has not been challenged because of the dogma that no new neurons are formed in the adult brain.

Exciting experiments during the past two decades have demonstrated that new neurons continually form in the brain of adult animals, including primates and humans. New neurons were first found in the brains of adult songbirds, in areas of the brain associated with song production. Then, new granule cells were found in the hippocampus of adult chickadees, then, in rats and primates.[28] The same pattern of neuronal generation has been found in the hippocampus of adult humans.[29] Recently, in monkeys, new neurons were found to be migrating to the neocortex from stem cells in the region of the ventricles.[30] Adult neurogenesis results in continual influx of neurons that are (temporarily) immature and therefore structurally plastic. The hope is that the immature cells can take on functions of mature, adult cells. Although this premise has not been verified yet, adult neurogenesis can have important implications for our understanding of the mechanisms of neural plasticity, in general, and recovery of function following brain lesions, in particular.[31]

In summary, the aforementioned effects of cell injury, DAI, and metabolic dysfunction contribute to the morbidity and severity of neurobehavioral outcomes. As the metabolic balance returns to premorbid levels and neuronal reorganization takes place, the patient's clinical picture begins to evolve and the long-lasting effects of the injury become evident. The following section presents general principles of cognitive theory and the effect of injury on those systems.

18.3 General Principles of Cognitive Systems

Perhaps the most influential guiding principle of modern cognitive neuroscience is the concept of modularity. Early in the history of cognitive psychology, modularity referred to the strong claim that specific faculties could be completely delineated into separate neural areas.[32] This very rigid view of local representation of function was contrasted with the neo-Lashley hypothesis that computation is distributed across large neural populations and that whole patterns of neural activity, modeled in devices referred to as *neural networks* or *parallel distributed processing systems*, constituted states of cognition.[33] When taken to the extreme, the distributed processing approach spawned a model of brain function that was holographic in nature.[34] The truth, not surprisingly, lies somewhere in between these two end points, and today, most cognitive neuroscientists adopt a "weak" modularity framework to describe cognitive processing in the brain. Weak modularity holds that the simple computations and their underlying neural substrates are relatively localized and loosely autonomous.[35] Responses of neurons within these systems are tuned to specific characteristics in the environment but that tuning is broad (i.e., the response of the cell falls off gracefully when the stimulus departs from the cell's preferred stimulus).[36] Complex cognitive activities are accomplished by the coordination and communication among these more specialized modules. Basic processing principles governing how processing takes place appear to hold across systems, and these principles may be formulated in terms of computational styles or strategies. That is, cognitive activities spanning a variety of tasks may be rule governed, similarity governed, or, through extensive experience or preexisting propensities, may be automatically accomplished. Characteristics of the environment, the task demands, and the individual all play into which processing strategies and systems are utilized.

The implication of this framework for cognitive psychology has been to redirect research to identifying and characterizing functional systems and their basic components. In addition, investigators now also search for basic processing principles that hold across different functional systems and may dictate how different situations lead the brain to recruit different processing strategies. Methodologies from both traditional cognitive psychology (involving behavioral measures of accuracy and response times) and modern cognitive neuroscience (utilizing brain imaging and lesion/damage dissociation logic) have been brought together in identifying major systems and their processing characteristics. The following sections review the basic cognitive systems (executive function and attention, memory, and language). Each of these may be broken down into even smaller functional units, as well. Examples of their coordinated deployment in higher cognitive tasks are provided to highlight the interactive processing so central to the weak modularity hypothesis.

18.3.1 Domains of Cognition

18.3.1.1 Attention

Clinicians and researchers have used a variety of tasks to assess attentional processes. Unfortunately, some of the tasks can be easily contaminated by heavy requirements on memory, verbal, math, and motor abilities in addition to attentional demands. Consequently, it is important that the measures used to assess attention processes do just that. Posner[37] identifies three qualitatively different anatomic and functional attention networks that are distinct from other cognitive systems: the orienting network, the executive network, and the arousal or alerting network. The existence of these three systems illustrates the principle of modularity that is central to the cognitive neuroscience approach: They can operate independently and be selectively influenced (e.g., impaired), but are usually coordinated in complex cognitive tasks. Also, each system individually expresses modularity in that each can be further decomposed into distinct computations subserved by distinct neural substrates.

18.3.1.1.1 Orienting Network

The goal of this system is to guide the sensory organs to relevant locations within the environment so that processing of information in those locations is enhanced. In vision, attentional orienting is closely tied to shifting the gaze of the eyes to that part of the visual field containing stimuli to which the organism must respond. The shift of attention, however, can be dissociated from the movement of the eyes, per se, in that processing of items in to-be-attended or cued locations has been shown to be facilitated even when the eyes do not move or when the items are no longer present in the visual field by the time the eyes reach their location, if they do move.[37] This suggests a spotlight metaphor to describe this covert (i.e., without eye movements) shift of attention, and recent evidence indicates that there may be more than one spotlight available.[38] The areas in the brain responsible for covertly orienting attention in vision include the posterior parietal lobe, the superior colliculus (and, possibly, other areas of the midbrain), and the pulvinar. An earlier model of the 1990s[39] suggested that the superior parietal lobe disengages attention from its current focus, after which the superior colliculus moves attention to the new location. The pulvinar then enhances processing at that location. More recent evidence suggests that, when an unexpected event occurs, a more posterior region, the temporal–parietal junction, is necessary for the disengagement of the current focus of attention to orient to the new event.[40] The superior parietal lobe appears to be more involved in voluntary movements of attention in response to some type of cue.[41] Damage to any one of these structures leads to deficits in their respective functions. One deficit, termed *visual neglect,* with core symptoms that are most commonly associated with damage to the temporal–parietal junction,[42] is characterized by the inability to attend to parts of visual space contralateral to the damage (especially, if the damage is located in the right hemisphere). The specific problem is an inability to disengage focal attention from currently attended targets so that it can be moved to somewhere else. This failure is attentional in nature (rather than perceptual) because it can be revealed in tasks requiring the participant to imagine rather than actually perceive scenes from different perspectives.[43]

Neglect often resolves into a condition known as *extinction,* in which the individual is unable to perceive or respond to an object in the visual field that is contralateral to the damage only when another object is simultaneously present in the opposite visual field (i.e., on the same side as or ipsilateral to the lesion). It is as if the object has been "extinguished," hence its name. One question that has dominated research on extinction is: To what extent, if any, is the unnoticed stimulus processed? Initially, it was believed that no perceptual processing of the neglected object took place—a view similar to the early selection theories of attention in general. Recently, research has revealed that a remarkable amount of detail regarding the neglected object is available in the perceptual system, including semantic information, and that the failure is that this information does not reach conscious awareness. Volpe et al.[44] and Farah et al.[45] demonstrated that patients could determine whether a stimulus in the contralateral field was the same or different as a stimulus in the intact, ipsilateral field although they could not identify the former. This implicit processing has also been demonstrated in a number of studies,[46] including those examining the effects of similarity on the strength of extinction and in priming studies similar to those used to study memory. In the former, extinction is found to be greater when the intact object is highly similar to the neglected object, and this accuracy improves with decreasing similarity. Ladavas et al.[47] asked a patient with right-hemisphere damage to identify words such as *nurse* presented in the intact (ipsilateral) field that were sometimes preceded by a semantically related prime, such as *doctor* briefly flashed in the neglected, field and found performance better than when the target was not preceded by a related prime. Clearly, then, some semantic processing of the neglected word occurred, enough to influence processing of the target word (in the ipsilateral field). Despite this priming, the patient was unable to detect, read aloud, or make judgments regarding the lexical status and meaning of the word presented in the neglected field.

18.3.1.1.2 *Executive Network*

Governing the bulk of cognitive processing, at least what is consciously available, is the executive system, also referred to as the *central executive in working memory,*[48] the *anterior attentional network,*[49] and *controlled processes of short-term memory* (as opposed to automatic processes).[50,51] This system is largely responsible for activating a dynamic mental representation of the current situation, ensuring that important relevant features of that situation are amplified,[52] and selecting the most appropriate response from among a set of competing alternatives. To work properly, the executive network must be flexible enough to switch attention to different aspects of the situation or change response selection strategies as environmental events change. This system is limited in that there is difficulty in attending to several mental events simultaneously. This limitation goes beyond the interference in attending to multiple aspects of a stimulus resulting from shared processing pathways in the perceptual system. This capacity, termed *working memory capacity*,[53,54] varies among and within individuals at different times. Factors such as age, mood, fatigue, and arousal contribute significantly to an individual's effectiveness with controlled operations.[55,56]

A growing body of evidence points to the importance of individual differences, especially in working memory capacity, for understanding performance in a variety of cognitive tasks. The individual differences perspective is not news in psychometric research areas such as intelligence and neuropsychological assessment. A significant body of work points to the clear relationship between one's ability to control cognitive resources and better performance on standard measures of intelligence. This perspective, that more working memory capacity is always better, may need to be modified in light of recent theories. Cognitive literature is currently concerned with understanding the multiple systems that could be deployed for any given task.[57] One theme that is beginning to emerge is that, not only do task demands recruit one system versus another to solve a particular problem, but that an individual's working memory capacity can bias performance to rely on different cognitive subsystems that may, or may not, be optimal in a given situation.[58,59] We comment on this peculiar result in Section 18.3.1.4. Apparently, an individual's working memory capacity is not related to individual differences in the orienting network.[60,61]

Not all cognitive processing requires the effortful attention of the executive network. Automatic operations place minimal demands upon the executive system's limited processing capacity and can take place in parallel with other cognitive activities. These processes are distinct from the controlled operations of executive function and, hence, are considered preattentive or nonattentional. Automatic processes can be hardwired, such as the easy perceptual event of detecting a loud sound, flash of light, or change in color. They can also develop through extensive practice, as in the case of reading (for literate individuals). With normal brain functioning and practice, action sequences become increasingly autonomous at the subcortical level, and the management role of the executive system diminishes. There does not seem to be evidence to suggest individuals differ with respect to the development of efficacy of automatic processes in the same way that individual differences exist in controlled attention.[62] TBI can cause diffuse cortical and subcortical lesions in the brain and may interrupt the efficient and automatic activation of neural pathways and routines. Activities that previously required little or no effort may require deliberate control and effort, resulting in reduced efficiency.[56] It also appears that patients with right frontal lobe lesions fair worse than patients with left frontal and posterior lesions.[63,64]

Damage specific to the frontal lobes disrupts executive functioning because this brain region is thought to subserve it.[12,65] Patients with frontal lobe lesions often exhibit perseveration, or a difficulty in changing behavior in the short run. Neuropsychological tests of frontal dysfunction, such as the Wisconsin Card Sorting Test, are designed to reveal this specific deficit. Patients learn a series of category structures that can be described as differing along a single critical dimension (e.g., color, shape, or numerosity). During the test, the rule that best separates the categories is switched so that learners will have to abandon the old rule to learn the new one. Individuals with damage to the frontal cortex cannot perform this necessary switch; the old rule cannot be inhibited so that the new one can be selected.

A relatively famous example of failure of executive inhibition found in normal functioning individuals is the classic Stroop effect.[66] In a typical Stroop task, an observer is required to identify the color of ink that is used in the printing of various words, which are, themselves, color names. Performance in this color-naming task is severely diminished relative to performance using noncolor nouns. The automatic process of reading the words is difficult to inhibit, thus leading to response interference in the color naming. Perseveration and inability of inhibition of competing responses can interfere with activities of daily living. As part of cognitive treatment, structured therapy tasks, as well as activities that foster social awareness, should/must be incorporated to improve self-regulation and self-inhibition, and reduce perseverative responses.

18.3.1.1.3 Alerting Network

The ability to maintain a state of alertness or arousal is, phylogenically, the earliest of attentional systems. In humans, it is studied by requiring observers to monitor the environment for an extensive period of time for the occurrence of a low-probability event. Sustained attention involves the right frontal areas of the brain, as well as the midbrain areas associated with the cortical distribution of norepinephrine, the main neurotransmitter required for alertness. TBI individuals who also sustain right frontal damage have difficulty in sustained attention tasks. Robertson et al.[67] looked at a sustained attention to response target task in brain-injured subjects compared with control subjects. They found that TBI patients showed a significantly reduced tendency to slow down their responding after an error when compared with control subjects, and had greater variability in response times. In addition, Robertson et al.[67] found that variance on the sustained attention to response target task strongly correlated with informant report of daily life attentional failures in the TBI group.

In summary, following TBI, increased attention requirements result in increased fatigue and errors much more so than in the noninjured population. These individuals may experience inability to maintain attention and discriminate in the presence of distracters (e.g., vigilance), as well as difficulty in shifting between targets. Clinical assessment will often reveal a pattern in functional inconsistencies. These inconsistencies in functioning may leave TBI patients with a sense of vulnerability to circumstances that they do not understand and cannot control, especially during periods of fatigue, pain, distractions, and excessive task demands.[56]

CR of attentional processes attempts to recognize and control potentially adverse personal and environmental conditions, and ultimately trains patients to become more resistive to distracting situations. TBI patients could be trained to recognize particular situations that may affect their performance and can learn to seek out environments that are more conducive to productivity. In addition to awareness training, another component of attention training is rehearsal. It has been observed that, with practice, the effort and attentional control required for a task will decrease as the task becomes more automatic and efficient.[56] Therefore, it is important to train a patient to perform functional tasks, rehearse them to improve accuracy and efficiency, and decrease the amount of mental effort. Attention retraining should also challenge the individual by systematically increasing the level of distracters to simulate real-life demands.

In the Attention Process Training (APT) program, a component of a hierarchically organized process-specific approach to cognitive retraining,[68] begin with sustained attention tasks. The APT program progresses, hierarchically, from sustained attention to selective, alternating, and divided attention activities. Attention training has reportedly resulted in improved memory performance in patients with TBI.[68] Refer to Sohlberg and Mateer[12,68,69] for further information regarding this training program. Attention training that focuses on strategy building, like the APT, seems to be appropriate during the postacute phase when the patient is oriented and able to remember day-to-day information.[70]

18.3.1.2 Memory Processes

Our current understanding of memory suggests that it is organized with respect to both time and contents.[71] On the basis of behavioral evidence[72,73] and neuropsychological data,[74] the distinction between a short-term and a long-term retention system was the first to be made.[50] Initially, the nature of the information handled within these time-delineated systems was thought to be unitary, but a variety of neuropsychological and behavioral findings argued for a content-based subdivision that incorporates multiple memory systems (see Schacter and Tulving[75] for a review). We present this organization here and discuss its implications for CR following TBI. It should be emphasized that the concept of system organization needs to be supplemented with considerations of memory processes operating across all subsystems, such as encoding and retrieval.[76] The executive network described earlier in the context of attention is deeply involved in these active memory-related processes. Hence, any disruption to the frontal lobes underlying executive function will produce impairments in memory tasks, in addition to attention tasks as described in the previous section. Table 18.1[77–79] lays out the current view of the organization of memory in the human (and possibly, mammalian) brain.

18.3.1.2.1 Short-Term/Working Memory

When information arrives via the sense organs (i.e., perceptually encoded), it is deposited into an immediate working memory[1] system that is divided into three subsystems

TABLE 18.1

Memory Systems in the Human Brain

System	Subsystems	Divisions	Function	Brain Structures
Working memory	Central executive		Control	Frontal lobes
	Visuospatial sketchpad		Hold visual information	Occipital–parietal
	Phonologic loop		Hold acoustic information	Left temporal–parietal
Long term	Explicit	Semantic	General facts	Temporal
		Episodic	Autobiographic experiences	Medial temporal (hippocampus) diencephalon
	Implicit	Procedural	Motor and cognitive skill	Basal ganglia/motor cortex
		Perceptual representation	Priming/perceptual encoding	Sensory cortex
		Simple associative/ classical conditioning		General, throughout central nervous system; cerebellum

Note: The term *working memory* has different meanings in different literature. For example, in animal learning research, working memory describes tasks in which the capacity to hold information across trails within a test session is necessary for performance, as in a radial maze navigation task.[77] Baddeley[78] argues that the concept of working memory in this literature probably involves long-term memory, as is conceived in human memory research. Yet another approach to the short-term versus long-term distinction argues that short-term, or working memory, refers to traces that are lost if consolidation via the medial temporal lobe system is prevented as a result of injury or insult.[79] The timescale for this (on the order of 30–40 minutes) is much longer than the very brief duration of short-term memory (on the order of seconds[73]) as considered in cognitive psychology. Within the consolidation point of view, a memory is short term if its availability still involves the hippocampus; it becomes long term as permanent corticocortical connections are formed.

specialized for different functions[80] a control system, the executive network of attention described earlier, and two slave systems, each handling different types of information. Visual (e.g., color and shape) and spatial (i.e., location) information is held and manipulated in a visuospatial sketchpad. Cortical areas that are involved in visual perception (the occipital lobe) and spatial orienting (the parietal areas, especially the right parietal lobe) subserve the operations of this sketchpad.[81,82] Sounds, especially auditory speech sounds, are stored and processed by the phonologic or articulatory loop, a term that emphasizes its prototypical activity of recycling acoustic information to keep it in conscious awareness. More recently, Baddeley and Wilson[83] proposed a memory buffer mechanism responsible for integrating information between the phonologic and visuospatial systems and storing information that exceeds the span capacities of the two subsystems. The neuroanatomic correlates of this additional system have not been confirmed, but it seems that the functions might be independent of the frontal lobe. The existence of this buffer accounts for the fact that some patients may demonstrate intact immediate recall abilities (including supraspan capacities) but impaired long-term memory functioning.[84]

Studies of the capacity of working memory often use a task in which a sequence of items (e.g., letters or digits) is presented to a subject who must reproduce them immediately from memory in the correct order. The length of the longest sequence (in terms of number of digits/letters) correctly produced, termed the *letter* or *digit span*, is an index of the size of short-term memory that some believe is correlated with IQ measures of intelligence.[85] However, others suggest that this span reflects the capacity of the phonologic loop rather than the entire working memory system, and the role of the phonologic loop in general cognitive function has been called into question.[54,78,86] True working memory capacity of the executive network that has been shown to relate to higher cognitive functioning[87] is better measured by tasks that require either dual processing or inhibiting prepotent responses, both activities that are the hallmark of flexible control of attention.[54,80–90] Tests that measure static spans (e.g., forward span of the Wechsler Memory Scale-III) are dissociable from those that measure the more active processes involved in attentional control, such as digit span backward and verbal learning paradigms like the Rey Auditory Verbal Learning Test or the California Verbal Learning Test.[54,84,91] The loop Wechsler Memory Scale-III appears to be necessary, however, for language acquisition, either the early childhood learning of a native language[92] or in adult learning of foreign languages.[93,94]

18.3.1.2.2 Long-Term Memory

Some incoming information undergoes the process known as *consolidation*, which results in it being stored in various long-term retention systems. The different routes to storage, together with the distinctions among the kinds of information permanently stored, define the various hierarchical subsystems of long-term memory. At the top level of the taxonomy adopted by many cognitive neuroscientists[75,95] is the divide between information that can be consciously declared to have been learned or experienced (explicit memory), and information whose learning is only reflected by changes in future behavior as a result of the prior experience without conscious remembrance (implicit memory). The kinds of items deemed declarative include general knowledge or facts about the world, termed *semantic memory*; and personal, autobiographic recollection of experiences, termed *episodic memory*. The exact locus of stored memories is not known,[96] but it has been suggested that various cortical sites involved in perception may hold perceptual memories regarding events, whereas general factual knowledge is likely to be represented at least in the temporal cortex.[97]

Both semantic and episodic memories are thought to require a functioning medial temporal lobe system (hippocampus, amygdala, and adjacent cortex, but especially the hippocampus) for their learning.[95,97] Individuals with medial temporal lesions typically show very little retrograde amnesia; they have excellent memory for most of the experiences that they have had prior to the brain injury with the exception of events immediately preceding insult, perhaps as a result of their lack of consolidation. However, these patients show profound anterograde amnesia in that they cannot recall new events that they experience after the lesion. They perform poorly on the standard measures of declarative memory, such as recognition and recall of previously studied material. The subject can recall a new experience for a few seconds, before it fades, reflecting an intact working memory. The role of the medial temporal system appears to be one of storage or consolidation of short-term memories rather than one of retrieval, given that amnesiacs can retrieve remote memories with little difficulty.

Explicit memories are not only vulnerable to disruption following medial temporal brain lesions and TBI, but are relatively vulnerable in healthy individuals, and episodic memories are typically more vulnerable than semantic memories. Most people could not remember the event during which they learned that Tokyo was the capital of Japan. Although semantic or factual memory appears to be strengthened with repeated exposure, especially in the presence of interfering or distracting information, episodic memory, by its nature, cannot undergo repeated exposure. It appears that most episodic memories fade unless they include or are accompanied by some emotionally significant experience.[79] Recent evidence actually suggests that semantic memory may not require an undamaged hippocampus whereas episodic memories do. Vargha-Khadem et al.[98] describe three patients with childhood hippocampal pathology who were able to perform normally in schoolwork and attain average levels of competence with fact knowledge and language development, yet could not recall their daily experiences. Tulving et al.[99] discuss a case study of an individual after a TBI who experienced a total loss of episodic memory, both retrograde and anterograde, yet maintained an intact semantic memory system as well as other forms of implicit memory. In the future, if more observations such as these occur, semantic memory may be reclassified as a kind of implicit memory that neither requires the conscious recollection of the learning event nor an intact medial temporal lobe system for its operation.

Implicit memory consists of a heterogeneous collection of various kinds of memory preserved in the loss of declarative memory ability. These systems are quite distinct from one another and rely on entirely different brain structures. The development of procedural memory is independent of the hippocampal formation, but appears to depend on the basal ganglia, especially the caudate nucleus.[100,101] Procedural memory is typically divided into two major subtypes, which, on their surface, appear to be quite different, but appear to depend on the integrity of similar brain systems. One of the major categories is motor skill memory; the other is cognitive skill or reference memory. If an individual learned how to ride a unicycle today, and her episodic memory is intact, tomorrow she will report having remembered the experience. However, even if she has no explicit memory of the experience (as a result of hippocampal damage), she will show intact motor skill memory as manifested by improved performance on unicycle riding. Subjects with lesions invading the motor and premotor areas of the neocortex frequently display difficulty in motor skill learning. Yet, if their hippocampus is intact, they will recall the experience of attempting to ride the unicycle.

Reference or cognitive skill memory, the memory of the procedures that are necessary to win a game or solve a problem, including some kinds of category learning (discussed later), constitutes the second kind of procedural memory. This form of memory does not refer to explicit declarative memory for the rules of the game, but refers to the acquisition of successful strategies. An individual with medial temporal lobe lesions could improve their skill at board games, such as checkers, without recalling that they had ever played the game before. Thus, the solution of some complex cognitive tasks does not require explicit memory, but rather repeated exposure to a specific situation and rules for solutions. Quite possibly, the learned strategies are a collection of observations of cause and effect that are reinforced according to the principles of operant or instrumental conditioning. Consequently, patients with TBI may benefit from the repetitive nature of certain activities in CR, and become more adapted and independent without necessarily demonstrating improvement in explicit memory tasks. Although both forms of procedural learning involve the basal ganglia, motor skill learning appears to be dependent on the integrity of the motor areas of the neocortex, including the premotor strip, and cognitive skill learning appears to be more dependent on sensory cortices in the parietal and occipital lobes.[100]

Another type of implicit memory is revealed in studies of priming phenomena. Priming refers to the facilitation in the processing, detection, or identification of an item as a consequence of its prior exposure in tasks not requiring conscious recollection.[102] A classic priming paradigm involves an initial study of items, such as a list of words, under the guise of some ruse instructions, which is then followed with a nonmemory task such as lexical decision ("Is this letter string a word or nonword?"), word identification ("What is this word?"), or word-stem completion ("wo_ _"). The typical finding is that lexical decisions and word identifications occur more quickly or require less stimulus energy to achieve a given level of performance for words previously seen. In the word-stem completion task, subjects tend to supply words seen from the earlier list to complete the partial words.[103] That priming is subserved by a different system than explicit memory is demonstrated by several observations (although a recent brain imaging study suggests some involvement of the hippocampus in priming).[104] Individuals with amnesia who fail traditional tests of explicit memory exhibit normal priming;[105–108] individuals with damage to perceptual areas, such as the occipital lobe, show normal performance on explicit measures of memory but do not evidence priming,[109] and performance on standard recognition and recall tasks can be dissociated from priming tasks in normal subjects.[110–113] Priming appears to be perceptual in nature because any surface change of the stimulus (e.g., font changes for word stimuli or changes in picture orientation for visual stimuli) from prior exposure to test can reduce it[114–118] and is mediated by the sensory cortices (visual priming in visual cortex, auditory priming in auditory cortex, and so forth). This system responsible for priming is referred to as the *perceptual representation system* in Schacter's framework[119] and is the system involved in the initial perception and encoding of a stimulus.

A final category of implicit memory includes simple classical conditioning and associative learning of the sort often studied in animal learning research. These simple forms of learning, evidenced even in invertebrates, may reflect principles of neuronal plasticity in general, such as Hebbian learning or long-term potentiation. However, there is evidence for the special role of the cerebellum in classical conditioning of discrete motor responses, such as eye blinks in the presence of air puffs.[96] It is unlikely that TBI would disrupt this form of learning if the patient exhibits any signs of consciousness or demonstrates basic cognitive functioning. Classical conditioning has been demonstrated in decorticate and decerebrate laboratory animals. We mention this type of memory here to provide a complete picture of what is known regarding memory systems.

18.3.1.2.3 The Role of Processes and Strategies in Memory

The previous sections describe different categories of memories emphasizing the nature of the memory content as revealed by dissociations of the effects of variables on performance using different types of tasks and materials. However, understanding memory performance requires consideration of the active strategies and processes implemented during the various memory tasks. Most forms of memory assessment, especially in clinical neuropsychological contexts, rely heavily on explicit measures[120,121] because this type of memory is most characteristic of human cognitive performance and seems to be most influenced by active memory strategies.

Early cognitive studies of memory formation focused on the stage model (consisting of encoding, storage, and retrieval) and argued that certain ways of organizing the to-be-remembered material led to more durable memory traces.[122] If the individual elaborated upon the deeper meaning of items, emphasizing connections to already learned material or involving visual imagery,[123,124] those items would be less subject to forgetting than items merely rehearsed by being recycled in the phonologic loop. This idea has been exploited in various prescriptions of strategies to improve memory performance in CR.[125–128]

This active elaboration clearly places demands on working memory, especially the executive control component responsible for the planning and sequencing of currently active mental operations. When subjects with CHI were presented with unclustered words (word lists that were randomly organized), they did not actively organize this information according to meaning as did control subjects, indicating a passive or shallow learning style.[129,138] Although normal immediate recall is observed in these patients, suggesting an intact auditory span, the reported passive learning style of the CHI subjects reflects an inability to acquire information successfully in the working memory buffer zone and, subsequently, move information from working memory to long-term memory. This difficulty is manifested during demanding tasks such as the Auditory Verbal Learning Test and the California Verbal Learning Test.[120,129–131] These aforementioned multitrial tasks provide an opportunity to assess various aspects of working memory processes involving frontal lobe function in addition to learning. Studies incorporating the California Verbal Learning Test and the Auditory Verbal Learning Test indicate that decreased performance can also be the result of inefficiency in guiding the retrieval process,[132] especially if the right frontal areas are damaged.[133]

Difficulty in transferring of information from working memory to long-term memory (i.e., consolidation) can be disrupted by the appearance of distracting or interfering material,[134] as well as failure to organize information appropriately. TBI patients seem to be most vulnerable to the debilitating effects of interference, possibly as a result of the insult to the frontal lobes, especially the left frontal[133] or the medial temporal lobe areas. Studies following TBI suggest that immediate recall (measured by span tasks) appears to be intact.[135,136] However, when interference is imposed, memory performance is significantly affected, indicative of difficulties in consolidating declarative information into long-term memory.[132,135] Interference can be introduced in the form of a delay or in the form of a competing stimulus.[136] Even a 10-second delay between stimulus presentation and response has been reported to affect recall performance.[137]

The current view of the organization of memory and its processes has been developed, in part, as a result of focal lesions, both in human and in animals, and their resulting effects on various memory tasks. TBI, however, rarely causes circumscribed lesions. Subsequently, multiple memory systems may be affected.[84,131,138]

Research suggests that patients with moderate to severe CHI are able to learn new information, but at a decreased rate, compared with normal subjects. Furthermore, the ability to recognize information is superior to their free recall skills.[130,132,139] Although, as a group, CHI subjects tend to have a more passive learning style, subgroups of patients that apply active memory strategies have been reported. These patients typically have better working memories in comparison with patient subgroups that do not use active memory strategies.[138]

Patients with moderate–severe TBI benefit from pictorial presentation of verbal material rather than auditory presentation of information.[130,137] In addition, the use of visual imagery as a remedial approach to facilitate verbal recall seems to be effective for patients with mild memory impairment in TBI.[140] However, elaborate visual imagery techniques are not effective after TBI as a result of increased mental effort demands.[125,141–143] Furthermore, patients with severe memory impairments benefit more from external memory aids and alerting devices for activities of daily living, provided that they receive extensive training for the use of the strategy/device.[70] Specific external memory strategies, such as the implementation of a memory notebook, may be beneficial for everyday (or prospective) memory functions, such as remembering important dates and appointments (see Sohlberg and Mateer[69] for extensive information on this approach).

Teaching domain-specific memory tasks as they pertain to a given job may be successful because they incorporate procedural memory, repetition, and routine building.[144,145] However, the application of that knowledge to novel situations and problems requires declarative knowledge of strategies, as well as intact executive abilities,[10] which are frequently impaired after moderate–severe TBI. The hierarchical perceptual tasks proposed later in this chapter are designed to facilitate working memory and executive abilities.

18.3.1.3 *Verbal Language*

The verbal/logical language system, collectively, is another important system that is related to higher cognitive function. For instance, strategies for successful encoding and retrieval of information and categorization techniques typically incorporate verbal language. Consequently, language is used routinely during neuropsychological testing for the assessment of cognitive abilities, such as working memory, semantic knowledge, reasoning, and problem solving.

TBI can affect language directly and indirectly. Direct focal damage to the language-dominant regions of the left hemisphere and disruption of language-specific networks, can result in aphasic symptomatology. The patient may have difficulty processing linguistic types of information and may experience decline with receptive and expressive language.

More often, though, TBI is not associated with traditional aphasic syndromes. Although aphasia may be present during the early stages of the recovery process because of direct lesions in language-specific networks of the left hemisphere, the clinical picture usually evolves and the primary language deficits center in the area of word finding and lexical retrieval. These can persist for at least a year postinjury.[146,147]

The neuropathology of TBI, as described earlier in the chapter, involves multifocal lesions. Recent evidence acquired during the past two decades indicates that multiple cortical and subcortical brain regions (in both hemispheres) are activated during language tasks, even though the left hemisphere demonstrates greater activation.[148] Hence, focal damage to cortical and subcortical brain structures in either hemisphere, such as the medial temporal lobes, the frontal and parietal lobes, the thalamus, and the fusiform gurus, may result in the disruption of various cognitive processes that support language (i.e., working memory and organization) and language-specific networks. Furthermore, diffuse axonal injury can result in generalized cognitive disruption that often affects complex linguistic abilities.

Difficulties in discourse organization and other extralinguistic difficulties are a result of impairments in cognitive nonlinguistic processes that support language. Damage, dysfunction, or disorganization of attention, memory, categorization, and executive control (including self-awareness) can hamper language abilities during discourse. These deficits can be manifested as problems in social communication. Oftentimes, the patient with TBI may lack verbal sensitivity, may be verbally impulsive, and may exhibit difficulty in using and interpreting humor, as well as interpreting nonverbal language cues. In addition, attention and memory problems may create difficulties in remembering names and events, and in processing large amounts of material during discourse. Consequently, deficits in language can create significant social burden for the patient with TBI. Linguistic–communication therapy in TBI focuses on discourse management skills (during individual and group therapy formats) and in treating the underlying cognitive deficits that contribute to the linguistic–communication impairment. The Categorization Program described later in this chapter is an example of an approach that begins with basic object description and progresses hierarchically into linguistic abstraction. For more information on the major brain areas involved in language functions, language networks, and their processing characteristics, and the effects of brain lesions on language functions, see Hillis,[148] Fromkin and Rodman,[149] and Benson and Ardilla.[150]

18.3.1.4 Categorization

In the hierarchy of cognitive function, complex or "higher" reasoning abilities, such as categorization (including object recognition and perception/action), problem solving, and decision making, are those that require the coordination of several of the basic systems. Because of the greater complexity inherent in these higher level tasks, understanding the alternative processing strategies and subsystems deployed by the executive system becomes important for modeling individual performance. When we categorize, we assign objects or events into groups. This may be done to support other types of activities or decisions that have to be made. That is, categorization itself is a process that serves as a subcomponent to other higher processes. For example, expert problem solvers must categorize the situation as a particular kind of problem before solutions are made available.

The research on categorization distinguishes between aspects of classifying and recognizing everyday objects and situations, and the learning of novel categories. These two processes can be dissociated in brain-damaged individuals[151] in that, sometimes, one can lose the ability to learn new categories (e.g., in Parkinson's disease) but not lose old familiar categories. The opposite pattern has been observed as well, with some deficits leading to the loss of specific highly learned categories[152,153] with no obvious general category-learning problems. An attempt to integrate these two distinct researches suggests that our knowledge of natural categories and common objects is likely to have been acquired through the use of a similarity-based system.[154,155]

18.3.1.4.1 Recognition and Categorization of Everyday Objects

The visual recognition and categorization of everyday objects involve two anatomically and functionally distinct pathways specialized for different kinds of information. As seen in Figure 18.1, the ventral pathway (through the temporal lobes) subserves passive recognition in which the object is perceived as a kind of thing that the observer has seen before.

This recognition includes all aspects of visual memory, such as form, function, the object's typical location, and many other associated memories. The dorsal pathway (through the parietal lobes) mediates visually guided behavior, such as reaching and grasping of objects and self-locomotion (Figure 18.1). The dorsal perception-and-action system is understood in terms of spatial attention, orienting, and motor control.[65]

Deficits in the passive object recognition system resulting from brain injury lead to dissociations in categorization ability as a function of the type of stimulus material. Most often, patients lose the ability to recognize living or animate objects whereas artifactual recognition is spared, although the opposite dissociation has been observed. Whether this pattern results from a semantic (memory) system that is organized along domain-specific modules,[156] or in terms of perceptual and function features,[157] is still open to debate. Recent views of the concept system based on object naming tasks suggest that both aspects of representation may be correct.[158–160] In their tripartite model of concept and lexical access, Damasio et al.[158–160] argue that concept representations are separable from the word form systems that reside in classical language areas. Mediating between the two in the left inferotemporal area is a neural structure that links the concept knowledge system to the word form system. They have provided evidence that this intermediary system is modality neutral, open to access through any sensory channel,[160] but is categorically organized in the manner suggested by Caramazza et al.,[156,161–163] who have argued for a semantic memory system organized into the categories of plants, animals, tools, and conspecifics.[158,164] The concept knowledge system, itself, broadly located throughout the right and left temporal lobes, is likely to be organized by properties and relevant object attributes.[165,166] There is clear evidence in vision of a hierarchical recognition process that begins with early feature processing (such as orientation, motion, and color) and leads to the processing and representation of objects and object classes in the inferotemporal cortex.[167] We propose that cognitive treatment should incorporate a systematic hierarchical protocol beginning with early feature identification to retrain the passive object recognition system. The tasks should consist of both animate and inanimate classes of objects to account for the possibility of domain specificity in the representation of visual memories.

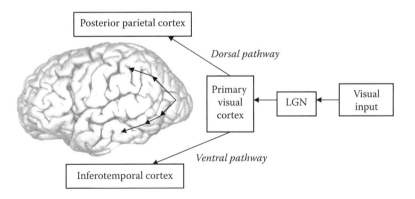

FIGURE 18.1
Pathways for recognition and categorization of everyday objects. Input from the retina traverses two major visual pathways in the primate brain. Information supporting visually guided action (e.g., reaching) is routed through the lateral geniculate nucleus (LGN), the primary visual cortex in the occipital lobe, and on to the posterior parietal regions (the dorsal pathway). Visual attributes that are necessary for the identification and recognition of an object and its related properties are processed in the ventral pathway, including the LGN and the primary visual cortex, ending in the inferotemporal cortex.

18.3.1.4.2 Recognition and Categorization of Novel Situations

When people are faced with having to learn to categorize novel objects or situations, current cognitive theory suggests they may be able to recruit one of three specialized systems for this purpose.[168] Two of these are "explicit" in the sense that their processes and outputs are consciously available to the category learner. The most important of these—the rule-based or rule-governed category system—involves the use of explicit rules that can be verbalized and hypothesis testing to determine category membership and, hence, relies heavily on executive functioning for its operation. The other explicit system requires significant episodic memory in that categorization is accomplished by the recall of previously experienced category members, or exemplars, that are similar to the current novel object.[169] Exemplar-based categorization likely draws upon brain structures known to underlie episodic memory performance—that is, the medial temporal lobe including the hippocampus. This type of process would be efficient only for categories of few members. When the number of category members exceeds the limits of working memory, other, more robust procedures are brought to bear.[170]

It has been observed that, even in the case of severe deficits in episodic memory and/ or in the case of category rules that cannot be verbalized, individuals can still learn to classify objects.[170–172] An example of the latter kind of category learning problem is the complex pattern recognition required in such cases as radiology or sonography in which the category boundaries are quite fuzzy and the elements in the pattern combine in nonlinear or interactive ways to specify identity. It is because of these observations, a third category system, recently described as a *procedural learning system*,[151,173] has been proposed. It is currently thought to rely on the structures of the basal ganglia and involve processes similar to that of procedural motor learning (see Section 18.3.1.2.2). Which system is recruited for a particular problem is a complex interaction of task characteristics, individual differences, and stage of learning.[174] A recent finding suggests that an individual's working memory capacity may be an important factor in determining which system—the explicit rule-governed one or the procedural learning system—gets recruited for a given category learning task.[59] Specifically, individuals with high working memory capacities will learn rule-based problems faster than they can learn problems requiring procedural learning strategy. Alternatively, individuals with lower working memory capacity learn category structures with mapping that cannot be verbalized faster than they learn those defined by rules. This suggests that understanding the relationship between individual neuropsychological characteristics, such as executive function or other reasoning-type processes, and performance in categorization retraining tasks may be important in the design of cognitive retraining tasks.[175]

Moderate to severe TBI seems to interfere with the patient's ability to use attributes to describe objects. In a preliminary study by Constantinidou and Kreimer,[176] subjects with moderate to severe brain injury provided significantly fewer attributes to describe common household objects compared with matched noninjured subjects. Subjects with brain injury were able to learn a list of eight core attributes, such as color, shape, composition, and weight. Finally, they were able to apply these attributes to describe another set of common objects more effectively compared with their spontaneous description. However, their performance was, at all times, significantly poorer than that of noninjured subjects. These findings support the need for a systematic rehabilitation program to improve the categorization abilities of patients with moderate to severe TBI. We discuss such a program later in Section 18.4.

18.3.1.5 Abstract Thought

Reasoning, making decisions, and solving problems are among the highest forms of cognition, and characterize what we think of as human intelligence. These complex processes emerge from the interaction of many of the more basic cognitive processes that have already been described. For example, a current model of expert decision making combines the executive network of attention, the function of which is to amplify the relevant features of the current situation, and an implicit categorization process that recognizes the current situation as similar to one that has been experienced before. Hence, a response or choice for action is automatically selected based on situation awareness.[177] Judgments of the probabilities of events are governed by heuristics such as representativeness in which the likelihood of an event is determined by how typical the event is of the category it represents.[178] Thus, there is a categorization process involved in making probability judgments. Similarly, models of problem solving rely on selective attention, memory, and categorization capabilities as crucial components.[179] Consequently, a deficit in any of these more elemental processes will disturb performance on tasks of higher order thinking.

18.4 Directions for Rehabilitation

The cognitive system is comprised of hierarchical processes and systems. Depending on specific task demands, different levels of processes are recruited for successful task completion. At infancy, the individual begins with basic concrete abilities, such as directing attention to a given object or person. Infants and young children learn features of objects (such as color, texture, and shape) in a predictable manner. These skills enhance their ability to learn categories, discriminate, and make generalizations.[180,181] As the cognitive system matures, attention capabilities become more sophisticated. Cognitively intact adults are able to direct attention, discriminate, shift, and sustain response sets in the presence of distraction. Brain injury causes a disruption of neuronal systems and interferes with the efficiency of the cognitive hierarchies. Consequently, postacute CR should implement systematic hierarchical treatment protocols that target attentional, memory, categorization, and abstract thinking tasks to restore impaired cognitive processes.[182,183] A systematic hierarchical approach has been suggested in the brain injury rehabilitation literature as a means to rehabilitate and reorganize cognitive systems, and to restore concept formation and cognitive function.[184–186]

Where should CR begin? One needs to consider that even the most minimal cognitive act, from input to output, involves recognition and categorization. In the previous edition of this book, we proposed that postacute CR should implement a hierarchical program beginning with basic levels of categorization, such as feature identification, with the ultimate goal to target higher processes, such as abstract thought, decision making, and problem solving. We developed a treatment model that integrated principles of cognitive theory and models of category learning,[187,188] language theory,[180,181] and rehabilitation[182,189] for the design of hierarchical tasks to treat the two aspects of categorization described earlier: (1) recognition and categorization of everyday objects, and (2) recognition and categorization of novel situations. The theoretical model was the basis for the Categorization Program.[190]

As seen in the Appendix, the first part of the Categorization Program begins with a very basic level of concept formation and thought productivity, which includes asking and training the person to express as many attributes as possible about a common object. Subjects progress through the various levels of the Categorization Program as they achieve the criterion at each level. Each level becomes increasingly demanding, requiring more cognitive effort. The stimuli begin with concrete objects (to minimize cognitive distance) and progress gradually to abstract ideas. Abstract reasoning, mental flexibility, and problem-solving abilities are the targets of the higher levels of this systematic perceptual training program.[9]

The Categorization Program integrates principles of cognitive neuroscience and rehabilitation, and designs hierarchical tasks for the similarity-based and the rule-governed systems described previously. The tasks begin with basic feature identification and feature extraction (such as color, shape, and size) and progress to higher levels of concept formation and abstraction (such as rule-based decision making). The Categorization Program is a systematic hierarchical training program consisting of eight levels. It provides a standardized approach to categorization training, yet it incorporates mastery criteria for each level to account for individual differences. Furthermore, it implements systematic cueing hierarchies and errorless learning to facilitate patient training and learning. A preliminary study with the Categorization Program[190] and a follow-up randomized, controlled trial[175] indicate that the Categorization Program is effective in improving categorization abilities in patients with TBI who are enrolled in postacute rehabilitation. Patients who were treated with the Categorization Program demonstrated greater gains on neuropsychological tests than those patients who received the standard treatment. Furthermore, the Categorization Program facilitated the generalizability of skills into new tasks that required the application of high-level categorization abilities, including mental flexibility. Research in patients with TBI who received this protocol during their postacute rehabilitation phase indicates that the Categorization Program helps patients improve their cognitive performance during neuropsychological tests, categorization tasks, and functional outcome measures.[175,190]

In summary, the remedial systematic hierarchical approaches are based on the fact that our cognitive system is comprised of systematic hierarchical components. All these basic and complex systems tie together in order for the individual to learn and adapt to the environment. The combination of hierarchical remedial (or restorative) therapy that follows a neurodevelopmental approach along with compensatory techniques could be used integratively to maximize the patient's level of functioning during the rehabilitation process.

18.5 Efficacy Research

Efficacy research in the area of CR is a relatively new science (i.e., about 20 years old). The proliferation of TBI outcomes research during the past decade is consistent with the 1998 consensus statement in TBI that calls for new and innovative research in the area of CR.[191] Yet, efficacy research in TBI CR causes a plethora of methodologic and ethical problems. Behavioral researchers are called to aspire to the "gold standard": the double-blind, randomized, controlled trial implemented in pharmacologic research. Although this type of elegant research protocol might work in a behavioral neuroscience laboratory, it is certainly not pragmatic for the daily life of the rehabilitation team, which is subjected to patient health problems that interfere with treatment, insurance funding cuts, staff turnover, and scheduling conflicts. Yet it is important that efficacy research demonstrates that CR treatment is both effective and efficacious. That is, treatment ought to cause a positive change to the targeted dependent variable in the setting that is designed to be implemented. Consequently, outcomes research that takes place in the actual clinical setting should be designed carefully to maximize experimental control and account for potential sources of variability that might compromise its results.

CR is an integral component of most TBI rehabilitation centers. Yet there is great variability in the treatment methodology implemented at the various centers across the United States and internationally. Groups like the Special Interest Group of the American Congress of Rehabilitation Medicine (BI-ISIG),[70] the special task force of the European Federation of Neurological Societies,[192] and the Academy of Neurologic Communication Disorders in the United States[193] have conducted extensive reviews of the literature to assess the evidence on CR and develop clinical practice guidelines.

As Malec[10] pointed out, scientific inquiry has a sequence of development and is a "slow process that frequently begins with uncontrolled naturalistic observations leading to single-case and other limited experiments that, in the long term, provide a basis for more sophisticated experimental designs."[p.232] Currently, the majority of CR research is classified as class III evidence (i.e., single subject with quantitative analyses and clinical series without concurrent control subjects). For instance, the BI-ISIG review[71] examined research articles published between 1998 and 2002. It included 17 class I (prospective randomized, controlled trials); 8 class II (prospective, nonrandomized cohort studies or multiple baseline, or retrospective, nonrandomized case–control studies); and 62 class III studies. In contrast, the first BI-ISIG review,[194] which included all peer-reviewed published studies on CR prior to 1997, identified 39 studies as class I studies. Therefore, the publication of 17 new class I studies in only 4 years is an indication of the development of CR research in brain injury.

Cicerone et al.[70] proposed that research should focus on standardized interventions (which we believe need to be based on theoretical models of human cognition and learning) and the identification of various components of complex interventions (i.e., active ingredients). Research protocols need to use sensitive measures to measure changes that directly relate to the hypothesis at hand and to the changes (or behaviors) that the study intends to measure. Furthermore, both functional and formal neuropsychological measures that are not only sensitive, but also have been validated with the TBI population need to be incorporated to assess changes as a result of specific treatment.

The most dramatic recovery following brain injury occurs during the first year postinjury, also known as the *spontaneous recovery stage*. Efficacy research may want to identify treatment strategies that enhance recovery during the first year postinjury. It is possible that certain treatment paradigms may yield different results depending on the time since injury.

In addition to chronicity, injury severity is another factor that needs to be investigated in relationship to rehabilitation outcomes. The length of impaired consciousness, the length of posttraumatic amnesia, and Glasgow Coma Scale scores have been traditionally used to determine injury severity. In the recent years, the presence of genetic markers, such as the apolipoprotein E4 allele, and elevated serum 100B protein have also been associated with poorer recovery.[195] Efficacy research may want to investigate whether certain treatment paradigms are more beneficial for patients with specific neuropsychological and biophysical profiles (i.e., Is technique A better than technique B in treating this population with X characteristics?) to design treatment paradigms that target patient needs more effectively.

18.6 Summary

Children learn new skills by attending, discriminating, categorizing, and acting upon their environment. The essence of CR following brain injury is to teach the patient new skills, remediate old skills, refine existing abilities, and teach compensatory strategies in an integrative manner to enhance and maximize the patient's level of functioning. Evidence presented in this chapter from cognitive theory, neurobiology, psychology, and clinical research supports the use of remedial techniques using systematic hierarchical programs targeting basic and complex cognitive systems. Evidence indicates that, in postacute brain injury rehabilitation, CR goals addressing attentional, language, categorization, visual processing, problem solving, and abstract skills may have lasting effects in patients with CHI.[70,183] The categorization tasks included in the Appendix are being used as examples of how a hierarchical treatment model of a standardized therapy modality might be developed.

Neurobiologic research on learning suggests that repetition enhances learning. We could assert that systematic, hierarchical restorative training, as part of a CR program, could facilitate adaptive neuronal sprouting occurring during the spontaneous recovery process. Furthermore, CR would provide environmental support and stimulation that will facilitate central nervous system functional reorganization as part of the recovery process. As neuroimaging techniques improve, future research may provide clear information on the extent of neuronal reorganization associated with CR after TBI.

Successful rehabilitation following brain injury is a complex process. The focus of this chapter was to apply cognitive theory and neurophysiologic principles of learning and recovery as they relate to the restoration of attention, memory, and categorization/perceptual skills following TBI. However, CR is part of the large umbrella of neuropsychological rehabilitation. As part of that, the person's psychosocial functioning, self-awareness, self-acceptance, emotional and environmental support mechanisms, and access to the community and services are necessary components for successful rehabilitation. When all these processes function in synergy, the outcome is greater than the sum of its parts, resulting in an optimal treatment outcome.

References

1. Squire, L. R., *Memory and Brain*, Oxford University Press, New York, 1987.
2. Coelho, C. A., DeRuyter, F., and Stein, M., Treatment efficacy: Cognitive communicative disorders resulting from traumatic brain injury in adults, *Journal of Speech and Hearing Research*, 39 (suppl.), S5–S17, 1996.
3. Ben-Yishay, Y., Silver, S. M., Plasetsky, E., and Rattock, J., Relationship between employability and vocational outcome after intensive holistic cognitive rehabilitation, *Journal of Head Trauma Rehabilitation*, 2(1), 35–48, 1987.
4. Caetano, C. and Christensen, A. L., The design of neuropsychological rehabilitation: The role of neuropsychological assessment, in L. León-Carrión (Ed.) *Neuropsychological Rehabilitation: Fundamentals, Innovations, and Directions*, GR/St. Lucie Press, Delray Beach, FL, 63–72, 1997.
5. Christensen, A. L. and Caetano, C., Luria's neuropsychological investigation in the Nordic countries, *Neuropsychology Review*, 9(2), 71–78, 1999.
6. Ben-Yishay, Y. and Prigatano, G. P., Cognitive rehabilitation, in M. Rosenthal, E. R. Griffith, M. R. Bond, and J. D. Miller (Eds.), *Rehabilitation of the Adult and Child with Traumatic Brain Injury*, 2nd ed., Davis, Philadelphia, 393–400, 1990.

7. Prigatano, G. P., *Principles of Neuropsychological Rehabilitation*, Oxford University Press, New York, 1999.
8. Ashley, M. J., Leal, R., and Mehta, Z., Cognitive disorders: Diagnosis and treatment in the TBI patient, in M. J. Ashley (Ed.), *Traumatic Brain Injury: Rehabilitative Treatment and Case Management*, 2nd ed., CRC Press, Boca Raton, FL, 367–402, 2004.
9. Constantinidou, F., Thomas, R., and Best, P., Principles of cognitive rehabilitation: An integrative approach, in M. J. Ashley (Ed.), *Traumatic Brain Injury: Rehabilitative Treatment and Case Management*, 2nd ed., CRC Press, Boca Raton, FL, 337–366, 2004.
10. Malec, J. F., Cognitive rehabilitation, in R. W. Evans (Ed.), *Neurology and Trauma*, W. B. Saunders, Philadelphia, PA, 231–248, 1996.
11. Mateer, C. and Raskin, S., Rehabilitation of attention, memory, and executive functions, in M. Rosenthal, E. Griffith, M. Bond, and J. Miller (Eds.), *Rehabilitation of the Adult and Child with Traumatic Brain Injury*, 3rd ed., F. A. Davis, Philadelphia, 254–270, 1999.
12. Sohlberg, M. M. and Mateer, C. A., *Cognitive Rehabilitation: An Integrative Neuropsychological Approach*, Guilford Press, New York, 2001.
13. Katz, D. I., Neuropathology and neurobehavioral recovery from closed head injury, *The Journal of Head Trauma Rehabilitation*, 7(2), 1–15, 1992.
14. Levin, H. S., Benton, A. L., and Grossmann, R. G., *Neurobehavioral Consequences of Closed Head Injury*, Oxford University Press, New York, 1982.
15. Viano, D. C., Biomechanics of head injury: Toward a theory linking head dynamic motion, brain tissue deformation, and neural trauma, Technical paper, Society of Automotive Engineers, Warrendale, PA, 1988.
16. Povlishock, J. T. and Katz, D. I., Update on neuropathology and neurological recovery after traumatic brain injury, *Journal of Head Trauma Rehabilitation*, 20(1), 76–94, 2005.
17. Povlishock, J. T. and Coburn, T. H., Morphopathological change associated with mild head injury, in H. S. Levin, H. M. Eisenberg, and A. L. Benton (Eds.), *Mild Head Injury*, Oxford University Press, New York, 37–53, 1989.
18. Verity, A. M., Povlishock, J. T., and Cheung, M., Brain cellular injury and recovery: Horizons for improving medical therapies in stroke and trauma, *The Western Journal of Medicine*, 148(6), 670–684, 1988.
19. O'Leary, D. D. M., Ruff, N. L., and Dyck, R. H., Development, critical period plasticity, and adult reorganization of mammalian somatosensory systems, *Current Opinions in Neurobiology*, 4(4), 535–544, 1994.
20. Hillerred, L., Vespa, P. M., and Hovda, D. A., Translational neurochemical research in acute human brain injury: The current status and potential future for cerebral microdialysis, *Journal of Neurotrauma*, 22(1), 1–34, 2005.
21. Hovda, D. A., The neurobiology of traumatic brain injury: Why is the brain so vulnerable after injury?, *Brain Injury Source*, 2(2), 22–25, 1998.
22. Yakolev, A. G. and Faden, A. I., Molecular strategies in central nervous system injury, *Journal of Neurotrauma*, 12(5), 767–777, 1995.
23. Bergsneider, M., Hovda, D. A., Shalmon, E., Kelly, D. F., Vespa, P. M., Martin, N. A., Phelps, M. E., et al. Cerebral hyperglycolysis following severe traumatic brain injury in humans: A positron emission tomography study, *Journal of Neurosurgery*, 86(2), 241–251, 1997.
24. Hall, E. D., Mohlberg, D. N., and Poole, R. M., Development of novel therapies for acute traumatic brain injury: Pharmaceutical industry perspective, *Brain Injury Source*, 2(2), 18–21, 1998.
25. Yoshino, A., Hovda, D. A., Kawamata, T., Katayama, Y., and Becker, D. P., Dynamic changes in local cerebral glucose utilization following cerebral concussion in rats: Evidence of a hyper- and subsequent hypermetabolic state, *Brain Research*, 561(1), 106–119, 1991.
26. Finger, S., Le Vere, T. E., Almi, C. R., and Stein, D. G., *Brain Injury and Recovery: Theoretical and Controversial Issues*, Plenum, New York, 1988.
27. Greenough, W. T. and Volkmar, F. R., Pattern of dendritic branching in occipital cortex of rats in complex environments, *Experimental Neurology*, 40(2), 491–504, 1973.

28. Cameron, H. A., Woolley, C. S., McEwin, B. S., and Gould, E., Differentiation of newly born neurons and glia in the dentate gyrus of the adult rat, *Neuroscience*, 56(2), 337–344, 1993.

29. Erickson, P. S., Perfilieva, E., Bjork-Eriksson, T., Alborn, A. M., Nordborg, C., Peterson, D. A., and Gage, F. H., Neurogenesis in the adult human hippocampus, *Nature Medicine*, 4, 1313–1317, 1998.

30. Gould, E., Reeves, A. J., Graziano, M. S. A., and Gross, C. G., Neurogenesis in the neocortex of adult primates, *Science*, 286(5439), 548–552, 1999.

31. Gould, E. and Gross, C. G., Neurogenesis in adult mammals: Some progress and problems, *Journal of Neuroscience*, 22(3), 619–623, 2002.

32. Fodor, J. A., *The Modularity of Mind*, MIT Press, Cambridge, MA, 1983.

33. Rumelhart, D. E., McClelland, J. L., and the PDP Research Group, *Parallel Distributed Processing: Explorations in the Microstructure of Cognition*, MIT Press, Cambridge, MA, 1986.

34. Eich, J. M., A composite holographic associative recall model, *Psychological Review*, 89(6), 627–661, 1982.

35. Kosslyn, S. M. and Koenig, O., *Wet Mind: The New Cognitive Neuroscience*, Free Press, New York, 1992.

36. Farah, M. J., *Visual Agnosia: Disorders of Object Recognition and What They Tell Us*, MIT Press, Cambridge, MA, 1990.

37. Posner, M. I., Attention in cognitive neuroscience: A overview, in M. S. Gazzaniga (Ed.), *The Cognitive Neurosciences*, MIT Press, Cambridge, MA, 615–624, 1995.

38. Awh, E. and Pashler, H., Evidence for split attentional foci, *Journal of Experimental Psychology: Human Perception and Performance*, 26(2), 834–846, 2000.

39. Posner, M. I. and Peterson, S. E., The attention system of the human, *Annual Review of Neuroscience*, 12, 25–42, 1990.

40. Corbetta, M. and Shulman, G., Control of goal-directed and stimulus-driven attention in the brain, *Nature Neuroscience Reviews*, 5(3), 201–215, 2002.

41. Corbetta, M., Kincade, J. M., Ollinger, J. M., McAvoy, M. P., and Shulman, G., Voluntary orienting is dissociated from target detection in human posterior parietal cortex, *Nature Neuroscience*, 3(3), 292–297, 2000.

42. Posner, M. I., Rueda, M. R., and Kanske, P., Probing the mechanisms of attention, in J. T. Cacioppo, L. G. Tassinary, and G. G. Berntson (Eds.), *Handbook of Psychophysiology*, 3rd ed., Cambridge University Press, New York, 2007.

43. Bisiach, E. and Luzzatti, C., Unilateral neglect of representational space, *Cortex*, 14(1), 129–133, 1978.

44. Volpe, B. T., LeDoux, J. E., and Gazzaniga, M. S., Information processing of visual stimuli in an "extinguished" field, *Nature*, 282(5740), 722–724, 1979.

45. Farah, M. J., Monheit, M. A., and Wallace, M. A., Unconscious perception of "extinguished" visual stimuli: Reassessing the evidence, *Neuropsychologia*, 29(10), 949–958, 1991.

46. Wallace, M. A., Implicit perception in visual neglect: Implications for theories of attention, in M. J. Farah and G. Ratcliff (Eds.), *The Neuropsychology of High-Level Vision*, Erlbaum, Hillsdale, NJ, 359–370, 1994.

47. Ladavas, E., Paladini, R., and Cubelli, R., Implicit associative priming in a patient with left hemisphere visual neglect, *Neuropsychologia*, 31(12), 1307–1320, 1993.

48. Baddeley, A. D., Working memory, *Science*, 255(5044), 556–559, 1992.

49. Posner, M. I. and Raichle, M. E., *Images of Mind*, Scientific American Library, New York, 1994.

50. Atkinson, R. C. and Shiffrin, R. M., Human memory: A proposed system and its control process, in K. W. Spence and J. T. Spence (Eds.), *The Psychology of Learning and Motivation*, Vol. 2, Academic Press, New York, 89–195, 1968.

51. Shiffrin, R. M. and Schneider, W., Controlled and automatic human information processing: II. Perceptual learning, automatic attending, and a general theory, *Psychological Review*, 84(2), 127–190, 1977.

52. Shimamura, A. P., Memory and frontal lobe function, in M. S. Gazzaniga (Ed.), *The Cognitive Neurosciences*, MIT Press, Cambridge, MA, 803–813, 1995.

53. Engle, R. W., Working memory capacity as executive attention, *Current Directions in Psychological Science*, 11(1), 19–23, 2002.

54. Conway, A. R. A., Kane, M. J., Bunting, M. F., Hambrick, D. Z., Wilhelm, O., and Engle, R. W., Working memory span tasks: A methodological review and user's guide, *Psychonomic Bulletin & Review*, 12(5), 769–786, 2005.

55. Eimer, M., An event related potential (ERP) study of transient and sustained visual attention to color and form, *Biological Psychology*, 44(3), 143–160, 1997.

56. Montgomery, G. K., A multi-factor account of disability after brain injury: Implications for neuropsychological counseling, *Brain Injury*, 9(5), 453–469, 1995.

57. Ashby, F. G. and O'Brien, J. B., Category learning and multiple memory systems, *Trends in Cognitive Sciences*, 9(2), 83–89, 2004.

58. Beilock, S. L. and Carr, T. H., When high-powered people fail: Working memory and "choking under pressure" in math, *Psychological Science*, 16(2), 101–105, 2005.

59. DeCaro, M. S., Thomas, R. D., and Beilock, S. L., Individual differences in category learning: Sometimes less working memory capacity is better than more, *Cognition*, 107(1), 284–294, 2008.

60. Fan, J., McCandliss, B. D., Sommer, T., Raz, M., and Posner, M. I., Testing the efficiency and independence of attentional networks, *Journal of Cognitive Neuroscience*, 14(3), 340–347, 2002.

61. Redick, T. S. and Engle, R. W., Working memory capacity and attention network test performance, *Applied Cognitive Psychology*, 20(5), 713–721, 2006.

62. Heitz, R. P., Unsworth, N., and Engle, R. W., Working memory capacity, attention control, and fluid intelligence, in O. Wilhelm and R. W. Engle (Eds.), *Handbook of Understanding and Measuring Intelligence*, Sage Publications, Thousand Oaks, CA, 61–77, 2005.

63. Glosser, G. and Goodglass, H., Disorders in executive control functions among aphasic and other brain damaged patients, *Journal of Clinical and Experimental Neuropsychology*, 12(4), 485–501, 1990.

64. Knight, R. T., Hillyard, S. A., Woods, D. L., and Neville, H. J., the effects of frontal and temporal–parietal lesions on the auditory evoked potential in man, *Electroencephalography Clinical Neuropsychology*, 50(1–2), 112–124, 1980.

65. Gazzaniga, M. S., Ivry, R. B., and Mangun, G. R., *Cognitive Neuroscience: The Biology of the Mind*, W. W. Morton, New York, 1998.

66. Stroop, J. R., Studies of interference in serial verbal reactions, *Journal of Experimental Psychology*, 18(6), 624–643, 1935.

67. Robertson, I. H., Manly, T., Andrade, J., Baddeley, B. T., and Yiend, J., Oops!: Performance correlates of everyday attentional functional to traumatic brain injured and normal subjects, *Neuropsychologia*, 35(6), 747–758, 1997.

68. Sohlberg, M. M. and Mateer, C. A., Effectiveness of an attentional training program, *Journal of Clinical and Experimental Neuropsychology*, 9(2), 117–130, 1987.

69. Sohlberg, M. M. and Mateer, C. A., *Introduction to Cognitive Rehabilitation*, Guilford Press, New York, 1989.

70. Cicerone, K. D., Dahlberg, C., Malec, J. F., Langenbahn, D. M., Felicetti, T., Kneipp, S., Ellmo, W., et al., Evidence-based cognitive rehabilitation: Updated review of the literature from 1998 through 2002, *Archives of Physical Medicine and Rehabilitation*, 86(8), 1681–1692, 2005.

71. Markowitsch, H. J., Anatomical basis of memory disorders, in M. S. Gazzaniga (Ed.), *The Cognitive Neurosciences*, MIT Press, Cambridge, MA, 765–779, 1995.

72. Brown, J. A., Some tests of the decay theory of immediate memory, *Quarterly Journal of Experimental Psychology*, 10(1), 12–21, 1958.

73. Peterson, L. R. and Peterson, M. J., Short-term retention of individual verbal items, *Journal of Experimental Psychology*, 58(3), 193–198, 1959.

74. Milner, B., Amnesia following operation on the temporal lobes, in C. W. M. Witty and O. L. Zangwill (Eds.), *Amnesia*, Butterworths, London, 109–133, 1966.

75. Schacter, D. L. and Tulving, E., *Memory Systems (1994)*, MIT Press, Cambridge, MA, 1994.

76. Tulving, E., Organization of memory: Quo vadis?, in M. S. Gazzaniga (Ed.), *The Cognitive Neurosciences*, MIT Press, Cambridge, MA, 839–847, 1995.

77. Olton, D. S., Becker, J. T., and Handlemann, G. E., Hippocampal function: Working memory or cognitive mapping, *Physiological Psychology*, 8(2), 239–246, 1980.

78. Baddeley, A., Working memory, in M. S. Gazzaniga (Ed.), *The Cognitive Neurosciences*, MIT Press, Cambridge, MA, 755–764, 1995.

79. McGaugh, J. L., Memory: A century of consolidation, *Science*, 287(5451), 248–251, 2000.

80. Baddeley, A. D., *Working Memory*, Oxford University Press, Oxford, 1986.

81. Farah, M. J., Is visual imagery really visual? Overlooked evidence from neuropsychology, *Psychological Review*, 95(3), 307–317, 1988.

82. Jonides, J., Smith, E. E., Koeppe, R. A., Awh, E., Minoshima, S., and Mintun, M. A., Spatial working memory in humans as revealed by PET, *Nature*, 363(6430), 623–625, 1993.

83. Baddeley, A. D. and Wilson, B. A., Prose recall and amnesia: Implications for the structure of working memory, *Neuropsychologia*, 40(10), 1737–1743, 2002.

84. Sanders, A., Nakase-Thomson, R., Constantinidou, F., Wertheimer, J., and Paul, D., Memory assessment on an interdisciplinary rehabilitation team: A theoretically based framework, *American Journal of Speech–Language Pathology*, 16(4), 316–330, 2007.

85. Kyllonen, P. C. and Christal, R. E., Reasoning ability is (little more than) working-memory capacity, *Intelligence*, 14(4), 389–433, 1990.

86. Unsworth, N. and Engle, R. W., On the division of short-term and working memory: An examination of simple and complex span and their relations to higher order abilities, *Psychological Bulletin*, 133(6), 1038–1066, 2007.

87. Salthouse, T. A., Relations between cognitive abilities and measures of executive functioning, *Neuropsychology*, 19(4), 532–545, 2005.

88. Colfesh, G. J. H. and Conway, A. R. A., Individual differences in working memory capacity and divided attention in dichotic listening, *Psychonomic Bulletin & Review*, 14(4), 699–703, 2007.

89. Kane, M. J. and Engle, R. W., The role of prefrontal cortex in working-memory capacity, executive attention, and general fluid intelligence: An individual-differences perspective, *Psychonomic Bulletin & Review*, 9(4), 637–671, 2002.

90. Kane, M. J. and Engle, R. W., Working-memory capacity and the control of attention: The contributions of goal neglect, response competition, and task set to Stroop interference, *Journal of Experimental Psychology: General*, 132(1), 47–70, 2003.

91. Kane, M. J., Hambrick, D. Z., Tuholski, S. W., Wilhelm, O., Payne, T. W., and Engle, R. W., The generality of working memory capacity: A latent variable approach to verbal and visuospatial memory span and reasoning, *Journal of Experimental Psychology: General*, 133(2), 189–217, 2004.

92. Gathercole, S. and Baddeley, A. D., Phonological memory deficits in language-disordered children: Is there a causal connection?, *Journal of Memory and Language*, 29(3), 336–360, 1990.

93. Baddeley, A. D., Papagno, C., and Valar, C., When long-term learning depends on short-term storage, *Journal of Memory and Language*, 27(5), 586–595, 1988.

94. Papagno, C., Valentine, T., and Baddeley, A. D., Phonological short-term memory and foreign language vocabulary learning, *Journal of Memory and Language*, 30(3), 331–347, 1991.

95. Squire, L. R. and Zola-Morgan, S., The medial temporal lobe memory system, *Science*, 253(5026), 1380–1386, 1991.

96. Thompson, R. F. and Krupa, D. J., Organization of memory traces in the mammalian brain, *Annual Review of Neuroscience*, 17, 519–550, 1994.

97. Squire, L. R. and Knowlton, B. J., Learning about categories in the absence of memory, *Proceedings of the National Academy of Sciences of the United States of America*, 92(26), 12470–12474, 1995.

98. Vargha-Khadem, F., Gadian, D. G., Watkins, K. E., Connelly, A., Van Paesschen, W., and Mishkin, M., Differential effects of early hippocampal pathology on episodic and semantic memory, *Science*, 277(5324), 376–380, 1997.

99. Tulving, E., Hayman, C. A. G., and MacDonald, C. A., Long-lasting perceptual priming and semantic learning in amnesia: A case experiment, *Journal of Experimental Psychology: Learning, Memory, and Cognition*, 17(4), 595–617, 1991.

100. Ewert, J., Levin, H. S., Watson, M. G., and Kalisky, Z., Procedural memory during posttraumatic amnesia in survivors of severe closed head injury, *Archives of Neurology*, 46(8), 911–916, 1989.

101. Ashby, F. G. and Waldron, F. G., The neuropsychological basis of category learning, *Current Directions in Psychological Science*, 9(1), 10–14, 2000.

102. Schacter, D. L., Understanding implicit memory: A cognitive neuroscience approach, *American Psychologist*, 47(4), 559–569, 1992.

103. Schacter, D. L., Implicit memory: History and current status, *Journal of Experimental Psychology: Learning, Memory, and Cognition*, 13(3), 501–518, 1987.

104. Beauregard, M., Gold, D., Evans, A. C., and Chertkow, H., A role for the hippocampal formation in implicit memory: A 3-D PET study, *Neuroreport*, 9(8), 1867–1873, 1998.

105. Jacoby, L. L. and Witherspoon, D., Remembering without awareness, *Canadian Journal of Psychology*, 36(2), 300–324, 1982.

106. Graf, P., Squire, L. S., and Mandler, G., The information that amnesic patients do not forget, *Journal of Experimental Psychology: Learning, Memory, and Cognition*, 10(1), 164–178, 1984.

107. Shimamura, A. P. and Squire, L. R., Paired-associate learning and priming effects in amnesia: A neuropsychological study, *Journal of Experimental Psychology: General*, 113(4), 556–570, 1984.

108. Schacter, D. L., Priming of old and new knowledge in amnesic patients and normal subjects, *Annals of the New York Academy of Sciences*, 444, 44–53, 1985.

109. Gabrieli, J. D. E., Fleischman, D. A., Keane, M. M., Reminger, S. L., and Morel, F., Double dissociation between memory systems underlying explicit and implicit memory in the human brain, *Psychological Science*, 6(2), 76–82, 1995.

110. Jacoby, L. L. and Dallas, M., On the relationship between autobiographical memory and perceptual learning, *Journal of Experimental Psychology: General*, 110(3), 306–340, 1981.

111. Graf, P., Mandler, G., and Haden, P., Simulating amnesic symptoms in normal subjects, *Science*, 218(4578), 1243–1244, 1982.

112. Tulving, E., Schacter, D. L., and Stark, H. A., Priming effects in word-fragment completion are independent of recognition memory, *Journal of Experimental Psychology: Learning, Memory, and Cognition*, 8(4), 352–373, 1982.

113. Graf, P. and Mandler, G., Activation makes words more accessible, but not necessarily more retrievable, *Journal of Verbal Learning and Verbal Behavior*, 23(5), 553–568, 1984.

114. Graf, P. and Ryan, L., Transfer-appropriate processing for implicit and explicit memory, *Journal of Experimental Psychology: Learning, Memory, and Cognition*, 16(6), 978–992, 1990.

115. Jacoby, L. L. and Hayman, C. A. G., Specific visual transfer in word identification, *Journal of Experimental Psychology: Learning, Memory, and Cognition*, 13, 456–463, 1987.

116. Roediger, H. L. and Blaxton, T. A., Retrieval modes produce dissociations in memory for surface information, in D. S. Gorfein and R. R. Hoffman (Eds.), *The Ebbinghous Centennial Conference*, Erlbaum, Hillsdale, NJ, 349–379, 1987.

117. Biederman, I. and Cooper, E. E., Priming contour-deleted images: Evidence for intermediate representations in visual object recognition, *Cognitive Psychology*, 23(5), 393–419, 1991.

118. Cave, C. B. and Squire, L. S., Intact and long-lasting repetition priming in amnesia, *Journal of Experimental Psychology: Learning, Memory, and Cognition*, 18(3), 509–520, 1992.

119. Schacter, D. L., Perceptual representation systems and implicit memory: Toward a resolution of the multiple memory systems debate, in A. Diamond (Ed.), *Development and Neural Bases of Higher Cognitive Functions*, New York Academy of Sciences, New York, 543–571, 1990.

120. Lezak, M. D., *Neuropsychological Assessment*, 3rd ed., Oxford University Press, Oxford, 1995.

121. Lezak, M. D., Howieson, D. B., and Loring, D. W., *Neuropsychological Assessment*, 4th ed., Oxford University Press, Oxford, 2004.

122. Craik, F. I. M. and Lockhart, R. S., Levels of processing: A framework for memory research, *Journal of Verbal Learning and Verbal Behavior*, 11(6), 671–684, 1972.

123. Paivio, A., *Imagery and Verbal Processes*, Holt, Rinehart & Winston, New York, 1971.

124. Paivio, A., Imagery in recall and recognition, in J. Brown (Ed.), *Recall and Recognition*, Wiley, New York, 103–129, 1976.

125. Crosson, B. and Buenning, W., An individualized memory retraining program after closed-head injury: A single-case study, *Journal of Clinical Neuropsychology*, 6(3), 287–301, 1984.

126. Goldstein, F. C., Levin, H. S., Boake, C., and Lohrey, J. H., Facilitation of memory performance through induced semantic processing in survivors of severe closed-head injury, *Journal of Clinical and Experimental Neuropsychology*, 12(2), 286–300, 1990.

127. Levin, H. S., Memory deficit after closed-head injury, *Journal of Experimental Psychology*, 12(1), 95–103, 1989.

128. Wilson, B. A., *Rehabilitation of Memory*, Guilford, London, 1987.

129. Levin, H. S. and Goldstein, F. C., Organization of verbal memory after severe closed-head injury, *Journal of Clinical and Experimental Neuropsychology*, 8(6), 643–656, 1986.

130. Constantinidou, F. and Neils, J., Stimulus modality and verbal learning in moderate to severe closed head injury, *Journal of Head Trauma Rehabilitation*, 10(4), 90–100, 1995.

131. Millis, S. R. and Ricker, J. H., Verbal learning patterns in moderate and severe traumatic brain injury, *Journal of Clinical Experimental Neuropsychology*, 16(4), 498–507, 1994.

132. Constantinidou, F., The effects of stimulus modality on interference and recognition performance following brain injury, *Journal of Medical Speech–Language Pathology*, 7(4), 283–295, 1999.

133. Nyberg, L., Cabeza, R., and Tulving, E., PET studies of encoding and retrieval: The HERA model, *Psychonomic Bulletin & Review*, 3(2), 135–148, 1996.

134. Waugh, N. C. and Norman, D. A., Primary memory, *Psychological Review*, 72(2), 89–104, 1965.

135. Brooks, D. N., Long-term and short-term memory in head injured patients, *Cortex*, 11(4), 329–340, 1975.

136. O'Donnell, J. P., Radtke, R. C., Leicht, D. J., and Caesar, R., Encoding and retrieval processes in learning-disabled, head-injured, and nondisabled young adults, *The Journal of General Psychology*, 115(4), 335–368, 1988.

137. Constantinidou, F., Neils, J., Bouman, D., Lee, L., and Shuren, J., Pictorial superiority during verbal learning tasks following moderate to severe close head injury: Additional evidence, *Journal of General Psychology*, 123(3), 173–184, 1996.

138. Constantinidou, F., Active memory strategies following moderate-to-severe head injury: In search of important components, *Hearsay*, 12(1), 20–26, 1998.

139. Spikman, J. M., Berg, I. J., and Deelman, B. G., Spared recognition capacity in elderly and closed-head injury subjects with clinical memory deficits, *Journal of Clinical and Experimental Neuropsychology*, 17(1), 29–34, 1995.

140. Kaschel, R., Sala, D. A., Cantagallo, A., Fahlbock, A., Laaksonen, R., and Kazen, M., Imagery mnemonics for the rehabilitation of memory: A randomized group controlled trial, *Neuropsychological Rehabilitation*, 12(2), 127–153, 2002.

141. Crovitz, H. F., Harvey, M. T., and Horn, R. W., Problems in the acquisition of imagery mnemonics: Three brain-damaged cases, *Cortex*, 15(2), 225–243, 1979.

142. Richardson, J. T., Mental imagery, human memory, and the effects of closed head injury, *British Journal of Social and Clinical Psychology*, 18(3), 319–327, 1979.

143. Richardson, J. T. and Barry, C., The effects of minor closed head injury upon human memory: Further evidence on the role of mental imagery, *Cognitive Neuropsychology*, 2(2), 149–168, 1985.

144. Glinsky, E. L., Computer-assisted instruction for patients with traumatic brain injury: Teaching of domain-specific knowledge, *Journal of Head Trauma Rehabilitation*, 7(3), 1–12, 1992.

145. Parente, R. and Anderson-Parente, J. K., Retraining memory: Theory and application, *Journal of Head Trauma Rehabilitation*, 4(3), 55–65, 1989.

146. Crosson, B., Cooper, P. V., Lincoln, R. K., Bauer, R. M., and Velozo, C. A., Relationship between verbal memory and language performance after blunt head injury, *The Clinical Neuropsychologist*, 7(3), 250–267, 1993.

147. Sarno, M. T., Verbal impairment after head injury, *Journal of Nervous and Mental Disease*, 172(8), 475–479, 1984.

148. Hillis, A. E., Aphasia progress in the last quarter of a century, *Neurology*, 69(2), 200–213, 2007.

149. Fromkin, V. and Rodman, R., *An Introduction to Language*, Harcourt Brace Publications, 1992.

150. Benson, F. D. and Ardilla, A., Human category learning, *Annual Review of Psychology*, 56(1), 149–178, 2005.

151. Ashby, F. G. and Maddox, W. T., Human category learning, *Annual Review of Psychology*, 56, 149–178, 2005.

152. Warrington, E. K. and McCarthy, R. A., Categories of knowledge: Further fractionations and an attempted integration, *Brain*, 110(5), 1273–1296, 1987.

153. Joseph, John, *Journey into the Vulnerable Brain*, Focus Education, Adelaide, Australia, 2001.

154. Lamberts, K., Category-specific deficits and exemplar models, *Behavior and Brain Sciences*, 24, 484–485, 2001.

155. Lamberts, K. and Shapiro, L., Exemplar models and category-specific deficits, in E. M. E. Forde, and G. W. Humphreys (Eds.), *Category Specificity in Brain and Mind*, Psychology Press, 291–314, 2002.

156. Caramazza, A. and Shelton, J. R., Domain-specific knowledge systems in the brain: The animate–inanimate distinction, *Journal of Cognitive Neuroscience*, 10, 1–34, 1998.

157. Farah, M. J. and McClelland, J. L., A computational model of semantic memory impairment: Modality specificity and emergent category specificity, *Journal of Experimental Psychology: General*, 120(4), 339–357, 1991.

158. Damasio, H., Grabowski, T., Tranel, D., Hichwa, R. D., and Damasio, A., A neural basis for lexical retrieval, *Nature*, 380(6574), 499–505, 1996.

159. Damasio, H., Tranel, D., Grabowskia, T., Adolphs, R., and Damasio, A., Neural systems behind word and concept retrieval, *Cognition*, 92(1–2), 179–229, 2004.

160. Tranel, D., Kemmerer, D., Adolphs, R., Damasio, H., and Damasio, A., Neural correlates of conceptual knowledge for actions, *Cognitive Neuropsychology*, 20(3–6), 409–432, 2003.

161. Caramazza, A. and Mahon, B. Z., The organization of conceptual knowledge: The evidence from category-specific semantic deficits, *Trends in Cognitive Sciences*, 7(8), 354–361, 2003.

162. Caramazza, A. and Mahon, B. Z., The organisation of conceptual knowledge in the brain: The future's past and some future directions, *Cognitive Neuropsychology*, 23(1), 13–38, 2006.

163. Laicona, M., Capitani, E., and Caramazza, A., Category-specific semantic deficits do not reflect the sensory/functional organization of the brain: A test of the "sensory quality" hypothesis, *Neuroscience*, 9(3), 221–231, 2003.

164. Caramazza, A., Neuropsychology: The brain's dictionary, *Nature*, 380(6574), 485–486, 1996.

165. Cree, G. S. and McRae, K., Analyzing the factors underlying the structure and computation of the meaning of chipmunk, cherry, chisel, cheese, and cello (and many other such concrete nouns), *Journal of Experimental Psychology: General*, 132(2), 163–201, 2003.

166. Humphreys, G. W. and Forde, M. E., Hierarchies, similarity, and interactivity in object recognition: "Category-specific" neuropsychological deficits, *Behavioral and Brain Sciences*, 24(3), 453–476, 2001, Discussion, 476–509, 2001.

167. Humphreys, G. W., Price, C. J., and Riddoch, M. J., From objects to names: A cognitive neuroscience approach, *Psychological Research*, 62(2–3), 118–130, 1999.

168. Ashby, F. G., Alfonso-Reese, L. A., Turken, A. U., and Waldron, E. M., A neuropsychological theory of multiple systems in category learning, *Psychological Review*, 105(3), 442–481, 1998.

169. Nosofsky, R. M., Exemplar-based approach to relating categorization, identification, and recognition, in F. G. Ashby (Ed.), *Multidimensional Models of Perception and Cognition*, Erlbaum, Hillsdale, NJ, 363–393, 1992.

170. Ashby, F. G. and Ell, S. W., The neurobiology of human category learning, *Trends in Cognitive Sciences*, 5(5), 204–210, 2001.

171. Knowlton, B. J. and Squire, L. R., The learning of natural categories: Parallel memory systems for item memory and category-level knowledge, *Science*, 626(5140), 1747–1749, 1993.

172. Maddox, W. T. and Ashby, F. G., Comparing decision bound and exemplar models of categorization, *Perception and Psychophysics*, 53(1), 49–70, 1993.

173. Mattox, W. T. and Ashby, F. G., Dissociating explicit and procedural-learning based systems of perceptual category learning, *Behavioural Processes*, 66(3), 309–332, 2004.

174. Thomas, R. D., Learning correlations in categorization tasks using large, ill-defined categories, *Journal of Experimental Psychology: Learning, Memory, and Cognition*, 24(1), 119–143, 1998.

175. Constantinidou, F., Thomas, R. D., and Haren, L., Benefits of categorization training in patients with TBI during post acute rehabilitation: Additional evidence from a randomized controlled trial, *Journal of Head Trauma Rehabilitation*, 23(5), 312–328, 2008.

176. Constantinidou, F. and Kreimer, L. T., Feature description and categorization of common objects after traumatic brain injury: The effects of a multi-trial paradigm, *Brain and Language*, 89(1), 216–225, 2004.

177. Klein, G. A., A recognition primed decision (RPD) model of rapid decision making, in G. A. Klein, J. Orasanu, R. Calderwood, and C. E. Zsambok (Eds.), *Decision Making in Action: Models and Methods*, Ablex, Norwood, NJ, 138–147, 1993.

178. Kahneman, D. and Tversky, A., Subjective probability: A judgment of representativeness, *Cognitive Psychology*, 3(3), 430–454, 1972.

179. Holyoak, K. J., Problem solving, in E. E. Smith and D. N. Osherson (Eds.,), *An Invitation to Cognitive Science*, (2nd ed.): *Thinking (vol. 3)*, MIT Press, Cambridge, MA, 267–296, 1995.

180. Braisby, N. and Dockrell, J., Why is color naming difficult? *Journal of Child Language*, 26(1), 23–47, 1999.

181. Younger, B. A. and Fearing, D. D., Parsing items into separate categories: Developmental changes in infant categorization, *Child Development*, 70(2), 291–303, 1999.

182. Adamovich, B. B., Henderson, J. A., and Auerbach, S., *Cognitive Rehabilitation of Closed Head Injured Patients: A Dynamic Approach*, College Hill Press, San Diego, CA, 1985.

183. Malec, J. F. and Basford, J. S., Postacute train injury rehabilitation, *Archives of Physical and Medical Rehabilitation*, 77(2), 198–207, 1996.

184. Bracy, O. L., Cognitive rehabilitation: A process approach, *Cognitive Rehabilitation*, 4(2), 11–16, 1986.

185. Levin, H. S., Neuropsychological rehabilitation of head injured patients: An appraisal of recent progress, *Scandinavian Journal of Rehabilitation Medicine*, 26(Suppl.), 14–24, 1992.

186. Luria, A. R., *Restoration of Function after Brain Injury*, Pergamon Press, Oxford, 1963.

187. Rosch, E. and Mervis, C. B., Family resemblances: Studies in the internal structure of categories, *Cognitive Psychology*, 7(4), 573–605, 1975.

188. Rosch, E., Simpson, E. J., and Miller, R. S., Structural bases of typicality effects, *Journal of Experimental Psychology*, 2(4), 491–502, 1976.

189. Parente, R. and Hermann, D., *Retraining Cognition: Techniques and Applications*, Aspen Publishers, Gaithersburg, MD, 1996.

190. Constantinidou, F., Thomas, R. D., Scharp, V. L., Laske, K. M., Hammerly, M. D., and Guitonde, S., Effects of categorization training in patients with TBI during post acute rehabilitation: Preliminary findings, *The Journal of Head Trauma Rehabilitation* 20(2), 143–157, 2005.

191. National Institutes of Health, Rehabilitation of persons with traumatic brain injury, *NIH Consensus Statement 1998 October 26–28*, 16(1), 1–41, 1999.

192. Cappa, S. F., Benke, T., Clarke, S., Rossi, B., Stemmer, B., and van Heugten, C. M., EFNS guidelines on cognitive rehabilitation report of an EFNS Task Force, *European Journal of Neurology*, 10(1), 11–23, 2003.

193. Sohlberg, M. M., Avery, J., Kennedy, M., et al., Practice guidelines for direct attention training, *Journal of Medical Speech Language Pathology*, 11(3), 19–39, 2003.

194. Cicerone, K. D., Dahlberg, C., Kramer, K., Langenbahn, D. M., Malec, J. F., Berquist, T. F., Felicetti, T., et al., Evidence-based cognitive rehabilitation: Recommendations for clinical practice, *Archives of Physical Medicine and Rehabilitation*, 81(12), 1596–1615, 2000.

195. Stranjalis, G., Korfias, S., Papapetrou, C., Kouyialis, A. T., Boviatsis, E. J., Psachoulia, C., and Sakas, D. E., Increased S-100b protein can predict short time failure to return to activities after mild head injuries, *Journal of Neurotrauma*, 21(8), 1070–1075, 2004.

Appendix

The Categorization Program is comprised of two parts and eight levels that are designed to retrain a series of categorization abilities. Each level, in both parts, builds on the skill set trained and applied during the previous level. Therefore, a range of concrete to abstract thinking abilities is targeted. The purpose, specific aspect of categorization trained, and the ultimate goal of each level are outlined here.

Part A

Level 1: Perceptual Feature Identification and Application

The purpose of this section is to train perceptual feature identification, thereby building a framework for cognitive structures. The retraining of basic categorization abilities will build the foundation for more abstract functions and will facilitate communication during word-finding difficulties. The goal is to have the patient learn eight perceptual features and then consistently apply all the features to describe common objects. Objects are presented via a range of stimulus types, including real objects, color photos, line drawings, written words, and spoken words.

Level 2: Similarities and Differences

The purpose of this level is to apply the eight perceptual features trained in level 1 to compare objects. Identification of similarities and differences between two objects of the same and of different categories using the eight perceptual features is utilized to train conceptual thinking. The process of applying the trained perceptual features is the next layer of the continuum of concrete to abstract functional abilities. Stimulus types include color photos, written words, and spoken words.

Level 3: Functional Categorization

The purpose of this task is to identify functional categories and maintain the delineations within that category. There are two specific foci in this level that require the consideration of the features of the objects trained and applied in levels 1 and 2: the application of retrieval strategies to generate novel items that belong in a given category and the mental flexibility required to generate alternate uses for the objects in a given category. This task enhances functional problem-solving abilities and mental flexibility.

Level 4: Analogies

The purpose of this level is to apply both the categorization abilities trained in levels 1 through 3 and inductive reasoning skills to identify and match the concepts represented in analogies. The analogies progress from concrete to abstract to train word abstraction. Stimulus materials include multiple-choice responses for each analogy that will aid in the training process of word abstraction as needed.

Level 5: Abstract Word Categorization

The purpose of this level is to develop concept formation and abstract conceptual thinking further. The goal is to identify similarities and differences in abstract verbal concepts. The generation of similar word pairs using synonyms that represent the relationship between the words is incorporated to enhance cognitive and linguistic flexibility.

Part B

The exercises in Part B are constructed to examine and train learning rule-based classification strategies. A core set of five conditions or rules is utilized in levels 6 through 8. The conditions, which stem from cognitive psychology, are affirmative, conjunctive, disjunctive, exclusive, and conditional. The stimulus for Part B range from concrete to abstract and include shapes (level 1), gauges (level 2), and written word groups (level 3). The goal of Part B is the formulation of the rule that governs the classification of each stimulus into either category A or category B. Errorless learning is implemented as a cueing technique to counter frustration and aid rule formulation. Ultimately, the tasks in the part will enhance decision-making and problem-solving abilities.

Level 6: Progressive Rule Learning 1

The stimuli for level 6 vary along two dimensions: shape and color. The nine stimuli include squares, circles, and triangles that are red, white, and black. Each stimulus is presented individually, and a formulation of the rule that classifies each stimulus into either category A or category B follows.

Level 7: Progressive Rule Learning 2

The stimulus presentation for level 7 of Part B are gauges that include two dials that must be interpreted as a single unit. This level forces generalization into a real-world situation by simulating the reading of gauges at a power plant. The determination of "operational" or "not operational" for each stimulus is utilized, and the cumulative interpretation of each judgment leads to the formulation of the rule that classifies the stimuli for each of the five conditions.

Level 8: Progressive Rule Learning 3

The final explicit rule task contains the same underlying structure as the earlier two levels; however, this time, a judgment is made using stimuli constructed from dimensions of language. This further abstracts the rule formulation and forces generalization of training to a real-world situation. The stimuli in this task consist of a summary of three laboratory tests (lung capacity, heart fluid, bone marrow count) and their orthogonal combination with two measurement adjectives (low, high).

19

Cognitive Disorders: Diagnosis and Treatment in Traumatic Brain Injury

Mark J. Ashley, Rose Leal, Zenobia Mehta, Jessica G. Ashley, and Matthew J. Ashley

CONTENTS

19.1 Introduction

Cognitive rehabilitation for people with acquired brain injury first became a clinical focus in the late 1970s. The sequelae of acquired brain injury were increasingly recognized as medical science became proficient at life-preserving practices following severe injury to the brain. Larger numbers of people survived traumatic and nontraumatic events alike that resulted in injury to the brain. Rehabilitation services were largely restricted to those rendered in an acute hospital setting, whereas available discharge settings consisted of the home, psychiatric hospitals, or skilled nursing facilities. The level of restitution of physical and communicative deficits achieved was not sufficient to allow for a return of many of these individuals to independent and productive lifestyles.

The significant limitations of available settings were soon recognized by the private funding sector that had a long-term financial responsibility for some of these people, as a result of the events surrounding their injuries. That is, workers' compensation and liability insurance carriers came to question whether further rehabilitative interventions might be developed to reduce the level of disability following discharge from acute rehabilitation hospitalization, thereby reducing the level of assistance for physical and cognitive deficits that might be required, and the lifetime costs ascribed thereto.

The field of postacute rehabilitation was born of this time, and with it, investigation into existing treatment interventions that had been developed for other neurologically impaired populations that might have applicability to persons with acquired brain injury. Physical disabilities were identified to be less disabling than cognitive disabilities, and this remains the case today. Cognitive disabilities continue to impose severe limitations on a person's ability to interact meaningfully and independently, as well as in an age-appropriate fashion within most aspects of society. This is not to diminish the tremendous obstacles faced by people with physical disability, but rather to point out that societal accommodation to physical disabilities has been greater to date, whereas accommodation of cognitive disabilities is both less prevalent and far more difficult to accomplish.

This chapter does not deal with the debate of payer coverage for cognitive rehabilitation, nor does it deal with the debate about the efficacy of cognitive rehabilitation. See the Blue Cross/Blue Shield Technical Evaluation Center report on cognitive rehabilitation as the primary determinant of noncoverage across the country.[1] The counterpoint arguments are provided by a number of literature reviews of the world literature that provide robust support for the efficacy of cognitive rehabilitation.[2–4] This chapter also will not provide a review of compensatory strategies for cognitive dysfunction or a review of the literature of cognitive rehabilitation. The sources noted earlier provide such information.

Neuroscience has a very broad concept of cognition. Cognition, as addressed in this chapter, will be more circumscribed, excluding some areas of cognition that might be encompassed in the view of the neuroscientist interested in computational modeling and the like. Chapter 17 reviews the neuroanatomic structures that serve information processing. The term *information processing* is used in a relatively narrow sense in this chapter, referring predominantly to the information processing that supports so-called *executive function*. Cognitive skills and processes are discussed and rehabilitative avenues reviewed insofar as they are the focus of[4] concern for persons with acquired brain injury.

This chapter addresses cognition from a particular vantage point. The information presented herein provides detailed insight into a particular approach to cognitive rehabilitation that has been used for almost three decades and has been found to be effective in restoration of improved cognitive function following brain injury. Analogous approaches have been systematically reviewed and published and are not covered here.[5,6]

19.1.1 Cognition

Cognition, in simple terms, refers to conscious mental activity such as thinking, remembering, learning, or using language. Cognition includes "awareness with perception, reasoning, judgment, intuition, and memory; the mental process by which knowledge is acquired."[7, p. 408] Coelho et al.[8] defined cognition to include such processes as attention; memory; reasoning; problem solving; and executive functioning (i.e., self-awareness and goal setting, planning, self-directing/initiating, self-inhibiting, self-monitoring, self-evaluation, flexible thinking). Reed and Seale[9] include attention, memory, visual–spatial skills, judgment, problem solving, awareness, comprehension, and psychomotor speed.

Cognition can be thought to include an individual's ability mentally to represent, organize, and manipulate the environment. Cognition is comprised of a group of "*processes* by which sensory input is transformed, reduced, elaborated, stored, recovered, and used."[10, p. 351]

Among these processes are: attending (alertness, awareness, attention span, selective attention), recognizing, discriminating among stimuli and identifying similarities and differences, maintaining the temporal order of stimuli and responses to them, learning and remembering (including retention span and immediate, recent, and remote memory), organizing (including categorizing, associating, and/or synthesizing stimuli), comprehending, thinking, reasoning, and problem solving. Essential to the most efficient use of these processes is an adequately developed *knowledge base* (including general information, linguistic knowledge, academic skills, knowledge of social rules and roles, and much more). This knowledge base forms the basis of implicit knowledge or information. Cognition also includes the *use* of these processes to (1) make decisions as to the most appropriate and functional ways of interacting with the environment, (2) execute those decisions, (3) monitor responses to determine the appropriateness and accuracy of those decisions, and (4) adjust behavior if it is determined to be inappropriate and/or inaccurate.[11]

A dimension of self-regulation of functional behavior is emphasized in the definition of cognition to promote a treatment focus on functional goals during cognitive interventions.[11]

Cognition entails specific skill sets (e.g., the ability to maintain a focus of attention) that, combined, form processes (learning, remembering, planning, problem solving). Interventions designed to improve overall cognitive function must, therefore, address both specific skill sets and processes. Because many cognitive skills combine to form processes of cognition, a review of the definitions just listed provides insight into the breadth and complexity of cognitive skills and processes. The American Congress of Rehabilitation Medicine[12] and the American Speech–Language–Hearing Association[11] guidelines combined provide the most comprehensive analysis of cognitive skills and processes. These include attention, alertness, awareness, attention span, selective attention, stimuli recognition, stimuli discrimination, maintenance of the temporal order of stimuli, learning, retention, memory, organizing, categorizing, association, synthesis of information, comprehension, thinking, problem solving, decision making, planning, insight, reasoning, learning ability, maintenance of sequential goal-directed behavior with self-correction of responses, and emotionality.

Tulving[13] pointed to the componential and hierarchical nature of memory. Neuroscience tends to support the view of a highly interrelated and integrated system of cognitive function being subserved by the basic physiology. Amaral[14] reviewed the neuroanatomic organization of information processing that supports Tulving's concept and stated: "A general principle of brain information processing is that it is carried out in a hierarchical fashion. Stimulus information is conveyed through a succession of subcortical and then cortical regions."[14, p. 338] Tulving's[13] concept of a hierarchical structure to memory systems included the idea that interventions that impacted a system at any particular level would necessarily impact the system as a whole. The hierarchical and interrelated nature of proposed memory systems, together with the underlying neuroanatomic and neurophysiologic substrates, become important in determining an approach to designing interventions for memory system problems following traumatic brain injury (TBI).

19.2 Attention

Attention is viewed as foundational to cognition overall. It is the most basic of cognitive skill sets and it impacts virtually all other cognitive skill sets. Posner[15] proposed the organization of three attention networks: a network for orienting to sensory stimuli, a network for activating ideas from memory, and a network for maintaining an alert state. Attention consists of both orienting and executive attention networks. Arousal and alertness are basic components of orienting, whereas executive processes involve information processing of a potentially higher order and include selective and divided attention. Selective attention incorporates focused and divided attention during which filtering relevant from irrelevant information is required. Divided attention requires the division or sharing of resources between two or more kinds of information, sources, or mental operations.[16] Focused attention requires selection of one source of information while withholding response to irrelevant stimuli. Attention also has a construct along two dimensions: intensity and selectivity. Intensity involves the state of receptivity to stimulation, response preparedness (alertness), and attentional activation for specific target appearance within a stream of otherwise irrelevant stimuli (vigilance).[17]

Supervisory attention skills are hypothesized as the mechanism by which attention resources are directed consciously and subconsciously by the individual, thereby exerting some measure of cognitive control.[18] Attention can be controlled and uncontrolled. Through exercise of various measures of control, attention can facilitate enhanced awareness of a perceptual attribute, facilitate conflict monitoring and resolution, and facilitate response selection.

Sensory information entering the central nervous system (CNS) makes its way to the brainstem with the exception of visual and olfactory stimuli. Visual and olfactory stimuli remain above the tentorium and only oculomotor responses involve the brainstem. The reticular activating formation receives cortical, auditory, tactile, proprioceptive, and vestibular input. In addition, the reticular formation receives input from the cerebellum, basal ganglia, hypothalamus, and the reticulospinal pathway. The ascending projectional systems send information from the brainstem reticular formation to the nonspecific thalamic nuclei,[19] the hypothalamus, and the reticulospinal pathway. The ascending projectional system reaches the cortex via the widely distributed thalamic projections arising from the nonspecific nuclei. A broad spectrum of structures in the neuraxis is involved in arousal and attention.

At the brainstem level, the mesencephalic reticular formation and its thalamic projections have been implicated in maintenance of arousal[20] and the orientation of attention.[21,22] In fact, substantial changes occur via the autonomic nervous system in relation to conscious direction of attention. These include changes in heart rate, vascular dilation, pupil size, and galvanic skin response.[23]

The basal ganglia project to the cortex indirectly via the thalamus. Bares and Rektor[24] studied the role of the basal ganglia in cognitive processing of sensory information and found the basal ganglia to be active in a contingent negative paradigm linked to a motor task. Experience in Parkinson's disease has resulted in the suggestion that dopamine might play a role in regulating attention.[25] The striata receive inputs from all cortical areas and projects principally to the prefrontal, premotor, and supplementary motor areas via the thalamus. These areas are involved in motor planning, shifting attentional sets, and in spatial working memory.[26] Nauta[27] notes the circuitous connections between the cerebral cortex, limbic system, and corpus striatum in the overall fluidity of attentional processes.

The thalamofrontal gating system is implicated in selective or controlled attentional processes.[28] Distractibility may occur following disturbance of the diffuse thalamic projection system. Difficulties with interference and integrative behaviors of judgment, planning, and socially appropriate behavior are found with damage to the thalamofrontal gating system. A fair amount of information processing occurs at the level of the thalamus. The purpose of the thalamofrontal gating system is to direct selected information up to cortical structures. Incoming stimuli are enhanced or attenuated by the facilitation or inhibition of transmission of neural impulses there. Attention can thus be directed to specific stimuli while other stimuli are suppressed. Perception of stimuli at the cortical level only occurs when the diffuse projection system is also active.[29]

At the cortical level, frontal, posterior parietal, and cingulate cortices are involved in attentional processing.[28,30–32] The neocortex is involved in response selection based upon cognitive or semantic dimensions.[33] The associative cortices appear most active in attentional processes.[34] One hypothesis suggests that a competition for neural resource is created when cells in associative cortex respond to a novel stimulus.[35] The number of cells available to respond to another stimulus is decreased proportionately to the number responding to the first stimulus. Experimental evidence supports this hypothesis in the finding that some pathways were facilitated by attention to a signal, whereas others were simultaneously inhibited.[36] Conscious processing of a stimulus causes a decrease in the ability to detect new stimuli.[37]

Information appears to be dealt with either reflexively or intentionally within the system. Schneider and Shiffrin[38] refer to automatic and controlled processing wherein automatic processing is almost of unlimited capacity and rate. Controlled processing is serial and is limited in both rate and capacity. Anderson[39] conceptualized these issues earlier as deliberate and automatic processing. Tasks that require conscious direction of attention take up attentional resources, slowing or preventing information processing of other stimuli. Repeated task completion, however, may allow for deliberate attentional resources to be decreased, changing over to automatic processing, thereby freeing system resources.[39]

It is easier to attend to different aspects of the same object than to attend to the same attributes in different objects. Some of these limitations are the result of similarity of perceptual information of the attended information. Information presented in the same modality is harder to attend to than information coming from different modalities. Duncan[40] demonstrated that ongoing cognitive processes, too, can interfere with the detection of new signals. These include storage of recently presented information, generation of ideas from long-term storage (LTS), and development of schema.

Posner[41] provided a description of the manner in which attention resources act upon events after biasing from the individual's mindset:

> Perhaps because of these limitations, much of perceptual input goes unattended while some aspects become the focus of attention. Attending, in this sense, is jointly determined by environmental events and current goals and concerns. When appropriately balanced, these two kinds of input will lead to the selection of information relevant to the achievement of goals and lends coherence to behavior. The system must, however, remain sufficiently flexible to allow goals and concerns to be re-prioritized on the basis of changing environmental events. This balance appears to be adversely affected by major damage to the frontal lobes.[41, p. 620]

Large amounts of information can be screened in the face of competing stimuli, such as in dichotic listening studies. Information retention appears to be based on specific features that are determined by the listener,[42] and evidence suggests that selective attention occurs during the early levels of processing for both visual and auditory attention.[43]

The existence of a brief visual sensory register was demonstrated by Spurling.[44] Visual stimulus was first referred to as an *icon*[10] and the auditory equivalent of *iconic* memory is referred to as *echoic* memory.[10,45,46] Sensory registers, such as iconic and echoic stores, allow for information to be entered without the subject paying attention to the source.[10] These sensory registers store information in a literal way, can be overwritten by further input in the same modality, are vulnerable to "washout," are modality specific, and have a moderately large capacity. Similar mechanisms have been identified for olfactory and haptic stimuli.[47,48]

Although sensory registers can store a great deal of information, information is initially stored for very brief periods of time (<60 seconds) in iconic and echoic store mechanisms. Information that is retained beyond this time period is thought to have been processed and integrated into other memory structures or other cognitive processes. Note the similarity between these concepts and those of post-tetanic potentiation, short-term potentiation, and long-term potentiation (LTP). Rate of forgetting has been shown to be 0.25 to 2 seconds for sensory stores and less than 30 seconds for short-term storage (STS). Rate of forgetting is very slow or does not occur in LTS.[49]

Sensory store mechanisms also have some limitations in capacity.[23,44] The size of sensory stores has been found to be dependent upon the nature of the information presented. Two different studies found that recall for words was between two and four words.[50,51] Crannell and Parrish[52] found sensory store memory span to be between five and nine items, depending upon whether the items were digits, letters, or words. In experiments during which words were strung together to form sentences, recall of up to 20 words was found.[53]

Deficits in attention are either rate or capacity of controlled processing related, or dysfunction of higher level processes, such as the supervisory attentional system. Divided attention deficits arise when controlled processing is limited and divided between two sources, resulting in overloading and relevant signals being missed.[54] Focused attention deficits occur when an automatic response interferes with the execution of a response produced by controlled processes.[54] Studies suggest that deficits in focused and divided attention occur largely as a result of speed of processing rather than interference by competing stimuli, inefficient sharing of resources, or switching of attention between tasks.[55] Longer reaction times in dual task loading suggest that selective attention impairments may be more evident when tasks load heavily on controlled processing or working memory.[55]

19.3 Perceptual Features

The human perceptual system is inherently designed to give priority to certain types of perceptual cues.[56] Perception of certain cues is facilitated by basic physiologic mechanisms. Others, however, are guided by experience. The visual system, for example, is physiologically predisposed to enable an individual to register the visual stimuli associated with a falling snowflake. However, only through experience could an individual gain an appreciation for different types of snow, although all the perceptual information required to allow such discrimination is present to the less experienced observer. Sensory stimuli from different sensory systems will, likewise, have both physiologic and experiential features. These features have been referred to as *perceptual attributes* or *features*. Some perceptual cues, particularly those arising from a physiologic predisposition, have been found to be represented in different languages and cultures in so-called *natural categories*.[57]

Perceptual features can be those that are descriptive of a physical characteristic (iconic) or those that are descriptive of functional characteristics (symbolic). The iconic features of a table may include that the table is made of wood, is 4 feet tall, is rectangular, weighs 200 pounds, is brown, and has a smooth surface. The symbolic features of the table may include that it is used as someplace to work or to eat. Perceptual features can also include "characteristics." For example, the characteristics of "pretty" or "fast" might be considered perceptual features of a car. Essentially, every noun, verb, preposition, adjective, and adverb can be a potential feature. Of course, perceptual features are not just limited to objects. Events also have perceptual features. A lecture, for example, might have the perceptual feature of "boring" or "interesting." Essentially, every object or event is comprised of its perceptual features.[57,58]

The encoding of memory has been described as a process of utilization of perceptual features in the establishment of an internal representation of an event.[59] Perceptual features of an event, which can include the context of the events (external context), are combined with perceptual features that may arise from the individual's previous experience (internal context or implicit knowledge) to encode the event in memory. Each perceptual feature can also be used for recall of an event. Only those perceptual features that are utilized during encoding can be used for recall. "The effectiveness of a retrieval cue depends on its compatibility with the item's initial encoding or, more generally, the extent to which the retrieval situation reinstates the learning context."[60] The memory trace, its coding characteristics, and persistence are by-products of perceptual processing.[61] Craik and Lockhart[60] suggest that trace persistence is a function of the depth of analysis and that deeper levels of analysis lead to stronger, longer lasting, and more elaborate memory trace persistence. As sensory stimuli are converted to mental representation in the form of memory, the actual input attributes may be purged.

The perceptual features that are encoded at the time of stimulus presentation will impact both long-term retention and recall. In addition, the integrity and nature of the organizational structure used or developed at the time of acquisition will impact long-term retention.[62,63] Long-term retention of information may be directly related to the depth of information processing of the sensory experience.

> Highly familiar, meaningful stimuli are compatible, by definition, with existing cognitive structures. Such stimuli (for example, pictures and sentences) will be processed to a deep level more rapidly than less meaningful stimuli and will be well-retained. . . . Retention is a function of depth, and various factors, such as the amount of attention devoted to a stimulus, its compatibility with the analyzing structures, and the processing time available, will determine the depth to which it is processed.[60]

Craik and Lockhart[60] proposed a *level of processing* framework designed to account for how information progressed from STS to LTS. The level of processing framework theorizes that information transfer from STS to LTS is impacted by the degree to which the stimulus is processed. Superficial processing results in lesser likelihood of transfer of information to LTS, whereas more in-depth processing more likely results in such a transfer.

Craik and Lockhart[60] proposed that attributes of encountered perceptual stimuli combine with the needs of the individual to determine both what information is recognized and to what degree it is stored. Much of the totality of sensory experience is lost in the earliest stages of information processing because it is either not deemed to be immediately relevant or it is "washed out" or overwritten by the early sensory store mechanism.[10] Information that is more familiar is processed more quickly and at a deeper level. Because of the individual's previous experiential encoding, a great deal more information becomes available compared with that available for relatively novel stimuli.

A perceptual assay is conducted beginning with the sensory registers. An overwhelming amount of information is available at any point in time to the system because both relevant and irrelevant information is being experienced. Stimuli with which the individual has experience will be recognized and processed more completely than novel stimuli unless the situation demands greater attention to the novel stimuli. The ability to discern perceptual features is physiologically quite keen. In studies when a novel stimulus is presented and habituation is allowed, a slight change in the perceptual characteristics of the stimulus following habituation results in changes in the autonomic nervous system and electroencephalographic recordings.[64]

Perceptual salience has been described by many authors.[65,66] Perceptual salience results when a particular perceptual feature becomes the focus of inordinate attention, sometimes to the exclusion of recognition of other features. Perceptual salience can be so strong that it interferes with other cognitive processing. Developmentally, perceptual salience appears to assist in the acquisition of certain concepts. Preschool-age children are more perceptually salient for variability than older children. Older children show no differential sensitivity between variability and constancy.[67] In fact, perceptual salience for variability leads 6 year olds to make more overdiscrimination errors resulting from attention paid to feature differences that were irrelevant.[68] Reflectivity has been noted to increase, and impulsivity decrease, with age.[69,70]

The degree to which an individual can move freely among perceptual attributes will impact that individual's creativity and problem solving. Frequently, problem solving requires a novel use of perceptual features. The chair's iconic features of construction and height can allow the chair to be used as a ladder. However, perhaps the most salient feature of a chair is the symbolic attribute (function) of "to sit on." To "problem solve" the use of a chair in place of a ladder, the individual must be able to survey the chair's iconic features, ignoring its typical symbolic feature (function), and determine whether the chair can be used safely to stand on. A chair on rollers might be deemed too unstable. After this is accomplished, the novel functional application as a ladder may become stored as simply another acceptable functional application of the chair.

Some perseverative behaviors following TBI may, in fact, be a manifestation of perceptual salience and a form of cognitive interference. Deficits in processing featural information have been noted in people with TBI,[71] with observed patterns of response showing a tendency to base decisions upon a single salient feature and a lesser likelihood of responding to complex multidimensional stimuli.

19.4 Categorization

Classification or categorization allows for large amounts of information to be managed.[72] Categorization is thought to be crucial to nearly all cognitive ability.[73] "In dealing with the world, people have a system for classifying objects into categories. The system makes these classifications on the basis of salient attributes like shape, size, function, and activity. . . . The systems for classifying and for naming are not really distinct."[74] Of course, categorical organization need not be restricted to objects but can include experiences. "Categorization may be what makes possible human perception, memory, communication, and thought as we know it."[75, p. 1013]

The ability to perceive, assay, and utilize perceptual features is crucial to categorization.[76] Perceptual features become categorical descriptors and, as has already been discussed, are critical for memory encoding and retrieval. During early developmental stages, perceptual salience for variability may support the individual's ability to encounter a broad spectrum of perceptual features. As experience with the environment increases and age advances, a tendency toward constancy emerges.[67] Experience with the environment allows efficiency in perception. That is to say, a novel experience with a chair requires maximal attentional and perceptual resources. As experience with the chair increases, the features of "chairness" become encoded, and future encounters with a chair place less demand on perceptual and attentional systems. Just as the specific perceptual features of a chair are grouped both to define the chair and to encode it, large amounts of information from the environment must be dealt with similarly. Rosch developed a paradigm depicting three levels of categorization: basic, superordinate, and subordinate.[77,78] Examples of each would be vehicles (superordinate), cars (basic), and dragsters (subordinate). One's experience with a category and level of expertise determines the level of categorization at which one interacts and the amount of detail one is able to discern in observing exemplars of any given category. This concept fits well with that proposed by Craik and Lockhart,[60] describe levels of processing that provide an explanation for the effects and efficiencies arising from prior experience during information processing.

Three styles of categorization have been identified as involved in information processing: *rule application, exemplar similarity,* and *prototype similarity.* Each categorical process involves distinct regions of the brain. Exemplar similarity categorization involves the medial temporal and diencephalic structures and requires explicit memory. Exemplar-based categorization probably involves reference to memory storage areas of the cortex that correspond to the nature of the information being referenced (e.g., picture recognition to the occipital regions, verbal recognition to the temporal regions, and so on). In addition, experiments in which category naming is involved show routine activation of the angular gyrus in the left hemisphere.[79] Finally, when the stimulus used is presented pictorially, activation is seen in the occipital cortex, not the angular gyrus.[80]

Frontal lobe damage has been noted to impact rule application but not exemplar similarity. Specifically, the dorsolateral prefrontal cortex (PFC) has been implicated in rule following as seen via the Wisconsin Card Sorting Test,[81] which requires discerning rules from observation and context relation. D'Esposito et al.[82] showed the dorsolateral PFC to be involved in rule-based categorization when the task required switching attention between mental processes. For rule application, the individual must (1) "selectively attend to each critical attribute"; (2) "for each attended attribute, determine whether the perceptual information instantiates the value specified in the rule"; and (3) "amalgamate the outcomes of Stage 2 so as to determine final categorization. . . . The first stage involves selective attention, the second involves the perceptual instantiation of abstract conditions, and the third requires the working-memory operations of storing and combining information."[83, p. 1017]

Prototype similarity categorization appears to call upon implicit representation. As such, use of prototype similarity categorization may be dependent upon the level of processing required to make categorical judgments based on available perceptual information or the lack of success in application of exemplar similarity-based strategies.

Utilization of perceptual features in categorization is referred to as the *featural approach of categorization.*[57,58,84–88] As a category is defined or created, category members vary in the degree to which they represent the category. In the category "birds," a robin is a fairly typical member of the category. Conversely, an emu would still be a member; however, it would not be a typical member. "Typicality" is quite important in categorization. Members of a category share many, although not all, perceptual features. A core group of perceptual features is required of all category members; however, other frequently shared perceptual features may only be "characteristic" of the category and not required for category inclusion.

Typicality bears on processing speed.[57,89] Defining features are those features that are necessary for an item to be included in a category. Characteristic features are those features that are commonly seen but need not be present for category inclusion.[90] The combination of defining and characteristic features, or lack thereof, impacts verification time for category inclusion/exclusion.[90]

Processing speed, as measured through reaction time studies, is dependent upon access to categorical information and differences in categorical complexity.[88] It has been suggested that naming is actually an act of categorization and that word-finding problems in aphasic individuals might be viewed as concept formation disturbances.[91] Speed of problem solving appears to be assisted by object labeling.[92]

Development of categorization skills follows an acquisition sequence: (1) piling, (2) key chaining, (3) iconic categorization, and (4) symbolic categorization.[93] Piling occurs when the individual places all items in a single group without regard for shared attributes. Key chaining (or edge matching[93]) involves a serial ordering of members of the category in which only a single feature is shared between adjacent members. Item 1 and item 2 might share color whereas item 2 and item 3 share shape. Item 1 and item 3 may not share any attributes. Difficulties with key chaining are often manifest in the communication patterns of people with TBI. Discourse analysis shows people with TBI have impairment of productivity, content, and cohesion.[94] A conversational topic is, in fact, a category. Language, on the other hand, is quite abstract and, consequently, tangential speech, or difficulties in maintaining topic cohesion, is most likely a manifestation of difficulty maintaining categorical boundaries.

In iconic categorization, iconic features or physical attributes are utilized for defining category members. Items are grouped on the basis of a shared iconic feature or features. Symbolic categorization requires that members of the category share a common symbolic feature or function.

Categories can be simple or rather complex, but categorization remains a binary process. The category "car" is fairly simple in that an item is either a car or is not. The category can be complicated by adding adjectives and adverbs such as "foreign" car or "fast foreign" car; however, the process remains a binary one.

Individuals with left-hemisphere lesions experience problems in categorizing fruit and vegetable items, but are able to categorize on the basis of perceptual features alone. Right-hemisphere lesions, however, produce a reverse effect. Lesions in the left posterior hemisphere cause individuals to have difficulty with weak categorical boundaries that can lead to reclassification, whereas those with left anterior hemisphere lesions evidence highly categorical responses and categorical boundary rigidity.[95] These findings are consistent with a loss of cognitive flexibility observed with injury to the PFC. Individuals with left posterior disease experience difficulty sorting words or pictures of objects into categories.[96,97]

Fluent aphasics have been found to have difficulty in the use of perceptual or contextual information and recognition naming.[98] People with Broca's aphasia and normals had no difficulty. In general, those with Broca's aphasia and individuals with right-hemisphere lesions are more competent in categorization than fluent aphasics, although categorization ability may not be normal.[99–101] Several studies have demonstrated that fluent aphasics have more or less difficulty with determination of category membership depending upon the "representativeness" or typicality of the stimulus.[99,102,103] A study evaluating the ability to verify category membership and generate exemplars involving both fluent and nonfluent aphasics found that both groups required extended verification time and had difficulty in generating atypical categorical exemplars.[104] Ability to generate typical category exemplars was better for both groups. The study concluded that subjects experienced diminished representations of boundaries around the category's referential field.

Verbal recall of categorized and noncategorized word lists was evaluated in epileptic individuals with left or right temporal lobectomies and normals. The left temporal group had poorer performance in recognition and recall compared with normals. There was no difference between normals and the right temporal group for recognition or recall. Performance was enhanced for both groups with word lists that were categorized.[105] Verbal learning in amnesiacs and individuals with frontal lobe damage was studied using "categorizable" word lists. Individuals with frontal lobe damage did not spontaneously categorize the word lists whereas amnesiacs did. When categorization was forced, those with frontal lobe damage showed improved performance.[106]

Categorization and its many manifestations cannot be ascribed to a single area of the brain. In fact, some of the most exciting work has been done utilizing positron emission tomographic scans, functional magnetic resonance imaging (fMRI), and electroencephalography. Naming actions and spatial relations have been shown to activate the left frontal inferior gyrus (frontal operculum), the left parietal lobe, and sectors of the left inferotemporal cortices.[107] Processing of familiar words involves the right PFC, posterior left parahippocampal gyrus, left medial parietal cortex, and the right superior temporal gyrus whereas novel words activated the left hippocampal region.[108] There appears to be an anterior–posterior functional differentiation involving the medial temporal lobe (MTL). The anterior MTL is crucial for processing of novel episodic information whereas the posterior MTL is involved in processing for familiar verbal information.[108] Visual confrontation naming shows activation of the left frontal, bilateral temporo-occipital junctions, and inferior temporal regions, with differential activation of the right inferior temporal cortex seen for living versus nonliving category items.[109] These few studies show how highly differentiated cortical structures are for categorical processes.

19.5 Cognitive Distance

Piaget[110] noted that, as individuals become better able to represent experience cognitively, they are better able to do so while being physically removed from the experience itself. Availability and accuracy of information about an object or experience varies with proximity to the object or experience. For example, available information about a "table" is greatest when the table is present. Information availability decreases as proximity to the object decreases. A color photograph of the same object provides less opportunity for direct sensory appreciation of attributes than does the actual object. Likewise, lesser information is available in a black-and-white photograph, progressing to a line drawing, to the written word "table," to the spoken word "table," and finally, to the concept of "table." As feature availability decreases to sensory mechanisms, reliance upon previously stored information increases. Such reliance is logically dependent upon the extent of previously stored information as well as the structural integrity of the underlying neural network allowing either direct or indirect access to stored information. The neural network must allow access to distributed information stored in various cortical regions (e.g., category naming in the left angular gyrus, pictorial information in the occipital cortices).

Information is input to as many sensory stores as the individual needs to recruit to "experience" the table. Visual sensory stores take in lines, angles, color, and may allow for estimation of dimensions of the table and recognition of the material from which it is constructed. If visual sensory input is inadequate to determine information of interest, other sensory mechanisms, such as touch and audition, can be recruited to identify additional attributes, or the individual may call upon experience-based stored knowledge to fill in missing attributes.

Because sensory information is first processed at primary sensory cortices, any amalgamation of multisensory information requires that information processing continue from primary sensory cortices to unimodal sensory cortices and on to higher order sensory (associational) cortices. Of course, in instances when the individual can rely upon exemplar or prototypic knowledge derived from previous experience with the object or event, information processing is impacted, usually more efficiently, although not necessarily.

> The semantic representation of an object is composed of stored information about the features and attributes defining that object, including its typical form, color, and motion, and the motor movements associated with its use. Evidence from functional brain imaging studies of normal individuals indicates that this information is represented in the brain as a distributed network of discrete cortical regions. Within this network, the features that define an object are stored close to the primary sensory and motor areas that were active when information about that object was acquired.[111, p. 1023]

The organization of the PFC for perceptual and executive function appears to follow a somewhat hierarchical neuroanatomic and neuropsychological ordering that enables progression from basic motor or sensory functions through higher order processes of increasing complexity, culminating in the highest order executive, perceptual, motor, linguistic, and cognitive function. Unlayering of the PFC through injury to structures within the PFC essentially impacts the higher order functions, although lesser order functions may also be impacted, or may remain intact.[112]

Figure 19.1 demonstrates both the organization of primary, secondary, and tertiary cortices in the depiction of the brain, and the imposition of lower and increasingly higher order skills.[7,112] The skills are segregated into pre- and postrolandic (central) fissure locations and functions. Sensory functions are represented in blue, whereas "executable" or "actionable" functions are depicted in red (Figure 19.1). This diagram helps to provide a visual representation of the concept of cognitive distance progressing bottom to top for both perceptual and executive memory functions.

Cognitive distance should be viewed as an important clinical entity for reestablishing the individual's ability not only to take in sensory information when it is readily available, but also to call upon information when available sensory information is reduced or, perhaps, absent. Burger and Muma[113] showed that cognitive distance was a factor in aphasic and elderly nonaphasic individuals when performance was enhanced with objects contrasted to performance with pictorials of the same objects. Muma[114] noted similar discrepancies in performance with learning-disabled, mentally retarded, and autistic children.

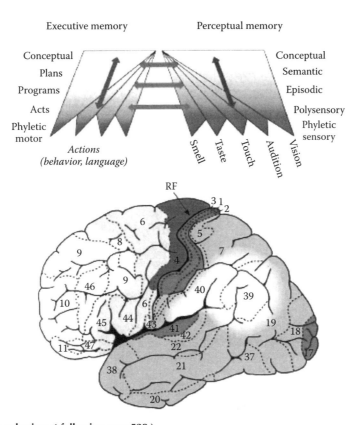

Executive memory   Perceptual memory

Conceptual   Conceptual

Plans   Semantic

Programs   Episodic

Acts   Polysensory

Phyletic   Phyletic
motor   sensory
                    Actions   Smell Taste Touch Audition Vision
              (behavior, language)

RF

FIGURE 19.1 (See color insert following page 528.)
General organization of cognitive representation in the human lateral cortex. (Top) Schema of the two major hierarchies of cortical memory. (Bottom) Distribution of memory networks indicated in broad outline by the same color code as in the upper figure. RF, Rolandic fissure. (From Fuster, J. M., *Neuron*, 30(2), 319–333, 2001. With permission.)

Muma[114] reported improved performance by an autistic child when play with items in a real house with a real kitchen was compared with play with items in a toy house. The ability to identify in an abstract manner features of objects or experiences that may be relevant to a situation depends upon both the ability to call upon stored featural information and the ability to use that information in both conventional and novel ways.

19.6 Intervention Techniques and Strategies

Individuals who have sustained TBI exhibit cognitive disorders in the areas of memory (long and short term), attention, processing speed, fluid reasoning, categorization, and shifting. A variety of formal measures has been utilized to determine the presence and extent of cognitive dysfunction, such as the Woodcock Johnson–III (Tests of Cognitive Abilities),[115] portions of the Scales for Cognitive Abilities for Traumatic Brain Injury,[116] Muma Assessment Program,[117] and the Ross Information Processing Assessment,[118] to name only a few. As a result of the nature of the brain injury, modifications to formal measures may be required if the assessment is to be a true measurement of the individual's cognitive skills. For example, time limits are often a part of the diagnostic tool. However, if the individual is processing information at a much slower rate, then it would be appropriate to allow for more processing time to complete tasks. In addition, test items may be enlarged or simplified to accommodate for visual or motor deficits. All modifications must be reported in the initial evaluation report.

19.7 Conditions for Cognitive Rehabilitation

A number of factors should be considered in determining whether the individual is able to benefit from cognitive rehabilitation. First, the CNS must be metabolically optimized to support rehabilitation efforts and learning properly. At the earliest stages after brain injury, metabolic function can be compromised by medications, cerebral swelling, glucose metabolism anomalies, neuromodulator, neuroendocrine, and biochemical imbalances. These factors, combined with other system involvement commonly seen following TBI,[119] raise questions about the influence of these systems on a recovering CNS. Pulmonary, infectious, renal, hepatic, or endocrine dysfunctions can all compromise cerebral function. General anesthesia and pharmacologic iatrogenic complications can delay recovery following TBI. Consequently, the overall medical stability of the individual should be considered. Metabolic function is an ongoing concern beyond the immediate days or weeks postinjury.

At the metabolic level, neuronal death within the CNS can be accompanied by the death of surrounding cells in the form of anterograde and retrograde axonal degeneration. Clearly, metabolic status impacts the extent of degenerative processes.[120] In some instances, cells in the vicinity of those that have died will enter a state of metabolic paralysis. These cells are only able to generate an action potential that is approximately one seventh the strength of a normal action potential. If metabolic compromise occurs while a cell is in a state of metabolic paralysis, these cells will likely succumb even to metabolic events that would not harm normally functioning cells.

Widespread/diffuse cortical traumatic axonal injury (TAI) is a component to nearly all TBI,[121] and TAI impacts not only neurons, but axons, dendrites, glial structures, and vascular supply.[122] As Povlishock and Katz[122] point out, TAI represents a progressive condition arising from activation of cysteine proteases, caspase, and calpain, which plays a role in proteolytic digestion of brain spectrin following TBI. Spectrin is a major component of the cytoskeletal network. In addition, overloading of calpains results in mitochondrial injury,[123] and mitochondria play a significant role in cellular necrosis and apoptosis. The end point of the progression of TAI is not yet clear.

Cellular death is also, in part, dependent upon the proximity of a sheared axon or dendrite to the cell body. Recovery from axonal shearing occurs via axonal sprouting and collateral sprouting, the latter of which is not dependent upon neuronal damage for elicitation.[124] Cortical representation is continuously modulated in response to activity, behavior, and skill acquisition in normal function. Environmental enrichment is known to bear positively on the density of dendritic, glial, and vascular structures.[125,126] Evidence suggests that similar processes occur following injury, either with adjacent areas taking over function or via use of alternative pathways.[127] Neuroanatomic changes that take place over long periods of time are represented by LTP, axonal regeneration and sprouting, and synaptic remodeling, at least. Rehabilitative therapy should represent such enrichment/demand and appropriately designed programs have been shown by fMRI to impact cortical reorganization.[128,129]

Neuroendocrine function as a precursor to cognitive function, in general, is increasingly being recognized as important. Neuroendocrine dysfunction arising from hypopituitarism following TBI has been found in up to 40% of persons tested.[130,131] Anterior pituitary function has been linked to cognitive outcome from TBI.[132] Growth hormone, sex hormones, leuteinizing and follicle-stimulating hormones, prolactin, thyroid, and cortisol function must be evaluated and treated prior to or during the undertaking of cognitive rehabilitation. This complex subject is addressed in Chapters 11, 12, and 14 in this volume.

Fatigue and depression can complicate cognitive function, and cognitive dysfunction arising from these complications is significantly different from that arising from brain injury. It is important to differentiate fatigue and depression and the cognitive dysfunction that can arise from each. Treating the underlying problem causing fatigue, such as neuroendocrine dysfunction or sleep disorder, will not only improve fatigue but also alleviate cognitive dysfunction arising from fatigue. Similarly, the cognitive dysfunction associated with depression should mitigate as depression improves. However, treatment of cognitive dysfunction arising from fatigue or depression with the techniques to be described herein cannot be reasonably expected to be successful.

Timing of rehabilitation intervention must be considered because it may impact the efficacy of treatment, because some interventions do not appear to be effective if undertaken too early after injury.[131] Interventions that are taken early during the course of recovery may be difficult to differentiate from the effects of spontaneous recovery, and it becomes important to clinicians to utilize procedures that will enable such assessment, whenever possible·

19.8 Therapeutic Intervention

The interventions that follow have been designed to be approached in a hierarchical order that is fashioned after the normal developmental sequences observed in linguistic and cognitive development. The approaches attempt to respect the underlying physiology and known neuroanatomic substrates of cognition. The techniques are restorative rather than compensatory in nature. There is relatively little evidence to support the undertaking of certain compensatory approaches, such as memory notebooks, and there is little clear physiologic rationale for such an approach if one desires to build skill sets necessary for a return to functionality, rather than simply means to overcome lack of such skill sets.

Three primary areas of cognition will be considered: attention, perceptual feature processing, and categorization. As previously noted, attention, although often presumed to be the most basic of skills, clearly impacts and underlies most, if not all, aspects of cognitive function. The ability to identify and interpret perceptual features effectively is instrumental, in turn, to building categorizing skills. Cognitive distance skills are accumulated and honed throughout the process of categorization. The assumption is that this collection of skills is foundational to most, if not all, other cognitive processes.

Given the interrelated nature of cognitive processing, it is important to conduct treatment in an organized and hierarchical fashion. All aspects of the treatment protocol to be outlined must be fulfilled in the proposed order and without omissions. Individuals who possess competencies in certain areas will progress through those modules very quickly but will nevertheless benefit from the developmentally oriented approach. Pre- and posttreatment testing using broad measures of neuropsychological function should be undertaken to document changes. Care should be taken in choosing test instruments to ensure that these tests do not measure specific skill sets being trained; instead, broader, more generalized measures should be used.

19.8.1 Attention

One of the major cognitive deficits following TBI is impaired attention. This can include complaints of inability to concentrate, sensitivity to perceptual noise, or difficulty with task completion or multitasking. Although therapists often recognize the manifestation of attentional deficits, the underlying cause may be difficult to identify precisely. For example, when an individual presents with "distractibility," the therapist acknowledges the need to simplify the environment; however, this does not adequately address the complex nature of the attentional disorder, nor does it afford any form of remedy for the underlying cause. Intervention techniques targeting only one aspect of the disorder will not result in true and consistent improvements of the disorder as a whole. What is instead required is a technique that addresses the impairment in attention itself rather than merely its manifestations. In addition, the same is true for individuals who display perseverative behaviors. The term *perseveration* does not adequately communicate the complex essence of the disorder.

A holistic approach to outlining the deficit is beneficial in the assessment and treatment process. A distractible individual finds directing and/or maintaining a focus of attention challenging. Therefore, the therapist must introduce activities designed to improve the individual's ability to direct and/or maintain a focus of attention. Concepts and techniques used to build attention skills include, but are not limited to, manipulation of environmental stimuli (auditory and visual); increasing complexity of tasks in a controlled, hierarchical fashion; and respecting and integrating a taxonomy of cognitive distance over time and when appropriate.

Although there are several ways in which to address attention, designing a bottom-up therapeutic program allows for a developmental approach to building attention skills. Taking this approach with all individuals exhibiting attentional deficits ensures that all skills have been acquired in a developmental and sequential fashion, setting the foundation for higher level cognitive processes. At the base of the hierarchy lies *focused attention*, the ability to direct one's attention to a specific stimulus. After the individual is capable of directing attention, the person must be able to sustain attention. Although treatment in an isolated setting is recommended early on, it does not allow for generalization of skills. Therefore, treatment should then shift to a higher level of attention skills, such as being able to attend to a specific stimulus selectively in the presence of numerous auditory and visual distractors, alternating attention between two or more tasks, and, finally, simultaneously attending to two or more tasks.

In keeping with this framework of attention, the environment must be modified to implement a stepwise progression through this hierarchy of attention. Therapy should initially be performed in a controlled and enclosed environment in which auditory and visual stimuli are minimal. The treatment area should be designed such that furnishings, therapy materials, lighting, and temperature can be managed. For example, an individual exhibiting a severe attentional deficit may require an environment with little visual and auditory stimuli present, such as a room without furniture, with low lighting, and temperature adjusted to their liking. It may be necessary for therapists to adjust their attire to decrease color stimuli from clothing, to remove jewelry, and so on.

After the individual can perform simple therapeutic tasks in the controlled environment, auditory and/or visual stimuli may be gradually introduced, moving from least to most salient and advancing in one sensory modality at a time. For example, therapy for an individual who enjoys rap/soul music may start with soft, relaxing music and then progress to more energetic music at louder levels, ending with the type of music the individual enjoys most and knows well. Similarly, initiating tasks in a sterile environment, one without furniture and other visual distractions, may be necessary. When the individual is able to perform tasks in simplified settings, visual stimuli can gradually be introduced. It may be necessary for all disciplines to conduct therapy in a sensory-controlled environment to achieve maximum therapeutic benefit.

An important part of the therapeutic process involves task complexing. Consistent with the framework of a bottom-up approach, tasks should start with physical activities and gradually progress to mental activities, utilizing a taxonomy of cognitive distance. Physical activities can include sorting/categorizing by iconic features such as color or size, whereas abstract activities might include symbolic categorization.

The principles of cognitive distance previously mentioned in this chapter must be taken into account. Treatment should begin with the utilization of objects because objects are most concrete. With an object, individuals have the ability to determine size, weight, color, texture, and so forth, physically. As cognitive distance increases, use of pictorials (color, black and white, line drawings, and photographs) is introduced.

Keeping these principles in mind when working with a severely impaired individual, tasks should initially target physical activities with the use of objects. Complexity is increased by adding more objects or lengthening the time required for engaging in tasks. For example, the individual may be required to attend to tasks for 10 seconds. After this is achieved, the individual should be required to perform this task consistently with 80% accuracy. The next level would involve increasing the length of time engaged in the activity. When working with severely impaired individuals, it is often necessary to perform a single therapeutic activity repeatedly for lengthy periods of time to build basic attention skills. It is important to monitor accuracy and response time to determine when it is appropriate to move the individual to the next level of difficulty.

Despite the degree of impairment, treatment should always be initiated in a stimulus-controlled environment and with a physical task. In this way, concentration is improved, adequately preparing the individual for increasingly cognitively distant tasks. When appropriate performance accuracy and response times are achieved in a stimulus-controlled environment, visual and auditory distractors can be gradually added, one modality at a time, to increase environmental complexity. The therapeutic environment should continually challenge the individual until, ultimately, activities are performed with satisfactory accuracy and sustained attention in a stimulus-rich environment. It is imperative to ensure that data are collected throughout the therapeutic process, including changes in environmental complexity. A general criterion for increasing task and environmental complexities for physical activities is 90% to 100% accuracy, whereas 80% accuracy is appropriate for mental activities. Time limits to perform tasks can be modified depending on the individual's physical limitations. For example, when analyzing the task completion time, the therapist should note whether processing speed was impacted by the existence of a physical impairment, such as the use of a nondominant hand.

There are various ways to alter activities systematically while regarding the three primary variables of environmental stimulus, task complexity, and cognitive distance. Table 19.1 shows the order of therapeutic task presentation, including variables such as level of task and environmental complexities. Treatment should begin with performing

TABLE 19.1

Order of Distractor Presentation

Task	No Distractor	Simple Auditory or Visual Distractor	Multisensory Distractor
Physical	1	2	3
Physical/mental	4	5	6
Mental	7	8	9

physical tasks in a controlled and enclosed environment, and ultimately progress to mental tasks in a stimulus-rich environment.

A hierarchy of varying levels of attention should be utilized to strengthen concentration skills. At the base of the hierarchy lies *sustained attention*. This is the individual's ability to direct and maintain focus with regard to a task across a period of time in a quiet environment. Therapeutic activities addressing categorization, memory, visual and auditory processing, direction following, shifting, and problem solving can be performed to address the development of attentional skills. Physical or concrete tasks, such as sorting, scanning, and direction following, should be initiated first. Individuals with very poor attention may start with simple auditory sustained attention or vigilance tasks. Such tasks require the individual to listen to a string of stimuli targeting a specific number, letter, or word for short periods of time. After attention and accuracy improve, the length of time may be extended. The same hierarchy can be utilized for visual sustained attention tasks. For example, the individual can sort picture cards or hardware pieces into different categories. Visual scanning or vigilance tasks can involve searching magazine articles for a target word. Again, after this task has been mastered, the addition of multiple targets further challenges attentional skills. Auditory scanning activities involve listening to stories or passages and indicating a targeted response for a designated word and then increasing the number of target words. Basic-level strategies to improve accuracy on concrete tasks include teaching systematic scanning, double-checking work, and increasing awareness of attention deficits.

After individuals demonstrate the ability to maintain attention with good accuracy on concrete tasks, more mental or abstract tasks can be implemented. Working memory tasks, such as reordering a string of random numbers from smallest to largest or in reverse order, are more cognitively challenging. Other potential working memory tasks include listening to sentences and reorganizing the words within the sentences in alphabetical, reverse alphabetical, and/or progressive word length order.[133] Mental math calculations can also be performed.[133] Higher level visual processing tasks, such as iconic store modules, may also be chosen. This task involves the individual viewing a card with three rows of letters for a brief period of time (2 seconds) and then being asked to recall a specified row. The generalization of quick visual processing can be facilitated through setting up a scene in a room and having the individual enter the room for a brief amount of time. Upon leaving the room, the individual would be required to recall as many details as possible. Several Attention Process Training[133] tasks involving attention, processing, and categorization may be initiated. These tasks involve listening to a string of words and identifying items that fit into a designated category (e.g., round objects, pairs, related words, opposite words, and so on).

The next level in the attentional hierarchy is *selective attention*. Consistency must be established prior to moving the individual to a higher distractor level. After the individual exhibits the ability to perform tasks consistently in a quiet and controlled environment, a hierarchy of distractors should be introduced. Initially, noise (e.g., a radio playing) should be presented in the controlled environment. Then, the individual can be moved from the controlled environment to a familiar environment with minimal distractors. This might simulate a person in a living or family room, providing the individual with the opportunity of a chance conversation and/or the presence of others nearby. To challenge the attentional system further, the next level should require the individual to perform tasks in a highly distractible, familiar setting (e.g., lobby, lounge, or gym areas). Finally, the individual should be placed in unfamiliar and high-traffic areas (e.g., mall, bowling alley, bus station) to provide a maximal distractor-laden environment.

The highest level of attention is *divided attention*, which requires the ability to attend to two or more different tasks simultaneously. Individuals divide their attention while driving, taking notes in class, performing household chores while watching television, and so forth. Divided attention can be addressed in a variety of ways, such as performing previously mentioned concrete and abstract tasks while simultaneously answering a series of questions differing in levels of complexity. For example, the individual may be required to sort hardware pieces into categories while simultaneously responding to yes/no or open-ended questions of varying complexity. The therapist can document response time to complete the sorting task, the percentage of correct responses, and any delay in responses to questions. In this way, processing speed can be monitored not only for task completion, but also for frequency of delayed responses.

Perseverative behaviors are another type of attentional deficit. A perseverative response may be characterized as an inability to shift a focus of attention among perceptual features. Therapeutic activities that decrease perceptual salience and establish the use of iconic and symbolic feature identification skills usually result in a reduction of perseverative responses. For example, the therapist may present an object to an individual and direct attention to various perceptual features of the object such as color, shape, construction, and so on. Some perseverative behaviors, however, may be a result of perceptual salience in other sensory domains, such as self-abuse as a result of sensory integration deficits. Treatment for improving perceptual salience is discussed later in this chapter.

Attentional deficits also include problems with *vigilance*, referring to the ability to sustain a focus of attention and regulate perception of incoming information for a particular set of features. For individuals to be successful, they must first be able to take in large amounts of visual and/or auditory information quickly, resisting distractions of extraneous stimuli, and then be able to filter that information for the preferred features. This process requires quick processing speed and increasingly abstract cognitive distance skills. Thus, therapy should address sustaining attention in a multisensory environment and building cognitive distance skills.

Cognitive shift refers to the ability to alternate attention from one activity to another with the least amount of interference to sensory stores, task sequencing, and task accuracy. This cognitive skill is hierarchically more complex and is often impaired in the individual with TBI. Basic-level attention should be relatively intact prior to addressing cognitive shift skills.

Cognitive shift activities should adhere to the concepts of task complexity and presentation of external sensory stimuli. Activities should begin with two simple physical tasks, requiring the individual to shift from one activity to the other and back. Data collection includes response time to shift between tasks and accuracy of task completion. After the individual demonstrates competency with physical tasks, task complexity should then progress to physical and mental, then to mental only. Tasks can be further complicated with the addition of external sensory stimuli. Table 19.1 presents the order of distractor presentation.

Physical tasks include simple rote motor tasks such as linking chains together or sorting objects by a designated iconic feature (e.g., color, shape, size, weight). Mental tasks include sorting picture or word cards by categories, sorting objects by a designated symbolic feature (e.g., things that provide light, things that are used for scooping, things that make noise), performing various math calculations, and so on. Recalling a sequence of shifts can be added for increased complexity. A telephone book scanning activity can be performed involving the individual locating addresses and phone numbers of businesses in a specified order. Other tasks addressing shifting can be located in the Attention Process Training kit.[2] For example, one task may be to listen to a string of words and alternate between identifying fruits and articles of clothing throughout the task. Higher level shifting tasks address memory, initiation, and time management by incorporating visual and self-regulating tasks into the treatment program.[2] Now, the individual no longer has an auditory cue from the therapist but rather is presented with a visual cue and/or a specified time interval to shift. Two or three sets of instructions are told to the individual. Visual tasks require the individual to shift when presented with a visual signal. For example, when performing a visual scanning activity, visual marks should be placed randomly throughout the page. When individuals arrive at a visual mark, they must first recognize the mark to be a symbol, recall which set of instructions to perform, and then initiate the task to be performed. Self-regulating tasks require the individual to self-initiate alternating between two tasks at specified time intervals by monitoring time on a stopwatch. For example, when provided with math worksheets, addition tasks are performed initially. The individual performs the math calculations while simultaneously monitoring time. After the established time interval (e.g., every 30 seconds), the individual must then recall and initiate the next set of instructions. These tasks can also be performed with the hierarchy of distractors presented in Table 19.1.

Throughout the progression of the attention hierarchy, impulse control should be in the forefront of the therapist's mind. Awareness of deficit and self-monitoring techniques should be explored and implemented. For example, prior to the initiation of a task, it would be appropriate to ask individuals to predict their success on the specific task. Following the completion of the task, any errors made should be reviewed and correlated to the individual's prediction. Based upon the difference between predicted and actual performance, strategies for improving attention can be discussed.

19.8.2 Feature Identification

A therapeutic tool known as the *Cognition Module* can be used to improve overall cognitive functioning in a structured and developmental manner. At the first level of feature identification, the individual is trained to attend to and identify different perceptual features of real objects. Perceptual features can be broken down into seven iconic and one symbolic feature. Iconic features consist of, but are not limited to, color, shape, construction, size, weight, texture, and detail. The symbolic feature requires the individual to identify the function of objects. The list of perceptual features reflects some of the "linguistic universals" referred to by Rosch.[58]

Cognitive distance is introduced at level I. The individual describes the iconic and symbolic features of real objects. Cognitive distance is built by moving the individual through a hierarchy of sublevels consisting of objects, color photographs of objects, black-and-white photographs of objects, line drawings of objects, written words, and, ultimately, spoken words. When objects are no longer physically represented, the individual is required to rely on mental representation of objects.

Initially, a checklist of the eight perceptual features may be required. After the individual begins to learn the features in an organized manner, the checklist can be phased out. Criteria for successful completion at this level is individually based. Although it is important to monitor accuracy at each sublevel, the therapist should keep in mind the broader scope of performance. Therefore, a comparison of the overall performance between sublevel objects and spoken words should determine whether the individual is ready to progress to the next level. For example, individuals may demonstrate difficulty at lower sublevels; however, through repetition, accuracy may improve at the spoken word sublevel. Because the individual has achieved greater task accuracy at a more cognitively distant task, it can be inferred that the individual's level of cognitive functioning has improved. Response time should be fairly quick; however, this should not be used as a criterion for progression to the next level, because individuals with brain injury commonly present with slower processing speed.

Level II requires the individual to expand feature identification skills. The individual must still identify the eight features one by one and must also provide an extended feature. For example, when describing a stop sign, the individual must verbalize that the stop sign is red and must identify another object which is also red, such as an apple. Responses provided must be different for each of the eight extended features, thereby maximizing categorization, word finding, and memory skills. In addition, the extended feature response should not be an object within the individual's visual field. The cognitive distance hierarchy ranging from real objects to spoken words should again be followed.

Level III focuses on abstract negation. The purpose of this section is to expand feature identification skills further through negative categorization. At this level, the individual is required to identify the eight perceptual features of the object in terms of what the object is not and then state another object which does not have the same characteristics. For example, when describing a stop sign, the individual must verbalize that the stop sign is not blue and must identify another object which is not blue, such as the sun. Again, the cognitive distance hierarchy ranging from real objects to spoken words should be followed.

It is often difficult for individuals with TBI to provide extended and negative feature identification secondary to decreased visual imagery skills. Visual imagery is important in everyday life to assist with episodic memory, abstract thinking, and problem solving. Often, individuals exhibit a limited repertoire of responses secondary to decreased visual imagery, word finding, and categorization skills. Several strategies can be used to assist with these skills. For example, visual imagery cues can assist with visualizing familiar places, such as different rooms in a house, playground, garage, mall, or office. If the individual is unable to verbalize an extended feature, further visual and/or semantic cues may be utilized. For example, if the individual was unable to visualize something in a kitchen that was also yellow, a cue to think of a fruit or something in a refrigerator may help trigger a response. With an increase in cognitive distance, for example, at the spoken word level, the inability to recall a target item is often observed. Cuing the individual to recall previous responses may be beneficial. However, providing structure to the task, such as having the individual state the name of the object prior to describing each feature, is usually more effective. Individuals with decreased word finding and visual imagery skills often repeat responses. In these cases, it is imperative that the therapist monitor responses and provide cues to generate novel responses, as needed.

Mental flexibility is another skill that is addressed throughout the Cognition Module. The ability to perform negative categorization is significantly impacted by the individual's mental flexibility, visual imagery, and cognitive distance skills. When provided with an object (e.g., a banana), the individual with reduced mental flexibility will often say "The color is not yellow." However, with cues, such as verbalizing colors other than yellow, and repetition of the task, mental flexibility is noted to improve.

19.8.3 Categorization

The next level of the Cognition Module requires the individual to identify iconic and symbolic features of objects grouped together. Each sublevel is divided into two parts. As suggested by the cognitive distance hierarchy, activities again begin with real objects—in this instance, arranged in three rows with three objects in each row. The first part requires the individual to identify one perceptual feature in common across the three rows. For example, if rows of red, yellow, and blue objects are set on a table, the individual must recognize the common perceptual feature as being "color." The next part of this level requires the individual to identify three different perceptual features. Therefore, each row targets a different feature. For example, the first row can consist of items of similar "color," such as a fork, spoon, and knife. Another row can consist of items of similar "shape," such as a ball, plate, and tire. The last row can consist of items of similar "function," such as a flashlight, candle, and penlight. To address mental flexibility further, the therapist can ask the individual to provide additional responses. For example, in addition to color, a fork, spoon, and knife have the same shape, construction, size, texture, detail, and function. To promote effective problem solving and impulse control, the rows of objects can be manipulated such that the individual is required to scan the three rows prior to committing to a response. At this level, the cognitive distance hierarchy progresses to written words and does not include spoken words. The strategy of process of elimination can also be taught to facilitate effective problem solving.

The next level of the Cognition Module requires symbolic categorization. For some individuals, symbolic categorization may be less difficult than iconic categorization. Research indicates that symbolic categorization may be more easily stored.[134] However, this may not be reflective of an intact feature processing system. Therefore, although it may appear that the individual has a basic understanding of symbolic features, this may only be a cursory understanding of common functional attributes of objects and not a true representation of proficiency in feature identification and categorization skills.

The purpose of this level is to develop the ability to categorize objects by function. This level consists of three steps and three levels of cognitive distance (color photographs of objects, black-and-white photographs of objects, and spoken word). If photographs are too abstract for an individual to begin with, it may be necessary first to use real objects. When shown a photograph of an object, the first two steps are to identify the traditional function of the object and the category to which it belongs. The next step involves verbalizing three alternate functions of the object. This includes functions the object can perform but that are not typically done with the object. For the last step, individuals must shift their perspective and identify three functions the object cannot be used to perform. At this level, the individual must integrate all iconic and symbolic features to think of alternative and negative functions of objects. For example, alternative functions of a fork may be to dig with, stir with, scratch with, use as a hair clip, use to poke holes with, or use as a screwdriver. To visualize these functions, analysis and synthesis of iconic and symbolic features must occur. Therefore, because the construction of the fork is strong and hard and it has a long, flat handle and sharp tines, it should be able to carry out the functions mentioned previously. For individuals who exhibit poor mental flexibility, it may be necessary to bring their attention to the eight features of the target object. The same cues may be used for identifying negative functions of objects. In addition, having the individual recall the traditional function of the object and then determine other objects that do not serve the same purpose may assist with negative categorization. Again, therapists should closely monitor individuals' responses to discourage for repetitive responses and facilitate a wide spectrum of responses instead.

A multisensory visualization task is next performed to enhance cognitive abilities further. The task requires the individual to describe a given experience using the five senses as well as generating emotionally based responses relevant to the situation. Initially, it may be necessary to target familiar experiences, such as a high school football game, a child's birthday party, Christmas Eve, hobbies, and so forth. In the football game example, a response might include, "I see two teams in different uniforms—blue and white, red and gold—on the field. The chalked lines are clean and fresh. It's cold and the wind is steady. I smell hot cocoa, and the hot dog being eaten by a friend. The crowd is cheering, following the lead of the cheerleading squad. The bench is hard, cold, and uncomfortable, with no back support. We use an old sleeping bag to spread over our legs for warmth. It's fun here with my friends and I am excited that our team may win this championship game." As the individual's visual imagery skills improve, increasing the cognitive distance by having the individual describe situations or experiences he or she is not familiar with can be used. Previously learned skills, including feature identification, categorization, cognitive distance, perceptual salience, and visual imagery, are inherent to the successful completion of this task. Because responses are subjective, the ability to express and support opinions can be concurrently addressed at this level, thus improving the expression of complex ideas.

Processing speed can be monitored by timing the individual's response times to the different levels of the Cognition Module. When progressing to higher levels or increasing the complexity of tasks, response times may become lengthier. However, it is expected that response times improve with repetition. When comparing performance on a lower sublevel to a higher sublevel (objects, spoken word), if response times maintain, it can be inferred that processing speed actually improved secondary to the increased cognitive demands of the higher sublevel. Other tasks to help improve processing speed include performing word fluency activities such as naming as many items within a concrete category (animals, modes of transportation, occupations, and so on) or an abstract category (naming words beginning with a specific letter of the alphabet).

The Cognition Module assists with the overall thought organization process in numerous ways. The initial task is to learn the iconic and symbolic features in an organized manner. Therefore, it is important to cue the individual consistently to a specific order, allowing for improved organization and efficiency of information processing. Cognitive skills, such as attention, feature identification, categorization, cognitive shift, and cognitive distance, are required simultaneously. Interference from perceptual salience (an excessive amount of attention to a particular perceptual feature) can be restricted through the use of seven iconic features and one symbolic feature. Categorization skills are optimized throughout the module by initially performing feature identification tasks using iconic and symbolic features. Each level consists of sublevels that address cognitive distance, requiring the individual to rely heavily on mental representation of objects by diminishing the amount of physical information presented.

The therapeutic tools reviewed in this chapter are designed to reestablish basic-level cognitive abilities. Higher level thought processes and memory cannot be adequately addressed if basic level cognitive skills are not first put into place. The Cognition Module is not meant to be the only treatment activity; rather, it is an essential part of the overall rehabilitation program. Different activities can be used to develop attentional and cognitive shift skills.

19.9 Neuroanatomy of the Cognition Module

In this section we will assign aspects of the cognitive interventions described to their respective neuroanatomic substrates, when possible. To begin, each of us has encountered a situation in which we needed to adapt an object or process to a purpose for which it was not designed to accomplish a given objective. In fact, in many ways, this ability is one of many in which human cognition differs significantly from that of lesser species. In effect, this is the heart of innovation, the recognition of salient attributes of a useful object or process that would serve the necessary function to accomplish a goal.

Both simple and complex examples of such situations abound in everyday life. A common, simple example might be one that has frustrated most of us at some point or another: when an item falls into the crevice between the seat and the console in an automobile such that it cannot be reached by the driver but must nevertheless be retrieved. There exists a multitude of possible solutions to this simple problem in theory, but in practical application, only a handful of these might be available in a particular instance because the available tools within the vehicle are likely to be limited. So the solution to the problem becomes one that must be derived, if possible, from the available tools or processes at the time. One such solution would be to use a pen to extend the reach of the driver and push the object free; another might be to have a child, whose smaller hand or arm could extend more readily into the narrow gap, reach for the object; a third might be to use an object tailored to the attributes of the fallen item, such as a magnet to retrieve keys or a piece of tape for a dollar bill; still another might be to reposition the seat forward or backward to reach the object more easily. We will return to this example in our examination of the Cognition Module as a therapeutic tool later.

First, it is worthwhile to point out that even the most complex problem solving relies on essentially the same elements as our simple one—namely, determination of the characteristics of the problem; identification of the necessary features or attributes of a solution; identification of a solution to the problem; followed or preceded by comparison of those attributes in relation to a specific object, process, or combination thereof; and subsequent application of the objects or processes as the solution to the problem. The modern concept of vaccination evolved via this process. In solving the problem of the smallpox epidemic, astute and observant scientists recognized that certain strains of the smallpox virus that did not result in severe disease had the attribute of conferring immunity to all other strains of the virus. These scientists recognized that this attribute could be used to prevent severe smallpox disease if the particular nonsevere (also referred to as *nonvirulent*) strains of the virus were administered systematically to healthy individuals. In effect, this formed the theoretical basis for attenuated live vaccinations and paved the way for all modern forms of vaccination.

Based upon the premise that the recognition of features or attributes of objects or processes, and subsequent application of this to problems underlies most, if not all, forms of problem solving, a logical target for therapeutic intervention would be to induce or improve this type of identification and categorization. In essence, the Cognition Module is directed at precisely this endeavor. The aim of this discussion is to explore the manner in which this is accomplished, using an example to highlight the various requirements of the Cognition Module from a functional standpoint, as well as the neuroanatomy and neurophysiology underlying these requirements, where this is known. Ultimately, we will return to the common problem mentioned in the opening of this section of the chapter, tying the use of the skill sets used in the Cognition Module to solving problems in everyday life. However, to begin, we will envision an individual beginning the Cognition Module at level I, with the object stimulus presented being a no. 2 pencil. One set of the many appropriate responses for the individual to give would be that the pencil is yellow, cylindrical, composed of wood and graphite, 8 inches long with a diameter of 0.25 inch, a few ounces in weight, smoothly textured, possessed of an eraser, and used for writing. The question relevant to this discussion is what cognitive processes are required to generate these responses and what are the neuroanatomic underpinnings of those processes.

One of the most basic cognitive processes requisite to success in completing the Cognition Module is attention. To perceive and identify features of an object adequately, it is first necessary to attend to that object in a selective fashion. This concept has been labeled *selective attention*. Specifically, in our therapy task, the individual would be required to attend to the stimulus presented (the pencil) selectively to the exclusion of various other stimuli that might be present. When addressing each specific feature identification task, the individual must selectively attend only to those stimuli that appear relevant to this task. This type of selective attention has been described as being determined by the processes of competitive selection and top-down sensitivity control.[135]

Attention, as a critical cognitive process, has been of great interest to cognitive neuroscientists, and many attempts have been made to elucidate its neuroanatomic and neurophysiologic correlates. The results of these studies have indicated that attention is a process that is mediated by widely distributed neural structures. Attention is dependent upon arousal/vigilance, which is subserved by the ascending reticular activating system. Selective attention appears to be mediated by the thalamofrontal gating system, the PFC, the anterior cingulate (executive attention, attention during auditory processing), the parietal lobe cortex (attention to location), and the occipitotemporal cortex (attention to color/form).[136–138] What has been traditionally referred to as *Treisman's spotlight* seems likely to be mediated by the pulvinar complex, a nucleus in the thalamus that has projections to the posterior parietal, temporal, and prefrontal cortices, in addition to secondary visual areas.[136,139] The hypothesis is that the pulvinar mediates a top-down influence on cells in various regions, specifically by imposing bias criteria upon cells that respond to a particular stimulus. The influence of the pulvinar has been most explored in relation to the visual and spatial attentional systems. However, the manner in which the pulvinar complex becomes tuned to a particular task demand remains unresolved. In addition to the pulvinar complex, the posterior parietal cortex also appears to be implicated in the process of competitive selection and is another area likely involved in top-down influences on attention.[135,140] Information about the relative salience of stimuli may be encoded elsewhere. Encoding of the relative salience of visual field stimuli, for example, appears to be located in the lateral intraparietal area.[135,141–143]

Thus, attention appears to be a widely distributed process anatomically. The PFC seems to be the most consistently activated region during attention tasks, but other regions mentioned may also be activated, depending upon the specific task at hand and the type of information involved with the task (e.g., visual, spatial, auditory, executive). There are also important neurophysiologic correlates for attention. Specifically, the catecholaminergic neurotransmitters dopamine and norepinephrine are thought to modulate processes of attention.[144] Further evidence that these neurotransmitters play an important role in attentional processes is the impact of noradrenergic and dopaminergic medications on attention.

Bringing the discussion back to the example introduced at the beginning of the section, the individual would be charged with the task of attending to the pencil in very particular ways to discriminate its perceptual features. In determining its shape, for example, top-down processes arising from such areas as the PFC, the pulvinar complex, and also from other regions or networks that have not yet been elucidated would establish the bias criteria for salience of information being presented. In this case, because the information refers to shape, the occipitotemporal cortex is likely to be involved in attending to this specific type of information. Based upon the bias criteria imposed, specific cells programmed to respond ideally to the form presented by the pencil would be preferentially selected for firing, thus making them more effective in competitive selection, and more likely to enter working memory as salient information to the task of determining the perceptual feature of shape for this object.

Working memory and attention are processes that are inextricably interrelated by virtue of their influence upon one another. Thus, no discussion of one can be complete in the absence of the other. Just as individuals must attend to the stimulus in a manner appropriate to the completion of each aspect of the feature identification task, so must they hold the information garnered in working memory for use in interpreting results, modifying a perceptual search pattern or strategy, or monitoring progress through the module. To be more explicit, individuals must hold the perceptual information acquired with regard to the specific stimulus of the pencil in working memory. They must simultaneously hold information about which perceptual feature is currently being identified, which features have already been identified, and which must still be identified. This information is then used not only for the generation of responses to the Cognition Module task, but also, obviously, must impact the attentional process as well.

Neuroanatomic substrates of working memory have been studied extensively in the field of cognitive neuroscience. The most frequently cited area of interest with regard to working memory is the PFC, and indeed, data from studies in both humans and nonhuman primates support the PFC as a relevant area of involvement.[136] However, additional areas also appear to be important in working memory and it is becoming increasingly recognized that working memory, like attention, is a widely distributed process and relies on such structures as the inferior temporal cortex and medial temporal cortical areas (including the hippocampus, and the parahippocampal, perirhinal, and entorhinal cortices), the posterior parietal cortex, the inferior parietal cortex, and higher order areas in the occipital cortex, in addition to the PFC.[135,145,146] Data from fMRI studies show that tasks involving working memory consistently activate both the dorsolateral PFC and the posterior parietal cortex, and that reciprocal pathways exist between these two areas.[135,146,147] The inferior temporal cortex has been demonstrated to be of importance with regard to short-term retention of visual object features.[145] The medial temporal cortical areas appear to be relevant to working memory, particularly in the maintenance of visual objects when distraction is present, as well as for complex novel objects, faces, or scenes.[145]

The processes of attention and working memory are not only interrelated, but also are mediated by many of the same neural structures or networks. This is consistent with the finding that damage to the frontal lobes impairs the ability to balance between environmental events and current goals, as this inability could, in essence, be a manifestation of disruption of either process.[41] An individual performing the tasks involved in the Cognition Module would require effective synergy between the interrelated processes of attention and working memory. Selective attention would be subject to modification via top-down processes influenced by working memory. To give a concrete example, if we suppose that the individual has responded to the perceptual feature of construction but not yet to size, then we can reason that within working memory must be information regarding the next perceptual feature to be described (size) as well as those that have already been described (color, shape, construction), in addition to the perceptual feature information that has been gathered about the object already (the object's name, its color, its shape, and its construction). Presumably, the influence of this information contained in working memory would serve via top-down processes to influence attention and provide a bias for those attributes of the object that would facilitate identification of the size. However, merely attending to and placing the perceptual information into working memory will not alone be sufficient for the individual to determine the features of the object accurately.

To identify the perceptual features accurately, the individual must also bring prior knowledge to bear, which leads to a discussion of long-term memory systems, including episodic and semantic memory.[148] In this case, the individual would need to draw from either episodic memory (e.g., a specific past experience with a pencil, the color yellow, a cylindrical shape, a wooden object) or semantic memory (e.g., generalized knowledge about pencils, the color yellow, cylinders, wood) to make sense of the perceptual information at hand. This is to say that mere perception alone is insufficient to produce the desired recognition of the perceptual features of the object. Rather, the individual must draw on some previously encoded information to convert the perceptual information to meaningful features. As discussed later, both episodic and semantic memory have implications for the process of categorization.

Episodic memories are encoded and retrieved through various neuroanatomic mechanisms. Most studies addressing encoding and retrieval have focused upon the PFC and the asymmetric involvement specific to these two processes. According to the hemispheric encoding retrieval asymmetry (HERA) model, the left-side PFC is more involved with encoding, whereas the right side is more involved with retrieval.[149] However, this has been called into question, because some studies have demonstrated bilateral activation during retrieval.[150] The retrieval of episodic memories appears to be distributed fairly widely throughout the brain. Areas of relevance in retrieval of episodic memories include the hippocampus and parahippocampal gyri, with some debate about lateralization; the parietal (specifically, the posterior medial parietal cortex), inferior temporal and occipital cortices; the cingulate cortex; and the thalamus.[150] The hippocampus appears to be important in topographic memory formation, memory for faces, and memory for complex colored pictures.

Semantic memory appears to be stored in various regions of the brain that are dependent upon the attributes of the particular unit of knowledge. Evidence for this stems from the recognition that injury to specific regions can produce relatively focal agnosias wherein specific types of semantic information cannot be readily accessed but other types of knowledge are unaffected. One such example is prosopagnosia, which follows damage to the fusiform face area.[151] Similarly, many other selective agnosias have been described, including apperceptive, finger, landmark, somatosensory, topographic, and visuospatial agnosias.[136] Particular regions appear to be critical to accessing stored semantic information. These regions are somewhat specific to type of information as well, and, in fact, some regions may underlie the specific agnosias, although the specific neuroanatomic correlates of the various agnosias mentioned have not been specifically identified. Among the regions implicated in semantic memory are the inferior parietal lobe, the fusiform gyrus, the middle temporal gyrus, the inferior frontal gyrus, the dorsal premotor cortex, and the retrosplenial cortex.[152] There is a general propensity for left-side involvement compared with right in terms of semantic retrieval. Brain imaging studies evaluating various domains or types of semantic knowledge have demonstrated different brain activation patterns. The most consistent difference in brain activation has centered upon the discrimination between living and nonliving stimuli. The results indicate that the semantic information pertaining to the living stimuli being correlated with activation in the lateral fusiform gyrus, whereas that correlated with the nonliving being localized to the medial fusiform gyrus.[152] Another distinction has been identified between motor-based knowledge and knowledge of abstract properties, with motor-based knowledge showing activation more in the left frontal parietal network (the intraparietal sulcus, inferior parietal lobe, dorsal premotor cortex), and abstract knowledge showing more activation in the retrosplenial and lateral anterior inferotemporal cortex.[152]

In addition to the neuroanatomic correlates of memory formation, there are important neurophysiologic mechanisms involved, including LTP. A detailed discussion of LTP is not warranted here, but a few points are highly relevant. LTP is involved with synaptic consolidation in the hippocampus, is dependent upon the N-methyl-D-aspartate receptor in many instances, and is impacted by the dopaminergic system.[153,154] Some therapeutic interventions aimed at improvement of memory function have attempted to exploit this mechanism using drugs that target the N-methyl-D-aspartate receptor, such as memantine, although the efficacy of these efforts has yet to be fully determined.

As the individual progresses through the levels of the Cognition Module, the stimulus presented for feature identification progresses from the tangible object presented in level I to a photograph, line drawing, written, and, finally, spoken word. Each of these transitions occurs to introduce cognitive distance, which forces the individual to rely to greater and greater extents upon visual imagery, prior semantic or episodic knowledge (as discussed previously), and, in some cases, working memory.

The neuroanatomic underpinnings of visual imagery are still poorly understood. The traditional understanding of visual imagery is that the image is displayed in the same sensory cortices in which it was perceptually processed. Thus, visual images have been traditionally thought to be displayed in the topographically organized visual cortices in the occipital lobe. However, there is some evidence that indicates that this picture is incomplete and suggests the involvement of other regions. Neuroimaging studies have demonstrated that visual imagery depends upon large networks that involve the frontal and parietal lobes as mediators of top-down influence upon the temporal lobe.[155] The area of the left temporal lobe appears to be of particular importance, and lesions in this area, when occipital cortex is spared, have produced cases of impaired visual imagery with relatively preserved perceptual function.[155] Given that the contrary dissociation has also been observed with pure occipital lesions leading to cortical blindness, or impaired perception with preserved visual imagery, the combination seems to indicate a likely dissociation in neuroanatomic bases for the two processes. There is also evidence that mental images are formed based upon categorical relations, stored predominantly in the left hemisphere, between particular features of the object, which are encoded diffusely, potentially according to the traditional view of imagery in the analogous regions to the initial perception of such an object. This evidence comes from a case of a split-brain patient who demonstrated impaired mental imagery for stimuli presented to the left hemisphere with relatively preserved imagery for stimuli presented to the right hemisphere.[156]

As the individual progresses through the Cognition Module, categorization becomes a critical component of performance. This requirement is introduced first in the form of naming additional objects in each feature identification task, then, eventually, by the generation of category names specifically. To give a specific example, the individual might be presented with nine objects, three of which are used for writing, such as a pencil, pen, and crayon; three of which are red, such as a stop sign, an apple, and a rose; and three of which are spherical, such as a baseball, an orange, and a globe. The individual's task would be to identify the similarities between the objects—namely, that they share function, color, and shape, respectively.

Categorization is also a process that is diffusely mediated. It is a complex process that has intricate interrelations with the other processes reviewed in this section. It is not surprising, then, to discover that many of the same regions are involved in this aspect of cognition. Evidence for the neuroanatomic correlates of categorization are based primarily upon lesion and image studies and are somewhat limited. A more detailed discussion of the theoretical models of categorization is provided elsewhere, but a limited review reveals several areas of importance to this discussion. Different types of categorization appear to be mediated by different anatomic constituents. Exemplar similarity categorization is dependent upon explicit memory and has been demonstrated to involve medial temporal and diencephalic structures.[75] The dorsolateral PFC has also been implicated in rule-based categorization, particularly when task switching is involved.[75,82] Category naming tasks demonstrate activation of the left-hemisphere angular gyrus[79] or, if they are presented in picture form, the occipital cortex.[80] Generally speaking, the left hemisphere appears to be important in categorization relative to the right hemisphere. Left anterior hemisphere lesions lead to rigid categorical boundaries consistent with impaired cognitive flexibility observed with injury to the PFC.[95] Left posterior hemisphere lesions lead to weak categorical boundaries[95] and inability to categorize pictures or words.[96,97]

Now that we have characterized the underlying neurobiologic systems that are implicated in the task of the Cognition Module, what follows is a theoretical discussion of how these structures relate to the goal of therapy—namely, problem solving. To explore this, we will return to the opening example and discuss the complex interplay between the various cognitive systems involved. This example is intended to be illustrative rather than complete, because this example could be discussed at length in this context.

In the case of an individual who has dropped an item—say, car keys—between the seats, it is easy to demonstrate the complicated manner in which these systems are involved, influence and are influenced by the other systems, and mediate everyday problem solving. Beginning at the outset of the event, attention must be directed to what has happened in order for a problem to be recognized. Attention to the event and the subsequent task of recovering the keys must be maintained throughout the process. In addition, attentional processes must be modified over the course of the recovery to adjust to different needs. For example, in the first case, working memory must be involved to store the properties of the various objects involved and their relationship to one another. The properties of the keys, for example, must be attended to and held in working memory so they may be assessed for salience. In this case, their size, weight, and construction might prove to be useful, and so they must be selectively attended to and then held in working memory. If the strategy for recovery were to include the use of a magnetic object, then construction would become a particularly salient feature. If the strategy were to lift or push the keys free, then the size and weight would become most salient. Information gathered by the individual that has importance for which of these strategies is preferable must also be held in working memory and would be used to modify the attentional process to refer to these particular perceptual features.

In this case, assume that the strategy chosen is to push or lift the keys free. In this scenario, what becomes necessary is to determine which attributes of an object would be required for success, assess the attributes of an object that might be used to achieve this task, and determine whether these attributes fulfill the criteria required for success. Specifically, the task involved here might require an object that is sufficiently long to reach the object, thin enough to fit in the space between the seats, and sturdy enough to lift or push the keys free. In determining this set of requirements, the individual must attend to and hold in working memory the salient perceptual features of the space between the seat and the center console as well as the keys themselves. When assessing a potential object, top-down attentional control systems must be used to modify the attentional system, increasing the salience of these features to the exclusion of other stimuli. Retrieval of semantic and episodic memories will also inform the individual of potential objects and their attributes that may not be directly available to the individual's sensorium. For example, the individual might recall from semantic memory stores that a pencil is long, thin, and relatively sturdy, and, from declarative memory, that one was placed in the glove box the day before. Obviously, visual imagery is inherent to some of these processes as well. Lastly, categorization could impact the process via the use of previous categorization to produce suitable (i.e. long, thin, sturdy) objects.

Throughout the problem-solving task, then, it is apparent that various cognitive systems are implicated, along with their various neuroanatomic and neurophysiologic counterparts. In reviewing these counterparts, it becomes clear that such a task involves widespread structures, not all of which have been clearly elucidated. What also seems reasonable then, is that a therapeutic intervention aimed at remediation of such processes should attempt to recapitulate the process in a systematic fashion. This would involve the various neuroanatomic structures and neurophysiologic mechanisms involved, and this, in fact, forms some of the theoretical basis for the Cognition Module as a therapeutic intervention.

19.10 Summary

Cognitive rehabilitation for people with TBI is a crucial component of the rehabilitative process. Although compensatory practices have some appeal as a result of the financial and length-of-stay constraints imposed upon treatment, remediative practices should be undertaken for cognitive deficits following TBI. Compensatory strategies should only be introduced as tools to supplement cognitive function. Remediative practices must be based upon sound theoretical constructs and be in harmony with known functional attributes of the neurologic system. Likewise, cognitive rehabilitation must be approached like any other acquired skill set—that is, hierarchically or developmentally. The interrelated nature of cognitive functions must be respected in undertaking therapeutic interventions. Finally, broadly based cognitive evaluation should be undertaken before and after treatment to evaluate and document improved function across cognitive domains.

References

1. Technology Evaluation Center, Blue Cross Blue Shield Association, Cognitive rehabilitation for traumatic brain injury in adults, *TEC Assessment Program*, 23(5), 1–28, 2008.
2. Cicerone, K. D., Dahlberg, C., Kalmar, K., Langenbahn, D. M., Malec, J. F., Bergquist, T. F., et al., Evidence-based cognitive rehabilitation: Recommendations for clinical practice, *Archives of Physical Medicine and Rehabilitation*, 81(12), 1596–1615, 2000.

3. Cicerone, K. D., Dahlberg, C., Malec, J. F., Langenbahn, D. M., Felicetti, T., Kneipp, S., et al., Evidence-based cognitive rehabilitation: Updated review of the literature from 1998 through 2002, *Archives of Physical Medicine and Rehabilitation*, 86(8), 1681–1692, 2005.

4. Rohling, M. L., Faust, M. E., Beverly, B., and Demakis, G., Effectiveness of cognitive rehabilitation following acquired brain injury: A meta-analytic reexamination of Cicerone et al.'s (2000, 2005) systematic reviews, *Neuropsychology*, 23(1), 20–39, 2009.

5. Constantinidou, F., Thomas, R. D., and Robinson, L., Benefits of categorization training in patients with traumatic brain injury during post-acute rehabilitation: Additional evidence from a randomized controlled trial, *Journal of Head Trauma Rehabilitation*, 23(5), 312–328, 2008.

6. Constantinidou, F., Thomas, R. D., Scharp, V. L., Laske, K. M., Hammerly, M. D., and Guitonde, S., Effects of categorization training in patients with TBI during postacute rehabilitation, *Journal of Head Trauma Rehabilitation*, 20(2), 143–157, 2005.

7. Thomas, C. L. (Ed.), *Taber's Cyclopedic Medical Dictionary*, 17th ed., F. A. Davis, Philadelphia, PA, 1993.

8. Coelho, C. A., DeRuyter, F., and Stein, M., Treatment efficacy: Cognitive–communicative disorders resulting from traumatic brain injury in adults, *Journal of Speech and Hearing Research*, 39(5), S5–S17, 1996.

9. Reed, K. M. and Seal, G. S., Neurocognitive remediation: What is it and who does it?, *The Journal of Care Management*, 4(5), 18–19, 21–22, 1998.

10. Neisser, U., *Cognitive Psychology*, Appleton, New York, 1967.

11. American Speech–Language–Hearing Association, Guidelines for speech–language pathologists serving persons with language, socio-communicative and/or cognitive–communicative impairments, *American Speech-Language-Hearing Association*, 32, 85–92, 1990.

12. Harley, J. P., Allen, C., Braciszeski, T. L., Cicerone, K. D., Dahlberg, C., Evans, S., et al., Guidelines for cognitive rehabilitation, *Neurorehabilitation*, 2(3), 62–67, 1992.

13. Tulving, E., How many memory systems are there?, *American Psychologist*, 40(4), 385, 1985.

14. Amaral, D. G., A functional organization of perception and movement, in E. R. Kandel, J. H. Schwartz, and T. M. Jessell (Eds.), *Principles of Neural Science*, 4th ed., McGraw-Hill, New York, 337–348, 2000.

15. Posner, M. I., Attention: The mechanisms of consciousness, *Proceedings of the National Academy of Sciences of the United States of America*, 91(16), 7398–7403, 1994.

16. Davies, D. R., Jones, D. M., and Taylor, A. (Eds.), *Selective and Sustained Attention: Individual and Group Differences*, Academic Press, New York, 1984.

17. Sturm, W. and Willmes, K., On the functional neuroanatomy of intrinsic and phasic alertness, *Neuroimage*, 14(1), S76–S84, 2001.

18. Norman, D. A. and Shallice, T., Attention to action: Willed and automatic control of behaviour, in R. Davidson, G. Schwartz, and D. Shapiro (Eds.), *Consciousness and Self-Regulation: Advances in Research and Theory*, Plenum Press, New York, 376–389, 1986.

19. Scheibel, M. E. and Scheibel, A. B., Structural organization of nonspecific thalamic nuclei and their projection toward cortex, *Brain Research*, 6(1), 60–94, 1967.

20. Gummow, L., Miller, P., and Dustman, R. E., Attention and brain injury: A case for cognitive rehabilitation of attentional deficits, *Clinical Psychology Review*, 3(3), 255, 1983.

21. Posner, M. I., Psychobiology of attention, in M. S. Gazzaniga and C. Blakemore (Eds.), *Handbook of Psychobiology*, Academic Press, New York, 441, 1975.

22. Goldberg, M. E. and Wurtz, R. H., Activity of superior colliculus in behaving monkey. II. Effect of attention on neuronal responses, *Journal of Neurophysiology*, 35(4), 560–574, 1972.

23. Kahneman, D., *Attention and Effort*, Prentice-Hall, Englewood Cliffs, NJ, 1973.

24. Bares, M. and Rektor, I., Basal ganglia involvement in sensory and cognitive processing: A depth electrode CNV study in human subjects, *Clinical Neurophysiology*, 112(11) 2022–2030, 2001.

25. Nieoullon, A., Dopamine and the regulation of cognition and attention, *Progress in Neurobiology*, 67(1), 53–83, 2002.

26. Herrero, M. T., Barcia, C., and Navarro, M., Functional anatomy of thalamus and basal ganglia, *Childs Nervous System*, 18(8), 386–404, 2002.

27. Nauta, W. J., Circuitous connections linking cerebral cortex, limbic system, and corpus striatum, in B. K. Doane and K. F. Livingston (Eds.), *The Limbic System: Functional Organization and Clinical Disorders*, Raven Press, New York, 43, 1986.

28. Trexler, L. E. and Zappala, G., Neuropathological determinants of acquired attention disorders in traumatic brain injury, *Brain and Cognition*, 8(3), 291–302, 1988.

29. Daube, J. R., Sandok, B. A., Reagon, T. J., and Westmoreland, B. F., *Medical Neurosciences: An Approach to Anatomy, Pathology, and Physiology by Systems and Levels*, Little, Brown, Boston, 1978.

30. Naatanen, R., Orienting and evoked potential, in H. D. Kimmel, E. H. Van Olst, and J. F. Orlebeke (Eds.), *The Orienting Reflex in Humans*, Wiley, New York, 61–75, 1979.

31. Watson, R. T., Heilman, K. M., Cauthen, J. C., and King, F. A., Neglect after cingulectomy, *Neurology*, 23(9), 1003–1007, 367–401, 1973.

32. Heilman, K. M. and Valenstein, E., Frontal lobe neglect in man, *Neurology*, 22(6), 660–664, 1972.

33. Goodglass, H. and Kaplan, E., Assessment of cognitive deficit in the brain-injured patient, in M. S. Gazzaniga (Ed.), *Handbook of Behavioral Neurobiology*, vol. 2, Plenum Press, New York, 1979.

34. Mesulam, M. M. and Geschwind, N., On the possible role of neocortex and its limbic connections in the process of attention and schizophrenia: Clinical cases of inattention in man and experimental anatomy in monkey, *Journal of Psychiatric Research*, 14(1–4), 249–259, 1978.

35. Thompson, R. F. and Bettinger, L. A., Neural substrates of attention, in D. L. Mostofsky (Ed.), *Attention: Contemporary Theory and Analysis*, Appleton, New York, 367–401, 1970.

36. Posner, M. I. and Snyder, C. R., Facilitation and inhibition in the processing of signals, in P. M. A. Rabbitt (Ed.), *Attention and Performance V*, Academic Press, New York, 669–698, 1975.

37. Kahneman, D., Remarks on attention control, *Acta Psychologica*, 33, 118–131, 1970.

38. Schneider, W. and Shiffrin, R. M., Controlled and automatic human information processing: II. Perceptual learning, automatic attending and a general theory, *Psychological Review*, 84(2), 127–190, 1977.

39. Anderson, J. R., *Cognitive Psychology and Its Implications*, W. H. Freeman, San Francisco, CA, 1980.

40. Duncan, J., The locus of interference in the perception of simultaneous stimuli, *Psychological Review*, 87(3), 272–300, 1980.

41. Posner, M. I., Attention in cognitive neuroscience: An overview, in M. S. Gazzaniga (Ed.), *The Cognitive Neurosciences*, MIT Press, Cambridge, MA, 615–624, 1995.

42. Treisman, A. M., Verbal cues, language, and meaning in selective attention, *American Journal of Psychology*, 77(2), 206–219, 1964.

43. Hillyard, S. A., Mangun, G. R., Woldorff, M. G., and Luck, S. J., Neural systems mediating selective attention, in M. S. Gazzaniga (Ed.), *The Cognitive Neurosciences*, MIT Press, Cambridge, MA, 665–681, 1995.

44. Spurling, G. A., The information available in brief presentation, *Psychological Monographs*, 74(11), 498, 1960.

45. Moray, N., Bates, A., and Barnett, T., Experiments on the four-eared man, *Journal of the Acoustical Society of America*, 38(2), 196–206, 1965.

46. Darwin, C. J., Turvy, M. T., and Crowder, R. G., The auditory analog of the Sperling partial report procedure: Evidence for brief auditory storage, *Cognitive Psychology*, 3(2), 255, 1972.

47. Galan, R. F., Weidert, M., Menzel, R., Herz, A. V. M., and Galizia, C. G., Sensory memory for odors is encoded in spontaneous correlated activity between olfactory glomeruli, *Neural Computation*, 18(1), 10–25, 2006.

48. Kaas, A. L., van Mier, H., and Goebel, R., The neural correlates of human working memory for haptically explored object orientations, *Cerebral Cortex*, 17(7), 1637–1649, 2007.

49. Shiffrin, R. M. and Atkinson, R. C., Storage and retrieval processes in long-term memory, *Psychological Review*, 76(2), 179–193, 1969.

50. Baddeley, A. D., Estimating the short-term component in free recall, *Quarterly Journal of Experimental Psychology*, 61(1), 13–15, 1970.

51. Murdock, B. B., Short-term memory, in G. H. Bower (Ed.), *Psychology of Learning and Motivation*, Academic Press, New York, 67–127, 1972.
52. Crannell, C. W. and Parrish, J. M., A comparison of immediate memory span for digits, letters, and words, *Journal of Psychology*, 44, 319–327, 1957.
53. Craig, F. I. M. and Masani, P. A., Age and intelligence differences in coding and retrieval of word lists, *British Journal of Psychology*, 60(3), 315–319, 1969.
54. van Zomerer, A. H. and Brouwer, W. H., *Clinical Neuropsychology of Attention*, Oxford University Press, New York, 1994.
55. Ziino, C. and Ponsford, J., Selective attention deficits and subjective fatigue following traumatic brain injury, *Neuropsychology*, 20(3), 383–390, 2006.
56. Olson, D. R., Language and thought: Aspects of a cognitive theory of semantics, *Psychological Review*, 77(4), 257–273, 1970.
57. Rosch, E., On the internal structure of perceptual and semantic categories, in T. Moor (Ed.), *Cognitive Development and the Acquisition of Language*, Academic Press, New York, 111–144, 1973.
58. Rosch, E., Universals and cultural specifics in human categorization, in R. W. Brislin, S. Bochner, and W. J. Lonner (Eds.), *Cross-Cultural Perspectives on Learning*, Wiley, New York, 177–206, 1975.
59. Voss, J. F., On the relationship of associative and organizational processes, in E. Tulving and W. Donaldson (Eds.), *Organization of Memory*, Academic Press, New York, 174, 1972.
60. Craik, F. I. and Lockhart, R. S., Levels of processing: A framework for memory research, *Journal of Verbal Learning and Verbal Behavior*, 11(6), 671–684, 1972.
61. Eidelberg, E. and Schwartz, A. S., Experimental analysis of the extinction phenomenon in monkeys, *Brain*, 94(1), 91–108, 1971.
62. Mandler, G., Organization and memory, in K. W. Spence and J. T. Spence (Eds.), *The Psychology of Learning and Motivation*, Academic Press, New York, 327–372, 1967.
63. Mandler, G., Pearlstone, Z, and Koopmans, H. S., Effects of organization and semantic similarity on recall and recognition, *Journal of Verbal Learning and Verbal Behavior*, 8, 410, 1969.
64. Sokovlov, E. N., *Perception and the Conditioned Reflex*, Macmillan, New York, 1963.
65. Odom, R. D. and Corbin, D. W., Perceptual salience and children's multidimensional problem solving, *Child Development*, 44(3), 425–432, 1973.
66. Caron, A., Discrimination shifts in three year olds as a function of dimensional salience, *Developmental Psychology*, 1, 333, 1969.
67. Odom, R. D. and Guzman, R. D., Problem solving and the perceptual salience of variability and constancy: A developmental study, *Journal of Experimental Child Psychology*, 9(2), 156–165, 1970.
68. Saltz, E. and Sigel, I. E., Concept over-discrimination in children, *Journal of Experimental Psychology*, 73(1), 1–8, 1967.
69. Kagan, J., Reflectivity–impulsivity and reading ability in primary grade children, *Child Development*, 36, 609, 1965.
70. Kagan, J., Developmental studies in reflectional analysis, in A. Kidd and J. Rivoire (Eds.), *Perceptual Developments in Children*, International University Press, New York, 487, 1966.
71. Wayland, S. and Taplin, J. E., Feature-processing deficits following brain injury. I. Overselectivity in recognition memory for compound stimuli, *Brain and Cognition*, 4(3), 338–355, 1985.
72. Tyler, S., *Cognitive Anthropology*, Holt, Rinehart and Winston, New York, 1969.
73. Bruner, J., Goodnow, J., and Austin, G., *A Study of Thinking*, Science Editions, New York, 1956.
74. Clark, H. and Clark, E., *Psychology and Language*, Harcourt, Brace & Jovanovich, New York, 1977.
75. Smith, E. E. and Jonides, J., The cognitive neuroscience of categorization, in M. S. Gazzaniga (Ed.), *The New Cognitive Neurosciences*, 2nd ed., MIT Press, Cambridge, MA, 1013–1022, 2000.
76. Bowerman, M., Semantic factors in the acquisition of rules for word use and sentence construction, in D. Morehead and R. Morehead (Eds.), *Normal and Deficient Child Language*, University Park Press, Baltimore, MD, 1976.

77. Rosch, E., Classification of real-world objects: Origins and representations in cognition, in P. N. Johnson-Lair and P. C. Watson (Eds.), *Thinking: Readings in Cognitive Science*, Cambridge University Press, Cambridge, MA, 212–277, 1976.

78. Rosch, E. and Mervis, C. B., Basic objects in natural categories, *Cognitive Psychology*, 8(3), 383–439, 1976.

79. Grossman, M., Robinson, K., and Jaggi, J., The neural basis for semantic memory: Converging evidence from Alzheimer's disease, *Brain and Language*, 55, 96–98, 1996.

80. Kosslyn, S. M., Alpert, H. M., and Thompson, W. L., Identifying objects at different levels of hierarchy: A positron emission tomography study, *Human Brain Mapping*, 3(2), 107–132, 1995.

81. Heaton, R. K., Chelune, G. J., Talley, J. L., Kay, G. G., and Curtiss, G., *Wisconsin Card Sorting Test Manual, Revised and Expanded*, Psychological Assessment Resources, Odessa, FL, 1993.

82. D'Esposito, M., Detre, J. A., Alsop, D. C., Shin, R. K., Atlas, S., and Grossman, M., The neural basis of the central executive system of working memory, *Nature*, 378(6554), 279–281, 1995.

83. Smith, E. E. and Jonides, J., The cognitive neuroscience of categorization, in M. S. Gazzaniga (Ed.), *The New Cognitive Neurosciences*, 2nd ed., MIT Press, Cambridge, MA, 1013–1022, 2000.

84. Rosch, E. and Mervic, C. B., Family resemblances: Studies in the internal structure of categories, *Cognitive Psychology*, 7(4), 573–605, 1975.

85. Rosch, E., Simpson, C., and Miller, R. S., Structural bases of typicality effects, *Journal of Experimental Psychology*, 2(4), 491–502, 1976.

86. Smitt, E. E., Shoben, E. J., and Rips, L. J., Structure and process in semantic memory: A featural model for semantic decisions, *Psychological Review*, 81(3), 214–241, 1974.

87. Rips, L. J., Inductive judgments about natural categories, *Journal of Verbal Learning and Verbal Behavior*, 14(6), 665–681, 1975.

88. Shoben, E. J., The verification of semantic relations in a same–different paradigm: An asymmetry in semantic memory, *Journal of Verbal Learning and Verbal Behavior*, 15(4), 365–379, 1976.

89. Rips, L. J., Shoben, E. J., and Smith, E. E., Semantic distance and the verification of semantic relations, *Journal of Verbal Learning and Verbal Behavior*, 12(1), 1–20, 1973.

90. Smith, E. E., Rips, L. J., and Shoben, E. J., Semantic memory and psychological semantics, in G. H. Bower (Ed.), *The Psychology of Learning and Motivation*, Academic Press, New York, 1974.

91. Bowleska, A., Some aspects of conceptual organization in aphasics with naming disturbances, *Zeitschrift fur Psychologie mit Zeitschrift fur angewandte Psychologie*, 189, 67, 1981.

92. Glucksberg, S. and Weisberg, R. W., Verbal behavior and problem solving: Some effects of labeling in a functional fixedness problem, *Journal of Experimental Psychology*, 71(5), 659–664, 1966.

93. Vygotsky, L., *Thought and Language*, MIT Press, Cambridge, MA, 1986.

94. Hartley, L. L. and Jensen, P. J., Narrative and procedural discourse after closed head injury, *Brain Injury*, 5(3), 267–285, 1991.

95. Grossman, M. and Wilson, M., Stimulus categorization by brain-damaged patients, *Brain and Cognition*, 6(1), 55–71, 1987.

96. Lhermitte, F., Derouesne, J., and Lecours, A. R., Contribution a l'etude des troubles semantiques dans l'aphasie [Contribution to the study of semantic disorders in aphasia], *Revue Neurologie (Paris)*, 125(2), 81–101, 1971.

97. Goldstein, K., *Language and Language Disorders*, Grune and Stratton, New York, 1948.

98. Caramazza, A., Berndt, R. S., and Brownell, H. H., The semantic deficit hypothesis: Perceptual parsing and object classification by aphasic patients, *Brain and Language*, 15(1), 161–189, 1982.

99. Grossman, M., The figurative representation of a superordinate's referents after brain damage, Presented at the meeting of the International Neuropsychological Society, San Francisco, CA, 1980, Feb.

100. Cavalli, M., De Renzi, E., Faglioni, P., and Vitale, A., Impairment of right brain-damaged patients on a linguistic cognitive task, *Cortex*, 17(4), 545–555, 1981.

101. Gainotti, G., Caltagirone, C., Miceli, G., and Masullo, C., Selective semantic–lexical impairment of language comprehension in right-brain-damaged patients, *Brain and Language*, 13(2), 201–211, 1981.

102. Grober, E., Perecman, E., Kellar, L., and Brown, J., Lexical knowledge in anterior and posterior aphasies, *Brain and Language*, 10(2), 318–330, 1980.

103. Grossman, M., The game of the name: An examination of linguistic reference after brain damage, *Brain and Language*, 6(1), 112–119, 1978.
104. Hough, M. S., Categorization in aphasia: Access and organization of goal-derived and common categories, *Aphasiology*, 7(4), 335–357, 1993.
105. Channon, S., Daum, I., and Polkey, C. E., The effect of categorization on verbal memory after temporal lobectomy, *Neuropsychologia*, 27(6), 777–785, 1989.
106. Hirst, W. and Volpe, B. T., Memory strategies with brain damage, *Brain and Cognition*, 8(3), 379–408, 1988.
107. Damasio, H., Grabowski, T. J., Tranel, D., Ponto, L. L., Hichwa, R. D., and Damasio, A. R., Neural correlates of naming actions and of naming spatial relations, *Neuroimage*, 13(6 Pt.1), 1053–1064, 2001.
108. Saykin, A. J., Johnson, S. C., Flashman, L. A., McAllister, T. W., Sparling, M., Darcey, T. M., et al., Functional differentiation of medial temporal and frontal regions involved in processing novel and familiar words: An fMRI study, *Brain*, 122(Pt. 10), 1963–1971, 1999.
109. Smith, C. D., Andersen, A. H., Dryscio, R. J., Schmitt, F. A., Kindy, M. S., Blonder, L. X., et al., Differences in functional magnetic resonance imaging activation by category in a visual confrontation naming task, *Journal of Neuroimaging*, 11(2), 165–170, 2001.
110. Piaget, J., *Play, Dreams, and Imitation in Childhood*, Norton, New York, 1962.
111. Martin, A., Ungerleider, L. G., and Haxby, J. V., Category specificity and the brain: The sensory/motor model of semantic representations of objects, in M. S. Gazzaniga (Ed.), *The New Cognitive Neurosciences*, 2nd ed., MIT Press, Cambridge, MA, 1023–1036, 2000.
112. Fuster, J. M., The prefrontal cortex—An update: Time is of the essence, *Neuron*, 30(2), 319–333, 2001.
113. Burger, R. A. and Muma, J. R., Cognitive distancing in mediated categorization in aphasia, *Journal of Psycholinguistic Research*, 9(4), 355–365, 1980.
114. Muma, J. R., *Language Handbook: Concepts, Assessment, Intervention*, Prentice-Hall, Englewood Cliffs, NJ, 1978.
115. Woodcock, R. W., McGrew, K., and Mathers, N., *Woodcock Johnson–III (Tests of Cognitive Abilities)*, The Riverside Publishing Company, Itasca, IL, 2001.
116. Adamovich, B. and Henderson, J., *Scales of Cognitive Ability for Traumatic Brain Injury*, Applied Symbolix, Chicago, IL, 1992.
117. Muma, J. R. and Muma, D. B., *Muma Assessment Program*, Natural Child Publishing Company, Lubbock, TX, 1979.
118. Ross, D., *Ross Information Processing Assessment*, Pro-Ed, Austin, TX, 1986.
119. Bontke, C. F., Lehmkuhl, L. D., Englander, J., Mann, N., Ragnarsson, K. T., Zasler, N. D., et al., Medical complications and associated injuries of persons treated in the traumatic brain injury model systems programs, *Journal of Head Trauma Rehabilitation*, 8(2), 34–46, 1993.
120. Becker, D. P., Verity, M. A., Povlishock, J., and Cheung, M., Brain cellular injury and recovery: Horizons for improving medical therapies in stroke and trauma, *The Western Journal of Medicine*, 148(6), 670–684, 1988.
121. Meythaler, J. M., Peduzzi, J. D., Eleftheriou, E., and Novack, T. A., Current concepts: Diffuse axonal injury-associated traumatic brain injury, *Archives of Physical Medicine and Rehabilitation*, 82(10), 1461–1471, 2001.
122. Povlishock, J. T. and Katz, D. I., Update of neuropathology and neurological recovery after traumatic brain injury, *Journal of Head Trauma Rehabilitation*, 20(1), 76–94, 2005, Jan-Feb.
123. Büki, A. and Povlishock, J. T., All roads lead to disconnection? Traumatic axonal injury revisited, *Acta Neurochirurgica*, 148(2), 181–194, 2006.
124. Crutcher, K. A., Anatomical correlates of neuronal plasticity, in J. L. Martinez and R. P. Kesner, (Eds.), *Learning and Memory: A Biological View*, Academic Press, San Diego, CA, 1991.
125. Sirevaag, A. M., Smith, S., and Greenough, W. T., Rats reared in a complex environment have larger astrocytes with more processes than rats raised socially or individually, *Society of Neurosciences Abstracts*, 14, 1135, 1988.

126. Black, J. E., Jones, A. L., Anderson, B. J., Isaacs, K. R., Alcantra, A. A., and Greenough, W. T., Cerebellar plasticity: Preliminary evidence that learning, rather than repetitive motor exercise, alters cerebellar cortex thickness in middle-aged rats, *Society of Neurosciences Abstracts*, 13, 1596, 1987.

127. Chen, R., Cohen, L. G., and Hallett, M., Nervous system reorganization following injury, *Neuroscience*, 111(4), 761–773, 2002.

128. Little, D. M., Klein, R., Shobat, D. M., McClure, E. D., and Thulborn, K. R., Changing patterns of brain activation during category learning revealed by functional MRI, *Cognitive Brain Research*, 22(1), 84–93, 2004.

129. Little, D. M. and Thulborn, K. R., Correlations of cortical activation and behavior during the application of newly learned categories, *Cognitive Brain Research*, 25(1), 33–47, 2005.

130. Kelly, D. F., Gonzalo, I. T., Cohan, P., Berman, N., Swerdloff, R., and Wang, C., Hypopituitarism following traumatic brain injury and aneurysmal subarachnoid hemorrhage: A preliminary report, *Journal of Neurosurgery*, 93(5), 743–752, 2000.

131. Lieberman, S. A., Oberoi, A. L., Gilkison, C. R., Masel, B. E., and Urban, R. J., Prevalence of neuroendocrine dysfunction in patients recovering from traumatic brain injury, *Journal of Clinical Endocrinology and Metabolism*, 86(6), 2752–2756, 2001.

132. Bondanelli, M., Ambrosio, M. R., Cavazzini, L., Bertocchi, A., Zatelli, M. C., Carli, A., et al., Anterior pituitary function may predict functional and cognitive outcome in patients with traumatic brain injury undergoing rehabilitation, *Journal of Neurotrauma*, 24(11), 1687–1698, 2007.

133. Sohlberg, M. M. and Mateer, C. A., *Attention Process Training*, Association for Neuropsychological Research and Development, Puyallop, WA, 1989.

134. Bruner, J., The course of cognitive growth, *American Psychologist*, 19(1), 1–15, 1964.

135. Knudsen, E. I., Fundamental components of attention, *Annual Review of Neuroscience*, 30, 57–78, 2007.

136. Kolb, B. and Whishaw, I. Q., *Fundamentals of Human Neuropsychology*, 5th ed., Worth Publishers, New York, 2003.

137. Corbetta, M., Miezin, F. M., Dobmeyer, S., Shulman, G. L., and Petersen, S. E., Selective and divided attention during visual discrimination of shape, color and speed: Functional anatomy by positron emission tomography, *Journal of Neuroscience*, 11(8), 2383–2402, 1991.

138. Corbetta, M., Miezin, F. M., Shulman, G. L., and Petersen, S. E., A PET study of visuospatial attention, *Journal of Neuroscience*, 13(5), 1202–1226, 1993.

139. Petersen, S. E., Robinson, D. L., and Morris, J. D., Contributions of the pulvinar to visual spatial orientation, *Neuropsychologia*, 25(1-A), 97–106, 1987.

140. Colby, C. L. and Goldberg, M. E., Space and attention in parietal cortex, *Annual Review of Neuroscience*, 22(1), 319–349, 1999.

141. Bisley, J. W. and Goldberg, M. E., Neuronal activity in the lateral intraparietal area and spatial attention, *Science*, 299(5603), 81–86, 2003.

142. Platt, M. L. and Glimcher, P. W., Responses of intraparietal neurons to saccadic targets and visual distractors, *Journal of Neurophysiology*, 78(3), 1574–1589, 1997.

143. Sugrue, L. P., Corrado, G. S., and Newsome, W. T., Choosing the greater of two goods: Neural currencies for valuation and decision making, *Nature Reviews Neuroscience*, 6(5), 363–375, 2005.

144. Vaidya, C. J. and Stollstorff, M., Cognitive neuroscience of attention deficit hyperactivity disorder: Current status and working hypotheses, *Developmental Disabilities Research Reviews*, 14(4), 261–267, 2008.

145. Ranganath, C., Working memory for visual objects: Complementary roles of inferior temporal, medial temporal, and prefrontal cortex, *Neuroscience*, 139(1), 277–289, 2006.

146. Curtis, C. E., Prefrontal and parietal contributions to spatial working memory, *Neuroscience*, 139(1), 173–180, 2006.

147. Schwartz, M. L. and Goldman-Rakic, P. S., Callosal and intrahemispheric connectivity of the prefrontal association cortex in rhesus monkey: Relation between intraparietal and principal sulcal cortex, *Journal of Comparative Neurology*, 226(3), 403–420, 1984.

148. Tulving, E., *Elements of Episodic Memory*, Oxford University Press, Cambridge, MA, 1983.

149. Habib, R., Nyberg, L., and Tulving, E., Hemispheric asymmetries of memory: The HERA model revisited, *Trends in Cognitive Science*, 7(6), 241–245, 2003.
150. Desgranges, B., Baron, J.- C., and Eustache, F., The functional neuroanatomy of episodic memory: The role of the frontal lobes, the hippocampal formation, and other areas, *Neuroimage*, 8(2), 198–213, 1998.
151. Barton, J. S., Press, D. Z., Keenan, J. P., and O'Connor, M., Lesions of the fusiform face area impair perception of facial configuration in prosopagnosia, *Neurology*, 58(1), 71–78, 2008.
152. Cappa, S. F., Imaging studies of semantic memory, *Current Opinion in Neurology*, 21(6), 669–675, 2008.
153. Wise, R. A., Dopamine, learning, and motivation, *Nature Reviews Neuroscience*, 5(6), 483–494, 2004.
154. Navakkode, S., Sajikumar, S., and Frey, J. U., Synergistic requirements for the induction of dopaminergic D1/D5-receptor-mediated LTP in hippocampal slices of rat CA1 in vitro, *Neuropharmacology*, 52(7), 1547–1554, 2007.
155. Bartolomeo, P., The neural correlates of visual mental imagery: An ongoing debate, *Cortex*, 44, 107–108, 2008.
156. Kosslyn, S. M., Aspects of a cognitive neuroscience of mental imagery, *Science*, 240(4859), 1621–1626, 1988.

20

The Use of Applied Behavior Analysis in Traumatic Brain Injury Rehabilitation

Craig S. Persel and Chris H. Persel

CONTENTS

20.1 Introduction

The issue of maladaptive behavior, as an associated consequence of traumatic brain injury (TBI), is one of the most important aspects in brain injury rehabilitation because behavior disorders often represent a significant barrier to effective rehabilitation and functional outcome.[1–3] Changes in personality and behavior are also familiar consequences of TBI.[4–9] During the acute stages of recovery from TBI, it is common for a person to exhibit a variety of behavior disorders.[10] Such behavioral disturbances are considered by many to be a phase of normal recovery of cognition.[11,12] When these behaviors continue beyond acute recovery, however, and begin to form standard patterns of interaction with others, genuine concern is warranted. Behavioral disorders are disturbing to families and staff,[13,14] disruptive to therapy,[15,16] and can jeopardize client safety[17]; thus, effective behavior analysis can be a powerful tool for teaching people more positive ways of interacting with their environment.

The purpose of this chapter is to illustrate clearly and simplify the concepts, techniques, and uses of applied behavior analysis with those suffering from TBI. Although it is assumed that you have some basic understanding and/or experience with applied behavior analysis, difficult technical terms have been avoided whenever possible. When only technical jargon will suffice to explain or label a particular concept or method effectively, the term is defined.

In keeping with the more practical nature of this chapter, a couple of areas related to applied behavior analysis will not be covered. First, single-subject research design will not be discussed. Although single-subject research is important to the scientific advancement of applied behavior analysis, we feel that it requires special attention that is beyond the scope of this chapter. Second, there will be no instruction for measuring interrater reliability. Substantiating agreement between independent observers is important in determining reliability of data, like single-subject research design, but it falls within the boundaries of research and not necessarily the practical application of behavior technology.

Included in this chapter are the tools necessary to organize and carry out effective behavior programming for people with TBI. The person with TBI represents a special challenge to rehabilitation professionals and family members. Maladaptive behavior is only one facet of a complex neurobehavioral picture. Cognitive, physical, and emotional changes resulting from brain injury must be taken into consideration in the overall behavioral treatment of the client with TBI. Behavioral treatment does not work alone. Behavioral programming is most effective when it is integrated with a comprehensive rehabilitation program. For example, as a client's information processing skills increase, so does the ability to deal with cognitively challenging situations. As adjustment to disability improves, the client becomes better equipped to face the loss of functional ability. As motor and perceptual skills develop, so does the opportunity to live more independently. Behavior programs provide a "metastructure" within which the various therapeutic disciplines are carried out.

The challenge is to rehabilitate people with TBI in the least restrictive setting possible.[18] Hopefully, this chapter will provide therapists, educators, family members, and other involved people with the materials and methods necessary to help clients with TBI regain their highest level of independence.

20.2 The Brain–Behavior Relationship

As many of you know, TBI can have many serious consequences. Physical, cognitive–communicative, functional, and psychological skills can be severely affected. Common areas of physical deficit are ambulation, balance and coordination, fine motor skills, strength, and endurance.[19,20] Cognitive deficits can encompass language and communication, information processing, memory, and perceptual skills.[21,22] Functional skills, such as hygiene and grooming, dressing, and money management, to name but a few, are usually affected.[23] A person's psychological status is also stressed. Depression, anxiety, adjustment to disability, and sexuality issues are frequently encountered by people with TBI.[24–28] Any or all of these difficulties may bear directly on the behavior of a client. Recent studies have even linked cognitive recovery with the degree of psychopathology.[11,29] Compound these with medical issues, such as location of damage, severity of injury, seizure disorders, as well as preinjury characteristics of personality,[30–32] intelligence,[33,34] substance abuse,[35] and learning style, and a complex neurobehavioral picture is created.

Brain injury can occur in a number of ways. TBIs, as opposed to stroke, Alzheimer's, Parkinson's, and so forth, typically result from accidents in which the head strikes an object (e.g., windshield, ground). This is the most common type of TBI. However, other acquired brain injuries, such as those caused by insufficient oxygen (e.g., cardiac arrest, near drowning, suffocation), poisoning (e.g., toxic fumes, chemicals), electrical shock, or infection (e.g., encephalitis, malaria), can cause similar deficits.[36–37] Many of the most severely behaviorally challenged clients we have worked with over the years were injured in these "less common" ways.

Mild TBI, another important category of brain injury, is characterized by one or more of the following symptoms: a brief loss of consciousness, loss of memory immediately before or after the injury, any alteration in mental state at the time of the accident, or focal neuro-logic deficits.[38] In many mild TBI cases, the person is only "dazed" yet continues to endure chronic functional, cognitive, and motor difficulties.[39,40] Some people sustain long-term effects, known as *postconcussive syndrome* (PCS).[41,42] Persons with postconcussive syndrome can experience subtle, yet significant, changes in cognition and personality [43,44] and even experience seizurelike symptoms.[45]

All of these brain injuries will influence behavior. The relationship between the brain and behavior is very complex and beyond the scope of this chapter to review comprehen-sively; however, it is important for those involved in behavioral programming to have at least a rudimentary understanding of this association because of its significant, underly-ing effect on behavior.[46] Problems such as denial, apathy, emotional lability, impulsivity, frustration, intolerance, lack of insight, inflexibility, perseveration, confabulation, lack of initiation, poor judgment and reasoning, and decreased social skills can often be linked to specific areas of brain damage.[47-52]

To begin with, most TBIs result in widespread damage to the brain. This is because the brain is "bounced" and "twisted" inside the skull during the impact of an accident. Nerve cells are torn from one another in what is known as *diffuse axonal injury*.[53-56] Localized damage also occurs when the brain is forced against the skull during the "acceleration–deceleration" phase of an accident. The brainstem, limbic system, frontal lobe, and tempo-ral lobes are particularly vulnerable in this type of injury.

The brainstem is located at the base of the brain near bony areas. Aside from regulating basic arousal and vegetative functions, the brainstem is involved in attention and, thus, short-term memory skills. Deficits to these areas can lead to disorientation, frustration, and anger. The limbic system, higher up in the brain, is associated with emotions and affect. Disorders of the limbic system can result in explosive rage.[57,58] Connected to the limbic system are the temporal lobes, which are involved in many cognitive skills such as memory, language, and sequencing. Damage to the temporal lobes, or seizures in this region, have been associated with a number of behavioral disorders.[59] A part of the anterior temporal lobe, the amygdala, has been implicated in social behavior. Lesions in this area have been associated with increased fear and anxiety, and may contribute to a number of social disorders.[60] The frontal lobe is almost always injured as a result of its size (taking up 29% of total cortical space) and its location near the front of the cranium.[61] The frontal lobe, like the temporal lobes, is involved in many cognitive functions. It is also considered our emotional control center and home of the personality.[62,63] Damage to this area, result-ing in what is sometimes called *frontal lobe syndrome,* can result in decreased judgment and increased impulsivity, irritability, and aggression.[64,65] Neuroendocrine damage after TBI is receiving increasing attention because of its potential effect on recovery, function, and behavior. Consequent hormone deficiencies can directly influence the brain and result in fatigue, depression, fear, and stress.[66,67]

20.3 Medication

It is now widely recognized that pharmacologic intervention for behavioral disorders with the postacute client with TBI is not necessarily the treatment of choice.[68,69] It is much more desirable to implement behavior programs that manipulate the environment and help the client develop self-control.[70,71] Many medications used in the past with other populations to combat behavior problems may elicit more agitation from the TBI person or confuse them at a time when attention and arousal are often already problematic.[72-75] Recent studies have indicated that disorientation, which can be compounded by medications, is closely related to both physical and verbal aggression with those with TBI.[76] Recent research has also indicated that the use of neuroleptics during the acute stages of recovery can have a negative impact on recovery of cognitive function.[77] Although a number of medications, such as haloperidol, amantadine, and propranolol, have proved useful in treating behavior problems during the early stages of recovery from TBI,[78-89] the brain-injured person may experience more cognitive confusion and react with increased agitation. The use of stimulants, such as methylphenidate, to reduce behavior problems has shown mixed results.[90-92] This is not to say that medications should never be used, but there should be careful monitoring of the interactive effects of medication with behavior, as well as awareness of the potential for oversedation, increased seizure activity and health risks,[93,94] or chronic overuse resulting in permanent side effects for the client, such as tardive dyskinesia, motor restlessness, and others.[95-97]

The treatment setting may be such that pharmacologic management is necessary. In those unfortunate circumstances, medications should be closely monitored because they can often lose effectiveness. The choice, then, may be between prescribing no medication, trial periods of alternative medications, or medication dosages to the point of sedation. After a person has progressed beyond acute hospitalization, many behavior medications can be tapered while closely observing the person's behavior within the structure of a behavior program.[69] This approach makes it much easier to reach an educated decision regarding continuation of the medication.

20.4 Ethics

Applied behavior analysis (sometimes referred to as *behavior modification*) has always been plagued by controversy. The mere mention of behavior modification is usually enough to elicit a strong response from professionals and the public alike. For many, the use of behavior modification principles and techniques is, in some way, "forcing" a person to change against his or her will. Deep-rooted concepts regarding democracy, free will, and humanism are threatened by the notion of applying scientific methods to change human behavior.

What many of us fail to realize is that our behavior is continuously being modified. Influences from politicians and parents to television and teachers help shape and pattern our behavior. Applying behavior analysis is not meant to assume an authoritarian position over a person, but to analyze the relationship between events and behavior. The goal is to increase, not decrease, personal freedom by expanding the behavioral options available to the person, thereby enhancing opportunities for community, social, and family interaction. Such opportunities are severely restricted for people with behavior problems. Applied behavior analysis is a structured technique for reducing behaviors that limit independence and increase behaviors that empower a person.

Of course, misuse of applied behavior analysis has occurred, and punishment techniques have been overused. However, the notion that applied behavior analysis should not be used or, more specifically, that punishment should be severely limited, is neither rational nor practical. The alternatives to applied behavior analysis are typically medication,[98] physical restraint,[99,100] or life in a locked institution,[101] all of which carry their own ethical ramifications.[102] Applied behavior analysis, used within proper guidelines, is an effective and humane method for reducing maladaptive behaviors and teaching new skills.

A number of authors and governmental agencies, such as the California Department of Developmental Services, have published guidelines for positive behavioral services and procedures. The Association for Behavior Analysis *Right to Effective Treatment* statement provides the following guidelines[103]:

- An individual has a right to a therapeutic environment. A physical and social environment that is safe, humane, and responsive to individual needs is a necessary prerequisite for effective treatment.

- An individual has a right to services with the overriding goal of personal welfare. Both the immediate and long-term welfare of an individual are taken into account through active participation by the client or an authorized proxy in making treatment-related decisions.

- An individual has a right to treatment by a competent behavior analyst. Professionals responsible for delivering, directing, or evaluating the effects of behavioral treatment possess appropriate education and experience.

- An individual has a right to programs that teach functional skills. The ultimate goal of all services is to increase the ability of individuals to function effectively in both their immediate environment and the larger society.

- An individual has a right to behavioral assessment and ongoing evaluation. Prior to the onset of treatment, individuals are entitled to a complete diagnostic evaluation to identify factors that contribute to the presence of a skill deficit or a behavioral disorder.

- An individual has a right to the most effective treatment procedure available. An individual is entitled to effective and scientifically validated treatment. In turn, behavior analysts have an obligation to use only those techniques that have been demonstrated by researchers to be effective, to acquaint consumers and the public with the advantages and disadvantages of these techniques, and to search for the most optimal means of changing behavior.

As the number of people with TBI increases, rehabilitation programs will face difficult ethical questions.[104] Accountability is the key. All facilities carrying out behavior programs should have clear goals, comprehensive data collection, and the ability to provide rationale for starting, continuing, and ending a behavior program. This includes a means of closely monitoring all the previously discussed guidelines to operate ethically sound behavior programs. Applied behavior analysis is a powerful tool for changing behavior. If used correctly, clients are given the opportunity to relearn many lost skills and to become as independent as possible in the shortest amount of time.

20.5 General Management Guidelines

The environmental conditions posed by treatment and care settings for people with TBI can have a significant impact on behavior. Organizing the therapeutic setting and carefully planning an approach to the client can increase opportunities for successful learning and decrease the chances of a behavioral episode. The following are 10 recommendations for structuring a positive learning environment for the person with TBI:

1. Allow for rest time. People with TBI, especially during the initial stages of recovery, can be extremely fatigued.[105,106] Monitor the person's behavior and schedule rest periods during those times related to an increased probability of problem behavior. A word of warning, though, do not forget to reduce these rest periods as the person recovers and gains endurance.

2. Keep the environment simple. People with TBI are easily overstimulated by their surroundings. The inability to filter out external stimuli can lead to confusion and increase the chances of a behavioral episode. Interruptions and distractions should be kept to a minimum and the therapy session format should be kept consistent.

3. Keep instructions simple. Instructions, prompts, and cues should be kept as concrete and simple as possible. This may mean writing down instructions as well as stating them. It may also mean keeping verbal prompts to a minimum. Many people with TBI have difficulty processing auditory information. Instead, try using nonverbal instruction techniques such as modeling (demonstrating) or gesturing.

4. Give feedback and set goals. Self-monitoring skills can be diminished in those with TBI,[107,108] who must rely on others to provide feedback until the ability is relearned.[109–111] Provide frequent and consistent positive feedback of success. Most people respond well to supportive encouragement. Setting goals helps clients predict where they are "going" with therapy and provides them with some incentive for completing therapeutic tasks.[112,113]

5. Be calm and redirect to task. People who cannot control their own behavior need others to demonstrate and produce a stable, nonthreatening environment. Remaining calm while the client is escalated can help reduce agitation and decrease the chances of inadvertently reinforcing the client with attention for acting out. A related method gaining widespread attention, "gentle teaching," uses a variation of this approach as a central technique.[114–116] It involves ignoring the exhibited behavior, redirecting the client to the task,[117] and rewarding successful performance. However, "gentle teaching's" rather unstructured approach, lack of scientific support, and philosophic assumptions contrast sharply with traditional behavior analysis.[118]

6. Provide choices. Research indicates that providing clients with choices can reduce serious behavior problems[119] and increase on-task behavior.[120] Giving them opportunities to choose tasks can be an effective technique when working with those with TBI. It allows clients an element of freedom and a measure of control over their environment. Some clients, however, require "limited" choices that decrease the range of decisions so that they are not overwhelmed or left with an open-ended opportunity to say no.

7. Decrease chance of failure. Do not work above the client's level of ability. This will only lead to frustration and increase the chance of a behavioral episode. Try to keep the success rate above 80%. This ensures that the client is challenged, while at the same time feeling successful. A variation of this technique is known as *behavioral momentum.* This procedure involves presenting tasks with which the client is likely to comply immediately before presenting tasks that are likely to be more problematic.[121] This establishes a high rate of performance (and, hopefully,

reinforcement) just prior to more difficult tasks, with the idea that compliance will be more likely to continue.

8. Vary activities. Although there is a need for consistency and repetition when working with the person with TBI, there is also a need to keep the session interesting. Therapy can become boring and frustrating if the same tasks are endlessly repeated. Vary the activities to maintain interest and increase success. Also, try interspersing easy tasks (those likely to be done correctly) among more difficult tasks. Studies have shown this procedure to be effective in reducing the likelihood of aggression.[122]

9. Overplan. Do not approach a session with only a few ideas or activities to complete. There will be days when the client finishes everything quickly and you are left with nothing else to do, or the client may be having a difficult time (e.g., more confused) and you need some alternate activities more suited to the functioning of the client that day. Be prepared for anything, and confronting a behavior problem will be less likely.

10. Analyze tasks. Try dividing a task into smaller steps. Each step can then be treated as a complete task. Functional skills, such as dressing, hygiene, grooming, and so forth, are particularly suited to this approach[123]; however, just about any activity or task can be divided into its component parts. Breaking down a task also increases the opportunity to reinforce the individual for participation and/or completion of the various steps.

20.6 Basic Principles

The basic principles of applied behavior analysis are relatively easy to understand. Within a short time, most of the fundamental concepts of behavior analysis, and what is termed *operant conditioning,* can be grasped. Simply put, behavior analysis focuses on the *behavior* of people and the environmental influences that precede and follow the behavior, as opposed to their thoughts and feelings. We can refer to these factors as a person's *behavioral condition.* The components of a person's behavioral condition are the *antecedent,* the *behavior,* and the *consequence.* Behavior analysis attempts to explain the relationship between these components. This relationship is referred to as a *contingency.* For example, reinforcers are delivered "contingent" upon performance of a certain behavior.

20.6.1 Antecedent

To begin with, all *target behaviors* (those behaviors to be modified) are preceded by some event in the person's environment. This preceding event is called the *antecedent.* This event can be a broad-based condition that influences behavior (the setting event) or a more specific stimulus (the stimulus event). In a manner of speaking, the setting event "sets" the stage for the occurrence of the behavior (e.g., fatigue resulting from lack of sleep may be a setting event for behavior problems the next day).[124] Stimulus events are more discrete. For example, a phone ringing means that a behavior (answering the phone) will be reinforced (talking to someone). The antecedent may be an event occurring externally to the person (e.g., lighting, noises, instructions) or internally to the person (e.g., headache, flu, seizure, medication). One word of caution: Even though one has to take into consideration internal antecedents to behavior, the focus of behavior analysis is always on those factors external to the person. Internal antecedents to behavior (e.g., vestibular sensitivity, headache) are best dealt with via medical and therapeutic disciplines within the rehabilitation regimen.

Recently, behavior analysts have increasingly used the term *motivating operations* to refer to environmental events (antecedents) that establish whether a behavior will be affected by a consequence.[125] These can include *establishing operations* that increase effectiveness of consequence and *abolishing operations* that decrease effectiveness of consequences. For example, if a person is hungry, he or she is more likely to engage in behavior that results in being fed (establishing operation). If the person is not hungry, he or she is less likely to engage in the behavior (abolishing operation).

It is important for staff members to realize that external antecedents are under staff control. Tone of voice, body language, therapeutic demands, and physical setting are some of the variables that staff can adjust to decrease the likelihood of a behavioral episode.[126–128]

Necessary tasks, however, should not be avoided simply because they can, at times, be antecedents to behavioral episodes. Continued progress toward independence is often reliant on the person's participation in such tasks at a very intense level of rehabilitation.[129,130] Avoidance of difficult therapy tasks to reduce "problem" behaviors can be very seductive to staff, but it may simultaneously teach the client to exhibit more negative behavior as a means of escaping the rigorous demands of therapy.[131] Therapists and behavioral programmers need to survey all environmental antecedents and weigh the advantages and disadvantages of the therapeutic regimen before eliminating or modifying any requirements. Lowering therapeutic expectations because of potential acting out by the person may negatively impact the person's long-term independence. In fact, behavior programs are not a separate treatment, rather they are integrated with the therapeutic plan and run simultaneous to rehabilitative treatment.

Likewise, internal antecedents should be evaluated for other potential treatments that may assist in the person's behavioral improvement. These should not be viewed as reasons to avoid implementation of a behavioral program. Let us say, for example, that a person has a vestibular lesion that causes him to be quite sensitive to motion. One day, after a motor vehicle trip, the person is not feeling well and, during therapy, is quite escalated and trying to avoid participation. He strikes a staff member. Some therapists would be inclined to believe that the individual did not feel well and that the therapist who was struck should not have persisted in treatment. Although this reasoning may seem sound, it is limited by the fact that under no circumstances is it acceptable to strike another person. Thus, the behavioral program would include recognition of the contribution of the vestibular component, but would also include a means for deescalating behavioral agitation and for responding to physical aggression.

20.6.2 Behavior

An antecedent event is followed by the occurrence of a behavior. If the behavior has been chosen for modification, either to increase or decrease, it is referred to as the *target behavior*. People with TBI can exhibit a wide variety of behaviors that require intervention. A target behavior must be observable and immediately recordable. The target behavior must also be very clearly defined in terms of observable actions.[132] This is known as an *operational definition*. Two therapists, for instance, can have very different ideas about what constitutes a behavior. For example, take the behavior of physical aggression. Does it include spitting or threatening? What about self-injurious behavior? Should throwing or breaking objects be included? Clear and concise definitions of target behaviors are critical to identifying the behaviors and to implementing programs consistently.

People with TBI can exhibit a number of maladaptive behaviors. Behavior disorders (Table 20.1) can be categorized as those of excess (occurring too often), those of deficit (not occurring often enough), and those of stimulus control (not occurring in the correct context).

Excess behaviors tend to be the most noticeable and, thus, receive the most attention from other persons. Examples of excess behavioral disorders typically seen in those with TBI are noncompliance,[133] angry language,[134] hoarding,[135] escaping,[136] physical aggression,[137] socially inappropriate talk,[138] impulsivity,[139] and tardiness.[140] Some other excess behaviors that may be exhibited are sexually aberrant behavior, perseveration, self-abuse, stealing, property destruction, and overfamiliarity. These behaviors can be disruptive to other clients, can frighten others, and/or can increase the risk of injury during treatment, thus increasing exposure to legal liability. If severe enough, they can result in a person not receiving proper therapeutic services or, worse yet, being isolated from family, friends, and community in an institutional setting.

Common deficit behaviors of people with TBI are activities of daily living,[141] communication,[142] social skills,[143,144] and initiation.[145] Rehabilitation of these skills is of paramount importance in a client's progress toward more independent living. It is also important that excess behaviors that have been eliminated or reduced through structured behavioral programming be replaced with more appropriate behaviors occurring at a proper rate. Such behaviors will allow the client access to a wider range of naturally occurring reinforcers, thereby increasing the opportunity for successful generalization and maintenance of skills.

Stimulus control disorders can occur with any behavior that occurs during the wrong situation (e.g., brushing teeth, hugging another person). For example, the behavior may occur at the wrong time or place, or with the wrong person. The problem of stimulus control as a behavioral disorder has not been fully explored in TBI literature, even though there are indications it is a very common problem with this population. Most people with

TABLE 20.1

Behavior Categories and Examples

Excess	Deficit	Stimulus Control
Noncompliance	Compliance	Overfamiliarity
Angry language	Self-control	Public sexual behavior
Socially inappropriate talk	Social skills	Public grooming behavior
Disinhibition	Timeliness	Public discussion of private events
Physical aggression	Initiation	Undressing in public
Escaping	Activities of daily living	
Hoarding		
Tardiness		
Impulsivity		
Sexually aberrant		
Perseveration		
Self-abuse		
Stealing		
Property destruction		
Overfamiliarity		

TBI are adults who have already acquired many life skills. Their injury does not necessarily result in loss of the skill but, seemingly, loss of knowledge of the more abstract "situation" in which the behavior should occur. Antecedent or stimulus control behavior programs are tailor-made to impact these disorders positively.

20.6.3 Consequence

Target behaviors are followed by a consequent event that is going to affect the future rate, duration, and/or intensity of the behavior. Consequences are either "reinforcing" or "punishing." Reinforcers will increase and punishers will decrease the future occurrence of the target behavior. Consequences do not inherently possess the quality of being either a reinforcer or a punisher. The effect of the consequent event on the frequency of a target behavior (i.e., whether it increases or decreases the target behavior) defines it as a reinforcer or a punisher. Let us use chocolate as an example. For a person who likes chocolate, its use after the occurrence of a behavior may increase the frequency of that behavior, thereby defining it as a reinforcer. For a person who dislikes chocolate, its use may actually decrease the frequency of a target behavior, thus defining it as a punisher.

There are two types of positive reinforcers: *primary* and *secondary*. Primary reinforcers do not require any type of special training to develop their value. Food and water are two examples of primary reinforcers. Secondary reinforcers have gained their value through learning. Examples of secondary reinforcers are praise and money. Secondary reinforcers can be developed by pairing them with a primary reinforcer. For example, if praise is not a reinforcer for a person and food is, food can be paired with praise during behavioral procedures until praise serves as a reinforcer. Food can then be discontinued as a reinforcer.

There are also two types of punishment. One type involves presenting an aversive event following the behavior and the other removes a positive event following the behavior. For example, getting a ticket for speeding can be an aversive event while having your driver's license taken away after three tickets is the removal of a positive event.

One of the most misunderstood concepts of behavior analysis is *negative reinforcement*. It is important that those who work with people with TBI understand this term. Negative reinforcement increases the occurrence of a behavior by eliminating the aversive event after the behavior has occurred.[146] In TBI rehabilitation, being allowed to "escape and avoid" therapeutic tasks is a common example of negative reinforcement.

Another basic principle of behavior analysis is *extinction*. Extinction does not involve either presenting or taking away consequences to behavior, but rather discontinues the reinforcement of a behavior. Not reinforcing the behavior eventually decreases or eliminates the occurrence of the behavior. "Ignoring" is probably the best example of an extinction procedure. Ignoring behaviors that were previously given attention (e.g., complaining, yelling) can be an effective technique when combined with reinforcement of positive behaviors.

It is recommended that reinforcement programs (or reinforcement combined with extinction) be attempted before implementing a punishment program. Reinforcement programs that teach people "what to do" are generally more effective for long-term maintenance of the desired behavior and do not elicit many of the negative side effects inherent to punishment programs.

20.6.4 Prompting and Fading

Teaching behaviors involves *prompting* to help initiate the behavior. Instructions, gestures, and modeling are all examples of prompting. The *self-efficacy theory* of Bandura[147] includes as one of its components *guided mastery,* which can include breaking down tasks into sub-tasks of easily mastered steps. They are antecedents to the target behavior. The way in which prompting is utilized can have significant impact on how easily a client learns. A person with language deficits will have difficulty following verbal prompts. In this case, using physical gestures and cues can be more effective. Different types of prompts can be combined to facilitate the desired behavior. Shaping and chaining procedures rely on competent use of various prompting techniques (e.g., backward and forward chaining) to teach new skills.

The goal is for the behavior to occur independently without prompting. The method for accomplishing this is called *fading.* Fading is the systematic and gradual removal of prompting. If prompting is ended too quickly, the behavior may not continue. A more gradual reduction in prompting is recommended until the behavior is performed independently or with as little prompting as possible. For example, teaching a person with TBI a showering sequence may start with actual physical guidance through many of the steps. Next, some of the physical cues can be reduced to gestures (e.g., pointing) and then to verbal cues. Later, a written checklist can be placed in the shower, listing each step of the showering sequence. The checklist can then be removed, allowing the client to perform the task independently.

20.6.5 Generalization

Like fading, *generalization* is an important procedure in developing the independence of a person with TBI or transferring responsibility to primary caregivers and other environments for long-term care, and so on.[148] There are two types of generalization: stimulus generalization and response generalization. Whereas fading involves decreasing a behavior's dependence on prompts, stimulus generalization reduces a behavior's dependence on the conditions under which it was learned. Most people would agree that rehabilitation takes place in a restricted environment. It is the goal of stimulus generalization that behaviors learned under these conditions be transferred to other settings. For instance, the goal of learning to read in a clinic setting is that it will generalize to reading the newspaper at home or the grocery list at the supermarket. Learning to control physical aggression in the clinic, to give another example, is not as important as the ability to control aggression in the community.

Response generalization involves behaviors rather than the conditions under which they occur. In other words, reinforcing or punishing a specific behavior will also affect similar behaviors. We have seen this occur with clients. A behavior treatment plan that focuses on reducing the most problematic behavior at the same time decreases other less severe behaviors. This experience lends support to the saying: *Worry about the big things and the little things will take care of themselves.* Target the most severe behaviors first and the small ones may never require treatment.

20.7 Behavioral Diagnostics

Prior to writing a behavioral treatment plan, it is essential that a comprehensive assessment of the client's history, current status, and future goals be performed. The success of a behavior program depends as much on an accurate evaluation of the client's behavior as on the intervention plan itself.[149] The evaluation must analyze all the potential factors contributing to a client's behavior. The three basic behavioral diagnostic tools are (1) a historical survey, (2) a current status evaluation, and (3) a functional assessment.

20.7.1 Historical Survey

Collecting historical information helps the behavior programmer understand how the client may respond to the rehabilitation process, and what he or she expects to gain from treatment.[150] The first half of a historical survey covers a range of demographic data. This includes information on age, sex, marital status, children, parents, friends, religious preference, living conditions prior to the injury, education, work history, and recreational interests. Information we have found to be particularly important is that concerning eating preferences, sleeping patterns, personal likes and dislikes, daily routines, and lifestyle characteristics. Many behavior problems can be averted with an understanding and appreciation of a client's lifestyle prior to the injury. Requiring the client to conform to unfamiliar schedules, foods, people, and situations that can be reasonably modified creates a potential setting event.[151,152] As we explained in the previous section, a setting event increases the likelihood of a problem behavior occurring. This can happen when facilities develop schedules that are easier or less expensive to manage. This inflexibility can contribute to unnecessary behavior problems that are actually more difficult and expensive to manage.

The second half of the historical survey concerns medical and rehabilitation history. It can be helpful for the behavior programmer to know the location and etiology of injury, the elapsed time since injury, and the course of treatment that has been provided. This furnishes the programmer with an idea of the client's rate of recovery.[153] In addition, knowledge of a client's medical history can be beneficial. For example, any diseases, major illnesses, or substance abuse problems that may have occurred before the injury may contribute to the client's current behavioral status and future prognosis.

Most of this information can be gathered from medical records, discussions with the previous treating staff, and an interview with the client and/or significant others, such as family and friends. Contact with prior treatment facilities provides insight into behaviors exhibited by the client since the injury, under what circumstances the behavior occurred, and staff response. Interviews with the client and/or significant others help to determine the client's preinjury behavior pattern that, in part, determines his or her response to the demands of rehabilitation and life after a TBI.

20.7.2 Current Status

TBI usually involves more than just damage to the brain. Many medical and psychological complications can result from TBI. These issues need to be clearly outlined in the behavior plan so that staff can be aware, because these complications can also be setting events for behavior problems. These complications can also be setting events for behavior problems. For example, if a person is in pain or constantly dizzy, his or her behavioral control will likely be diminished. This is why a comprehensive evaluation of a client's current status is important.

A current status evaluation reviews a client's medical and psychological status and therapeutic testing results and examines the relationship of these to behavioral issues. A comprehensive review of the medical status involves looking at the cardiac, vascular, and respiratory systems; orthopedic and muscular capability; the sensory system; bowel and bladder functioning; and other areas of physiologic functioning. Of all possible medical problems, medication usually has the most direct relationship to behavior. Medications can profoundly affect behavior; thus, programmers need to be educated and informed on the subject.

A TBI has an impact not only on the client, but on family and friends as well. It is important that programmers understand the dynamics between the client and significant others. After discharge from rehabilitation, family or friends may be required to carry out behavioral procedures with their loved one or, at the very least, maintain an environment that is conducive to continued learning and development.

One of the most important assessments of current status is a functional skills evaluation. How well is the client able to perform activities of daily living such as hygiene, grooming, dressing, and toileting? Is the client able to cook meals and clean the house? What about community mobility, driving, and shopping? Is the client able to manage his money? All of these issues are fundamental to levels of independent functioning. They will prescribe the type of living arrangement and level of assistance the client will require. Also, relearning functional skills can help to replace maladaptive behaviors while reducing the need for aversive procedures.

A review of therapeutic testing results completes the current status evaluation. Standard therapeutic testing includes cognitive, physical, and psychological evaluations, as well as a neuropsychological examination. A client's cognitive level can dictate the type of behavioral procedure that is implemented. Clients with severe cognitive impairment, for instance, will probably not participate in a "contracting" program because it requires more abstract thinking. Physical issues can also directly affect the treatment plan. For example, overcorrection or contingent restraint procedures can be especially ill suited for clients with orthopedic concerns. The neuropsychological examination brings all the client's skills and deficits into focus, helping the behavior programmer to design an appropriate treatment plan.

20.7.3 Functional Assessment

A functional assessment is central to the design of the treatment plan. Its purpose is to identify the function that each target behavior serves.[154] A functional assessment can be composed of three parts: (1) describing the behavior and its surrounding events, (2) predicting the factors that control the behavior, and (3) testing the predictions by manipulating the identified factors.

A descriptive analysis begins by describing the behavior. This is accomplished by interview and/or direct observation. Direct observations should constitute the primary source of information because anecdotal reports from interviews can be clouded by subjective perceptions. The observations should also occur in a wide range of settings and situations. Nevertheless, in cases when direct observations are not possible, interviews may be the only method for gathering the information needed to start a treatment plan. Interviews are conducted with those who have direct contact with the client, such as family members, caregivers, therapists, or paraprofessionals. The interview consists of identifying the target behavior, the conditions under which it normally takes place (antecedent or setting events), what events occur following the behavior (consequence), and what function the behavior serves (e.g., communicating needs). Some behavior problems can be reduced by simply improving the function that the behavior is attempting to perform.[155] If behavior problems are being caused by an inability to communicate one's needs effectively, for example, then improving a client's communication skills may decrease the problem behaviors. Although indirect assessments, such as interviews, are important to functional assessment, if possible, they should be a secondary source of information.

Functional assessment is usually based on direct observations. The most precise method for collecting observational data is by recording the events surrounding behavioral episodes. An excellent form for organizing this information was designed by O'Neill et al.[156] Figure 20.1 is a modified version of this form. It includes a place to write in the time of each behavioral event; possible setting events (e.g., difficult task, demands); the perceived function of the behavior (e.g., attention, avoiding activity); and the consequence to the behavior. The completed form can then be analyzed for patterns of behavior and the conditions in which they most frequently occur. From this analysis, hypotheses can be formulated regarding conditions maintaining the behavior.

The last step is a functional analysis to test the conclusions drawn from the interviews and direct observations.[157] This involves manipulating specific conditions and observing

Functional Assessment	Time					
Behaviors						
Antecedent/Setting Events						
Demand/Request						
Difficult Task						
Perceived Functions						
Get/Obtain						
Attention						
Desired item/activity						
Escape/Avoid						
Demand/Request						
Activity						
Person						
Consequences						

FIGURE 20.1
Functional analysis form.

the level of the behavior occurrences. The idea is that, by changing the consequences to a behavior, one may be able to determine the condition maintaining the behavior. After the conditions have been identified, then a treatment plan can be developed. For example, if physical aggression occurs with a client 25% of the time while in therapy, but only during 5% of the time before starting therapy, one may try allowing the client "alone time" after completing a specified amount of therapy.

Of course, the time and financial constraints of rehabilitation may make it difficult to always complete this last step of a functional analysis before implementing a treatment plan. However, identifying the conditions that maintain behavior and monitoring the effects of changing these conditions can, at the very least, be utilized during the treatment plan.

20.8 Behavior Plan Format

A behavior treatment program includes seven major components: (1) short- and long-term goals, (2) precautions, (3) operational definitions of target behaviors, (4) rationale, (5) data collection system and materials needed, (6) staff procedures, and (7) contraindications (Figure 20.2). The behavior programmer must synthesize diagnostic data (historical information, current status, and functional analysis) with goals of the client, family, treating staff, and payer to create an individualized treatment program. The treatment plan should be written as clearly as possible and in an "easy-to-follow" structure. The programmer has to strike a balance between including all the necessary information and, at the same time, presenting it in a way that is concise and readable. The degree of staff behavioral training will dictate the level of sophistication with which the program can be written and followed with consistency. However, the reality of most rehabilitation environments, whether acute, postacute, or in the home, is that there is a wide range of behavioral competence. The Behavior Analyst Certification Board (or BACB)* was created to develop, promote, and implement a voluntary national certification program for behavior analyst practitioners. However, even after extensive training, there are significant differences in the degree of "natural" ability among staff to carry out effective behavioral treatment. Differences in natural ability can be the result of difficulty in controlling one's own behavior, lower sensitivity to nonverbal signs exhibited by a patient, and personal attitudes about the patient and/or behavior program. This being the case, a "step-by-step" procedural outline, combined with close monitoring of staff performance, is the most practical format with which to run behavior treatment plans.

20.8.1 Goals

Behavior treatment goals are separated into short- and long-term goals. Short-term goals are objectives that define the desired measurable change in the target behavior. A specific time frame for accomplishing the objective should be clearly stated. For example, physical aggression (the target behavior) will be reduced to 5% of the total recorded intervals within 30 days. Short-term goals help the client and staff focus on tangible achievements while continuing to strive toward long-term goals.

Long-term goals, on the other hand, describe the projected functional outcome of the treatment plan. For example, the client will increase independent living to a minimal

---

* The trademarks Behavior Analyst Certification Board, Inc., BACB, Board Certified Behavior Analyst, BCBA, Board Certified Associate Behavior Analyst, and BCABA are owned by the Behavior Analyst Certification Board, Inc. All rights reserved. Copyright 2002 by BACB™.

BEHAVIOR TREATMENT PLAN

Client Name: C. G.
Program Start Date: 11-30-03
Implemented By: Clinical therapists and staff aides.

GOALS:

Short-Term Goal: To decrease physical aggression by 5% of total intervals from last month.
Long-Term Goal: To increase Independent Living Scale (ILS) score to more than 80/100 pts. (min–mod. supervision).
Evaluation of Goals: Weekly summary of interval data.

TARGET BEHAVIORS:

Primary:

Physical Aggression (PA) - attempting to and/or striking out with an object or body part; may include hitting, kicking, pinching, grabbing without permission, scratching, throwing items at someone, etc.; includes attempted or actual contact; does not include verbal threats or invasion of personal space.

Property Destruction (PD) - ramming, throwing, tearing, striking, or breaking property (even if accidental; or attempts to do so), property does not have to be damaged.

No Cooperation (None) - did not participate in therapy at all and exhibited at least one target behavior. May be in therapy area, yet did not attempt any activities.

Secondary:

Angry Language (AL) - cursing, yelling, threats, hostile language, demands delivered with increased volume (above conversational level) lasting more than two seconds.

Refusal to Work (R) - active or passive statements or actions meant to evade start, interrupt, or stop therapy tasks or directives; must be more than one minute; does not include slow processing time or lack of ability.

Escaping (E) - attempted to and/or left place of required activity.

Partial Cooperation (Part) - attempted and/or completed some therapy tasks as directed. Displayed one or more target behavior(s), but was able to be redirected to task or attempted the task prior to any behavior episode.

Full Cooperation (Full) - attempted and/or completed all therapy tasks as directed. No target behaviors displayed.

MATERIALS AND DATA COLLECTION:

1. 15-minute interval data sheet.
2. Two-minute Therapy Chart.
3. Two-minute board with countdown timer.

TREATMENT PROCEDURES:

Outline - This program will consist of several key components including: 1) a two-minute fixed interval DRO, 2) primary target behaviors of PA and PD, 3) a reward contingent upon completion of the five, two minute blocks of therapy with no occurrence of the target behaviors, 4) a graduated guidance program contingent on the occurrence of non-compliance, and 4) relaxation practice each hour.

Relaxation - Begin each hour with two minutes of timed relaxation practice. Tell C. G. to "take a couple of minutes to relax." Ask him to close his eyes, take a deep breath, and let his mind and muscles relax. Make every effort to keep the surrounding therapy area quiet during his relaxation time.

FIGURE 20.2
Example of a behavior treatment plan.

TREATMENT PROCEDURES:

DRO - Following the relaxation period, post the two-minute board on a straight back chair near the task area where C. G. can see it clearly. Inform him that when each of the boxes has an "X" in it, he can go outside. Set the timer for two minutes and begin therapy. Each time the timer sounds and C. G. has not exhibited a primary target behavior, "X" out a box on the board, quickly reset the timer, and continue therapy. Try and keep therapy tasks flowing comfortably while maintaining awareness of the timer. Immediately after the final (fifth) box has been "X'd", state to C. G. "Great, you stayed calm; we can go now" and take him for a short walk outside. Have C. G. walk himself during the walk unless he asks for assistance. Reflect to him that this is his time and he has earned it. After about 3–5 minutes, redirect C. G. back to therapy. Do not allow him to manipulate or slow his return to therapy. Assist as needed. Immediately reset the timer and repeat the above sequence.

Graduated Guidance - If C. G. displays non-compliance (i.e., refusing to start a task), **immediately** provide hand-over-hand guidance. Have tasks available that C. G. can be physically guided through. For example, tasks requiring pointing, reaching, touching, etc. As soon as non-compliance begins, start prompting the current task or immediately switch to an activity requiring motor involvement. Provide guidance until C. G. begins complying, then fade physical prompting. Once guidance has been discontinued, return to the task and/or approach used before the behavior occurred.

FIGURE 20.2 (continued)

supervision level (group home) or will be able to work in a part-time volunteer employment position. Long-term goals are to be defined by the client, family, caregivers, funding source, and other responsible parties.

All goals and objectives should include three parts: (1) how they will be assessed, (2) how often they will be reviewed, and (3) what type of report will be generated. Many accrediting or regulating agencies, such as the Commission on Accreditation of Rehabilitation Facilities (or CARF), require these guidelines for accreditation. The assessment of goals can be accomplished by many public or in-house rating systems. For example, long-term goals of disability level can be gauged by the Disability Rating Scale.[158] Short-term goals can be evaluated by a standard data collection system (e.g., frequency count, time sampling). Short- and long-term goals should include a statement concerning the frequency of review (e.g., weekly, biweekly, monthly) and what type of report will be produced.

20.8.2 Target Behavior

Target behaviors are the focus of the treatment plan. They are the behaviors that are interrupting therapy, impeding progress, endangering others, disrupting activities, or otherwise interfering with a person's ability to live independently in the community. They can be behaviors of excess (e.g., physical aggression); deficit (e.g., hygiene and grooming); or stimulus control (e.g., public sexual behavior).

Each target behavior must be operationally defined. The operational definition describes what the behavior "looks like" in objective, observable terms. For example, labeling a target behavior "physical aggression" without an operational definition leaves it wide open to interpretation. The more interpretation is allowed in a behavior program, the less consistent it will be. Not only does an operational definition describe what a behavior *is*, it also describes what it *is not*. For example, physical aggression could be defined as any attempted or actual hit, strike, kick, pinch, or grab by the client, not including spitting.

Operational definitions sometimes require that the context in which the target behavior will occur be identified. For example, "hand waving" is only a problem when it interferes with writing activities. The definition may also need to include the duration or rate at which the behavior must occur before it is considered a target behavior. For example, refusing to participate in therapy for more than 30 seconds may be the minimum criteria for "noncompliance."

20.8.3 Rationale

This section briefly outlines the reasons why an individual may require a behavior treatment program. Information such as a review of assessment and/or baseline data results, direct observations, and interviews with relevant caregivers and family can be discussed. It may be important to describe the behaviors of concern and the impact these behaviors may have on the individual's future access to social reintegration. A summary statement regarding why the program has been developed will help those implementing the program better understand what led to the plan.

20.8.4 Materials and Data Collection

The fourth section of a behavior treatment plan outlines all the materials required to carry out the prescribed procedures, and the data collection system for tracking the rate and/or duration of the target behavior. Many behavior treatment plans require specific materials for implementing procedures. For example, a stopwatch may be needed for a "differential reinforcement of other behavior" program that calls for reinforcing the client after a specified period of time in which the target behavior does not occur. Any supplies or items that are used to implement the treatment plan (e.g., timer, tokens, tape recorder) need to be described in this section.

The second half of this section describes the data collection system. All behavior programs should have a procedure for gathering information that will be used to determine the effect of the treatment plan. The data collection and graphing section of this chapter details methods for systematically recording and analyzing behavioral data. Without consistent data collection, it is difficult to ascertain whether the program is working. Anecdotal reports (i.e., verbal feedback from staff) are usually not reliable enough, because of their subjectivity, to make important decisions concerning the effectiveness of behavior programming. Frequency, interval, duration, or time-sampled data of operationally defined target behaviors gives the behavior programmer ample information that, together with staff feedback, will allow for better treatment decisions.

20.8.5 Treatment Procedures

The procedures section of the treatment plan describes the steps of the behavior program. It outlines the staff's response to the target behavior (consequence) and arranging of environmental conditions prior to the behavior (antecedent). The section on behavior plan procedures details a variety of behavior treatment plans.

The treatment plan describes each step a staff member is to take before and after the occurrence of the target behavior. Every step needs to be described in clear, concrete terms that can be understood by a wide range of people, including the client, staff, and family. More often than not, the success of a program rests on the ease with which the procedures can be followed. Figure 20.2 is an example of a completed treatment plan.

20.8.6 Contraindications

Behavior programs are not without "side effects." As programs are implemented, individuals may react in a numbers of ways. This section is the programmer's opportunity to consider what reactions may be anticipated and how staff can best respond. Frustration, reactive aggression, elopement, and verbal agitation may occur during implementation of the program. It is important to consider how the individual may behave so those providing the treatment are less surprised and can anticipate how to respond to maintain program integrity.

20.9 Behavior Plan Procedures

The staff member responsible for writing behavior programs has many designs from which to choose (Table 20.2). The types of behaviors exhibited by the client, the setting for implementing the program, and the level of staff skills and experience are all factors to be considered in choosing the most suitable behavior program. After these factors have been identified and weighed, one can then choose a treatment procedure that is *accelerative* (designed to increase the frequency or duration of a target behavior), *decelerative* (designed to decrease the frequency or duration of a target behavior), or *complex* (having characteristics of both accelerative and decelerative programs). Combinations of these procedures, in a multicomponent approach, can also be used simultaneously to increase the speed of and maintain behavioral change.[159]

We will outline procedures for the most common behavior programs and provide illustrations (for most procedures) of actual cases encountered in behavioral treatment. Some of the techniques we will not be covering in this chapter are group-based programs, peer-administered contingencies, biofeedback, and cognitively based treatment (e.g., stress reduction, problem-solving skills, self-statements). These methods are either not often used, not practical for people with TBI (e.g., group-based programs, peer-administered contingencies), or fall more into the realm of counseling (e.g., cognitively based treatment).

20.9.1 Accelerative Programs

20.9.1.1 Positive Programming

Positive programming is nothing more than teaching individuals new skills through the use of reinforcing consequences.[160] Activities of daily living, functional communication, and social skills training are all examples of positive programming. This technique is

TABLE 20.2

Behavior Program Treatment Procedure Designs

Accelerative	Decelerative	Complex	Other
Positive programming	DRI	Contracting	NCR
Shaping and chaining	DRO	Stimulus control	
	DRL	Token economy	
	Overcorrection		
	Stimulus change		
	Stimulus satiation		
	Time-out		

DRI, differential reinforcement of incompatible behaviors; DRL, differential reinforcement of low rates of behavior; DRO, differential reinforcement of other behaviors; NCR, noncontingent reinforcement.

familiar to most of us, because we have been exposed to learning new skills (e.g., reading) and being rewarded for our performance (e.g., grade).

An advantage of positive programming is that it is constructive in nature. It teaches people "how to do something." Positive programming helps to reduce undesirable behaviors that are incompatible with the new skill (e.g., the social skill of shaking hands is incongruous with hitting).[161] Generalization and maintenance of skills taught through positive programming are also often supported by naturally occurring contingencies (e.g., learning to verbalize allows one to express and receive one's needs).

A disadvantage of positive programming can be its lack of quick results; positive programming takes time. Because of the tremendous costs involved in rehabilitation of people with TBI, pressures are exerted on rehabilitation programs to bring about behavioral change as quickly as possible. This does not infer that positive programming should be excluded; rather, efficient programming must be developed to meet the needs of payers. To help accomplish this, positive programming can be integrated with other behavior programs that focus on decreasing undesirable behaviors. The result should be increased efficiency and rate of behavioral change.

20.9.1.1.1 Case Illustration

H.H. was a 32-year-old male injured in a motor vehicle accident. H.H.'s physical and cognitive skills were severely impaired. Expressive language, in particular, was extremely difficult. Most of his severe behavior, which included physical aggression and self-injurious behavior, occurred when his wife would leave for home at the end of his day at the clinic. When she would inform him she was leaving, he would start yelling, attempt to attack her or anyone intervening, and throw himself out of his chair. On one occasion, he even stabbed himself with a pencil that was lying nearby.

The program for reducing his aggressive behavior was to replace it with more appropriate social and communication skills. H.H. was taught to wave goodbye to his wife before she departed for the evening. This was accomplished by having the client, during counseling sessions, practice saying goodbye to a videotaped presentation of his wife. If he completed the sequence correctly, and without any negative behavior, he was allowed to color in one section of a black-and-white drawing of his house. The drawing was divided into seven sections. When he completed coloring in the seven sections, he earned a supervised weekend home visit. Once he succeeded at the videotape presentation, and earned a visit home, the client practiced saying goodnight to his wife in person. The same reinforcement procedure was used again. Seven successful trial sessions resulted in a weekend home. H.H. successfully completed both training procedures within approximately 30 days and never presented the problem again during the rest of his stay in rehabilitation. The more appropriate social skills of saying goodnight and waving goodbye had replaced the maladaptive behaviors of physical aggression and self-injurious behavior.

20.9.1.2 Shaping

Shaping refers to the reinforcement of gradual approximations to a target behavior and is generally used with behaviors that do not require urgent change. For example, if a therapist wants a client to remain seated during the therapy session, she may start by reinforcing the client for remaining seated for 5 continuous minutes at a time. After the client is able to accomplish this consistently, the time can be increased to 10 minutes, and so on, until the client remains seated the entire session. Although shaping is used primarily for skill building (e.g., learning a single step of a dressing procedure, such as pulling one's shirt all the way down), it can also be used to modify maladaptive behaviors. For example, if a client is constantly late for therapy, he or she could be reinforced for approximating closer correct arrival times to therapy.

20.9.1.3 Chaining

Chaining, often confused with shaping, involves teaching a sequence of steps to a task.[162] The basic sequences in which such a task may be taught are termed *forward chaining, backward chaining*, and *whole task method*.[163] For example, putting on a pullover shirt would involve teaching a person the steps of (1) putting his arms through the sleeves, (2) pulling the shirt over his head, and (3) pulling the shirt down over his body. In forward chaining, one would begin teaching with the first step (putting arms through the sleeves), then combine steps 1 and 2, and finally connect the sequence of steps 1 through 3. In backward chaining, one actually begins teaching the last step first (e.g., pulling the shirt down), then combines step 3 and 2wo, and finally steps 3 through 1. In whole task method, the most common teaching technique, the entire sequence (step 1 to step 3) is taught each time. Evidence is not clear regarding which of these methods is most effective; however, backward and forward chaining is usually used if one is trying to reduce the number of errors produced by the client during learning.

20.9.1.3.1 Case Illustration

K.T. was a 38-year-old female who was injured in a motor vehicle accident. The injury left K.T. with severe cognitive and behavioral problems. Her most difficult behavior was an intense motor restlessness and inability to sustain attention. She was constantly moving her legs and arms and would exit from therapy every few minutes. A shaping program was introduced to try to increase her ability to sit in a chair and participate in therapy. The procedure started with having K.T. sit on the floor for 30 seconds. If she completed this successfully, she was allowed up and a poker chip token was placed in a circle on a board with 10 total circles. When all 10 circles were filled with a token, K.T. was taken for a walk around the clinic or outside. After she mastered floor sitting for 30 seconds with minimal failures, she was instructed to sit in a chair for 30 seconds. The same procedure was repeated. The 30-second time period was systematically increased over several weeks, with the structured introduction of "tabletop" activities, until she could sit at a therapy table for 45 minutes and work on therapeutic tasks without exiting. K.T.'s ability to sit quietly and work on cognitive activities had been shaped to a length commensurate with most clients participating in rehabilitation. The same program was used with K.T. in her living environment to help her sit at the dining table and finish eating a meal.

20.9.2 Decelerative Programs

20.9.2.1 Differential Reinforcement of Incompatible Behaviors (DRI)

DRI involves reinforcing behaviors that are *topographically* different from, or incompatible with, the target behavior.[164] For example, the behavior of keeping one's hands in the lap or to the side is topographically different from hitting oneself. The production of the topographically different behavior actually competes with, or disallows, the production of the target behavior. Thus, reinforcing the client for keeping his hands in his lap or to his side is said to reinforce an incompatible behavior differentially.

Careful monitoring of behaviors during a DRI program is required to make certain that the target behavior is actually decreasing and not only that incompatible behaviors are increasing. Using the previous example, one could imagine that the client's time with hands in his lap or to this side (incompatible behaviors) could increase, and self-hitting (target behavior) could remain unchanged. If this occurs, use of a differential reinforcement of other behaviors (DRO) program may be more effective.

20.9.2.1.1 *Case Illustration*

E.N. was a 43-year-old male who was injured in a motor vehicle accident. E.N. exhibited a variety of ticlike behaviors. He would touch or pick at his nose and face and grab his crotch area constantly throughout the day. As you can probably guess, social interaction with others was severely limited by these behaviors. DRI was implemented to help reduce these socially unacceptable behaviors. During therapy sessions, E.N. was reinforced with tokens for keeping his hands either on the table or engaged in hand-involved therapeutic tasks. The tokens were exchangeable for certain privileges in his living environment. Over a period of several months, E.N.'s "ticlike" behaviors decreased to a socially acceptable level. His inappropriate behavior (i.e., touching nose, face, or crotch) had been replaced by incompatible behaviors (i.e., hands on the table or engaged in a task). It was not possible for E.N. to exhibit both behaviors at the same time.

20.9.2.2 Differential Reinforcement of Other Behaviors (DRO)

DRO is defined as reinforcing any behavior other than the target behavior for a specific interval of time.[165,166] For example, if the target behavior is physical aggression, the therapist would reinforce the client at the end of every designated time interval in which the physical aggression was not exhibited. One can keep the time intervals *absolute* (e.g., every 15 minutes) or *relative* (e.g., resetting the clock after every occurrence of the target behavior). If the client exhibits physical aggression, the clock is reset for another 15 minutes. When there is an increase in the number of intervals in which aggression does not occur or when it is occurring at a predetermined lower rate, the interval size can be systematically lengthened and eventually eliminated.

There are, however, a few precautions to take when implementing a DRO program. DRO programs are not designed to reduce high-rate behaviors. High-rate behaviors do not allow enough time to reinforce the client between episodes of the targeted inappropriate behavior. Also, by their nature, DRO programs reinforce any other occurring behaviors. Therapists need to be aware that they may inadvertently reinforce another undesirable behavior.[167] As with many decelerative programs, DRO procedures do not teach people new skills and, thus, are more effective if implemented in concert with positive programming.

20.9.2.2.1 *Case Illustration*

C.I. was a 27-year-old male who was injured in an industrial explosion. As a result of the accident, C.I. had severe cognitive deficits and could not ambulate independently. He also had severe aggressive behavior problems that were significantly interfering with all rehabilitative therapy. C.I. exhibited hitting, kicking, biting, yelling, exiting, and noncompliance in therapy. A DRO program was started to reduce these behaviors. C.I. was required to participate in the therapy task for a total of 2 minutes without any of the target behaviors. If he was successful, an "X" was marked over one of five squares on an erasable dry ink board. A picture of an outdoor scene was attached to the board at the end of the five-square sequence. Any time C.I. displayed one of the target behaviors, the clock was reset to zero and a new 2-minute interval would begin. As soon as five squares were marked, C.I. was taken for a walk outside the clinic (the identified reinforcer). When he was able to complete 2-minute intervals approximately 80% of the time without resetting, the time was increased to 5 minutes, and then to 10 minutes. Eventually, C.I. was able to participate in therapy for a full 45 minutes before taking a break. He was being reinforced for any behaviors "other" than the target behaviors.

20.9.2.3 Differential Reinforcement of Low Rates of Behavior (DRL)

DRL programs provide reinforcement if a specified interval of time has elapsed since a target behavior last occurred or if a specified number of occurrences of the target behavior have occurred during the interval.[168] For example, if the target behavior is yelling, a DRL program may state that a client is to be reinforced for each 15-minute interval of time that passes since yelling last occurred or for each time interval in which the target behavior occurs below a certain rate (e.g., five occurrences or less of yelling every 15 minutes). The time intervals can then be lengthened (e.g., from 15 minutes to 30 minutes) or the number of occurrences allowed can be decreased (e.g., five occurrences to two occurrences every 15 minutes) until the target behavior is eliminated or reduced to an acceptable level. Baseline data must be collected to determine either the initial time interval length or the initial number of occurrences to be allowed for the client to receive a reinforcer. For example, if a behavior is occurring four times per hour, an appropriate interval length may be 15 minutes, or reinforcement for every 15 minutes that the behavior occurs only once. This interval length will ensure initial success by the client and help develop reinforcer strength.

Some of the advantages of DRL programs are that interval times can be adapted to fit therapy sessions (e.g., 45-minute sessions can be divided into 15-minute intervals) and high-rate behaviors, for which DRO programs are not designed, can be systematically reduced. Like DRO programs, however, DRL programs do not teach new skills. Instead, the focus is on reduction of maladaptive behaviors. DRL programs therefore should be supplemented with positive programming of some type.

20.9.2.3.1 Case Illustration

K.C. was a 36-year-old male who was injured when the bicycle he was riding was hit by a car. K.C. presented several behavior problems, including verbal and physical aggression. If he displayed any target behavior, the DRL program stated he must go to his kitchen and remove one of four keys hanging on a cork board. If, at the end of 3 days, he still had one key remaining, he could unlock a box and choose one of several available reinforcers (e.g., $10). When K.C. was able to earn his 3-day reinforcer three consecutive times, the reinforcer period was increased to 4 days, and so on, until it reached a 1-week reinforcer time period. The number of keys was then reduced until only two keys were available. This meant he could only exhibit one target behavior per week and still earn a reinforcer. K.C.'s target behaviors had been systematically reduced to lower rates.

20.9.2.4 Overcorrection

There are two types of overcorrection procedures: *restitutional* and *positive-practice* overcorrection.[169] Restitutional overcorrection requires that a person returns the environment (e.g., therapy room) to a state better than before the behavioral episode. For example, if an agitated client knocks over a chair, he or she is required to pick up not only that chair, but to straighten all other chairs in the room as well.

Positive-practice overcorrection requires repeated practice of an appropriate behavior. For example, if a client walks with poor posture, he or she may be asked to practice walking with upright posture for specified periods of time.

Overcorrection can be an alternative to other, more punitive punishment procedures. The disadvantages are that overcorrection can be time-consuming and can elicit aggression during circumstances in which overcorrection requires physical guidance to obtain compliance.

20.9.2.4.1 Case Illustration

O.H. was a 42-year-old female who was injured in a motor vehicle accident. She had spent approximately 1 year in a locked psychiatric institute on multiple psychoactive medications prior to admission for rehabilitation. She exhibited behaviors of yelling, hitting, stripping, exiting, and noncompliance with therapy. Although continent of bowel and bladder, O.H. would periodically urinate small amounts on furniture during therapy. A restitutional overcorrection program was implemented to reduce this behavior. If O.H. urinated on a chair, she was required to change her clothing, put the dirty clothes in the wash, clean the chair that was soiled, and wipe off all other chairs in the room. O.H.'s inappropriate urination ended within a few weeks.

20.9.2.4.2 Case Illustration

S.D. was a 29-year-old female who fell into a diabetic coma and suffered anoxia. S.D. displayed yelling and noncompliance to therapy, and was also incontinent of bladder. A positive-practice overcorrection program was started to reduce her incontinence. If S.D. was incontinent between her scheduled bathroom visits, she was required to go to the bathroom and practice a series of five correct "toileting" sequences (i.e., adjust clothing, sit on toilet, clean self, get up, adjust clothing, wash hands). After several months, S.D. was continent of bladder and able to live in a supervised group home.

20.9.2.5 Stimulus Change

Stimulus change is the sudden introduction of an unrelated (nonfunctional) stimulus, or change in stimulus conditions, that results in a temporary reduction of the target behavior.[170] For example, clapping loudly once while a client is engaged in yelling, or suddenly shouting the client's name if he is engaged in aggressive behavior, may cause a lapse in the behavior.

An advantage of stimulus change programs is that their effectiveness can be determined very quickly. There is no need for any long-term assessment of the program. The disadvantage of a stimulus change program is that its effect may be temporary (startle effect) and/or the client may quickly adapt to the stimulus event and return to the maladaptive behavior. Stimulus change programs are almost exclusively used as "emergency" programs to stop destructive behavior quickly.

20.9.2.6 Stimulus Satiation

Stimulus satiation programming allows unrestricted access to the reinforcer of an undesirable behavior.[171] The unconditional availability of the reinforcer will eventually weaken its relationship to the target behavior. Stimulus satiation weakens the reinforcer through the process of satiation (complete satisfaction) and deprivation of other reinforcers.[172]

20.9.2.6.1 Case Illustration

C.F. was a 32-year-old male who, while working on a rooftop, was electrocuted and fell. C.F. exhibited a number of severe behavior problems; however, one unusual behavior was his obsession with staying on the toilet. When cued to leave the bathroom, C.F. would become extremely agitated and start yelling. If anyone tried to help him out, he would become physically aggressive. His time in the bathroom was becoming increasingly longer and his behavior more severe. A stimulus satiation program was implemented to reduce his time in the bathroom. The program allowed the client to stay in the bathroom, and on the toilet, for as long as he desired. Over a period of 2 weeks, C.F.'s time on the toilet increased to over 19 consecutive hours in 1 day. The following 2 weeks saw his time in the bathroom decrease gradually to what would be considered "normal" lengths of time. Unlimited access to "toilet time" eventually weakened its reinforcement quality (i.e., satiation).

20.9.2.7 Time-Out

Time-out procedures[173] (also known as *contingent withdrawal*) can be either nonseclusionary or exclusionary. Nonseclusionary time-out involves withdrawing attention from a person while remaining in his or her presence. Exclusionary time-out consists of removing the person from a reinforcing environment following the occurrence of a target behavior. For example, when a client exhibits verbal threats, one can either ignore the statements (nonseclusionary) or remove the client from the area (exclusionary). Time-out procedures are more effective if the reinforcer sustaining the behavior is attention from others. A third type of time-out procedure, seclusionary, involves the use of a time-out room when the client exhibits a specific target behavior. Strict guidelines need to be followed to operate seclusionary time-out procedures safely.[174]

- The duration of seclusionary time-out should be as brief as possible (e.g., 1–5 minutes).
- The room should be well lit, ventilated, and free of dangerous objects (e.g., light fixtures).
- The room should have provisions for visually monitoring the person.
- The room should not be locked, only latched.
- Records should be kept for each use of the time-out room. At a minimum, records should include the client's name, description of the behavioral episode, and start/end time of the procedure.

An advantage of time-out procedures is that they are easy for staff to understand. The disadvantage is that, in reality, time-out procedures can be very difficult for staff to implement. It is extremely difficult for staff to ignore a client's target behavior completely (e.g., threats, cursing) 100% of the time. If the target behavior is not ignored, it can be inadvertently intermittently reinforced. Intermittently reinforced behavior is actually strengthened. Also, a client should not be removed from the therapy area as part of an exclusionary time-out procedure if the behavior is to escape and avoid therapy. Time-out procedures should always be combined with positive, skill-building procedures (e.g., positive programming, shaping) to develop functional skills to replace the behavior being extinguished.

20.9.2.7.1 Case Illustration

L.I. was a 24-year-old male who was injured in a motor vehicle accident. L.I. exhibited behaviors of verbal aggression, threatening behavior, and noncompliance. He had sustained a mild TBI. If L.I. did not want to participate in a therapeutic activity, he began by arguing, then escalated to yelling and threatening physical aggression. A nonseclusionary time-out procedure was started to reduce his aggressive behavior and increase his compliance with therapy. Attention from staff was the identified reinforcer. Any time that L.I. began arguing and refusing to follow instructions, therapists were instructed to inform L.I. that they were going to their office and would return when he was ready to stop yelling and cooperate. Other staff members were also instructed to ignore L.I. if he was not with his therapist during therapy time. Cooperation increased to an acceptable level over a 2-week period.

20.9.3 Complex Programs

20.9.3.1 *Contracting*

Contracting is a technique that involves a written agreement between the client and another person.[175] A key to behavioral contracting is that the elements of the contract are agreeable and understandable to both parties. Contracting can shift the focus of therapy away from the demands of a therapist to one of cooperative problem solving. Clients may be more likely to follow therapeutic guidelines when they feel part of the decision-making process and can see behavioral steps and reinforcers outlined in a written format. Contracting should include a definition of the target behavior or goal, how the behavior or goal will be measured or monitored, rewards for following the contract, and the signatures of both parties. Contracting can work well for behaviors such as tardiness, cooperation, and quality of performance, which are typically thought of as involving "higher" levels of self-control.

20.9.3.1.1 *Case Illustration*

T.K. was a 36-year-old female who, while working as a junior high teacher, was injured when hit in the head by a student. T.K. was diagnosed as having "mild" head injury. Most of her symptoms were related to psychological functioning and high-level abstract thinking. One specific symptom that caused her difficulty was a sensitivity to light. Following the injury, she could not tolerate bright light, including indoor florescent lighting. She developed a habit of wearing dark glasses, both outdoors and indoors. As therapy progressed, she still felt the need to wear dark glasses indoors. T.K. stated that she wanted to stop wearing dark glasses inside; however, she could never fully cooperate. Various procedures were attempted to reduce her dependence on dark glasses, but none worked. Contracting was finally adopted. T.K. signed a contract stating she would cooperate with systematically reducing her time wearing glasses based on gradually increasing periods without "dark glasses on." After the goals were outlined and the contract signed, full cooperation from T.K. was achieved. She completed her rehabilitation and was discharged without the need to wear dark glasses indoors.

20.9.3.2 *Stimulus Control*

Stimulus control programming involves bringing the target behavior under the control of a specific stimulus or set of conditions.[176] Many behaviors are deemed acceptable, or unacceptable, based on the circumstances under which they occur. Sexual intimacy, for example, is considered an acceptable behavior if it occurs between consenting adults in the privacy of their home. If it occurs at the supermarket or on a public bus, however, it would not be considered acceptable. The goal of stimulus control programs, then, is to bring behaviors that may be occurring at the wrong time, place, or frequency into more appropriate, or more easily controlled, stimulus conditions.[177] Behaviors are brought under stimulus control by reinforcing the target behavior at the time and/or location where the behavior should naturally or acceptably occur (e.g., masturbating in the bedroom rather than in public). Behaviors can also be brought under a specific stimulus control that is then progressively reduced, decreasing the frequency of the behavior as access to the stimulus decreases. Stimulus control programs are considered positive in nature because the behavior is being reinforced, in most cases, for occurring in a more appropriate environment or time.

It is not recommended that stimulus control programs be used with more violent or destructive behaviors (e.g., physical aggression, self-injurious behavior). Severe behaviors are potentially dangerous to the client and others and, thus, are not acceptable even at low rates of occurrence or in selected settings.

20.9.3.2.1 Case Illustration

D.K. was a 37-year-old male who was injured in a motor vehicle accident. As a result of severe brain injury, D.K. displayed physical and verbal aggression, exiting, and noncompliance with therapy. His verbal behavior (i.e., threats, cursing, and yelling) was his predominant problem. A stimulus control program was implemented to reduce verbal agitation. A therapy room was set aside as the stimulus control environment. A lamp, with a blue incandescent light bulb, was placed on the table to increase the uniqueness of the room. To begin with, all therapy sessions were done in this room. If D.K. exhibited any verbal target behaviors, he was reinforced with a variety of edibles and verbal praise. To ensure a high reinforcer rate, if D.K. did not exhibit a target behavior within 60 seconds, he was prompted by the staff to "please yell." In contrast, when D.K. was outside of the room (for walks, bathroom breaks, and so forth), all target behaviors were ignored. After 3 weeks of using the stimulus control room exclusively for therapy, D.K. was systematically moved to conventional rooms at a rate of one per week. Again, he was reinforced for exhibiting target behaviors only in the stimulus control room, whereas target behaviors were ignored in all other conditions.

20.9.3.3 Token Economies

Token economies require the use of secondary reinforcers (tokens) that a person has earned and that can be traded later for something of value to the person.[178] For example, plastic poker chips are commonly used as tokens that are earned for positive behaviors such as compliance with therapy. Clients can then trade in the chips daily, weekly, and so forth (depending on the reinforcement interval length required) for any activity, privilege, or item identified as a reinforcer (e.g., dining out, movies, money). One can also include a response–cost aspect to a token program. This involves losing tokens for exhibition of specific behaviors. For example, a client may earn tokens for compliance with therapy and lose tokens for exhibiting any physical aggression.

The most difficult aspect of a token program is deciding the value of each token and how often the client can earn it. Baseline data on the frequency of the target behavior is necessary to determine the potential earning power of the client. Token programs should be neither too easy nor too difficult for a client. An earning rate of about 70% to 80% is probably a good rule of thumb. Advantages of token programs are that they provide for structure; concrete feedback; delay of gratification; and ease of use across many settings (e.g., therapy room, community, home).

20.9.3.3.1 Case Illustration

S.X. was a 28-year-old male who was hit by a motorist while working as a motorcycle highway patrolman. S.X. suffered a severe brain injury that left him with significant cognitive and physical deficits. With the exception of physical therapy, S.X. was limited to using a wheelchair for mobility. Although sitting, S.X. would let his head fall forward and begin drooling.

He would also let his left hand pull up to his chest, instead of keeping it in a more neutral position on his lap. A token program was started to decrease these behaviors. He could also earn bonus tokens for each 15-minute interval in which he added inflection to his "monotone" voice. A response–cost element was added to decrease his habit of transferring out of the wheelchair without supervision. He was given a "transfer ticket," which cost him tokens if anyone witnessed him transferring without another person present. Tokens were earned on a 15-minute interval basis (determined by baseline data on the rate of target behaviors) and could be cashed in for food outings and extra walking time. By time of discharge, S.X.'s drooling and hand position had been resolved, and he was placed in a semi-independent living environment and a part-time position with the police force as an office clerk.

20.9.4 Other Programs

20.9.4.1 Noncontingent Reinforcement (NCR)

NCR procedures involve the delivery of reinforcers on a time schedule that is not contingent upon the subject's behavior.[179] This is different from a traditional, contingency-based model of reinforcement. For instance, if "attention from others" is the identified reinforcer, attention will be delivered to the client on a fixed schedule (e.g., every 15 minutes), independent of the client's behavior. Whether the client acts inappropriately or appropriately, the reinforcer "attention" will be given to the client every 15 minutes.

NCR has some advantages over other reinforcement programs. It requires little in the way of monitoring, whereas other programs require constant observation of the client's behavior. This can be an important factor in situations in which staffing levels are less intensive, such as long-term care environments or programs that do not offer one-to-one therapy-to-client treatment ratios.

20.9.4.1.1 Case Illustration

C.I. was a 40-year-old male with TBI participating in a long-term care program. C.I. sustained a brain injury as a result of a motor vehicle accident 13 years prior to his admission. Although suffering from severe cognitive deficits, C.I.'s aggressive behavior toward others and himself was of primary concern. C.I. participated in structured individual and group-oriented activities during the day and in a residential setting during the evenings and weekends, relearning activities of daily living.

Physical aggression and self-injurious behavior were identified as the target behaviors, and "attention" as the maintaining reinforcer. Attendants delivered attention every 30 minutes, independent of behavior, for the client's waking hours. The attention sequence consisted of spending 3 minutes in social conversation with C.I., after which he was redirected to an activity. Implementation of the NCR program resulted in physical aggression occurring four times less often and self-injurious behavior two and a half times less often than prior to the program.

20.9.5 Summary

The design of an effective behavioral program may require combining a number of the procedures just described. No single design can be used universally. Consequently, it is often necessary to begin with one procedure and switch to another when the first plan fails or loses its effectiveness.

Recent studies have also stressed the importance of *contextual control* in choosing treatment plans.[180] Contextual control recognizes the role that context (stimulus setting) plays in altering the effect of behavior programs. A treatment plan designed to modify behavior in one environment may not be effective in another.[181]

20.10 Data Collection and Graphing

Behavior programming requires a procedure for systematically recording and graphing behavior data. Decisions regarding the effectiveness of treatment plans should be data based, and this demands comprehensive data collection. When possible, collect data throughout the entire day and evening, not just in structured settings. Behavior data from the home and community are just as important as those from a school or rehabilitation facility. Long-term maintenance is questionable if behavior changes do not generalize to other, more natural environments. This section will cover methods of data collection, graphing, and analysis of data, and the use of computer technology to assist in data management. Although comprehensive data collection and graphing can be time-consuming and somewhat rigorous to implement, there are a number of important reasons to collect data on a consistent basis.

- Provide baseline information prior to starting a behavior program. Before beginning any behavior program, it is recommended that data be collected on the person's target behaviors. Baseline data provide the behavior programmer and staff with a clear picture of the frequency of maladaptive behaviors being exhibited by the person. This information bears directly upon the design of the treatment plan. For example, if, after baseline data analysis, it is determined that the target behavior rate is extremely high, then one would not choose to implement a DRO program, which is suited for low-rate behaviors

- Method for judging the ongoing effectiveness of the behavior program. Systematic collection and graphing of data are important in tracking the progress of a treatment plan. Trends in data can be analyzed to support any changes necessary to the initial program. Modifications to the program should be "data driven" and not based on anecdotal staff reports alone.

- Feedback to family, staff, payers, and client. Behavior data provide important information to those responsible for the client's well-being and/or funding. People typically respond more favorably to observationally recorded data of behavior, rather than statements such as, "She is behaving better." Graphs, based on collected data, help the client, staff, and others visualize and understand the impact of the behavioral intervention plan. Graphs can also assist the client in developing self-monitoring skills.

- Valuable information for research and program development. If the person is in a school or rehabilitation program, systematic collection of behavior data assists those responsible for clinical research, conference presentations, preparation of professional manuscripts, and program development. These activities require the support of reliably collected data.

20.10.1 Data Collection

There are many methods for collecting data. The three most common and practical methods are *event recording, interval recording,* and *time-sample recording.* These three data collection methods are known as *direct observational recordings* (Table 20.3).

TABLE 20.3

Direct Observational Data Collection Methods

Method	Definition	Considerations
Event recording	Tally *each* occurrence of target behavior.	Requires constant observation. Difficult to judge beginning and end of behavior.
Interval recording	Record each occurrence or nonoccurrence of target behavior *during* each interval.	Requires constant observation. Results in approximations of behavior duration and frequency.
Time-sample recording	Record occurrence or nonoccurrence of target behavior at the *end* of each interval.	Broad approximation of behavior duration and frequency.

20.10.1.1 Event Recording

Event recording (Figure 20.3) is probably the easiest direct observational recording system. The only requirement is to mark on a piece of paper each time a specific target behavior occurs. Hand-held devices, such as golf counters, can be used to make counting easier for high-frequency behaviors. The drawback to event recording is that it can be difficult to judge when one occurrence of a behavior ends and another occurrence begins. In tallying angry

Client Name: **John Williams**	Date: **4-14-03**	Time: **1–2 pm**	
Therapist Name: **Mary Smith**		Therapy: **OT**	
Instructions: Tally the *number of occurrences* of each target behavior.			
Target Behaviors		**Tallies**	**Total**
1. Physical Aggression Definition - attempting to and/or actual striking of an individual with an object or body part.		I	1
2. Angry Language Definition - cursing, threats, or any hostile language delivered with increased volume.		IIIII	5
3. Property Destruction Definition - attempting to and/or actual damaging of property.		I	1
4. Refusal Definition - not starting, interrupting, or stopping therapy or instructions > 60 seconds.		IIIIIII	7
5. Escaping Definition - attempting to and/or leaving the place of required activity.		III	3

FIGURE 20.3

Example of an event recording sheet.

language, for example, if a person is yelling for several minutes, it would be difficult to judge how many instances of angry language actually occurred. The person recording would have to decide whether to count the entire period as one event or try to tally each statement as a separate occurrence. In addition, high-frequency and long-duration behaviors are more difficult to count because of the amount of attention required. Event recording requires constant observation of the client so all occurrences of the target behavior are recorded, thus making it one of the most time-consuming of the data collection procedures.

20.10.1.2 Interval Recording

Interval recording (Figure 20.4) eliminates the task of judging the beginning and ending of behavioral episodes and tallying high-frequency or long-duration behaviors. Instead, interval recording divides the therapy session (or observation period) into equal time intervals (e.g., 15-minute periods) and requires the person recording to mark whether the target behavior occurred during each interval. It does not matter how many times the behavior occurred during the interval, only that it occurred at least once. Interval recording requires choosing an appropriate interval size. Time intervals should approximate the frequency rate of the behavior. High-rate behaviors require short time intervals (e.g., 5 minutes) and low-rate behaviors need long time intervals (e.g., 15 minutes). For example, if a person uses angry language approximately once every 10 minutes, an observation interval of 10 or 15 minutes would capture most of the variability in the behavior. If the interval size is too long, the rate of behavior may change and not be reflected in a measurement of percent of interval change. When the intervals are extremely short (e.g., 30 seconds), every other interval should be used for marking the data sheet. This achieves greater accuracy because the observer does not miss occurrences of behavior while attending to the recording sheet. If several target behaviors are being tracked simultaneously, the use of behavioral codes is recommended to simplify the procedure. At the end of each interval, the person recording marks the behavioral code (e.g., PA, physical aggression) for those behaviors that occurred during the interval. As in event recording, interval recording requires the undivided attention of the person recording. It is necessary to track both interval time and occurrence of target behaviors.

20.10.1.3 Time-Sample Recording

The last data collection method to be covered is time-sample recording (Figure 20.5). Time-sample recording is similar to interval recording except that it does not require constant attention by the person recording. Behavior is only periodically sampled. A therapy session (or observation period) can be divided into equal or variable (random) periods at the end of which (during a brief time sample) the person recording marks the occurrence or nonoccurrence of the target behavior. The advantage of this method is that the person recording does not have to monitor the client's behavior continuously and it is minimally intrusive on any activities, which also makes it ideally suited for monitoring high-frequency behaviors. It does require a device such as a timer to signal the end of each time period. The disadvantage is that time-sample recording results in an even broader approximation of behavior frequency than interval recording.

20.10.1.4 Computer Management of Data

With the advent of powerful and affordable personal computers, a number of spreadsheet programs have been made available that are well suited to managing and

Client: **John Williams**	Day: **Monday**		Date: **4/14/03**

Instructions: *Every 15 minutes you are to mark any* **target behaviors***, and level of* **cooperation***, listed below that occurred during that period by circling the letter corresponding to the behavior. The interval begins at the listed time (e.g., mark in the 2:00 period behaviors seen from 2:00 to 2:15). Note any observations and* **comments** *in the space provided.*

Target Behaviors: PA = Physical Aggression, AL = Angry Language, PD = Property Destruction, R = Refusal to Work, E = Exiting

Cooperation: None = No cooperation (with behavior), Part = Partial cooperation (with behavior), Full = Full cooperation (no behavior)

Therapy SP	9:00 a.m.	9:15 a.m.	9:30 a.m.	9:45 a.m.
Target Behaviors >	PA AL PD R E	PA AL PD R E	PA AL PD R E	PA AL PD R E
Cooperation >	None Part Full	None Part Full	None Part Full	None Part Full
Comments/Other >				

Therapy OT	10:00 a.m.	10:15 a.m.	10:30 a.m.	10:45 a.m.
Target Behaviors >	PA AL PD R E	PA AL PD R E	PA AL PD R E	PA AL PD R E
Cooperation >	None Part Full	None Part Full	None Part Full	None Part Full
Comments/Other >				

Therapy ED	11:00 a.m.	11:15 a.m.	11:30 a.m.	11:45 a.m
Target Behaviors >	PA AL PD R E	PA AL PD R E	PA AL PD R E	PA AL PD R E
Cooperation >	None Part Full	None Part Full	None Part Full	None Part Full
Comments/Other >				

Therapy PT	1:00 p.m.	1:15 p.m.	1:30 p.m.	1:45 p.m.
Target Behaviors >	PA AL PD R E	PA AL PD R E	PA AL PD R E	PA AL PD R E
Cooperation >	None Part Full	None Part Full	None Part Full	None Part Full
Comments/Other >				

Therapy RT	2:00 p.m.	2:15 p.m.	2:30 p.m.	2:45 p.m.
Target Behaviors >	PA AL PD R E	PA AL PD R E	PA AL PD R E	PA AL PD R E
Cooperation >	None Part Full	None Part Full	None Part Full	None Part Full
Comments/Other >				

Therapy SP	3:00 p.m.	3:15 p.m.	3:30 p.m.	3:45 p.m
Target Behaviors >	PA AL PD R E	PA AL PD R E	PA AL PD R E	PA AL PD R E
Cooperation >	None Part Full	None Part Full	None Part Full	None Part Full
Comments/Other >				

FIGURE 20.4
Example of an interval recording sheet.

graphing behavior data. If a facility handles a fair number of clients with behavior difficulties, it is highly recommended that one of these programs be used. Organizing data is a time-consuming task that can be streamlined with the help of computer technology. Spreadsheet programs, such as Excel®, are very useful for this purpose. They typically include both spreadsheet functions and graphing capabilities. Figure 20.6 is an example of a computer summary sheet covering 1 week of interval data. It includes columns for the date, day, each target behavior (e.g., PA, physical aggression), and the

Client Name: **John Williams**			Date: **4-14-03**		Time: **2-3 pm**
Therapist Name: **Mary Smith**			Therapy: **OT**		

Instructions: At the times listed in the left column, observe the client for 30 seconds then put an X under *Yes* if the target behavior occurred, or under *No* if the target behavior did not occur.

Target behavior			Definition		
Angry Language			Cursing, threats, yelling, or any hostile language delivered with increased volume.		
Time	Yes	No	Time	Yes	No
9:00	X		9:32		X
9:03		X	9:35	X	
9:10		X	9:40	X	
9:15	X		9:47		X
9:23		X	9:51		X
9:25		X	9:56	X	

Data Calculation:

Total Yes's = 5
Total No's = 7   Total Yes's/ Total Samples = **5/12**
Total Samples = 12   = **42%** of time-samples

FIGURE 20.5
Example of a time-sample recording sheet.

total number of intervals recorded. All that is required is to write simple formulas for each of the percent calculations and design a master form that can be retrieved for each new client.

Another option, especially for high-volume data collection, is electronic forms. Most of us are familiar with survey forms and questionnaires that we receive in the mail. After we fill them out, we either fax or mail the completed forms to the survey company. Behavior data can be collected in the same fashion. Behavior data sheets can be created in an available program, such as Scantron's Cognition® automated forms processing software, and the results scanned and organized electronically.

20.10.2 Graphing

As a result of its single-case structure, behavior analysis does not lend itself to statistical procedures to judge the effectiveness of treatment interventions. Graphs are the traditional means of accomplishing this task. They provide an overall visual impression of behavior that is easy for staff, families, clients, and others to understand. Because it is common for behavior problems to accelerate before decreasing after the introduction of the treatment

PA = Physical Aggression, AL = Angry Language, PD = Property Destruction, R = Refusals,
E = Exiting, T = Total Intervals

John Williams

Week 1		PA	AL	PD	R	E	T
	4/10	1	5	0	2	1	24
	4/11	0	2	0	1	0	20
	4/12	3	5	1	3	1	24
	4/13	1	1	0	0	0	20
	4/14	2	4	1	2	1	24
Total		7	17	2	8	3	112
Percent		6.25	15.18	1.79	7.14	2.68	

FIGURE 20.6
Example of a computer summary data sheet.

intervention, graphs are an easy way to track learning curves. Graphs can be produced by hand or with one of the numerous commercially available computer graphics programs or with a spreadsheet program, such as Excel.

There are two fundamental concepts to remember when graphing. First, what information goes with the vertical line (ordinate, or y-axis) of the graph and, second, what information goes with the horizontal line (abscissa, or x-axis) of the graph. Figure 20.7 labels all the basic components of a graph.

For event-recorded data, the ordinate indicates the number of occurrences of the target behavior (e.g., physical aggression) and the abscissa indicates the time across which the

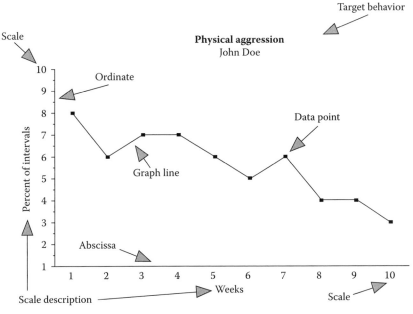

FIGURE 20.7
Components of a graph.

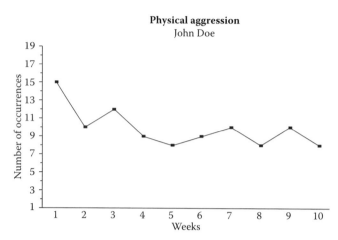

FIGURE 20.8
Example of an event graph.

behavior was recorded (e.g., days, weeks). For example, if one were graphing the number of occurrences of physical aggression on a weekly basis, the graph would look something like that in Figure 20.8.

In addition, choose the maximum value for the ordinate scale based on a number that is slightly higher than the highest frequency that has occurred with the person. For example, if the highest number of occurrences of physical aggression in a week was four, then choose five as your maximum value for the ordinate scale.

For interval or time-sample recording, the ordinate of the graph indicates the percentage of intervals (or time samples) during which the target behavior has occurred. The abscissa of the graph represents the time period during which the behavior was recorded. For example, if one were graphing the percentage of intervals for physical aggression on a weekly basis, the graph would look something like that in Figure 20.9.

Choose the maximum percentage for the ordinate scale based on a slightly higher percentage than the maximum that has occurred with the person. For example, if the highest

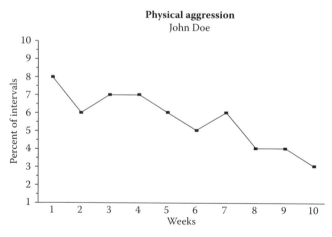

FIGURE 20.9
Example of an interval or time-sample graph.

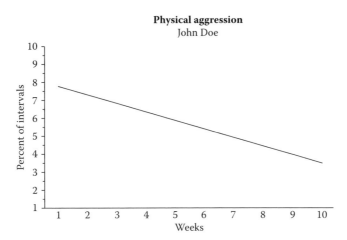

FIGURE 20.10
Example of a trend graph.

percentage of intervals with physical aggression in a week was 20%, then choose 25% as your maximum value for the ordinate scale.

Interpreting graphs can sometimes be very difficult. Behavior that is either highly variable or changes very little can make analysis a challenging proposition. One can look for a general trend or slope, or one can begin grouping data and comparing means (averages) to help detect changes in behavior.

A graphing technique we have found to be extremely useful in situations in which interpretation is difficult is called *trend* graphing. This graph is tedious to complete by hand, but most spreadsheet programs now have the ability to calculate a "line-of-best-fit" graph. If we take a behavior (e.g., physical aggression) and create a trend graph, it will show us the future projected change of physical aggression based upon the current observed rate of change. Figure 20.10 is an example of a trend graph. It clarifies the effect of the treatment and indicates when a target behavior might be expected to reach a projected goal. Of course, there are numerous variables that can have an impact on goal attainment, so care must be taken when interpreting trend graphing.

20.11 Crisis Prevention and Intervention

Assaultive behavior, such as physical aggression, is common in the field of TBI rehabilitation.[33] All the planning and programming described in the previous sections cannot always prevent or predict the occurrence of assaultive behavior by a client. In some cases, behavioral programming may even elicit aggression when it exerts control over sensitive aspects of a client's environment. Assaultive situations can be a frightening experience. People can be combative during the acute phase of recovery as they reorient themselves to the world around them and during postacute rehabilitation (i.e., when a person has reached medical stability) as they develop awareness of functional deficits. Severe behavior is a reality of the rehabilitation process and staff can learn to take measures, when possible, to prevent its occurrence. However, if a crisis situation does occur, staff should also be equipped with techniques to de-escalate the client and decrease the likelihood of injury to the client and others.

This section will cover some basic models of the assault cycle, common reasons for assaultive episodes, techniques for preventing the development of crisis situations, and useful interventions if a crisis cannot be prevented. However, this chapter is not a replacement for a certified course in crisis intervention or management of assaultive behavior. There are a number of training programs available to train staff directly or to certify staff members as instructors. We highly recommend that all facilities, schools, or families that work with people with TBI with behavior problems incorporate this training as standard practice. The content, structure, and training methodology of these courses, including the practice of self-defense and restraint techniques, are effective means of comprehensively equipping a person to handle assaultive situations safely.

20.11.1 Models of Assault

Paul Smith,[182] founder of *Professional Assault Crisis Training and Certification* (Pro-ACT)®, has proposed two categories and seven models of assaultive behavior. The first category is identification models and includes Stress Model, Communication Model, Environmental Model, Developmental Model, and Basic Needs Model. The second category is response models, which includes Common Knowledge Model and Legal Model. We will only concern ourselves here with five of the models. The Developmental Model and Basic Needs Model are not as clearly related to the field of TBI rehabilitation.

20.11.1.1 Identification Models

20.11.1.1.1 Stress Model

The stress model views assaultive behavior as a reaction to extreme stress. The rehabilitation process, as we know, is an extremely stressful situation for a person. When a client perceives a threat to his well-being (e.g., daily confrontation of deficits), he can either fight or flee from the situation. In TBI rehabilitation, we see both of these responses. Some clients try to escape the stress of their condition by either escaping or avoiding therapy. Others become combative when stressed. Each client has specific responses to stress, which can be detected and recognized as predictable patterns. A common tool for visualizing these response patterns is the assault cycle graph (Figure 20.11). It is divided into five separate phases: (1) triggering event, (2) escalation, (3) crisis, (4) recovery, and (5) postcrisis depression.

The triggering event is any stimuli or event that exceeds the client's tolerance for stress (e.g., demands for compliance, being touched). This begins the assault cycle. Any prevention techniques (e.g., arranging of environment, level of demands) would have to occur before the triggering event. The escalation stage is characterized by increasing levels of agitation or changes in the normal (i.e., baseline) behavior of the client. Deescalation techniques are used during this phase to try to help the client return to a baseline level of behavioral activity. The sooner deescalation techniques are used during this stage, the less likely more restrictive measures will have to be implemented. The crisis stage is characterized by the client's physically "acting out." At this point, deescalation techniques have failed and physical intervention may be necessary. During the recovery phase, the client's level of activity is decreasing. After the person regains self-control, decrease any external control that may have been introduced. The last stage, postcrisis depression, is characterized by activity that falls below baseline levels. The client may require a short period of rest or less active tasks until recovery occurs.

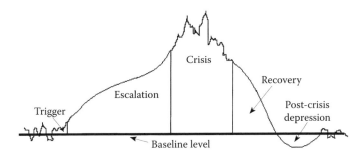

FIGURE 20.11
The assault cycle. (From Smith, P., Professional Assault Response Training Workshop Syllabus, 1983. With permission.)

20.11.1.1.2 Communication Model

The communication model focuses on the balance of communication between the therapist and client. On one end of the spectrum is "withdrawal" and on the other end, "assault." Smith[182] believes that the best means for achieving a "balance" that decreases the chances of triggering an assaultive cycle is with assertive communication. Smith[182] states that the communication model takes into account client manipulation and intimidation. When staff members respond with either intimidating aggressiveness or submissive nurturing, they contribute to an imbalance of communication and increase the opportunity for an assaultive situation. Smith[182] emphasizes that, "by using assertive communication, employees (or clients) reduce the chance that an assault will occur" (Ch.4, p. 13).

20.11.1.1.3 Environmental Model

Smith[182] describes the environmental model from the perspective that assaultive behavior is, for the most part, a product of the circumstances in which it occurs. This is the model that most closely fits the fundamental philosophy of behavior analysis. Although Smith does not discuss consequences to behavior as part of his model, he does emphasize the role of antecedents and setting events in triggering or setting the stage for assaultive behavior. Such things as weather conditions, level of sound, crowding, and scheduling of activities are given as examples of events that can "predispose people to assaultive behavior." The important point to make concerning the environmental model is that staff is in control of most environmental antecedents to behavior. Schedules, noise level, tone of voice, and so forth, are usually under the control of the staff. Staff can take advantage of this opportunity to prevent "trigger events" and minimize assaultive behavior.

20.11.1.2 Response Models

20.11.1.2.1 Common Knowledge Model

Smith[182] believes that the underlying reasons why people attempt to injure one another are relatively simple and that one can apply intervention techniques to respond effectively to these events. He states that assaultive incidents can be reduced to four common motives: *fear, frustration, manipulation,* and *intimidation.*

When people are afraid, or feel that their safety is threatened, their behavior may escalate to physical aggression as a means of defending themselves. To reduce fear, staff can respond to the client with a relaxed posture; use slow and natural gestures; keep a safe distance from the client; stand off to the side; position oneself below the client's eye level; use a firm, yet reassuring voice; stay logical; and encourage calm reflection.

When a client's behavior escalates as a result of frustration, staff members need to follow different guidelines than those used with a fearful client. Staff should demonstrate control with a more commanding posture, use forceful gestures such as pointing, stay directly in front of the person but just out of reach, keep the tone of voice quiet, yet forceful and confident, and repeat commands.

If a client is escalating behaviorally as a means of manipulation, a role of "detachment" is the technique recommended by Smith.[182] This method involves maintaining a closed, yet relaxed, posture, mild gestures of disapproval (e.g., finger tapping), positioning far enough away from the client to show noninvolvement, turning slightly away from the client, using a detached, slightly "bored" tone of voice, and quiet, repetitive commands.

If the client is attempting to intimidate through escalated behavior, the technique Smith[182] advises is "identifying consequences." The basic premise is that clear communication of the consequences of an assaultive act will reduce the probability that the episode will occur. Staff should be poised and ready to react (without giving the impression of fear), keep gestures to a minimum, position oneself for protection (e.g., behind a chair or desk), maintain a monotone, emotionless tone of voice, and give clear and direct statements of consequences.

20.11.1.2.2 *Legal Model*

Assaultive behavior can be separated into legal categories. They are (1) simple assault, (2) assault and battery, and (3) aggravated assault. The staff can legally protect itself against these varying degrees of assault, but is limited to using only "reasonable force." As Smith[182] states, "A reasonable amount of force is just enough for effective self-protection" (p. 5-2). For example, with simple assault (i.e., threatening gestures or speech), communication techniques would be the maximum force that could be legally applied. With assault and battery (i.e., use of physical force and threats), evasive self-defense would probably be the maximum reasonable force allowed. If aggravated assault (i.e., attempt to cause serious bodily harm) occurs, a controlling self-defense (i.e., restraint) and physical intervention would be reasonable. The use of physical techniques for self-defense and other interventions requires intensive training. Unless staff members have completed this training, they should have limited contact with clients exhibiting severe behavior disorders.

20.11.2 General Techniques and Methods

There are many techniques for preventing a crisis situation or intervening after it has started. We have covered many of those methods in the previous section. Smith's[182] recommendations regarding body posture, tone of voice, content of speech, and use of gestures are invaluable aids to dealing effectively with a crisis episode. There are other techniques that can be added to this list.

To help prevent a crisis situation from being "triggered," review the guidelines outlined Section 20.5 of this chapter, General Management Guidelines. These included (1) increasing rest time for the client, (2) keeping the environment simple, (3) keeping instructions simple, (4) giving feedback and setting goals, (5) staying calm and redirecting the client to task, (6) providing choices, (7) decreasing chances of task failure, (8) varying the type of activities, (9) overplanning, and (10) utilizing task analysis procedures. If one can implement these environmental controls and combine them with sensitivity to patterns of interaction and sharpened observational skills, most assaultive events can be prevented. For those that are unavoidable, intervention techniques for deescalating the client must be used.

After the escalation phase of an assault cycle has begun, measures by staff change from one of prevention to one of intervention. The intervention techniques used during the escalation stage are an attempt to deescalate the client before the cycle reaches the crisis stage. The earlier the intervention, the less restrictive the measures needed to be to control the situation. If the client progresses to the crisis stage, deescalation techniques will not be useful and may, in fact, prolong the crisis. Physical intervention by staff, unfortunately, becomes likely.

Some of the most effective deescalation techniques staff can utilize are *active listening, orientation, setting limits, redirection, withdrawal of attention,* and *contracting.*

- Active listening, a technique incorporating a variety of listening skills.[183] Active listening begins on a "nonverbal" basis. The staff member should make eye contact with the client, maintain a relaxed posture that shows interest, and use natural gestures. After this nonverbal basis has been established, verbal statements can be utilized. These consist of *paraphrasing, clarifying,* and *perception checking.* Paraphrasing is a method of restating the client's message in fewer words. Its purpose is to indicate to the client that you are trying to understand his message. Clarifying focuses on the more abstract messages from the client. The staff member admits confusion about a statement and tries a restatement or asks for clarification—for example, "'I'm confused. Is what you are saying . . . ?" Perception checking involves asking the client for verification of your perception. For example, "You seem to be very mad at me. Is that correct?"

- Orientation. Memory deficits are one of the most common consequences of a TBI. People can experience periods of severe disorientation. Disorientation has been found to be a key factor in the severe behavior of people with TBI. Orienting a client to the time, to his location, and to whom he is with can sometimes help to deescalate a client. It helps the client feel less threatened by the environment when he can understand where he is and why he is there.

- Setting limits. As stated earlier, setting limits can be a useful technique. This is especially true for clients who are trying to intimidate staff by threatening severe behavior. Although these can be frightening experiences, escalation can be curtailed if the staff member remains calm and confident, and outlines the consequences of the threatened behavior. For example, "If you throw that chair at me, you will be restrained by four other staff members until you are calm."

- Redirection. Also known as *topic dispersal,* redirection is useful when a client is in the early stages of escalation. Staying calm and redirecting a client to another task or activity can interrupt the escalation phase and refocus the client on something else. It also decreases the opportunity for inadvertently reinforcing the client with attention that may be the behavior problem's maintaining reinforcer.

- Withdrawal of attention. This technique is the opposite of active listening. Although active listening provides undivided attention to the client during escalation, withdrawal of attention discontinues any attention during escalated behavior. Withdrawal of attention is usually more effective with "manipulative" types of behavior. Clients exhibiting this type of behavior thrive on attention from others. Withdrawing attention for brief periods of time when they begin to escalate helps establish a relationship between "attention" and cooperative, calm behavior.

- Contracting. Like other deescalation techniques, this is a skill that takes some practice. The reason, however, is that contracting has the potential for being misused.

If used incorrectly, it becomes a method of "buying" good behavior that may lead to further behavior problems from the client. For example, if a client is escalated over completing an unpleasant task and you "contract" with him that he does not have to finish the task if he calms down, you have set yourself up for future problems when the client does not want to complete a task. You may have reinforced the escalated behavior. A more constructive response may be to tell the client that he can switch to another task for the moment and finish the difficult task later in that session. This teaches the client that he can let you know when he has reached his limit of frustration with an activity and would like to work on something else for a while.

The models of assault, as outlined by Smith,[182] provide us with a structure in which to view crisis episodes. Techniques for prevention should be the first line of defense in dealing with severe behavior problems. Behavior treatment plans should always include instructions for controlling antecedents and setting events to help prevent problem behaviors from occurring. If they do occur, the treatment plan outlines the consequences to the behavior and provides procedures for staff to follow. All crisis situations, however, cannot be predicted or prevented by a behavior program. This is why it is important for staff to be trained in techniques and methods of crisis intervention. Hopefully, the techniques described in this section, although not a substitute for direct training, will at least assist staff and family members with basic approaches to crisis intervention.

Recommended Training

Pro-ACT, Inc.	Crisis Prevention Institute, Inc. (CPI)
PO Box 5979	3315-H North 124th Street
San Clemente, CA 92674-5979	Brookfield, WI 53005
(949) 498-5700	(800) 558-8976 or (262) 783-5787
proact@cox.net	info@crisisprevention.com
www.parttraining.com	www.crisisprevention.com

20.12 Staff and Family Training

A fundamental component to the implementation of a sound behavioral treatment plan is staff training. To be successful in treating people with TBI with behavioral difficulties, rehabilitation facilities must be committed to providing adequate staff training and support. This commitment is not only one of allocating the time and financial resources for training but also of providing philosophical support of behavioral principles, use of its techniques, and sufficient staffing levels to carry out behavior programs effectively. Without this foundation, it would be very difficult for a facility to realize the full benefit of behavioral programming. These issues aside, training consists of the following steps:

- Basic principles. Training must begin with an understanding of basic behavioral principles. Staff should be able to identify environmental influences (antecedents and setting events) and responses (consequences) that help to maintain target behaviors. It is especially important for staff and families to understand the importance of consistency in implementing treatment plans and in responding to client behavior.

- Data collection. Staff members require training to enable them to observe client behavior accurately and record data reliably. This can include training to criteria. For example, staff can observe client behavior on videotape and fill out data sheets until they are within 90% agreement of preestablished scoring.

- Behavior procedures. It is important for staff and families to understand the structure of behavior treatment design, for example, the differences between accelerative programs (e.g., positive programming), decelerative programs (e.g., DRO), and complex programs (e.g., token economy). Staff members are better able to follow programs consistently that they understand.

- Ethical issues. It is recommended that staff and families be informed of current ethical issues and guidelines regarding the use of behavior programs. Applied behavior analysis can be a powerful and controversial intervention for behavioral change. The procedures must be implemented with great care, understanding, and sensitivity.

- Environmental validity and generalization. Staff and families need to understand the concept of environmental validity (the teaching of skills at the proper time and in a natural setting) and generalization (the transfer of skills from one setting to another). Skills are not useful if they cannot be performed in the correct context or cannot be transferred from a clinical setting to the home and community. For example, being able to dress in a clinic treatment room at 11 AM is not the same as being able to dress at 7 AM in your own bedroom.

- Team approach. Training should emphasize the importance of a team approach to applied behavior analysis. Assisting one another in crisis situations or helping when a client or staff member is not "having a good day" are just a couple of situations that illustrate the need for staff to act as a team. Staff members are more confident at implementing behavior programs when they know that others are there to help if the circumstances warrant it.

- Management of assaultive behavior. Even the most effective behavior programs may not always prevent a crisis situation. Several courses provide training in management of aggressive behavior and crisis intervention. They typically include methods of observation, deescalation, self-defense, and physical restraint. This training, in our experience, affords one of the best means for instilling confidence in staff to work effectively with behaviorally difficult clients. It provides for a systematic approach to aggression and a structure in which all behavioral interactions and interventions can be gauged. These courses tend to emphasize early intervention in the client's "assault cycle," before it reaches a crisis stage that requires physical intervention. This training also provides a useful means for ensuring adherence to the legal requirements of balancing the restraint of clients and self-defense.

- Behavior "staffings." Staff members require a forum to openly address and discuss current behavioral issues. Staff can, at times, be hesitant to discuss client behavior, so may require assertive questioning by the facilitator to draw out details of behavioral episodes and the surrounding factors that might be influencing the behavior. Frequent behavior staffings are also necessary for keeping abreast of the latest behavioral concerns, as well as providing an excellent venue for continuing staff education on behavior methodology.

- Family training. Many clients continue to have behavior problems that persist after being discharged from a facility. Those people who will play a significant role in the client's life after rehabilitation will need training in the proper use of behavior analysis and access to behavior specialists for ongoing support. Facilities can provide families with the same training as their staff. Family members can practice behavior procedures (with the client) under the guidance of the facility. Without this training, behavioral stability after discharge from a facility is less likely to be maintained.

20.13 Putting It All Together

This chapter has described the basic components of effective behavior program design. However, each component does not stand alone. All of the steps are integrated and must be systematically completed in order to reach the desired behavioral outcome.

- Perform *behavioral diagnostics*. First, a thorough assessment must be performed. This consists of reviewing historical information about the client that helps the behavior programmer understand how the client may respond to rehabilitation and what he or she expects to gain from treatment. It involves evaluating the client's current functional skills and analyzing clinical test results that can dictate the type of behavioral procedure that is implemented. Most important, a thorough behavioral assessment includes a functional analysis that identifies the function served by each target behavior.
- Identify potential conditions maintaining the behavior. The result of behavioral diagnostics should be the identification of conditions that might be supporting the target behavior. Is there an antecedent or setting event to the behavior? Are there responses to the behavior that are reinforcing? What function might the behavior be serving? The three parts of a functional analysis are (1) identification of the target behavior and its surrounding events, (2) predicting the factors that control the behavior, and (3) testing of the behavioral hypothesis by manipulating those factors.
- Collect baseline data. After the assessment is complete, the target behavior defined, and the maintaining conditions identified, baseline data can be collected. Baseline data will provide valuable information concerning the frequency and duration of the target behavior and a means for judging the effectiveness of the treatment procedure. The behavior programmer can choose an event, interval, or time-sample recording method based on the characteristics of the target behavior. Event recording is better suited to discrete behaviors (i.e., those with a clearly defined beginning and end). Time-sample recording is more appropriate for high-rate behaviors that are ill suited to constant observation, and interval recording works for general-purpose data collection.
- Design and implement treatment procedures. After baseline data have been collected, a treatment plan can be designed and implemented. The behavior program

should include short- and long-term goals, rationale, clear operational definitions of the target behavior, a list of any materials needed, contraindications, a description of the data collection system, and procedures for staff to follow. Procedures can be accelerative (designed to increase the target behavior), decelerative (designed to decrease the target behavior), or complex (having characteristics of both accelerative and decelerative programs). Effective behavioral programming may even require combining more than one of these procedures simultaneously.

- Continue data collection. After the treatment plan has started, data collection should continue as a means of monitoring the progress of the client. Data recording sheets should be completed on a daily basis in as many environments and conditions as possible. Systematic data collection allows the programmer, staff, client, family, and others to be kept abreast of the client's progress. People typically respond more favorably to observationally recorded data of behavior than statements such as "She is behaving better."

- Graph and analyze behavior data. Behavior data should be routinely summarized and graphed. Graphing is one of the best means for analyzing the effect of a treatment plan. It provides an overall visual impression of behavior that is easy to understand and, also, is an effective way of tracking learning curves. The behavior programmer can then base any modifications to the treatment plan on more objective data rather than anecdotal reports.

- Modify treatment procedures. Treatment procedures should be altered only when there is sufficient evidence in the data to indicate a failure in the procedure's effectiveness, or when the data indicate a need for a transition to a less structured approach. This can happen when the original behavior problem has been resolved. In this situation, the use of *trend* graphing can be useful. Trend graphs show the future projected change in a behavior based on the current observed rate of change.

- Plan for generalization and maintenance of changed behavior. Treatment plans are not successful if a behavioral change is not generalized to other environments and conditions, and maintained over time. As treatment and recovery progress, procedures require modification—for example, thinning a reinforcement schedule or decreasing dependence on prompts. If the client will be living with others after rehabilitation, training of these individuals in basic principles and treatment procedures is essential for a successful outcome. Long-term maintenance of behavior changes can hinge on the ability of family and friends to continue the treatment plan after a client has been discharged from a facility.

20.14 Summary

As the field of TBI rehabilitation continues to evolve, behavioral treatment procedures are being recognized as an essential component of successful client outcome. Applied behavior analysis provides the structure and consistent feedback required by people with TBI. Although many facilities understand the concepts of behavior analysis and recognize the need for its implementation, we have seen too few facilities actualize this ideal. Usually, this is a result of a division between a behavioral approach on the one hand and a therapeutic approach on the other. Behaviorally oriented staff focus primarily on the behavior of a client, whereas therapists' main concern is with recovery of lost cognitive and physical skills. Both need to work together, recognizing shared goals and the contribution each makes to the total rehabilitation of the client. The result of any such division is that behaviorally challenged clients are undertreated, not able to progress to their highest level of independence, and, in many cases, placed in a long-term restrictive environment.

Emphasizing positive programming while minimizing aversive procedures is the current mantra of behavior analysis. Legal and ethical concerns related to the use of aversive procedures make these programs increasingly more difficult to implement, which is understandable, but at the same time can potentially generate unfortunate and impractical consequences. The full spectrum of behavior technology, properly utilized with comprehensive ethical guidelines and monitoring, can maximize treatment efficiency and positive outcome for the client.

Applied behavior analysis is an essential component in helping people with TBI rebuild their lives. Helping these individuals reintegrate into the home, community, and work settings presents a great challenge to the field of rehabilitation. Behavior analysis provides an effective means of achieving this goal.

References

1. Slifer, K. J., Cataldo, M. D., Babbitt, R. L., Kane, A. C., Harrison, K. A., and Cataldo, M. F., Behavior analysis and intervention during hospitalization for brain trauma rehabilitation, *Archives of Physical Medicine and Rehabilitation*, 74(8), 810–817, 1993.
2. Bogner, J. A., Corrigan, J. D., Fugate, L., Mysiw, W. J., and Clinchot, D., Role of agitation in prediction of outcomes after traumatic brain injury, *American Journal of Physical Medicine and Rehabilitation*, 80(9), 636–644, 2001.
3. Lequerica, A. H., Rapport, L. J., Loeher, K., Axelrod, B. N., Vangel, S. J., Jr., and Hanks, R. A., Agitation in acquired brain injury: Impact on acute rehabilitation therapies, *Journal of Head Trauma Rehabilitation*, 22(3), 177–183, 2007.
4. DiCesare, A., Parente, R., and Anderson-Parente, J., Personality changes after traumatic brain injury: Problems and solutions, *Journal of Cognitive Rehabilitation*, 8(2), 1–18, 1990.
5. Denny-Brown, D., Disability arising from closed head injury, *Journal of the American Medical Association*, 127(8), 429–436, 1945.
6. Max, J. E., Robertson, B. A., and Lansing, A. E., The phenomenology of personality change due to traumatic brain injury in children and adolescents, *The Journal of Neuropsychiatry and Clinical Neurosciences*, 13(2), 161–170, 2001.
7. Prigatano, G. P., Personality disturbances associated with traumatic brain injury, *Journal of Consulting and Clinical Psychology*, 60(3), 360–368, 1992.
8. Hilton, G., Behavioral and cognitive sequelae of head trauma, *Orthopedic Nursing*, 13(4), 25–32, 1994.
9. Warriner, E. M. and Velikonja, D., Psychiatric disturbances after traumatic brain injury: Neurobehavioral and personality changes, *Current Psychiatry Reports*, 8(1), 73–80, 2006.
10. Levin, H. S. and Grossman, R. G., Behavioral sequelae of closed head injury. A quantitative study, *Archives of Neurology*, 35(11), 720–727, 1978.
11. Corrigan, J. D., Mysiw, W. J., Gribble, M. W., and Chock, S. K. L., Agitation, cognition, and attention during post-traumatic amnesia, *Brain Injury*, 6(2), 155–160, 1992.
12. Corrigan, J. D. and Mysiw, W. J., Agitation following traumatic head injury: Equivocal evidence for a discrete stage of cognitive recovery, *Archives of Physical Medicine and Rehabilitation*, 69(7), 487–492, 1988.

13. Montgomery, P., Kitten, M., and Niemiec, C., The agitated patient with brain injury and the rehabilitation staff: Bridging the gap of misunderstanding, *Rehabilitation Nursing,* 22(1), 20–23, 39, 1997.

14. Riley, G. A., Stress and depression in family carers following traumatic brain injury: The influence of beliefs about difficult behaviours, *Clinical Rehabilitation,* 21(1), 82–88, 2007.

15. Riedel, D. and Shaw, V., Nursing management of patients with brain injury requiring one-on-one care, *Rehabilitation Nursing,* 22(1), 36–39, 1997.

16. Levy, M., Berson, A., Cook, T., Bollegala, N., Seto, E., Tursanski, S., Kim, J., et al., Treatment of agitation following traumatic brain injury: A review of the literature, *Neurorehabilitation,* 20(4), 279–306, 2005.

17. Brooke, M. M., Questad, K. A., Patterson, D. R., and Bashak, K. J., Agitation and restlessness after closed head injury: A prospective study of 100 consecutive admissions, *Archives of Physical Medicine and Rehabilitation,* 73(4), 320–323, 1992.

18. Peters, M. D., Gluck, M., and McCormick, M., Behaviour rehabilitation of the challenging client in less restrictive settings, *Brain Injury,* 6(4), 299–314, 1992.

19. Duncan, P. W., Physical therapy assessment, in M. Rosenthal, E. R. Griffith, M. R. Bond, and J. D. Miller (Eds.), *Rehabilitation of the Adult and Child with Traumatic Brain Injury,* F. A. Davis, Philadelphia, PA, 1990, 264.

20. Rinne, M. B., Pasanen, M. E., Vartianen, M. V., Lehto, T. M., Sarajuuri, J. M., and Alaranta, H. T., Motor performance in physically well-recovered men with traumatic brain injury, *Journal of Rehabilitation Medicine,* 38(4), 224–229, 2006.

21. Adamovich, B. L. B., Cognition, language, attention, and information processing following closed head injury, in J. S. Kreutzer and P. H. Wehman (Eds.), *Cognitive Rehabilitation for Persons with Traumatic Brain Injury: A Functional Approach,* Paul H. Brookes Publishing, Baltimore, MD, 1991, 75.

22. Ponsford, J., *Cognitive and Behavioral Rehabilitation: From Neurobiology to Clinical Practice,* Guilford Press, New York, 2004.

23. McNeny, R., Activities of daily living, in J. Kreutzer, E. Griffith, B. Pentland, and M. Rosenthal (Eds.) *Rehabilitation of the Adult and Child with Traumatic Brain Injury,* F. A. Davis, Philadelphia, PA, 1999, 242.

24. Armstrong, C., Emotional changes following brain injury: Psychological and neurological components of depression, denial, and anxiety, *Journal of Rehabilitation,* 57(2), 15–21, 1991.

25. Simpson, G., Blaszczynski, A., and Hodgkinson, A., Sex offending as a psychological sequela of traumatic brain injury, *Journal of Head Trauma Rehabilitation,* 14(6), 567–580, 1999.

26. Kersel, D. A., Marsh, N. V., Havill, J. H., and Sleigh, J. W., Psychosocial functioning during the year following severe traumatic brain injury, *Brain Injury,* 15(8), 683–696, 2001.

27. Rogers, J. M. and Read, C. A., Psychiatric comorbidity following traumatic brain injury, *Brain Injury,* 21(13–14),1321–1333, 2007.

28. Draper, K., Ponsford, J., and Schoenberger, M., Psychosocial and emotional outcomes 10 years following traumatic brain injury, *The Journal of Head Trauma Rehabilitation,* 22(5), 278–287, 2007.

29. MacNiven, E. and Finlayson, M. A. J., The interplay between emotional and cognitive recovery after closed head injury, *Brain Injury,* 7(3), 241–246, 1993.

30. Kim, S. H., Manes, F., Kosier, T., Baruah, S., and Robinson, R. G., Irritability following traumatic brain injury, *The Journal of Nervous and Mental Disease,* 187(6), 327–335, 1999.

31. Max, J. E., Castillo, C. S., Bokura, H., Robin, D. A., Lindgren, S. D., Smith, W. L., Jr., Sato, Y., and Mattheis, P. J., Oppositional defiant disorder symptomatology after traumatic brain injury: A prospective study, *The Journal of Nervous and Mental Disease,* 186(6), 325–332, 1998.

32. Greve, K. W., Sherwin, E., Stanford, M. S., Mathias, C., Love, J., and Ramzinski, P., Personality and neurocognitive correlates of impulsive aggression in long-term survivors of severe traumatic brain injury, *Brain Injury,* 15(3), 255–262, 2001.

33. Morris, P. G., Wilson, J. T., Dunn, L. T., and Teasdale, G. M., Premorbid intelligence and brain injury, *British Journal of Clinical Psychology,* 44(2), 209–214, 2005.

34. Kesler, S. R., Adams, H. F., Blasey, C. M., and Bigler, E. D., Premorbid intellectual functioning, education, and brain size in traumatic brain injury: An investigation of the cognitive reserve hypothesis, *Applied Neuropsychology*, 10(3), 153–162, 2003.

35. Walker, R., Hiller, M., Staton, M., and Leukefeld, C. G., Head injury among drug abusers: An indicator of co-occurring problems, *Journal of Psychoactive Drugs*, 35(3), 343–353, 2003.

36. Bendiksen, M. and Bendiksen, I., A multi-dimensional intervention for a toxic solvent injured population, *Journal of Cognitive Rehabilitation*, 10(3), 20–27, 1992.

37. McMillan, T. M., Papadopoulos, H., Cornall, C., and Greenwood, R. J., Modification of severe behaviour problems following herpes simplex encephalitis, *Brain Injury*, 4(4), 399–406, 1990.

38. Mild Traumatic Brain Injury Committee of the Head Injury Interdisciplinary Special Interest Group of the American Congress of Rehabilitation Medicine, Definition of mild traumatic brain injury, *Journal of Head Trauma Rehabilitation*, 8(3), 86–87, 1993.

39. Alexander, M. P., Neuropsychiatric correlates of persistent postconcussive syndrome, *Journal of Head Trauma Rehabilitation*, 7(2), 60–69, 1992.

40. Sosnoff, J. J., Broglio, S. P., and Ferrara, M. S., Cognitive and motor function are associated following mild traumatic brain injury, *Experimental Brain Research*, 187(4), 563–571, 2008.

41. Harrington, D. E., Malec, J., Cicerone, K., and Katz, H. T., Current perceptions of rehabilitation professionals towards mild traumatic brain injury, *Archives of Physical Medicine and Rehabilitation*, 74(6), 579–586, 1993.

42. Bigler, E. D., Neuropsychology and clinical neuroscience of persistent post-concussive syndrome, *Journal of the International Neuropsychological Society*, 14(1), 1–22, 2008.

43. Boake, C., Bobetic, K. M., and Bontke, C. F., Rehabilitation of the patient with mild traumatic brain injury, *Neurorehabilitation*, 1(3), 70–78, 1991.

44. Sterr, A., Herron, K. A., Hayward, C., and Montaldi, D., Are mild head injuries as mild as we think? Neurobehavioral concomitants of chronic post-concussion syndrome, *BMC Neurology*, 6(1), 7, 2006.

45. Verduyn, W. H., Hilt, J., Roberts, M. A., and Roberts, R. J., Multiple partial seizure-like symptoms following "minor" closed head injury, *Brain Injury*, 6(3), 245–260, 1992.

46. Mysiw, W. J. and Sandel, M. E., The agitated brain injured patient. Part 2: Pathophysiology and treatment, *Archives of Physical Medicine and Rehabilitation*, 78(2), 213–220, 1997.

47. Swiercinsky, D. P., Price, T. L., and Leaf, L. E., *Traumatic Head Injury: Cause, Consequence, and Challenge*, The Kansas Head Injury Association, Shawnee Mission, KS, 1987.

48. Oder, W., Goldenberg, G., Spatt, J., Podreka, I., Binder, H., and Deecke, L., Behavioural and psychosocial sequelae of severe closed head injury and regional cerebral blood flow: A SPECT study, *Journal of Neurology, Neurosurgery, and Psychiatry*, 55(6), 475–480, 1992.

49. Tate, R. L., Executive dysfunction and characterological changes after traumatic brain injury: Two sides of the same coin?, *Cortex*, 35(1), 39–55, 1999.

50. Hanten, G., Wilde, E. A., Menefee, D. S., Li, X., Lane, S., Vasquez, C., Chu, Z., et al., Correlates of social problem solving during the first year after traumatic brain injury in children, *Neuropsychology*, 22(3), 357–370, 2008.

51. Schmitz, T. W., Rowley, H. A., Kawahara, T. N., and Johnson, S. C., Neural correlates of self-evaluative accuracy after traumatic brain injury, *Neuropsychologia*, 44(5), 762–773, 2006.

52. Cazalis, F., Feydy, A., Valabregue, R., Pelegrini-Issac, M., Pierot, L., and Azouvi, P., fMRI study of problem-solving after severe traumatic brain injury, *Brain Injury*, 20(10), 1019–1028, 2006.

53. Katz, D. I., Neuropathology and neurobehavioral recovery from closed head injury, *Journal of Head Trauma Rehabilitation*, 7(2), 1–15, 1992.

54. Adams, J. H., Doyle, D., Ford, I., Gennarelli, T. A., Graham, D. I., and McLellan, D. R., Diffuse axonal injury in head injury: Definition, diagnosis, and grading, *Histopathology*, 15(1), 49–59, 1989.

55. Povlishock, J. T. and Katz, D. I., Update of neuropathology and neurological recovery after traumatic brain injury, *Journal of Head Trauma Rehabilitation*, 20(1), 76–94, 2005.

56. Farkas, O. and Povlishock, J. T., Cellular and subcellular change evoked by diffuse traumatic brain injury: A complex web of change extending far beyond focal damage, *Progress in Brain Research*, 161, 43–59, 2007.

57. Coutant, N. S., Rage: Implied neurological correlates, *Journal of Neurosurgical Nursing*, 14(1), 28–33, 1982.
58. Crompton, M. R., Hypothalamic lesions following closed head injury, *Brain*, 94(1), 165–172, 1971.
59. Elliott, F. A., The neurology of explosive rage: The dyscontrol syndrome, *Practitioner*, 217(1297), 51–60, 1976.
60. Amaral, D. G., The amygdala, social behavior, and danger detection, *Annals of the New York Academy of Sciences*, 1000, 337–347, 2003.
61. Grafman, J., Sirigu, A., Spector, L., and Hendler, J., Damage to the prefrontal cortex leads to decomposition of structured event complexes, *Journal of Head Trauma Rehabilitation*, 8(1), 73–87, 1993.
62. Goldman-Rakic, P. S., Specifications of higher cortical functions, *Journal of Head Trauma Rehabilitation*, 8(1), 13–23, 1993.
63. Max, J. E., Levin, H. S., Schachar, R. J., Landis, J., Saunders, A. E., Ewing-Cobbs, L., Chapman, S. B., and Dennis, M., Predictors of personality change due to traumatic brain injury in children and adolescents six to twenty-four months after injury, *The Journal of Neuropsychiatry and Clinical Neurosciences*, 20(1), 118–119, 2008.
64. Hart, T. and Jacobs, H. E., Rehabilitation and management of behavioral disturbances following frontal lobe injury, *Journal of Head Trauma Rehabilitation*, 8, 1–12, 1993.
65. Slachevsky, A., Pena, M., Perez, C., Bravo, E., and Alegria, P., Neuroanatomical basis of behavioral disturbances in patients with prefrontal lesions, *Biological Research*, 39(2), 237–250, 2006.
66. Behan, L. A., Phillips, J., Thompson, C. J., and Agha, A., Neuroendocrine disorders after traumatic brain injury, *Journal of Neurology, Neurosurgery, and Psychiatry*, 79(7), 753–759, 2008.
67. Schulkin, J., *The Neuroendocrine Regulation of Behavior*, Cambridge University Press, Cambridge, UK, 1998.
68. Cantini, E., Gluck, M., and McLean, A., Jr., Psychotropic-absent behavioural improvement following severe traumatic brain injury, *Brain Injury*, 6(2), 193–197, 1992.
69. Fleminger, S., Greenwood, R. J., and Oliver, D. L., Pharmacological management for agitation and aggression in people with acquired brain injury, *Cochrane Database of Systematic Review*, 1 Jan 2006 (4), CD003299, 2006.
70. Rose, M. J., The place of drugs in the management of behavior disorders after traumatic brain injury, *Journal of Head Trauma Rehabilitation*, 3(3), 7–13, 1988.
71. Carnevale, G. J., Anselmi, V., Johnston, M. V., Busichio, K., and Walsh, V., A natural setting behavior management program for persons with acquired brain injury: A randomized controlled trial, *Archives of Physical Medicine and Rehabilitation*, 87(10), 1289–1297, 2006.
72. Yablon, S. A., Posttraumatic seizures, *Archives of Physical Medicine and Rehabilitation*, 74(9), 983–1001, 1993.
73. Sandel, M. E., Olive, D. A., and Rader, M. A., Chlorpromazine-induced psychosis after brain injury, *Brain Injury*, 7(1), 77–83, 1993.
74. Stanislave, S. W., Cognitive effects of antipsychotic agents in persons with traumatic brain injury, *Brain Injury*, 11(5), 335–341, 1997.
75. Harmsen M., Geurts, A. C., Fasotti, L., and Bevaart, B. J., Positive behavioural disturbances in the rehabilitation phase after severe traumatic brain injury: An historic cohort study, *Brain Injury*, 18(8), 787–796, 2004.
76. Galski, T., Palasz, J., Bruno, R. L., and Walker, J. E., Predicting physical and verbal aggression on a brain trauma unit, *Archives of Physical Medicine and Rehabilitation*, 75(4), 380–383, 1994.
77. Mysiw, W. J., Bogner, J. A., Corrigan, J. D., Fugate, L. P., Clinchot, D. M., and Kadyan, V., The impact of acute care medications on rehabilitation outcome after traumatic brain injury, *Brain Injury*, 20(9), 905–911, 2006.
78. Rao, N., Jellinek, H. M., and Woolston, D. C., Agitation in closed head injury: Haloperidol effects on rehabilitation outcome, *Archives of Physical Medicine and Rehabilitation*, 66(1), 30–34, 1985.
79. Chandler, M. C., Barnhill, J. L., and Gualtieri, C. T., Amantadine for the agitated head-injury patient, *Brain Injury*, 2(4), 309–311, 1988.

80. Brooke, M. M., Patterson, D. R., Questad, K. A., Cardenas, D., and Farrel-Roberts, L., The treatment of agitation during initial hospitalization after traumatic brain injury, *Archives of Physical Medicine and Rehabilitation*, 73(10), 917–921, 1992.

81. Stanislav, S. W. and Childs, A., Evaluating the usage of droperidol in acutely agitated persons with brain injury, *Brain Injury*, 14(3), 261–265, 2000.

82. Maryniak, O., Manchanda, R., and Velani, A., Methotrimeprazine in the treatment of agitation in acquired brain injury patients, *Brain Injury*, 15(2), 167–174, 2001.

83. Chatham-Showalter, P. E. and Kimmel, D. N., Agitated symptom response to divalproex following acute brain injury, *Journal of Neuropsychiatry and Clinical Neurosciences*, 12(3), 395–397, 2000.

84. Mysiw, W. J., Jackson, R. D., and Corrigan, J. D., Amitriptyline for posttraumatic agitation, *American Journal of Physical Medicine and Rehabilitation*, 67(1), 29–33, 1988.

85. Meythaler, J. M., Depalma, L., Devivo, M. J., Guin-Renfroe, S., and Novack, T. A., Sertraline to improve arousal and alertness in severe traumatic brain injury secondary to motor vehicle crashes, *Brain Injury*, 15(4), 321–331, 2001.

86. Stanislav, S. W., Fabre, T., Crismon, M. L., and Childs, A., Buspirone's efficacy in organic-induced aggression, *Journal of Clinical Psychopharmacology*, 14(2), 126–130, 1994.

87. Chatham-Showalter, P. E., Carbamazepine for combativeness in acute traumatic brain injury, *Journal of Neuropsychiatry and Clinical Neurosciences*, 8(1), 96–99, 1996.

88. Azouvi, P., Jokic, C., Attal, N., Denys, P., Markabi, S., and Bussel, B., Carbamazepine in agitation and aggressive behaviour following severe closed-head injury: Results of an open trial, *Brain Injury*, 13(10), 797–804, 1999.

89. Wroblewski, B. A., Joseph, A. B., Kupfer, J., and Kalliel, K., Effectiveness of valproic acid on destructive and aggressive behaviours in patients with acquired brain injury, *Brain Injury*, 11(1), 37–47, 1997.

90. Mooney, G. F. and Haas, L. J., Effect of methylphenidate on brain injury-related anger, *Archives of Physical Medicine and Rehabilitation*, 74(2), 153–160, 1993.

91. Speech, T. J., Rao, S. M., Osmon, D. C., and Sperry, L. T., A double-blind controlled study of methylphenidate treatment in closed head injury, *Brain Injury*, 7(4), 333–338, 1993.

92. Siddall, O. M., Use of methylphenidate in traumatic brain injury, *The Annals of Pharmacotherapy*, 39(7–8), 1309–1313, 2005.

93. Michals, M. L., Crismon, M. L., Roberts, S., and Childs, A., Clozapine response and adverse effects in nine brain-injured patients, *Journal of Clinical Psychopharmacology*, 13(3), 198–203, 1993.

94. Alban, J. P., Hopson, M. M., Ly, V., and Whyte, J., Effect of methylphenidate on vital signs and adverse effects in adults with traumatic brain injury, *American Journal of Physical Medicine and Rehabilitation*, 83(2), 131–137, 2004.

95. Silver, J. M. and Yudofsky, S. C., Pharmacologic treatment of neuropsychiatric disorders, *Neurorehabilitation*, 3(1), 15–25, 1993.

96. Wilkinson, R., Meythaler, J. M., and Guin-Renfroe, S., Neuroleptic malignant syndrome induced by haloperidol following traumatic brain injury, *Brain Injury*, 13(2), 1025–1031, 1999.

97. Fowler, S. B., Hertzog, J., Wagner, B. K., and Johnson, R. W., Pharmacological interventions for agitation in head-injured patients in the acute care setting, *Journal of Neuroscience Nursing*, 27(2), 119–123, 1995.

98. Cope, D. N., Legal and ethical issues in the psychopharmacological treatment of traumatic brain injury, *Journal of Head Trauma Rehabilitation*, 4(1), 13–21, 1989.

99. Edlund, M. J., Goldberg, R. J., and Morris, P. L., The use of physical restraint in patients with cerebral contusion, *International Journal of Psychiatry in Medicine*, 21(2), 173–182, 1991.

100. Gregory, H. H., Jr. and Bonfiglio, R. P., Limiting restraint use for behavior control: The brain injury rehabilitation unit as a model, *Maryland Medical Journal*, 44(4), 279–283, 1995.

101. Colantonio, A., Stamenova, V., Abramowitz, C., Clarke, D., and Christensen, B., Brain injury in a forensic psychiatry population, *Brain Injury*, 21(13–14), 1353–1360, 2007.

102. Kant, R., Bogyi, A. M., Carosella, N. W., Fishman, E., Kane, V., and Coffey, C. E., ECT as a therapeutic option in severe brain injury, *Convulsive Therapy*, 11(1), 45–50, 1995.

103. Van Houten, R., Axelrod, S., Bailey, J. S., Favell, J. E., Foxx, R. M., Iwata, B. A., and Lovaas, O. I., The right to effective behavioral treatment, *Journal of Applied Behavior Analysis*, 21(4), 381–384, 1988.

104. Scofield, G. R., Ethical considerations in rehabilitation medicine, *Archives of Physical Medicine and Rehabilitation*, 74(4), 341–346, 1993.

105. LaChapelle, D. L. and Finlayson, M. A., An evaluation of subjective and objective measures of fatigue in patients with brain injury and healthy controls, *Brain Injury*, 12(8), 649–659, 1998.

106. Cantor, J. B., Ashman, T., Gordon, W., Ginsberg, A., Engmann, C., Egan, M., Spielman, L., Dijkers, M., and Flanagan, S., Fatigue after traumatic brain injury and its impact on participation and quality of life, *Journal of Head Trauma Rehabilitation*, 23(1), 41–51, 2008.

107. Bergquist, T. F. and Jacket, M. P., Awareness and goal setting with the traumatically brain injured, *Brain Injury*, 7(3), 275–282, 1993.

108. Hart, T., Seignourel, P. J., and Sherer, M., A longitudinal study of awareness of deficit after moderate to severe traumatic brain injury, *Neuropsychological Rehabilitation*, 19(2), 161–176, 2009.

109. Schlund, M. W. and Pace, G., Relations between traumatic brain injury and the environment: Feedback reduces maladaptive behaviour exhibited by three persons with traumatic brain injury, *Brain Injury*, 13(11), 889–897, 1999.

110. Davis, P. K. and Chittum, R., A group-oriented contingency to increase leisure activities of adults with traumatic brain injury, *Journal of Applied Behavior Analysis*, 27(3), 553–554, 1994.

111. McGraw-Hunter, M., Faw, G. D., and Davis, P. K., The use of video self-modeling and feedback to teach cooking skills to individuals with traumatic brain injury: A pilot study, *Brain Injury*, 20(10), 1061–1068, 2006.

112. Miller, D. L. and Kelly, M. L., The use of goal setting and contingency contracting for improving children's homework performance, *Journal of Applied Behavior Analysis*, 27(1), 73–84, 1994.

113. Joyce, B. M., Rockwood, K. J., and Mate-Kole, C. C., Use of goal attainment scaling in brain injury in a rehabilitation hospital, *American Journal of Physical Medicine and Rehabilitation*, 73(1), 10–14, 1994.

114. Jones, R. S. and McCaughey, R. E., Gentle teaching and applied behavior analysis: A critical review, *Journal of Applied Behavior Analysis*, 25(4), 853–867, 1992.

115. McGee, J. J., Gentle teaching's assumptions and paradigm, *Journal of Applied Behavior Analysis*, 25(4), 869–872, 1992.

116. Aylott, J. and Sell, I., Gentle teaching as an empowering approach to challenging behaviour, *British Journal of Nursing*, 6(8), 442–446, 1997.

117. Yuen, H. K. and Benzing, P., Treatment methodology: Guiding of behaviour through redirection in brain injury rehabilitation, *Brain Injury*, 10(3), 229–238, 1996.

118. Bailey, J. S., Gentle teaching: Trying to win friends and influence people with euphemism, metaphor, smoke, and mirrors, *Journal of Applied Behavior Analysis*, 25(4), 879–883, 1992.

119. Dyer, K., Dunlap, G., and Winterling, V., Effects of choice making on the serious problem behaviors of students with severe handicaps, *Journal of Applied Behavior Analysis*, 23(4), 515–524, 1990.

120. Tasky, K. K., Rudrud, E. H., Schulze, K. A., and Rapp, J. T., Using choice to increase on-task behavior in individuals with traumatic brain injury, *Journal of Applied Behavior Analysis*, 41(2), 261–265, 2008.

121. Mace, F. C. and Belfiore, P., Behavioral momentum in the treatment of escape-motivated stereotype, *Journal of Applied Behavior Analysis*, 23(4), 507–514, 1990.

122. Horner, R. H., Day, H. M., Sprague, J. R., O'Brien, M., and Heathfield, L. T., Interspersed requests: A nonaversive procedure for reducing aggression and self-injury during instruction, *Journal of Applied Behavior Analysis*, 24(2), 265–278, 1991.

123. Wheeler, A. J., Miller, R. A., Duke, J., Salisbury, E. W., Merritt, V., and Horton, B., *Murdoch Center C & Y Program Library: A Collection of Step-By-Step Programs for the Developmentally Disabled*, Murdoch Center, Butner, NC, 1977.

124. Kennedy, C. H. and Itkonen, T., Effects of setting events on the problem behavior of students with severe disabilities, *Journal of Applied Behavior Analysis*, 26(3), 321–327, 1993.

125. Michael, J., Implications and refinements of the establishing operation concept, *Journal of Applied Behavior Analysis*, 33(4), 401–410, 2000.

126. Fluharty, G. and Glassman, N., Use of antecedent control to improve the outcome of rehabilitation for a client with frontal lobe injury and intolerance for auditory and tactile stimuli, *Brain Injury*, 15(11), 995–1002, 2001.

127. Slifer, K. J., Tucker, C. L., Gerson, A. C., Sevier, R. C., Kane, A. C., Amari, A., and Clawson, B. P., Antecedent management and compliance training improve adolescents' participation in early brain injury rehabilitation, *Brain Injury*, 11(12), 877–889, 1997.

128. Pace, G. M., Dunn, E. K., Luiselli, J. K., Cochran, C. R., and Skowron, J., Antecedent interventions in the management of maladaptive behaviours in a child with brain injury, *Brain Injury*, 19(5), 365–369, 2005.

129. Cifu, D. X., Kreutzer, J. S., Kolakowsky-Hayner, S. A., Marwitz, J. H., and Englander, J., The relationship between therapy intensity and rehabilitative outcomes after traumatic brain injury: A multicenter analysis, *Archives of Physical Medicine and Rehabilitation*, 84(10), 1441–1448, 2003.

130. Dumas, H. M., Haley, S. M., Carey, T. M., and Ni, P. S., The relationship between functional mobility and the intensity of physical therapy intervention in children with traumatic brain injury, *Pediatric Physical Therapy*, 16(3), 157–164, 2004.

131. Pace, G. M., Ivancic, M. T., and Jefferson, G., Stimulus fading as treatment for obscenity in a brain-injured adult, *Journal of Applied Behavior Analysis*, 27(2), 301–305, 1994.

132. Fugate, L. P., Spacek, L. A., Kresty, L. A., Levy, C. E., Johnson, J. C., and Mysiw, W. J., Definition of agitation following traumatic brain injury: I. A survey of the Brain Injury Special Interest Group of the American Academy of Physical Medicine and Rehabilitation, *Archives of Physical Medicine and Rehabilitation*, 78(9), 917–923, 1997.

133. Tate, R. L., Behaviour management techniques for organic psychosocial deficit incurred by severe head injury, *Scandinavian Journal of Rehabilitation Medicine*, 19(1), 19–24, 1987.

134. Turner, J. M., Green, G., and Braunling-McMorrow, D., Differential reinforcement of low rates of responding (DRL) to reduce dysfunctional social behaviors of a head injured man, *Behavioral Residential Treatment*, 5(1), 15–27, 1990.

135. Lane, I. M., Wesolowski, M. D., and Burke, W. H., Teaching socially appropriate behavior to eliminate hoarding in a brain injured adult, *Journal of Behavior Therapy and Experimental Psychiatry*, 20(1), 79–82, 1989.

136. Youngson, H. A. and Alderman, N., Fear of incontinence and its effects on a community-based rehabilitation programme after severe brain injury: Successful remediation of escape behaviour using behaviour modification, *Brain Injury*, 8(1), 23–36, 1994.

137. Zencius, A., Wesolowski, M. D., and Burke, W. H., Comparing motivational systems with two noncompliant head-injured adolescents, *Brain Injury*, 3(1), 67–71, 1989.

138. Giles, G. M., Fussey, I., and Burgess, P., The behavioural treatment of verbal interaction skills following severe head injury: A single case study, *Brain Injury*, 2(1), 75–79, 1988.

139. McHugh, L. and Wood, R. L., Using a temporal discounting paradigm to measure decision-making and impulsivity following traumatic brain injury: A pilot study, *Brain Injury*, 22(9), 715–721, 2008.

140. Hegel, M. T., Application of a token economy with a non-compliant closed head-injured male, *Brain Injury*, 2(4), 333–338, 1988.

141. Giles, G. M. and Clark-Wilson, J., The use of behavioral techniques in functional skills training after severe brain injury, *American Journal of Occupational Therapy*, 42(10), 658–665, 1988.

142. Zencius, A. H., Wesolowski, M. D., Burke, W. H., and McQuade, P., Antecedent control in the treatment of brain-injured clients, *Brain Injury*, 3(2), 199–205, 1989.

143. Braunling-McMorrow, D., Lloyd, K., and Fralish, K., Teaching social skills to head injured adults, *Journal of Rehabilitation*, 52(1), 39–44, 1986.

144. Blair, D. C. and Lanyon, R. I., Retraining social and adaptive living skills in severely head injured adults, *Archives of Clinical Neuropsychology*, 2(1), 33–43, 1987.

145. Kelly, G., Brown, S., Todd, J., and Kremer, P., Challenging behaviour profiles of people with acquired brain injury living in community settings, *Brain Injury*, 22(6), 457–470, 2008.

146. Steege, M. W., Wacker, D. P., Cigrand, K. C., Berg, W. K., Novak, C. G., Reimers, T. M., Sasso, G. M., and DeRaad, A., Use of negative reinforcement in the treatment of self-injurious behavior, *Journal of Applied Behavior Analysis*, 23(4), 459–467, 1990.

147. Bandura, A., Self-efficacy, in V. S. Ramachaudran (Ed.), *Encyclopedia of Human Behavior*, Academic Press, San Diego, CA, 1998, 71.

148. Lloyd, L. F. and Cuvo, A. J., Maintenance and generalization of behaviours after treatment of persons with traumatic brain injury, *Brain Injury*, 8(6), 529–540, 1994.

149. Yody, B. B., Schaub, C., Conway, J., Peters, S., Strauss, D., and Helsinger, S., Applied behavior management and acquired brain injury: Approaches and assessment, *Journal of Head Trauma Rehabilitation*, 15(4), 1041–1060, 2000.

150. Jacobs, H. E., *Behavior Analysis Guidelines and Brain Injury Rehabilitation: People, Principles, and Programs*, Aspen Publications, Gaithsburg, MD, 1993.

151. Wahler, R. G. and Fox, J. J., Setting events in applied behavior analysis: Toward a conceptual and methodological expansion, *Journal of Applied Behavior Analysis*, 14(3), 327–338, 1981.

152. Chandler, L. K., Fowler, S. A., and Lubeck, R. C., An analysis of the effects of multiple setting events on the social behavior of preschool children with special needs, *Journal of Applied Behavior Analysis*, 25(2), 249–263, 1992.

153. Ashley, M. J. and Persel, C. S., Traumatic brain injury recovery rates in post-acute rehabilitation of traumatic brain injury: Spontaneous recovery or treatment?, *Journal of Rehabilitation Outcomes Measurement*, 3(4), 15–21, 1999.

154. Iwata, B. A., Vollmer, T. R., and Zarcone, J. R., The experimental (functional) analysis of behavior disorders: Methodology, applications, and limitations, in A. C. Repp and N. N. Singh (Eds.), *Perspectives on the Use of Nonaversive and Aversive Interventions for Persons with Developmental Disabilities*, Sycamore Press, Sycamore, IL, 1990, 301.

155. Durand, M. V. and Carr, E. G., Functional communication training to reduce challenging behavior: Maintenance and application in new settings, *Journal of Applied Behavior Analysis*, 24(2), 251–264, 1991.

156. O'Neill, R. E., Horner, R. H., Albin, R. W., Storey, K., and Sprague, J. R., *Functional Analysis of Problem Behaviors: A Practical Assessment Guide*, Sycamore Press, Sycamore, IL, 1990.

157. Derby, K. M., Wacker, D. P., Peck, S., Sasso, G., DeRaad, A., Berg, W., Asmus, J., and Ulrich, S., Functional analysis of separate topographies of aberrant behavior, *Journal of Applied Behavior Analysis*, 27(2), 267–278, 1994.

158. Rappaport, M., Hall, K. M., Hopkins, K., Belleza, T., and Cope, D. N., Disability Rating Scale for severe head trauma: Coma to community, *Archives of Physical Medicine and Rehabilitation*, 63(3), 118–123, 1982.

159. Carr, E. G. and Carlson, J. I., Reduction of severe behavior problems in the community using a multicomponent treatment approach, *Journal of Applied Behavior Analysis*, 26(2), 157–172, 1993.

160. LaVigna, G. W. and Donnellan, A. M., *Alternatives to Punishment: Solving Behavior Problems with Non-Aversive Strategies*, Irvington Publishers, New York, 1986.

161. Ducharme, J. M., A conceptual model for treatment of externalizing behaviour in acquired brain injury, *Brain Injury*, 13(9), 645–668, 1999.

162. Schwartz, S. M., Adults with traumatic brain injury: Three case studies of cognitive rehabilitation in the home setting, *American Journal of Occupational Therapy*, 49(7), 655–667, 1995.

163. Walls, R. T., Zane, T., and Ellis, W. D., Forward and backward chaining and whole task methods, Behavior *Modification*, 5(1), 61–74, 1981.

164. Mulick, J. A., Leitenberg, H., and Rawson, R. A., Alternative response training, differential reinforcement of other behavior, and extinction in squirrel monkeys (*Saimiri sciureus*), *Journal of the Experimental Analysis of Behavior*, 25(3), 311–320, 1976.

165. Reynolds, G. S., Behavioral contrast, *Journal of the Experimental Analysis of Behavior*, 4, 57–71, 1961.

166. Hegel, M. T. and Ferguson, R. J., Differential reinforcement of other behavior (DRO) to reduce aggressive behavior following traumatic brain injury, *Behavior Modification*, 24(1), 94–101, 2000.

167. Cowdery, G. E., Iwata, B. A., and Pace, G. M., Effects and side effects of DRO as treatment for self-injurious behavior, *Journal of Applied Behavior Analysis*, 23(4), 497–506, 1990.

168. Skinner, B. F., *The Behavior of Organisms*, Appleton-Century-Crofts, New York, 1938.

169. Azrin, N. H. and Foxx, R. M., A rapid method of toilet training the institutionalized retarded, *Journal of Applied Behavior Analysis*, 4(2), 89–99, 1971.

170. Azrin, N. H., Some effects of noise on human behavior, *Journal of the Experimental Analysis of Behavior*, 1(2), 183–200, 1958.

171. Ayllon, T., Intensive treatment of psychotic behavior by stimulus satiation and food reinforcement, *Behaviour Research and Therapy*, 1(1), 53–61, 1963.

172. Alderman, N., The treatment of avoidance behaviour following severe brain injury by satiation through negative practice, *Brain Injury*, 5(1), 77–86, 1991.

173. McClellan, C. B., Cohen, L. L., and Moffett, K., Time out based discipline strategy for children's non-compliance with cystic fibrosis treatment, *Disability and Rehabilitation*, 31(4), 327–336, 2009.

174. Czyzewski, M. J., Sheldon, J., and Hannah, G. T., Legal safety in residential treatment environments, in F. J. Fuoco and W. P. Christian (Eds.), *Behavior Analysis and Therapy in Residential Programs*, Van Nostrand Reinhold, New York, 1986, 194.

175. DeRisi, W. J. and Butz, G., *Writing Behavioral Contracts: A Case Simulation Practice Manual*, Research Press, Champaign, IL, 1975.

176. Catania, A. C. (Ed.), *Contemporary Research in Operant Behavior*, Scott-Foresman, Glenview, IL, 1968.

177. Teichner, G., Golden, C. J., and Giannaris, W. J., A multimodal approach to treatment of aggression in a severely brain-injured adolescent, *Rehabilitation Nursing*, 24(5), 207–211, 1999.

178. Ayllon, T. and Azrin, N. H., *The Token Economy: A Motivational System for Therapy and Rehabilitation*, Appleton-Century-Crofts, New York, 1968.

179. Persel, C. S., Persel, C. H., and Ashley, M. J., The use of noncontingent reinforcement and contingent restraint to reduce physical aggression and self-injurious behavior in a traumatically brain injured adult, *Brain Injury*, 11(10), 751–760, 1997.

180. Baer, D. M., Wolf, M. M., and Risley, T. R., Some still current dimensions of applied behavior analysis, *Journal of Applied Behavior Analysis*, 20(4), 313–328, 1987.

181. Haring, T. G. and Kennedy, C. H., Contextual control of problem behavior in students with severe disabilities, *Journal of Applied Behavior Analysis*, 23(2), 235–243, 1990.

182. Smith, P., *Professional Assault Response Training (PART)*, Workshop Syllabus, Citrus Heights, CA, 1993.

183. Brammer, L. M., *The Helping Relationship: Process and Skills*, Prentice Hall, Englewood Cliffs, NJ, 1973.

21

Neuropsychological Interventions Following Traumatic Brain Injury

Theodore Tsaousides and Wayne A. Gordon

CONTENTS

21.1 Introduction

Traumatic brain injury (TBI) often results in a myriad of complex physical, cognitive, and emotional impairments that can disrupt individuals' capacity to live independently, to perform social and occupational roles successfully, and to attain their preinjury quality of life.[1] These negative effects are rarely transient, and often persist for the remainder of a person's life, especially when he or she remains untreated. As a result, a relatively high rate of neuropsychiatric challenges are evident among individuals with TBI several years postinjury.[2-4] Given the complexity and duration of the difficulties that are secondary to TBI, a multitude of treatment approaches and interventions have been developed to address the broad impact of the injury on physical, cognitive, and psychosocial functioning. Overall, the aim of TBI rehabilitation is to improve physical, cognitive, and psychosocial functioning; to engender independence; and to facilitate community reintegration.[5]

Neuropsychological rehabilitation is the aspect of TBI rehabilitation that focuses on the diagnosis and treatment of brain–behavior impairments. Neuropsychological interventions address the cognitive, emotional, and psychosocial consequences of TBI and consist of a variety of clinical approaches that are aimed at improving a person's ability to perform cognitive tasks more effectively, to cope with affective distress, and to increase self-awareness and self-esteem, all of which are aimed at improving the person's sense of well-being.

The purpose of this chapter is to provide an overview of neuropsychological rehabilitation; briefly review the research demonstrating its efficacy; identify recurrent and often unresolved themes in the relevant literature; present an overview of prevalent neuropsychological interventions for cognition, emotion, and self-awareness; and discuss future directions of neuropsychological rehabilitation for TBI.

21.2 Neuropsychological Rehabilitation

Neuropsychological rehabilitation refers to a broad range of interventions designed to improve cognitive and psychosocial functioning. These interventions include cognitive rehabilitation, psychotherapy, psychoeducation, family involvement, and vocational training.[6] Neuropsychological rehabilitation has a relatively brief history, and in a short period of time, it has resulted in advances in the treatment of individuals with TBI, leading to functional improvements and increased engagement in productive and meaningful activities in several spheres of life, including employment, social, and community participation. Since the emergence of the first comprehensive and coordinated efforts to address the impairments resulting from TBI more than 30 years ago, neuropsychological rehabilitation has spurred significant research interest, which grew out of the need to distinguish therapeutic activities of significant outcome value from those that made no clinically meaningful contribution to functional improvement.[7] Despite the strong evidence for the effectiveness of these interventions, most third-party payers still do not reimburse patients for these services.

Neuropsychological rehabilitation interventions are applicable to all stages of brain injury rehabilitation (i.e., acute, subacute, and postacute).[8] During the acute stage, neuropsychological interventions consist mainly of initiation of cognitive interventions to improve basic skill function (e.g., attention, orientation) and neurobehavioral approaches for the management of emotional and behavioral symptoms.[4] During the subacute stage, the range of applicable interventions includes managing neurobehavioral symptoms, especially when the severity of the injury prevents or delays participation in more intensive types of treatment.[8] A variety of neuropsychological interventions is available during the postacute treatment stage as well, some of which are described in the following sections. The plethora of these interventions renders rehabilitation likely to begin at any time postinjury. In other words, it is never too late to begin treatment.

21.2.1 Principles of Neuropsychological Rehabilitation

Prigatano[6] developed a set of guidelines that is useful in guiding the practice of clinicians who are likely to enhance the therapeutic experience of the patient and to maximize the patient's potential benefit from treatment. He delineated 13 principles that pervade neuropsychological rehabilitation. In summary, these principles address, among other issues, the importance of understanding the individual's subjective experience of the injury, the interaction of premorbid cognitive and personality characteristics with presenting symptomatology, the impairments in self-awareness and the need to address them in treatment, the inclusion of retraining and management of cognitive deficits, psychotherapy and coping skill building for emotional distress, and support for families and staff to handle their own affective responses during the rehabilitation process. In addition, Prigatano[6] underscored the dynamic nature of neuropsychological rehabilitation, which is fluid and constantly informed and transformed by scientific efforts, phenomenologic approaches, as well as the clinical judgment of the therapist.

21.2.2 From Isolation to Integration: The Evolution of Comprehensive Treatment

Over time, the repertoire of interventions that constitute neuropsychological rehabilitation for TBI has evolved.[6] At the core of neuropsychological treatment is cognitive rehabilitation. Frequently used interchangeably with the term *cognitive remediation*,[9] cognitive rehabilitation was originally conceptualized as a cluster of interventions designed to equip individuals with TBI with a set of skills and strategies to enable them to complete cognitively oriented tasks, the completion of which was hampered by the cognitive impairments resulting from the injury. Over time, as cognitive remediation interventions proliferated, treatment needs of individuals with TBI were better understood, and evidence for the additional benefits of milieu treatment for deficits related to TBI became available,[8,10,11] these interventions began to be administered in concert with other therapeutic activities and treatments that are designed to address brain–behavior deficits.[9,12] Cognitive rehabilitation that purely targeted specific cognitive skills in isolation, although effective,[7,11] did not have a direct impact on patients' quality of life and functional performance or ability in real-life settings.[13–15] What, then, could link skill training to positive psychosocial outcomes? Integrating interventions that addressed multiple skills was one way to address this issue. Sohlberg and Mateer[16] suggested expanding the term *cognitive rehabilitation* to "rehabilitation of individuals with cognitive impairments"[p.3] to capture the breadth of the treatment needs of individuals who sustained brain injuries that extend beyond retraining and managing the cognitive difficulties, to include management of affective and behavioral symptoms, and, ultimately, improvement in psychosocial functioning and reintegration in the community. This emerging definition of cognitive rehabilitation resulted in the convergence of the terms *cognitive rehabilitation* and *neuropsychological rehabilitation*.

During the mid 1970s, treatment programs were developed that combined different interventions, the effectiveness of which was further enhanced by their complementarity, as each one targeted different skills.[10] Ben-Yishay[10] was the first to develop a comprehensive holistic day treatment program for individuals with brain injuries that incorporated a combination of individuals and group treatment approaches, as well as community activities. This innovative, comprehensive intervention received rapid recognition, was adapted by a variety of settings and applied in many iterations, and has become standard of care in neuropsychological rehabilitation.[6] The defining characteristics of a comprehensive holistic day treatment program include neuropsychological interventions to improve cognitive skill function, increase awareness, and address interpersonal, social, and emotional concerns in individual and group sessions; a transdisciplinary treatment approach with clearly defined and regularly monitored treatment goals; opportunities for involvement of significant others; independent living and/or vocational trials; and assessment of outcomes.[8]

21.3 The Imminent Question: Is There Evidence That Cognitive Rehabilitation Is Effective?

Theoretical and conceptual developments; technologic advances in imaging, measurement, and treatment applications; invaluable clinical observations; and significant improvements in research methodology have resulted in the accumulation of knowledge and evidence that rendered possible the evaluation of cognitive rehabilitation and neuropsychological interventions. The tool kit of cognitive rehabilitation interventions has grown rapidly during the past three decades. Interventions have been developed to improve visual–perceptual skills,[17] language,[18–20] attention,[21–23] memory,[24–27] and executive functioning following TBI.[28–30] Parallel to the emergence of a multitude of interventions, the need to validate empirically the effectiveness of these interventions grew as well, as most of these interventions were developed in clinical settings and were based on clinical observations. Responsiveness to the research needs resulted in accumulation of evidence supporting the clinical effectiveness of cognitive rehabilitation, heightened awareness of the need for methodologic rigor in the area of TBI rehabilitation, and identification of treatment-related issues that need further investigation, such as the interaction between demographic, injury, and treatment variables on outcome.

The evidence amassed has supported the efficacy of cognitive rehabilitation interventions. As early as the late 1970s, research in this field revealed the effectiveness of these interventions on improving cognitive functioning.[7,9] Two systematic reviews were published in 2000 and 2004 conducted by the Cognitive Rehabilitation Task Force of the Brain Injury–Interdisciplinary Special Interest Group of the American Congress of Rehabilitation Medicine.[7,11] These reviews evaluated the literature on cognitive rehabilitation interventions for TBI and stroke. The conclusions based on these reviews revealed that (1) cognitive rehabilitation was effective over traditional types of treatment, (2) studies that showed no advantage were comparing one cognitive rehabilitation treatment with another, and (3) in no study was cognitive rehabilitation less effective than alternative treatment.[7,11] Hence, a growing body of evidence became available supporting the efficacy of cognitive rehabilitation interventions for individuals with TBI. Interestingly, the review by Cicerone et al.,[7] in 2000, which spanned almost 25 years of research, yielded 171 studies (29 of which were class I), whereas the 2004[11] review, which spanned 5 years, included 87 studies (17 of which were class I). The relatively larger per-year yield illustrates the responsiveness to the need for evidence, as well as the improvements in methodologic rigor. Nevertheless, Cicerone et al.[11] caution that the quest for evidence should now shift from validating the effectiveness of cognitive rehabilitation treatments to understanding the nuances in treatment and patient characteristics that maximize the clinical benefits.

21.4 Recurrent Themes in Neuropsychological Rehabilitation

In reviewing the literature on clinical interventions, whether empirical or descriptive, certain themes become evident that pertain to different trends and unresolved issues within the field. Three issues are discussed in the following sections: the dichotomy between restorative and compensatory interventions, the selection of appropriate outcome measures, and the timing of the intervention.

21.4.1 The Dichotomy between Restorative and Compensatory Interventions

Cognitive rehabilitation interventions are commonly classified as either restorative or compensatory. The goal of restorative approaches is to "restore" or strengthen a particular cognitive function through training and practice utilizing that particular function. Restorative interventions include practice drills and repetitious exercises.[16,31,32] For example, in the memory domain, restorative approaches are based on memory exercises, verbal and written rehearsals, and repetitive practice and drills. The goal of compensatory approaches is to increase task competence in a cognitive domain, without using the cognitive functions of that domain directly.[32] Compensatory approaches rely on circumventing the dysfunctional cognitive domain by utilizing external aids, such as using checklists with step-by-step procedures on how to accomplish a task, or using a notebook to record things to avoid memory problems.

Concerns were raised about the value of restorative approaches to cognitive remediation, because evidence failed to show significant gains made in cognitive functioning through intensive practice involving the affected cognitive domain.[32] Advances, however, in other areas of rehabilitation have demonstrated the value of restorative approaches, especially when examining the treatment of motor function. More specifically, the application of *forced-use* techniques has resulted in functional gains, particularly in upper extremity motor function.[33] Taub[33] reviewed the evidence that has emerged from studies in primates and humans suggesting functional reorganization of the brain occurs after injury. He stated that "learned nonuse" of a limb is a learned response, the effects of which can be reversed through preventing the compensatory mechanisms from taking place. *Forced use* is induced by constraining the functional limb to necessitate the use of the affected limb, and results in brain plasticity, especially for motor deficits of organic origin. Thus, the person is forced to use the impaired extremity because the unimpaired extremity is constrained. Hart[32] pointed out that evidence for recovery of affected limbs may challenge the belief that spontaneous recovery of a cognitive function is only possible within a certain time interval following injury, after which no further improvement is attainable without the application of compensatory mechanisms. The use of compensatory strategies, however, leads to behavioral changes that may, in turn, lead to functional and structural changes in the brain, making the distinction between compensation and restoration blurry. In an innovative study, Gauthier et al.[34] observed not only functional improvement in motor ability in a group of stroke patients, but, more important, structural changes in the brain were observed and manifested as gray matter increases in sensory and motor cortical areas and in the hippocampus.

A critical conclusion to be drawn from this study[34] is that behavioral changes (in this case, use of an affected extremity) lead to structural changes in the brain (increase in gray matter in sensory and motor cortical areas and the hippocampus). This causal relationship raises concerns about the common classification of neuropsychological interventions as either restorative or compensatory. This distinction might be, at best, not helpful and, at worst, arbitrary and impractical. All neuropsychological interventions lead to behavioral changes, which enable individuals to function more successfully in their daily lives. Although evidence has not accrued yet, the emergence of new technologies that depict brain anatomy and activity will permit further investigation of the reciprocity between restoration and compensation.

21.4.2 The Selection of Appropriate Outcome Measures

The goal of rehabilitation after TBI is to improve function. The multifaceted nature of neuropsychological rehabilitation, with the diverse interventions and the multiple treatment goals, renders it more challenging to determine how to assess appropriately the impact of participation in treatment and to identify at which level (cognitive, emotional, behavioral, functional) changes have occurred. Ultimately, the goal of rehabilitation is to improve an individual's ability to perform social roles and functions at a competent level. Accomplishing this requires addressing the emotional issues related to the losses and the affective response to emerging awareness of the potential impact of the injury. Finally, the treatment focuses on regaining functional independence, which can range from ability for self-care to ability to support self and others financially, and to participate in meaningful and productive activities, such as gainful employment, recreation, volunteerism, and education. Given the diversity and complexity of these goals, how can it be demonstrated that neuropsychological interventions lead to positive changes?

Traditionally, the interventions for the rehabilitation of individuals with TBI were focused on improving the function of specific cognitive skills (e.g., memory, attention, motor speed), and measures were selected to assess specific neurocognitive functions in each of these domains being treated. The effectiveness of such isolated cognitive interventions is measured by (1) measuring performance on the specific task in which instruction took place, (2) administering standardized neuropsychological tests, and (3) using self-report measures of day-to-day function and participation. Measuring outcome by comparing an individual's performance on a task that is identical or similar to the task that was used during training is particularly prevalent in single-case or small sample multiple baseline designs. The legitimate question is: How does specific skill training improve the person's ability to function in "real life?" For example, a study evaluated the ability of individuals with severe memory and executive functioning impairments to learn a stepwise procedure for using e-mail by counting the number of correct procedural steps achieved when attempting to send e-mail.[24] After training was completed, participants were able to use the original and a slightly altered version of the e-mail interface successfully, but their performance on a computer memory game did not improve, suggesting minimal generalization across domains. For studies with larger samples and objectives that are broader than learning a single task, neuropsychological measures are often used to evaluate effectiveness. For example, the effectiveness of interventions to improve attention might include measures like the digit span subtest of the Wechsler Adult Intelligence Scale, the Paced Auditory Serial Addition Test, the Verbal Paired Associates from the Wechsler Memory Scale, Auditory Consonant Trigrams, Trail-Making Test, and the Continuous Performance Task.[21–23, 35,36] However, once again, the question can be raised regarding how improvement on tests relates to improved day-to-day function. Finally, attempts to capture changes in performance are often based on self-report questionnaires, such as the Attention Rating and Monitoring Scale to assess changes in experienced attention difficulties,[21] the Dysexecutive Questionnaire to assess problems with executive functioning, and the Beck Depression Inventory to assess depression. The validity of the self-report questionnaires in individuals with TBI may be confounded by the cognitive impairments per se (e.g., not remembering pertinent information) as well as lack of awareness of the deficits (e.g., not being cognizant of the frequent lapses in attention during a conversation). Hence, the validity of self-report measures when applied to individuals with TBI is a complex issue.

Nevertheless, as Cicerone et al.[11] point out in their review of the cognitive rehabilitation literature, there is an assumption that interventions that lead to the reduction in impairments, as manifested by changes in test scores, are also effective in improving functioning in other contexts. This is a leap of faith because the relationship between everyday function and neuropsychological test scores is, at best, tenuous. What is evident in the review by Cicerone et al.[11] is that the neuropsychological measures that are frequently used as outcome measures may not accurately reflect the effects of the intervention in reducing disability and increasing psychosocial functioning, in addition to reducing impairments. In fact, research regarding the relationship between neuropsychological test scores and functional outcome is inconclusive, with some studies showing support,[5,37,38] and others showing no relationship between neuropsychological test scores and functional improvement.[8,13–15] Rattok et al.,[39] for instance, found that although including cognitive remediation in group treatment for TBI resulted in some advantages in performance on neuropsychological tests, it did not show additional gains in measures of behavioral, interpersonal, and vocational functioning. Quemada et al.,[40] in their review of rehabilitation interventions for memory deficits, stated that there was no relationship between performance on tests of memory dysfunction and ability to carry out activities of daily living, or reports from family members regarding memory failures in daily living.

A trend exists among milieu-oriented programs to use measures other than neuropsychological tests to evaluate the effectiveness of intervention and to assess meaningful changes in the individuals' ability to perform successfully in relevant contexts. A majority of the studies investigating the effects of comprehensive–holistic day treatment programs have incorporated functional measures in their outcome assessment procedures. For instance, to measure the frequency of participation in activities following TBI, several programs have used the Community Integration Questionnaire, a 15-item questionnaire that assesses home integration, social integration, and productive activities.[5,41–43] Ability, adjustment, and participation have frequently been measured with the Mayo-Portland Adaptability Inventory.[44–47] Other functional measures have included independence in personal and domestic activities of daily living,[48] staff ratings or work readiness/eagerness,[13] emotional and psychosocial adjustment,[49] adaptation to community skills, self-care, involvement with others, regulation of affect, performance on vocational trials,[39] and return to and longevity of productive activities, including gainful employment and enrollment in school or other training programs.[13,50,51] Incorporating functional measures in intervention research is critical because the ultimate goal of any intervention is to improve function in real-life settings.

A related issue is that of skill transfer and generalizability.[52] Typically, rehabilitation occurs within a structured setting (i.e., a facility that is staffed with professionals experienced in treating individuals with TBI). Hence, training and learning occur in a specific context (the treatment setting) and within a specific domain of functioning (e.g., going grocery shopping). Skill transfer refers to using a specific learned skill in a similar situation. For example, if cognitive training targeted creating a grocery-shopping and step-by-step plan on how to obtain the groceries, skill transfer occurs when the individual is able to use the list and the plan to go grocery shopping to the neighborhood supermarket independently. However, creating lists and step-by-step plans may not generalize to other activities (i.e., it will not be used to complete other tasks that involve a procedure, such as preparing a meal). Generalization refers to the ability to use and apply a learned strategy to a variety of novel situations. Consistent with the goals of rehabilitation, the skills learned during treatment are expected to be applied outside of treatment. To measure the success of the learning that occurred during rehabilitation, either the ability to perform the same task or the ability to perform other tasks that incorporate one or more of the learned skills could be assessed. Neuropsychological tests measure domain-specific learning and skill transfer when a cognitive domain different from the one trained is assessed following treatment. Functional measures, in contrast, measure generalization of learning to real life situations.

21.4.3 The Timing of the Intervention

Another important issue that has been raised in the neuropsychological intervention literature pertains to the timing of the intervention. The positive effects of cognitive rehabilitation treatment for individuals with TBI are indisputable.[7,11] What has not been clearly addressed in the literature is whether there is a critical period during which neuropsychological interventions are more effective and are more likely to produce gains, especially during the postacute stage. The majority of studies in this area include patients who are relatively recently injured, rarely exceeding 2 years postinjury. The overinclusion of individuals who are closer to their injury may be attributed to the ease of access to this population, because of their continuous or recent involvement with a rehabilitative system of care, and the limited access of researchers to individuals at a later stage postinjury. There is often an implicit or explicit assumption that the effects of rehabilitation are attenuated unless interventions are administered soon after the onset of the injury. The first 2 years postinjury are usually considered the most critical in terms of neurologic recovery, after which the rate of neurologic recovery is expected to plateau.[53] This information is often presented to clients and their families without further qualification and is met with a sense of haste, urgency, and pessimism, creating a belief that, unless treatment is received within that "critical" window, improvement will be hampered. The evidence regarding the chronicity of the intervention is divided. Some studies declare early rehabilitation more beneficial.[54–57] For instance, Malec et al.[54] reported more positive vocational outcomes for individuals beginning treatment within a year postinjury compared with those who began more than a year postinjury. Nevertheless, in this study, both groups benefitted from treatment, suggesting that effective interventions are beneficial at any stage. Other studies comparing early and late onset of neuropsychological rehabilitation treatment have shown no differences in psychosocial outcome,[53,58] independence and community integration,[42] and even performance on neuropsychological tests.[59] The lack of strong and conclusive evidence and the persistent need for further research in this area notwithstanding, there is no *critical window* for new learning. Thus, there is no ceiling on when learning occurs, and thus, intervention can begin at any point postinjury and with no limit to the degree of benefit the person can obtain from treatment. Hence, it is critical for clinicians, as well as individuals with TBI, to be aware that appropriate interventions could lead to improvements in cognitive, emotional, and psychosocial functioning regardless of how much time has elapsed since the injury.

21.5 Neuropsychological Interventions: Some Highlights

21.5.1 Interventions for Cognition

21.5.1.1 Attention

Interventions for attention deficits vary as a function of the particular attention component or system they target. For example, several interventions have been developed to improve working memory that range from simple tasks, such as using flash cards to improve orientation,[60] to more complex tasks, such as mental arithmetic, anagram solutions, *n-back* procedures, and other serial logic verbal tasks.[21,22,61]

One of the most popular interventions for improving attention has been developed by Sohlberg and Mateer.[62] Their Attention Process Training (APT-I and APT-II) program consists of a variety of visual and auditory tasks organized hierarchically in terms of difficulty and is designed to remediate different components of attention (focused, selective, sustained, divided, alternating). The APT-II was developed by Sohlberg and Mateer[62] as an extension of the training provided by the APT-I, in response to feedback from clinicians that individuals with mild brain injuries, whose attention deficits interfere in daily functioning in more subtle ways and remain unaddressed by APT-I, would benefit additionally from tasks that were higher in complexity and intensity. There are several advantages to the APT. It is evidence based, it is an easy-to-implement clinical tool, and it is expected to generalize to activities beyond the treatment session.[62,63] To accomplish the latter, Sohlberg and Mateer[62] have incorporated generalization tasks within the interventions, which are hierarchically implemented and monitored. Treatment is typically conducted in individual sessions, with feedback provided to the patient consistently throughout the session. The ease of implementing the treatment notwithstanding, clinical skill is always important and necessary, as with any intervention. The role of the clinician is indispensable, and the APT is a good tool insofar as it is applied by therapists with a good understanding of the needs of persons with brain injury.

21.5.1.2 Memory

Impairments in memory are common after TBI. Memory deficits interfere significantly with a person's ability to function independently. Memory problems could also interfere with treatment because they may prevent the learning and recall of the recently learned material. Improvements in other cognitive domains may be further hampered because of difficulties in learning and recalling new material, difficulties remembering when and how to use the tools and strategies associated with improved memory function, and difficulty maintaining a high level of motivation in both the patient and the clinician, resulting from the extensive time and effort required to notice improvements.[64] Memory problems could also be exacerbated by deficits in attention.

Given the prevalence of deficits in memory following TBI, there has been a proliferation of interventions focused on improving different aspects of memory functioning, including face–name associations, memory for past events, enhancing the ability to recall appointments and other future events, and facilitating learning of new information. Both restorative and compensatory approaches have been used in treating memory deficits. Restorative approaches have included word-list learning, paragraph listening, visual imagery, and use of mnemonic strategies.[31,65] Compensatory tools include memory notebooks, date books, and other paper-and-pencil methods of recording and tracking information, and, more recently, technology-based tools, such as personal computers, portable electronic devices, voice recorders, and pagers.[66–69] A widely used and researched compensatory tool for memory rehabilitation is the memory book.

21.5.1.2.1 The Memory Book

Unequivocally one of the most effective tools in memory rehabilitation, the memory notebook is widely implemented in rehabilitation settings across different populations. To render the use of the memory book more systematic, and hence more effective in terms of learning how to use it, using it efficiently, and generalizing its use across different settings, Sohlberg and Mateer[65] presented a method of developing a memory book that is personally relevant to the individual, and a set of training procedures to facilitate the use of the memory book. In determining the contents of the memory book, Sohlberg and Mateer[65] suggest reviewing the person's living and work environment, as well as current and anticipated level of cognitive functioning. Potential sections include orientation, memory log, calendar, things to do, transportation, feelings log, names, today at work. Training in the use of a memory book consists of three phases: acquisition, which refers to increasing familiarity with the sections and purpose of the notebook; application, which refers to training to use the memory book in simulated settings; and adaptation, which refers to training to use the memory book in naturalistic settings, with the goal of skill transfer. Using the pioneering work of Sohlberg and Mateer[65] as a springboard, Donaghy and Williams[64] developed a protocol for memory journal training to assist clinicians working with individuals with memory deficits increase the successful use of the memory book by their clients. Successful use of a memory notebook should include the ability to schedule future events (prospective memory) and track past events, a note-keeping system that makes retrieval effortless, and ease of use that fosters independence.

Despite the overwhelming evidence for the effectiveness of the memory book in addressing memory deficits,[70–73] inconsistent use prevents maximizing its benefits. McKerracher et al.[74] identified several barriers that interfere with successful use of external memory aids. Among them they listed personal characteristics (lack of awareness, which leads to failure to see the need for aid; reluctance to use strategies that draw attention to problems; perceiving use of aid as "cheating"; belief that aids will reduce the chance of natural recovery; severity of memory impairment; and presence of other cognitive problems, such as executive impairments), simplicity of the diary, (low) level of demand in person's environment, and the method by which it is introduced, which is relevant to clinicians. Memory notebooks may require memory and executive function to be used effectively, may be cumbersome to use in some environments, may be viewed as "demeaning," and may not be easy to use to enhance memory for certain events (e.g., conversations).[69]

21.5.1.2.2 Prospective Memory

Considerable efforts have been made during the last decade to develop cognitive rehabilitation interventions to address issues of prospective memory. *Prospective memory* refers to the ability to remember to carry out a certain action at a specified time in the future or in response to a specific future event.[75] Einstein and McDaniel[76] identify two components to prospective memory: remembering what actions are to be carried out and the cue for implementing the action, and recall and initiation of the action at a given time, following a particular cue. This type of memory is vital to maintaining successful performance in employment, social, and daily living situations. Failures in prospective memory surpass failures in retrospective memory (the ability to recall information) among individuals with TBI.[75] Prospective memory has been enhanced significantly with the use of electronic aids.[20,28,66–68,77,78]

21.5.1.3 Executive Function

The term *executive function* refers to a broad range of abilities that include planning, initiation, organization, and monitoring.[11] Additional abilities identified as part of executive function have included anticipation, action sequencing, cognitive flexibility,[79] problem solving,[80–82] and emotional and behavioral regulation.[32] Despite definitional problems, there is little disagreement that disruption in the cognitive functions underlying goal-directed behavior has widespread impact on emotional, behavioral, and social outcomes of acquired brain injury.[16,80] Consequently, the treatment of executive dysfunction has received significant attention in the literature. Interventions have been based on explicit theoretical models of executive function,[81,83,84] comprehensive holistic day treatment programs that emphasize cognitive operations such as self-awareness and daily problem solving,[5,13,46,80,85,86] and specific interventions focused on improving problem solving,[80,87–89] goal management,[29] and self-regulation.[80,87,90]

Improvement in executive functioning is typically facilitated via the use of *metacognitive strategies*.[80,87,91,92] Metacognitive strategies aim at improving self-regulation by increasing self-awareness, which promotes the formation of feasible and personally relevant goals; self-monitoring, which enables individuals to assess their performance and reduce or prevent errors; and self-control, which initiates action and behavioral change.[91] In a systematic review of the literature on executive functioning following TBI, Kennedy et al.[91] identified *metacognitive strategy instruction* as a common intervention among several studies, including randomized clinical trials.[29,87] Metacognitive strategy instruction includes using and internalizing step-by-step procedures intended to enhance problem solving, planning, organization, and multitasking by increasing the capacity for self-regulation.[91]

Gordon et al.[80] are currently investigating the effectiveness of a metacognitive strategy instruction intervention to improve executive function. The intervention entails learning a step-by-step problem-solving procedure, in individual and group sessions, to facilitate identification of problems, reduction to more elemental components, generation of alternatives, initiation of action, and self-monitoring, while simultaneously dealing appropriately with the emotional reactions elicited in different situations. Generalization to multiple settings is achieved by incorporating repetition and feedback throughout the treatment. Preliminary results for this intervention are expected to be available within the next few months.

21.5.2 Interventions for Emotion

There are two types of emotional consequences following TBI: emotional symptoms that are directly related to brain dysfunction, and emotional reactions to the personal loss and disability. Emotional symptoms that are related to brain injury have been associated with damage to the prefrontal and limbic structures[93,94] and include affective disinhibition, emotional blunting, decreased initiative, emotional lability, poor temper control, aggression, impatience, misperception of emotional cues, lack of empathy, and pathologic laughing and crying.[95–100] Emotional symptoms that are reactions to the sequelae of the injury include depression, anxiety, posttraumatic stress disorder, feelings of grief and loss, low self-esteem, social isolation, loneliness, agitation, and suicide risk.[3,97,101]

Interventions for the first type of emotional symptoms have included metacognitive strategies to increase emotional self-regulation and prevent impulsive, damaging behaviors,[80,87,102] as well as training in emotion recognition and correct interpretation of emotional cues.[95,103] These interventions have yielded promising results with respect to the management of emotion perception and regulation.

Several psychological interventions have been adapted to address the second type of emotional symptoms—namely, the emotional distress experienced by individuals with TBI. Cognitive behavioral therapy (CBT) provides a good framework and has been used extensively as a first-line treatment option in the treatment of post-TBI depression,[104] posttraumatic stress disorder,[105–107] anxiety,[108,109] irritability and aggression,[110] and anger.[90] A critical factor in adapting CBT for individuals with TBI is incorporating principles of cognitive remediation to address diverse cognitive deficits that may thwart treatment success[111,112] (e.g., problems in attention and concentration, word finding, processing speed, memory, learning skills, and/or disrupted executive functioning).

Other models of psychotherapy have been introduced as potential interventions for individuals with TBI. Coetzer[113] applied Orlinsky and Howard's Generic Model of

Psychotherapy, which is based on nonspecific factors of psychotherapy, to elicit therapeutic change. In a similar vain, we have developed two models of psychotherapy for depression—a CBT-based intervention and a supportive psychotherapy intervention based on nonspecific factors and adapted for individuals with TBI. The two models are currently under investigation as part of a randomized, clinical trial.

21.5.3 Interventions for Self-Awareness

Increasing awareness is an essential goal of neuropsychological rehabilitation.[6,114] Diminished self-awareness may interfere with treatment and has been related to poor rehabilitation outcome.[114,115] In contrast, improved self-awareness may result in psychological distress. Self-awareness of deficits, often referred to as *anosognosia* in the TBI literature, refers to lack of awareness of neurologic and neuropsychological impairments that are evident to care providers and significant others.[115] Several models exist that explain impaired self-awareness resulting from TBI. Crosson et al.[116] introduced the pyramid model of awareness that distinguishes between intellectual awareness (the ability to understand that there are certain deficits in functioning), emergent awareness (the ability to recognize a functional problem as it occurs), and anticipatory awareness (the ability to predict that an area of deficit may lead to problems in functioning). Other models include Langer and Padrone's[117] tripartite model of unawareness (unawareness of information, unawareness of implications, and psychological denial); Fleming and Ownsworth's[114] model of awareness of objective knowledge, awareness of the functional implications of the deficits for daily activities, and the ability to set realistic goals; and Ruff and Niemann's[49] model, which includes the ability to attend to, encode, and retrieve information about the self, the ability to compare current with premorbid functioning, and willingness to report self-perception to another person. Finally, Giacino and Cicerone[118] identified three sources for limited awareness: cognitive impairment (especially attention, memory, and self-monitoring); psychogenic denial; and failure of higher order cognitive systems to recognize deficits and incorporate them in self-knowledge. In addition to the neurocognitive and psychological sources of unawareness that are typically described in these models, Fleming and Ownsworth[114] identified social–environmental factors that contribute to diminished awareness. These factors include minimal opportunities to obtain information or to observe deficits in a social context, reluctance to disclose information about the deficits resulting from concerns about how the information will be used, and the interference of cultural values with the neuropsychological rehabilitation process.

In their review of the literature, Fleming and Ownsworth[114] identified several types of interventions focused on addressing self-awareness deficits. Neuropsychological interventions include milieu-oriented treatment programs aimed at increasing awareness via peer, staff, and family feedback; psychoeducation; and psychotherapy[6,119,120] and cognitive remediation interventions that use techniques such as therapist feedback, monitoring and recording performance, and generating lists of strengths and weaknesses.[121] These interventions are based on the interaction between impaired self-awareness of a neurologic origin (unilateral vs. bilateral injury) and of a psychogenic origin (defensive vs. nondefensive coping styles).[6,122] In a randomized clinical trial to improve executive function that was described in a previous section,[80] the investigators observed significant improvements in self-awareness. Although still anecdotal, the investigators attribute the observed improvement to a combination of the comprehensive nature of treatment, a mixture of individual and group sessions that provides an opportunity to share challenges and improve insight (i.e., "What he is saying has also happened to me"), and instruction in the use of a meta-cognitive strategy.

Psychotherapeutic interventions are aimed at exploring the meaning of loss following TBI and ameliorating the effects by developing meaningful and realistic goals. Langer and Padrone's[117] tripartite model of unawareness provides a useful framework for developing psychotherapeutic interventions to raise awareness. Within this model, interventions to increase awareness of deficits include psychoeducation and feedback about the individual's TBI-related impairments, interventions to increase awareness of the implications include building a supportive structure to allow the individual to learn compensatory strategies to avoid failures, and interventions to address the psychological denial include assessing the client's readiness to be confronted with awareness of deficits and the implications and to strengthen his or her ego function. Interventions based on the pyramid model of Crosson et al.[116] have included psychoeducation, feedback, planned failures, and emotional support to increase intellectual awareness, feedback during and after task completion to increase emergent awareness, and helping the individual create plans and anticipate problems to raise anticipatory awareness. Self-determination[123] is an approach based on the pyramid model that includes education, practice in safe and structured environments, and application in real-life situations.

Other interventions to increase self-awareness have included structured experiences, direct feedback, support groups, and game format. Structured experiences are preplanned exercises that are tailored to the individual's mastery level to increase self-efficacy, online awareness, and metacognitive knowledge. Techniques including anticipation of obstacles, self-prediction, self-checking, self-questioning and self-evaluation, time monitoring, and role reversal are used in the duration of the structured experience. Direct feedback involves the therapist's commentary on the individual's task performance. Direct feedback is beneficial when it is specific, timely, consistent, and respectful, and when the unawareness is neurologic rather than psychogenic. Finally, support groups and the utilization of games (e.g., board games) in treatment are methods used to facilitate improvements in awareness.[114]

21.6 Future Directions in Neuropsychological Rehabilitation

21.6.1 Technology and Neuropsychological Rehabilitation

Technological aids have been used in the treatment of individuals with cognitive deficits since the early developmental stages of cognitive remediation. Use of computers to project visual and verbal stimuli to provide training in attention, memory, processing speed, and problem solving became common after computers were available. Over time, the use of technology in neuropsychological rehabilitation progressed from using computers as passive tools to facilitate cognitive training, to active training tools that could expand the scope of training, as well as compensatory tools or *cognitive orthotics*[12] that could be utilized in naturalistic settings to facilitate functioning. Examples of the use of technology as training tools include the use of computers in the training of memory,[124–126] attention,[124,127] problem solving,[124] and job simulation.[128] The advantage of using technology as a training tool is that it permits the administration of tasks that would otherwise be impossible to administer. However, when the gains of computer-assisted training are compared with therapist-assisted training, they show no superiority.[124,127]

The use of technology to develop compensatory tools has resulted in the creation of devices that, on the one hand, facilitate the performance of cognition-dependent tasks, such as prospective memory or executive functioning tasks,[66–69] and, on the other hand, result in significant improvements in psychosocial functioning,[129] rendering individuals with TBI more competent in task completion, time management, and record keeping, while bolstering their self-efficacy. LoPresti et al.[12] provide an extensive review of the existing technologic aids, which he divides into technologies for memory and executive function impairments and technologies for information processing impairments. Devices for memory and executive function compensation range from digital watches and alarms to more sophisticated devices like voice organizers (some of which will replay a message aloud at a prespecified time), mobile phone–computer interactive systems, and handheld devices, like personal digital assistants. Devices for information processing impairments include use of a keyboard for typing instead of writing, software that alters the features of text (e.g., size, color) on a computer screen to facilitate reading, and speech output/speech recognition software.

An additional use of technology includes teletherapy. Bell et al.[130] tested the effectiveness of telephone interviews on behavioral outcomes. The content of the phone call was a mixture of counseling, motivational interviewing, and psychoeducation. Results showed that there were significant improvements in functional measures in the participants that received telephone counseling compared with those who did not, suggesting that telephone counseling may be an effective, low-cost, easily accessible alternative intervention. Melton and Bourgeois,[131] who assessed the effectiveness of a learning and memory intervention over the telephone, identified three advantages to applying the intervention over the telephone: (1) it facilitates generalization because the skill learning occurs in the individual's living environment; (2) it renders effective interventions accessible to individuals with TBI who, because of practical difficulties (e.g., limited transportation, financial constraints, mobility issues, considerable distance from treatment providers) would be unable to receive treatment; and (3) it has the potential to reduce absenteeism.

Given consumer satisfaction with the use of technologic devices[132] and the encouraging results from small-scale studies, it is expected that during the next few years, several improvements and adjustments will be made to create portable electronic devices that will facilitate functioning in naturalistic settings even further for individuals with TBI. The transition from paper-and-pencil tools (such as the memory notebook) may be rugged and met with resistance, especially for older individuals and those less familiar with technology, but it is a necessary one because of the pervasiveness of technology in all aspects of daily living. Consistent use of external aids is prevented by a variety of reasons, including inconvenience, reluctance, and concern that external aids minimize the probability of improvement.[69,74] Use of technologic aids may render the use of compensatory tools more consistent and make it more attractive, especially to younger individuals, who may be more reluctant to use tools that would draw attention to their brain injury. State-of-the-art portable electronic organizers may be much more amenable tools to own and use consistently.

Although the use of technology in TBI rehabilitation is expected to increase during the next few years, technologic aids are not invented or intended to replace a therapist, but to augment the therapeutic experience. Findings from studies showing no advantage of computer-assisted interventions over traditional interventions[124,127] highlight the importance of the clinician as an active participant in the treatment. Therapists set and maintain the structure, determine treatment needs and readiness, provide feedback and guidance, teach and reinforce the use of tools, and process emotional reactions. Training in the consistent use of compensatory tools is necessary to render the use of tools effective and habitual.[64,66–69] Most important, a positive working alliance between therapist and client facilitates treatment and contributes to successful treatment outcome.[6,133,134]

21.7 Summary

Neuropsychological rehabilitation is a dynamic intervention that is continually evolving. It is an area of study in which theories are refined and new theories are developed, yet a grand unifying theory of treatment has not been developed. It is a field that diligently generates research questions and answers based on remarkable scientific labor. Ylvisaker[135] points out that there has been a paradigm shift from more traditional approaches (the goal of which is to "fix" the cognitive problem) to more contextualized approaches (the goal of which is to enable individuals to live a fuller life by minimizing the hindrance caused by the cognitive problems). Wilson[136] stated:

> We have moved on from the early days of cognitive rehabilitation with its emphasis on drills and exercises to try to reduce basic impairments, to a more individualized approach addressing the everyday manifestations of these impairments, i.e., disabilities and handicaps. . . . Cognitive rehabilitation should focus on real-life, functional problems; it should address associated problems such as mood and behavioral problems in addition to the cognitive difficulties and it should involve the person with the brain injury, relatives and others in the planning and implementation of cognitive rehabilitation.(p.98–99)

The balance between these two paradigms is the underlying dynamic behind several of the unresolved issues, such as the issue of appropriate measurement, the distinction between domain-specific training and generalization, or the contrast between restoration and compensation. It also seems to be the dialectic from which we draw our ideas, through which we express our creativity, and by which we continue the quest for better ways to help individuals with TBI pick up the fabric of their lives.

Acknowledgments

This work was supported by grants from the National Institute for Rehabilitation Research (H133B040033 and H133A070033) and from the Centers for Disease Control and Prevention (1R49CE001171-01).

References

1. Ashman, T. A., Gordon, W. A., Cantor, J. B., and Hibbard, M. R., Neurobehavioral consequences of traumatic brain injury, *Mt. Sinai Journal of Medicine*, 73(7), 999–1005, 2006.
2. Ashman, T. A., Spielman, L. A., Hibbard, M. R., Silver, J. M., Chandna, T., and Gordon, W. A., Psychiatric challenges in the first 6 years after traumatic brain injury: Cross-sequential analyses of axis I disorders, *Archives of Physical Medicine and Rehabilitation*, 85(4 Suppl. 2), S36–S42, 2004.

3. Hibbard, M. R., Uysal, S., Kepler, K., Bogdany, J., and Silver, J., Axis I psychopathology in individuals with traumatic brain injury, *Journal of Head Trauma Rehabilitation*, 13(4), 24–39, 1998.

4. Niemeier, J. P., Kreutzer, J. S., and Taylor, L. A., Acute cognitive and neurobehavioural intervention for individuals with acquired brain injury: Preliminary outcome data, *Neuropsychological Rehabilitation*, 15(2), 129–146, 2005.

5. Cicerone, K. D., Mott, T., Azulay, J., and Friel, J. C., Community integration and satisfaction with functioning after intensive cognitive rehabilitation for traumatic brain injury, *Archives of Physical Medicine and Rehabilitation*, 85(6), 943–950, 2004.

6. Prigatano, G. P., *Principles of Neuropsychological Rehabilitation*, Oxford University Press, New York, 1999.

7. Cicerone, K. D., Dahlberg, C., Kalmar, K., Langenbahn, D. M., Malec, J. F., Berqquist, T. F., Felicetti, T., et al., Evidence-based cognitive rehabilitation: Recommendations for clinical practice, *Archives of Physical Medicine and Rehabilitation*, 81(12), 1596–1615, 2000.

8. Malec, J. F. and Basford, J. S., Postacute brain injury rehabilitation, *Archives of Physical Medicine and Rehabilitation*, 77(2), 198–207, 1996.

9. Gordon, W. A. and Hibbard, M. R., Cognitive rehabilitation, in J. M. Silver, T. W. McAllister, and S. C. Yudofsky (Eds.), *Textbook of Traumatic Brain Injury*, American Psychiatric Publishing, Washington, DC, 655–660, 2005.

10. Ben-Yishay, Y., Reflections on the evolution of the therapeutic milieu concept, *Neuropsychological Rehabilitation*, 6(4), 327–343, 1996.

11. Cicerone, K. D., Dahlberg, C., Malec, J. J., Langenbahn, D. M., Felicetti, T., Kneipp, S., Ellmo, W., et al., Evidence-based cognitive rehabilitation: Updated review of the literature from 1998 through 2002, *Archives of Physical Medicine and Rehabilitation*, 86(8), 1681–1692, 2005.

12. LoPresti, E. F., Mihailidis, A., and Kirsch, N., Assistive technology for cognitive rehabilitation: State of the art, *Neuropsychological Rehabilitation*, 14(1/2), 5–39, 2004.

13. Klonoff, P. S., Lamb, D. G., Henderson, S. W., and Shepherd, J., Outcome assessment after milieu-oriented rehabilitation: New considerations, *Archives of Physical Medicine and Rehabilitation*, 79(6), 684–690, 1998.

14. Mills, V. M., Nesbeda, T., Katz, D. I., and Alexander, M. P., Outcomes for traumatically brain-injured patients following postacute rehabilitation programmes, *Brain Injury*, 6(3), 219–228, 1992.

15. Teasdale, T. W., Hansen, H. S., and Christensen, A. G., Neuropsychological test scores before and after brain injury rehabilitation in relation to return to employment, *Neuropsychological Rehabilitation*, 7(1), 23–42, 1997.

16. Sohlberg, M. M. and Mateer, C. A., *Cognitive Rehabilitation: An Integrative Neuropsychological Approach*, Guilford Press, New York, 2001.

17. Bouwmeester, L., Heutink, J., and Lucas, C., The effect of visual training for patients with visual field defects due to brain damage: A systematic review, *Journal of Neurology, Neurosurgery, and Psychiatry*, 78(6), 555–564, 2007.

18. Coelho, C. A., McHugh, R. E., and Boyle, M., Semantic feature analysis as a treatment for aphasic dysnomia: A replication, *Aphasiology*, 14(2), 133–142, 2000.

19. Dahlberg, C. A., Cusick, C. P., Hawley, L. A., Newman, J. K., Morey, C. E., Harrison-Felix, C. L., and Whiteneck, G. G., Treatment efficacy of social communication skills training after traumatic brain injury: A randomized treatment and deferred treatment controlled trial, *Archives of Physical Medicine and Rehabilitation*, 88(12), 1561–1573, 2007.

20. Kirsch, N. L., Shenton, M., Spirl, E., Simpson, R., Lopresti, E., and Schreckenghost, D., An assistive-technology intervention for verbose speech after traumatic brain injury: A single case study, *Journal of Head Trauma Rehabilitation*, 19(5), 366–377, 2004.

21. Cicerone, K. D., Remediation of "working attention" in mild traumatic brain injury, *Brain Injury*, 16(3), 185–195, 2002.

22. Serino, A., Ciaramelli, E., Santantonio, A. D., Malagù, S., Servadei, F., and Làdavas, E., A pilot study for rehabilitation of central executive deficits after traumatic brain injury, *Brain Injury*, 21(1), 11–19, 2007.

23. Sohlberg, M. M., McLaughlin, K. A., Pavese, A., Heidrich, A., and Posner, M. I., Evaluation of attention process training and brain injury education in persons with acquired brain injury, *Journal of Clinical and Experimental Neuropsychology*, 22(5), 656–676, 2000.

24. Ehlhardt, L. A., Sohlberg, M. M., Glang, A., and Albin, R., TEACH-M: A pilot study evaluating an instructional sequence for persons with impaired memory and executive functions, *Brain Injury*, 19(8), 569–583, 2005.

25. Kaschel, R., Dalla Sala, S., Cantagallo, A., Fahlboeck, A., Laaksonen, R., and Kazen, M., Imagery mnemonics for the rehabilitation of memory: A randomised group controlled trial, *Neuropsychological Rehabilitation*, 12(2), 127–153, 2002.

26. Pitel, A. L., Beaunieux, H., Lebaron, N., Joyeux, F., Desgranges, B., and Eustache, F., Two case studies in the application of errorless learning techniques in memory impaired patients with additional executive deficits, *Brain Injury*, 20(10), 1099–1110, 2006.

27. Raskin, S. A. and Sohlberg, M. M., The efficacy of prospective memory training in two adults with brain injury, *Journal of Head Trauma Rehabilitation*, 11(3), 32–51, 1996.

28. Fish, J., Evans, J. J., Nimmo, M., Martin, E., Kersel, D., Bateman, A., Wilson, B. A., and Manly, T., Rehabilitation of executive dysfunction following brain injury: "Content-free" cueing improves everyday prospective memory performance, *Neuropsychologia*, 45(6), 1318–1330, 2007.

29. Levine, B., Robertson, I. H., Clare, L., Carter, G., Hong, J., Wilson, B. A., Duncan, J., and Stuss, D. T., Rehabilitation of executive functioning: An experimental–clinical validation of goal management training, *Journal of the International Neuropsychological Society*, 6(3), 299–312, 2000.

30. Manly, T., Hawkins, K., Evans, J., Woldt, K., and Robertson, I. H., Rehabilitation of executive function: Facilitation of effective goal management on complex tasks using periodic auditory alerts, *Neuropsychologia*, 40(3), 271–281, 2002.

31. Sohlberg, M. M., White, O., Evans, E., and Mateer, C., Background and initial case studies into the effects of prospective memory training, *Brain Injury*, 6(2), 129–138, 1992.

32. Hart, T., Cognitive rehabilitation, in R. G. Frank, M. Rosenthal, and B. Caplan (Eds.), *Handbook of Rehabilitation Psychology*, 2nd ed., American Psychological Association, Washington, DC, in press.

33. Taub, E., Harnessing brain plasticity through behavioral techniques to produce new treatments in neurorehabilitation, *The American Psychologist*, 59(8), 692–704, 2004.

34. Gauthier, L. V., Taub, E., Perkins, C., Ortmann, M., Mark, V. W., and Uswatte, G., Remodeling the brain: Plastic structural brain changes produced by different motor therapies after stroke, *Stroke*, 39(5), 1520–1525, 2008.

35. Middleton, D. K., Lambert, M. J., and Seggar, L. B., Neuropsychological rehabilitation: Microcomputer-assisted treatment of brain-injured adults, *Perceptual and Motor Skills*, 72(2), 527–530, 1991.

36. Park, N. W., Proulx, G. B., and Towers, W. M., Evaluation of the Attention Process Training programme, *Neuropsychological Rehabilitation*, 9(2), 135–154, 1999.

37. Ownsworth, T. L. and Mcfarland, K., Memory remediation in long-term acquired brain injury: Two approaches in diary training, *Brain Injury*, 13(8), 605–626, 1999.

38. Thickpenny-Davis, K. L. and Barker-Collo, S. L., Evaluation of a structured group format memory rehabilitation program for adults following brain injury, *Journal of Head Trauma Rehabilitation*, 22(5), 303–313, 2007.

39. Rattok, J., Ben-Yishay, Y., Ezrachi, O., Lakin, P., Piasetsky, E., Ross, B., Silver, S., Vakil, E., Zide, E., and Diller, L., Outcome of different treatment mixes in a multidimensional neuropsychological rehabilitation program, *Neuropsychology*, 6(4), 395–415, 1992.

40. Quemada, J. I, Muñoz Céspedes, J. M., Ezkerra, J., Ballesteros, J., Ibarra, N., and Urruticoechea, I., Outcome of memory rehabilitation in traumatic brain injury assessed by neuropsychological tests and questionnaires, *Journal of Head Trauma Rehabilitation*, 18(6), 532–540, 2003.

41. Goranson, T. E., Graves, R. E., Allison, D., and La Freniere, R., Community integration following multidisciplinary rehabilitation for traumatic brain injury, *Brain Injury*, 17(9), 759–774, 2003.

42. High, W. M., Jr., Roebuck-Spencer, T., Sander, A. M., Struchen, M. A., and Sherer, M., Early versus later admission to postacute rehabilitation: Impact on functional outcome after traumatic brain injury, *Archives of Physical Medicine and Rehabilitation*, 87(3), 334–342, 2006.

43. Seale, G. S., Caroselli, J. S., High, W. M., Jr., Becker, C. L., Neese, L. E., and Scheibel, R., Use of Community Integration Questionnaire (CIQ) to characterize changes in functioning for individuals with traumatic brain injury who participated in a postacute rehabilitation programme, *Brain Injury*, 16(11), 955–967, 2002.

44. Constantinidou, F., Thomas, R. D., Scharp, V. L., Laske, K. M., Hammerly, M. D., and Guitonde, S., Effects of categorization training in patients with TBI during postacute rehabilitation: Preliminary findings, *Journal of Head Trauma Rehabilitation*, 20(2), 143–157, 2005.

45. Harradine, P. G., Winstanley, J. B., Tate, R., Cameron, I. D., Baguley, I. J., and Harris, R. D., Severe traumatic brain injury in New South Wales: Comparable outcomes for rural and urban residents, *The Medical Journal of Australia*, 181(3), 130–134, 2004.

46. Malec, J. F., Impact of comprehensive day treatment on societal participation for persons with acquired brain injury, *Archives of Physical Medicine and Rehabilitation*, 82(7), 885–895, 2001.

47. Malec, J. F. and Degiorgio, L., Characteristics of successful and unsuccessful completers of 3 postacute brain injury rehabilitation pathways, *Archives of Physical Medicine and Rehabilitation*, 83(12), 1759–1764, 2002.

48. Ponsford, J., Harrington, H., Olver, J., and Roper, M., Evaluation of a community-based model of rehabilitation following traumatic brain injury, *Neuropsychological Rehabilitation*, 16(3), 315–328, 2006.

49. Ruff, R. M. and Niemann, H., Cognitive rehabilitation versus day treatment in head-injured adults: Is there an impact on emotional and psychosocial adjustment?, *Brain Injury*, 4(4), 339–347, 1990.

50. Parente, R. and Stapleton, M., Development of a cognitive strategies group for vocational training after traumatic brain injury, *Neurorehabilitation*, 13(1), 13–20, 1999.

51. Klonoff, P. S., Lamb, D. G., and Henderson, S. W., Milieu-based neurorehabilitation in patients with traumatic brain injury: Outcome at up to 11 years postdischarge, *Archives of Physical Medicine and Rehabilitation*, 81(11), 1535–1537, 2000.

52. Parente, R. and Anderson-Parente, J. K., Retraining memory: Theory and application, *Journal of Head Trauma Rehabilitation*, 4(3), 55–65, 1989.

53. Coetzer, R. and Rushe, R., Post-acute rehabilitation following traumatic brain injury: Are both early and later improved outcomes possible?, *International Journal of Rehabilitation Research*, 28(4), 361–363, 2005.

54. Malec, J. F., Smigielski, J. S., DePompolo, R. W., and Thompson, J. M., Outcome evaluation and prediction in a comprehensive-integrated postacute outpatient brain injury rehabilitation programme, *Brain Injury*, 7(1), 15–29, 1993.

55. Tobis, J. S., Puri, K. B., and Sheridan, J., Rehabilitation of the severely brain-injured patient, *Scandinavian Journal of Rehabilitation Medicine*, 14(2), 83–88, 1982.

56. Cope, D. N. and Hall, K., Head injury rehabilitation: Benefit of early intervention, *Archives of Physical Medicine and Rehabilitation*, 63(9), 433–437, 1982.

57. Mackay, L. E., Bernstein, B. A., Chapman, P. E., Morgan, A. S., and Milazzo, L. S., Early intervention in severe head injury: Long-term benefits of a formalized program, *Archives of Physical Medicine and Rehabilitation*, 73(7), 635–641, 1992.

58. Teasdale, T. W., Christensen, A. L., and Pinner, E. M., Psychosocial rehabilitation of cranial trauma and stroke patients, *Brain Injury*, 7(6), 535–542, 1993.

59. Laatsch, L. and Stress, M., Neuropsychological change following individualized cognitive rehabilitation therapy, *Neurorehabilitation*, 15(3), 189–197, 2000.

60. Zencius, A. H., Wesolowski, M. D., and Rodriguez, I. M., Improving orientation in head injured adults by repeated practice, multi-sensory input and peer participation, *Brain Injury*, 12(1), 53–61, 1998.

61. Parente, R., Kolakowsky-Hayner, S. A., Krug, K., and Wilk, C., Retraining working memory after traumatic brain injury, *Neurorehabilitation*, 13(3), 157–163, 1999.

62. Sohlberg, M. M. and Mateer, C. A., Effectiveness of an attention-training program, *Journal of Clinical and Experimental Neuropsychology*, 9(2), 117–130, 1987.
63. Park, N. W. and Ingles, J. L., Effectiveness of attention rehabilitation after an acquired brain injury: A meta-analysis, *Neuropsychology*, 15(2), 199–210, 2001.
64. Donaghy, S. and Williams, W., A new protocol for training severely impaired patients in the usage of memory journals, *Brain Injury*, 12(12), 1061–1076, 1998.
65. Sohlberg, M. M. and Mateer, C. A., Training use of compensatory memory books: A three stage behavioral approach, *Journal of Clinical and Experimental Neuropsychology*, 11(6), 871–891, 1989.
66. Wilson, B. A., Evans, J. J., Emslie, H., and Malinek, V., Evaluation of NeuroPage: A new memory aid, *Journal of Neurology, Neurosurgery, and Psychiatry*, 63(1), 113–115, 1997.
67. Wilson, B. A., Emslie, H. C., Quirk, K., and Evans, J. J., Reducing everyday memory and planning problems by means of a paging system: A randomised control crossover study, *Journal of Neurology, Neurosurgery, and Psychiatry*, 70(4), 477–482, 2001.
68. Wilson, B. A., Emslie, H., Quirk, K., Evans, J., and Watson, P., A randomized control trial to evaluate a paging system for people with traumatic brain injury, *Brain Injury*, 19(11), 891–894, 2005.
69. Hart, T., Hawkey, K., and Whyte, J., Use of a portable voice organizer to remember therapy goals in traumatic brain injury rehabilitation: A within-subjects trial, *Journal of Head Trauma Rehabilitation*, 17(6), 556–570, 2002.
70. Schmitter-Edgecombe, M., Fahy, J. F., Whelan, J. P., and Long, C. J., Memory remediation after severe closed head injury: Notebook training versus supportive therapy, *Journal of Consulting and Clinical Psychology*, 63(3), 484–489, 1995.
71. Zencius, A., Wesolowski, M. D., Krankowski, T., and Burke, W. H., Memory notebook training with traumatically brain-injured clients, *Brain Injury*, 5(3), 321–325, 1991.
72. Zencius, A., Wesolowski, M. D., and Burke, W. H., A comparison of four memory strategies with traumatically brain-injured clients, *Brain Injury*, 4(1), 33–38, 1990.
73. Freeman, M. R., Mittenberg, W., Dicowden, M., and Bat-Ami, M., Executive and compensatory memory retraining in traumatic brain injury, *Brain Injury*, 6(1), 65–70, 1992.
74. McKerracher, G., Powell, T., and Oyebode, J., A single case experimental design comparing two memory notebook formats for a man with memory problems caused by traumatic brain injury, *Neuropsychological Rehabilitation*, 15(2), 115–128, 2005.
75. Roche, N. L., Moody, A., Szabo, K., Fleming, J. M., and Shum, D. H., Prospective memory in adults with traumatic brain injury: An analysis of perceived reasons for remembering and forgetting, *Neuropsychological Rehabilitation*, 17(3), 314–334, 2007.
76. Einstein, G. O. and McDaniel, M. A., Normal aging and prospective memory, *Journal of Experimental Psychology: Learning, Memory, and Cognition*, 16(4), 717–726, 1990.
77. van den Broek, M. D., Downes, J., Johnson, Z., Dayus, B., and Hilton, N., Evaluation of an electronic memory aid in the neuropsychological rehabilitation of prospective memory deficits, *Brain Injury*, 14(5), 455–462, 2000.
78. Wright, P., Rogers, N., Hall, C., Wilson, B., Evans, J., Emslie, H., and Bartram, C., Comparison of pocket-computer memory aids for people with brain injury, *Brain Injury*, 15(9), 787–800, 2001.
79. Rieger, M. and Gauggel, S., Inhibition of ongoing responses in patients with traumatic brain injury, *Neuropsychologia*, 40(1), 76–85, 2002.
80. Gordon, W. A., Cantor, J., Ashman, T., and Brown, M., Treatment of post-TBI executive dysfunction: Application of theory to clinical practice, *Journal of Head Trauma Rehabilitation*, 21(2), 156–167, 2006.
81. Luria, A. R., *Higher Cortical Functions in Man*, Oxford University Press, New York, 1966.
82. Sbordone, R. J., The executive functions of the brain, in G. Groth-Marnat (Ed.), *Neuropsychological Assessment in Clinical Practice: A Guide to Test Interpretation and Integration*, Wiley, New York, 2000, 437–456.
83. D'Zurilla, T. J. and Goldfried, M. R., Problem solving and behavior modification, *Journal of Abnormal Psychology*, 78(1), 107–126, 1971.
84. Shallice, T. and Burgess, P., The domain of supervisory processes and temporal organization of behaviour, *Philosophical Transactions of the Royal Society of London, Series B, Biological Sciences*, 351(1346), 1405–1411, 1996.

85. Scherzer, B. P., Rehabilitation following severe head trauma: Results of a three year program, *Archives of Physical Medicine and Rehabilitation*, 67(6), 366–374, 1986.

86. Ben-Yishay, Y., Rattock, J., Lakin, P., Piasetsky, E. B., Ross, B., Silver, S., Zide, E., and Ezrachi, O., Neuropsychological rehabilitation: Quest for a holistic approach, *Seminars in Neurology*, 5(3), 252–259, 1985.

87. Rath, J. F., Simon, D., Langenbahn, D. M., Sherr, R. L., and Diller, L., Group treatment of problem-solving deficits in outpatients with traumatic brain injury: A randomised outcome study, *Neuropsychological Rehabilitation*, 13(4), 461–488, 2003.

88. Foxx, R. M., Martella, R. C., and Marchand-Martella, N. E., The acquisition, maintenance, and generalization of problem solving skills by closed head injured adults, *Behavior Therapy*, 20(1), 61–76, 1989.

89. von Cramon, D. Y., Matthes-von Cramon, G., and Mai, N., Problem-solving deficits in brain injured patients: A therapeutic approach, *Neuropsychological Rehabilitation*, 1(1), 45–64, 1991.

90. Medd, J. and Tate, R. L., Evaluation of an anger management therapy programme following acquired brain injury: A preliminary study, *Neuropsychological Rehabilitation*, 10(2), 185–201, 2000.

91. Kennedy, M. R., Coelho, C., Turkstra, L., Ylvisaker, M., Moore-Sohlberg, M., Yorkston, K., Chiou, H. H., and Kan, P. F., Intervention for executive functions after traumatic brain injury: A systematic review, meta-analysis and clinical recommendations, *Neuropsychological Rehabilitation*, 18(3), 257–299, 2008.

92. Marshall, R. C., Karow, C. M., Morelli, C. A., Iden, K., Dixon, J., and Cranfill, T., Effects of interactive strategy modeling training on problem-solving by persons with traumatic brain injury, *Aphasiology*, 18(8), 659–673, 2004.

93. Behan, L. A., Phillips, J., Thompson, C. J., and Agha, A., Neuroendocrine disorders after traumatic brain injury, *Journal of Neurology, Neurosurgery, and Psychiatry*, 79(7), 753–759, 2008.

94. Kelly, D. F., McArthur, D. L., Levin, H., Swimmer, S., Dusick, J. R., Cohan, P., Wang, C., and Swerdloff, R., Neurobehavioral and quality of life changes associated with growth hormone insufficiency after complicated mild, moderate, or severe traumatic brain injury, *Journal of Neurotrauma*, 23(6), 928–942, 2006.

95. Bornhofen, C. and McDonald, S., Emotion perception deficits following traumatic brain injury: A review of the evidence and rationale for intervention, *Journal of the International Neuropsychological Society*, 14(4), 511–525, 2008.

96. Henry, J. D., Phillips, L. H., Crawford, J. R., Ietswaart, M., and Summers, F., Theory of mind following traumatic brain injury: The role of emotion recognition and executive dysfunction, *Neuropsychologia*, 44(10), 1623–1628, 2006.

97. McAllister, T. W., Evaluation of brain injury related behavioral disturbances in community mental health centers, *Community Mental Health Journal*, 33(4), 341–358, 1997, Discussion, 359–364.

98. Tateno, A., Jorge, R. E., and Robinson, R. G., Pathological laughing and crying following traumatic brain injury, *The Journal of Neuropsychiatry and Clinical Neurosciences*, 16(4), 426–434, 2004.

99. Tateno, A., Jorge, R. E., and Robinson, R. G., Clinical correlates of aggressive behavior after traumatic brain injury, *The Journal of Neuropsychiatry and Clinical Neurosciences*, 15(2), 155–160, 2003.

100. Wood, R. L. and Williams, C., Inability to empathize following traumatic brain injury, *Journal of the International Neuropsychological Society*, 14(2), 289–296, 2008.

101. Gaylord, K. M., Cooper, D. B., Mercado, J. M., Kennedy, J. E., Yoder, L. H., and Holcomb, J. B., Incidence of posttraumatic stress disorder and mild traumatic brain injury in burned service members: Preliminary report. *Journal of Trauma*, 64(Suppl. 2), S200–S205, 2008, Discussion, S205–S206.

102. Alderman, N., Fry, R. K., and Youngson, H. A., Improvement of self-monitoring skills, reduction of behaviour disturbance, and the dysexecutive syndrome: Comparison of response-cost and a new programme of self-monitoring training, *Neuropsychological Rehabilitation*, 5(3), 193–221, 1995.

103. Guercio, J. M., Podolska-Schroeder, H., and Rehfeldt, R. A., Using stimulus equivalence technology to teach emotion recognition to adults with acquired brain injury, *Brain Injury*, 18(6), 593–601, 2004.

104. Payne, H. C., Traumatic brain injury, depression and cannabis use: Assessing their effects on a cognitive performance, *Brain Injury*, 14(5), 479–489, 2000.

105. McMillan, T. M., Williams, W. H., and Bryant, R., Post-traumatic stress disorder and traumatic brain injury: A review of causal mechanisms, assessment, and treatment, *Neuropsychological Rehabilitation*, 13(1–2), 149–164, 2003.

106. Williams, W. H., Evans, J. J., and Wilson, B. A., Neurorehabilitation for two cases of posttraumatic stress disorder following traumatic brain injury, *Cognitive Neuropsychiatry*, 8(1), 1–18, 2003.

107. Blanchard, E. B., Hickling, E. J., Devineni, T., Veazey, C. H., Galovski, T. E., Mundy, E., Malta, L. S., and Buckley, T. C., A controlled evaluation of cognitive behavioural therapy for posttraumatic stress in motor vehicle accident survivors, *Behaviour Research and Therapy*, 41(1), 79–96, 2003.

108. Williams, W. H., Evans, J. J., and Fleminger, S., Neurorehabilitation and cognitive–behaviour therapy of anxiety disorders after brain injury: An overview and a case illustration of obsessive–compulsive disorder, *Neuropsychological Rehabilitation*, 13(1–2), 133–148, 2003.

109. Soo, C. and Tate, R., Psychological treatment for anxiety in people with traumatic brain injury, *Cochrane Database of Systematic Reviews (Online)*, (3), CD005239, 2007.

110. Alderman, N., Contemporary approaches to the management of irritability and aggression following traumatic brain injury, *Neuropsychological Rehabilitation*, 13(1–2), 211–240, 2003.

111. Hibbard, M. R., Grober, S. E., Gordon, W. A., and Aletta, E. G., Modification of cognitive psychotherapy for the treatment of poststroke depression, *Behavior Therapist*, 1, 15–17, 1990.

112. Hibbard, M. R., Gordon, W. A., and Kothera, L., Traumatic brain injury, in F. M. Dattilio and A. Freeman (Eds.), *Cognitive–Behavioral Strategies in Crisis Intervention*, 2nd ed., Guilford Publications, New York, 219–242, 2000.

113. Coetzer, R., Psychotherapy following traumatic brain injury: Integrating theory and practice, *Journal of Head Trauma Rehabilitation*, 22(1), 39–47, 2007.

114. Fleming, J. M. and Ownsworth, T., A review of awareness interventions in brain injury rehabilitation, *Neuropsychological Rehabilitation*, 16(4), 474–500, 2006.

115. Cheng, S. K. and Man, D. W., Management of impaired self-awareness in persons with traumatic brain injury, *Brain Injury*, 20(6), 621–628, 2005.

116. Crosson, B., Barco, P. P., Velozo, C. A., Bolesta, M. M., Cooper, P. V., Werts, D., and Brobeck, T. C., Awareness and compensation in postacute head injury rehabilitation, *Journal of Head Trauma Rehabilitation*, 4(3), 46–54, 1989.

117. Langer, K. G. and Padrone, F. J., Psychotherapeutic treatment of awareness in acute rehabilitation of traumatic brain injury, *Neuropsychological Rehabilitation*, 2(1), 59–70, 1992.

118. Giacino, J. T. and Cicerone, K. D., Varieties of deficit unawareness after brain injury, *Journal of Head Trauma Rehabilitation*, 13(5), 1–15, 1998.

119. Ben-Yishay, Y., Silver, S. M., Piasetsky, E., and Rattok, J., Relationship between employability and vocational outcomes after intensive holistic cognitive rehabilitation, *Journal of Head Trauma Rehabilitation*, 2(1), 35–48, 1987.

120. Sherer, M., Bergloff, P., Levin, E., High, W. M., Jr., Oden, K. E., and Nick, T. G., Impaired awareness and employment outcome after traumatic brain injury. *Journal of Head Trauma Rehabilitation*, 13(5), 52–61, 1998.

121. Klonoff, P. S., O'Brien, K. P., Prigatano, G. P., Chiapello, D. A, and Cunningham, M., Cognitive retraining after traumatic brain injury and its role in facilitating awareness. *Journal of Head Trauma Rehabilitation*, 4(3), 37–46, 1989.

122. Prigatano, G. P. and Klonoff, P. S., A clinician's rating scale for evaluating impaired self-awareness and denial of disability after brain injury, *The Clinical Neuropsychologist*, 12(1), 56–67, 1998.

123. DeHope, E. and Finegan, J., The self-determination model: An approach to develop awareness for survivors of traumatic brain injury, *Neurorehabilitation*, 13(1), 3–12, 1999.

124. Chen, S. H. A., Thomas, J. D., Glueckauf, R. L., and Bracy, O. L., The effectiveness of computer-assisted cognitive rehabilitation for persons with traumatic brain injury, *Brain Injury*, 11(3), 197–209, 1997.

125. Dou, Z. L., Man, D. W., Ou, H. N., Zheng, J. L., and Tam, S. F., Computerized errorless learning-based memory rehabilitation for Chinese patients with brain injury: A preliminary quasi-experimental clinical design study, *Brain Injury*, 20(3), 219–225, 2006.

126. Goldstein, G., Beers, S. R., Shemansky, W. J., and Longmore, S., An assistive device for persons with severe amnesia, *Journal of Rehabilitation Research and Development*, 35(2), 238–244, 1998.

127. Batchelor, J., Shores, E. A., Marosszeky, J. E., Sandanam, J., and Lovarini, M., Cognitive rehabilitation of severely closed-head injured patients using computer assisted and noncomputerized treatment techniques, *Journal of Head Trauma Rehabilitation*, 3(3), 78–85, 1988.

128. Kirsch, N. L., Levine, S. P., Lajiness-O'Neill, R., and Schnyder, M., Computer-assisted interactive task guidance: Facilitating the performance of a simulated vocational task, *Journal of Head Trauma Rehabilitation*, 7(3), 13–25, 1992.

129. Gentry, T., Wallace, J., Kvarfordt, C., and Lynch, K. B., Personal digital assistants as cognitive aids for individuals with severe traumatic brain injury: A community-based trial, *Brain Injury*, 22(1), 19–24, 2008.

130. Bell, K. R., Temkin, N. R., Esselman, P. C., Doctor, J. N., Bombardier, C. H., Fraser, R. T., Hoffman, J. M., Powell, J. M., and Dikmen, S., The effect of a scheduled telephone intervention on outcome after moderate to severe traumatic brain injury: A randomized trial, *Archives of Physical Medicine and Rehabilitation*, 86(5), 851–856, 2005.

131. Melton, A. K. and Bourgeois, M. S., Training compensatory memory strategies via the telephone for persons with TBI, *Aphasiology*, 19(3–5), 353–364, 2005.

132. Hart, T., Buchhofer, R., and Vaccaro, M., Portable electronic devices as memory and organizational aids after traumatic brain injury: A consumer survey study, *Journal of Head Trauma Rehabilitation*, 19(5), 351–365, 2004.

133. Schönberger, M., Humle, F., Zeeman, P., and Teasdale, T. W., Working alliance and patient compliance in brain injury rehabilitation and their relation to psychosocial outcome, *Neuropsychological Rehabilitation*, 16(3), 298–314, 2006.

134. Wampold, B. E., Mondin, G. W., Moody, M., Stich, F., Benson, K., and Ahn, H., A meta-analysis of outcome studies comparing bona fide psychotherapies: Empirically "all must have prizes," *Psychological Bulletin*, 122(3), 203–215, 1997.

135. Ylvisaker, M., Hanks, R., and Johnson-Greene, D., Perspectives on rehabilitation of individuals with cognitive impairment after brain injury: Rationale for reconsideration of theoretical paradigms, *Journal of Head Trauma Rehabilitation*, 17(3), 191–209, 2002.

136. Wilson, B. A., Towards a comprehensive model of cognitive rehabilitation, *Neuropsychological Rehabilitation*, 12(2), 97–110, 2002.

22

Management of Residual Physical Deficits

Velda L. Bryan, David W. Harrington, and Michael G. Elliott

CONTENTS

22.1 Introduction: A Historical Perspective

Since World War II, an internationally scattered group of occupational therapists (OTs) and physical therapists (PTs) have developed and advocated theories and treatment procedures to address sensorimotor deficits in the neurologically impaired patient.[1-7] However, until the early 1980s, training and practice of these techniques were usually found only in specialty clinics and in advanced professional workshops. The majority of general practice therapists were neither trained in nor practiced a therapeutic approach based on neurophysiologic or developmental principles. Among those with training, some therapists were strong advocates of only one approach, whereas others were applying bits and pieces of all the then-known treatment approaches. Their patients were usually those with cerebral palsy, stroke, multiple sclerosis, and other neurologic etiologies.

Survivors of traumatic brain injury (TBI) prior to the 1970s were encouraged to use functional extremities, were put into wheelchairs and braces, and were eventually sent home or to an institution. Treatment was usually dictated by medical personnel who were not rehabilitation oriented. An early entry into the therapy department was rare and usually awaited the TBI patient's ability to respond or cooperate.

Most intensive care units were not familiar territory for therapists until the mid 1980s, when it was realized that early consistent range of motion (ROM) and positioning would later enhance general care and rehabilitation outcome. As early as the 1960s, Bobath[1] advocated that nurses and therapists should develop cooperative relationships at the intensive care unit and acute floor levels. Building a bridge of understanding and cooperation between nurses and therapists required careful diplomacy and patience.

The "brain injury unit," as an important, separate, and distinct unit, was not prevalent in general or acute rehabilitation hospitals prior to the 1980s. A focused, comprehensive team approach was absent, and vital supportive components were missing. The various therapy departments represented distinct territories, each treating a designated anatomic portion of the person. Speech and occupational therapists often bickered over the territory of oral feeding programs. Physical and occupational therapists did battle over the upper extremity, and some were concerned when a speech therapist would attempt to ambulate or transfer a person during a session.

Physical rehabilitation essentially focused on strengthening the "good" side and rarely challenged the impaired or "bad" side. We neglected the potential of the person as a "whole." Bobath[1] warned of the inherent failure of this "compensatory rehabilitation" approach. Many therapists made assumptions about a person's skills from the narrow view of the clinical setting rather than from a broader real-world perspective.

Severe cognitive and perceptual deficits and inappropriate behaviors often overwhelmed the physical rehabilitation effort, and these people were usually discharged as a result of "lack of progress," "lack of motivation," or because they were "uncooperative." Behavior modification training to support the treating staff was nonexistent. Therapies were frequently further hindered by use of psychoactive medications. People with TBI were often discharged to nursing homes or to locked psychiatric hospitals, or without other options, many were discharged to frightened families. TBI was puzzling and many wrong assumptions were made about the sequelae of brain injury. In the process, the notion that the person with acquired brain injury could not appreciably benefit from rehabilitation was perpetuated.

Meanwhile, emergency neurotrauma and neurosurgical technology dramatically improved as a result of the Korean Conflict and the Vietnam War. By the mid 1970s, the TBI survivor population was increasing, and institutionalization became more and more unacceptable. Although early, aggressive involvement of therapists in the acute facility had not yet captured great enthusiasm, therapists began to question the old points of view and began to be truly challenged by people with TBI. By the late 1970s, a handful of therapists dedicated themselves to organizing a TBI rehabilitation environment. These people knew inherently that they could expand horizons for this special population, and soon, their vision became a reality. A chance for "life after head injury" was coming into view through the lens of a new rehabilitation concept: postacute neurologic rehabilitation involving a comprehensive therapeutic environment with both clinical and residential/community care.

During the early 1980s, professional attendance at the first TBI conferences and response to initial publications revealed an intensified international interest. Jennett and Teasdale[8] and Rosenthal et al.[9] brought the broad scope of TBI into clearer view and the idea of continuity of care to our attention. During this time, many postacute brain injury rehabilitation admissions presented with unnecessary contractures, unattended heterotopic ossification, misdiagnosed or ignored vestibular and oculomotor deficits, poorly defined cognitive deficits, and polypharmacy for aggressive behaviors. Until the mid 1980s, many TBI patients lost valuable time, at tremendous expense, because of the fact that they required "reconstructive therapy." This loss ultimately reflected a less than optimal outcome. Although it was a frustrating time for patients and therapists, many knew that more could be accomplished.

During this time, it was also recognized that an interim step may be needed by some patients who were slower to recover from the minimally responsive phase and did not meet criteria for an acute rehabilitation phase. The subacute rehabilitation concept became a reality during the early 1980s and, through this aggressive approach, many slow-to-recover patients graduated on to an acute rehabilitation phase and then into a postacute rehabilitation phase. However, there were some who were able to transition from the subacute phase directly into a postacute phase. A continuity of neurologic rehabilitation care was established. Many therapists began to reflect on the seemingly obscure lessons of the past. New enthusiasm for Bobath's[1] teachings and Ayres'[7] concept of sensory integration emerged. The notion of hierarchical development in the human being was revisited. Therapeutic intervention was noted to be more successful when directed in the appropriate developmental order. The complex nature of TBI residuals required, and was recognized to benefit from, an organized, integrated, progressive approach that utilizes theories and treatments from all rehabilitation disciplines.[10] Alternative views regarding posture and movement control emerged and gave therapists fresh avenues through which to evaluate and treat balance and movement deficits.[7,11–14]

By 1990, increasing involvement of therapists during the acute stage was evidenced. Recent authors point out that *good preventative care must begin at the acute level* for the severely brain-injured patient.[15–17] As a result, early consistent positioning, use of inhibitory and facilitatory techniques, and orienting activation of the TBI patient are now provided.[18,19] Greater focus is placed on treatment team communication and cooperation. The "brain injury unit" offers a more structured and less distracting rehabilitation environment within the acute setting. Supportive systems to address aggressive and other inappropriate behaviors now assist staff in the acute rehabilitation facility. The results of all these efforts are reflected in the patient's subsequent improved status when discharged from the acute phase and admitted to the postacute neurologic rehabilitation program.

Sazbon and Groswasser[20] reviewed TBI sequelae in relationship to the length of postcomatose unawareness (PCU) relative to physical rehabilitation. The review of 72 patients with postcomatose unawareness periods of more than 1 month showed that approximately 33% of all patients achieved full ambulation, 38.9% achieved aided ambulation, and 27.8% required wheelchairs for mobility. The patients were classified, according to length of PCU, into four groups. Of those patients in PCU for 31 to 60 days, 55.2% progressed to full ambulation, 34.2% to aided ambulation, and 10.5% to wheelchair mobility. Conversely, of those patients who fell into the PCU group of 91 to 180 days, only 10% progressed to full ambulation, 20% to aided ambulation, and 70% to wheelchair mobility. Because PCU is, essentially, a manifestation of severity of injury, it can be seen that the more severely injured individuals were, not surprisingly, the individuals most likely to present in physical therapy and occupational therapy departments with ongoing neurorehabilitation needs. These patients were also the most likely to have significant problems with aphasia, speech disorders, visual deficits, behavior disturbances, and cognitive disturbances.

It has become common practice for PTs and OTs to consult with physicians about medications administered to their patients. With feedback from therapists about the positive or negative impact of medications on therapeutic efforts, physicians have been able to make better choices. For example, they have found that, in many situations, the sedating effect of antispasticity or psychoactive medications can be avoided with appropriate treatment approaches by well-trained and supported therapists,[18,21] except in cases of severe spasticity, flaccidity, or behavioral disturbance. Severe spasticity, which is not amenable to therapeutic or conventional pharmacologic management, may respond well to intrathecal baclofen (Lioresal, Watson Laboratories, Corona, CA) management.[22] Flaccidity may be treated successfully with conventional techniques, electromyography (EMG)/biofeedback,[23] and, in some cases, administration of dopaminergic medications such as Sinemet (Dupont Pharma, Wilmington, DE)[24–26] (see Chapter 4, this volume). Cooperative effort between physicians, nurses, psychologists, and therapists has greatly enhanced patient progress.

As people with TBI are provided excellent early acute rehabilitative care, they move into the postacute phase with greater potential for progress. Now the level of expectation of both the therapist and the patient with TBI has been raised. The therapeutic approach (how) and the environment (where) become influential factors to successful outcomes. During this process, the ultimate exchange occurs as the patient learns and teaches as much as the therapist teaches and learns.

The neurorehabilitation experience is at its best when provided in environmentally valid settings with comprehensive neurorehabilitation-experienced teams working with the patient and family toward a common goal. With a broader and more realistic scope of treatment settings, therapists are allowed to challenge their patients more fully. Intensified treatment, with graded structure and proper generalization of skills, translates into shorter lengths of stay, reduced costs, and more favorable outcomes.[27–29]

22.1.1 Purpose and Focus

A truly experienced comprehensive TBI rehabilitation program is qualified to admit a broad range of patients, and therapists must treat patients with severe, moderate, or mild levels of disability. A severely impaired patient may have significant sensorimotor, perceptual, visual, vestibular, language/communication, and cognitive deficits, and may be wheelchair-bound, have a gastrostomy, and be incontinent, along with multiple other deficits. A severe level of disability can also include the ambulatory, physically functioning patient who is significantly confused and behaviorally difficult. The moderately impaired individual may have some perceptual, visual, vestibular, and cognitive deficits while being capable of independent ambulation and performance of simple activities of daily living (ADLs) with supervision.

The person suffering sequelae from mild traumatic brain injury (MTBI) may not routinely appear as an early referral to the TBI rehabilitation program. It is more likely that this patient will be first referred to and treated by an orthopedic therapist for commonly associated musculoskeletal complaints. Comments about changes in routines or bizarre complaints regarding symptoms should be questioned. Subtle changes in daily routines occur as a result of unrecognized deficits. For example, driving habits may change in response to deficits in visual and cognitive processing. Driving at night may be gradually avoided and more lighting used in the house after sundown. An astute therapist will pick up on these clues from the patient and will recommend referral for appropriate assessments to define the core cause and to direct effective treatment. This cooperative effort will prevent a comparatively minor injury from becoming a catastrophic one.

Brain-injured persons may be 2 weeks or 2 years, or more, postinjury upon admission to neurorehabilitation programming. They may be directly admitted from the acute hospital or may come from home, a psychiatric hospital, a nursing home, or another program. TBI may be combined with various levels of spinal cord injuries, unresolved orthopedic/neurologic injuries, and diseases or dysfunctions of various systems. Consequently, the evaluative process and the management of residual physical deficits need to be thorough and capable of addressing neurologic, musculoskeletal, psychological, visual, vestibular, cognitive, and behavioral influences to physical functioning.

The purpose of this chapter is to offer some practical information to PTs and OTs treating TBI patients at the rehabilitation level. The focus is to address the continuum of evaluation and management of residual physical deficits that complicate recovery. Although it may appear that specific areas of evaluation and treatment have been designated to the PT or the OT, there is no intent to imply that these designations are, necessarily, as described. The important point is that every area must be appropriately evaluated and aggressively treated by the best therapist for the task.

22.2 The Evaluative Process

The purpose of a complete evaluation is to identify both obvious and subtle deficits to set the stage for an effective continuum of treatment and achievement of realistic goals. It is important not only to evaluate problem areas, but to evaluate all systems for proper identification and treatment of specific deficits within those systems.[10] The therapist must be able to identify which parts are missing during the patient's attempt to perform a task or what is interfering with the patient's ability to complete the task. It is not uncommon in the TBI population to encounter persons with seemingly more advanced skills than are actually present. A good example can be found in the person who is able to ambulate reasonably well when certain challenges are not present; however, when balance is challenged, delayed protective reactions may be revealed. Such a person is in greater jeopardy for reinjury following a loss of balance or a fall.

In an efficient admission to the TBI rehab program, the therapeutic team will be informed in advance about the patient's injury, and medical and early rehabilitation histories, and will be given a glimpse into the preinjury history and lifestyle prior to the commencement of the individual's therapy. Recommendations, pertinent factors to explore, and discussion of possible discharge options should be reviewed prior to admission. The collection and presentation of this information should be provided by experienced field evaluators (see Chapter 27, this volume, on field evaluation).

All therapists should be able to recognize the influence of various cognitive deficits that impact the patient's ability to solve problems, organize, and sequence motor acts. The rehabilitation team needs to understand impairments in perception and integration of the senses influencing movement, balance, and position in space.

Agitation or other inappropriate behaviors can seriously hinder progress. Therefore, proper staff training and effective approaches to behavior management should be expected in a comprehensive TBI program (see Chapter 20, this volume, on applied behavior analysis). Behavioral deficits are a fairly common sequelae in TBI. Many persons are tactilely defensive and/or easily overstimulated by even modest amounts of stimuli. Disorientation adds to the likelihood that verbal or physical aggression or withdrawal from treatment will occur. The proximity of physical and occupational therapy treatments, together with the factors mentioned earlier, makes it quite likely that therapists in physical rehabilitation will require skills in behavioral intervention.

Behavioral programming should be superimposed on treatment in either physical or occupational therapy. Application of defined behavioral strategies and programs can be best achieved in tandem with physical rehabilitation programming. Occasionally, it will be necessary for behavioral programming to supplant other programming; however, careful monitoring should be conducted to ensure that rehabilitation programming is undertaken as soon as possible. It is neither realistic nor necessary for behavioral issues to be completely resolved prior to initiation or continuation of rehabilitation programming. In fact, there are very few instances when rehabilitation programming should be deemed "unfeasible" as a result of behavioral deficits.

Emotional problems may manifest in problems with cooperation or motivation. Hopefully, a team member is available to assist in the address of such problems; however, the PT or OT may become the *de facto* counselor to the brain-injured person. Often, the intimacy of the physical rehabilitation treatment setting allows for the breakdown of psychological defense mechanisms or allows the development of a level of trust and understanding that will allow access to the person's emotional status. Overall, discussion among team members will allow for all aspects of the clinical presentation to be shared and treatment approaches to be developed by the appropriate discipline.

As patients enter the initial physical and occupation therapy evaluation sessions, the therapist should explore them as a whole. There should be no assumptions made about functional skills despite the report of previous diagnoses, treatment records, or initial appearances. Such premature assumptions can lead to inappropriate or absent treatment.[30]

Evaluation should be performed in a variety of clinical, residential, and community settings. Although personal lifestyle and medical histories were introduced in the preadmission information, the initial session should still allow time for getting acquainted. During this interaction, trust and understanding should be nurtured. To signify respect, the therapist should attempt to explain the purpose of each test or exercise and relate it to tasks in daily life. Most patients will respond to this type of interaction and will probably attempt to rise to a realistic level of expectation. A vital aspect of the therapist's role is that of motivator.

The evaluation should be thorough and well documented in quantitative and qualitative terms. Utilization of videotape is an excellent tool to assist in recording the person's performance progress from evaluation throughout treatment to discharge. If the person is unable to follow directions or is uncooperative, document observations of how the individual functions. For example, in an evaluation of a person who was heavily medicated, depressed, and unable to respond to usual evaluative techniques, the person was asked to tie his shoe. After a significant delay, presumably for processing, the individual sat down in a chair, slowly brought his left leg to his right knee, and tied the shoe. Observation allowed for comment about probable ROM impairments, at least, for the observed joints in movement, dexterity, trunk flexibility, strength of the left hip and knee flexors, fine and gross motor coordination, visual–motor integration, proprioception, and antigravity muscle groups during standing. There were no obvious impairments of gait, other than speed. Flexibility of the trunk was demonstrated by reaching to tie the shoe during sitting. Obvious impairments of dexterity, possibly related to medication, were observed as well. It was also obvious that the individual was able to respond to a verbal command, was able to follow through, did not demonstrate evidence of apraxia, and was cooperative within his capabilities. When the ability to respond becomes more appropriate, more conventional testing can be performed and documented.[31–34]

The neurologic rehabilitation field is currently responding to an increasing demand for assessment tools to provide better documentation of functional skills and outcomes.[32,35,36] Such assessments as the Barthel Index,[37] the Disability Rating Scale,[38] the Tuft's Assessment of Motor Performance,[39] the Tinetti Performance-Oriented Assessment of Mobility,[40] and the Functional Independence Measurement[41] have been utilized. More recently, "functional status measurements" are being developed to measure performance during daily activity, which includes cognitive, social, and psychological functioning.[30] Therapists should be acquainted with a variety of measurement tools and should choose the most appropriate tool for the level of patient and the information desired. Rating systems provide ongoing comparative data to review the flow of progress. Computerized programs are available not only to document but to graph an ongoing view of the course of treatment. By interval reviews of graphs or other visual aids, such as videotaping, the therapist provides a concrete tool for the patient to determine whether progress is being made. The therapist can take that opportunity to either encourage the patient to continue good effort or explore an alternative approach toward the desired goal.

Additional information can be obtained from pertinent family members.[42,43] Their insights about the individual's previous lifestyle and their perception of changes since the injury can reveal information that may help the therapist to understand and, perhaps, enhance motivation. Also, in appropriate situations, the family can be included in treatment sessions to educate and prepare them as potential participants in the person's future discharge environment.

During the initial interview, the therapist may wish to expand upon preadmission information by exploring the person's perception of the accident. Indications of retrograde or anterograde amnesia may be detected. If available, family members may provide their perceptions or additional insights for a confused or otherwise noncommunicative person. Documentation should include review of preinjury and postinjury history of fractures, surgeries, medications, and visual and/or auditory dysfunctions.

The subjective review should also include the individual's perception of current symptoms and any changes in activity levels that may be related to endurance, musculoskeletal complaints, sensorimotor deficits, pain, or vestibular dysfunction as they impact the person's quality of life. The person should also be asked to provide the therapist with an understanding of both short- and long-term goals for treatment. As the individual relates problems in a given area, it may be helpful to provide a checklist, such as the Vestibular Symptoms Checklist (Figure 22.1), to elicit further information about the nature of the problem prior to evaluation. Additional research has been performed to develop comprehensive patient-centered methods for recording goals. The Canadian Occupational Performance Measure is one such interview procedure that focuses on the individual's different occupational goals based on the arenas of self-care, productivity, and leisure skills.[44]

22.2.1 Range of Motion, Flexibility, and Dexterity

A thorough evaluation and documentation of active and passive hip, knee, ankle, and cervical/lumbar spine ranges of motion must be conducted. Evaluation should also review upper extremity ranges of motion, including the shoulders, elbows, wrists, and fingers. Documentation of flexibility (Figure 22.2) should include an assessment of the hamstrings, the gastrocnemius (with the knee extended), Thomas test, long sitting, trunk extension in the prone position, and trunk flexion from a seated position. Assessment of iliotibial band flexibility should be included.

When evaluating upper extremity and hand function, hand dominance should be documented. Observe the person's ability to control gross grasp and release and perform lateral pinch, tripod pinch, and palmar prehension. Upper extremity and hand function are further observed for the ability to hold, stabilize, and carry a variety of both light and heavy objects. Gross motor coordination of the upper extremity can be documented during timed performance testing via the Box and Block Test of Manual Dexterity.[45]

Fine motor coordination and selective movements are assessed during timed performance tests (e.g., the Nine-Hole Peg Test[46]) and through functional task observation. Such tests as the Purdue Pegboard[47] and the Minnesota Rate of Manipulation[48] can be used for advanced patient testing. If desired, additional prevocational assessments of dexterity, cognitive, and perceptual functions can be attained with such tests as the Crawford Small Parts Dexterity Test[49] and the Bennett Hand Tool Dexterity Test.[50] Objects that are pertinent to the patient's lifestyle should be used in the functional task evaluation (e.g., razors, toothbrushes, combs, buttons, zippers, eating utensils, pencils/pens, kitchen tools,

A. Vestibular symptoms checklist

   1. Current symptoms: _____

     _____

   2. Activity level change: _____

     _____

   3. Rate baseline dizziness on a scale of 0–10: _____

     _____

   4. Do any of the following activities make you dizzy?

Yes	No	
_____	_____	riding on escalators
_____	_____	riding in elevators
_____	_____	walking up/down stairs
_____	_____	walking in the dark
_____	_____	walking on a busy street
_____	_____	walking on grass or thick carpet
_____	_____	driving in a car
_____	_____	bending over
_____	_____	grocery shopping
_____	_____	making the bed
_____	_____	getting into or out of bed
_____	_____	rolling over in bed
_____	_____	reaching up

   5. Do you have a history of becoming motion sick prior to your injury?

     Yes   No

B. Self-perception:

   1. Self-Reported Deficits: _____

     _____

     _____

   2. Self-Reported Goals: _____

     _____

     _____

C.   Other pertinent information: _____

     _____

     _____

     _____

FIGURE 22.1

The Vestibular Symptoms Checklist is used to collect initial evaluative information about the nature of problems from the patient's perspective.

Flexibility Evaluation		
	Left	Right
A. Hamstring	_____	_____
B. Thomas test	_____	_____
C. Gastrocnemius (knee extended)	_____	_____
D. Long sit test	_____	
E. Prone trunk extension	_____	
F. Seated flexion	_____	
G. Iliotibial band (ITB)	_____	_____

FIGURE 22.2
The Flexibility Evaluation form is used to document information about the lower extremities and trunk.

cards, work tools). Any complaints of pain, or observations of edema, tremors, or changes in muscle tone should be documented.

22.2.2 The Neurologic Examination

Although the comprehensive neurologic examination takes place during the initial field evaluation and, subsequently, by other treatment professionals, this does not relieve the need for further assessment by the OT and the PT. A focused neurologic examination is necessary to look at those components that will eventually be addressed by the OT and the PT.

22.2.2.1 Sensation and Proprioception

Although the structure of documentation varies in each clinical setting, a complete sensory evaluation should be performed (Figure 22.3). Tactile sensation is tested for light/firm and sharp/dull discrimination and hot/cold temperature discrimination. Responses should be recorded as intact or hyper-/hyposensitive. Proprioception testing includes the ability to name movements, mirror movements, and detect vibration. Graphesthesia (the ability to identify numbers written on the skin by the examiner's finger) and stereognosis (the ability to identify objects by touch) should be tested and documented. Record responses to proprioceptive testing as intact or impaired.

22.2.2.2 Deep Tendon Reflexes and Pathologic Reflexes

These reflexes influence responses to movement. Record responses to the patellar, Achilles, biceps, brachioradialis, and triceps reflex tests as hyper (3+), normal (2+), hypo (1+), and absent (0) (Figure 22.4). The Babinski reflex should also be tested and recorded as present or absent.

22.2.2.3 Cerebellar Tests

Cerebellar reflexes have significant influence on the performance of smooth movements. Tests should include (1) finger-to-finger, (2) finger-to-nose, and (3) heel-to-shin performance.

Neurologic Evaluation				
I. Sensation				
	Upper Extremity		Lower Extremity	
	Left	Right	Left	Right
A. Light/Firm	Intact	Intact	Intact	Intact
	Hyper	Hyper	Hyper	Hyper
	Impaired	Impaired	Impaired	Impaired
B. Sharp/Dull	Intact	Intact	Intact	Intact
	Hyper	Hyper	Hyper	Hyper
	Impaired	Impaired	Impaired	Impaired
C. Hot/Cold	Intact	Intact	Intact	Intact
	Hyper	Hyper	Hyper	Hyper
	Impaired	Impaired	Impaired	Impaired
II. Proprioception				
	Upper Extremity		Lower Extremity	
	Left	Right	Left	Right
A. Naming Movements	Intact	Intact	Intact	Intact
	Impaired	Impaired	Impaired	Impaired
B. Mirroring Movements	Intact	Intact	Intact	Intact
	Impaired	Impaired	Impaired	Impaired
C. Vibration	Intact	Intact	Intact	Intact
	Impaired	Impaired	Impaired	Impaired
D. Graphesthesia	Intact	Intact	Intact	Intact
	Impaired	Impaired	Impaired	Impaired
E. Stereognosis	Intact	Intact	Intact	Intact
	Impaired	Impaired	Impaired	Impaired

FIGURE 22.3

The Neurologic Evaluation form is used to document sensory and proprioceptive functions.

Record findings as normal, hypermetric, ataxic, or with intention tremor (Figure 22.5). Diadochokinesis is tested symmetrically and asymmetrically and is recorded as normal, ataxic, or unable.

Melnick[13] reported that the "little brain," located under the occipital lobe, has "more neurons than the rest of the brain put together."[p. 834] When the cerebellum and its connections are disrupted by traumatic or nontraumatic events, multiple deficits may be manifested. The most significant deficit is loss of motor learning. There is disorganization in rapid alternating movements and decreases in balance and central postural control. Intention tremor greatly impacts the ability to conduct daily activities. Other functions negatively impacted by cerebellar damage include speech and control of eye movement and gaze.

Urbscheit[14] discussed the frustration encountered by many therapists in the evaluation and treatment of cerebellar deficits. Many therapists are unable to diagnose and treat

Reflex Testing				
I. Deep tendon eflexes				
A. Patellar				
Left	Hyper (3+)	Normal (2+)	Hypo (1+)	Absent (0)
Right	Hyper (3+)	Normal (2+)	Hypo (1+)	Absent (0)
B. Achilles				
Left	Hyper (3+)	Normal (2+)	Hypo (1+)	Absent (0)
Right	Hyper (3+)	Normal (2+)	Impaired	Absent (0)
II. Pathological reflexes				
A. Babinski reflex				
Left	Absent	Present		
Right	Absent	Present		

FIGURE 22.4
The Reflex Testing form is used to document reflex testing information.

cerebellar dysfunction adequately. Swaine and Sullivan[51] reviewed interrater reliability for measurement of clinical features of finger-to-nose testing and reported fairly poor inter-rater reliability for determination of the presence of dysmetria. The therapist working with this population must become proficient in cerebellar evaluation and treatment.

The individual must be observed for hypotonicity, dysmetria, difficulty with rapid alternating movements, and movement decomposition. These deficits may be observed in gait, pace of gait, and ADLs (e.g., brushing teeth, stirring food, eating, trying to walk at a fast pace). Complaints of difficulties with vision while the individual is in motion may be related to cerebellar dysfunction as well as vestibular dysfunction.

Cerebellar Tests				
A. Finger - Finger				
Left	Normal	Hypermetric	Ataxic	Int. Tremor
Right	Normal	Hypermetric	Ataxic	Int. Tremor
B. Finger - Nose				
Left	Normal	Hypermetric	Ataxic	Int. Tremor
Right	Normal	Hypermetric	Ataxic	Int. Tremor
C. Heel - Shin				
Left	Normal	Hypermetric	Ataxic	Int. Tremor
Right	Normal	Hypermetric	Ataxic	Int. Tremor
D. Diadochokinesis				
Symmetrical	Normal	Hypermetric	Unable	
Asymmetrical	Normal	Hypermetric	Unable	

FIGURE 22.5
The Cerebellar Tests form is used to document cerebellar functions.

Rapid Alternating Movement Evaluation (# repetitions in 10 seconds)		
	Left	Right
I. Heel-toe:	_____	_____
II. Seated side steps:	_____	_____
III. Standing side steps:	_____	_____

FIGURE 22.6
The Rapid Alternating Movements form provides a simple format for documenting rapid alternating movements.

22.2.3 Rapid Alternating Movement Evaluation

While seated, alternate floor touching with the heel and toe and seated sidesteps are observed for the number of repetitions performed in 10 seconds. The number of repeated standing sidesteps are also recorded for a 10-second period. Note quality of performance (Figure 22.6). These simple tasks can be good indicators of asymmetries or the ability to mimic a motor pattern, as well as coordination of the lower limbs.

22.2.4 The Manual Muscle Test

The technique for manual muscle testing is well known by all qualified OTs and PTs. This assessment is performed not only to evaluate a muscle group's ability to produce force against gravity, but also the person's ability to isolate a muscle's movement and force. Manual muscle tests document strength in the musculature of the neck, shoulders, arms, hands, hips, knees, ankles, abdominals, and trunk extensors. In some situations, the manual muscle test may not be appropriate. For example, in the presence of spasticity, a forcefully opposing muscle group will increase muscle tone and assessment of the ability to perform an isolated muscle contraction will not be valid.

22.2.5 Muscle Tone

Most neurorehabilitation clinicians will point to abnormal muscle tone as one of the major physiologic barriers to a full achievement of rehabilitation goals. Normal muscle tone allows the extremities and trunk to move through available ranges of motion from joint to joint. Abnormal muscle tone may be hypertonic or hypotonic. Hypotonia may result from a lower motor neuron or peripheral nerve injury. Hypotonia may also be a residual of TBI involving the cerebellum. Hypotonic muscles are less firm to touch and demonstrate a lower resistance to passive stretch than normal. There is a limpness in the limb during passive ranging. Flaccidity is differentiated from hypotonicity by the absence of voluntary, postural, and reflex movements with a loss of resistance to passive stretch.

Assessment of hypotonia starts with palpation of muscles and testing deep tendon reflexes. As mentioned, the hypotonic muscle lacks firmness. A pendular movement is seen when testing the deep tendon reflexes. Sitting posture at rest appears asymmetric or limp. An object held in the hand may be dropped when the person is distracted. All fingers on the hand will flex when the individual attempts to flex only one at a time. A wet footprint is wider on the involved side.

Hypertonia, a term used interchangeably with *spasticity,* is one component of an upper motor neuron injury and may be a residual deficit from TBIs. Spasticity, as defined by Lance,[52] is an increase in muscle tone resulting from hyperexcitability of the stretch reflex. Consideration must be given to the differentiation between spasticity and rigidity in an effort to determine the best treatment approach. Although spasticity is characterized by a velocity-dependent increase in tonic stretch reflexes, the increased tonic stretch reflexes in rigidity are not velocity dependent. Spasticity typically involves a muscle on one side of a joint but rigidity affects the muscles on both sides of a joint. Both hypertonia and hypotonia become problematic when the patient is unable to regulate the amount of muscle tone needed when activating various muscle groups. The residual problem is often very one sided, either hyperreflexive or hyporeflexive, resulting in mobility deficits at specific joints that interfere with functional activities.

Many scales to assess spasticity following neurologic injury have been proposed over the years. However, there has been some controversy regarding the determination of the most reliable assessment format. Many studies examined these scales for appropriateness. Pros and cons of the Modified Ashworth Scale and the Modified Tardieu Scale were studied, but no clear decision was made about which scale should be used. To add to the confusion, Burridge et al.[53] reported that appropriate methods for use in the research of the mechanism of spasticity did not satisfy the needs of the clinician. They proposed that there was a need for an objective but clinically applicable tool and standardized protocols.

The Ashworth Scale for Grading Spasticity was proposed by Ashworth in 1964.[54] In 1987, the Modified Ashworth Scale was proposed by Bohannon and Smith.[55] The "modified" scale is the currently accepted tool for the initial and ongoing reevaluation of spasticity. The difference between the original Ashworth Scale and the Modified Ashworth Scale is that the original scale measures movement of a limb through *full* passive ROM and the modified scale measures limb movement through *partial* passive ROM at a specific joint without specifying speed of motion. Resistance was then graded according to a numeric scale. Graded references using the Modified Ashworth Scale are as follows:

0 = No increase in muscle tone
1 = Slight increase in muscle tone, manifested by slight catch and release or by minimal resistance at end of ROM when affected parts are moved in flexion or extension
1+ = Slight increase in muscle tone, manifested by slight catch and release or by minimal resistance throughout the remainder (less than half) of ROM
2 = More marked increase in muscle tone through most of ROM, but affected parts easily moved
3 = Considerable increase in muscle tone, passive movement difficult
4 = Affected parts rigid in flexion or extension

During initial observations, many people may seem to have minimal to nil abnormal tone. However, the individual should be closely observed during active functional movements. This is another reason for evaluating the individual while performing functions in various environments. The evaluation should begin with an analysis of the motor control present in each extremity.

Observations pertaining to lack of movement or minimal movement, in particular, in cases where the dopaminergic system may have been impacted by the injury, may suggest the application of dopaminergic medication to enhance motor function. Conversely, persons who present with significant spasticity will generally not benefit from such an approach. The response of spasticity to stretching, relaxation, positioning, and medication will need to be explored, together with an appraisal of the likelihood of response to chemical neurolysis and casting. Spasticity should be differentiated from rigidity in the hypertonic patient. Rigidity may respond to dopaminergic drugs, whereas spasticity may be worsened. The PT and OT can provide quite valuable information to the physician in these arenas. The influence of emotion, pain, fatigue, and varying demands of motion and posture should be considered in evaluation of movement.

22.2.6 Muscle and Cardiovascular Endurance

Muscle endurance of the trunk and lower extremities is assessed by the PT. Trunk endurance (Figure 22.7) testing documents the maximum number of sit-ups performed in 1 minute and the maximum number of push-ups the individual is able to produce. Bridging and hyperextension are each sustained as long as possible (Figure 22.7). Acceptable performance is considered to be 1 minute for bridging and 30 seconds for hyperextension. Cardiovascular endurance can be tested with a standard or modified Bruce Test[56] (Figure 22.8 and Figure 22.9), based on the individual's level of conditioning. It is very important to monitor heart rate and blood pressure during this exercise. Do not forget to document the patient's current medications, which may affect vital signs at rest and during exercise. Advanced endurance testing, such as a physical capacity evaluation, may be performed to address back-to-work potential.

Differential diagnosis of cardiorespiratory endurance problems and vestibular dysfunction cannot be undertaken completely at this point in the evaluation; however, findings of nystagmus or other indicators during testing may point to vestibular dysfunction and should be noted for consideration during subsequent vestibular testing.

22.2.7 Mobility, Posture, and Gait Evaluations

Although the majority of severely disabled TBI persons may have become quite mobile during the acute rehabilitation stay, there will be an occasional need for full evaluation of bed mobility, transfers, tub/shower, and wheelchair skills. In the residential setting, most

Muscle Endurance		
1. Trunk endurance		
Sit-Ups	_____ repetitions	(1 minute)
Push-Ups	_____ repetitions	(maximum)
Bridging	_____ seconds	(norm: 1 minute)
Hyperextension	_____ seconds	(norm: 30 seconds)
2. Lower extremity endurance		
Wall slide (90°/90°)	_____ seconds	(norm: 1 minute)

FIGURE 22.7
The Muscle Endurance form is used to document trunk, lower extremity, and cardiovascular endurance.

Cardiovascular Endurance									
Bruce's low level treadmill test (Modified Shefield-Bruce Submaximal Protocol™)									
Stage	Time	Speed	Grade	Mets	Date	Date	Date	Date	Date
Rest HR	xxxxx	xxxxx	xxxxx	xxxxx					
Rest BP	xxxxx	xxxxx	xxxxx	xxxxx					
Stage 1	min 1 min 2 min 3	1.7 mph	0%	2.3					
Stage 2	min 4 min 5 min 6	1.7 mph	5%	3.5					
RPE	xxxxx	xxxxx	xxxxx	xxxxx					
Stage 3	min 7 min 8 min 9	1.7 mph	10%	4.6					
Stage 4	min 10 min 11 min 12	2.5 mph	12%	6.8					
RPE	xxxxx	xxxxx	xxxxx	xxxxx					
Recovery _____ min	xxxxx	xxxxx	xxxxx	xxxxx					
Recovery _____ min	xxxxx	xxxxx	xxxxx	xxxxx					
Recovery _____ min	xxxxx	xxxxx	xxxxx	xxxxx					

FIGURE 22.8
The Cardiovascular Endurance form is used to document Bruce's Low-Level Treadmill Test.

people will be able to sleep in standard double-size (or larger) bed. Bathrooms should be an appropriate size and equipped for wheelchair, walker, or cane mobility.

Beyond the expected physical components for bed mobilization and bed/tub/toilet transfers, other areas that impact mobility, such as cognitive abilities, safety judgment, impulsivity, visual deficits, and systems impacting postural control, should be observed and documented. The evaluation should document the person's ability to perform the tasks independently or with assistance and include notation of the quality of performance.

Bed mobility (Figure 22.10) explores scooting up and down as well as to the right or left sides. Is the person able to turn to either side and attain sitting and supine positions? A useful method to provide objective measurement of bed mobility is to time the task and document any observation of asymmetries between right and left sides. Note if the individual includes the hemiparetic side or is using compensatory strategies during movements. Is the person using some aspect of abnormal tone to achieve movement? For example, extensor

Cardiovascular Endurance									
Bruce's standard treadmill protocol									
Stage	Time	Speed	Grade	Mets	Date	Date	Date	Date	Date
Rest HR	xxxxx	xxxxx	xxxxx	xxxxx					
Rest BP	xxxxx	xxxxx	xxxxx	xxxxx					
Stage 1	min 1 min 2 min 3	1.7 mph	10%	4–5	hr				
Stage 2	min 4 min 5 min 6	2.5 mph	12%	6–7	hr				
RPE	xxxxx	xxxxx	xxxxx	xxxxx					
Stage 3	min 7 min 8 min 9	3.4 mph	14%	8–10	hr				
Stage 4	min 10 min 11 min 12	4.2 mph	16%	11–13	hr				
Stage 5	min 13 min 14 min 15	5.0 mph	18%	14–16	hr				
Stage 6	min 16 min 17 min 18	6.0 mph	20%	17–19	hr				
RPE	xxxxx	xxxxx	xxxxx	xxxxx					
Recovery _____ min HR BP	xxxxx	xxxxx	xxxxx	xxxxx					
Recovery _____ min HR BP	xxxxx	xxxxx	xxxxx	xxxxx					
Recovery _____ min HR BP	xxxxx	xxxxx	xxxxx	xxxxx					

FIGURE 22.9
The Cardiovascular Endurance form is used to document Bruce's Standard Treadmill Protocol.

Mobility Evaluation		

I. Bed mobility — Assist — Quality

	Assist	Quality
A. Scooting	_____	_____
1. Up	_____	_____
2. Down	_____	_____
3. Left	_____	_____
4. Right	_____	_____
B. 1/2 Rolls		
1. Left	_____	_____
2. Right	_____	_____
C. Attain Sitting	_____	_____
D. Attain Supine	_____	_____

II. Wheelchair mobility

	Assist	Quality
A. Even Surfaces	_____	_____
B. Uneven Surfaces	_____	_____
C. Inclines	_____	_____
D. Declines	_____	_____
E. Doorways	_____	_____
F. Curbs _____ inches	_____	_____

III. Transfers

	Assist	Quality
A. Preparation	_____	_____
B. Wheelchair to level surface	_____	_____
C. Wheelchair to elevated surface	_____	_____
D. Wheelchair to floor	_____	_____
E. Floor to wheelchair	_____	_____

IV. Ambulation

	Assist	Quality
A. Sit to stand	_____	_____
B. Assistive device	_____	_____
C. Indoors	_____	_____
D. Outdoors	_____	_____
E. neven terrain	_____	_____
F. Inclines/declines	_____	_____
G. Curbs	_____	_____
H. Stairs	_____	_____

FIGURE 22.10

The Mobility Evaluation form is used to collect information on bed, wheelchair, transfer, and ambulation activities.

thrust may be used to complete rolling. Note differences in bed mobilization abilities on a gym mat versus a soft bed in the residential setting. Quality of movement should be emphasized. Wheelchair mobility (Figure 22.10) assessments include the patient's ability to mobilize on even and uneven surfaces, inclines and declines, through doorways, and over curbs. Note the approximate height of the curb and time to cover specific distances.

Document the person's preparation for transfer (Figure 22.10). Record any need for verbal and/or physical cues, as well as the need for physical assistance. Note performance in transferring from the wheelchair to a level surface, an elevated surface, the floor, and floor to wheelchair.

Observations of the general ability to ambulate should document (Figure 22.10) whether the individual has detectable mobility problems or appears quite normal. The evaluation should include observations from clinical, residential, and community settings. Observe and document ambulation indoors, outdoors, on uneven terrain, on inclines and declines, and negotiating curbs and stairs. Document the ability to rise from sitting to standing. Note the need for assistance and the use of any supportive devices. The Timed "Up and Go" Test[57] is a quick and objective gait test (Figure 22.11).

When evaluating ambulatory skills, an initial impression of minimal or no obvious abnormalities may change when the situation moves from a well-lit, even-surfaced, clinical setting to a less ideal environment with low light and uneven terrain (e.g., darkened room with plush carpeting or evening time on grassy/rocky terrain). Impairments in sensorimotor and/or vestibular system-related performance may be revealed under more realistic and demanding circumstances. The evaluation may even be extended to include movement onto or off of escalators and into or out of elevators. Watch for a tendency to avoid or complain about tasks in noisy or busy environments. Subtle changes in fluidity of body movement during ambulation can point to vestibular, cerebellar, or oculomotor problems.

During ambulation evaluations, document reduced or absent reciprocal arm swing, slowed pace of walking, reduced head turning or visual scanning, drifting or "wall walking," and slight or obvious hesitancy when changing directions. It is also important to note subjective complaints of dizziness, nausea, or feelings of drunkenness or

Timed "Up and Go" Test	
Equipment:	Chair (without arms) and stop watch.
Criteria:	Individuals must be able to ambulate at least 200 feet with/without any type of assistive device.
Description:	Individuals are asked to rise from a chair (without arms) on the signal "Go," walk 10 feet, turn, walk back to chair, turn, and sit down. The total time to complete the test is recorded in seconds. The goal is to complete the test in the shortest time possible.
Scoring:	Practice Trial: _____ Test Trial 1: _____ Test Trial 2: _____ Test Trial 3: _____ Mean Time: _____
Interpretation of Results: 1. <20's 2. 20's–30's 3. >30's	Functionally independent in basic ADLs "Grey area," variable functional abilities Functionally dependent in basic ADLs

FIGURE 22.11
The Timed "Up and Go" Test.

light-headedness when walking. These may be additional indicators of visual and/or vestibular disturbances.

Notations should be made regarding the patient's posture during sitting and standing activities, as well as any gait deviations.[58] Observations should also note apparent influences from muscle weakness; leg length discrepancies; pain; vestibular, cerebellar, or ocular dysfunctions; cognitive/perceptual deficits; poor endurance; loss of flexibility; and impairments in somatosensory functions.[12,14,18,59,60]

As emphasized in neurodevelopmental theory (NDT),[1,61] observations of postures should include the position of the scapula, pelvis, rib cage, and spinal column. Position of the trunk may vary greatly, so also note the conditions under which observations are made. For example, is the individual sitting on a solid surface or on a bed or standing? Note if the person is able to recognize and maintain midline with head and trunk positions.

22.2.8 Neurodevelopmental Sequence Evaluation

To gather a baseline on a variety of movement patterns, the neurodevelopmental sequence is a good place to start. Assessment of the motorically intact individual is just as important as assessing the motorically impaired person. Omission of this evaluation for people functioning at a high level may prevent observations of subtle deficits in sensorimotor integration. Observe closely for inefficient movement patterns.

The ability to perform independently or with assistance is recorded as well as the quality of performance. Video recording of this initial evaluation further documents quality of performance. Of course, recording is repeated at various intervals throughout the treatment process.

The evaluation follows a very basic sequence of movement patterns (Figure 22.12). It begins with logrolling to both sides. Next, observe the ability to assume and maintain a prone-on-elbows position, followed by the quadruped, or all-fours, position. Contralateral (Figure 22.13A) and ipsilateral (Figure 22.13B) positions are assumed next, and the maintained positions are timed. Reciprocal crawling is observed forward and backward. Tall-kneel position is observed for the ability to assume and maintain the position as well as the ability to weight shift. Knee walking is also observed forward and backward. The half-kneel position is assumed and maintained for both sides. The half-kneel-to-stand position is also observed from both sides.

22.2.9 Vestibular Evaluation

It has already been pointed out that an important aspect of the evaluation is to identify subtle deficits impacting ADL task performance because proper identification of the core cause leads to a better choice of treatment avenues. The therapist should be trained in the assessment and treatment of various vestibular dysfunctions, although much of the training in this subject is available primarily through postgraduate courseware.[11,12,62–64] Lingering problems related to balance, postural control, and spatial orientation can disable any TBI patient. See Chapter 6 in this text on vestibular dysfunction by Roland and Blau, where assessment and treatment approaches are reviewed and demonstrated and, therefore, not are discussed in this chapter.

Additional tools for the therapist include the Motion Sensitivity Quotient[65] (Figure 22.14) and the Functional Reach Test[66] (Figure 22.15). Despite the fact that the Functional Reach Test was developed for the geriatric population, it provides a quick and easy balance test for most age groups. Age-appropriate norms for both male and female populations are included.

Neurodevelopmental Sequence Evaluation			
		<u>Assist</u>	<u>Quality</u>
I.	Log rolling		
	A. Left	_____	_____
	B. Right	_____	_____
II.	Prone on elbows		
	A. Assume	_____	_____
	B. Maintain	_____	_____
III.	Quadruped		
	A. Assume	_____	_____
	B. Maintain	_____	_____
IV.	Contralateral balance		
	A. Left Knee	_____	_____ sec.
	B. Right Knee	_____	_____ sec.
V.	Psilateral balance		
	A. Left Knee	_____	_____ sec.
	B. Right Knee	_____	_____ sec.
VI.	Reciprocal crawling		
	A. Forward	_____	_____
	B. Backward	_____	_____
VII.	Tall kneel		
	A. Assume	_____	_____
	B. Maintain	_____	_____
	C. Weight Shift	_____	_____
VIII.	Knee walk		
	A. Forward	_____	_____
	B. Backward	_____	_____
IX.	Half kneel		
	A. Assume Left Knee	_____	_____
	Right Knee	_____	_____
	B. Maintain Left Knee	_____	_____
	Right Knee	_____	_____
X.	Half kneel to stand		
	A. Left Foot	_____	_____
	B. Right Foot	_____	_____

FIGURE 22.12
The Neurodevelopmental Sequence Evaluation form is used to document information on various movements through the sequence.

22.2.10 Sensorimotor Integration and Dynamic Balance Evaluations

In a normal central nervous system, purposeful activity of the extremities depends upon the stabilization of the trunk. When postural control is maintained, significant influence is exerted on limb tone, ROM, and control.[58] However, the individual with moderate to severe sensorimotor impairment may find that extremity movement is less than functional

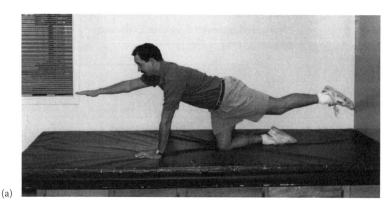

(a)

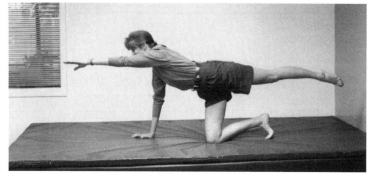

(b)

FIGURE 22.13

(a) Illustration of the contralateral position in the neurodevelopmental sequence. (Courtesy of James E. Eaton.) (b) Illustration of the ipsilateral position in the neurodevelopmental sequence. (Courtesy of Lynda R. Eaton.)

when selective movement is reduced to gross movement patterns influenced by primitive reflexes.

The ability to maintain standing balance in static or dynamic conditions requires the complex interaction of several systems—vision, vestibular, and somatosensory. However, these systems must be coupled with appropriate motor programs, muscle contractions, body alignment, and ROMs to allow for smooth and well-coordinated, purposeful movements.

The sensorimotor integration evaluation considers the manner in which postural control, reflexes, and feedback from vision, vestibular, and proprioceptive systems impact upon motor control and programming. The evaluation should therefore document postural control in sitting and standing (Figure 22.16). With the patient in the sitting position, observe body alignment, then note responses to weight shifting in lateral and anterior/ posterior directions. While the individual orients the head, rights the trunk, or resumes the vertical position, note the direction of shift. Notice responses of dizziness, disequilibrium, and protective responses.

The Tinetti Performance-Oriented Assessment of Mobility[40] allows assessment of balance deficits in more impaired patients during movement in functional tasks. The assessment calls for observation of the patient during sitting, arising, standing, and walking. Balance reactions are also observed while the individual turns around (360 degrees), sits down, and attempts single-foot support. The test provides a scoring system

Motion Sensitivity Quotient			

Client Name: _____   Date: _____

Baseline Symptoms: _____

Intensity Score	Duration Score		Intensity Score
0–least	0–5 sec.	= 0	+
5–most	6–10 sec.	= 1	Duration Score
	11–30 sec.	= 2	
	>30 sec.	= 3	

Movement	Intensity	Duration	Score (I+D)
1. Sit to supine			
2. Supine to right side			
3. Supine to left side			
4. Supine to longsit			
5. Right Hallpike			
6. Return to sit			
7. Left Hallpike			
8. Return to sit			
9. Sitting – nose to right knee			
10. Return to vertical			
11. Sitting – nose to left knee			
12. Return to vertical			
13. Head rotation × 5			
14. Head flex/ext. × 5			
15. Standing 180 degree turn right			
16. Standing 180 degree turn left			

MSQ = Total Score × number of provoking positions divided by 20.48.	Total Score: _____
	MSQ: _____

Score Key:	0–10% = Mild	11–30% = Moderate	.30% = Severe.

FIGURE 22.14
Motion Sensitivity Quotient.

Functional Reach Norms		
Norms	Men (inches)	Women (inches)
20–40 years	16.7+/−1.9	14.6+/−2.2
41–69 years	14.9+/−2.2	13.8+/−2.2
70–87 years	13.2+/−1.6	10.5+/−3.5

FIGURE 22.15
Functional Reach Norms.

Sensorimotor Integration Evaluation

I. Postural control

  A. Sitting:

    1. Alignment:

    _____

    _____

    2. Weight shifts:

		Eyes Open			Eyes Closed	
		Lateral	Ant/Post		Lateral	Ant/Post
a. Shifts Weight:		+ −	+ −		+ −	+ −
b. Head Oriented:		+ −	+ −		+ −	+ −
c. Trunk Righted:		+ −	+ −		+ −	+ −
d. Resume Vertical:		+ −	+ −		+ −	+ −
e. Dizziness:		+ −	+ −		+ −	+ −
f. Dysequilibrium:		+ −	+ −		+ −	+ −
g. Protective Response:		+ −	+ −		+ −	+ −

  B. Standing:

    1. Active weight shifts:

a. Anterior/posterior:	Ankle	Hip	Stepping	Other
b. Lateral:	Ankle	Hip	Stepping	Other
c. Dizziness:	Yes	No		
d. Comments:_____				

    2. Induced weight shifts:

a. Anterior/posterior:	Ankle	Hip	Stepping	Other
b. Lateral:	Ankle	Hip	Stepping	Other
c. Dizziness:	Yes	No		
d. Comments:_____				

    3. Standing One-Foot Balance: A = Ankle   H = Hip   S = Stepping   O = Other

	Left		Right	
	Time	Strategy	Time	Strategy
Trial 1	_____	_____	_____	_____
Trial 2	_____	_____	_____	_____

    4. Sensory Organization:

	Time	Sway
a. Eyes Open, Firm Surface	_____	_____
b. Eyes Open, Foam Surface	_____	_____
c. Eyes Closed, Firm Surface	_____	_____
d. Eyes Closed, Foam Surface	_____	_____

FIGURE 22.16

The Sensorimotor Integration Evaluation form is used to document postural control in sitting and standing positions.

for comparative data. As patients reach scoring criteria, they can be advanced to more appropriate tests.

People without severe impairments to postural control and balance/coordination may also benefit from an evaluation of sensorimotor integration (Figure 22.16).[67,68] With the patient in the standing position, balance skills can be evaluated through observation of postural control strategies used during both active and induced weight shifts as well as standing one-foot balance evaluation. Observation of active weight shifts (initiated by the person) to anterior/posterior and lateral positions assesses the use of ankle, hip, stepping, or other types of postural control strategies. Presence or absence of dizziness is noted. Induced weight shifts (imposed by the examiner) measure the same positions.

Standing one-foot balance is measured by the length of time maintained, and the postural control strategy utilized (i.e., ankle, hip, stepping, or other) should be noted. Undertake two to three trials and average the times. Sensory organization (the integration of proprioceptive and vestibular input) is measured by timing and the amount of sway with eyes open and eyes closed on a firm surface and on a foam surface. Care should be taken to disallow any potential for orientation that might be available from a continuous light or sound source during balance and sensorimotor testing (Figure 22.16).

The dynamic balance evaluation (Figure 22.17) again documents the type of postural control strategy (ankle, hip, stepping, falls) used in dynamic gait activities, heel–toe ambulation, balance beam ambulation, winding strip ambulation, and step-ups. The dynamic gait activity task involves walking forward for 12 feet to an abrupt stop. Note the postural control strategy utilized and complaints of dizziness. Next, have the individual walk forward for 12 feet and then sharply pivot to the right. Repeat to the left. Note the strategy utilized and any complaint of dizziness. The final dynamic gait activity task involves walking with the head first repeatedly rotating horizontally (right/left) and then walking with the head repeatedly moving vertically (up/down). Note the strategy utilized and any complaint of dizziness.

Heel–toe and balance beam ambulation evaluation should document required assistance levels and the quality of performance for going forward, backward, sideways, and during Carioca or braiding step maneuvers. The winding strip ambulation test (heel–toe walking following a piece of string or fabric laid out in a curvilinear fashion on the floor; Figure 22.18) is conducted for forward, backward, and sideways walking. Step-ups are repeated 20 times, first leading with the left, and then with the right. Note the time needed to perform this task. The careful notation of the times will provide a window on the progress of the improvement as it occurs.

22.2.11 Quick Reciprocal Movement Evaluation

For evaluation of higher level balance and coordination disorders, movements to be assessed include straddle jumps, straddle crosses, reciprocal jumping, pendulum, slalom (forward/backward), four-point, shuffling (left/right), running Carioca (left/right), skipping, and reciprocal marching (forward/backward; Figure 22.19).

With regard to higher level balance and coordination skills, the admonition "never assume" comes into play. We have observed many patients who initially present as very functional in mobility assessments but show significant deterioration of skill performance when higher level demands are requested. The importance of going a step further to assess higher levels of balance is related to the hopeful achievement of as near-premorbid levels

Dynamic Balance Evaluation		

I.   Dynamic gait activities:

       Strategy: A = Ankle   H = Hip   S = Stepping   F = Falls

	Strategy	Dizziness
A. Walk 12 ft., stop abruptly	_____	_____
B. Walk 12 ft., pivot sharply		
1. Left	_____	_____
2. Right	_____	_____
C. Walk with head motion		
1. Horizontal	_____	_____
2. Vertical	_____	_____

II. Heel-toe ambulation:	Assist	Quality
A. Forward	_____	_____
B. Backward	_____	_____
C. Sideways	_____	_____
D. Carioca	_____	_____

III. Balance beam ambulation:	Assist	Quality
A. Forward	_____	_____
B. Backward	_____	_____
C. Sideways	_____	_____
D. Carioca	_____	_____

IV. Winding strip ambulation:	Assist	Quality
A. Forward	_____	_____
B. Backward	_____	_____
C. Sideways	_____	_____

V. Step-ups (20 repetitions)	Assist	Time
A. Left	_____	_____
B. Right	_____	_____

FIGURE 22.17
The Dynamic Balance Evaluation form is used to document performance during dynamic activities.

of functioning as possible. These quick movement demands arise in various sports activities or in certain driving conditions. The same requirement for high-level coordination skills may arise in various vocational duties involving coordinated quick upper and lower extremity movements.

22.2.11.1 Straddle Jump

The *straddle jump* is performed beginning in a standing position with the feet together. The individual jumps from the feet-together position and lands with the feet separated via hip abduction, as in a jumping-jack exercise (Figure 22.20).

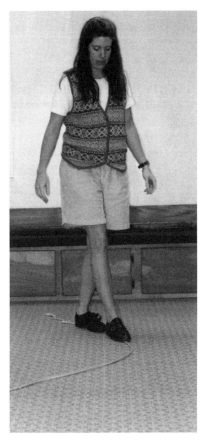

FIGURE 22.18
An illustration of the Winding Strip Ambulation Test. (Courtesy of Caryn Murphy.)

22.2.11.2 Straddle Cross

The *straddle cross* is performed beginning in the same position as the straddle jump; however, rather than separating the feet, while in the air, the individual crosses the feet and lands in a legs-scissored position. The second straddle cross reverses the front leg position with the back leg position (Figure 22.21).

22.2.11.3 Reciprocal Jumping

Reciprocal jumping is accomplished by beginning in a standing position with the feet together. The individual jumps and lands with one foot outstretched in a forward, hip-flexed position, whereas the other foot is in a backward, hip-extended position. The arm swing should be reciprocal as in normal walking. The second reciprocal jump reverses the leg and arm positions (Figure 22.22).

22.2.11.4 Pendulum

The *pendulum* maneuver is accomplished by beginning in the standing, feet-together position. The individual jumps, kicking one leg into hip abduction, keeping the foot in the air,

Quick Reciprocal Movement Evaluation		
	Assist	Quality
I. Straddle jumps:	_____	_____
II. Straddle crosses:	_____	_____
III. Reciprocal jumping:	_____	_____
IV. Pendulum:	_____	_____
V. Slalom:		
A. Forward	_____	_____
B. Backward	_____	_____
VI. 4-POINT:	_____	_____
VII. Shuffling:		
A. Left	_____	_____
B. Right	_____	_____
VIII. Running carioca:		
A. Left	_____	_____
B. Right	_____	_____
XI. Skipping:	_____	_____
X. Reciprocal marching:		
A. Forward	_____	_____
B. Backward	_____	_____

FIGURE 22.19

The Quick Reciprocal Movement Evaluation form is used to document performance of quick reciprocal movements.

and landing on the opposite foot. The second pendulum swing is accomplished by jumping and reversing leg/foot positions (Figure 22.23).

22.2.11.5 Slalom

The *slalom* exercise begins with standing in the feet-together position. The feet are kept together as the individual jumps and lands. The first jump places the feet off to the left and the second places the feet off to the right, while maintaining an upright torso. The knees should be flexed and pointed forward. The feet positions are similar to those used in parallel turns while downhill skiing (Figure 22.24).

22.2.11.6 Four-Point

The *four-point* jump is initiated in the standing, feet-together position. The individual jumps using both feet, but moves one foot forward, via hip flexion, to toe-touch the floor in front of the individual in harmony with the other foot returning to the floor. On the next jump,

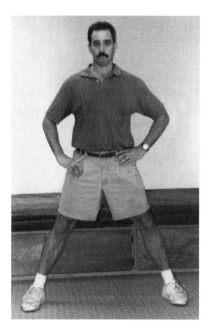

FIGURE 22.20
Illustration of the beginning and ending position of the straddle jump. (Courtesy of James E. Eaton.)

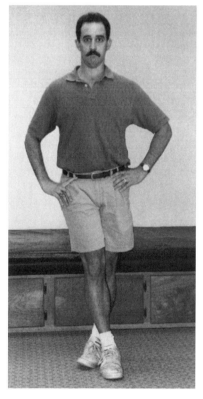

FIGURE 22.21
Illustration of the cross position of the straddle cross. (Courtesy of James E. Eaton.)

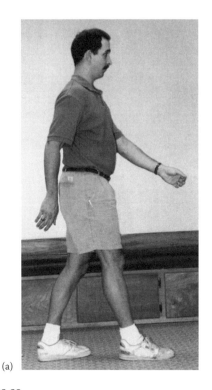 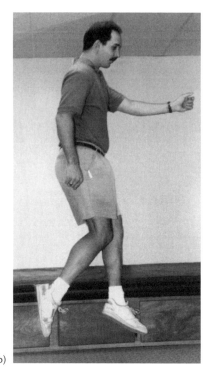

(a)   (b)

FIGURE 22.22
(a) Illustration of the beginning position of the reciprocal jump. (b) Illustration of the change of leg positions during the midjump phase of the reciprocal jump. (Courtesy of James E. Eaton.)

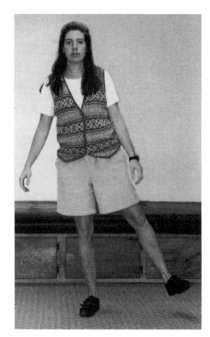

FIGURE 22.23
Illustration of the pendulum position. (Courtesy of Caryn Murphy.)

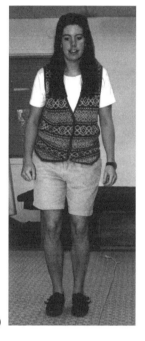 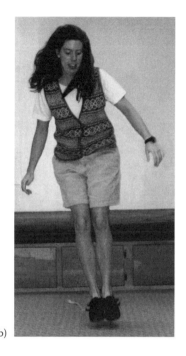 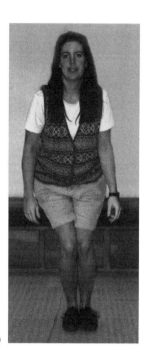

(a)   (b)   (c)

FIGURE 22.24
(a) Illustration of position no. 1 of the slalom activity. (b) Illustration of position no. 2 of the Slalom activity. (c) Illustration of position no. 3 of the Slalom activity. This sequence (a–c) is then repeated a specified number of times. (Courtesy of Caryn Murphy.)

the foot that was moved to the forward toe-touch position is moved to the side toe-touch position via rotation of the hip to a hip-abducted position. On the third jump, the foot is moved to the rear toe-touch position, via hip rotation to a hip-extended position. The final jump brings the feet back together. The exercise is performed to each side (Figure 22.25).

22.2.11.7 Shuffling

The *shuffling* maneuver is initiated with feet together in a standing position. Separations of the feet are accomplished via hip abduction followed by quick return to the feet-together position via hip adduction to produce a rapid sideways shuffle. The maneuver should produce sideways movement and should be conducted in both directions.

22.2.11.8 Running Carioca

Running Carioca is a rapid production of the grapevine step or cross step.

22.2.11.9 Skipping

Skipping should be self-explanatory.

22.2.11.10 Reciprocal Marching

The *reciprocal march* is an exaggerated march step with large arm swing and exaggerated hip and knee flexion during the march.

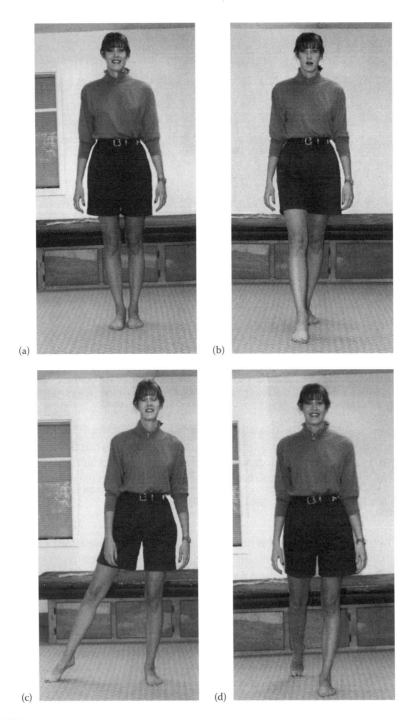

(a)   (b)

(c)   (d)

FIGURE 22.25

(a) Illustration of the starting position of the four-point, which is followed by a jump to the next position. (b) Illustration of the second position of the four-point with a foot forward. (c) Illustration of the third position of the four-point with the foot adducted to the side. (d) Illustration of the fourth position of the four-point with the foot posterior to midline. The next jump returns to the starting position (a), and the sequence is repeated a specified number of times. (Courtesy of Lynda R. Eaton.)

Each of these exercises is repeated until the evaluator has a good understanding of the person's abilities. Measure assistance required and quality of performance.

22.2.12 Assessment of Smell and Taste

It is imperative that assessments of olfactory (smell) and gustatory (taste) senses are included in the overall evaluations by the OT or PT. Impairment or absence of smell can occur in mild to severe TBIs depending upon the focus of injury. It is estimated that disturbances in smell function occurs in approximately 20% of head traumas with damage to cranial nerve I (olfactory nerve) or in the orbitofrontal area of the frontal lobe.[69] Some patients may not be aware of change in these senses. However, the individual who is aware may have no understanding of the implications of such an impairment on daily life. For this reason, the patient and family must be educated about hazards related to impaired function in taste and smell.

Changes in the ability to detect smells may occur with or without fracture injuries to the bony structure of the face. Fracture injuries may result in shearing of some or all of the olfactory axons that protrude through the cribriform plate of the ethmoid bone above the nasal cavity posterior to the bridge of the nose. As odor is taken up the nose, the olfactory axons capture and transmit the odor signal above the cribriform plate and into olfactory bulbs of the olfactory nerve. The odor signal may be transmitted along the olfactory nerve through branches into the thalamus or other areas of the internal capsule before being relayed into the olfactory cortex (orbitofrontal cortex). Factors involved in emotion and motivation may be impacted when olfactory signals mediated through the amygdala and hypothalamus are impaired. An inability to discriminate odors occurs when lesions are found in the orbitofrontal cortex.[70]

The complete loss of smell (anosmia) occurs when bulb shearing has occurred. An altered or distorted perception of odors (dysosmia) may occur when damage is in the orbitofrontal cortex. A favorite food may be perceived as smelling foul (parosmia).

Taste is detected by taste cells in the mouth involving the tongue, palate, pharynx, epiglottis, and upper third of the esophagus. Taste buds on the tongue detect molecules on the anterior two thirds of the tongue through the taste fibers of cranial nerve VII (facial nerve). The afferent portion of cranial nerve IX (glossopharyngeal nerve) controls the sense of taste for the posterior third of the tongue. The palate taste buds are innervated by a branch of cranial nerve VII, and the epiglottis and esophagus by branches of cranial nerve X (vagus nerve). Taste sensory fibers enter the medulla of the brainstem and transmit into the thalamus. Gustatory functions detect four basic stimuli: bitter, salty, sour, and sweet. Taste buds responding to each of the four basic stimuli are found in all regions of the tongue. Most of food flavors are derived from information coming through the olfactory system. Molecules are sent into the back of the nasal cavity by cheeks, tongue, and throat movements.

The University of Connecticut Health Center's Taste and Smell Clinic (www.uchc.edu) estimates that approximately 0.5% of the TBI population experiences loss of taste. In terms of rehabilitation interest, the focus of attention is typically given to the sense of smell. Olfactory dysfunction may have gone undetected until the individual reaches the postacute phase of treatment. Anosmia is thought to occur in approximately 5.5% of the TBI population, whereas more than a third of TBI patients have dysosmia.[71,72] As many as a third of people with TBI may have difficulty with olfactory naming and recognition. Questions should be raised by complaints of smelling foul odors, poor appetite, or unawareness of body odor or various household smells, including burning or spoiled foods.

Following a chemosensory screening by the OT or PT, alterations in function should be examined in light of the original injury. The patient's medical history should be explored to consider any type of respiratory problem or allergies. In some cases, a loss or partial loss of smell may be transitory in nature. An easy manner to assess smell function can be obtained by presenting some familiar odors to the patient. Unlabeled items such as vanilla, coffee, chocolate, and lemon are often used for this rough assessment. A very quick estimate of sense of smell can be obtained by placing an alcohol pad under the patient's nose.

A more extensive and quantitative assessment of smell function can be obtained with The Smell Identification Test, developed by the University of Pennsylvania.[73] The test consists of four packets, each containing 10 "scratch-and-sniff" odorant strips. Above each strip is a multiple choice of four possible responses. A test booklet lists the correct answers and provides a table to determine the degree of olfactory loss based on the age and sex of the patient in addition to the number of correct responses.

The individual will require awareness and education in ways to detect smoke, gas, other toxic fumes, and spoiled foods.[74,75] A chemosensory screening may also indicate the necessity to refer for additional clinical examinations by an otorhinolaryngologist or neurosurgeon.

22.2.13 Evaluation of Vision

The incidence of visual dysfunction following TBI is fairly high. Schlageter et al.[76] reviewed 51 patients within days of admission. They found that 30 (59%) were impaired in one or more of the following: pursuits, saccades, ocular posturing, stereopsis, extraocular movements, and near/far eso-/exotropia. Because the acute rehabilitation experience has become increasingly shorter in duration for this population, relatively little attention is paid to visual–motor and visual perceptual remediative efforts. As a consequence, these deficits are frequently evidenced in rehabilitation settings.

A thorough occupational therapy evaluation should include a complete vision screening test.[77] Prior to the vision screening, preliminary information is collected via the Visual Symptoms Checklist (Figure 22.26). This questionnaire not only collects subjective responses but provides an opportunity for objective documentation. For example, the individual may be aware of symptoms. However, the therapist may observe head tilting, squinting, or closing an eye; difficulty reading; or bumping into walls or furniture on one side.

The screening should include visual attentiveness, near and distance acuities, ocular pursuits, saccades, near point convergence, eye alignment, stereopsis, color identification, and peripheral fields. Changes in acuities may be reflected in difficulty performing tasks requiring near vision (e.g., shaving or putting on makeup) or difficulty recognizing environmental cues (e.g., facial expressions).

Smooth ocular pursuits are required for such tasks as reading a line of print or a column of words or numbers. Saccades provide a rapid but accurate shift of the eye in such visual tasks as reading to the end of a line of print and rapidly shifting leftward to the beginning of the next line. The King-Devick Test[78] measures scanning and saccadic function required to read detailed and structured formats (e.g., reading a bus or train schedule). Evaluation of visual system integrity may raise suspicion of vestibular or cerebellar dysfunction. Impairment in near point convergence is another tracking deficit that may be manifested in double or blurred vision and decreased depth perception.

Visual Symptoms Checklist

Prescription glasses:　　　　　Yes _____　　No _____

　　　If yes:　　Were glasses worn prior to injury? _____

　　　　　　　　Since the injury only? _____

　　　　　　　　Last vision examination? _____

　　　　　　　　New prescription? _____　　Date: _____

Answer **yes** or **no** to the following questions:　　　　　　　　　Yes　　　　　　No

1.　Do you have blurred or double vision?　　　　　　　　　　_____　　　_____

2.　Do you tilt your head to see more clearly?　　　　　　　　_____　　　_____

3.　Do you squint or close an eye to see?　　　　　　　　　　_____　　　_____

4.　Do you get a headache while reading, watching television, riding in or　　_____　　　_____
　　driving a car? Other? _____

5.　Do your eyes feel "tired"?　　　　　　　　　　　　　　　_____　　　_____

6.　Do you lose your place while reading?　　　　　　　　　　_____　　　_____

7.　Do you hold objects or reading material close to see?　　　_____　　　_____

8.　Do you avoid reading or not read as often as you did before the injury?　_____　　　_____

9.　Do you miss words, letters, or numbers while reading?　　_____　　　_____

10.　Do you have difficulty distinguishing colors?　　　　　　_____　　　_____

11.　Do you avoid dark areas or avoid driving after dark?　　　_____　　　_____

12.　Do you sometimes confuse which direction is right or left?　_____　　　_____

13.　Do you reverse letters, numbers, or words?　　　　　　　_____　　　_____

14.　Do you have difficulty recognizing road or street signs before it is too　_____　　　_____
　　late to turn?

15.　While you are standing still, do objects seem to jump or move?　_____　　　_____

16.　While you are walking, do objects seem to jump around?　_____　　　_____

17.　Do you bump into objects on one side or the other?　　　_____　　　_____

FIGURE 22.26
The Visual Symptoms Checklist is used to collect information on vision from the patient.

Strabismus may result in double or blurred vision as the eyes move through the visual sphere. The ability to scan visually may be impaired in such tasks as reading, writing, grocery shopping, driving, or reviewing a map. Eye alignment measures horizontal and vertical alignments to detect possible deviations.

Deficits in stereopsis impact many functions requiring depth perception. The ability to judge spatial relationships in such eye–hand tasks as threading a needle, targeting food on a plate, or negotiating stairs is affected by this deficit.

Peripheral and central vision are required for a full field of vision. A loss of the peripheral fields will impact safety for ambulation, awareness of environment, and safe driving, and will require the patient's awareness and ability to compensate with appropriate head turning.

Following the vision screening, appropriate referrals to the neuro-ophthalmologist or neuro-optometrist may be required for further in-depth assessments. (Refer to Chapters 7 and 9 in this text by in-depth discussion of evaluative and treatment options.)

People with TBI may or may not complain of visual disturbances. However, behavioral evidence of oculomotor deficits may be seen in problems with reading, writing, driving, playing video games, or watching television. As the therapist asks more specific questions, patients may report that words "jump" around on the page or that they frequently lose their place while reading. They may complain that they can read for only short periods of time. They may relate that images move in strange ways while watching television or while driving. They may experience dizziness, headaches, or nausea during these activities. Head position adjustments can foretell oculomotor problems, as can observation of dysfluencies of gait, especially in uneven terrain such as curbs, uneven sidewalks, stairs, or multilevel surfaces. Often, a person will complain of neck and shoulder problems that might actually be a vision-driven versus purely orthopedic difficulty.

The field of vision therapy represents a valuable evaluation and treatment process that has been practiced by too few over the years. It is now being incorporated more routinely into the clinical practice of neurologic rehabilitation.[77–80]

22.2.14 Visual Perception and Perceptual Motor Evaluation

Following the vision evaluation, perceptual motor assessments should proceed. Deficits may impact upon the patient's ability to perform normal daily living tasks adequately. Observations and documentation should be taken from clinical and other environments.[81–83] Clinical assessments may include information from tests performed by both the OT and the neuropsychologist.

Visual perception examines visual figure–ground, form constancy, spatial awareness or position in space, depth perception, visual memory, visual sequential memory, visual–motor integration, and spatial relationships. *Visual figure–ground* is the ability to distinguish foreground from background, and *form constancy* explores the ability to perceive subtle variations in form. *Position in space* is the ability to manage such spatial concepts as in/out, up/down, and front/behind. *Spatial relationships* examines the individual's ability to perceive positioning of two or more objects in relation to themselves or other objects. It is easy to understand how frequently the patient requires these functions in everyday living.

Clinical evaluations of visual perception should include such tests as the Motor-Free Visual Perception Test—Vertical Format (MVPT-V).[84] The Motor-Free Visual Perception Test measures the time it takes to process visual information and react to that information. In vertical, it helps to eliminate errors that may be caused by hemianopsia or visual neglect. This information applies to such tasks as reading comprehension, depth perception for ambulation, and driving. Standardized scores are compared among individuals without head injuries, individuals with head injuries but not visual neglect, and those with a head injury and visual neglect.

Advanced standardized perceptual tests, such as The Test of Visual–Perceptual Skills (nonmotor)-Revised,[85] greatly enhance previously available detail and precision. The norms were based on developmental ages for perceptual skills.

The Hooper Visual Organization Test[86] examines the ability to organize visual stimuli by showing pieces of an object. These skills are needed to locate items in a grocery store, refrigerator, or in a cupboard. The Hooper Visual Organization Test is useful in detecting deficits in the right hemisphere and will determine actual perceptual deficits, aside from performance.

An evaluation of the ability to perform purposeful movements on command or praxis is important for all people with TBI. Apraxia or dyspraxia may be obvious or subtle and may influence physical performance. Even in the person with MTBI, initiation and sequencing of functional motor acts need close observation for potential disorganization.[87] Skills required to produce a design in two and three dimensions (e.g., assemble various items from written or illustrated instructions) relate to constructional praxis and block design. Form perception is assessed via the form board and examines the ability to differentiate variations in form.

Difficulties in identifying body parts or right/left discrimination impact perception of body self or scheme. The OT can assess these abilities with the Draw-a-Person, Body Part Identification, and Body Puzzle tests.[88]

Lezak[89] warned that observations must distinguish between perceptual failures, apraxias, spatial confusions, motivation, or attention problems. Therapists have, more recently, responded to this need for clearer definition of deficits and better direction for treatments. In this regard, Bowler[82] noted that two assessments are beginning to be utilized to define perceptual skills and other neurologic skills that contribute to overall function. The Rivermead Perceptual Assessment Battery[90] assesses deficits in visual perception and was developed for adults with brain injury. The Lowenstein Occupational Therapy Cognitive Assessment[91] examines orientation, perception, visual–motor organization, and cognition, and provides baseline information for treatment. Although some areas of assessment overlap, the combined tests view each function from a variety of perspectives to define deficits more distinctly.

22.2.15 Assessment of Activities of Daily Living

The OT is able to gather quite meaningful information from observations during actual daily tasks in the residential treatment setting or the person's home. The structure of some programs allows a trained rehabilitation assistant to gather appropriately documented data of several specific tasks over several days during the initial assessment. This documentation continues throughout the program for the purpose of reassessment or as feedback data. For example, observations of the manner in which the individual organizes and sequences tasks and manages time can be documented while the person plans the meal, shops for items, and prepares the meal. This continually collected data directs the OT along a progression of therapeutic focus, clinically and residentially (Figure 22.27).

ADL assessment may also include an evaluation of the living environment where the person resides. Home modifications, environmental controls, and adaptive equipment needs should be addressed to maximize independence and safety. Training and education may be provided concerning energy conservation techniques, transfers within the home, and emergency alert systems. An evaluation of the community is also helpful to identify resources for vocational or leisure exploration. Community transportation needs may also be addressed.

Take careful note of potential dependency behaviors. The family or others may fail to recognize that tasks are innocently assisted or completely performed by them for the injured person. If possible, assess ADL skills in a normal living environment, independent

Activities of Daily Living Checklist

Assistance levels

0 = No assistance required to initiate, continue, or complete task
1 = Minimal verbal cues or gestural prompts
2 = Intermittent verbal cues or gestural prompts
3 = Minimal physical prompts
4 = Intermittent physical prompts
5 = Guided performance
6 = Unable

Dressing   Date: _____

                                            Level   Comments

1.   Don shirt/blouse/dress   _____   _____
2.   Doff shirt/blouse/dress   _____   _____
3.   Don underwear   _____   _____
4.   Doff underwear   _____   _____
5.   Don pants   _____   _____
6.   Doff pants   _____   _____
7.   Buttoning (small, large)   _____   _____
8.   Zipping (tops, pants)   _____   _____
9.   Buckle/unbuckle belt   _____   _____
10. Don/doff socks/hose   _____   _____
11. Don/doff brace/splint   _____   _____
12. Accessories on/off   _____   _____
13. Shoe on/off   _____   _____

Grooming/hygiene   Date: _____

                                            Level   Comments

1.   Use faucets   _____   _____
2.   Wash face/hands   _____   _____
3.   Use handkerchief/tissue   _____   _____
4.   Apply/remove glasses   _____   _____
5.   Brush teeth/clean dentures   _____   _____
6.   Brush/comb hair   _____   _____
7.   Shampoo hair   _____   _____
8.   Style hair   _____   _____
9.   Shave face/legs   _____   _____
10. Apply deodorant   _____   _____
11. Apply make-up   _____   _____
12. Care for nails   _____   _____
13. Manage clothes at toilet   _____   _____
14. Cleans self at toilet   _____   _____
15. Manages feminine hygiene   _____   _____
16. Bathe/towel dry entire body   _____   _____
17. Skin inspection   _____   _____

FIGURE 22.27
The Activities of Daily Living Checklist is used to document daily performance of ADLs. This information is used by staff to produce weekly and monthly reports of the patient's progress.

Household cleaning		Date: _____
	Level	Comments
1. Change sheets/make bed	_____	_____
2. Pick up objects from floor	_____	_____
3. Dust	_____	_____
4. Sweep/mop/vacuum	_____	_____
5. Transport pail of water	_____	_____
6. Wring out mop	_____	_____
7. Clean windows	_____	_____
8. Clean refrigerator/stove	_____	_____
9. Put out garbage	_____	_____

Laundry		Date: _____
	Level	Comments
1. Sort clothes	_____	_____
2. Use washer/dryer	_____	_____
3. Use detergent	_____	_____
4. Hand launder	_____	_____
5. Put clothes on hangers	_____	_____
6. Fold clothes	_____	_____
7. Put clothes away	_____	_____
8. Iron clothes	_____	_____

Meal planning		Date: _____
	Level	Comments
1. Plan balanced meals	_____	_____
2. Scan kitchen for necessary items	_____	_____
3. Compile grocery list	_____	_____
4. Estimate amount of money needed	_____	_____
5. Get to/from store	_____	_____
6. Locate items in store	_____	_____
7. Retrieve items from shelves	_____	_____

Meal preparation/cleanup		Date: _____
	Level	Comments
1. Read recipe/directions	_____	_____
2. Follow recipe/directions	_____	_____
3. Remove food from refrigerator	_____	_____
4. Remove items from cupboard	_____	_____
5. Organize and transfer items to work area	_____	_____
6. Open packages/cans/bottles	_____	_____
7. Handle pots/pans/utensils	_____	_____
8. Use faucets	_____	_____
9. Pour liquids (hot/cold)	_____	_____
10. Use microwave	_____	_____
11. Use stove	_____	_____
12. Use oven	_____	_____
13. Peel/cut vegetables	_____	_____
14. Break eggs	_____	_____
15. Stir	_____	_____
16. Measure	_____	_____
17. Use timer/clock	_____	_____
18. Set table/clear table	_____	_____
19. Transfer food/liquids to table	_____	_____
20. Wash/dry dishes	_____	_____
21. Load/unload/use dishwasher	_____	_____
22. Wipe stove/microwave/table	_____	_____
23. Put dishes away	_____	_____

FIGURE 22.27 (continued)

of family interaction. This approach should help to identify true problem areas and can be a good time to educate the individual and family about observed deficits and needed intervention for same.

22.2.16 Concomitant Injuries

22.2.16.1 Orthopedic and Spinal Cord

Therapists will encounter people with TBI who have accompanying orthopedic and/or spinal cord injuries. Special orthopedic issues, such as heterotopic ossification, must be appropriately addressed.[92] Regardless of the possibility that surgical intervention may or may not be involved, the PT and the OT will play a vital role. In a postoperative situation, therapeutic follow-up will be necessary to prevent loss of flexibility and function. Botte and Moore[93] describe, in detail, the methods for acute orthopedic management of extremity injuries. They point out the importance of anticipation of uncontrolled limb movement, avoidance of joint immobilization, and avoidance of prolonged traction methods. In the majority of cases, the acute orthopedic issues will have received adequate attention from medical staff.

At the acute level, musculoskeletal injuries are missed diagnoses in approximately 10% of individuals arriving at head trauma units.[94] As people are moved at an increasing pace through the acute phases of treatment, therapists are faced with greater demands for orthopedic management. Monitoring of proper positioning, modalities, splinting/casting, sensation, mobility, and pain management is necessary. The therapists will need to educate the injured person, the family, and other therapeutic staff in the possible adjustments required to allow an optimum of function.

Review of frequency of musculoskeletal injury[93] shows that the shoulder girdle, radius, and ulna are among the most common upper extremity injuries. The elbow must be watched because of frequent spasticity around the joint, development of heterotopic ossification, and possible ulnar neuropathy. Fractures of the humerus are relatively rare. In the lower extremities, fracture of the femur is most common, followed by fracture of the tibia. Pedestrian accidents will often involve the pelvis. Injuries to the acetabulum and hip are comparatively rare.

There are occasions when a traumatic event involves both brain injury and spinal cord injury. The subject of spinal cord injury assessment and treatment is not discussed in this chapter; however, the point to be made involves the occasion of moderate to severe TBI and concomitant spinal cord injury. In the acute phase of care, the potential for significant complications is present. However, as neuromedical stability occurs, the patient will be a candidate for acute rehabilitation to address both spinal cord and brain injury residuals. The next expected phase will be a transition into a postacute neurorehabilitation program experienced in the postacute treatment needs of the patient with the dual diagnosis of spinal cord and brain injury. This ensures that the cognitive, behavioral, and psychological aspects will be addressed along with the physical aspects of living with paraplegia or quadriplegia. A normalized residential setting provides environmental validity while the patient adjusts and transitions toward a new lifestyle. From the beginning, every neurorehabilitation discipline must be involved as a united team with three goals: (1) a thorough assessment of all functions, (2) a well-managed treatment approach to advance the individual's ability to function at the highest possible level, and (3) preparation for a smooth transition to the discharge environment.

In some cases, the traumatic event results in spinal cord injury but without initial evidence of significant cerebral injury. However, as the individual becomes activated, evidence of MTBI may appear. Such problems as memory, concentration, vision, spatial orientation, behavioral changes, or others may be observed. In this regard, additional assessments may lead to a diagnosis of MTBI. Those working in the postacute neurorehabilitation setting have the advantage of experience to recognize the more subtle features of MTBI and to be proactive in treatment.

22.2.16.2 Temporomandibular Joint Dysfunction

Another frequent concomitant injury is that of the temporomandibular joint (TMJ). TMJ dysfunction may arise from an associated facial injury or cervical myofascial injury.[95] Mechanisms of injury associated with MTBI can produce minor to severe TMJ dysfunction. TMJ problems may be manifested by headaches (described as fan shaped in radiation in proximity to the joint), jaw, neck, or back pain; eating problems; or subtle postural disorders. As a matter of awareness and thoroughness in the evaluation process, the physical therapy evaluation should include a TMJ screening assessment. If the neurologic therapist is not trained in treatment of TMJ dysfunction, appropriate referrals can be made for indepth examinations and potential treatment. Some PTs are trained and work with dentists in assessment and treatment of TMJ-related problems. Although pain behavior related to this dysfunction can represent a hindering factor to an efficiently addressed TBI rehabilitation program, TMJ dysfunction is often ignored. It is important to keep in mind that visual and vestibular deficits may be associated with TMJ pain; therefore, careful screening in all areas is needed to address these complaints fully.

22.2.16.3 Pain

Pain behaviors, in general, are seen more frequently in the person with MTBI than the more severely injured person. In fact, the existence of mild brain injury can actually be hidden by pain behaviors.[96] Headaches are a common focus of the MTBI patient.[97] Pain—whether real, exaggerated, or imagined—is pain and, along with companion emotional issues, can become a large obstacle to progress.

Perhaps the most frequent complaint of pain arises from headache.[97] Headache, though, can arise from a number of etiologies.[98] It is important to differentiate headaches arising from TMJ dysfunction from those arising from sinusitis. Injuries to the head often include injury to the sinuses. These headaches typically localize around the eyes and maxillary region in a masklike distribution. Headaches that are occipitally and/or frontally located may represent tension headaches arising from muscular tension in the neck and shoulder musculature. The patient who complains of daily headache may benefit from review of medications or substances that are known to cause rebound headache.

Headaches that arise from muscular tension or TMJ dysfunction may be improved by physical therapy for those problems. Of course, the etiology for the muscular tension must be determined in terms of whether it arises from musculoligamentous strain, orthopedic injury, visual disturbances, or compensatory reaction to vestibular hypersensitivity.

In management of pain, utilize a system that allows for the patient to rate the pain experience throughout the day. In addition, concomitant recording of the degree to which pain impacts the person's ability to function is useful. These reference points can be utilized by the treating physician and team to determine appropriate medication and therapeutic approaches. Therapeutic approaches available include thermal treatments, ultrasound, massage, flexibility exercises, strengthening exercises, and relaxation. In some cases, pain management may be enhanced by involvement of psychological services for the individual to explore relaxation or hypnosis as potential avenues of treatment. Fortunately, the vast majority of pain management programs for TBI respond well to conservative modalities of treatment, either in isolation or in combination.

It should be understood that the brain-injured person may tend to perseverate on a painful extremity, cast, and so forth. The therapist must be sympathetic and pursue appropriate investigations into potential causes and treatments; however, the therapist should also be aware that the problem may appear to be larger than it truly is. It is for this reason that behavioral observation of activity restriction caused by pain can be useful in addition to the person's report.

22.2.17 Driving

Driving is the most complex and dangerous ADL. It requires a person to process, plan, and respond while managing the moving components of the car, which is constantly moving through a dynamic environment of potential hazards. The ability to drive can be dramatically impacted by impairments in or damage to interconnections between the vestibular, ocular, physical, and psychoemotional systems. The rate at which the car and the environment change will demand immediate and accurate visual, vestibular, cognitive, physical, and behavioral responses. Lack of adequate integration and responses from these systems can result in death or life-long disability.

Driving is not viewed as a privilege in our society, rather as a right. It is symbolic of independence. It reduces the barriers to community integration, including meaningful activities outside of the home. Restrictions in driving have a profound social impact on a person. Without access to driving, a person may experience financial implications by absence from a job, isolation, and diminished ability to assimilate into a community. Restricted drivers may rely on family or friends who are able to assist for the short term, but perhaps not for the long term.

Many inaccurate perceptions about driving exist among individuals with brain injury and their families. They may believe that the mere physical possession of a license indicates that driving privileges have not been revoked or suspended after injury. Health professionals may fail to inform the Department of Motor Vehicles (DMV). Therefore, the injured person may have the perception that he is safe or cleared to drive and may lack the insight to restrict him-/herself. Family or friends may clearly see that driving will pose significant problems for the injured person and others. For this reason, interviews during rehabilitation assessments should not be limited to the injured person but should include family members and/or friends.

Information regarding driving behavior may be revealing. For example, are there times of day or night or certain areas that the individual avoids driving? Does the person get lost more often than usual? Does the driving behavior show impulsiveness and poor safety awareness or judgment? Does dizziness occur? Is anxiety increased when driving? Confusing visual perceptions, movement imperceptions, and spatial disorientation can produce frightening and disabling effects.[77,99–101] An interview of the injured person may not be adequate when the traumatic injury has involved the frontal lobes. Poor insight or loss of insight is a frequent deficit exhibited after frontal lobe injury and the person may fail to recognize the functional implications because they believe they have the necessary skills to drive. Studies have reported that 39% to 46% of those who sustained a severe brain injury return to driving; however, only 24% to 37% of those who returned to driving participated in a formal driving assessment.[102,103]

Return to driving after acquired or TBI mandates a comprehensive evaluation by multiple disciplines. Evaluative information is collected by an ancillary team involving the individual's family and friends, OT, occupational therapy assistant, speech/language pathologist, PT, neuropsychologist or psychologist, audiologist, therapeutic recreation specialist, social worker, nurses, physicians, orthotist, prosthetist, seating specialist, developmental optometrist, ophthalmologist, and the DMV at the state level.[104]

The actual driving component is then addressed by the primary team involving the injured individual and caregivers, an OT–driving specialist, a vehicle modifier, physicians, and case manager. A comprehensive driver screening must be completed prior to attempting a behind-the-wheel evaluation. This screening should include a complete review of the medical history. Current medications should be reviewed to identify salient problems or to anticipate any issues potentially related to pharmacologic agents. The interview should include the individual and any family members or friends who can provide insight.

Following review of the medical records, assessments of vision, physical, cognitive, and psychological components should be performed. Visual screening should include components of the optic system (eye and motility), primary visual system (optic nerve, chiasm, tract, and radiations), and the secondary visual system (visual perception). Within the optic system, assessments include distant and near acuities. Ocular motility is assessed for pursuits, saccades, convergence, and divergence. Refined coordination of the 12 eye muscles is necessary to point the eyes in a rapid, accurate manner to obtain visual information to react to the dynamic environment. Accommodation from distant to near vision and the speed at which a person accommodates is essential. Accommodation speed is necessary because the person is constantly changing focus from distant to near as the driver looks at the odometer and glances at the distance to anticipate the upcoming environment as well as the immediate environment. The accommodation convergence reflex must be rapid and well coordinated. Pupillary responses must be intact for necessary changes to dimly lit areas (e.g., shaded areas or tunnels) and to brightly lit areas. Eye alignment impacts diplopia or may cause blurring, particularly as fatigue increases, and impacts the driver's ability to read signs, perceive depth and distance, and have proper lane positioning.

Visual fields, suppression, and visual neglect must be evaluated. Discriminating between deficits related to visual fields, suppression, and neglect is necessary for predriving therapy, anticipation of problems behind the wheel, and implications for driving training strategies. Deficits in visual fields, binocular vision, or neglect often occur without the driver's awareness, which impacts the driver's ability to obtain information from a visual field. Binocular vision is not necessarily a prerequisite for driving. A driver with a known visual field cut may be trained to scan toward the limited visual field, whereas a suppressor may not have been trained to scan into the suppressed area. Suppression may not only affect how much information a driver captures but will also impact accurate depth perception. Visual perception skills must be adequate to interpret our environment properly, particularly form constancy, visual memory, visual closure, and visual discrimination. Accuracy must be coupled with rapid visual processing speed. Color discrimination and contrast sensitivity are also important in the vision assessment process.

The physical assessment should explore ROM restrictions throughout lower and upper extremities, trunk, and cervical spine to ensure adequate range to operate the steering wheel, manage foot pedals, and look over the shoulders into the blind spot. Limitations can be accommodated with various modifications ranging from simple to complex. The driver must also have adequate strength and endurance for pushing a gas pedal and brake pedal, grasping the steering wheel, and sustained contraction without fatigue. Visual–motor coordination must be refined. Coordination of lower and upper extremities for gross movements and rapid fine movements, as well as eye–hand–foot coordination, should be evaluated. Alertness is a prerequisite for sedentary cognitive and visual tasks, and is imperative for driving. Adequate balance reactions and trunk coordination with the visual and proprioceptive system are necessary for steering around corners or clover-leaf configurations on many freeway systems. Vestibular function, in coordination with the visual and proprioceptive system, must be intact to provide a proper sense of position, linear acceleration, or deceleration.

The patient's cognitive status must be assessed on several levels. As a foundation to cognition, attention is a prerequisite for further processing and must be intact to drive safely. Attention must also be sustained for protracted lengths of time, shifted and divided between various environmental stimuli, such as an ambulance, as speed is monitored, or occurrences in the car. Cognitive processing speed should be assessed thoroughly, particularly in a visually and auditorily distracting environment, as processing speed may slow in a dynamic environment. Basic pathfinding and topographic orientation should be assessed to project the patient's anticipated skills while behind the wheel. There must also be an assessment of psychosocial, emotional, and behavioral functioning. This may include frustration tolerance, conflict management, behavior in overstimulating environments, and coping strategies.

After the assessment is complete, a compilation of overall strengths and weaknesses must be completed and discussed with the primary and ancillary treatment teams. It may be that the patient has areas of weakness but still participates in a driving assessment. Driving skills behind the wheel may be better than anticipated, depending on the driver's prior experience. It may also be an opportunity to educate the driver with poor insight to deficits and the family on the concrete risks of driving, and to explore other means of community transportation.

If the patient is cleared to participate in a driving evaluation, a visit to the DMV may be required to obtain a temporary permit. This process may include an interview with a safety officer, as well as a written test. Presence of therapy staff is beneficial to advocate on the patient's behalf or to present concerns from the clinical staff. If the driver's license has not been suspended, it is still important for the person to obtain a behind-the-wheel assessment. This assessment team includes an OT and a driving rehabilitation specialist (either an OT specializing in driving or a certified driver specialist).

A typical evaluation should grade intervention from simple to complex environments, such as beginning in residential areas and moving to a congested downtown business district. Begin in a parking lot or isolated area to address basic skills, such as steering control, backing up, using mirrors, managing the controls, and accelerating and decelerating with control. Drive into a residential setting to look at lane position, approach to an uncontrolled intersection, and speed control. Transition to a business district with increased traffic, one-way streets, and greater visual stimuli and distractions. The freeway should be driven to look at control, speed, and merging onto and off of the freeway. The evaluators look for scanning, intersection approaches, good control over the car, appropriate speed, including acceleration and braking, attention and distractibility, including radio and conversation. The OT and driving rehabilitation specialist should collaborate on the assessment outcomes and make recommendations to the DMV if it is necessary to regain a license, educate the patient, and inform the family. Further driving instruction is often necessary to address weaknesses and to increase the patient's comfort and self-efficacy.

Driving is a reflection of a person's independence. Although most people are unwilling to relinquish their driver's licenses voluntarily, it requires a committed staff whom the patient trusts to assist remediation of driving skills, protect the patient, and ensure safety for the community. Given the complexity and dangers of driving, it is an ADL that all providers should consider.

22.2.18 Functioning at Heights

Falls are the primary cause of TBI. Regardless of whether the initial injury was caused by a fall, many people have a fear of returning to heights after injury. However, they may not consider a kitchen stool, chair, or ladder as a risk. It is important to consider impairments related to visual, proprioceptive, and vestibular systems and emotional control. These problematic areas may place the individual at greater risk of falling and exacerbating the existing injury. Repositioning some overhead objects to easily reachable heights reduces the need to use a step stool. Special consideration must be given to those individuals with the potential to return to vocations requiring use of tall A-frame or extension ladders or climbing telephone poles or working on roofs.

A thorough evaluation of balance should be completed. This evaluation includes balance with a narrowed base of support, proprioception, visual perception, balance reactions, coordination, and strength. Components of the evaluation must include issues related to ladder safety involving proper placement, ground surfaces, and harness equipment. The actual height assessment should include graduated levels ranging from small kitchen ladders to 6-foot A-frame ladders to 15-foot extension ladders. The patient should be required to carry a small toolbox or occupation-specific objects up and down the ladder, work overhead, and look in all directions. The evaluator should note changes in balance, inaccurate steps, complaints or signs of dizziness, fearfulness, safety judgment, and problem solving. Despite all these considerations, it is generally recommended that, following a TBI (even an MTBI), the individual should not be required to work at heights.

22.3 Management of Residual Physical Deficits

After the evaluative process has been completed and the treatment team has shared their findings, the individual rehabilitation program begins to take shape. The purpose of treatment is to facilitate relearning and continue the momentum of improvement in skills, thus reducing dependence. The development of a management plan begins with understanding the factors that limit adequate performance. As is evidenced by the complexity of the evaluative process, the management program can be expected to be equally complicated.

Neurologic rehabilitation differs from other types of rehabilitation in that people who have sustained neurologic damage frequently evidence multiple areas of impairment in addition to those areas that require physical restoration of function. These individuals often cannot be left alone to undertake therapy exercises. They require attention for safety, follow-through, motivation, documentation, and ongoing evaluation. Treatment is best conducted in one-to-one treatment settings. Therapists must possess adequate knowledge of evaluative and treatment techniques and must also have a repertoire of interpersonal skills that will enable them to motivate the unmotivated, calm the agitated, or educate the person in denial. There will be times when a therapy session is nearly consumed by education or counseling, and others when the session focuses exclusively on prescribed exercises.

The treatment environment should be such that the treatment can be segregated from high-stimulus environments that distract the individual. Attentional deficits that accompany brain injury can make it quite difficult to focus on the treatment session. Overstimulation can lead to behavioral problems.

Rehabilitation of physical function requires maximal repetition. As such, the therapist should attempt to treat in blocks of time that allow for ample repetition of a wide array of therapeutic tasks that will be required in most treatment plans. Newly emerging positive responses should be focused upon until they are reliably reproducible, even if this means continuing a treatment session beyond scheduled times.

The therapist should develop the ability to approach treatment exercises hierarchically, utilizing task analysis when necessary, to break larger tasks into smaller ones to accentuate the learning experience. TBI results in changes in the manner in which a person acquires new information, so physically restorative therapies may be expected to take longer in the neurologically impaired population compared with other populations. To this end, quantitative measurement of treatment exercises that have been broken into smaller, more readily learned components can give a clearer picture of slowly progressing improvement.

22.3.1 Therapeutic Measurement

It is now more widely accepted that continued rehabilitation with the TBI person can bring about substantial reduction in disability, improvement in living status, and improvement in occupational status.[105–110] This was not always the case, however. When rehabilitation for this population was largely restricted to the acute rehabilitation experience, it was necessary to develop methods of measurement that would allow both the therapist and the consumer access to critical review of the therapeutic process. Progress could no longer be viewed through the subjectivity of the therapists' eyes, but instead, a new period of accountability was emerging. Qualitative summaries of patient performance were no longer acceptable. Many therapists found the expectation for quantitative analysis to be difficult, but, once accomplished, the improved objectivity about therapist–patient performance, over time, allowed for some major therapeutic advances. In fact, quantitative measurement allowed therapists to acquire new perspectives about breaking therapeutic tasks into hierarchical components as a means of teaching skills better to a learning-impaired patient. Therapy became easier to implement and monitor, and patients were better able to benefit from treatment.[10,14]

To understand most accurately whether a patient is benefiting from treatment, the therapist must reduce the therapeutic task to its hierarchical components, which can be operationally defined and objectively measured. For example, in evaluating ambulatory skills and progression therein, the therapist should refrain from characterization of skills as follows: "Mr. Smith is able to ambulate short distances with a hemicane." Rather, the therapist should characterize Mr. Smith's performance by a statement such as, "Mr. Smith is able to walk 100 feet, with a hemicane, in a mean of 2 minutes. This is an improvement from a mean of 3.5 minutes for the same distance last week."

Quantification can generally be achieved fairly readily. The therapist can count repetitions of a task, document specific amounts of weight or resistance being used, time performance, and/or count accurate versus inaccurate performance to obtain a percentage performed correctly. Of course, there remains room for subjective observations as well, but therapy that is quantitatively approached is far easier for all parties to participate in, enhancing cooperation, motivation, consistency of treatment, and, ultimately, progress.

The therapist should keep in mind that the brain-injured person has a number of special needs. In today's environment of managed care, it is important to keep the therapeutic focus on tasks that will translate, quickly and efficaciously, to good functional improvement. At the same time, the very measurement that is advocated herein may become the data utilized to justify continued treatment toward a longer term goal of improved functional capability. Outcomes are being viewed, increasingly, from the perspective of financial risks and benefits. Ashley et al.[105] address the idea that rehabilitation outcome translates to dollar savings for long-term care costs. These savings have their beginnings with the daily therapeutic sessions undertaken by the PT, the OT, and their allied health associates. Another study by Spivack et al.[111] demonstrated a clear relationship between treatment intensity and rehabilitative outcome. Thus, to advocate best for the TBI person, quantification of treatment will be of critical importance.

During treatment, the therapist must teach other pertinent clinical and residential staff methods that they can use to maximize the individual's learning throughout the entire day. Management of physical injury residuals cannot be performed in a vacuum apart from other therapeutic disciplines or from environments within which the person will be expected to function. Therefore, an important daily goal is to generalize skills into actual activities in residential and community environments.[32,34] This is where environmentally valid learning takes place. Maximized repetition and structure, performed in sequence and in realistic situations, maximizes the derived rehabilitation benefit.

Another factor to take into consideration is that the person with TBI is not passively traveling through the rehabilitation process. In physical and psychological terms, therapy is difficult work for the person with TBI. Confronting one's weaknesses is never easy. Early review of the individual's personal history and lifestyle can provide key information to fuel motivation. Perception of purpose and realization of goal achievement are enhanced by the therapist's ability to present concrete, appropriately sequenced tasks within the scope of the individual's interests. Progress requires a constant series of challenges. The therapist must be a creative motivator.

22.3.2 Mobility

Normal movement cannot be built on abnormal tone, and normal behaviors do not sequence from abnormal ones.[1,10,61] The primary treatment approach toward normalizing functional mobilization is NDT.[1,2] Postgraduate training courses are available to therapists throughout the United States and other parts of the world. This technique, often referred to as the *Bobath approach*, was originated by the husband and wife team of Karl and Berta Bobath in Sweden in 1943. The initial population served with this treatment approach was children with cerebral palsy. It is now an accepted treatment for individuals with acquired brain injury, including stroke and other neurologic disorders.

NDT is a means of treating the person with brain injury at, or above, the brainstem level. Treatment principles emphasize a holistic approach, which requires constant interdisciplinary communication. Analysis of normal and abnormal movement is always important. Trained therapists are able to identify problems interfering with function. The training enables the therapist to utilize handling techniques to inhibit abnormal tone while assisting the person in acquiring functional skills. The focus with hemiparesis is to incorporate the affected side into virtually every ADL. Instead of being satisfied with compensatory movements or learned nonuse of limbs, the person is assisted in recovery of symmetry.

Functional mobilization may be influenced by such injury residuals as fractures, peripheral nerve injuries, general weakness, pain, sensory impairments, visual impairments, balance and coordination deficits, as well as cognitive and behavioral factors. Each must be addressed to allow progress to more advanced performance levels. The goal is to facilitate and normalize movement, which will gradually advance into daily mobilization. ROM and adequate strength to move are among the fundamental requirements that can usually be conventionally addressed.

Significant motor impairments may require immediate treatment for ongoing hypertonicity or a movement disorder (i.e., ataxia), which will be discussed later. Hypertonicity may refer to spasticity or rigidity. Although these problems are often addressed and resolved during the acute rehabilitation phase, the therapist will have occasion to treat these impairments. These issues may be addressed via both a medical consultant and the therapist. Approaches can range from stretching and positioning to serial casting and chemical neurolysis. Orthopedic management of spasticity can be efficacious in obtaining temporary relief from spasticity.[112] Diagnostic blocks can be utilized to eliminate pain and muscle tone temporarily to ascertain the degree of motor control present and the amount of fixed contracture. Therapy is frequently enhanced by application of chemical neurolysis in that the treatment can focus on nontreated muscles groups, obtaining isolated contractions in those groups, enhancing awareness of control of those groups, and allowing for strengthening of those groups. Many quadriplegics from spinal cord or brainstem injury suffer severe global spasticity. Some have benefitted from a trial of localized antispasticity medication via intrathecal baclofen pump placement. The advantage of local application of medication into the thecal sac surrounding the spinal cord is that it helps to avoid the systemic effect of sedative properties of antispasticity medications when taken by mouth.

In the 1980s, many patients entered postacute rehabilitation with contractures resulting from lack of aggressive treatment at the acute level of care. Valuable rehabilitation time was lost at great expense while treatment focused on contracture reduction. Twenty years later, the early application of inhibitory techniques, such as weight bearing on joints impacted by hypertonic muscles, was found beneficial in reducing increased tone and reducing the number of joint contractures before arrival at the postacute facility.

In recent years, many OTs and PTs began to utilize a taping technique along with established splinting techniques for their neurologically compromised patients. The technique called *kinesiotaping* originated from the field of kinesiology or science of movement (www.kinesiotaping.com, www.kinesioworld.com, www.kinesiotape.ca). For some time, kinesiotaping has been used by practitioners in the treatment of peripheral injuries of athletes. The special elastic quality of the kinesiotape allows movement through a ROM without restriction to circulation. It is typically applied with the muscle in a stretched position. Placement of the tape is specific to the desired result for hypertonic or hypotonic muscle groups. When muscle support or facilitation is desired, the tape is applied from muscle origin to muscle insertion. The reverse is used when muscle inhibition is desired. Although evidence of efficacy from this technique has yet to be determined, some patients have benefitted from proprioceptive feedback during taping. Some have found benefit in the use of kinesiotape for repositioning an upper extremity when subluxation at the shoulder joint has occurred.

Mobility can be impacted by reductions in ROM. ROM can be reduced as a result of neuromuscular deficits or restriction of the joint resulting from contractures or heterotopic ossification. Decerebrate or decorticate posturing during coma or neuromuscular deficits seen most commonly after cortical or brainstem injury that result in spasticity will frequently result in the development of joint limitations. Restrictions arising from musculoligamentous contracture should be treated through a multimodal program. Lehmkuhl et al.[16] advocate early use of such a program to include passive and active ROM, positioning, serial inhibitive casting, bivalved casts, motor point blocks, and antispasticity medication. Elbows and knees were noted by Lehmkuhl et al.[16] to respond most quickly to therapeutic intervention, with elbows benefiting most. Increases in joint ROM can be expected to endure for at least 6 to 9 months. Of course, it should be expected that joint limitation improvements will be maximized by long-term use of the full ROM achieved through daily functional activity.[113]

It is imperative that mobility be taught in an appropriate progression from bed mobility to transfers to ambulation. Mobility skills will improve through intense repetition appropriate to the developmental sequence of movement. The neurodevelopmental sequence (previously described in this chapter) can become an exercise routine that can be practiced at any level required. For example, the therapist may begin with segmental rolling to improve body awareness and enhance movement. Rolling should progress to assuming prone-on-elbows and, eventually, the quadruped position until each is performed independently. The sequence continues to be practiced, component to component, through tall-kneel, half-kneel, and standing. Treatment of any difficulty within each component of the sequence may come from the therapist's choice of a variety of treatment approaches (e.g., proprioceptive neuromuscular facilitation and NDT).[1,4] The individual continues to practice, component to component, as the motor tasks are gradually progressed from the simple to the complex. Besides movement, strength, and flexibility, very basic balance skills are practiced within the sequenced exercises. The exercises may appear simple, although they can be quite challenging. Do not skip over sequential components. Do not assume competence at any level until performance is demonstrated.

An emerging gait training strategy uses the concept of partial body weight support. The individual is secured in a harness that provides 0% to 50% of support of body weight. The system may be used on a level ground surface or suspended over a treadmill. The harness system eliminates risk of falling and the person is able, gradually, to accept an increasing amount of his or her own body weight during standing and/or ambulation. With no fall risk, gait training can begin earlier during the rehabilitation process.[114–116] In addition, the therapist's hands are free to facilitate normal movement while the person is in the upright position. A critical component in this treatment technique is the physical cues provided by a therapist. These cues include weight shifting, stabilizing the trunk, rotating the pelvis, advancing the affected limb, and so on. Use of the body weight support technique during gait training in hemiplegia produced better results in regard to functional balance, motor recovery, walking speed, and endurance compared with gait training with full body weight.[115] Research has shown that ambulation was improved with partial weight-bearing protocol, including reduced stance time on the unaffected limb, increased weight acceptance on the affected limb, increased gait velocity, and improved gait symmetry.[116,117]

Studies of people with spinal cord injury have shown that, when provided with the proprioceptive input of weight bearing during gait, the lumbosacral spinal cord can generate rhythmic locomotor EMG patterns, even in the absence of supraspinal influences.[118] This indicates that control of the flexion/extension pattern of walking is in the spinal cord and, in the case of damage to the brain, these central program generators can be activated to facilitate and improve ambulation. Research on gait training with body weight support system in the TBI population is extremely limited and is an area in need of further attention.[118]

Treatment of mobility skills is greatly enhanced by daily practice of these skills in the residential setting. Bed mobility can be practiced every day in the environmentally valid routines of getting up and going to bed. Trained staff should be present to assist in additional home exercises, which should be designed by the clinical staff to ensure the use of proper techniques. The same is applied to all transfers, toileting, bathing, and early ambulatory routines. The individual advances through these daily routines from the clinic to the residence to the community until greater independence is accomplished.

22.3.3 Pain

In management of pain, it is very important to utilize a system that allows for the person to rate the pain experience throughout the day. A pain diary provides a way to document and rate pain. A rating scale of 0 to 10 points (0 point, none; 10 points, most severe) is a simple scale for the person to use. Headaches or neck and back pain in the brain-injured person can become a distracting somatic focus, and perseveration on pain may hinder progress in several aspects of the TBI program. An assumption that pain is exaggerated should not be made until complaints of pain are explored to rule out potential causes that may respond to treatment.

It is important to keep a concomitant recording of the degree to which pain impacts the person's ability to function. These reference points can be utilized by the treating physician and team to determine appropriate medication and therapeutic approaches. The physician must review all medications taken by the patient and determine what modifications, if any, should be made. Dosage and frequency of medication taken should be included in a diary. The physician may elect to utilize a controlled reduction of dosages with combined pain medications. Consultation with an experienced pain management physician may be required in some cases.

The therapist will have a major impact upon the individual's understanding of the various causes of pain. The individual who anticipates pain from movement develops increased anxiety and muscle tension and, therefore, the potential for chronic pain and stiffness. A kinesiologic orientation in the initial exercise program may be an effective tool to reduce this anxiety-produced pain and allow the patient to begin to move through and beyond pain. This approach teaches normalizing posture and improving body mechanics with more efficient movements to reduce pain.

Conventional therapeutic modalities include thermal treatment, ultrasound, transcutaneous electrical nerve stimulation, massage, aquatic therapy, flexibility exercises, and strengthening exercises. Pain management is best enhanced by involvement of psychological services for the individual to explore relaxation or hypnosis as potential avenues of treatment. The best approach to pain management is to address all deficit areas while unifying the physician, the treating therapist, and treating psychological team.

22.3.4 Postural Control and Balance

Fisher[58] describes postural deficits commonly seen in people with TBI and contrasts their postural abilities to normal people. In general, the individual with TBI can be observed to tend toward the relaxed sitting posture of normals, however, on a habitual basis. Trunk movements tend not to be incorporated into arm movements and, even when attempting to assume an erect sitting posture, truncal musculature strength and coordination may make achieving the erect position quite difficult. Not only do truncal weaknesses impact upper extremity function, but transfers can also be impacted. In preparation for rising from sitting to standing, postural deficits frequently will maintain weight so far posteriorly as to make the attempt to rise ineffective.

Effective treatment of postural deficits focuses on strengthening of the truncal musculature. In cases when there is concomitant cerebellar dysfunction, strengthening may not be indicated so much as learning selective utilization of muscle groups with slow, controlled muscle activation. In cases, however, when a cerebellar component is not present, strengthening exercises such as bridging, sit-ups or crunches, or resistive lateral bending can be helpful. It is important to achieve stabilization at the hips, back, neck, and shoulders. Activities such as hippotherapy (therapeutic horseback riding) are also excellent ways to retrain the postural system and impact balance along with visual, psychological, and vestibular enhancement. For detail regarding treatment of balance impairments related to vestibular dysfunction, see Chapter 6 in this volume.

22.3.5 Cerebellar Dysfunction

Many therapists struggle with movement disorders related to cerebellar dysfunction. Frustrations with ataxia or tremors in the extremities and/or trunk are compounded by the short period allowed for treatment and often lead a therapist to teach compensatory techniques (i.e., using the more functional limb or mobilizing from a wheelchair). Minimal to no time is then spent in therapeutic confrontation of the issue.

When undertaking cerebellar rehabilitation, it is important to keep several important factors in mind. The first is that muscle strengthening activities can result in exacerbation of tremor, causing the degree of tremor excursions to increase. The second point is that the individual must learn to relax selective muscle groups on command to reduce the excursion of tremor. Tremor results from agonist/antagonist muscle groups firing rhythmically. The individual must learn to turn on one muscle selectively while maintaining relative electrical silence in the antagonistic muscle. EMG/biofeedback training can be quite effective in teaching people to control muscles and even specific motor units.[23,119] The third point has to do with the importance of a progression of stabilization of the trunk, to the neck and head, to the proximal extremities, to the distal extremities. In severe cerebellar dysfunction, postural tremors may be so severe that they necessitate treatment commencing in a supine position. It is useful not only to retrain truncal control in this position, but also to approach proximal extremity musculature control as well. The utilization of selective muscular relaxation and activation can be particularly helpful at this stage, with positioning helpful in teaching the ability of selective relaxation and activation.

Diminished ability with rapid alternating movements, dysmetria, hypotonicity, and/or movement decomposition are manifestations of cerebellar damage that influence performance in ADLs (e.g., feeding, brushing teeth, dressing, or gait functions). OTs have begun to use a product from Nintendo to assist patients during practice of functional movements required in food preparation. The Wii (www.wii.com) product has a virtual reality program that allows a person to practice such movements as chopping or cutting foods without using a real knife. Movements are practiced until the patient has reached a safe level of movement control to begin using a real knife. The therapist monitors transition into the patient's home kitchen as the desired level of independence is realized. Reading, or other skills that require accuracy in visual scanning ability, can be impacted by oculomotor deficits related to cerebellar injury. A spastic hemiparesis may further complicate an ipsilateral or bilateral ataxia in one or more limbs. Acquiring a degree of movement control and normalizing functions can be frustrating. However, the therapist should pursue proper identification of the dysfunction and aggressively pursue appropriate treatment.[14,120]

Establishment of a stable base of support is the initial focus of treatment. For example, the performance of any task requiring an ataxic extremity to extend away from the body requires trunk stabilization. Therefore, goals of treatment are postural stability and accuracy in extremity movement during functional activities. Treatment must be pursued in a sequential manner until the individual is independent in each component. That is to say, head and trunk control must be addressed and established prior to sitting or ambulatory activities.

If poor head control is evident, initiate treatment with prone-on-elbows positioning or seated at a table, feet firmly planted on the floor, with weight on the forearms. If there is poor trunk control, bolsters, wedges, or pillows will assist with support in the prone position. The neck extensors can be briefly brushed with ice, no more than 5 seconds, followed by a stretch and then heavy resistance to the extensors. This is followed by downward compression on the shoulders. The goal is to maintain the head in a steady upright position.

Progression to management of trunk control will require a graduated removal of the pillow supports, and an increased demand will be placed on the elbows and shoulders. Approximation through the shoulders should be provided. Weight shifting should be practiced until the individual is able to sustain support on one elbow. Additional mat activities can include the quadruped position combined with joint approximation through the shoulders and hips, and weight shifting. During this phase, trunk rolling and supine/prone-to-sit exercises can be practiced with graduated mild resistance given by the therapist. The person should progress to crawling activity to challenge balance, strength, and weight shifts in reciprocal patterns.

As head and trunk control improve, sitting can then be addressed. Sitting on surfaces without benefit of structural supports (e.g., the edge of a mat or chairs without arms or backs) should be used. Stabilization is promoted by joint approximation at the hips and shoulders. Weight shifting should be practiced. Another mat activity can include the tall-kneel position. The therapist should provide approximation through the shoulders and hips, and weight shifting can be practiced. Contact support can be initially provided by the therapist. As stabilization and balance improve, support is gradually reduced.

During progress in sitting and tall-kneel activities, the upper extremities should be extended from the body to challenge trunk stability. Head and trunk rotations and bending from the hips can be practiced with one or both arms extended overhead, laterally, or forward. Realistic movements should be practiced (i.e., reaching for objects overhead, to the side, or from the floor). Functional upper extremity activities may be practiced while sitting or tall-kneeling at a table. To progress stabilization, weight may be shifted from one forearm to the other while the opposing extremity is active. This support is gradually reduced until two-hand activities can be practiced. Mild resistance to the trunk and extremities for feedback is initially helpful to the patient during movements. This can be provided manually by the therapist or by light wrist weights.

As head and trunk stabilization improves in sitting, supine/prone-to-sit, and tall-kneeling, the individual should practice transfers. Initiate transfers from the most stable position (i.e., sliding surface to surface) and graduate in degrees of difficulty until the person is safely independent.

Much of the previously noted activity prepares the person for standing and ambulation. Rolling, assuming and maintaining the quadruped position, crawling, and tall-kneeling are the basic neurodevelopmental sequence positions necessary prior to standing. Overall strength, endurance, and balance must be adequate to launch into the demands of the upright position. The person should repeatedly practice moving through foot placement, sliding forward, flexing from the hips, and pushing upward with a sense of center of gravity and balance. Manual guidance from the therapist and visual feedback from a mirror can initially assist the individual as extension of the hips and knees move the individual to the upright position.

After stability in standing is accomplished, the ambulatory phase can be initiated. A front-wheeled walker may be the first support device required for ambulation practice. On occasion, weighted walker legs may be necessary to assist stabilization. If appropriate, tall poles can be quite effective in developing a sense of rhythm, pace, and reciprocal movement.

Past-pointing or dysmetria will benefit from various techniques such as biofeedback,[119] proprioceptive neuromuscular facilitation,[4] and Frenkel's exercises.[121] EMG biofeedback can be useful during practical activities (e.g., combing hair, brushing teeth). Aquatic/pool exercises may be beneficial for relaxation of the person with ataxia.

22.3.6 Sensory Function

There is a therapeutic opportunity to address the sensory impairment of an extremity as the person is exposed to treatment in clinical, residential, and community activities. Yekutiel and Guttman[122] documented that somatosensory deficits in the plegic hand can significantly improve with intensive sensory retraining that incorporates functional tasks. The performance of basic self-care skills requires an integration of perceptual, cognitive, sensory, and motor functions. The ability to perform a motor task will depend upon the interactions of the residual components that are functioning throughout these systems.

An intensive effort should be made to stimulate sensory functions to normalize tactile sensitivity.[61,83] Keenan and Perry[123] noted that the sensory functions necessary for hand function included awareness of pain, light touch, temperature, proprioception, and two-point discrimination of less than 10 mm. Assessments will determine the specific deficits to be addressed. Treatment requires adequate time and opportunities to maximize repetition of stimuli. Also, incorporate visual input into treatment sessions to increase awareness.

If a significant motor impairment accompanies the sensory deficit, improvement of the motor function is usually addressed first. Tactile stimulation, however, can, and should be, incorporated into the initial treatment sessions. Weight bearing on the impaired extremity, through the palmar surface, on a variety of textured surfaces (e.g., carpet, sand, smooth metal) will facilitate motor function, proprioception, and touch. As improvement occurs in motor and sensory functions, progress to functional two-handed tasks. These tasks may include weight bearing on dirt or sand while gardening, holding down paper while writing, or weight bearing on the extremity while eating with the functional extremity.

Deficits in touch are addressed by providing a strong stimulus to the extremity. Initial sessions open with stimulus via rubbing various textures over the extremity. If possible, have the individual actively move the textured material over his or her own extremity with the unimpaired hand. Make the person aware of any abnormal positions in the extremity or hand during activities. This should be immediately corrected to stimulate a sense of normal touch during movements. Functional tasks in repetitive daily routines can include washing, rinsing, and drying the hands; dusting; cleaning windows; making the bed; or folding laundry.

Individuals who have hypersensitivity or sensory defensiveness may be appropriate for sensory integration techniques such as the Willbarger Protocol.[124] The protocol involves establishing a set sensory routine that encompasses deep proprioceptive input with active physical proprioceptive activity. Special training courses are offered to learn and teach the technique.

It is important to encourage the use of both hands in as many tasks or activities throughout the day as possible. A goal of treatment is to increase spontaneous use of the impaired side. It stands to reason that, if the impaired extremity is not spontaneously used, then overuse of the unimpaired side occurs. Eggers[61] suggests a remedy by having the patient wear a glove on the unimpaired hand, which should reduce overuse of the unimpaired extremity and facilitate increased use of the impaired extremity. This therapeutic approach is known as *constraint-induced movement therapy* (CIMT). Protocols for its use were established primarily for the stroke population. The EXCITE Multicenter Trial evaluated chronic stroke patients after using CIMT. In 2006, the study published results showing evidence of "statistically significant and clinically relevant improvements" in motor ability and use of a paretic upper extremity compared with patients receiving usual and customary treatment.[125] In 2008, Sawaki et al.[126] published results from the first multicenter study to measure cortical reorganization induced by CIMT in stroke patients during the subacute phase of recovery. The study used transcranial magnetic stimulation for evaluation at baseline, 2 weeks after baseline, and at 4 months in follow-up. Results from the study showed evidence that CIMT produced "statistically significant and clinically relevant" improvements in arm motor function in patients who had a stroke within the previous 3 to 9 months. Corresponding enlargement of transcranial magnetic stimulation motor maps appeared to indicate an important role in CIMT-dependent plasticity. Many therapists have reported that difficulty with the procedure typically involves behavioral compliance and cognitive ability to comprehend the treatment.

Proprioceptive deficits should be addressed while performing motor functions. The impaired extremity is initially guided by the therapist. This is progressed to the individual moving the impaired extremity through tasks with his or her own unimpaired extremity. If grip and strength are available, two-handed activities should then be incorporated to include lifting and movement of various objects (e.g., cans, plastic bottles, a brush). Engage activities that will include resistance (e.g., sanding or pushing objects). ADL tasks offer numerous opportunities to maximize therapeutic input for proprioceptive impairments. For example, dressing with a proprioceptively impaired upper extremity should begin with the practice of moving the extremity through sleeves or tubular materials. Have the person guide the extremity with the unimpaired hand and emphasize visual input as a reference. Progress to functional activities such as dressing. Practice should initiate with tasks in front of the body and overhead with visual input. As sensory function improves, progress to tasks without visual reference (e.g., tucking in a shirt, reaching for a wallet behind the back, or reaching for objects under a table).

22.3.7 Smell and Taste

In cases when impairment of smell or taste is irreversible, the individual and family need to be made aware of social, dietary, and safety implications of impaired smell and taste. The person with TBI who will be living and/or working independently in the community will require training in management of perishable foods and toxic materials. Food preparation training must include visual monitoring of food while cooking and identification of altered seasoning practices that may not be healthy. Structure should be established to assist by labeling and dating perishable foods. Pet care, if applicable, should be undertaken systematically. Toxic materials should be moved to a safe place and labeled. Smoke, carbon monoxide, and gas detectors within the home should be considered and can be assisted by current electronic detection technology.[75]

The workplace must, likewise, be considered when treating for olfactory/gustatory deficits. Education of the employer and coworkers may allow the candidate for vocational placement a chance to return to work with reduced risk. The vocational rehabilitation counselor should take these types of deficits into consideration while looking or planning for vocational placement.[75]

22.3.8 Visual Perception and Perceptual Motor Functions

Areas frequently requiring therapeutic intervention are visual inattention, gross ocular deficits, scanning, figure–ground, visuospatial perception, visual memory, and visual–motor skills.

Appropriately trained rehabilitation assistants can augment the clinical program by undertaking home exercises, as well as through functional application. Visual perception deficits, such as figure–ground, can be practiced via homework with worksheets and home exercises, such as word searches or community scans. It may be helpful to teach organizational skills and energy conservation techniques to help compensate for residual deficits. Puzzles, form boards, parquetry blocks, and other appropriate games can keep the patient's interest while being therapeutic. Visual scanning while reading or working word puzzles may be useful. Data should be collected and reviewed over time for progress.

Neistadt[127,128] has indicated that there is an association between functional and constructional skills. The presence of constructional apraxia and visuoconstructive disorders has been shown to impact independent living by difficulties with meal preparation, dressing, changing a tire, or assembling an object. Bouska et al.[77] discuss the importance of teaching the individual to approach a visuoconstructive task via sequential planning. For example, the task should begin first by visually and physically organizing the parts, followed by construction of the object. The person with apraxia benefits from physical guidance to initiate and carry out a simple task. With intense repetition, the ability to wash, groom, and feed should normalize. On higher levels, dyspraxia requires the same touch and guidance to accomplish more complex activities requiring the ability to plan, arrange, and build.

The neurodevelopmental approach to improving perceptual motor skills has been found to be effective and provides a guideline to the progression of treatment as the individual advances. Intensive practice is vital and should be pursued with functionally meaningful tasks in normal living environments. For additional therapeutic approaches to visual impairments, see Chapter 9 in this volume.

22.3.9 Driving

Independence, in terms of driving skills, can be enhanced through visual therapy and perceptual training.[100] Exercises to address visual attention and scanning, visuospatial relationships, oculomotor skills, eye–hand–foot coordination, and response times are some of the components required to drive a vehicle safely. As mentioned earlier in the evaluation of skills required for driving, retraining should include behind-the-wheel time with a professionally trained driving instructor in a dual-equipped vehicle.

Computer programs to address perceptual skills have become quite popular during the past decade. Many rehabilitation programs have depended heavily upon this tool as a therapeutic base. Although "computer-assisted therapy" is a useful and motivating approach, it does not provide stimulus to, or require responses from, other systems (e.g., vestibular, motor, other perceptual responses).[77] Any dysfunction in the perceptual realm may be impacted by concomitant vestibular and/or cerebellar deficits.[60] Again, the importance of hands-on therapy to reintegrate multiple systems into efficiently coordinated responses requires more than one evaluative or therapeutic approach. If driving skills are not adequate at evaluation, it may well be possible to enhance skills via training. It may be necessary to undertake drivers' retraining with both classroom and behind-the-wheel instruction to improve driving skills.

All therapeutic disciplines should be polled regarding potential limitations that may be experienced prior to the driving evaluation. This information should be reviewed by the treating physician, and a determination should made about the propriety of the driving evaluation. This information will be invaluable to the driving evaluator as the assessment is undertaken.

22.3.10 Cardiovascular Fitness

As major sensorimotor deficits are improved and general mobility advances to higher levels, it may be appropriate to initiate an aerobic and conditioning program. These programs can be developed to fit into the person's lifestyle by gradually transferring the exercise routine from the clinical setting to a community gym. The initial exercises must be performed with the therapist's close supervision and medical clearance.

An aerobic and conditioning program can be created for individuals with and without significant motor impairments. Stretching should also be taught to start any exercise routine. An exercise program can be developed with stationary bicycles (standard or recumbent), treadmills, and weights. Muscle conditioning may utilize isometric exercise or full-range exercise with weights, elastic exercise bands, free weights, or exercise machines. Low-impact aerobic exercise routines can be developed with walking, swimming, bicycling, and aerobic classes.

As the person becomes more independent and community reentry is developed, the therapist may assist in the choice of, and transfer to, a community-type exercise routine (e.g., a local gym or fitness center). Independent aerobic exercise routines can be established in walking, swimming, or bicycling as well as a maintenance stretching and muscle toning exercise program (e.g., sit-ups, push-ups). Many PTs are incorporating yoga stretching techniques and "short-form" Tai Chi into treatment sessions. These techniques also provide an additional benefit from balance exercises and various forms of breathing exercises for relaxation. As the benefits of conditioning renew the individual's sense of well-being and enhance overall functional status, the continuation of exercise as an enjoyable routine may allow a gradual reduction of supervision.

Motorically and cognitively impaired individuals also gain great benefit from a fitness program. Aside from endurance and stamina, it has been demonstrated that thinking ability and emotional status improve with physical fitness.[129,130] As a result, there are enhanced levels of energy, feelings of well-being, and independence for most people with TBI.

22.3.11 Leisure

The intent of the postacute neurorehabilitation setting is to provide an environment within which the individual is assisted in regaining a normal rhythm of living. Although the clinical aspects of the treatment program focus on rehabilitating specific skills impaired from injury, it is in the residential/community aspect that those skills are practiced in real-time ADLs. Each time the patient engages in a treatment session, he or she comes face to face with his or her disability, and the intensity of this bombardment can be overwhelming. In that regard, we must not forget the role that leisure plays in rebuilding a new life path. Many patients with brain injury have lost the ability to plan and initiate socialization or have fun. The patient with a significant motor impairment may feel that they are no longer able to participate in any type of leisure activities requiring physical skills. However, the creative therapist is able to find activities that will challenge deficits while the patient is having fun.

Although community outings are usually designed to be therapeutic, a sense of enjoyment should be the reward from doing the task. There are many creative tools available for therapists to rehabilitate leisure skills for their patients with brain injury. A leisure outing can range from going to the movies, shopping, going to parks and museums to playing a variety of games. Music is a potent tool to engage the patient in movement. The virtual reality products of Wii from Nintendo (www.wii.com) engage not only in motor activities but challenge cognitive skills. Games include such activities as virtual bowling, golf, baseball, yoga, balance, skiing, and tennis. Recent versions involve playing virtual musical instruments. A Wii activity can be enjoyed individually or in a group, which engages the patient in a social situation.

Kleiber et al.[131] considered the role of leisure in coping with and adjusting to disability after brain injury in postacute neurorehabilitation settings. Leisure activities are distractions from a daily focus on the negative aspects of disability. A "generation of optimism" helps to break from continual emotional pain after disability. The view is changed and the "emotional uplift provides the cognitive space for positive reappraisal."[131, p. 323] Some sense of self is restored. Cheryl Mattingly,[132] an OT and medical anthropologist, created a term for the clinician's role in assisting patients to reconstruct their life story, their identity: *therapeutic emplotment.* Pieper[133] put it well by stating that "leisure is an attitude of nonactivity, of inward calm, of silence; it means not being 'busy' but letting things happen.... Leisure is not the attitude of mind of those who actively intervene, but of those who are open to everything ... of those who leave the reins loose and who are free and easy themselves."[pp. 51–52]

22.3.12 Pool/Aquatic Therapy

Although the healing elements of water have been used for centuries, organized therapeutic protocols for the neurologically impaired have emerged only during the past decade. Current programs for musculoskeletal injuries (e.g., neck and back) are widely accepted by therapists and well received by those being treated. In this regard, the use of a pool program is a positive aspect to the physical rehabilitation for the person with MTBI. Aquatic therapy can address difficulties with balance and coordination, muscle weakness, poor endurance, and sensory dysfunctions. The buoyancy and warmth of the water, together with use of appliances to introduce resistive exercises, make a good combination for therapeutic application. Subtle vestibular impairments may manifest in aquatic activities, because water reduces proprioceptive feedback, making balance functions more dependent upon visual and vestibular feedback. Precautions for cardiac or other medical considerations should be taken prior to introduction of an aquatic program.

The more motorically impaired person can have quite positive responses to a pool program. Abnormal muscle tone, motor control, gait patterns, and ROM deficits can be addressed by utilizing the characteristics of water. This approach can add an element of fun and should be relaxing. As usual, normal precautions must be taken for cardiac, incontinence, and swallowing issues.[134,135]

22.4 Summary

This chapter presents a historical review of the integration of physical rehabilitation services into the developing field of head trauma rehabilitation. It provides a comprehensive review of evaluative and management protocols in areas that are most commonly observed to be problematic on a long-term basis for the person with TBI. The reader has been encouraged to adopt an expectation for continued improvement associated with continued treatment beyond acute hospitalization. Physical and occupational therapists should understand the tremendously complicated clinical presentation often associated with TBI and become familiar with the ever-evolving treatment strategies that can be used either individually or in tandem to treat the physical residuals associated with TBI.

References

1. Bobath, B., *Adult Hemiplegia: Evaluation and Treatment*, 2nd ed., rev., William Heinemann Medical Books, London, 1978.
2. Bobath, K. and Bobath, B., Cerebral palsy: Part 1: The neurological approach to treatment, in P. H. Pearson and C. E. Williams (Eds.), *Physical Therapy Services in the Developmental Disabilities*, Charles C. Thomas, Springfield, IL, 114, 1980.
3. Stockmeyer, S. A., An interpretation of the approach of Rood to the treatment of neuromuscular dysfunction, *American Journal of Physical Medicine*, 46(1), 900–961, 1967.
4. Knott, M. and Voss, D. E., *Proprioceptive Neuromuscular Facilitation: Patterns and Techniques*, Harper & Row, New York, 1956.
5. Brunnstrom, S., *Movement Therapy in Hemiplegia: A Neurophysiological Approach*, Harper & Row, New York, 1970.
6. Brunnstrom, S., *Mechanical Principles: Application to the Human Body in Clinical Kinesiology*, F. A. Davis, Philadelphia, PA, 1972.
7. Ayres, A. J., *Sensory Integration and Learning Disorders*, Western Psychological Services, Los Angeles, CA, 1972.
8. Jennett, B. and Teasdale, G., *Management of Head Injuries*, F. A. Davis, Philadelphia, PA, 1981.
9. Rosenthal, M., Griffith, E. R., Bond, M. B., and Miller, J. D., *Rehabilitation of the Head Injured Adult*, F. A. Davis, Philadelphia, PA, 1983.
10. Umphred, D. A., Conceptual model: A framework for clinical problem solving, in D. A. Umphred (Ed.), *Neurological Rehabilitation*, 2nd ed., C. V. Mosby, St. Louis, MO, 1990.
11. Horak, F. B. and Shumway-Cook, A., Clinical implications of posture control research, in P. W. Duncan (Ed.), *Balance, Proceedings of the APTA Forum*, American Physical Therapy Association, Alexandria, VA, 1990.
12. Shumway-Cook, A. and Olmscheid, R., A systems analysis of postural dyscontrol in traumatically brain-injured clients, *Journal of Head Trauma Rehabilitation*, 5(4), 51–62, 1990.
13. Melnick, M. E., Clients with cerebellar dysfunction, in D. A. Umphred (Ed.), *Neurological Rehabilitation*, 5th ed. C. V. Mosby, St. Louis, MO, 834–856, 2007.
14. Urbscheit, N. L., Cerebellar dysfunction, in D. A. Umphred (Ed.), *Neurological Rehabilitation*, C. V. Mosby, St. Louis, MO, 1990.
15. Boughton, A. and Ciesla, N., Physical therapy management of the head injured client in the intensive care unit, *Topics in Acute Care Trauma Rehabilitation*, 1, 1, 1986.

16. Lehmkuhl, L., Thoi, L., Baize, C., Kelley, C., Krawczyk, L., and Bontke, C., Multimodality treatment of joint contractures in clients with severe brain injury: Cost effectiveness and integration of therapies in the application of serial/inhibitive casts, *Journal of Head Trauma Rehabilitation*, 5, 23–42, 1990.

17. Murdock, K., Physical therapy in the neurologic intensive care unit, *Neurology Report*, 16(3), 17–24, 1992.

18. Smith, S. S. and Winkler, P. A., Traumatic head injuries, in D. A. Umphred (Ed.), *Neurological Rehabilitation*, C. V. Mosby, St. Louis, MO, 347, 1990.

19. Umphred, D. A. and McCormack, G. L., Classification of common facilitatory and inhibitory treatment techniques, in D. A. Umphred (Ed.), *Neurological Rehabilitation*, C. V. Mosby, St. Louis, MO, 1990.

20. Sazbon, L. and Groswasser, Z., Time-related sequelae of TBI in clients with prolonged postcomatose unawareness (PC-U) state, *Brain Injury*, 5(1), 3–8, 1991.

21. Glenn, M. B. and Wroblewski, B., Update of pharmacology: Antispasticity medications in the client with traumatic brain injury, *Journal of Head Trauma Rehabilitation*, 1, 71, 1986.

22. Abel, N. A. and Smith, R. A., Intrathecal baclofen for treatment of intractable spinal spasticity, *Archives of Physical Medicine and Rehabilitation*, 75(1), 54–58, 1994.

23. Schleenbaker, R. E. and Mainous, A. G., Electromyographic biofeedback for neuromuscular reeducation in the hemiplegic stroke client: A meta-analysis, *Archives of Physical Medicine and Rehabilitation*, 74(12), 1301–1304, 1993.

24. Rao, N. and Costa, J. L., Recovery in nonvascular locked-in syndrome during treatment with Sinemet, *Brain Injury*, 3(2), 207–211, 1989.

25. Lal, S., Merbitz, C. T., and Grip, J. C., Reply to Eames, *Brain Injury*, 3, 321, 1989.

26. Haig, A. J. and Ruess, J. M., Recovery from vegetative state of six month's duration associated with Sinemet (levodopa/carbidopa), *Archives of Physical Medicine and Rehabilitation*, 71(13), 1081–1083, 1990.

27. Blackerby, W. F., Intensity of rehabilitation and length of stay, *Brain Injury*, 4(2), 167–173, 1990.

28. Spivak, G., Spetell, C. M., Ellis, D. W., and Ross, S. E., Effects of intensity of treatment and length of stay on rehabilitation outcomes, *Brain Injury*, 6(5), 419–434, 1992.

29. Cifu, D. S., Kreutzer, J. S., Kolakowsky-Hayner, S. A., Marwitz, J. H., and Englander, J., Relationship between therapy intensity and rehabilitative outcomes after traumatic brain injury: A multicenter analysis, *Archives of Physical Medicine and Rehabilitation*, 84, 1441–1448, 2003.

30. Wilkerson, D. L., Batavia, A. I., and DeJong, G., Use of functional status measures for payment of medical rehabilitation devices, *Archives of Physical Medicine and Rehabilitation*, 73(2), 111–120, 1992.

31. Lewis, A. M., Documentation of movement patterns used in the performance of functional tasks, *Neurology Report*, 16, 13, 1992.

32. McCulloch, K. L. and Novack, T. A., Upper extremity functional assessment in traumatic brain-injured clients, *Journal of Head Trauma Rehabilitation*, 5, 1, 1990.

33. Kloos, A. D., Measurement of muscle tone and strength, *Neurology Report*, 16, 9, 1992.

34. Cardenas, D. D. and Clawson, D. R., Management of lower extremity strength and function in traumatically brain-injured clients, *Journal of Head Trauma Rehabilitation*, 5, 43, 1990.

35. Keith, R. A., Functional assessment measures in medical rehabilitation: Current status, *Archives of Physical Medicine and Rehabilitation*, 8, 74, 1984.

36. McCulloch, K., Functional assessment for adults with neurologic impairment, *Neurology Report*, 16, 4, 1992.

37. Mahoney, F. I. and Barthel, D. W., Functional evaluation: Barthel Index, *Maryland State Medical Journal*, 14, 61–65, 1965.

38. Rappaport, M., Hall, K. M., Hopkins, K., Belleza, T., and Cope, D. N., Disability Rating Scale for severe head trauma: Coma to community, *Archives of Physical Medicine and Rehabilitation*, 63(3), 118–123, 1982.

39. Gans, B. M., Haley, S. M., Hallenberg, S. C., Mann, N., et al., Description and interobserver reliability of the Tufts Assessment of Motor Performance, *American Journal of Physical Medicine and Rehabilitation*, 67(5), 202–210, 1988.

40. Tinetti, M. E., Performance-oriented assessment of mobility problems in elderly patients, *Journal of the American Geriatric Society*, 34(2), 119–126, 1986.

41. Hamilton, B. B., Granger, C. V., Sherwin, F. S., Zielezny, M., and Tashman, J. S., A uniform national data system for medical rehabilitation, in M. J. Fuhrer (Ed.), *Analysis and Measurement*, Brookes Publishing, Baltimore, MD, 1987.

42. Gronwall, D., Cumulative and persisting effects of concussion on attention and cognition, in H. S. Levin, H. M. Eisenberg, and A. L. Benton (Eds.), *Mild Head Injury*, Oxford University Press, New York, 1989.

43. Rutherford, W. H., Postconcussion symptoms: Relationship to acute neurological indices, individual differences, and circumstances of injury, in H. S. Levin, H. M. Eisenberg, and A. L. Benton (Eds.), *Mild Head Injury*, Oxford University Press, New York, 1989.

44. Law, M., Baptiste, S., Carswell, A., McColl, M. A., Polatajko, H., and Pollock, N., *Canadian Occupational Performance Measure Manual*, Ottawa: CAOT Publications ACE, 2nd ed., 1994.

45. Mathiowetz, V., Volland, G., Kashman, N., and Weber, K., Adult norms for the Box and Block Test of Manual Dexterity, *American Journal of Occupational Therapy*, 39(6), 386–391, 1985.

46. Sharpless, J. W., The Nine Hole Peg Test of finger–hand coordination for the hemiplegic client, in J. W. Sharpless (Ed.), *Mossman's A Problem Oriented Approach to Stroke Rehabilitation*, Charles C. Thomas, Springfield, IL, 470, 1982.

47. Tiffin, J., *Purdue Pegboard Test*, Lafayette Instrument Company, Lafayette, IN, 1968.

48. Ziegler, W. A., *Minnesota Rate of Manipulation Tests*, American Guidance Service, Circle Pines, MN, 1969.

49. Crawford, J. E. and Crawford, D. M., *Crawford Small Parts Dexterity Test*, The Psychological Corporation, New York, 1956.

50. Bennett, G. K., *Bennett Hand Tool Dexterity Test*, rev. ed., The Psychological Corporation, New York, 1981.

51. Swaine, B. R. and Sullivan, S. J., Relation between clinical and instrumented measures of motor coordination in traumatically brain injured persons, *Archives of Physical Medicine and Rehabilitation*, 73(1), 55–59, 1992.

52. Lance, J. W., Symposium synopsis, in R. G. Feldman, R. R. Yound, and W. P. Koella (Eds.), *Spasticity: Disordered Motor Control*, Year Book Medical, Chicago, IL, 485–494, 1980.

53. Burridge, J. H., Wood, D. R., Hermens, H. J., Voerman, G. E., Johnson, G. R., van Wijck, F., Platz, T., Gergoric, M., Hitchcock, R., and Pandyan, A. D., Theoretical and methodological considerations in the measurement of spasticity, *Disability Rehabilitation*, 27(1–2), 69–80, 2005.

54. Ashworth, B., Preliminary trial of carisoprodol in multiple sclerosis, *The Practitioner*, 192, 540–542, 1965.

55. Bohannon, R. W. and Smith, M. B., Interrater reliability of a modified Ashworth scale of muscle spasticity, *Physical Therapy*, 67(2), 206–207, 1987.

56. American College of Sports Medicine (Franklin, B. A., Whaley, M. H., Howley, E. T., et al.), *ACSM's Guidelines for Exercise Testing and Prescription*, 6th ed., Lippincott Williams & Wilkins, Philadelphia, PA, 2002.

57. Podsiadlo, D. and Richardson, S., The timed "Up and Go:" A test of basic functional mobility for frail elderly persons, *Journal of the American Geriatric Society*, 39(2), 142–148, 1991.

58. Fisher, B., Effect of trunk control and alignment on limb function, *Journal of Head Trauma Rehabilitation*, 2(2), 72–79, 1987.

59. Nutt, J. G., Marsden, C. D., and Thompson, P. D., Human walking and higher-level gait disorders, particularly in the elderly, *Neurology*, 43(2), 268–279, 1993.

60. Farber, S. D. and Zoltan, B., Visual–vestibular systems interaction: Therapeutic implications, *Journal of Head Trauma Rehabilitation*, 4(2), 9–16, 1989.

61. Eggers, O., *Occupational Therapy in the Treatment of Adult Hemiplegia*, Aspen Publishers, Rockville, MD, 1987.

62. Herdman, S. J., Treatment of vestibular disorders in traumatically brain-injured clients, *Journal of Head Trauma Rehabilitation*, 5, 63, 1990.
63. Shumway-Cook, A. and Horak, F. B., Assessing the influence of sensory interaction on balance: Suggestions from the field, *Physical Therapy*, 66(10), 1548–1550, 1986.
64. Weber, C. M. and Verbanets, J., Assessing balance performance in moderate head injury, *Topics in Acute Care Trauma Rehabilitation*, 1, 84, 1986.
65. Shepard, N. T., Telian, S. A., and Smith-Wheelock, M., Habituation and balance retraining therapy. A retrospective review, *Neurologic Clinics*, 8(2), 459–475, 1990.
66. Duncan, P. W., Weiner, D. K., Chankler, J., and Studenski, S., Functional reach: A new clinical measure of balance, *Journal of Gerontology*, 45(6), M192–M197, 1990.
67. Shumway-Cook, A. and Horak, F. B., Rehabilitation strategies for clients with vestibular deficits, *Neurologic Clinics*, 8(2), 441–457, 1990.
68. Flores, A. M., Objective measurement of standing balance, *Neurologic Report*, 6, 26, 1992.
69. Vytopil, M. and Jones, H. R., Cranial nerve I: Olfactory, in *Netter's Neurology*, Icon Learning Systems, Teterboro, NJ, 96, 2006.
70. Buck, L. B., Smell and taste: The chemical senses, in E. R. Kandel, J. H. Schwartz, and T. M. Jessell (Eds.), *Principles of Neural Science*, 4th ed., McGraw-Hill, New York, 625–647, 2000.
71. Levin H. S., High, W. M., and Eisenberg, H. M., Impairment of olfactory recognition after closed head injury, *Brain*, 108(Pt. 3), 579–591, 1985.
72. Costanzo, R. M. and Becker, D. P., Smell and taste disorders in head injury and neurosurgery clients, in H. L. Meiselman and R. S. Rivlin (Eds.), *Clinical Measurements of Taste and Smell*, Macmillan, New York, 1986.
73. Doty, R. L., *The Smell Identification Test Administration Manual*, Sensonics, Inc., Haddon Heights, NJ, 1995.
74. Doty, R. L., Diagnostic tests and assessments, *Journal of Head Trauma Rehabilitation*, 7, 47, 1992.
75. Zasler, N. D., McNeny, R., and Heywood, P. G., Rehabilitative management of olfactory and gustatory dysfunction following brain injury, *Journal of Head Trauma Rehabilitation*, 7(1), 66–75, 1992.
76. Schlageter, K., Gray, B., Hall, K., Shaw, R., and Sammet, R., Incidence and treatment of visual dysfunction in traumatic brain injury, *Brain Injury*, 7(5), 439–448, 1993.
77. Bouska, M. J., Kauffman, N. A., and Marcus, S. E., Disorders of the visual perceptual system, in D. A. Umphred (Ed.), *Neurological Rehabilitation*, C. V. Mosby, St. Louis, MO, 705, 1990.
78. Leiberman, S., Cohen, A., and Rubin, J., NYSOA-K-D test, *Journal of the American Optometric Association*, 54, 631, 1983.
79. Gianutsos, R. and Ramsey, G., Enabling the survivors of brain injury to receive rehabilitative optometric services, *Journal of Vision Rehabilitation*, 2, 37, 1988.
80. Strano, C. M., Effects of visual deficits on ability to drive in traumatically brain-injured population, *Journal of Head Trauma Rehabilitation*, 4(2), 35–43, 1989.
81. Baum, B. and Hall, K., Relationship between constructional praxis and dressing in the head injured adult, *American Journal of Occupational Therapy*, 35(7), 438–442, 1981.
82. Bowler, D. F., Perceptual assessment, *Neurologic Report*, 16, 26, 1992.
83. Titus, M. N., Gall, N. G., Yerxa, E. J., Roberson, T. A., and Mack, W., Correlation of perceptual performance with activities of daily living in stroke clients, *American Journal of Occupational Therapy*, 45(5), 410–418, 1991.
84. Mercier, L., Hebert, R., Colarusso, R. P., and Hammill, D. D., *The Motor-Free Visual Perception Test: Vertical Format*, Academic Therapy Publications, Novato, CA, 1997.
85. Gardner, M. F., *Test of Visual-Perceptual (nonmotor)—Revised*, Psychological and Educational Publications, Burlingame, CA, 1996.
86. Hooper, H. E., *The Hooper Visual Organization Test Manual*, Western Psychological Services, Los Angeles, CA, 1958.
87. Miller, N., *Dyspraxia and Its Management*, Aspen Publishers, Rockville, MD, 1986.
88. Zoltan, B., Jabri, J., Panikoff, L., and Ryckman, D., *Perceptual Motor Evaluation for Head Injured and Other Neurologically Impaired Adults*, Rev. ed., Santa Clara Valley Medical Center, Occupational Therapy Department, San Jose, CA, 1987.

89. Lezak, M. D., *Neuropsychological Assessment*, Oxford Press, New York, 1976.
90. Whiting, S., Lincoln, N., Bhavnani, G., and Cockbun, J., *RPAB–Rivermead Perceptual Assessment Battery Manual*, Nfer-Nelson Publishing, Windsor Berks, UK, 1985.
91. Itzkovich, M., Elazar, B., and Averbuch, S., *LOTCA Lowenstein Occupational Therapy Cognitive Assessment Manual*, Maddak, Pequahnock, NJ, 1990.
92. Garland, D. E. and Varpetian, A., Heterotopic ossification in traumatic brain injury, in M. J. Ashley (Ed.), *Traumatic Brain Injury: Rehabilitative Treatment and Case Management*, 2nd ed., CRC Press, Boca Raton, FL, 119–134, 2004.
93. Botte, M. J. and Moore, T. J., The orthopedic management of extremity injuries in head trauma, *Journal of Head Trauma Rehabilitation*, 2, 13, 1987.
94. Garland, D. E. and Bailey, S., Undetected injuries in head-injured adults, *Clinical Orthopedics and Related Research*, 155, 162–165, 1981.
95. Grummons, D., Stabilizing the occlusion: Finishing procedures, in S. L. Kraus (Ed.), *TMJ Disorders: Management of the Craniomandibular Complex*, Churchill Livingstone, New York, 1988.
96. Anderson, J. M., Kaplan, M. S., and Felsenthal, G., Brain injury obscured by chronic pain: A preliminary report, *Archives of Physical Medicine and Rehabilitation*, 71(9), 703–708, 1990.
97. Zasler, N., Mild traumatic brain injury: Medical assessment and intervention, *Journal of Head Trauma Rehabilitation*, 8, 13, 1993.
98. Pearce, J. M., Headache, *Journal of Neurology, Neurosurgery, and Psychiatry*, 57(2), 134–143, 1994.
99. Page, N. G. and Gresty, M. A., Motorist's vestibular disorientation syndrome, *Journal of Neurology, Neurosurgery, and Psychiatry*, 48(8), 729–735, 1985.
100. Sivak, M., Hill, C. S., Henson, D. L., Butler, B. P., Silber, S. M., and Olson, P. L., Improved driving performance following perceptual training in persons with brain damage, *Archives of Physical Medicine and Rehabilitation*, 65(4), 163–167, 1984.
101. Katz, R. T., Golden, R. S., Butler, J., Tepper, D., Rothke, S., Holmes, J., and Sahgal, V., Driving safely after brain damage: Follow-up of twenty-two patients with matched controls, *Archives of Physical Medicine and Rehabilitation*, 71(2), 133–137, 1990.
102. Coleman, R. D., Rapport, L. J., Ergh, T. C., Hanks, R. A., Ricker, J. H., and Millis, S. R., Predictors of driving outcome after traumatic brain injury, *Archives of Physical Medicine and Rehabilitation*, 83(10), 1415–1422, 2002.
103. Rapport, L. J., Hanks, R. A., and Bryer, R. C., Barriers to driving and community integration after brain injury, *Journal of Head Trauma Rehabilitation*, 21(1), 34–44, 2006.
104. Pellerito, Jr., J. M. and Davis, E. S., *Screening Driving and Community Mobility Status: A Critical Link to Participation and Productive Living*, American Occupational Therapy Association, Washington, DC, 2006.
105. Ashley, M. J., Krych, D. K., and Lehr, Jr., R. P., Cost/benefit analysis for postacute rehabilitation of the traumatically brain-injured client, *Journal of Insurance Medicine*, 22(2), 156–161, 1990.
106. Ashley, M. J., Persel, C. S., and Krych, D. K., Changes in reimbursement climate: Relationship between outcome, cost, and payer type in the postacute rehabilitation environment, *Journal of Head Trauma Rehabilitation*, 8(4), 30–47, 1993.
107. Haffey, W. J. and Abrams, D. L., Employment outcomes for participants in a brain injury work reentry program: Preliminary findings, *Journal of Head Trauma Rehabilitation*, 6(3), 24–34, 1991.
108. Ben-Yishay, Y., Silver, S. M., Piasetsky, E., and Rattok, J., Relationship between employability and vocational outcome after intensive holistic cognitive rehabilitation, *Journal of Head Trauma Rehabilitation*, 2(1), 35–48, 1987.
109. Cope, D. N., Cole, J. R., Hall, K. M., and Barkan, H., Brain injury: Analysis of outcome in a post-acute rehabilitation system. Part 1: General analysis, *Brain Injury*, 5(2), 111–125, 1991.
110. Cope, D. N., Cole, J. R., Hall, K. M., and Barkan, H., Brain injury: Analysis of outcome in a post-acute rehabilitation system. Part 2: Subanalysis, *Brain Injury*, 5(2), 127–139, 1991.
111. Spivack, G., Spettell, C. M., Ellis, D. W., and Ross, S. E., Effects of intensity of treatment and length of stay on rehabilitation outcomes, *Brain Injury*, 6(5), 419–434, 1992.

112. Keenan, M. E., The orthopedic management of spasticity, *Journal of Head Trauma Rehabilitation*, 2(2), 62–71, 1987.

113. Griffith, E. R. and Mayer, N. H., Hypertonicity and movement disorders, in M. R. Rosenthal, E. R. Griffith, M. R. Bond, and J. D. Miller (Eds.), *Rehabilitation of the Adult and Child with Traumatic Brain Injury*, F. A. Davis, Philadelphia, 1990.

114. Finch, T. and Barbeau, H., Hemiplegic gait: New treatment strategies, *Physiotherapy Canada*, 38(1), 36–41, 1986.

115. Visintin, M., Barbeau, H., Korner-Bitensky, N., and Mayo, N., A new approach to retrain gait in stroke clients through body weight support and treadmill stimulation, *Stroke*, 29(6), 1122–1128, 1998.

116. Wilson, D. J. and Swaboda, J. L., Partial weight-bearing gait training for persons following traumatic brain injury: Preliminary report and proposed assessment scale, *Brain Injury*, 16(3), 259–268, 2002.

117. Pilar, T., Dickstein, R., and Smolinski, Z., Walking reeducation with partial relief of body weight in rehabilitation of patients with locomotor disabilities, *Journal of Rehabilitation Research and Development*, 28(4), 47–52, 1991.

118. Dobkin, B., Harkema, S., Requejo, P., and Edgerton, R., Modulation of locomotor-like EMG activity in subjects with complete and incomplete spinal cord injury, *Journal of Neurologic Rehabilitation*, 9(4), 183–190, 1995.

119. Duckett, S. and Kramer, T., Managing myoclonus secondary to anoxic encephalopathy through EMG biofeedback, *Brain Injury*, 8(2), 185–188, 1994.

120. Roller, P. and Leahy, P., Cerebellar ataxia, *Neurologic Report*, 15, 25, 1991.

121. Kottke, F. J., Stillwell, G. K., and Lehmann, J. F. (Eds.), *Krusen's Handbook of Physical Medicine and Rehabilitation*, 3rd ed., W. B. Saunders, Philadelphia, PA, 423, 1982.

122. Yekutiel, M. and Guttman, E., A controlled trial of the retraining of the sensory function of the hand in stroke clients, *Journal of Neurology, Neurosurgery, and Psychiatry*, 56(3), 241–244, 1993.

123. Keenan, M. E. and Perry, J., Evaluation of upper extremity motor control in spastic brain-injured patients using dynamic electromyography, *Journal of Head Trauma Rehabilitation*, 5(4), 13–22, 1990.

124. Wilbarger, P. L. and Wilbarger, J. L., *Sensory Defensiveness: A Comprehensive Approach*, Avanti Educational Programs, Panorama City, CA, 2001.

125. Wolf, S. L., Winstein, C. J., Miller, J. P., Taub, E., Uswatte, G., Morris, D., Giuliani, C., Light, K. E., and Nichols-Larsen, D., Effect of constraint-induced movement therapy on upper extremity function 3 to 9 months after stroke: The EXCITE randomized clinical trial, *Journal of the American Medical Association*, 296(17), 2095–2104, 2006.

126. Sawaki, L., Butler, A. J., Leng, X., Wassenaar, P. A., Mohammad, Y. M., Blanton, S., Sathian, K., et al., Constraint-induced movement therapy results in increased motor map area in subjects 3 to 9 months after stroke, *Neurorehabilitation and Neural Repair*, 22(5), 505–513, 2008.

127. Neistadt, M. E., Normal adult performance on constructional praxis training tasks, *The American Journal of Occupational Therapy*, 43(7), 448–455, 1989.

128. Neistadt, M. E., The relationship between constructional and meal preparation skills, *Archives of Physical Medicine and Rehabilitation*, 74(2), 144–148, 1993.

129. Hayden, R. M. and Allen, G. J., Relationship between aerobic exercise, anxiety, and depression: Convergent validation by knowledgeable informants, *The Journal of Sports Medicine and Physical Fitness*, 24(1), 69–74, 1984.

130. Tomporowski, P. D. and Ellis, N. R., Effects of exercise on cognitive processes: A review, *Psychological Bulletin*, 99, 338–346, 1986.

131. Kleiber, D. A., Reel, H. A., and Hutchinson, S. L., When distress gives way to possibility: The relevance of leisure in adjustment to disability, *Neurorehabilitation*, 23(4), 321–328, 2008.

132. Mattingly, C., The concept of therapeutic "emplotment," *Social Science and Medicine*, 38(6), 811–822, 1994.

133. Pieper, J., *Leisure: The Basis of Culture*, Random House, New York, 1963.
134. Hurley, R. and Turner, C., Neurology and aquatic therapy, *Clinical Management*, 11(1), 26–29, 1991.
135. Morris, D. M., The use of pool therapy to improve the functional activities of adult hemiplegic clients, *Forum Proceedings: Forum on Physical Therapy Issues Related to Cerebrovascular Accident*, Neurology Section of the American Physical Therapy Association, Alexandria, VA, 45, 1992.

23

Vocational Rehabilitation

Mark J. Ashley, Joe Ninomiya, Jr., Amy Berryman, and Karen Rasavage

CONTENTS

23.1 Introduction

Return to work (RTW) following a traumatic brain injury (TBI) represents a pinnacle achievement for both the injured individual and those professionals working with the individual. The United Nations General Assembly produced "The Standard Rules on the Equalization of Opportunities for People with Disabilities" in 1993.[1] This report consists of 22 rules that are intended to serve as a guide in policy making for member states. Rule 2 states that "[s]tates should ensure the provision of effective medical care to persons with disabilities." Rule 3 indicates that "[s]tates should ensure the provision of rehabilitation services to persons with disabilities in order for them to reach and sustain their optimal level of independence and functioning." Finally, Rule 7 notes "[s]tates should recognize the principle that persons with disabilities must be empowered to exercise their human rights, particularly in the field of employment. In both rural and urban areas, they must have equal opportunities for gainful employment in the labour market." Taken together, the United Nations member states call for states to ensure that maximal disability reduction is achieved through access to medical treatment and rehabilitation culminating in gainful employment whenever feasible.[1]

Work is highly linked to identity and has significant meaning for most people. The meaning of work after TBI often changes, however, and can have a unique impact on quality of life.[2] Work provides structure to daily routines and provides purpose. The social aspect of work allows for community participation and provides opportunities for building relationships. Work can be a means of returning to a "normal" life and is perceived as a strong and effective means of rehabilitation. Essentially, the ultimate measure of rehabilitative success is life satisfaction; vocational success bears significantly on its achievement. Self-directed vocational participation as an adult is promoted from a very early age through young adulthood as a means of securing social and financial stability. TBI frequently deprives an individual of the ability to participate meaningfully in life through vocational and social involvement, in keeping with the rest of society.

Melamed et al.[3] reviewed gratification of basic needs, physical well-being, emotional security, and family, social, economic, and vocational needs 1 to 2 years following discharge from rehabilitation for 78 people with TBI. Those individuals who were employed in the open labor market, lived active lives, and had higher degrees of acceptance of disability reported the highest satisfaction. Lower satisfaction was associated with unemployment, with employment in protected conditions, and with passive, uninvolved lifestyles. These findings are supported by other authors who report life satisfaction associated with employment and degree of social integration.[4,5] Heinemann et al.[6] completed a survey designed to measure the unmet needs of persons with TBI. Responses from 895 respondents indicated that two of the three greatest needs—improving memory or problem-solving skills (51.9%), increasing income (50.5%), and improving job skills (46.3%)—were vocationally related.

Ironically, although rehabilitation endeavors to assist individuals to achieve maximal recovery so they will have the opportunity to participate fully in life, a societal predisposition exists toward insufficient effort in returning people to the workforce. This is manifest by restricted vocational rehabilitation benefits under various workers' compensation statutes across the United States, as well as by lack of provision of benefits for vocational rehabilitation services in any accident and health insurance coverage. Vocational rehabilitation services provided by publicly funded sources, such as state departments of vocational rehabilitation, are often ill-prepared to deal with the complexity of problems presented by persons with TBI.[7–9]

The General Accounting Office of the United States reviewed differences in RTW strategies comparing the United States with Germany and Sweden.[10] Public expenditures for vocational rehabilitation were two times higher in Germany and 2.6 times higher in Sweden as a percentage of gross domestic product. The General Accounting Office cited conflict created by divergent goals of Social Security's eligibility and provision of benefits and vocational rehabilitation agencies. It was concluded that differences also existed in the availability of vocational rehabilitation services, timing of vocational referral (later in the United States), and level of financial incentive involved in RTW.

Vocational rehabilitation services have been available since the 1970s,[11] with funding provided by the public sector in the form of state departments of vocational rehabilitation or the private sector as a benefit under workers' compensation. The primary thrust of vocational rehabilitation (i.e., returning an individual to work) is accomplished by careful evaluation of work responsibilities and comparison of the physical requirements of those responsibilities with the individual's capabilities following injury. Very few conditions present the complexity of deficits seen with TBI, however. People with TBI present with far more complicated problems, including behavioral, cognitive, communicative, psychological, emotional, social, and physical disabilities. The success of vocational rehabilitation therefore is highly dependent upon the degree of disability present in the individual. To the extent that medical rehabilitation has been truncated, individuals are left with higher levels of disability and with little recourse for additional medical rehabilitation services. As rehabilitation hospital lengths of stay continue to decline and as access to postacute rehabilitation is increasingly restricted,[12,13] fewer people will receive adequate medical rehabilitation to maximize disability reduction and to ready an individual for vocational rehabilitation.

Provision of vocational rehabilitation services is not uniformly applied to all individuals who sustain TBI.[14,15] RTW following TBI is difficult for many individuals regardless of the level of severity of injury[14,16] and is made more difficult by a lack of appropriate funding,[17] a lack of understanding regarding the proper undertaking of vocational rehabilitation services,[7,8] and a lack of awareness on the injured person's part, or the care provider's, of the applicability of vocational rehabilitation services.[15] Reported rates of RTW vary considerably in the literature, depending upon the population studied and limitations of individual study methodologies.[18] RTW is reported to range from 20% to 100%.[19–22]

Vocation serves a tremendously important role in life, yet vocational rehabilitation is one of the least understood and least delivered services for people with TBI. This chapter will address the provision of vocational rehabilitation services to individuals with TBI.

23.2 Employment Trends Following TBI

RTW following TBI is not easily accomplished and may not be accomplished by some individuals. Rates of RTW vary throughout the literature and are impacted by both the definition of "work" and the nature of the population studied. Rates of RTW have emotional, financial, and social implications. In a study by Johnstone et al.,[23] TBI was associated with an estimated $642 million in lost wages, $96 million in lost income taxes, and $353 million in increased public assistance secondary to unemployment 1 year postinjury. Corrigan et al.[24] report that review of 2004 annual findings from the Traumatic Brain Injury Model Systems national data set for the United States showed competitive employment at 1 year after injury for 27% of individuals and 29% at 5 years postinjury. Review of the Traumatic Brain Injury Model Systems data set for collected case data through 2007 showed competitive employment at 1 year for 28% and 33% at 2 years postinjury.[25]

Rao et al.[26] conducted a follow-up study on 79 consecutively admitted patients over a 2-year period. Subjects ranged in age from 17 to 66 years with a median age of 29 years. Preinjury, 90% were employed and 10% were students. Fifty-four percent had some high school education or had completed high school and 34% had some college education or had completed college. Median length of inpatient rehabilitation stay was 49 days with a range of 1 to 155 days. Median follow-up time from discharge was 16.5 months, ranging from 2 to 26 months. Computed tomographic (CT) scan findings were classified as normal (12.7%), evidence of unilateral damage (40.5%), and evidence of bilateral damage (46.8%). Posttraumatic amnesia in the severe, very severe, and extremely severe ranges had been present in 97% of subjects. A total of 66% returned to work or school and 34% failed to do so. Those who returned to work had an average of 13 consecutive months of employment, and 65% returned to work at an equivalent skill level to their preinjury vocational status. Those who returned to work or school were more likely to be younger, have a normal CT scan or unilateral damage, have a shorter coma duration, and have a shorter length of stay in inpatient rehabilitation.

McMordie et al.[27] reviewed RTW for 177 individuals averaging 6.7 years postinjury and belonging to the Iowa Head Injury Association who responded to a questionnaire. Severity of injury was by self-report and consisted of length of loss of consciousness. The study reported RTW along dimensions similar to those used in vocational rehabilitation in general (i.e., full-time, part-time, work/training, sheltered workshop, volunteer, and no work). Overall, 31 (17.5%) individuals achieved vocational outcomes of full- or part-time work. Another three individuals returned to homemaker responsibilities on a part- or full-time basis. The balance of working individuals were distributed as follows: work training, 2.8%; sheltered workshop, 13%; and volunteer work, 10.2%. McMordie et al.[27] suggest the population may have been biased by membership in the Iowa Head Injury Association, perhaps toward greater severity of injury. More than half the individuals (54.8%) remained unemployed.

Gonser[28] followed 122 people with severe head injury for 2 to 4 years postinjury. Of these, 43% were found to be without "employment handicap."

Felmingham et al.[29] assessed 55 individuals with TBI age 16 years and older. Mean Glasgow Coma Scale (GCS) score and mean length of posttraumatic amnesia (PTA) were 7 points and 33.5 days, respectively. Of these, 22% who were employed at 6 months were unemployed at 24 months. Psychological impairments were reported as the main reason for unemployment. Of those, 29% who were unemployed at 6 months were employed at 24 months.

Van der Naalt et al.[22] reported on a 1-year follow-up for 70 people with TBI in the Netherlands who originally sustained mild to moderate TBI. Mild head injury was defined as an initial GCS score of 13 to 14 points and moderate head injury as an initial GCS score of 9 to 12 points and duration of PTA of longer than 1 hour. Subjects with PTA longer than 28 days were excluded. The entire group of subjects returned to work by 1 year postinjury, although those with more severe injury did so on a more protracted basis over the course of time from injury to the 1-year postinjury point. Average RTW time for mild head injury was 2.7 months and for moderate head injury was 4.1 months. This did not necessarily mean return to full capacity, however. Return to full capacity averaged 5.6 months for the mild head injury group and 7.8 months for the moderate head injury group. Only 73% had resumed previous work and 84% complained of continuing problems. The prevalence of complaints during follow-up was reported for 1, 3, 6, and 12 months. At 1 year, physical complaints consisted of headache, dizziness, balance disorders, tinnitus, hearing loss, drowsiness, and fatigue. Cognitive complaints included forgetfulness, poor concentration, and slowness. Affective complaints included irritability, reduced tolerance for noise, and anxiety.

At the other end of the chronicity and severity spectrums, Englander et al.[30] followed 77 individuals age 15 years and older with mild TBI as measured by GCS scores of 13 to 15 points and PTA of less than 48 hours who were admitted to the hospital from the emergency room and discharged to home within 3 days. Subjects were contacted via telephone between 1 and 3 months postinjury. Among these, 88% had returned to work or school and 16% of those returning to work or school did so with some continuing symptoms. Overall, 74% reported no ongoing problems from the injury, whereas 26% reported difficulties. At an average of 56 days postinjury, subjective complaints were as follows: tire more easily, 70%; headaches, 70%; memory, 65%; change in sleep pattern, 65%; longer to process information, 65%; upset or frustrated easily, 60%; anxiety, 60%; muscle twitching, 60%; cannot get words out, 50%; muscle weakness, 50%; dizziness, 50%; depression, 50%; less recreation, 45%; and temper, 45%.

The timing of vocational rehabilitation involvement may impact RTW.[31,32] Individuals for whom vocational rehabilitation services were provided within a year of injury had a better rate of RTW than those who received services after 1 year.[32] Reid-Arndt et al.[33] reviewed differences between early-referral vocational rehabilitation candidates with TBI and late-referral candidates. Early referral candidates averaged 10.6 months from injury, with 40% being within 90 days of injury, and were enrolled an average of 19.4 months in the program. Late-referral candidates averaged 58.1 months and were enrolled an average of 29.9 months. The early-referral group reported significantly more hours of competitive pay per week and more weeks of competitive employment. Both groups, however, reported very low numbers: 5.11 paid hours per week and 7.85 weeks per year for the early-referral group and 4.18 paid hours per week and 2.19 weeks per year for the late-referral group.

RTW by an individual following TBI can also be complicated by difficulty in maintaining employment. The previous studies note a number of individuals who had returned to work but did not disclose the nature of difficulties encountered while at work or in maintaining the vocational placement. Sale et al.[34] followed 29 people with moderate to severe TBI and studied reasons for job separations. Average age at injury was 25.65 years and average age at the time of the study was 33.07 years, at an average of 7.42 years postinjury. Coma duration for the group averaged 48.2 days. Educational level achieved was as follows: some high school, $n = 7$; high school graduate, $n = 8$; some college, $n = 10$; college graduate, $n = 3$; and unknown, $n = 1$. Only medically stable individuals and those who were not actively abusing substances were included in the study. This group experienced 38 individual job separations. The mean length of employment noted before job separation was 5.8 months, with a range observed of 0.2 to 27.6 months. Fully two thirds of all job separations came within the first 6 months of employment. The most frequently cited reason for job separation was interpersonal relationship difficulties. These included displays of anger, inappropriate social interaction, and overfamiliarity. Additional reasons for job separation included economic layoffs, substance abuse, criminal activity, and mental health problems. Employment tends to decline over time as a consequence of these problems.

Ben-Yishay et al.[16] reviewed a group of 94 individuals with diffuse brain injuries. Average age was 27 years (range, 15–60 years), education level averaged 14 years (range, 8–20 years), coma duration averaged 34.40 days (range, 1–120 days), and time from injury to admission averaged 36.46 months (range, 4–207 months). Eligibility for program admission required a verbal or performance IQ of at least 80, ambulatory capability, no required physical restraints, and ability to reliably engage in two-way verbal communication. Patients were excluded if they had a history of a previous brain injury, significant psychiatric history, or significant history of drug/alcohol abuse. Ben-Yishay et al.[16] found a drop from 64% competitive employment immediately following program completion to 50% at 3 years postdischarge. A similar decline was noted in noncompetitive employment placements, from 30% at discharge to 22% by year 3. Principal causes of a lack of work stability were (1) social isolation manifest by alcohol abuse, disinhibition phenomena, and temporary psychiatric complications; (2) forgetting to use acquired strategies, which manifest as ill-advised attempts to resume high-level academic studies and counterproductive and obsessive quests for remediating intractable deficits, and (3) financial disincentives to work manifest by extravagant spending binges of settlement funds and anticipation of large settlement proceeds from pending litigation.

West[35] reviewed 37 individuals who were placed in supported employment. Only 19 (51%) of these individuals retained their jobs at 6 months. In a comparison of those individuals who remained employed with those who lost employment, there was no significant difference found between the groups with reference to race, marital status, highest educational level achieved, residential situation, community type, cause of injury, injury severity, work status prior to injury, or work status prior to referral to the supported employment project. Although there was a difference in average age, with the younger group tending toward employment retention, the difference was not statistically significant. Almost all the participants were employed in entry-level unskilled or semi-skilled positions. The study reviewed the integration of the individual into the job site, workforce position, and monetary benefits associated with employment. Inequities of the workplace and opportunities for monetary and nonmonetary benefits were found to be factors in job retention of supported individuals. Job retention outcomes appeared to be better for those individuals placed in positions offering fringe benefits, opportunities for raises and advancement, formal and informal support, and opportunities for socialization.

Wall et al.[36] reviewed 31 individuals with TBI and 7 with acquired brain injury arising from cardiovascular accident or chronic neurologic conditions who participated in a community-based training program. Injury severity was not provided. Mean time since injury was 10 years, and since diagnosis was 8.91 years. Median number of years of education was 12.0 and mean preinjury work history was 31.44 months. Fifty-eight percent received income from a federally funded program, averaging $439 monthly. Thirty-seven percent were working at injury or onset of illness. The average program duration was 10.54 weeks, with 58% completing the program. Those who completed the program differed only in that they had a longer duration of disability and longer preinjury work histories. A total of 67% of persons who completed the program retained their job at 60 days and 59% at about 18 months out. Mean starting salary was $5.68 per hour. Approximately half of those who did not complete the program reported substance abuse.

As can be seen, difficulties with employment following TBI are a common finding in both short- and long-term studies. The nature of the neurologic injuries sustained, inadequacies of vocational rehabilitation programming, and shortcomings of medical rehabilitation programming resulting in failure to provide adequate assistance in recovery from TBI contribute to reemployment difficulties. It is safe to assume that the neurologic injuries sustained impact the degree to which recovery can be expected. Comparatively less research has focused on the latter two factors. It appears, however, that competitive employment after TBI is difficult for most and impossible for many. Programmed interventions appear to be successful at improving the overall RTW rate and, to a lesser degree, job retention. Great care must be taken in review of the RTW literature in TBI because of the tremendous variability in the manner in which this topic is reported.

23.3 Prognosticating Return to Work

Recovery from TBI can occur over protracted periods of time.[37–39] Consequently, no reliable means of determining exactly when vocational rehabilitation services should be undertaken exists. Unfortunately, however, injured individuals, families, and professionals share a common concern for identifying the long-term, perhaps ultimate, recovery potential following injury. These questions begin very soon after injury and persist for many months, if not years. RTW is impacted both by the nature of the sequelae from the TBI as well as noninjury-related factors.

An awareness of prognostic variables impacting individuals with TBI can help determine the intensity and type of vocational rehabilitation services to be delivered.[40] Gonser[28] reviewed both cognitive and physical disabilities as prognostic factors in vocational return and suggested that neuropsychological impairment was the single most important factor in the prognostication of the vocational return. Machamer et al.[41] followed 165 workers with mild to severe TBI and found that higher neuropsychological functioning 1 month postinjury, combined with higher premorbid functioning and lower severity of injury, resulted in higher stability of employment. Ruff et al.[42] also found neuropsychological function to be important in RTW. They reviewed predictors of outcome following severe head injury and found age, Wechsler Adult Intelligence Scale-Revised (WAIS-R) vocabulary score, and selective attention speed combined to classify correctly 88% of subjects in a category of either productive or nonproductive work.

Age at injury has been well documented as a prognostic variable in RTW.[29,40,42–45] Most studies support the idea that a direct correlation exists between age and RTW.[29,40,42–45] Individuals who are younger at the time of injury are more likely to progress to RTW than individuals who are older.[40] Preinjury employment status and educational level have been demonstrated to be strong predictors of RTW.[40] Individuals who were employed at the time of injury and individuals with higher educational achievement were more likely to return to work than individuals who were unemployed at the time of injury, had poor employment history, or had lesser educational achievement. Keyser-Marcus et al.[40] found individuals who were employed at the time of injury were three to five times more likely to be employed postinjury. A partial explanation for this finding may be that, following brain injury, information that was well learned at the time of injury is more readily called upon by the individual, in contrast to information that must be acquired following injury and reliance upon new learning skills. This can be of great assistance in returning an individual to work—in particular, in instances when the work to be performed by the individual relies upon old information and has little demand for new learning. As such, rote tasks will be largely more successful in RTW scenarios than those tasks that require a high dependence on new learning. Conversely, some positions require much greater reliance on new information processing and will not benefit from dependence upon rote tasks.[46]

Coma duration has been documented as a prognostic variable for overall outcome following TBI and for RTW. Shorter coma durations are associated with greater likelihood of RTW. Similarly, duration of PTA has been correlated to RTW,[47] as has duration of acute rehabilitation treatment.[40,48] Again, in both instances, shorter periods are associated with a greater likelihood of RTW. Rao et al.[26] noted that fewer positive findings on CT scan correlated with RTW.

Length of stay has been studied as a potential predictor variable to vocational outcome. Keyser-Marcus et al.[40] reported that rehabilitation length of stay predicted RTW at 1 year postinjury. Shorter length of stay was associated with RTW. Although it might be argued that length of stay is an indirect measure of injury severity, more direct measures of injury severity, such as GCS score and duration of PTA, were not predictive of RTW. These findings support those of Gollaher et al.[18] and Ip et al.[19] GCS score has not been found to be highly predictive of outcome, in particular, for those individuals who are in the moderate range of severity of injury.[49] The utility of PTA for long-term functional prediction has also been questioned.[50] Gollaher et al.[18] utilized a functional outcome measure, the Disability

Rating Scale (DRS),[51] which is based upon the GCS, but further discriminates higher functional levels. Educational level, admission DRS score, discharge DRS score, and preinjury productivity allowed correct classification of 84% for employed subjects, 66% for unemployed subjects, and 75% across both groups. Leung and Man[52] also determined that the DRS, in combination with the Cognistat (Neurobehavioral Cognitive Status Examination), and premorbid occupation were significant predictors of RTW that allowed correct classification of 65.8% of subjects in a 79-subject study.

Ip et al.[19] reviewed RTW for 90 individuals with TBI age 17 to 64 years and ranging in severity of injury from severe to mild. Subjects who could not complete the WAIS-R, Wechsler Memory Scale, Grooved Pegboard Test, Trail-Making Test, Grip Strength Test, and Finger Tapping Test of the Halstead-Reitan Neuropsychological Test Battery were excluded, potentially biasing the population to lesser severity. Seventy of the 90 were randomly selected, RTW rates were identified, and a predictive RTW equation was generated. The generalizability (external validity) of the equation was tested using data from the remaining 20 subjects. Return to work/school (RTW/S) was defined as full- or part-time RTW or school following discharge from the hospital. Forty-two percent of subjects returned to work or school whereas 58% failed to do so. Age, marital status and reported alcohol abuse were significantly associated with RTW/S. Those who were younger, never married, and had no alcohol abuse were most likely to return to work/school. Gender; preinjury occupational status (professional, skilled, laborer, or student); educational status; chronicity; GCS score; coma duration; and CT scan findings were not associated with RTW/S. Physical impairment was not associated with RTW/S, but cognitive functioning was. Performance IQ score of the WAIS-R, Visual Memory Index of the Wechsler Memory Scale-Revised (WMS-R), Trail Making A and B, and Grooved Pegboard of the nondominant hand were associated with RTW/S. Performance on all tests was worse for those who did not return to work/school. Performance IQ score of the WAIS-R was found to be the most significant predictor of RTW/S.

The relationship between severity of injury and the vocational outcome is not linear.[53] Generally speaking, when impairment level at 24 hours postinjury is related to productivity at follow-up, a relationship is found that more severe impairment leads to less productivity. Some notable exceptions exist, however, in that some individuals who are severely impaired at 24 hours postinjury achieve good outcomes, whereas comparatively less severely impaired individuals experience poorer outcomes. In a study by Sherer et al.,[54] initial severity of injury did not significantly predict postinjury productivity. Individuals in their sample ranged from mild to severe TBIs and all were involved in postacute rehabilitation programs. Education level, preinjury substance abuse, need for behavioral supervision, and need for physical supervision all correlated with productivity status. Interestingly, when adjusting for the effects of all other predictors, preinjury substance abuse emerged as the only significant predictor of productivity. Substance abuse has emerged as a predictor in several other studies as well.[34,54–56] Sherer et al.[54] cited possible selection bias in the study compared with other studies in which severity of injury was found to be indicative of RTW. The fact remains, however, that many moderately to severely injured individuals were found to be unable to return to work successfully when evaluated some 2 years postinjury.[57] Felmingham et al.[29] agreed that severity of injury impacted outcome, but only when paired with age.

Dawson et al.[58] investigated determinants and correlates of return to productivity postinjury in 46 individuals with TBI. Injury severity was found to be a significant predictor for return to productivity, as well as physical, psychological, and spiritual factors. It is important to note that psychological well-being is often a subjective experience and is a noted predictor of RTW status. Because of this, collecting subjective information related to mood, fatigue, and behavior, may be more valuable, at times, in predicting RTW than objective measures.[59] These factors can often become amplified following acute rehabilitation, and can enhance prognostic predictability. Felmingham et al.[29] found that adding postdischarge predictors to acute variables improved the ability to predict work status 2 years after rehabilitation, particularly regarding psychological well-being. Those noted to have better adjustment tended to perform better in the workforce. In a similar vein, some have noted that individuals who have difficulty with awareness and acceptance of deficits associated with TBI are less likely to experience vocational success.[60,61] Felmingham et al.[29] concluded that severity of injury (only when paired with age), age at the time of injury, premorbid employment status or work status at 6 months postinjury, and level of psychological distress 6 months postdischarge from a rehabilitation hospital setting were significant predictors of RTW. Devitt et al.[62] also suggest comprehensively assessing pre- and postinjury predictors to predict occupational performance. Ownsworth and McKenna[63] reviewed the literature to determine factors most consistently related to employment outcomes in TBI pre- and postinjury. They concluded that preinjury occupational status, functional status at discharge, global cognitive functioning, perceptual ability, executive functioning, involvement in vocational services, and emotional status were most likely to impact RTW.

Rao and Kilgore[55] reviewed 57 consecutive admissions of individuals with severe TBI averaging 30.8 years of age. All but five were gainfully employed outside the home or were full-time students prior to injury. However, between 14 and 26 months postinjury, 38 (67%) had returned to gainful competitive employment or school. Employment may not have been with a previous employer/job and return to school was defined as mainstreamed into the school environment with a maximum assistance of special education services that were routinely available at the school. A regression equation was developed that predicted RTW with 73.5% to 84.4% accuracy. Social factors such as substance abuse, family and community supports, and financial need to return to work were factors in cases when inaccurate prediction of RTW status occurred.

In summary, the research literature implicates age, severity of injury, coma duration, duration of acute rehabilitation, duration of PTA, postacute adjustment, awareness and acceptance of deficits, substance abuse, premorbid work status, educational attainment, and functional status in the prognostication of RTW. It is clear that no single variable has predictive power sufficient to be used independently of the others. Many of these variables essentially implicate the overall severity of injury, although not all. There are, nonetheless, notable exceptions in instances when persons with less severe injuries face difficulty in RTW, and when psychosocial circumstances or issues such as substance abuse and family and community supports, or financial need to return to work, intervene. Regardless of the factors involved, comprehensive rehabilitation with vocational services can improve outcomes.[61]

23.4 Industry-Related Factors Influencing Return to Work

Individuals with TBI may not be familiar with vocational rehabilitation services, and vice versa. In a survey of 620 TBI individuals who were 1 year postinjury, only 34% were aware of the existence of vocational rehabilitation services.[15] Those involved in outpatient or postacute rehabilitation and those who were employed preinjury were more likely to be aware of available services. Ironically, Vocational Rehabilitation Counselors (VRCs) appear to be similarly unaware of the needs of people with TBI. Hallauer et al.[7] found that most VRCs lack experience with TBI. Most counselors surveyed had work experience with fewer than 10 TBI clients. Counselors tended to overattribute problems in memory dysfunction, even in the absence of supportive test findings.

In a survey that involved the New York State Office of Vocational Rehabilitation,[8] the vocational rehabilitation program success for 47 individuals with TBI was reviewed. Only 8.5% of the individuals who received services were ultimately placed in jobs. The VRCs, as a group, reported factual unawareness for the need for cognitive remedial services for this population. These professionals were keenly aware that they did not have specific programs developed to address the needs of the individual with TBI.

The need to bring VRCs and medical rehabilitation teams together has been suggested by a number of authors.[64–66] Each of these groups provides coordinated interdisciplinary care. The knowledge base of the VRC can be materially increased in this manner.[66] An additional mismatch can be found between the perceptions of VRCs and employers.[67] Employers' primary concerns had to do with whether the individual could actually fulfill the job responsibilities. Concerns of VRCs, however, tended to focus on workplace accommodations. Lastly, one study indicated failed vocational rehabilitation programs tended to be too short in duration or too long postinjury to be effective.[68]

Lack of availability of rehabilitation services, division of responsibility for rehabilitation between several governmental and private sector agencies, economic decline, employer's fitness requirements, disability discrimination, delayed or ineffectual management of treatable diseases and conditions, and disability compensation benefits can all contribute to failure to return to work.[69–75] Numerous articles have suggested the potential contribution of compensation in failure to return to work in the general population.[10,72–76] Although care must be taken in interpreting these ideas, there are clearly some discrepancies in RTW that are difficult to explain—namely, those found in RTW of people with mild to moderate TBI. There are differences in RTW rates for those people receiving disability and social security benefits and those who do not,[72,74] and some find vocational rehabilitation to be a potentially destabilizing threat to their financial status and eligibility for public health care coverage, such as Medicaid or Medicare.[73]

In summary, at the point of involvement of vocational rehabilitation, the individual with TBI may, or may not, have participated in medical rehabilitation. Participation in medical rehabilitation cannot be guaranteed, especially for those individuals who might be referred to departments of vocational rehabilitation without adequate documentation of the previous TBI. Once involved in the vocational rehabilitation process, placement may not be achieved or maintained as a result of (1) inadequate resolution of sequelae of the TBI; (2) awareness by individuals with TBI, their families, medical rehabilitation professionals, or vocational rehabilitation professionals of the need for vocational rehabilitation services; (3) knowledge on the part of the VRC regarding how to pursue job placement for individuals with TBI; (4) failure of the job placement to meet the esteem and financial needs of the injured worker; (5) socially inappropriate or unacceptable behaviors; (6) a mismatch between the focus of the VRC and the needs of the employer; (7) financial disincentives to RTW; or (8) a societal predisposition toward continued unemployment resulting from divergent agency goals or insufficient public expenditures to support RTW efforts. This list is by no means exhaustive or complete and, as such, points to the tremendous complexity of returning an individual with TBI to work.

23.5 Vocational Rehabilitation Prerequisites

Readiness for vocational rehabilitation, of course, involves identification and treatment of deficits following TBI—and more. In many jurisdictions, state legislatures have enacted rules that must be followed, in particular, when individuals are injured during the course of their employment. The VRC and, in some instances, medical rehabilitation providers should be familiar with reporting requirements and be able to comply with the various filings that may be required.

Ideally, the vocational rehabilitation process begins during the medical rehabilitation of individuals with TBI. The VRC should be familiar with the goals and plans of the medical rehabilitation team from an early point in the rehabilitation process. Likewise, the medical rehabilitation team can obtain insight from the VRC regarding the injured individual's personality, social status, educational attainment, socialization skills, and vocational aptitudes, all of which may bear upon medical rehabilitation goal setting. Rehabilitation teams often focus on "functional" capabilities, and achievement of a "functional" level of independence may not be sufficient to allow successful RTW.

An early review of an individual's deficits may allow a VRC timely recognition of those barriers to RTW that are likely to be overcome and those that are less likely. In instances when the individual is unlikely to return to a previous vocational setting, introduction of this idea to the injured individual and the family may allow for professional assistance with adjustment and better financial planning for the family. Adjustment to disability can be quite difficult and some people with TBI are reluctant to accept that their level of functioning may not be sufficient to allow a return to a previous level of employment.[29,60,77] Often, clients are unwilling to shift their expectations for RTW and can be resistant to rehabilitation plans that move in a direction other than return to previous employment. Medical rehabilitation providers can be quite helpful in assisting with adjustment issues and creatively addressing barriers to employment or development of vocational alternatives. The interplay between the vocational and medical rehabilitation professionals with the individual and his or her family can best ensure that the highest levels of independence and life satisfaction are incorporated into goal setting.

The VRC should work with medical rehabilitation professionals to conduct prevocational testing. Prevocational testing can be invaluable in identifying barriers to RTW for all parties. A host of standardized and subjective assessments can be utilized in this pursuit, and detailed information can be obtained that spells out deficits that will impact RTW. The allied health disciplines of occupational therapy, physical therapy, speech therapy, therapeutic recreation, educational therapy, clinical psychology, and neuropsychology can also provide insight into likely problem areas. Situational assessment to confirm test findings should be considered during prevocational testing.[78] Additionally, a review of a thorough job description, together with functional observation and the comprehensive interview, should accompany neuropsychological evaluation as the VRC attempts to discern vocational readiness and aptitude.[43] Care must be taken in evaluating people with TBI to avoid an overreliance on standardized testing. One study suggested that 38% of VRCs surveyed relied, either moderately or very heavily, on standardized testing.[8] A learning-style evaluation during prevocational testing may be helpful in determining optimal and nonoptimal strategy development for presentation of new learning.[43,79] To that end, the degree to which an intended vocational placement relies upon rote activities versus new learning should be considered. Based on prevocational testing results, attainment of further rehabilitative treatment may be necessary to prepare people better for success in the workplace.

23.6 Injury-Related Factors Influencing Return to Work

Introduction of vocational rehabilitation services typically occurs at a time determined by medical rehabilitation professionals. Although, on the surface, this may seem logical, the approach is problematic in those instances when well-meaning, although poorly informed, professionals believe that the medical rehabilitation has, in fact, resulted in a readiness for vocational rehabilitation. Unfortunately, all too often, this is not the case, and individuals with TBI are prematurely returned to work and are subjected unnecessarily to failure. This is clearly demonstrated in the literature reviewed thus far.

The typical approach taken in vocational rehabilitation is to attempt to achieve medical stability prior to undertaking vocational rehabilitation services. Recovery from TBI, however, seldom finds an individual at a point at which a clear demarcation exists between the end of medical treatment and readiness for vocational rehabilitation. The complexity of deficits seen following TBI complicates the delineation of the starting point for vocational rehabilitation.

The constellation of deficits seen following TBI can include motor, cognitive, communicative, psychosocial, psychological, and behavioral impairments.[5,80] Some of these deficits will persist in some fashion despite the best efforts at medical rehabilitation. Cognitive deficits, physical deficits, and personality changes contribute to failure in RTW.[5,14,20,27,81–83] Of course, severity of injury may impact both the number of deficits and their persistence, although there is not, necessarily, a direct relationship between severity of injury and likelihood of RTW.[29,40,55]

23.6.1 Physical Deficits

Given the shortened time frames in rehabilitation of people with TBI,[84–86] therapists are forced to focus on functional capabilities for performance of basic self-care and daily routines as a primary goal. Rarely will goals beyond these be a consideration early in the rehabilitation of a person with TBI, largely as a result of funding and utilization review constraints. Although the world has become much more "accessible" for people with physical disabilities, optimization of physical functioning following TBI via extended therapy can be quite important in RTW. Wehman et al.[45] discerned that an individual's level of functional limitations impacted the likelihood of RTW. Just as physical and cognitive limitations would impair functional capabilities with reference to self-care skills, these limitations appeared to culminate ultimately in difficulties in RTW as well. Physical limitations can bring about significant challenges to self-concept, body image, and social interactions, all of which are likely to impact RTW.[87] The VRC is in a unique position to advocate for such additional interventions.

The VRC must consider mobility, balance, coordination, vestibular function, extremity strength and range of motion, muscular and cardiorespiratory endurance, dexterity, vision, audition, and smell. The individual must be able to move about the workplace freely and safely. The highest level of ambulation with the least reliance upon aids should be sought. Canes, walkers, and wheelchairs, although designed to enhance environmental access, unfortunately, may contribute to workplace biases about an individual's inherent abilities. More pragmatically, such devices can raise questions in an employer's mind regarding safety.

Balance, coordination, and vestibular function must be such that the person is not experiencing dizziness that could impede the ability to move about the workplace or complete various job tasks.[88] Chamelian and Feinstein found that dizziness can cause significant emotional distress postinjury, and may be an independent predictor of failure to RTW.[89] Dehail et al.[90] reviewed 68 consecutive admissions of individuals with TBI to a vocational rehabilitation program compared with 52 healthy, age-matched control subjects. Mean age of the TBI group was 33.2 years with a mean chronicity since injury of 55.2 months. GCS score for the group averaged 6.6 points; however, the GCS score was less than 8 points for 60 of the 68 individuals. One third of the individuals with severe TBI complained of vertigo, dizziness, or balance instability at admission. Clinical examination found impairments in 17 of these and none in 9. Of those who had no complaints of vertigo, dizziness, or balance instability, clinical examination showed impairments in 19 cases. There were no demonstrable correlations between any posturographic parameter and age, gender, scores on cognitive tests, brain magnetic resonance imaging or CT abnormality, or psychotropic treatment. There were no correlations for those with or without complaints. It was clear that visual deprivation contributed strongly to posturographic findings. Individual awareness of deficits could not be relied upon for either confirmation of deficits of balance or for a lack thereof. The findings of Dehail et al.[90] bear significantly on risks associated with RTW, in particular for reinjury. Individuals who may need to work in low-light conditions may be particularly vulnerable. Individuals cannot be relied upon to report deficits accurately that may place them and their employer at risk. Confirmation of a lack of balance problems should be obtained by the VRC. Of course, such impairments may preclude return to certain jobs, such as those that require climbing ladders or working at heights. Physical therapy and medical treatment can be quite beneficial in improving functional capacity for balance disorders following TBI and can improve protective reactions. Care should be taken to avoid reliance solely upon medications that reduce the experience of dizziness because these medications act only to reduce the symptoms rather than improve the underlying condition. Consequently, impaired protective reactions continue to be present, thereby increasing the likelihood of reinjury. Information about vestibular dysfunction can be found in this text in the Chapter 6.

Perceptual deficits in either vision or hearing can also impact successful job task completion, socialization, communication, and safety. (See Chapters 7, 8, and 9 on vision, and Chapter 10 on audiology.) In some workplaces, the sense of smell is important to safety (e.g., in working with combustible liquids or gases) and may be integral to actual job task completion (e.g., in food preparation or storage responsibilities).

Muscular and cardiorespiratory endurance will materially impact job performance and mental acuity. Fatigue is a frequently reported component of TBI impairment.[5] Deconditioning following prolonged disability is common and should be assessed and addressed prior to RTW. Most jobs require a fairly high level of manual dexterity. As such, dexterity must be considered, as well as adaptations that may be appropriate to a specific job description. Further detailed information about treatment of physical deficits can be found in Chapter 22.

Finally, it is important to address the impact of fatigue on RTW. Up to 73% of people with TBI experience fatigue 5 years after injury. The long-standing effects of fatigue impact both physical and psychological functioning. In a study of 223 people with mild to severe TBI, Cantor et al.[91] found that postinjury fatigue negatively impacted subjective reports of quality of life. They also found, however, that fatigue did not negatively impact participation in desired life activities, meaning that fatigue was not stopping people from participating in life, but negatively impacted the quality of participation. Ziino and Ponsford[92] found that fatigue reduced the quality of performance on selective attention tasks and other complex cognitive tasks independent of mood. These types of tasks are common in the workplace.

With appropriate rehabilitation and structured routines, fatigue in the workplace can be managed to allow for improved quality of participation. Strategies for fatigue management include controlling cognitive processing demands by practicing tasks until they are well learned, reducing cognitive processing demands by simplifying tasks,[92] and scheduling frequent rest breaks.

23.6.2 Psychological and Behavioral Issues

TBI can cause significant disruption of function in the psychological/psychiatric realm, resulting in deficits in interpersonal, social, and occupational function.[93] Thorough rehabilitation for people with TBI may include psychiatric, psychological, and neuropsychological evaluation and interventions. Personality and neuropsychological testing that utilizes input from the client, family, friends, and coworkers will provide the greatest level of understanding for all rehabilitation professionals involved. Care should be taken, however, to avoid overreliance on neuropsychological test results for the determination of vocational aptitude or readiness.[78,94] Neuropsychological findings are best used in conjunction with observation of function in real-world settings. It is not uncommon following TBI to need to provide psychological interventions for awareness of and adjustment to disability,[95–97] motivation, sexuality, stress management, fear, interpersonal relationship management, depression,[98,99] substance abuse,[98] lifestyle changes, irritability and loss of temper,[5] family issues, parenting,[100] coping style,[101] spousal relationships,[102] anxiety,[98] and goal setting. The VRC may play a role in many of these areas, either in providing some of the counseling or providing insight into some of these areas to other psychology staff.

Evaluative tools, such as the Minnesota Multiphasic Personality Inventory II (MMPI-II),[103] the Taylor-Johnson Temperament Analysis,[104] the Fundamental Interpersonal Relations Orientation–Behavior Scale,[105] and the Beck Depression Scale,[106] can be useful in understanding variables that may be barriers to RTW. Care should be taken in interpretation of the MMPI-II because deficits following TBI can, fairly predictably, elevate specific scales, such as depression, hypochondriasis/somatization, schizophrenia, and psychosis.[107] Some have suggested that scoring of the MMPI for this population should be altered for this reason.[108–110] The tool can be useful, nonetheless, in a careful consideration of its findings coupled with information from the clinical observations of allied health professionals and family.

TBI is overwhelming in its impact upon the individual, and coping with the seemingly total change in one's abilities and lifestyle is arduous and grueling. Adaptation to such profound changes in one's life can take a lifetime, yet rehabilitation demands such accommodation in months. The VRC should have sufficient background to be able to identify when phases of the vocational rehabilitation process will be too challenging or likely to elicit maladaptive responses or adjustment opportunities. For example, a person placed in an employment position by a vocational rehabilitation counselor who knows the placement will fail may yield either an improved awareness of remaining areas of deficit to be worked on in therapy or a humiliation that strips the individual of all motivation. The difference between these two outcomes should be predicted by the VRC who is aware of the psychological status of the injured worker. Prevocational counseling allows for such insight to be gained by the counselor. The counselor may be in a position to recommend the involvement of a counselor or psychologist for rigorous investigation and treatment of issues pertaining to attitudes toward RTW, motivation, adjustment to disability, and so on. Given the pervasive and all-encompassing nature the impact of TBI has on one's life, all but the rarest of individuals will benefit from some assistance in handling the psychological burden.

Participation in therapy following TBI is difficult and some people suffer from motivational challenges to continue therapeutic endeavors. The appropriately designed vocational rehabilitation plan can be helpful to some in coming to an understanding of why seemingly useless therapy tasks will benefit them when they return to work. Conversely, although the proper timing of RTW has been emphasized, there are some instances when motivation to complete therapy tasks and goals can be enhanced by engaging the person in some part-time, perhaps lower level, RTW that is meaningfully associated with or drawn from their intended final vocational placement. Participation in the workplace exercises, in effect, all the skills that are the focus of therapeutic endeavors. Such placements, conducted coincidentally with therapy, can allow the individual to realize limitations and the relationship between those limitations gradually, successful completion of therapy tasks to address those limitations, and success in the workplace.

The individual's financial needs and status must be well understood prior to undertaking vocational rehabilitation.[71–75] This includes a review of all sources of income, including income that may derive from pending legal proceedings. The individual's financial well-being should be considered, together with the benefits that come from independence and self-reliance. An ethical quagmire can readily emerge in these considerations and the VRC should be well versed in both legal requirements that may impact vocational planning and ethical issues that ought to guide the counselor's approach to a case. An excellent review of ethical issues can be found in Chapter 30.

Motivational concerns that may present as challenges to a successful vocational plan can arise from both questionable and legitimate issues. In a study of 37 individuals with TBI in supported employment settings, West[111] concluded that a primary factor distinguishing those who retained employment after 6 months from those who did not could be found in whether the positions in which individuals were placed offered fringe benefits, opportunities for raises and advancement, formal and informal support, and opportunities for socialization with other employees. There were no statistically significant differences between the two groups in race, marital status, highest educational level achieved, residential status, community type, cause or severity of injury, work status prior to injury or prior to referral to supported employment, or age. The small size of the subject pool, however, is an important consideration. West[111] pointed out that career development differs from job placement, alone. The degree to which both are driven by the individual's goals and motivation will heighten the likelihood that positions that will hold the individual's interest inspire good work skills and behaviors, thereby promoting long-term success. As indicated earlier, the primary reasons for job separation from the first and second employment opportunities are related to interpersonal skills. Maintenance of personal boundaries can be difficult for the person with TBI. This includes respecting personal space, identifying body language that signals continued or waning interest in a conversational topic, respecting overt requests for changes in topic or cessation of a discussion, engaging in appropriate social pleasantries, respecting professional relationships and avoiding overly familiar behaviors, using proper manners, controlling emotional lability, and executing impulse control.

Social skills are acquired over a lifetime and are continuously updated. Social judgment is crucial in the workplace because it represents a primary source of socialization for most people. Social skills used on the job are considerably different than those used in the home environment and there is a clear demarcation of expectations between these two environments. TBI often impairs a person's ability to pick up on social cues, such as body language, facial expression, and subtle linguistic cues, that may be given. Failure to identify these cues will readily result in social isolation and failure, which obviously will impact both the injured person's ability to complete job tasks successfully and his or her derivation of personal satisfaction and self-esteem from the workplace.

Differences in level of socialization have been identified with different types of supported employment environment.[112] Individual, enclave, and work crew-supported employment environments were analyzed for the amount of contact between disabled and nondisabled workers. Individual and enclave environments showed substantially more interaction between coworkers than work crew environments. Individual and enclave environments might be more conducive to social integration, a key component in job retention and life satisfaction. Because job separations are common following TBI, and RTW occurs for only a portion of those injured, care must be taken not to jeopardize availability of financial support from such sources as Social Security, disability insurance policies, or permanent disability payments from workers' compensation claims. Dikmen et al.[113] reported on the earnings of 31 individuals with moderate to severe brain injury followed 2 years postinjury. Although the group was no different than a control group in earnings prior to injury, earnings were substantially below those of the control group at 1 year. Earnings improved slightly by year 2, although they remained substantially below the control group. Ashley et al.[114] conducted a follow-up study of 332 people with TBI who averaged 7.1 years postinjury and 5.3 years postdischarge. The group was heavily biased in that all participants had access to treatment funding from workers' compensation, accident and health, or liability insurance coverage. The study showed that only 83.9% of respondents reported they were financially "getting by or better." The estimated mean of monthly income loss per family was $1,058 in 1997 dollars, whereas the mean household earnings was decreased by about $402, suggesting that others in the family had become employed or changed employment to higher paying positions.

TBI regularly places families below the median income level and often into poverty levels. In the study by Ashley et al.,[114] 16.1% of respondents reported increased indebtedness and 7.4% required public assistance for medical costs. These numbers can be reasonably assumed to be much higher for the TBI population in general.

Income stability can become an issue in the case of people who were employed in seasonal positions. Those people who are covered by workers' compensation may acquire a more stable income source following injury. In some cases, prolonged medical disability translates to prolonged maintenance of immigration status. In still others, psychological benefits accrue from being dependent upon a spouse or parent or, conversely, spouses or other family members may derive some psychological or financial benefit from continued levels of dependency, such as when family members are paid for care of an injured person.

23.6.3 Cognitive Deficits

Cognitive rehabilitation following TBI represents one of the greatest challenges facing allied health professionals and people with TBI. Cognitive function impacts all aspects of daily living, social interaction, psychological function and adjustment, communication, and, of course, work. Rehabilitative efforts in cognition can be both compensatory and remediative.[115–117] Rehabilitation of cognitive function requires medical stability and a great deal of therapeutic effort. The most successful cognitive rehabilitation takes place over months, rather than weeks. Compensatory strategies may be developed, in some instances, to support the injured worker in job performance; however, some levels of cognitive dysfunction are less amenable to compensatory approaches. A realistic appraisal of the likelihood of success is crucial.

Cognitive deficits, such as problems with attention, concentration, persistence, problem solving, judgment, reasoning, memory, and self-regulation of behavior, will all detrimentally affect the injured worker's ability to perform on the job. Such deficits can be present in people without any obvious physical impairments and can be camouflaged by intact expressive language skills. Bjerke[118] found a lack of correspondence between neuropsychological tests results and levels of reported memory function for people with TBI. Severity of injury did not correspond linearly to reported memory function. The VRC must carefully investigate allied health professionals' assessment and documentation of cognitive skills, and determine the degree to which they will impact job performance. Various jobs have different cognitive demands; for example, the cognitive requirements for professional and technical positions are greater and will require more attention to higher level cognitive function.[46]

A primary indicator of success may be found in the individual's attention skills. Mateer and Sira[119] relate five components of attention: arousal, sustained attention, working attention, selective attention, and divided/alternating attention. The person must be able to maintain a focus of attention without undue interference or loss of information (sustained attention and vigilance). They must also be able to shift attention readily between two or more activities and do so efficiently without undue delay or loss of information or accuracy (divided/alternating attention). Melamed et al.[120] found that attentional capacity for shifting between dual task performance correlated with likelihood of RTW. Internal distractions can pose a problem for the individual. Techniques, such as thought-stopping exercises and learning to manage one's reactions to error, can reduce internal distractions.[119]

Mateer and Sira[119] suggest that education, rehabilitation, and environmental support can be effective for higher levels of attention, such as sustained attention, working memory, selective attention, and divided/alternating attention.[119] These include

1. Reduction of distractions
2. Selection of facilitating environments
3. Reduced visual clutter
4. Posted reminders
5. Labels
6. Message centers
7. Use of external aids (written calendars, personal data assistants)

They also suggest the utilization of task management strategies, such as doing one thing at a time, using earplugs, using answering machines or voice mail to reduce interruptions, and selecting nonpeak activity times to engage in certain aspects of one's work when the activity level of the environment can be expected to be lesser. Other strategies include

1. Pacing
2. Alternating an easy task with a difficult task
3. Taking breaks
4. Slowly increasing the amount of time on a task
5. Taking enough time to finish a task

Metacognitive strategies, such as encouraging the development of awareness of attentional failures and the reasons for them, can be helpful.[119] The individual's sense of self-control and his or her ability to manage his or her emotional response may improve with such awareness, positively impacting self-esteem.

Memory impairments clearly pose great difficulty in RTW. In some circumstances, the individual may not have been given access to or benefitted from cognitive rehabilitation services that resulted in improved memory function. Internal compensatory memory strategies can be effective in that they are always available to the individual. However, they can be limited in effectiveness as a result of difficulties the individual has in recognizing a need for a particular strategy or difficulty remembering to use a strategy.[119] External memory aids can be considered and may be more pragmatic, depending upon the nature of the information to be remembered or aided. External or environmental supports include

1. Environmental modification
2. Posted lists
3. Labeling
4. Calendars
5. External reminders
6. Aids such as
    A. Alarms
    B. Timers
    C. Beeping watches
    D. Computer-based reminders
    E. Pagers
    F. Cell phones
    G. Key finders
    H. Medication organizers
    I. Personal data assistants
    J. Voice recorders
    K. Calendars/memory books
    L. To-do lists
    M. Contacts list

In the end, even these techniques can fail as a result of the individual forgetting to use them, difficulty in operating devices, failure to use a technique systematically, or simple embarrassment.[119] Finally, the creation of task-specific routines can be useful in the form of checklists that enable the individual to be systematically reminded on how to complete a routine in the same manner every time.

Executive function is critical to overall success in RTW. The individual must be able to initiate, set goals, plan, organize, exercise judgment, and self-monitor and modify plans and/or behaviors according to feedback received.[95,119] The end product of job performance may not be immediately apparent in many vocations in which the work of an individual contributes to a large process and delayed production or emergence of a work product. In these instances, deficits in discriminating response–consequence relations[121] may impact an injured person's understanding of the impact of a failure to execute his or her job responsibilities properly or his or her ability to identify social cues within the workplace. Further detail regarding cognitive function and rehabilitation can be found in Chapter 18 and Chapter 19 in this volume.

RTW may be most successful in cases when job performance relies heavily upon previously learned information and skills and when physical impairments are relatively minor or can be minimized by adaptation of the workplace. Job performance that relies heavily upon new learning or rapid information assimilation will pose far greater challenges to the person with cognitive deficits following TBI.

23.6.4 Communicative Deficits

Some of the more common communicative deficits seen following TBI include oral dysarthria,[122–124] impairments of voice production and volume,[125–129] impairments of the prosodic features of speech,[130] impairments in auditory processing speed and accuracy,[131] and impairments in communicative pragmatics.[132–135]

Oral dysarthria presents with a slurred, thickened speech and can imbue the speaker with unflattering attributes to the uninformed listener. The speaker can appear to be under the influence of alcohol or drugs or can appear less intelligent than is truly the case. Because understanding dysarthric speech requires much more time and effort on the part of the listener, communication on the job may be diminished to unacceptable levels. Couple this with the logical impact on socialization, and a formula for isolation is present. A negative spiral beginning with difficult communication can progress to a reluctance to engage in appropriate clarification of details for a job task, reluctance in allocation of job tasks to the injured worker, frustration for the injured worker and supervisor at task failure, and arrival at a conclusion that the injured worker cannot complete the necessary job tasks to maintain employment.

Likewise, other communicative deficits can bring about deterioration of communicative events within a workplace. Inability to engage in communicative pragmatics, such as appropriate conversational turn-taking or maintenance of the topic of conversation among a group of coworkers, will discourage others from approaching and engaging the injured worker in either job-related or social discourse. People with TBI often have difficulty getting the point from figurative or metaphoric expressions, knowing the alternate meanings of ambiguous words, deriving inference, conveying the communicative intent of a speaker to another, and resolution of communicative ambiguity.[136] They will often produce speech that is shorter in length, less complex, and with less cohesion than people without TBI.[137] These tendencies will complicate communication on the job and require attention prior to and after RTW. Understanding the communicative intent of a speaker is heavily dependent upon interpretation of the prosodic nature of the communicative act and accompanying cues can be found in facial expression and body language. Failure to detect the facial and body language expressions of coworkers or employers often manifests as failure to identify and respect social boundaries. This can have devastating impact on communication and interpersonal relationships. Ability to perceive and remember facial expression has been demonstrated to be impaired in some people with TBI.[138,139]

Any communicative disorder must be considered for the potential to bring about effects upon the workplace as described earlier. Disorders of prosody, such as speaking with a monotone voice or speaking too loudly or softly, can cause tremendous confusion of the communicative intent. A person who speaks in a monotone voice can appear disinterested or unmotivated. Speaking too loudly may make it difficult for coworkers or employers to have confidence that the injured worker can handle sensitive issues in an appropriately discreet fashion. The speaker may be confused to be angry or upset when speaking too loudly. Dysfluency or stuttering sometimes occurs following TBI.[140,141] The general public historically misunderstands the dysfluent person, thinking him or her shy, unconfident, or difficult to listen to. Often, the dysfluent person is reluctant to speak because of the effort required and the embarrassment experienced.

The VRC may be able to impact the workplace by education of the nature of a particular communicative disorder, by adaptation of the workplace, or by encouraging continued remedial therapeutic efforts. Hearing problems may be addressed by medical intervention, amplification, environmental noise reduction, or written communication. In some instances, sign language may be used to some degree. Visual or language deficits may preclude reliance upon written communication, however. As such, graphic skills must also be evaluated for both their potential as a means of expressive communication and as a job requirement for task documentation or interoffice communication. Dexterity may impact the person's ability to write legibly or to use a keyboard for electronic communication.

23.7 Return to Work Models

Several models for RTW after TBI evolved in the 1980s, including the *cognitive remediation* model,[97] the *work hardening* model,[142] and the *supported employment* model.[143] Of these models, the most efficacious model appeared to be the supported employment model. In the supported employment model, "job coaches" are assigned to individuals to work alongside the injured worker in the workplace. Their primary function is to teach the job, monitor performance, and provide feedback for the individual and other rehabilitation professionals regarding job completion and quality.[144,145] Compensatory strategies may be implemented on the job as identified and designed by the job coach. West et al.[145] describe the role of job coach as having an advocacy component and an active role in job retention by provision of assessment of social skills and productivity. These authors and others[46] suggest that job coaching be both intensive and of sufficient duration to ensure proper RTW and job retention. Wehman et al.[146] reported that an average of 291 hours of job coaching was used to secure and maintain job placement in a population of people with TBI who averaged 7 years postinjury and 53 days of unconsciousness. Haffey and Abrams[147] reported a mean of only 85 hours per client for job coaching; however, their population was much closer to date of injury. Catalano et al.[148] reported an average case expenditure for successfully vocationally rehabilitated individuals of $4,809 over a much longer program that averaged 27.51 months. Clearly, interventions, such as job coaching, could not have been extensively used. Expenditures appear to have been related to job support, such as counseling, miscellaneous services, and college training costs.

Utilization of job coaching, however, is not without its disadvantages. The injured worker can be stigmatized by the presence of the job coach. It may be difficult to transition the job coach out of the work environment. Lastly, the job coach may impact the manner in which other employees behave and interact with the injured worker.[149] Consequently, it may be advisable to look for opportunities to use coworkers in a supportive role with the injured worker, although care must be taken to time the transition from a job coach to a coworker properly when the relative workload warrants such a change.

Wehman et al.[150] reported on vocational outcomes for 59 individuals with moderate to severe TBI. Individuals' injuries were classified as moderate to severe if coma duration was greater than 24 hours or if GCS score was less than 13 points. Average age was 32.6 years. The majority of individuals had a high school education or greater (76.9%) and 71.4% were employed full-time prior to injury, 3.6% part-time, and 1.8% were students who also worked. Individuals who returned to work averaged 42.58 months of employment with an average salary of $26,129.74 per year. The average cost of employment services was $10,349.37. Cumulative earnings for the group equaled $1,489,395 and cumulative program costs equaled $491,032.

Some authors suggest that supported employment may not be the most efficient model for successful vocational rehabilitation of people with TBI.[151] Models involving job coaches can be costly, reportedly $9,000 to $10,000,[152] and, consequently, such services may not be made available to people with less financial support for recovery. As a consequence, less expensive models have been used with the TBI population. These models include the *clubhouse* model,[153] *community-based training* model,[36] and the *empowerment* model.[151]

- The *clubhouse* model uses community-based training and natural supports. "Clubhouses" are "work units" that provide various work samples for clients to identify their particular interests and relative strengths. Support, training, and employment opportunities drive this model. An estimated 18% to 23% of those involved in the clubhouse model ultimately participate in competitive employment.[153]

- The *community-based training* model incorporates supported employment and work adjustment training to address economic disadvantages, job retention, and identification of meaningful and satisfying employment. These programs allow for equal input from the individual, program staff, and training/work site with an RTW plan developed. Individuals obtain work skills in an unpaid work setting. When the employment opportunity begins, the job coach is introduced to assist the person during transition into competitive employment by providing suggestions for work modifications, assistive devices, and strategies for improved work performance.[36] Community-based training models greatly challenge strategy development and enhance the opportunity for generalized work skills.[36]

- The *empowerment* model was designed to consist of several elements sequentially performed to include intake of personal information, vocational evaluation, work samples, work hardening, vocational counseling, job skills training, development of job skills, job training placement, and counseling for continued support.[151] Abrams et al.[151] followed 106 people involved with this type of vocational rehabilitation. Within 1 year, 92% were employed and 24% returned to the previous employment. They emphasized coordination of services based on individual need rather than mandatory programmatic requirements for people with TBI.

In summary, models of vocational rehabilitation currently in use for people with TBI achieve the best outcomes when they consider the unique challenges of this population and utilize integrative approaches over appropriate time durations and with appropriate supports. As these models become more widely implemented, it will be possible to conduct research to determine whether the programs are less expensive and involve more clients in the vocational rehabilitation system and to determine which approaches yield the best outcomes for subgroups of the TBI population.

23.8 Formalized Vocational Rehabilitation in TBI

The literature supports the idea that disincentives for RTW exist and negatively impact RTW rates. Of interest is the idea that RTW is higher for those without such disincentives. The need to work can be financial, social, or emotional. Although workers' compensation benefits often include some provision for vocational rehabilitation, accident and health insurance plans have no such provision. So, although vocational rehabilitation may be accessible under workers' compensation plans, the individual with private health insurance coverage will require other options. The need to integrate vocational rehabilitation services into medical rehabilitation planning and programming, and the improved outcomes associated with early versus late vocational interventions creates a dilemma for professionals. It can be difficult to bring about such vocational planning integration and prolonged vocational rehabilitation programming as is often required following brain injury. Hence, it may be useful to consider roles to be played by professionals of the treatment team. The scope of practice for occupational therapy includes "work," which encompasses employment-related and volunteer activities. Consequently, it is clearly acceptable for occupational therapy to assist in all processes related to RTW and may serve as an important option in the face of restricted benefits for vocational rehabilitation counseling specifically. The need for integration of vocational rehabilitation services provided by public agencies into the medical rehabilitation planning and programming presents yet another considerable challenge to be considered.

23.8.1 Prevocational Counseling

Prevocational counseling is a process during which the client's readiness to return to work becomes an active focus of treatment. The client's readiness and expectations must be reviewed and, perhaps, adjusted. Adjustment to disability can stand as a significant barrier to RTW, especially in instances when the individual may not be able to return to preinjury employment. It may be necessary to return to a lesser position within an employment setting, a part-time position, or a different position and employer altogether. For some, return to competitive employment may be questionable and only attainable after an extended period of work hardening. Finally, some individuals may be unable to return to work in any capacity, or may have sheltered work placement as a long-term outcome. Given the degree to which work impacts self-esteem and self-concept,[87] changes in work status following injury can have tremendous impact upon the individual, his or her family, and his or her social interaction.

In the prevocational counseling process, information is collected regarding historical matters, such as level of educational attainment and achievement. Previous work positions, employers, pay scales, and relevant vocational information are collected. It can be helpful to determine the nature of positions that exist with the employer of injury as well as contacts that family and friends may have. Previous employers can be helpful in RTW, especially in instances when the person was well-regarded. As historical information is collected and considered, it must be combined with information of known or anticipated limitations that may arise resulting from physical, cognitive, behavioral, psychological, social, communicative, or emotional factors. For example, an individual with an extensive roofing installation background who has vestibular and visual deficits is unlikely to return to roofing installation. However, the person's extensive knowledge base may facilitate work in the roofing field as an estimator, sales person, or supervisor.

23.8.2 Vocational Rehabilitation Plan Development

The vocational plan begins during the prevocational counseling process as the counselor attempts to piece together options for the various phases of RTW that may be necessary for the client. Requisite phases will vary from client to client. In many instances, development of a formal vocational rehabilitation plan will be required for submission to workers' compensation agencies or other funding sources for approval. In others, the formal vocational rehabilitation plan and all the attendant filing of forms may not be needed. Nonetheless, the formal vocational rehabilitation plan is integral to the process of returning an injured worker to work.

Plans developed for different individuals will vary considerably in the amount of time needed, the cost, and the process as a result of the tremendous individuality of each person with TBI. The plan must be developed in congruence with the interests, goals, aptitudes, and abilities of the injured worker, as well as consideration of the labor market and job availability. Ninomiya et al.[154] developed a list of issues that should be considered during the development of a rehabilitation plan. They include

- Actual versus stated motivation for the client's RTW
- The individual's cognitive abilities
- The individual's emotional profile
- Physical deficits and limitations
- Family support and interactions
- Financial gain/need
- Litigation
- Self-esteem and self-concept
- Work ethic
- Work history
- Preinjury work characteristics
- Current and preinjury personality factors
- Adjustment to disability
- Transferable skills
- Age
- The general employment index in the geographic area of the intended discharge
- Employer prejudices regarding brain injury and other disabilities
- General medical stability
- The presence or absence of a seizure disorder or other neurologic deficits
- Potential areas of conflict arising from various secondary gain issues

Vocational plans traditionally encompass one of the following seven outcomes: *RTW, modified work, alternative work, direct placement, on-the-job training, formalized schooling or training,* and *self-employment.* The order listed suggests a hierarchy of desirability. The *RTW* outcome is achieved when injured workers return to their former employment, in the same position, the same number of hours, and the same workplace. A *modified work* outcome consists of a return to the former employer, although modifications have been made to the work process or work site to accommodate for physical, cognitive, or other limitations.

An *alternative work* placement also occurs with the former employer, although the injured worker is placed in a different position altogether. The new position may have been identified via transferable skills analysis and is consistent with any limitations. *Direct placement* consists of a new position with a new employer or a similar position to the position of pre-injury employment, again using transferable skills. *On-the-job training* occurs with a new position and a new employer. The employer provides a training environment and some or all of the training. Responsibility for compensation can be shared between employer and a workers' compensation carrier. Insurance or employer benefits may continue until a successful long-term placement is assured. *Formalized schooling or training* plans involve enrollment in a vocational or academic schooling setting for the purpose of achieving vocational placement upon completion. The *self-employment* outcome is used when the plan is to establish a new, independent business that the injured worker will operate. Each of these plans assumes a competitive employment outcome. Occasionally, during execution of a plan, the VRC and injured worker may determine that the plan is not going to be successful. They may opt to modify the rehabilitation plan and establish a different outcome as the goal of the new plan.

The VRC will need to explore creative vocational options with the client, the employer, and family and friends, as well as medical rehabilitation providers. The process can require great diplomacy and careful planning. Although many employers are eager to be helpful in returning an individual to work, there may be other circumstances in which the employer is less willing. For example, the individual may have had a poor work record or may have been injured shortly after hiring. He or she may have been difficult to get along with. The employer may be fearful of reinjury or customer reaction to the injured worker. Some employers are angry with injured workers, either for the damage done to themselves or others, or for the financial losses incurred. Conversely, employers can be unrealistically optimistic about the person's recovery and, in their efforts to be supportive and encouraging, promote an RTW that is neither likely nor reasonable.

Care must be taken to avoid premature RTW or RTW that is ill-suited to the person's skills. A well-meaning family, employer, medical rehabilitation provider, or client can bring about an RTW that is doomed to failure as a result of poor matching of the job requirements and the person's residual and recovered skills. Vocational failure brings about embarrassment, humiliation, disappointment, and withdrawal of support. The employer of injury may represent an excellent final job placement, but a poor initial work hardening placement. The employer of injury and coworkers have intimate knowledge of the injured worker. Despite the best preparation, these parties will often be quite surprised at the differences they find in the injured worker. Their reaction may be so profound as to cause fear about safety, doubt about recovery, and reluctance to allow sufficient time and opportunity for progression through an extended work hardening, on-the-job training, and job coaching process before arriving at a final job placement. The injured worker, too, may be keenly aware of colleagues' watchfulness, and the extra social pressure can be unduly difficult.

Consequently, the prevocational counseling process should include an orientation for the client and family regarding these potential pitfalls. The plan should evolve to identify and avoid as many of them as possible. Education regarding the prolonged nature of vocational intervention and description of the process as a "therapy" rather than job placement can be helpful in arriving at a good understanding of the need to effect appropriate opportunities for transition into the RTW process.

After a vocational plan is established, it is often necessary to educate financially interested parties regarding the need to follow a protracted vocational rehabilitation course for people with TBI because most claims adjusters and case managers will have little experience with TBI. Their usual experience with vocational rehabilitation will be such that they will expect a comparatively short and simple process. They may expect that the medical file be closed and the client determined to be "permanent and stationary" or at "maximum medical improvement" before allowing formal vocational rehabilitation involvement. As discussed earlier, it is imperative in TBI that vocational and medical rehabilitation be better coordinated early during the recovery process. Determination of "permanent and stationary" or at "maximum medical improvement" status can be made shortly before final job placement and need not precede the commencement of vocational rehabilitation.

The VRC must evaluate the degree of awareness the medical rehabilitation professionals have regarding the likely job requirements for which they must attempt to prepare the injured person. The counselor may choose to develop job requirements for several possible job descriptions and meet with medical rehabilitation staff to review the position demands. Medical and therapeutic planning can be quite different when knowledge of such requirements is introduced. These differences can range from alteration of timing for various elective or planned surgical interventions to whether or how long therapy continues and to what goals.

23.8.3 Vocational Counseling

The VRC should begin vocational rehabilitation counseling with adequate disclosure of each party's roles and responsibilities. Expectations for the vocational process should be evaluated and clarified. Most people do not have a clear idea regarding what vocational rehabilitation entails, and so it is quite important to undertake a clear discussion of what is expected of the injured worker, an employer, and the VRC. Most states have requirements for provision of vocational rehabilitation benefits. Some insurance carriers and some states have published materials that explain available benefits to the injured worker. Because memory function may be impaired, it may be advisable to include a family member in the discussion of benefits to be sure that all their questions are answered and that the information can be reliably presented to the injured worker, in case aspects of the discussions are forgotten. Provision of available benefits in writing can facilitate this process.

The VRC may face obstacles posed by misinformation that an injured worker or his or her family has obtained from friends or family who had experience with vocational rehabilitation for a different injury or in a different state. The existence of such experience should be actively investigated because it will most likely influence receptivity to vocational rehabilitation.

The VRC must learn the vocational goals and expectations the injured worker and his or her family have. There may be discordance within a family or between the injured worker's desires and his or her abilities. Vocational counseling should undertake a supportive and coordinated educational process to attempt to align expectations and goal setting from the outset and before progression on the plan. The VRC will need to include medical rehabilitation professionals, case managers, claims adjusters, attorneys, and staff of state departments of vocational rehabilitation in these discussions to arrive at a vocational rehabilitation plan that has attainable goals that are agreed upon by all interested parties. Given the large number of interested parties and their respective roles, reaching concordance is crucial, although difficult.

Assessment of dependency must be undertaken in the vocational counseling process. Dependency can take many forms and is fostered, to some degree, through the medical rehabilitation process. The injured worker may need some assistance in overcoming learned dependence and moving toward independence and self-reliance once again. Dependency can be psychological, financial, social, or medical in nature. Psychological dependencies include having learned to be more comfortable having things done for one, rather than doing for oneself, having developed a dislike of a particular job or distrust of an employer, deriving some emotional benefit from medical treatment or the disabled status, or having developed a fear of failure that precludes consideration of reentry into the workplace as an independent person. Financial dependence can include the idea that it is easier not to work than to work for a minor discrepancy in income, income stability resulting from regular income payments rather than income derived from seasonal work, or acceptance of the idea that injury deserves compensation even though a Social Security or workers' compensation payment is not designed as such. Social dependency can occur when immigration status is dependent upon medical status or when cultural mores are such that injury is viewed as permanent and, consequently, as an entitlement rather than as something that is temporary and amenable to change. Medical dependency can include substance abuse that may, or may not, have preceded the injury.[155,156] After dependencies and their etiologies are identified, the VRC can work with a counselor or psychologist to address the dependencies and attempt to reverse them. Some dependencies, however, will not be amenable to reversal, and vocational rehabilitation plan success will be negatively affected.

23.9 Vocational Testing, Work Evaluation, and Work Hardening

Vocational testing can include interest inventory testing, vocational aptitude testing, utilization of standardized work samples, and utilization of work samples to assess specific skills. Many interest inventory and vocational aptitude tests are commercially available.[147–160] These tools are often helpful in identifying alternative employment options that may be of interest and within the capabilities of an injured worker who cannot return to preinjury employment. Results of these tests facilitate discussion and exploration of vocational options, although some care must be taken in that the universe of options is opened to the individual. This can be problematic because some options may require extended vocational or educational training that is not practical. Similarly, some options may entail self-employment. Given the nature of limitations experienced following TBI, formalized schooling and self-employment plans are less likely to be successful. In fact, it has been demonstrated that formalized schooling plans in vocational rehabilitation with other populations are less successful than nonschooling plans.[161]

Vocational evaluation may require a protracted timeline to complete properly.[162] Work evaluation consisting of situational[78,162] or community-based assessments, functional evaluation, simulated work, and work samples[163] might be included to identify potential barriers to employment that may not have been identified. Work evaluation can be helpful in determining whether a work adjustment or work hardening experience is warranted. Standardized work samples can be used that allow comparison of the person's function with a normal population. These work samples can be used to evaluate ability to use small tools,[164] size discrimination,[165] numeric sorting,[166] upper extremity range of motion,[167] clerical comprehension and aptitude,[168] independent problem solving,[169] multilevel sorting,[170] simulated assembly,[171] whole body range of motion,[172] trilevel measurement,[173] eye–hand–foot coordination,[174] and soldering and inspection.[175] Work samples designed to assess specific work skills can also be derived from an employment setting. Information is collected about the usual method of completion, time to complete, and job outcome, which is then compared with the skills demonstrated by the injured worker.

Work hardening placement is used to develop physical, cognitive, social, and job skills for a specific position, although the plan might intend that those skills will ultimately transfer to other job placements. Strength and endurance can be gradually improved by using a graded number of hours per day for the work schedule. An advantage to a work hardening placement is that it is disposable. That is, mistakes made on this type of placement can be used as learning experiences and are not likely to be noted by friends and coworkers. Gradual improvement in work productivity is the key to work hardening placement. It is sometimes useful to utilize more than one work hardening placement because of information gleaned from the first. The individual may demonstrate skills, or a lack thereof, that were not identified during testing. Accommodation to the workplace and all its demands can be accomplished by transition built into the work schedule and work responsibilities. Development of positive worker characteristics is an early focus. Continued monitoring by the VRC or job coach can provide excellent information to therapists for additional emphasis on identified areas or for compensatory approaches to be developed. The VRC must ensure that the work hardening experience provides good feedback to the injured worker and must work to maintain an employer's willingness to continue to provide access to the work hardening setting. Work hardening experiences need not be paid positions to be valuable. Some people benefit from protracted volunteer experiences, gradually improving endurance, positive worker characteristics, and job skills. On the other hand, work hardening experiences may progress within an employer's setting and culminate in an actual job placement. Obtaining a job placement from an initial work hardening experience may be as dependent upon the VRC's management of the entire process as it is upon the injured worker's skills and progress.[34]

The VRC must be certain to file all appropriate paperwork on behalf of the injured worker, insurer, or employer, as required by law. Continued monitoring of progress in the medical rehabilitation occurs until the proper time for administration of prevocational counseling and vocational testing is identified. As the injured worker nears completion of the medical rehabilitation plan, vocational evaluation begins.

As the medical rehabilitation process winds down, part-time work hardening placement or situational assessment can be used to reintroduce the injured worker to the workplace, and to assess and reestablish good basic worker characteristics, such as appropriate dress, punctuality, and job task completion. Work hardening placement may be progressive either in the amount of time spent on the job, in the nature of the work undertaken on a given job, or in changing from one job description to a more demanding one. Extensive job coaching should be used in the work evaluation and work hardening processes.

Success in work hardening placement leads to job placement in what may become the final placement for the injured worker. Job coaching should continue as needed and be transitioned out of the job site according to success. Continued monitoring should be undertaken for 6 to 12 months before case closure is achieved. Sale et al.[34] reported that placements often failed as result of a number of events occurring on the job rather than a single event, suggesting a role for VRC intervention. Finally, the VRC should always compare the original vocational goals and predicted vocational outcome with the final achievement to attempt to derive ways of improving personal effectiveness.

To summarize, in the general course of vocational rehabilitation for TBI, the VRC enters the process by monitoring the medical rehabilitation status and progress. A job analysis and description of the employment at the time of injury should be obtained and shared with the medical rehabilitation team. Likewise, a work history that reviews all past employment should be collected and shared. As this information is considered, the VRC and medical rehabilitation team can begin to discuss the RTW process and bring about the establishment of appropriate expectations for RTW among themselves and with the injured worker and family, review prognostic variables that may impact RTW, and review funding options and programs that will be available.

23.10 Follow-Up

The role of follow-up cannot be overstated. Given the instability in job maintenance following TBI, planned follow-up conducted over a lengthy period of time is only logical.[16,176] Unfortunately, though, completion of follow-up activities requires the approval of the client, the employer, and possibly an insurance carrier, in addition to the willingness of the VRC. Objectives for the follow-up visits should be clearly delineated in advance with all interested parties as part of the vocational rehabilitation plan.

The primary purpose of follow-up is to determine whether the individual is experiencing any problems on the job site that can be rectified before they culminate in job separation. The injured worker may, or may not, be aware and forthcoming about problems, as may be the employer. Consider tardiness, absenteeism, social interaction, and task completion at a minimum. Careful interview with the injured worker, family, coworkers, and the employer may reveal small or emerging problems that can be addressed. The VRC should review current job duties and compare with original responsibilities. Any changes that are noted should be reviewed to determine whether they are compatible with known skills and aptitudes of the injured worker.

The VRC must also investigate whether events have transpired that might jeopardize placement that may not be work site related. These include motor vehicle infractions or accidents, hospitalization, substance abuse, family or marital discord, or failure to comply with prescribed medical or therapeutic treatment plans. It may be advisable to contact the local department of motor vehicles (DMV) to check for infractions, accidents, or substance abuse.

The VRC must collate the collected information at follow-up and determine the best manner to approach addressing identified areas of concern. The goal must be to conduct follow-up frequently enough to allow early identification and resolution of problems, thereby ensuring job retention.

23.11 Summary

Successful vocational rehabilitation represents, perhaps, the highest achievement of return to life to be achieved after TBI. Formal vocational rehabilitation is challenged by societal predispositions that often preclude the initiation or successful completion of such efforts.

The process is extremely complicated and requires a thoughtful, adaptable, and progressive approach to restoration of the ability to work. Stability of medical rehabilitation outcomes and overall life satisfaction can be positively impacted by collaboratively undertaking the hard work involved in returning a person with TBI to work.

References

1. United Nations General Assembly, *The Standard Rules on the Equalization of Opportunities for Persons with Disabilities*, United General Assembly, 48th Session, Resolution 48/96, Annex, 1993. 20.
2. Johansson, U. and Tham, K., The meaning of work after acquired brain injury, *American Journal of Occupational Therapy*, 60(1), 60–69, 2006.
3. Melamed, S., Groswasser, Z., and Stern, M. J., Acceptance of disability, work, involvement and subjective rehabilitation status of traumatic brain-injured (TBI) patients, *Brain Injury*, 6(3), 233–243, 1992.
4. Corrigan, J. D., Bogner, J. A., Mysiw, W. J., Clinchot, D., and Fugate, L., Life satisfaction after traumatic brain injury, *Journal of Head Trauma Rehabilitation*, 16(6), 543–555, 2001.
5. Tennant, A., MacDermott, N., and Neary, D., The long-term outcome of head injury: Implications for service planning, *Brain Injury*, 9(6), 595–605, 1995.
6. Heinemann, A. W., Sokol, K., Garvin, L., and Bode, R. K., Measuring unmet needs and services among persons with traumatic brain injury, *Archives of Physical Medicine and Rehabilitation*, 83(8), 1052–1059, 2002.
7. Hallauer, D. S., Prosser, R. A., and Swift, K. F., Neuropsychological evaluation in the vocational rehabilitation of brain injured clients, *Journal of Applied Rehabilitation Counseling*, 20(2), 3–7, 1989.
8. Burns, P. G., Kay, T., and Pieper, B., *A Survey of the Vocational Service System as it Relates to Head Injury Survivors and Their Vocational Needs*, Grant no. 0001229, New York State Head Injury Association, 1986.
9. Goodall, P., Lawyer, H. L., and Wehman, P., Vocational rehabilitation and traumatic brain injury: A legislative and public policy perspective, *Journal of Head Trauma Rehabilitation*, 9(2), 61–81, 1994.
10. Sim, J., Improving return-to-work strategies in the United States disability programs, with analysis of program practices in Germany and Sweden, *Social Security Bulletin*, 62(3), 41–50, 1999.
11. Rubin, S. E. and Roessler, R. T., *Foundations of the Vocational Rehabilitation Process*, 3rd ed., Pro-Ed, Austin, TX, 1987.
12. Mellick, D., Gerhart, K. A., and Whiteneck, G. G., Understanding outcomes based on the post-acute hospitalization pathways followed by persons with traumatic brain injury, *Brain Injury*, 17(1), 55, 2003.
13. Ottenbacher, K. J., Smith, P. M., Illig, S. B., Linn, R. T., Ostir, G. V., and Granger, C. V., Trends in length of stay, living setting, functional outcome, and mortality following medical rehabilitation, *Journal of the American Medical Association*, 292(14), 1687–1695, 2004.
14. Greenspan, A. I., Wrigley, J. M., Kresnow, M., Branche-Dorsey, C. M., and Fine, P. R., Factors influencing failure to return to work due to traumatic brain injury, *Brain Injury*, 10(3), 207–218, 1996.
15. Sykes-Horn, W., Wrigley, M., Wallace, D., and Yoels, W., Factors associated with awareness of vocational rehabilitation services after traumatic brain injury, *Archives of Physical Medicine and Rehabilitation*, 78(12), 1327–1330, 1997.
16. Ben-Yishay, Y., Silver, S. M., Piasetsky, E., and Rattok, J., Relationship between employability and vocational outcome after intensive holistic cognitive rehabilitation, *Journal of Head Trauma Rehabilitation*, 2(1), 35–48, 1987.

17. Klonoff, P. S. and Shepherd, J. C., Management of individuals with traumatic brain injury, in C. Simkins (Ed.), *Analysis, Understanding, and Presentation of Cases Involving Traumatic Brain Injury*, National Head Injury Foundation, Washington, DC, VII, 107–124, 1994.

18. Gollaher, K., High, W., Sherer, M., Bergloff, P., Boake, C., Young, M. E., et al., Prediction of employment outcome one to three years following traumatic brain injury (TBI), *Brain Injury*, 12(4), 255–263, 1998.

19. Ip, R. Y., Dornan, J., and Schentag, C., Traumatic brain injury: Factors predicting return to work or school, *Brain Injury*, 9(5), 517–532, 1995.

20. Brooks, N., McKinlay, W., Symington, C., Beattie, A., and Campise, L., Return to work within the first seven years of severe head injury, *Brain Injury*, 1(1), 5–19, 1987.

21. Jacobs, H. E., The Los Angeles Head Injury Survey: Procedures and initial findings, *Archives of Physical Medicine and Rehabilitation*, 69(6), 425–431, 1988.

22. Van der Naalt, J., van Zomeren, A. H., Sluiter, W. J., and Minderhoud, J. M., One year outcome in mild to moderate head injury: The predictive value of acute injury characteristics related to complaints and return to work, *Journal of Neurology, Neurosurgery, and Psychiatry*, 66(2), 207–213, 1999.

23. Johnstone, B., Mount, D., and Schopp, L. H., Financial and vocational outcomes 1 year after traumatic brain injury, *Archives of Physical Medicine and Rehabilitation*, 84(2), 238–241, 2003.

24. Corrigan, J. D., Lineberry, L. A., Komaroff, E., Langlois, J. A., Selassie, A. W., and Wood, K. D., Employment after traumatic brain injury: Differences between men and women, *Archives of Physical Medicine and Rehabilitation*, 88(11), 1400–1409, 2007.

25. *The Traumatic Brain Injury Model System of Care: A project funded by the U.S. Department of Education*, National Institute on Disability and Rehabilitation Research, 2008.

26. Rao, N., Rosenthal, M., Cronin-Stubbs, D., Lambert, R., Barnes, P., and Swanson, B., Return to work after rehabilitation following traumatic brain injury, *Brain Injury*, 4(1), 49–56, 1990.

27. McMordie, W. R., Barker, S. L., and Paolo, T. M., Return to work (RTW) after head injury, *Brain Injury*, 4(1), 57–69, 1990.

28. Gonser, A., Prognose, Langzeitfolgen und berufliche Reintegration 2–4 Jahre nach schwerem Schadel-Hirn Trauma [Prognosis, long-term sequelae and occupational reintegration 2–4 years after severe craniocerebral trauma], *Nervenarzt*, 63(7), 426–433, 1992.

29. Felmingham, K. L., Baguley, I. J., and Crooks, J., A comparison of acute and postdischarge predictors of employment 2 years after traumatic brain injury, *Archives of Physical Medicine and Rehabilitation*, 82(4), 435–439, 2001.

30. Englander, J., Hall, K., Stimpson, T., and Chaffin, S., Mild traumatic brain injury in an insured population: Subjective complaints and return to employment, *Brain Injury*, 6(2), 161–166, 1992.

31. Malec, J. F. and Moessner, A. M., Replicated positive results for the VCC model of vocational intervention after ABI within the social model of disability, *Brain Injury*, 20(3), 227–236, 2006.

32. Buffington, A. L. and Malec, J. F., The vocational rehabilitation continuum: Maximizing outcomes through bridging the gap from hospital to community-based services, *Journal of Head Trauma Rehabilitation*, 12(5), 1–13, 1997.

33. Reid-Arndt, S. A., Schopp, L., Brenneke, L., Johnstone, B., and Poole, A. D., Evaluation of the traumatic brain injury early referral programme in Missouri, *Brain Injury*, 21(12), 1295–1302, 2007.

34. Sale, P., West, M., Sherron, P., and Wehman, P. H., Exploratory analysis of job separation from supported employment for persons with traumatic brain injury, *Journal of Head Trauma Rehabilitation*, 6(3), 1–11, 1991.

35. West, M. D., Aspects of the workplace and return to work for persons with brain injury in supported employment, *Brain Injury*, 9(3), 301–313, 1995.

36. Wall, J. R., Rosenthal, M., and Niemczura, J. G., Community-based training after acquired brain injury: Preliminary findings, *Brain Injury*, 12(3), 215–224, 1998.

37. Gray, D. S. and Burnham, R. S., Preliminary outcome analysis of a long-term rehabilitation program for severe acquired brain injury, *Archives of Physical Medicine and Rehabilitation*, 81(11), 1447–1456, 2000.

38. Eames, P., Cotterill, G., Kneale, T. A., Storrar, A. L., and Yeomans, P., Outcome of intensive rehabilitation after severe brain injury: A long-term follow-up study, *Brain Injury*, 10(9), 631–650, 1996.
39. Wood, R. L., McCrea, J. D., Wood, L. M., and Merriman, R. N., Clinical and cost effectiveness of post-acute neurobehavioural rehabilitation, *Brain Injury*, 13(2), 69–88, 1999.
40. Keyser-Marcus, L. A., Bricout, J. C., Wehman, P., Campbell, L. R., Cifu, D. X., Englanger, J., et al., Acute predictors of return to employment after traumatic brain injury: A longitudinal follow-up, *Archives of Physical Medicine and Rehabilitation*, 83(5), 635–641, 2002.
41. Machamer, J., Temkin, N., Fraser, R., Doctor, J. N., and Dikmen, S., Stability of employment after traumatic brain injury, *Journal of the International Neuropsychological Society*, 11(07), 807–816, 2005.
42. Ruff, R. M., Marshall, L. F., Crouch, J., Klauber, M. R., Levin, H. S., Barth, J., et al., Predictors of outcome following severe head trauma: Follow-up data from the Traumatic Coma Data Bank, *Brain Injury*, 7(2), 101–111, 1993.
43. Kowalske, K., Plenger, P. M., Lusby, B., and Hayden, M. E., Vocational re-entry following TBI: An enablement model, *Journal of Head Trauma Rehabilitation*, 15(4), 989–999, 2000.
44. Isaki, E. and Turkstra, L., Communication abilities and work re-entry following traumatic brain injury, *Brain Injury*, 14(5), 441–453, 2000.
45. Wehman, P., Kregel, J., Sherron, P., Nguyen, S., Kreutzer, J., Fry, R., et al., Critical factors associated with the successful supported employment placement of patients with severe traumatic brain injury, *Brain Injury*, 7(1), 31–44, 1993.
46. Brantner, C. L., Job coaching for persons with traumatic brain injuries employed in professional and technical occupations, *Journal of Applied Rehabilitation Counseling*, 23(3), 3–14, 1992.
47. van Zomeren, A. H. and van den Burg, W., Residual complaints of patients two years after severe head injury, *Journal of Neurology, Neurosurgery, and Psychiatry*, 48(1), 21–28, 1985.
48. Cattelani, R., Tanzi, F., Lombardi, F., and Mazzucchi, A., Competitive re-employment after severe traumatic brain injury: Clinical, cognitive and behavioural predictive variables, *Brain Injury*, 16(1), 51–64, 2002.
49. Young, B., Rapp, R. P., Norton, J. A., Haack, D., Tibbs, P. A., and Bean, J. R., Early prediction of outcome in head-injured patients, *Journal of Neurosurgery*, 54(3), 300–303, 1981.
50. Levati, A., Farina, M. L., Vecchi, G., Rossanda, M., and Marrubini, M. B., Prognosis of severe head injuries, *Journal of Neurosurgery*, 57(6), 779–783, 1982.
51. Rappaport, M., Hall, K. M., Hopkins, K., Belleza, T., and Cope, D. N., Disability rating scale for severe head trauma: Coma to community, *Archives of Physical Medicine and Rehabilitation*, 63(3), 118–123, 1982.
52. Leung, K. L. and Man, W. K. D., Prediction of vocational outcome of people with brain injury after rehabilitation: A discriminant analysis, *Work*, 25(4), 333–340, 2005.
53. Vogenthaler, D. R., Smith, Jr., K. R., and Goldfader, P., Head injury, an empirical study: Describing long-term productivity and independent living outcome, *Brain Injury*, 3(4), 355–368, 1989.
54. Sherer, M., Bergloff, P., High, Jr., W., and Nick, T. G., Contribution of functional ratings to prediction of long-term employment outcome after traumatic brain injury, *Brain Injury*, 13(12), 973–981, 1999.
55. Rao, N. and Kilgore, K. M., Predicting return to work in traumatic brain injury using assessment scales, *Archives of Physical Medicine and Rehabilitation*, 73(10), 911–916, 1992.
56. Kolb, C. L. and Woldt, A. L., The rehabilitative potential of a Gestalt approach to counseling severely impaired clients, in W. A. McDowell, S. A. Meadows, R. Crabtree, and R. Sakata, (Eds.), *Rehabilitation Counseling with Persons Who Are Severely Disabled*, Marshall University Press, Huntington, WV, 48–58, 1976.
57. Dikmen, S., Machamer, J., and Temkin, N., Psychosocial outcome in patients with moderate to severe head injury: 2-Year follow-up, *Brain Injury*, 7(2), 113–124, 1993.
58. Dawson, D. R., Schwartz, M. L., Winocur, G., and Stuss, D. T., Return to productivity following traumatic brain injury: Cognitive, psychological, physical, spiritual, and environmental correlates, *Disability & Rehabilitation*, 29(4), 301–313, 2007.

59. McCrimmon, S. and Oddy, M., Return to work following moderate-to-severe traumatic brain injury, *Brain Injury*, 20(10), 1037–1046, 2006.
60. Ezrachi, O., Ben-Yishay, Y., Kay, T., Diller, L., and Rattok, J., Predicting employment in traumatic brain injury following neuropsychological rehabilitation, *Journal of Head Trauma Rehabilitation*, 6(3), 71–84, 1991.
61. Shames, J., Treger, I., Ring, H., and Giaquinto, S., Return to work following traumatic brain injury: Trends and challenges, *Disability & Rehabilitation*, 29(17), 1387–1395, 2007.
62. Devitt, R., Colantonio, A., Dawson, D., Teare, G., Ratcliff, G., and Chase, S., Prediction of long-term occupational performance outcomes for adults after moderate to severe traumatic brain injury, *Disability & Rehabilitation*, 28(9), 547–559, 2006.
63. Ownsworth, T. and McKenna, K., Investigation of factors related to employment outcome following traumatic brain injury: A critical review and conceptual model, *Disability & Rehabilitation*, 26(13), 765–783, 2004.
64. Pampus, I., [Rehabilitation of brain-injured patients: Demonstrated with the help of a successfully performed individual rehabilitation plan], I. Pampus (Trans.), *Rehabilitation (Stuttg)*, 18(2), 51–55, 1979. [Article in German.]
65. Hackspacher, J., Dern, W., and Jeschke, H. A., [Interdisciplinary cooperation in rehabilitation: Problem solving following severe craniocerebral injury], *Rehabilitation (Stuttg)*, 30(2), 75–79, 1991. [Article in German.]
66. Jellinek, H. M. and Harvey, R. F., Vocational/educational services in a medical rehabilitation facility: Outcomes in spinal cord and brain injured patients, *Archives of Physical Medicine and Rehabilitation*, 63(2), 87–88, 1982.
67. Michaels, C. A. and Risucci, D. A., Employer and counselor perceptions of workplace accommodations for persons with traumatic brain injury, *Journal of Applied Rehabilitation Counseling*, 24(1), 38–46, 1993.
68. Johnson, R., Employment after severe head injury: Do the Manpower Services Commission schemes help?, *Injury*, 20(1), 59, 1989.
69. Grahame, R., The decline of rehabilitation services and its impact on disability benefits, *Journal of the Royal Society of Medicine*, 95(3), 114–117, 2002.
70. Glaussen, G., Rehabilitation efforts before and after tightening eligibility for disability benefits in Norway, *International Journal of Rehabilitation Research*, 20(2), 139–147, 1997.
71. Swales, K., *A Study of Disability Living Allowance and Attendance Allowance Awards*, Analytical Services Division, Department of Social Security, London, 1988.
72. Better, S. R., Fine, P. R., Simison, D., Doss, G. H., Walls, R. T., and McLaughlin, D. E., Disability benefits as disincentives to rehabilitation, *Milbank Memorial Fund Quarterly, Health and Society*, 57(3), 412–427, 1979.
73. Schlenoff, D., Obstacles to the rehabilitation of disability benefits recipients, *Journal of Rehabilitation*, 45(2), 56–58, 1979.
74. Drew, D., Drebing, C. E., Van Ormer, A., Losardo, M., Krebs, C., Penk, W., et al., Effects of disability compensation on participation in and outcomes of vocational rehabilitation, *Psychiatric Services*, 52(11), 1479–1484, 2001.
75. Tate, D. G., Workers' disability and return to work, *American Journal of Physical Medicine and Rehabilitation*, 71(2), 92–96, 1992.
76. Guerin, F., Kennepohl, S., Leveille, G., Dominique, A., and McKerral, M., Vocational outcome indicators in atypically recovering mild TBI: A post-intervention study, *Neurorehabilitation*, 21(4), 295–303, 2006.
77. Zuger, R. R., Vocational rehabilitation counseling of traumatic brain injury: Factors contributing to stress, *Journal of Rehabilitation*, 59(2), 28–30, 1993.
78. LeBlanc, J. M., Hayden, M. E., and Paulman, R. G., A comparison of neuropsychological and situation assessment for predicting employability after closed head injury, *Journal of Head Trauma Rehabilitation*, 15(4), 1022–1040, 2000.
79. Parente, R., Stapleton, M. C., and Wheatley, C. J., Practical strategies for vocational reentry after traumatic brain injury, *Journal of Head Trauma Rehabilitation*, 6(3), 35–45, 1991.

80. Ashley, M. J. and Krych, D. K., (Eds.), *Traumatic Brain Injury Rehabilitation*, CRC Press, Boca Raton, FL, 1995.
81. Humphrey, M. and Oddy, M., Return to work after head injury: A review of post-war studies, *Injury*, 12(2), 107–114, 1980.
82. Fraser, R., Dikmen, S., McClean, A., Miller, B., and Temkin, N., Employability of head injury survivors: First year post-injury, *Rehabilitation Counseling Bulletin*, 31(4), 276–288, 1988.
83. Lezak, M. D. and O'Brien, K. P., Longitudinal study of emotional, social, and physical changes after traumatic brain injury, *Journal of Learning Disabilities*, 21(8), 456–463, 1988.
84. Ashley, M. J., Persel, C. P., and Krych, D. K., Changes in reimbursement climate: Relationship among outcome, cost, and payer type in the postacute rehabilitation environment, *Journal of Head Trauma Rehabilitation*, 8(4), 30–47, 1993.
85. Kreutzer, J. S., Kolakowsky-Hayner, S. A., Ripley, D., Cifu, D. X., Rosenthal, M., Bushnik, T., et al., Charges and lengths of stay for acute and inpatient rehabilitation treatment of traumatic brain injury 1990–1996, *Brain Injury*, 15(9), 763–774, 2001.
86. U.S. Department of Education, National Institute on Disability and Rehabilitation Research, Traumatic brain injury facts and figures, *The Traumatic Brain Injury Model Systems National Data Center*, 5(1), 2000.
87. Marinelli, R. P. and Dell Orto, A. E., *The Psychological and Social Impact of Physical Disability*, 2nd ed., Springer Publishing, New York, 1984.
88. Jury, M. A. and Flynn, M. C., Auditory and vestibular sequelae to traumatic brain injury: A pilot study, *New Zealand Medical Journal*, 114(1134), 286–288, 2001.
89. Chamelian, L. and Feinstein, A., Outcome after mild to moderate traumatic brain injury: The role of dizziness, *Archives of Physical Medicine and Rehabilitation*, 85(10), 1662–1666, 2004.
90. Dehail, P., Petit, H., Joseph, P. A., Vuadens, P., and Mazaux, J. M., Assessment of postural instability in patients with traumatic brain injury upon enrollment in a vocation adjustment programme, *Journal of Rehabilitation Medicine*, 39(7), 531–536, 2007.
91. Cantor, J. B., Ashman, T., Gordon, W., Ginsberg, A., Engmann, C., Egan, M., et al., Fatigue after traumatic brain injury and its impact on participation and quality of life, *Journal of Head Trauma Rehabilitation*, 23(1), 41–51, 2008.
92. Ziino, C. and Ponsford, J., Selective attention deficits and subjective fatigue following traumatic brain injury, *Neuropsychology*, 20(3), 383–390, 2006.
93. Rao, V. and Lyketsos, C. G., Psychiatric aspects of traumatic brain injury, *The Psychiatric Clinics of North America*, 25(1), 43–69, 2002.
94. Sbordone, R. J., Limitations of neuropsychological testing to predict the cognitive and behavioral functioning of persons with brain injury in real-world settings, *Neurorehabilitation*, 16(4), 199–201, 2001.
95. Prigatano, C. P., Fordyce, D. J., Zeiner, H. K., Roueche, J. R., Pepping, M., and Wood, B. C., Neuropsychological rehabilitation after closed head injury in young adults, *Journal of Neurology, Neurosurgery, and Psychiatry*, 47(5), 505–513, 1984.
96. Ben-Yishay, Y. and Diller, L., Cognitive remediation in traumatic brain injury: Update and issues, *American Journal of Physical Medicine and Rehabilitation*, 74(2), 204–213, 1993.
97. Ciacino, J. T. and Cicerone, K. D., Varieties of deficit unawareness after brain injury, *Journal of Head Trauma Rehabilitation*, 13(5), 1–15, 1998.
98. Koponen, S., Taiminen, T., Portin, R., Himanen, L., Isoniemi, H., Heinonen, H., et al., Axis I and II psychiatric disorders after traumatic brain injury: A 30-year follow-up study, *American Journal of Psychiatry*, 159(8), 1315–1321, 2002.
99. Leon-Carrion, J., De Serdio-Aria, M. L., Cabezas, F. M., Roldan, J. M., Dominguez-Morales, R., Martin, J. M., et al., Neurobehavioural and cognitive profile of traumatic brain injury patients at risk for depression and suicide, *Brain Injury*, 15(2), 175–181, 2001.
100. Uysal, S., Hibbard, M. R., Robillard, D., Pappadopulos, E., and Jaffe, M., The effect of parental traumatic brain injury on parenting and child behavior, *Journal of Head Trauma Rehabilitation*, 13(6), 57–71, 1998.

101. Bryant, R. A., Marosszeky, J. E., Crooks, J., Baguley, I., and Gurka, J., Coping style and post-traumatic stress disorder following severe traumatic injury, *Brain Injury*, 14(2), 175–180, 2000.

102. Kravetz, S., Gross, Y., Weiler, B., Ben-Yakar, M., Tadir, M., and Stern, M. J., Self-concept, marital vulnerability and brain damage, *Brain Injury*, 9(2), 131–139, 1995.

103. Butcher, J. N., Dahlstrom, W. G., Graham, J. R., Tellegen, A., and Daemmer, B., *Minnesota Multiphasic Personality Inventory-2*, University of Minnesota Press, Minneapolis, MN, 1989.

104. Nash, L., (Ed.), *Taylor-Johnson Temperament Analysis Manual*, Western Psychological Services, Los Angeles, 1980.

105. Gluck, G. A., *Psychometric Properties of the FIRO-B: A Guide to Research*, Consulting Psychologists Press, Palo Alto, CA, 1983.

106. Beck, A. T., Ward, C. H., Mendelson, M., Mock, J., and Erbaugh, J., An inventory for measuring depression, *Archives of General Psychiatry*, 4(6), 561–571, 1961.

107. Gass, C. S., MMPI-2 interpretation and closed head injury: A correction factor, *Psychological Assessment*, 3(1), 27–31, 1991.

108. Van Balen, H. G., de Mey, H. R., and van Limbeek, J., A neurocorrective approach for MMPI-2 use with brain-damaged patients, *International Journal of Rehabilitation Research*, 22(4), 249–259, 1999.

109. Gass, C. S. and Wald, H. S., MMPI-2 interpretation and closed-head trauma: Cross-validation of correction factor, *Archives of Clinical Neuropsychology*, 12(3), 199–205, 1997.

110. Artzy, G., Correlation factors for the MMPI-2 in head injured men and women, *Dissertation Abstracts International: Section B: The Sciences & Engineering*, 57(4), 2935, 1996.

111. West, M. D., Aspects of the workplace and return to work for persons with brain injury in supported employment, *Brain Injury*, 9(3), 301–313, 1995.

112. Storey, K. and Horner, R. H., Social interactions in three supported employment options: A comparative analysis, *Journal of Applied Behavior Analysis*, 24(2), 349–360, 1991.

113. Dikmen, S., Machamer, J., and Temkin, N., Psychosocial outcome in patients with moderate to severe head injury: 2-Year follow-up, *Brain Injury*, 7(2), 113–124, 1993.

114. Ashley, M. J., Persel, C. S., and Krych, D. K., Long-term outcome follow-up of postacute traumatic brain injury rehabilitation: An assessment of functional and behavioral measures of daily living, *Journal of Rehabilitation Outcomes Measurement* 1(4), 40–47, 1997.

115. Carney, N., Chesnut, R. M., Maynard, H., Mann, N. C., Patterson, P., and Helfand, M., Effect of cognitive rehabilitation on outcomes for persons with traumatic brain injury: A systematic review, *Journal of Head Trauma Rehabilitation*, 81(12), 1596–1615, 2000.

116. Cicerone, K. D., Dahlberg, C., Kalmar, K., Langebahn, D. M., Malec, J. F., Bergquist, T. F., et al., Evidence-based cognitive rehabilitation: Recommendations for clinical practice, *Archives of Physical Medicine and Rehabilitation*, 81(12), 1596–1615, 2000.

117. Cicerone, K. D. and Giancino, J. T., Remediation of executive function deficits after traumatic brain injury, *Neurorehabilitation*, 2(3) 12–22, 1992.

118. Bjerke, L. G., Hukommelsesfunksjon etter hodeskader [Memory function after head injuries], *Tidsskr Nor Laeqeforen*, 109(6), 684–686, 1989.

119. Mateer, C. A. and Sira, C. S., Cognitive and emotional consequences of TBI: Intervention strategies for vocational rehabilitation, *Neurorehabilitation*, 21(4), 315–326, 2006.

120. Melamed, S., Stern, M. J., Rahmani, L., Groswasser, Z., and Najenson, T., Attention capacity limitation, psychiatric parameters and their impact on work involvement following brain injury, *Scandinavian Journal of Rehabilitation Medicine*, 12, 21–26, 1985.

121. Schlund, M. W., The effects of brain injury on choice and sensitivity to remote consequences: Deficits in discriminating response–consequence relations, *Brain Injury*, 16(4), 347–357, 2002.

122. Krauss, J. K. and Jankovic, J., Head injury and posttraumatic movement disorders, *Neurosurgery*, 50(5), 927–939, Discussion 939–940, 2002.

123. Menon, E. B., Ravichandran, S., and Tran, E. S., Speech disorders in closed head injury patients, *Singapore Medical Journal*, 34(1), 45–48, 1993.

124. Blumberger, J., Sullivan, S. J., and Clement, N., Diadochokinetic rate in persons with traumatic brain injury, *Brain Injury*, 9(8), 797–804, 1995.

125. Theodoros, D. G., Shrapnel, N., and Murdoch, B. E., Motor speech impairment following traumatic brain injury in childhood: A physiological and perceptual analysis of one case, *Pediatric Rehabilitation*, 2(3), 107–122, 1998.

126. McHenry, M. A., Vital capacity following traumatic brain injury, *Brain Injury*, 15(8), 741–745, 2001.

127. McHenry, M. A., Acoustic characteristic of voice after traumatic brain injury, *The Laryngoscope*, 110(7), 1157–1161, 2000.

128. Aronson, A. E., Laryngeal–phonatory dysfunction in closed-head injury, *Brain Injury*, 8(8), 663–665, 1994.

129. Jaeger, M., Frohlich, M., Hertrick, I., Ackermann, H., and Schonle, P. W., Dysphonia subsequent to severe traumatic brain injury: Comparative perceptual, acoustic and electroglottographic analyses, *Folio Phoniatrica et Logopaedica*, 53(6), 326–337, 2001.

130. Wymer, J. H., Lindman, L. S., and Booksh, R. L., A neuropsychological perspective of aprosody: Features, function, assessment, and treatment, *Applied Neuropsychology*, 9(1), 37–47, 2002.

131. Kewman, D. G., Yanus, B., and Kirsch, N., Assessment of distractibility in auditory comprehension after traumatic brain injury, *Brain Injury*, 2(2), 131–137, 1988.

132. Snow, P., Douglas, J., and Ponsford, J., Conversational discourse abilities following severe traumatic brain injury: A follow-up study, *Brain Injury*, 12(11), 911–935, 1998.

133. Galski, T., Tompkins, C., and Johnston, M. V., Competence in discourse as a measure of social integration and quality of life in persons with traumatic brain injury, *Brain Injury*, 12(9), 769–782, 1998.

134. Coelho, C. A., Liles, B. Z., and Duffy, R. J., Impairments of discourse abilities and executive functions in traumatically brain-injured adults, *Brain Injury*, 9(5), 471–477, 1995.

135. Biddle, K. R., McCabe, A., and Bliss, L. S., Narrative skills following traumatic brain injury in children and adults, *Journal of Communication Disorders*, 29(6), 447–468, 1996.

136. Dennis, M. and Barnes, M. A., Knowing the meaning, getting the point, bridging the gap, and carrying the message: Aspects of discourse following closed head injury in childhood and adolescence, *Brain and Language*, 29(3), 428–446, 1990.

137. Hartley, L. L. and Jensen, P. J., Narrative and procedural discourse after closed head injury, *Brain Injury*, 5(3), 267–285, 1991.

138. Hopkins, M. J., Dywan, J., and Segalowitz, S. J., Altered electrodermal response to facial expression after closed head injury, *Brain Injury*, 16(3), 245–257, 2002.

139. Prigatano, G. P. and Pribram, K. H., Perception and memory of facial affect following brain injury, *Perceptual and Motor Skills*, 54(3), 859–869, 1982.

140. Helm-Estabrooks, N., Yeo, R., Geschwind, N., Freedman, M., and Weinstein, C., Stuttering: Disappearance and reappearance with acquired brain lesions, *Neurology*, 36(8), 1109–1112, 1986.

141. Bijleveld, H., Lebrun, Y., and van Dongen, H., A case of acquired stuttering, *Folia Phoniatrica and Logopaedia*, 46(5), 250–253, 1994.

142. Thomsen, I. V., Late outcome of very severe blunt head trauma: A 10-15 year second follow-up, *Journal of Neurology, Neurosurgery, and Psychiatry*, 47(3), 260–268, 1984.

143. Wehman, P., Kreutzer, J., Stonnington, H. H., Wood, W., Sherron, P., Diambra, J., et al., Supported employment for persons with traumatic brain injury: A preliminary report, *Journal of Head Trauma Rehabilitation*, 3(4), 82–94, 1988.

144. Kreutzer, J. S., Wehman, P., Morton, M. V., and Stonnington, H. H., Supported employment and compensatory strategies for enhancing vocational outcome following traumatic brain injury, *International Disability Studies*, 13(4), 162–171, 1991.

145. West, M., Fry, R., Pastor, J., Moore, G., Killam, S., Wehman, P., et al., Helping postacute traumatically brain injured clients return to work: Three case studies, *International Journal of Rehabilitation Research*, 13(4), 291–298, 1990.

146. Wehman, P. H., Kreutzer, J., West, M. D., Sherron, P. D., Zasler, N. D., Groah, C. H., et al., Return to work for persons with traumatic brain injury: A supported employment approach, *Archives of Physical Medicine and Rehabilitation*, 71(13), 1047–1052, 1990.

147. Haffey, W. J. and Abrams, D. L., Employment outcomes for participants in a brain injury work re-entry program: Preliminary findings, *Journal of Head Trauma Rehabilitation*, 6(3), 24–34, 1991.

148. Catalano, D., Pereira, A. P., Wu, M., Ho, H., and Chan, F., Service patterns related to successful employment outcomes of persons with traumatic brain injury in vocational rehabilitation, *Neurorehabilitation*, 21(4), 279–293, 2006.

149. Nisbet, J. and Hagner, D., Natural supports in the workplace: A re-examination of supported employment, *Journal of the Association for Persons with Severe Handicaps*, 13(4), 260–267, 1988.

150. Wehman, P., Kregel, J., Keyser-Marcus, L., Sherron-Targett, P., Campbell, L., West, M., et al., Supported employment for persons with traumatic brain injury: A preliminary investigation of long-term follow-up costs and program efficiency, *Archives of Physical Medicine and Rehabilitation*, 84(2), 192–196, 2003.

151. Abrams, D., Barker, L. T., Haffey, W., and Nelson, H., The economics of return to work for survivors of traumatic brain injury: Vocational services are worth the investment, *Journal of Head Trauma Rehabilitation*, 8(14), 59–76, 1993.

152. Fraser, R. T. and Wehman, P., Traumatic brain injury rehabilitation: Issues in vocational outcome, *Neurorehabilitation*, 5(1), 39–48, 1995.

153. Jacobs, H. E. and DeMello, C., The clubhouse model and employment following brain injury, *Journal of Vocational Rehabilitation*, 7(3), 169–179, 1997.

154. Ninomiya, Jr., J., Ashley, M. J., Raney, M. L., and Krych, D. K., Vocational rehabilitation, in M. J. Ashley and D. K. Krych, (Eds.), *Traumatic Brain Injury Rehabilitation*, CRC Press, Boca Raton, FL, 367–395, 1995.

155. Kolakowsky-Hayner, S. A., Gourley, E. V., Kreutzer, J. S., Marwitz, J. H., Meade, M. A., and Cifu, D. X., Post-injury substance abuse among persons with brain injury and persons with spinal cord injury, *Brain Injury*, 16(7), 583–592, 2002.

156. Kreutzer, J. S., Witol, A. D., and Marwitz, H. J., Alcohol and drug use among young persons with traumatic brain injury, *Journal of Learning Disabilities*, 29(6), 643–651, 1996.

157. Knapp, R. R. and Knapp, L., *COPS 9 (California Occupational Preference System) Interest Inventory*, EdITS, San Diego, CA, 1982.

158. Langmuir, C. R., *Oral Directions Test*, The Psychological Corporation, New York, 1974.

159. Bennett, G. K., Seashore, H. G., and Wesman, A. G., *Differential Aptitude Test (DAT): Administrator's Manual*, Harcourt, Brace, Jovanovich, New York, 1982.

160. Kanpp, L. and Knapp, R. R., *CAPS (Career Ability Placement Survey) Technical Manual*, EdITS, San Diego, CA, 1984.

161. Drury, D., Vencill, M., and Scott, J., *Rehabilitation and the California Injured Worker: Findings from Case File Reviews: A Report to the Rehabilitation Presidents' Council of California*, Berkeley Planning Associates, Berkeley, CA, 1988.

162. Fraser, R. T., Vocational evaluation, *Journal of Head Trauma Rehabilitation*, 6(3), 46–58, 1991.

163. Bullard, J. A. and Cutshaw, R., Vocational evaluation of the closed head injury population: A challenge of the 1990's, *Vocational Evaluation & Work Adjustment Bulletin*, 24(1), 15–19, 1991.

164. Brandon, T. L., Button, W. L., Rastatter, C. J., and Ross, D. R., *Manual for Valpar Component Work Sample 1: Small Tools (Mechanical)*, Valpar Corporation, Tucson, AZ, 1974.

165. Brandon, T. L., Bujtton, W. L., Rastatter, C. J., and Ross, D. R., *Manual for Valpar Component Work Sample 2: Size Discrimination*, Valpar Corporation, Tucson, AZ, 1974.

166. Brandon, T. L., Bujtton, W. L., Rastatter, C. J., and Ross, D. R., *Manual for Valpar Component Work Sample 3: Numeric Scoring*, Valpar Corporation, Tucson, AZ, 1974.

167. Brandon, T. L., Bujtton, W. L., Rastatter, C. J., and Ross, D. R., *Manual for Valpar Component Work Sample 4: Upper Extremity Range of Motion*, Valpar Corporation, Tucson, AZ, 1974.

168. Brandon, T. L., Bujtton, W. L., Rastatter, C. J., and Ross, D. R., *Manual for Valpar Component Work Sample 5: Clerical Comprehension and Aptitude*, Valpar Corporation, Tucson, AZ, 1974.

169. Brandon, T. L., Bujtton, W. L., Rastatter, C. J., and Ross, D. R., *Manual for Valpar Component Work Sample 6: Independent Problem Solving*, Valpar Corporation, Tucson, AZ, 1974.

170. Brandon, T. L., Bujtton, W. L., Rastatter, C. J., and Ross, D. R., *Manual for Valpar Component Work Sample 7: Multi-level Scoring*, Valpar Corporation, Tucson, AZ, 1974.

171. Brandon, T. L., Bujtton, W. L., Rastatter, C. J., and Ross, D. R., *Manual for Valpar Component Work Sample 8: Simulated Assembly,* Valpar Corporation, Tucson, AZ, 1974.

172. Brandon, T. L., Bujtton, W. L., Rastatter, C. J., and Ross, D. R., *Manual for Valpar Component Work Sample 9: Whole Body Range of Motion,* Valpar Corporation, Tucson, AZ, 1974.

173. Brandon, T. L., Bujtton, W. L., Rastatter, C. J., and Ross, D. R., *Manual for Valpar Component Work Sample 10: Tri-Level Measurement,* Valpar Corporation, Tucson, AZ, 1974.

174. Brandon, T. L., Bujtton, W. L., Rastatter, C. J., and Ross, D. R., *Manual for Valpar Component Work Sample 11: Eye–Hand–Foot Coordination,* Valpar Corporation, Tucson, AZ, 1974.

175. Brandon, T. L., Bujtton, W. L., Rastatter, C. J., and Ross, D. R., *Manual for Valpar Component Work Sample 12: Soldering and Inspection (Electronic),* Valpar Corporation, Tucson, AZ, 1974.

176. Rubenson, C., Svensson, E., Linddahl, I., and Björklund, A., Experiences of returning to work after acquired brain injury, *Scandinavian Journal of Occupational Therapy,* 14(4), 205–214, 2007.

24

Therapeutic Recreation in Traumatic Brain Injury Rehabilitation

Sam S. Andrews, Kenneth A. Gerhart, Kenneth R. Hosack, and Jill Stelley Virden

CONTENTS

24.1 Brief History of Therapeutic Recreation

Therapeutic recreation traces its beginnings to 400 BC, when Socrates and Plato first considered the relationship between physical health and mental health. Centuries later, one of the signers of the U.S. Declaration of Independence, Benjamin Rush, MD, advocated for recreation in the Pennsylvania Hospital, a psychiatric facility in Philadelphia. In 1810, Rush said of the individuals hospitalized there, "certain kinds of labor, exercise, and amusements should be contrived for them, which should act, at the same time, upon their bodies and minds."[1] As such, recreational therapy had its roots in vocational and occupational therapy in psychiatric facilities for about the next 100 years, during which time crafts, amusements, drama, and hospital occupations were believed to be valuable for those involved in such typically long hospitalizations. Even as late as the beginning of the 20th century, the terms *occupational* and *recreational* were virtually synonymous.

It was during the early 1900s, however, that occupational and recreational therapies began to separate slowly and differentiate themselves. In 1908, in Chicago's Hull House, classes were offered in occupations and amusements for hospital attendants. In 1911, William Dunton, the "father of occupational therapy" and a staff psychiatrist at Sheppard Enoch Pratt Asylum in Baltimore, taught a series of classes on occupation and recreation for nurses at Sheppard Enoch Pratt Asylum, and, soon after, created a new department by the same name.[1] The first National Recreation Congress was conducted in 1918, and recreation therapy became more widespread in general hospitals and centers for people with visual impairments. Around that same time, the federal government first began to recognize and support therapeutic recreation. The first federal Recreation Act was passed in 1926 (44 Stat. 741) and the U.S. Works Progress Administration began to distribute Recreation Division funds to recreational leaders at various institutions in 1934.

Therapeutic recreation expanded to serve various disability groups, including persons with developmental disabilities, visual impairments, and amputations, as well as geriatric populations. Therapeutic recreation continued to be codified as a discrete discipline, and in 1935, Dr. John Davis wrote a text entitled *Recreational Therapy, Play, and Mental Health*.[1] A year later, he and Dunton coauthored another text called *Principles and Practice of Recreational Therapy*.[1]

Therapeutic recreation continued to develop during World War II, when there was heightened interest in mobilizing and restoring soldiers to maximum health and productivity. The Federal Vocational Act was passed in 1943 and the Veterans' Administration Recreation Service was established in 1945. Three years later, the American Recreation Society created a Hospital Recreation Section. In the early 1950s, colleges and universities began to offer bachelor's and master's programs in physical education and recreation in rehabilitation. By 1955, the first hospital recreation personnel standards were published, dividing personnel into three titles: hospital recreation director, hospital recreation leader, and hospital recreation aide.

During the 1950s and 1960s, the profession of therapeutic recreation experienced significant growth, as three separate phenomena within health care were integrated. First, hospitals and other service providers furthered their treatment efforts by grouping individuals according to specific diagnoses or etiologies, such as those with spinal cord injury, developmental disabilities, and amputations, to offer more specialized rehabilitation services. Second, efforts to humanize institutions were underway and became part of the societal movement to "habilitate" people with disabilities and to enhance their functional skills. The third phenomenon, which was closely related to the second, was the societal movement toward deinstitutionalization, normalization of living, and community integration. Those who were still institutionalized, or those who needed to be so, gradually became recipients of more respectful and considerate treatment. This movement toward "normalization" continued to increase emphasis on progressively restoring functional activities of common daily life. Recreation personnel played a key role in providing those normal life activities.

During the past 40 years, therapeutic recreation has continued to grow and develop as a profession. One of the first formal definitions of therapeutic recreation, offered by Dunton, described therapeutic recreation as "any free, voluntary, and expressive activity, motor, sensory, or mental, vitalized by the expansive play spirit, sustained by deep-rooted pleasurable attitudes and evoked by wholesome emotional release, prescribed by medical authority as an adjuvant in treatment."[1]

That definition, along with the profession it describes, has continued to evolve. Today, the National Council for Therapeutic Recreation Certification provides the professional designation and titles of certified therapeutic recreation specialist and certified therapeutic recreation assistant. The O*Net, which has recently replaced the *Dictionary of Occupational Titles*, now defines recreation therapists as individuals who "plan, direct, or coordinate medically approved recreation programs for patients in hospitals, nursing homes, or other institutions. Activities include sports, trips, dramatics, social activities, and arts and crafts. May assess a patient condition and recommend appropriate recreational activity."[2]

24.2 Therapeutic Recreation for Persons with Traumatic Brain Injury

Therapeutic recreation programs specifically for individuals with severe traumatic brain injury (TBI) were further developed in the 1960s and 1970s as specialty-diagnosis rehabilitation programs continued to evolve. The Vietnam War brought on rapid advances in emergency trauma systems, and neuroradiologic and neurosurgical advances that resulted in a dramatic increase in the number of survivors of TBI. In 1981, the newly formed National Head Injury Foundation[3] coined the phrase "silent epidemic" to describe this rapid increase in the number of TBI survivors. Categorical brain injury rehabilitation programs grew dramatically during the 1980s, and therapeutic recreation became a part of the interdisciplinary teams with those programs. In 1985, therapeutic recreation for persons with brain injury was first included in the *Standards Manual for Facilities Serving People with Disabilities* by the Commission on Accreditation of Rehabilitation Facilities (CARF). This established the recreation therapist as a member of the primary core team of allied health professionals.[4] Between 1985 and 2002, CARF continually refined its standards to include additional components through the continuum of care, from acute through community integration, and therapeutic recreation continued to be one of the disciplines recommended for TBI, as determined by individual patient assessment and progress.[5]

24.3 Effectiveness of Therapeutic Recreation for Persons with Disabilities

Research specifically for survivors of TBI is sparse; therefore, what follows is a review of studies that discuss the effectiveness of therapeutic recreation with various disability groups that are the most relevant to individuals with TBI. One of the most significant efforts was made in 1991 by Coyle et al.[6] Through the support of a grant from the U.S. Department of Education's National Institute on Disability Rehabilitation and Research, Coyle et al.[6] convened panels of expert therapeutic recreation practitioners and educators with extensive experience and skill in treating a wide array of people with disabilities, and compiled the results of research, interventions, and outcomes. This panel, called the *National Consensus Conference on the Benefits of Therapeutic Recreation in Rehabilitation*, concluded that therapeutic recreation does hold substantial value for people with disabilities. Areas of benefit that have been identified by this panel,[6] and others, include

- Physical health and health maintenance (e.g., improvement in general physical and perceptual motor functioning in individuals with disabilities)
- Cognitive functioning (e.g., improved short- and long-term memory)

- Mental and psychosocial health (e.g., improved coping skills, self-control, sense of self, social skills, cooperation, growth and personal development, reduction of inappropriate behavior, and increased acquisition of developmental milestones)
- Personal and life satisfaction (e.g., community integration, productivity, and increased life and leisure satisfaction)

24.3.1 Physical Health

Improving and maintaining physical health and functioning is a goal of all rehabilitation, and therapeutic recreation is extremely valuable in this area. Connolly and Garbarini[7] report that therapeutic recreation reduces the risk of physical complications secondary to disability. One of the primary ways therapeutic recreation does this is by promoting participation in leisure activities that foster physical activity and exercise. Santiago et al.[8] report that recreation programs that improve aerobic fitness, for example, do enhance health. Although the effect of exercise on health in nondisabled people is well documented and does not need to be reviewed, a review of a few disability-specific and therapeutic recreation-specific findings may prove useful. Exercise and physical activity in disabled persons have direct effects on muscle strength, endurance, flexibility, and balance. They also reportedly reduce health risk factors[9] and help prevent secondary complications for people with disabilities.[8,10] Exercise can prevent or forestall such secondary complications as contractures, bladder complications, decubitus ulcers, cardiovascular disease, osteoporosis, and obesity.[11,12] Stotts[11] found that a group of spinal cord-injured persons who participated in wheelchair athletics had three times fewer hospital admissions than comparable nonparticipants. Indeed, among disabled persons who participate in sports, lower levels of obesity have already been reported, along with decreased incidences of skin breakdown, greater levels of respiratory endurance, higher levels of health maintenance, and a reduced frequency of rehospitalization overall.[9,11,12] Conversely, others have reported that physical inactivity can contribute to progressively decreasing health in adults with physical disabilities.[13] In perhaps the most significant finding, activity level was one of the most prominent predictors of survival itself among people with spinal cord injury.[14]

For many individuals—and certainly for people with TBI—recreational activities may be more motivating, more desirable, and more tolerable than mere exercise. As such, therapeutic recreation has been shown to be an extremely effective means of addressing the previously noted health issues and goals. Moreover, it is frequently a valuable adjunct to physical therapy, bringing many of physical therapy's goals and skills into real-world application.[15] For example, wheelchair handling skills taught in the hospital's physical therapy department can be put to use in a wheelchair basketball tournament or tennis game. Strengthening exercises or balance activities, practiced with the physical therapist, can translate to rowing, sailing, skiing, or jogging. Therapeutic recreation activities can often go beyond what physical therapy has to offer with respect to fitness and endurance building. Individuals struggling through initial rehabilitation have sometimes argued that the routines of activities of daily living (ADLs) were all the exercise they needed, but research has shown that this is not the case. In a group of individuals with paraplegia, researchers found that performance of ADL and self-care activities alone were not enough to maintain fitness.[16–18] Conversely, fitness through therapeutic recreation can enhance the performance of ADL. Exercise and leisure activities that increase fitness levels can also lead to increases in the ability to do work and to meet the demands of everyday life.[16,19] In other words, fitness can lead to increased productivity.

24.3.2 Cognitive Functioning

Relevant to those with severe TBI are reports that therapeutic recreation has positive effects on cognitive functioning and decreases confusion and disorientation.[7] It can engage individuals with TBI in interesting but simplified activities that place few functional demands upon them.[15] This is particularly important early during the rehabilitation process because it allows the therapeutic recreation specialist to address such areas as attention span, selective attention, recognition of things and events, and figure–ground discrimination. In addition, therapeutic recreation can be an important way of engaging individuals with TBI in cognitive and physical rehabilitation within an activity they enjoy, particularly when they have deficits in self-awareness and may not be able to understand or comply with traditional therapy.

Many of the mental and cognitive benefits of therapeutic recreation also appear to be related to the positive effects of the physical activity and exercise that it promotes. In a study of people with severe mobility impairments, investigators found that mental alertness and cognitive activity increased following exercise.[20] Cognitive function was also found to improve when elderly people with mental illnesses underwent fitness training.[21] Activity may also strengthen the ability to cope.

For example, several years ago, an individual who had been an aircraft mechanic was hospitalized in a low level of responsiveness following a TBI. After attempting several strategies to improve arousal, he was taken to an aircraft maintenance facility to be exposed to the familiar environment of the people, aircraft, sights, smells, and sounds of the facility. The experience was successful and he returned to the hospital substantially more responsive than when he left. Although the experience was not strictly recreational in nature, therapeutic recreation resources were utilized to facilitate the trip. The increased responsiveness might have occurred anyway, but the experience seemed to accelerate the rate of improvement.

24.3.3 Mental Health

Therapeutic recreation also has a positive effect on mental health. Researchers report that depression and depressive symptomatology decrease with exercise and activity,[7,9,10] and that depression may actually be caused by lack of activity.[13] Moreover, the overall mental health of adults has been reported to be dramatically influenced by their satisfaction with their leisure activities, often more so than by their satisfaction with work and health itself.[22]

Depression, stress, and other negative mental states adversely affect quality of life.[23] However, therapeutic recreation has the potential to impact these. Depressive symptoms are less in people who exercise, including people with disabilities.[10,24,25] Others have also reported that, following recreation, participants have less tension; better temperament; more energy; less confusion; better coping; less anxiety, fatigue, confusion, and anger; as well as lower levels of stress.[7,24,26,27] All of these are particularly relevant to those with TBIs.

In addition to the areas described here, all of which relate to psychosocial health, a key area for people with TBI is restoration of their self-image and sense of self. Many different elements contribute to an individual's sense of self. A few of them include developing a sense of mastery, controlling stress, seeing one's life as productive and meaningful, developing a positive body image, and having a positive attitude toward one's (and others') disabilities.[15] Although most of these will be discussed in detail in other sections, one

particular element that has been shown to be vital for a positive sense of self—the development of a sense of mastery—merits consideration here.

A sense of mastery often results when the individual experiences the feeling of having
performed successfully and effectively. Many therapeutic recreation activities can lead to
a sense of mastery. Sports, athletics, outdoor activities, and even creative endeavors can all
have an impact. However, the mastery experience is particularly enhanced when the risk
or difficulty of the activity continually increases so that the individual faces ongoing and
increasing challenges.[28] Actual increases in self-efficacy have been demonstrated following disabled individuals' participation in two different outdoor activities: rugged terrain
hiking and camping.[29,30]

The implications for the individual with the TBI are profound. Mastery of *old* activities
(that now may be difficult and, perhaps, overwhelming) can potentially lead to a sense
of mastery. Winning a billiard game, mastering a computer game (like Nintendo's Wii),
getting back to bicycling or using a hand cycle, successfully using public transportation,
or going to a public sporting event can represent "risk" to the TBI survivor and, as such,
can create opportunities for mastery. More important, such mastery generalizes to other
life areas. Hedrick[31] found that wheelchair tennis skills significantly increased disabled
teens' perceptions of their physical competence. Similarly, others report that skills taught
and activities experienced in rehabilitation generalize into individuals' postrehabilitation
life (e.g., people with TBIs who participated in a fishing experience prior to discharge were
likely to continue with outdoor activities in the community).[32]

24.3.4 Psychosocial Health

Leisure activities, by their very nature, encourage socialization and interaction with others.[33] They are a vehicle for getting involved in the community and for achieving community integration.[34] The effective use of leisure is what therapeutic recreation is about;
the impact of therapeutic recreation on community integration is clear, and the role of
the therapeutic recreation specialist in enhancing community integration seems obvious. Frequently, leisure is an effective vehicle for community involvement, and those
who are engaged in leisure activities view themselves as productive and having purpose.
Therapeutic recreation helps prevent social isolation and may prevent the individual from
becoming withdrawn. It may increase the hospitalized individual's will to survive and
help him or her embrace the rehabilitation program.[15] Later, the skills therapeutic recreation teaches continue to counteract the tendency for isolation. Activities, sports, and leisure pursuits all decrease isolation by increasing interaction with others in groups, on
teams, and in the community. Therapeutic recreation experiences can enhance not only
social interaction but also the *desire for* social interaction as well.[15] A particular therapeutic
exercise program actually increased the participants' social contacts *outside* the program
by 25% in one study of nonbrain-injured adults.[25] Finally, there is also evidence that socialization and community integration affect health. Disabled people who are inactive and
socially isolated (as evidenced by increased TV watching) have more medical complications and less leisure satisfaction.[35]

Sports activities, in particular, may foster community integration. Disabled athletes are
perceived by the general population as having higher social status and integration. For the
participant, sports decrease isolation, whereas for those who observe them—particularly
nondisabled people—they provide education, positive profiles of athletes, and ultimately
may promote healthier attitudes toward disability and individuals with disabilities.[36] Sir
Ludwig Guttman is generally credited with utilizing sports as a fundamental component

of the rehabilitation process for physically disabled World War II veterans in the United Kingdom.[37] Although Sir Ludwig's role at Stoke Mandeville was as a neurosurgeon and a master influence of the facility, he insisted that those he cared for actively participate in sports because of his strong belief in their physical and psychosocial benefit. Modern therapeutic recreation, in many ways, reflects those same principles today, but it does so for a broader spectrum of people and with a scope that extends far beyond sports.

In addition to sports activities, social interaction and community integration can occur through arts, music, horticulture, and volunteerism of many kinds. Therapeutic outings, as part of the rehabilitation experience, provide individuals and their families with exposure to familiar community venues and potential future activities. They also provide an opportunity to experience possible attitudinal and physical barriers in a supportive milieu.

24.3.5 Personal Satisfaction and Satisfaction with Life

Out of the sense of mastery described earlier grows a feeling of purposefulness and productivity. Both are key elements in a satisfying life. Although we typically associate productivity with productive work or employment, this is a very limited view of a concept that should also include productive avocational activities and leisure, family role and productive relationships, community service, and learning and education.[38] Moreover, a limited, employment-focused view of productivity too often can relegate rehabilitation consumers, particularly TBI survivors, to hopeless "unproductivity." Physical limitations, reduced endurance, and cognitive disabilities, as well as a highly competitive workplace and numerous work disincentives that exist on a societal level, may make returning to work an unrealistic, impractical, and unlikely outcome. People with disabilities seem to know this and have taken a different look at "work."

Often, leisure, recreation, and relationships with others take on greater importance.[39] (Others have reported similar findings.) Riddick,[22] for example, reports that satisfaction with leisure is frequently more important than satisfaction with work—and even with health—in determining well-being. Godbey[40] writes that it is the ability of people with disabilities "to use leisure in satisfying and appropriate ways which determines their fate as surely as their ability to do useful work."

Clearly, therapeutic recreation interventions frequently impact productivity in all of its conceptualizations. The benefits already mentioned (i.e., the ability of meaningful activity to improve physical and mental health, cognitive functioning, and functional carryover, and the successful mastery of new challenges) all carry over to other potentially productive life areas. For those who are able to work, the benefits are obvious; for those who are not, leisure is often thought of as a replacement for work.[15] Moreover, even among those who do work, leisure has been shown to compensate, at least in part, for lacking job satisfaction.[41] Others have found that work is not a factor in successful community reintegration, whereas leisure and recreation are factors.[42] Thus, therapeutic recreation teaches skills and builds the confidence and successes necessary to be productive in a variety of life areas.

Finally, participation in leisure and leisure satisfaction has been more directly linked to quality of life.[9,17,40] Both have been found to correlate with higher life satisfaction.[17,43]

Of direct application to brain injury is the work of Niemi et al.[44] They studied a group of individuals who had survived strokes 4 years earlier and found that poorer leisure functioning was a major factor preventing them from returning to their prestroke quality of life. Similarly, in another study of 700 adults with physical disabilities, researchers found that the participants' satisfaction with their leisure activities was one of the strongest predictors of overall life satisfaction. This prompted the researchers to recommend that time be allotted during rehabilitation to help hospitalized persons understand how their disabilities impacted their leisure involvement.[41] That this same study found leisure satisfaction to be lowest among those with newly acquired disabilities further suggested that leisure adjustment and education could not only enhance the rehabilitation process but might improve future life satisfaction as well.

In summary, therapeutic recreation improves physical and mental health, cognitive functioning, psychosocial functioning, and life satisfaction. Being active and engaged in the community through strategic and appropriate recreational interventions can result in better self-esteem, less depression, less stress, greater productivity, and better overall health. All of these result in decreased health care utilization and less subjective burden and expense for survivors, their families, and those who pay their medical bills.

24.4 Models of Service Delivery

The following section describes a model of therapeutic recreation service delivery within a categorical brain injury rehabilitation program at Craig Hospital that has proved to be effective for more than 35 years for people with TBIs and their families. First, any model of therapeutic recreation must emphasize movement from a high level of dependence along a continuum toward a reduced level of dependence, or independence. At the far end of the continuum of service delivery and outcome, the therapist should provide as little intervention and control as possible. This conceptual framework is supported by Gunn and Peterson,[45] who divide therapeutic recreation service into three general phases. The first phase of intervention on the continuum involves a high degree of control by the therapeutic recreation specialist and constrained obligatory behavior of the participant. The second phase is characterized by skill building in a variety of areas. The final phase is achieved when participation in recreation becomes a reality lifestyle and there is little or no control by the therapist except for provision of opportunity. The individual is independent, self-regulated, and his or her behaviors are intrinsically rewarding.[45] The health promotion model, constructed by Austin and Crawford,[46] depicts a similar movement by the individual through a continuum starting with poor health in an unfavorable environment and culminating in optimal health in a favorable environment. Although total success is not always possible, some movement through the continuum as described here is almost always possible.

Common concepts in most models of therapeutic recreation service delivery and intervention are

- A continuum of growth and intervention
- Belief in the strengths and abilities of the individual
- Increasing freedom and self-determination
- Decreasing therapist control
- Increasing involvement and participation or inclusion in the "natural" community[37]

Exposing individuals with TBI to familiar, practical, and measured activity is an effective tool during early intervention. As they move through the continuum, gradual and strategic exposure provides the opportunity to measure progress, evaluate the effectiveness of interventions, and prepare them to actualize life skills, functionality, social connection, and quality of life.

Therapeutic recreation for people with TBI should be delivered within the context of an interdisciplinary team, and collaborative activities should be created that maximize functional independence, provide education, and help educate and enhance involvement with family and friends.

Therapeutic recreation provides ecological validity to the findings and recommendations of other team members. Therapy in a protected hospital setting often requires therapists to make inferential assumptions about how an individual will function outside the hospital. Therapeutic recreation is the discipline specifically charged with verifying the validity of such assumptions. Therapeutic recreation is the functional integration of physical, cognitive, emotional, and psychosocial skills in real world-settings, and is invaluable to a valid rehabilitation process.

24.4.1 Assessment

Assessment should occur early following injury with the individual, family, and significant others, and should include a thorough history. Although the individual may change drastically in a very short time, early and accurate information about his or her preinjury life is essential in developing a treatment plan. Information regarding social, educational, vocational, and recreational history is the cornerstone for development of therapeutic recreation treatment strategies. The value of recreation *prior* to injury should serve as a reference for the therapeutic recreation specialist as he or she implements "already-familiar" activities early in the rehabilitation program. Communication with family and members of other clinical disciplines with respect to early treatment goals helps the therapeutic recreation specialist formulate a collaborative intervention strategy with other treating disciplines so that appropriate therapeutic intervention in the most appropriate therapeutic environment can be established from the beginning.

A critical part of assessment of the person with TBI is the therapists' understanding of the brain, brain anatomy and physiology, types of brain injury, and common functional sequelae of brain injury. For each individual, therapists must understand the key roles of initiation, planning, problem solving, self-awareness, and so forth, and how these cognitive skills and deficits may impact the individual's recreational treatment plan. The therapeutic recreation specialist can establish goals and intermediate objectives that illuminate these aspects of behavior, set milestones for measurement of progress, and offer the opportunity for creation of activity that provides optimal condition for the individual's advancement.

One formal instrument that is particularly useful to the therapeutic recreation specialist is the Leisure Competence Measure (LCM).[47] This standardized tool is similar in function, validation, and application to the Functional Independence Measure,[48] and is used widely throughout the rehabilitation field to measure functioning over time, to guide goal setting and intervention, and to assess progress and measure recreational therapy outcomes.[47,49] As such, the LCM is readily understood by all other members of the multidisciplinary rehabilitation team as well as payers, researchers, and others, and meets accountability standards of such organizations as the Joint Commission on Accreditation of Healthcare Organization and CARF.[49] The LCM uses eight subscales: (1) leisure awareness, (2) leisure attitude, (3) leisure skills, (4) cultural/social behaviors, (5) interpersonal skills, (6) community integration skills, (7) social contact, and (8) community participation. It has been shown to be both valid and reliable.[49] As a part of that continuum, the LCM can also be used to provide valuable information—in concrete and universal terms—to community entities (e.g., adaptive recreation community programs, independent living skills trainers, or home care providers) that may ultimately become involved in treating and accommodating the individual.

Another instrument that can be of great use is some form of leisure interest survey to gain vital information regarding individuals' values and interests. From this information, the therapeutic recreation specialist can determine needs based on interest and values, and then formulate a plan of intervention that will address and, as completely as possible, meet those needs.

24.4.2 Treatment

Information is compiled and presented at the first patient/family conference, along with other information the treating team has to share. This conference typically occurs within the first 2 weeks following admission and is designed to provide information and align expectations regarding diagnosis, condition, and short-term rehabilitation goals. The first conference is ideal for explaining the planned therapeutic recreation intervention and rationale, and for emphasizing the importance of continuing active recreation and leisure activity after discharge. This is also an excellent time to establish a therapeutic alliance formally and a relationship based on collaboration with the individual with the TBI (if possible) and family, and to obtain their input into the care plan. Communication with family, staff, and case managers, when appropriate, continues on an ongoing basis, both formally and informally.

The most effective approach to providing therapeutic recreation service is to bring it to the individual as an integral part of the interdisciplinary team intervention. In collaboration with the individual, his or her family, and members of other treating disciplines, the therapeutic recreation specialist can, more effectively, create and schedule therapeutic activities that

- Augment the therapeutic activities other members of the treating team have initiated
- Extend the individual's exposure to opportunity for therapeutic intervention
- Appropriately intensify specific therapeutic exercises and skill training activities
- Increase the individual's opportunity to operate in a more familiar environment
- Increase the opportunity to operate in a more realistic setting
- Give family an appropriate venue for involvement in the treatment process

Involving the entire family in the recreational goals and activities often is a very effective way for them to participate in the rehabilitation process when other opportunities may be few. However, caution must be taken to avoid overinvolvement of family. Family members, in their understandably heightened emotional state, may overreact or underreact to the medical condition of their loved one. There is often fear, confusion, and misunderstanding of the individual's condition. Realistic activity involvement with the TBI survivor and family together gives family the opportunity to be actively involved in a more appropriate environment, one that the therapeutic recreation specialist can monitor and moderate. Thus, the family member (or friend) who tends to be overly involved can be guided into a more subdued level of interaction. At the other end of the spectrum, underinvolved families, in the comfort of familiar activity and surroundings, can be encouraged, and any concerns they might have about how their efforts might place their loved one in jeopardy can be alleviated. In either case, appropriate involvement can give the family a more realistic perspective and can more accurately illustrate the abilities and limitations of the person with TBI.

Indeed, as often occurs after TBI, when the perceptions of limitations held by the injured person and the staff differ, family insight and involvement may be crucial. In particular, when the individual with the TBI is unable to make legally competent decisions about therapeutic activities, some of which may involve risk, the family will need to increase its understanding of capabilities, risks, and potential benefits. With the therapeutic recreation specialist's guidance and input, they are better able to decide when to hang on and when to let go.

24.4.3 Cotreatment with Other Members of the Rehabilitation Team

Cotreating is a very effective tool for treatment. It allows the physical, speech, or occupational therapist, for example, and the therapeutic recreation specialist to address multiple therapeutic issues, often with more than just one or two persons in a group. Recreation activity is frequently an excellent opportunity to evaluate the individual's progress when all the clinical efforts of the treating team are incorporated into activity.

Examples of productive cotreatment goals and activities include balance and coordination, attentional/distractibility groups, sensory integration, sequential memory exercise, and rekindling of skills and abilities. Commonly used activities are frequently drawn from those the individual participated in prior to injury, such as shooting baskets, jogging, swimming, shopping, going out to eat or to concerts, and the like. Often, life skill activities such as cooking, community integration outings, social skills groups, scavenger hunts, music activities, use of animals, exercise, and horticulture activities are also conducted with therapists from multiple disciplines. Interventions like these provide mutual validation of the therapists, enhanced recognition of the therapists by the individual with TBI, consistency in treatment techniques, and greater application of expertise toward the individual's progress. Even more important, such activities give a taste of life in the postrehabilitation world. The list of possible activities that can translate to real-life skills is endless and, in a good rehabilitation program that focuses on community reintegration, that list is, in fact, *comprised* of real-life activities. Anything that individual might have done, or might do in the future, regardless of whether it is adapted is fair game for a therapeutic intervention, functional activity, and skill-building experience. The bottom line: Only the potential therapeutic value should be considered in selecting an activity. This is a tried-and-true therapeutic recreation concept that dates back more than 150 years. Introduced by Amariah Brigham, then superintendent of the Utica State Hospital in New York, it remains a guiding principal even today.[1]

In addition, in the hospital setting, it is often therapeutic recreation that offers the other disciplines a more accurate picture of real-world behaviors, performance, and capabilities. In a notable example, one individual's discharge goals were totally revamped when treatment in the greenhouse and recreation room yielded a completely different level of cooperation and motivation than the physical and occupational therapists were able to obtain in their more clinical, and seemingly more threatening and controlled, settings. In fact, what the individual was truly capable of in a more informal setting was so clearly and dramatically demonstrated to the entire team that a discharge to the home occurred rather than institutionalization. Unquestionably, a monumental difference was made in long-term care costs and personal quality of life in this instance.

This example illustrates another important point: Without *meaningful* activities that incorporate all the myriad clinical goals (e.g., behavior, cognitive function, perception, executive function, gross and fine motor skills, speech, attention span), the treating team has to guess how effective its combined therapeutic efforts have been. A more realistic and accurate evaluation can be made following the application of real-life skill exposure, social activity, proper stimulation, and, in some cases, appropriate use of diversion. Clearly, recreation in the rehabilitation setting is far more than "entertainment." Although a big "menu" of activities is helpful, the goals and context of those activities are more important. Therapeutic recreation should never be thought of as something that merely keeps people with disabilities from being bored, nor should it be presented as "stuff" to fill up their evenings and weekends.

24.4.4 Translating Therapeutic Recreation to the Real World: Community Integration

Therapeutic recreation must "set the stage" for the individual to access the community or, more likely, the community to reach out to the individual. Exposure to equipment and materials during rehabilitation greatly enhances the probability that individuals and families will access resources subsequent to discharge. Advocacy, practical assertiveness training, education leading to reasonable accommodation, and education on seeking and accessing resources in the community are vital subjects to be addressed. These topics must be covered thoroughly and accurately if individuals with TBI or their family members are to have any semblance of success in accomplishing social integration. Understanding these areas is equally important for families who hope to gain any effective form of respite from the sometimes overwhelming day-to-day maintenance and essential survival tasks.

Despite the best efforts of the entire interdisciplinary staff, major barriers to social and community integration exist. One such barrier is merely making the transition from safety and security to uncertainty. Although many therapeutic activities within the health care institution provide opportunity, they are initially unfamiliar to the consumer and, therefore, may not be as initially effective as they could. However, as time goes by, it is the rehabilitation setting itself that becomes secure and familiar, and the outside world becomes threatening. Thus, the therapeutic recreation specialist must work with the individual to again make that world familiar. Transitional events or settings must be used to provide exposure to the real-life venues that are likely to be encountered after discharge from the health care facility.

Transportation is generally another barrier that presents major challenges, especially because so many individuals with TBI have serious difficulty utilizing transportation on an independent basis. They either have enough difficulty with orientation that they are unable to travel throughout the community or they are legitimately fearful of using public transportation. Consequently, transportation is an issue the therapeutic recreation specialist needs to address thoroughly. Moreover, it is an issue that may need to be readdressed over time as the needs, interests, and abilities of the person with a disability change.

A third barrier is social isolation. Among those TBI survivors who are able to move about the community, some may, nonetheless, reject the idea of participation in specialized community programs provided for people with similar disabilities. Others may be reluctant to participate in regular events and activities because of inabilities they may have, or perceive themselves as having, in social functioning. They may encounter so many negative experiences that they give up attempts to access their community, and become isolated and socially deprived. Often, the social deprivation is even more exasperating because of the individual's strong desire for intimate relationships, which, for many, are very difficult to achieve. Those who make effective social connections usually do so as the result of the efforts of a significant other. This can be an independent living skills trainer, advocate, or any other dedicated individual who consistently intervenes on the individual's behalf.

Clearly, the possibility of isolation after discharge must be anticipated and addressed. Every possible effort must be made to prevent social isolation. A progressive approach of exposure to achievable and realistic situations is a must. Connecting the individuals and their families with activities that augment, if not replicate, other therapeutic activities by other disciplines brings about better understanding and enhanced self-esteem even when only a small amount of success can be achieved. It has been frequently observed that almost everyone functions more effectively in an environment in which they perceive a greater level of comfort. This is doubly true of the person with TBI, and the role of the therapeutic recreation specialist in facilitating a clear transition to home and community is an obvious and vital one.

The therapeutic recreation specialist's involvement with other key friends, family members, and facilitators is necessary for a smooth return to the community. Indeed, the therapeutic recreation specialist must pay attention not only to the individual with TBI but also to the person or persons who can be there to facilitate social interaction on a consistent and long-term basis. Independent living skills trainers, recreation center staff members, teachers, team members, and others can be effective resources to assist the individual toward improved function. Others may need to be sought out as the individual's situation and needs dictate. It is likely that the therapeutic recreation specialist and the discharging health care institution will need to orchestrate and channel individuals and their families to community activities and events that they can participate in. At the very least, this will be necessary during the transitional period as they begin their exploration of other activities that are available beyond the rehabilitation setting. This task becomes more challenging if the individual is being discharged to a community distant from where the rehabilitation program takes place. The therapeutic recreation specialist then must give increased effort to identifying and simulating activities available in the community to which the individual will return, and to identifying local experts and mentors. Clearly, additional effort must be made to make contact with resource entities in that community.

Despite the goal of autonomy and self-determination for many individuals, some persons may require continuous connection with support systems, be they individuals or organizations. In some cases, family members of the individual may have to support and help initiate community activity continually for the major part of the individual's life. The therapeutic recreation specialist should educate family regarding the scope of the family members' own abilities to cope with the demanding support role they will face. Coping mechanisms and resource exploration on their behalf are very important as well.

There is almost always a need for a significant other to encourage, to help with initiation, to moderate the individual's emotional reactions, to arrange for transportation, to intervene when a given situation becomes untenable, and to search out new and appropriate resources. In many cases, this effort takes a tremendous physical and emotional toll on family. Consequently, family members must have the skills and resources necessary to protect themselves, to the best extent possible, from exhaustion and exasperation, which may diminish or curtail their ability to intervene effectively. It is important that family members or significant others have skill in caring for themselves. They should be *encouraged* and *enabled* to do so, and should attend to their own needs, as well as their loved one's, so that they can maintain their efforts over a prolonged period, possibly even an entire lifetime. Respite, delegation of responsibilities, and measured effort across the entire lives of the person with the disability and his or her family must be common and frequently utilized tools.

24.4.5 Anticipation of Noncompliance with Medical Advice

Practicality of actual experience can be of value, especially when it can be reasonably expected that the individuals may not always follow directives or advice of staff or physicians. There is frequently a perception that individuals with TBI have lost a great deal of freedom and self-determination. Often, they may not have a realistic view of what abilities or limitations they may have. They perceive some restrictions as unnecessary, especially in light of how much they feel medical personnel and family have already taken away. A common comment may be, "I have no idea why they are making me do things this way," or "I do not see why I have to be here; I am just fine!" They, at the same time, may not be able to find the nearest restroom, even with directions. Restrictions are often documented in the medical record or mandated by law. Clearly, the physician can write into the chart at the time of discharge that the individual is not cognitively and/or physically capable of driving safely. In most states, this is sufficient to preclude most individuals from driving or attempting to obtain a license to drive. However, as an example, many of those same individuals face no government restriction in the use of firearms and can be out in a field with a loaded gun, completely unaware of the seemingly obvious safety issues or consequences. Even with a physician's strongly documented opinion that the individual must not take up hunting activities, the common mentality of many is, "They can take away a lot of things from me, but they are not taking away my hunting." The recreation assessment is absolutely critical in establishing if an issue such as this might arise. If there is the slightest suspicion by staff that the individual might return to hunting, it might make a great deal of sense to put the individual and a family member through progressive competency exercises. Only then can deficiencies in the ability to enter safely into a hunting situation become clear to all concerned. "Not going there," more often than not, is seen as tacit approval, and of course, could produce a deadly outcome. Therapeutic recreation specialists should take their intervening roles very seriously in cases like this. They must ensure that proper exploration of any issues of this nature takes place. If the therapist does not have the desire or expertise to do so, appropriate referral should be made.

The same issues and consequences can apply to biking, skiing, piloting a boat, operating farm equipment, fishing along a stream, or other adventure activities. If the therapeutic recreation specialist does not have the expertise or resources to provide competency evaluation in any such activity, appropriate referral should be made.

24.4.6 Conclusion

Independence and success are relative and dynamic throughout the life of an individual who has sustained a TBI. Therapeutic recreation is a vital piece of that success, and it is a piece that has been shown to be effective in maintaining physical health, improving mental health and cognitive functioning, increasing community integration and productivity, and enhancing life satisfaction. As such, the therapeutic recreation specialist is in an enviable position to impact the postrehabilitation outcome of a survivor of TBI.

Along with other members of the other clinical disciplines, he or she must make a concerted effort to educate the individual and any significant persons in that individual's life about the importance of preparation for the real-life issues the TBI will force them to face. A guided, gradual exposure to all that recreation and leisure have to offer will help all those dealing with a TBI to move from a position of dependence and isolation to one of increased independence and autonomy. The temptation to ignore quality-of-life issues is very great when there is so much to be done medically and functionally. However, if quality of life is not addressed, one might legitimately ask: What was the purpose of going through the medical motions? Therapeutic recreation professionals gain satisfaction from helping people with disabilities progress to the point that they can experience success in regaining functionality and in restoring purpose, self-esteem, and joy to their lives. In these modern, technology-saturated times, there is an unlimited amount of stuff available, but the lack of expertise on how to utilize that "stuff" as a viable resource remains problematic. The role of the therapeutic recreation specialist is to fill that gap in expertise to give people with disabilities a much better chance at maximizing the rehabilitation experience and returning to as high a quality of life as possible.

24.5 The Future of Therapeutic Recreation and TBI

The field of therapeutic recreation faces serious challenges in the future. Despite the fact that therapeutic recreation is widely valued, therapeutic recreation has not sufficiently convinced the medical and insurance communities that therapeutic recreation is "medically necessary," and therefore is not a covered benefit in many insurance policies. This is, in part, a result of a failure to view recreation as part of a holistic health and wellness model. Therapeutic recreation, historically, has not taken the time and resources to conduct and disseminate respected scientific research addressing its efficacy and cost-saving potential. The fact that therapeutic recreation is not included as a benefit in insurance policies creates a dilemma for rehabilitation providers. Even though hospital and rehabilitation administrators may recognize the value of therapeutic recreation, difficult economic times often make them unable to offer such services or force them to cut back on them, unless they have some philanthropic resource to fund recreation staff and programs. In the recent past, the number of therapeutic recreation specialists in rehabilitation facilities has declined as a result of economic pressures on institutional budgets. This action is seen as a measure to reduce operating expenses while exacting little perceived negative effect on the rehabilitation outcomes of individual consumers. Ideally, a case load in an inpatient rehabilitation setting caring for those with new catastrophic injuries would be five to six individuals, which is similar to a typical case load of a physical or occupational therapist. A caseload of 10 to 12 per therapist is possibly manageable, but not ideal. These ratios are predicated on the consideration that the therapeutic recreation specialist is experienced and is a functional part of an interdisciplinary treatment team. Unfortunately, these ratios are generally not the case today because many rehabilitation programs have significantly reduced their recreation departments or eliminated the departments entirely.

However, it is strongly argued that eliminating or cutting recreation resources may, in fact, add expenses and create more burden on rehabilitation programs. First, the physical, cognitive, psychosocial, and life satisfaction needs of people with disabilities and their families will continue to exist in the absence of therapeutic recreation. Without recreation resources, those needs simply spill over to physicians, nurses, psychologists, therapists, and other members of rehabilitation teams. Recent observations in one institution were that the absence of therapeutic recreation resulted in a significant increase in nurse call-light activity. Counselors, nurses, and psychologists experienced substantial increases in patient and family needs, increased incidents of customer dissatisfaction, and staff stress. This ultimately forced the institution to hire more staff and take steps to repair damage to its marketing efforts. Therefore, the absence of recreational options and time in rehabilitation programs creates a higher consumer and family demand and appears to offer little or no financial relief to the institution in the long run.

Beyond the rehabilitation hospital, the greater concern is the deterioration of postrehabilitation outcomes without recreation. In the absence of a therapeutic recreation program, persons with TBI may be discharged with significant unresolved issues and unmet needs, and may face a community without the skills and knowledge to master their future. These unmet needs almost certainly arise as serious barriers that prevent or impede a return to as functional a lifestyle as can be reasonably expected. Rehabilitation, without therapeutic recreation intervention, of a person who has sustained a TBI is incomplete and sometimes risky. The most important component of the rehabilitation process, next to medical improvement for which physicians, counselors, and therapists strive, is functionality. Competent therapeutic recreation service is a vital component to restoring that functionality and the greatest possible lifestyle quality that can be reasonably expected.

References

1a. Dixon, C. C., Recreational therapy—Beginning to 1885, Therapeutic Recreation Directory, http://www.recreationtherapy.com/history/rhistory1.htm (access January 11, 2010).

1b. William Rush Dunton, Jr, and John Davis. *Principles and Practice of Recreational Therapy for the Mentally Ill*, AS Barnes & Co., NY, 1936.

 2. O*Net Resource Center, Summary report for 29-1125.00-recreational therapists, O*Net Online, http://online.onetcenter.org/link/summary/29-1125.00 (accessed January 11, 2010).

 3. National Head Injury Foundation, Silent epidemic, *NHIF Newsletter*, 6(3–4), 1986–1987.

 4. Commission on Accreditation of Rehabilitation Facilities, *Standards Manual for Facilities Serving People with Disabilities,* Author, Tucson, AZ, 1985.

 5. Commission on Accreditation of Rehabilitation Facilities, *2002 Medical Rehabilitation, Standards Manual,* Author, Tucson, AZ, 2002.

 6. Coyle, C. P., Kinney, W. B., Riley, B., and Shank, J. W., *Benefits of Therapeutic Recreation. A Consensus View*, Idyll Harbor, Ravensdale, WA, 1991.

 7. Connolly, P. and Garbarini, A., Certified recreation specialists carve a niche in geriatric rehabilitation, *Journal of Long-term Care Administration*, 23(3), 34–35, 1995.

 8. Santiago, M. C., Coyle, D. P., and Kinney, W. B., Aerobic exercise effect on individuals with physical disabilities, *Archives of Physical Medicine and Rehabilitation*, 74(11), 1192–1198, 1993.

 9. Sorensen, B. and Luken, K., Improving functional outcomes with recreational therapy, *Case Manager*, 10(5), 49–52, 1999.

10. Compton, D. M., Eisenman, P. A., and Henderson, H. L., Exercise and fitness of persons with disabilities, *Sports Medicine,* 7(3), 150–162, 1989.

11. Stotts, K. M., Health maintenance: Paraplegic athletes and nonathletes, *Archives of Physical Medicine and Rehabilitation*, 67(2), 109–114, 1986.

12. Valliant, P. M., Bezzubyk, I., Daley, L., and Asu, M. E., Psychological impact of sport on disabled athletes, *Psychological Reports*, 56(3), 923–929, 1985.

13. Coyle, C. P. and Santiago, M. C., Aerobic exercise training and depressive symptomatology in adults with physical disabilities, *Archives of Physical Medicine and Rehabilitation*, 76(7), 647–652, 1995.

14. Krause, J. S. and Crewe, N. M., Prediction of long-term survival of persons with spinal cord injury, *Rehabilitation Psychology,* 32(4), 205–213, 1987.

15. Berryman, D., James, A., and Trader, B., The benefits of therapeutic recreation in physical medicine, in *Benefits of Therapeutic Recreation: A Consensus View*, Coyle, C. P., Kinney, W. B., Riley, B., and Shank, J. W., Eds., Idyll Harbor, Ravensdale, WA, Chap. 7, 261, 1991.

16. Hjetnes, H. and Vocak, Z., Circulatory strain in everyday life in paraplegics, *Scandinavian Journal of Rehabilitation Medicine,* 11(2), 67–73, 1979.
17. Knuttson, E., Lewenhaupt-Olsson, E., and Thorsen, M., Physical work capacity and physical conditioning in paraplegic patients, *Paraplegia*, 11(3), 205–216, 1973.
18. Hooker, S. P. and Wells, C. L., Effects of low and moderate intensity training in spinal cord injured persons, *Medicine and Science in Sports and Exercise,* 21(1), 18–22, 1989.
19. Jochheim, K. A. and Strokendhl, H., The value of particular sports of the wheelchair-disabled in maintaining health of the paraplegic, *Paraplegia*, 11(2), 173–178, 1973.
20. Krebs, P., Eickelberg, W., Krobath, H., and Barcfh, I., Effects of physical exercise on peripheral vision and learning in children with spinal bifida manifested, *Perceptual and Motor Skills,* 68(1), 167–174, 1989.
21. Folkins, C. H. and Sime, W. E., Physical fitness training and mental health, *American Psychologist*, 36(4), 373–389, 1981.
22. Riddick, C. C., Leisure satisfaction precursors, *Journal of Leisure Research*, 18(4), 259–265, 1986.
23. Gerhart, K. A., Weitzenkamp, D. A., Kennedy, P., Glass, C. A., and Charlifue S. W., Correlates of stress in long-term spinal cord injury, *Spinal Cord*, 37(3), 183–190, 1999.
24. Greenwood, C. M., Dzewattowski, D. A., and French R., Self-efficacy and psychological well-being of wheelchair tennis participants and wheelchair nontennis participants, *Adapted Physical Activity Quarterly*, 7(1), 12–21, 1990.
25. Weiss, C. and Jamieson, N., Hidden disabilities: A new enterprise for therapeutic recreation, *Therapeutic Recreation Journal*, 22(4), 9–17, 1988.
26. Hanrahan, S. J., Grove, J. R., and Lockwood, R. J., Psychological skills training for the blind athlete: A pilot program, *Adapted Physical Activity Quarterly,* 7(2), 143–155, 1990.
27. Katz, J. F., Adler, J. C., Mazzarella, N. J., and Inck, L. P., Psychological consequences of an exercise training program for a paraplegic man: A case study, *Rehabilitation Psychology*, 530(1), 53–58, 1985.
28. Bandura, A., *Social Learning Theory*, Prentice Hall, Englewood Cliffs, NJ, 1977.
29. Austin, D. R., Recreation and persons with physical disabilities: A literature synthesis, *Therapeutic Recreation Journal,* 21(1), 36–44, 1987.
30. Robb, G. M. and Ewert, A., Risk recreation in persons with disabilities, *Therapeutic Recreation Journal*, 21(1), 58–69, 1987.
31. Hedrick, B. N., The effect of wheelchair tennis participation and mainstreaming upon the perceptions of competence of physically disabled adolescents, *Therapeutic Recreation Journal*, 19(2), 34–46, 1985.
32. Trader, B., Nicholson, L., and Anson C., Effectiveness of a model leisure education program for use in SCI, Unpublished report to Research Review Committee, Shepherd Spinal Center, Atlanta, GA, 1991.
33. Hisek, D. D., Recreation planning for a nursing home, *Therapeutic Recreation Journal,* 12(2), 26–29, 1968.
34. Salzberg, C. L. and Langford, C. A., Community integration of mentally retarded adults through leisure activity, *Mental Retardation*, 19(3), 127–131, 1981.
35. Anson, C. and Shepherd, C., A survey of postacute spinal cord patients: Medical, psychological, and social characteristics, *Trends: Research News from Shepherd Spinal Center*, Atlanta, GA, 1990.
36. Jackson, R. W. and Davis, G. M., The value of sports and recreation for the physically disabled, *Orthopedic Clinics of North America,* 14(2), 301–315, 1983.
37. Bullock, C. C. and McMahon, M. J., *Introduction to Recreation Services for People with Disabilities*, Sagamore Publishing, Champaign, IL, 318, 1997.
38. Trieschmann, R. B., Vocational rehabilitation: A psychological perspective, *Rehabilitation Literature*, 45(11–12), 345–348, 1985.
39. Weitzenkamp, D. A., Gerhart, K. A., Charlifue, S. W., Whiteneck, G. G., Glass, C. A., and Kennedy, P., Ranking the criteria for assessing quality of life after disability: Evidence for priority shifting among long-term spinal cord injury survivors, *British Journal of Health Psychology*, 5(1), 57–69, 2000.

40. Godbey, G., *Leisure in Your Life: An Exploration*, Venture, State College, PA, 1990.
41. Kinney, W. B. and Coyle, C. P., Predicting life satisfaction among adults with physical disabilities, *Archives of Physical Medicine*, 73(9), 863–869, 1992.
42. Bruinniks, R. H., Chen, T. H., and Lakin, C., Components of personal competence and community integration for persons with mental retardation in small residential programs, *Research in Developmental Disabilities*, 13(5), 463–479, 1992.
43. Ragheb, M. G. and Griffith C. A., The contribution of leisure participation and leisure satisfaction to life satisfaction of older persons, *Journal of Leisure Research*, 14(4), 295–306, 1982.
44. Niemi, M., Laaksonen, R. R., Kotila, M., and Waltim, O., Quality of life four years after stroke, *Stroke*, 19 (Suppl.), 1101–1107, 1988.
45. Peterson C. A. and Gunn, S. L., *Therapeutic Recreation Program Design: Principles and Procedures*, 2nd ed., Prentice Hall, Englewood Cliffs, NJ, 1984.
46. Austin, D. R. and Crawford, M. E., *Therapeutic Recreation: An Introduction*, Allyn & Bacon, Needham Heights, MA, 1996.
47. Kloseck, M. and Crilly, R. G., *Leisure Competence Measure: Adult Version. Professional Manual and Users' Guide*, Leisure Competence Measure Data System, London, Ontario, Canada, 1997.
48. Uniform Data System for Medical Rehabilitation, Functional Independence Measure (FIM), State University New York, Buffalo, NY, 2009.
49. Leisure Competence Measure, Idyll Arbor, Inc., http://www.idyllarbor.com/cgi-bin/SoftCart.exe/assessme/A182.HTM?E_scstore (accessed June 22, 2002).

25

Children and Adolescents: Practical Strategies for School Participation and Transition

Roberta DePompei and Janet Siantz Tyler

CONTENTS

> No head injury is too severe to despair of nor too trivial to ignore.

> —**Hippocrates, 4th Century,** BC

25.1 Introduction

Children and adolescents sustain traumatic brain injuries (TBIs) of many types and severities. Regardless of the etiology, severity level, or progress made in acute care, the challenges of returning to home, school, and community are reported to be some of the least organized and poorly supported experiences for the child/adolescent and family.[1–7] DiScala et al.[5,8] found that many children and adolescents who are hospitalized at the time of injury are not referred to inpatient rehabilitation. When children and adolescents are reported to have three or less disabilities (e.g., problems with walking, eating, talking, dressing), 80% are discharged to home and community and, when there are four disabilities or more reported, 60% are discharged to home and community. Bedell et al.[6,9] reported that even the children and adolescents who were provided inpatient rehabilitation were less well prepared to participate in age-appropriate activities at discharge. The result is that the majority of rehabilitation for children and adolescents is completed within the community, and the school is often the primary provider of services.

We have traditionally approached the medical, educational, and community living aspects of service provision by referring to a continuum of care. DePompei[10] suggested that viewing treatment and rehabilitation from a traditional continuum of care (Figure 25.1) that says that treatment begins in the hospital and ends in the community may not be the most beneficial perspective and may, itself, be responsible for the lack of smooth transition among hospital, school, family, and community. This traditional continuum of care begins with emergency medical services caring for the injured child and transporting him or her to a hospital where trauma teams and medical teams in the acute care hospital provide specialized medical interventions. When stabilized, rehabilitation teams are involved in the process of treatment. At a point where the child/adolescent is showing progress and is medically able to return home, the medical team discharges the child to home, school, and community. The responsibility then rests with community resources and parents to provide additional rehabilitation and education services and to prepare the child/adolescent for transition to community living.

DePompei[10] believes that the continuum of care is insufficient to explain the concepts surrounding the injury and reintegration to community. It is, in and of itself, responsible

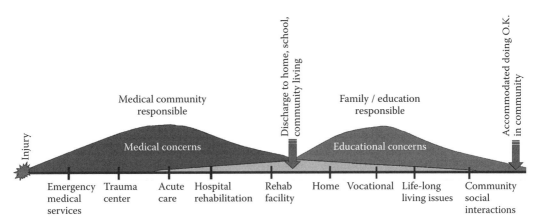

FIGURE 25.1
Continuum of care for youth with acquired brain injury (ABI). (From Blosser, J. and DePompei, R., *Pediatric Traumatic Brain Injury: Proactive Intervention*, 2nd ed., Delmar, New York, 2002, Ch. 2. With permission.)

for the false dichotomy of medical–educational systems treating these children. An alternative to thinking about a continuum of care can be found in Condalucci's[7,11–15] model of community interdependence. The interdependence concept suggests that there must be an interconnection or interrelationship among two or more entities. In our case, medical, family, educational, and community entities should be responsible to one another as points of contact on the circle. The circle of community interdependence (Figure 25.2) is not a linear model, as is suggested by the continuum of care, but a circular concept that begins and ends in the community.

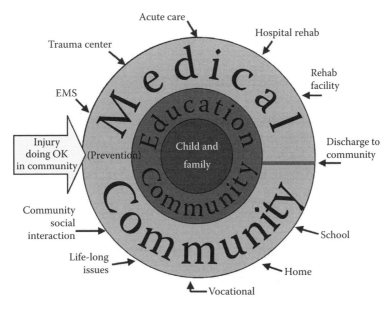

FIGURE 25.2
Circle of community interdependence. EMS, emergency medical services. (From Blosser, J. and DePompei, R., *Pediatric Traumatic Brain Injury: Proactive Interventions*, 2nd ed., Delmar, New York, 2002, Ch. 2. With permission.)

In this concept, the beginning point is not emergency medical service. The injury or illness begins in the community where the child/adolescent is a living, contributing member. Treatment of the child's brain injury then engages experts in medicine, education, community, and the family who collaborate with the same goal: to return the child to where he or she began—the community. Because this concept is based on a circle, any point on the circle may be the beginning point of care. For example, the child with a mild brain injury may not be seen first in the medical community, but may remain in the educational community for several months or years until the problem is recognized. It is at this later point that the child may be referred to the medical community for services. The circle of interdependence, therefore, accounts for all aspects of service equally within the community. This concept is supported heavily in the literature.[4,16–23]

If we provide services from a community of interdependence concept, we should assume responsibility for the entire circle of care regardless of which part we play in the circle. Thus, we, in the medical community, provide the treatment we are trained to provide. But treatment is provided with consideration of the eventual return of this child to the community; and we, in the educational and lifelong living community, receive the child/adolescent with an appreciation of the complex and unique medical and behavioral aspects that will affect learning by this child. Using this thought process, we are better able to focus on the total needs of the child/adolescent to function within the community.[2]

We acknowledge that some who work from a medical perspective regard TBI as a disease to be managed whereas those who work in the community regard TBI as an educational and community participation issue. Both perspectives are valid and represent means for obtaining financial and social supports, and agency services for these children and adolescents. Our belief is that both concepts are valid in the particular settings in which the children and adolescents are treated.

In this chapter, we operate from two concepts: (1) that the majority of rehabilitation for children and adolescents occurs at school and in the community and (2) that there is a circle of community care that should guide the interventions. If these perspectives are accepted, we can begin to plan, interactively and proactively, for this population. This chapter focuses on the following:

- Describing the cognitive–communicative behaviors a student may exhibit after TBI
- Suggesting how the cognitive–communicative challenges will affect learning and behaving in the classroom
- Outlining strategies for learning in school
- Discussing laws and regulations that affect education, provision of services, and transition issues
- Providing methods to affect seamless transitions throughout the educational lifetime of the student

25.2 Cognitive–Communicative Challenges after Traumatic Brain Injury

Many cognitive processes can be affected after sustaining a TBI. These processes can impact learning and behaving in the classroom. The processes of attention, processing speed, short- and long-term memory, organization, and problem solving are often challenged. In addition, impulsive behaviors and receptive, expressive, and pragmatic language skills are potentially problematic.[3,4,22,24,25] When developmental issues are also considered, challenges to learning are further confounded.

Classroom behaviors often reflect problems the student is experiencing with the previously mentioned cognitive–communicative processes. Unfortunately, many teachers attempt to alter the behaviors without considering the underlying processes that are affecting the behaviors. If these underlying processes are considered in the educational process, classroom behaviors and learning can be modified. Table 25.1 outlines the cognitive processes, describes how a process can be challenged in a student with TBI, and gives examples of how these behaviors may appear in the classroom and may be

TABLE 25.1

Cognitive Processes, Challenges to a Student with TBI, and Possible Classroom Behaviors

Underlying Cognitive Process	How Process Can Be Affected after TBI	Possible Classroom Behaviors
Attention	Unable to sustain or maintain attention to complete tasks or activities.	Fussing with books, papers, pencils; looking out a window; bothering a neighbor; daydreaming; moving about the classroom; calling for teacher's attention about a different matter.
Delayed processing speed	Much slower to respond to written or verbal directions, questions, requests; difficulty with rate and amount of complexity of information presented.	Unable to formulate a response to a question in usual time allotted for students to respond, even though he or she may know the correct response or behavior; speaking out; throwing paper or pencil; ceasing attempt to participate; bolting from classroom.
Short-term memory	Information is not held long enough to respond to it.	Unable to follow directions to locate certain page in text, sequence several requests at once, or respond to request to change an activity spontaneously.
Long-term memory	Information is unable to be stored for retrieval when needed; information that is stored cannot be accessed when required.	Recognizes memory strategies, such as rehearsal, but cannot use spontaneously; vocabulary learned for health on one day is not recalled the next; poor test-taking skills.
Organization	Unable to move through the day in a logical manner; planning for events or tasks is sporadic and uneven, lacking a methodologic means to achieve an end; inability to plan how to attack a job or assignment in a logical order.	Does not recall order of the classroom day and is unprepared for class assignments or locations; begins an assignment but does not finish; offers to do a task, such as collect and sort classroom papers, but becomes lost in the details before completing the task.
Problem solving	Often cannot locate alternative methods to solve a problem (believes there is only one way to approach a dilemma); disorganized in planning how to solve a problem; unable to sequence behaviors to resolve a challenge.	Insists there is no solution to a problem; tries to solve a problem in exactly the same way for long periods of time; does not recognize suggestions of the teacher for changing a way to work a problem.

(continued)

TABLE 25.1 (continued)

Cognitive Processes, Challenges to a Student with TBI, and Possible Classroom Behaviors

Underlying Cognitive Process	How Process Can Be Affected after TBI	Possible Classroom Behaviors
Impulsivity	Speaks or acts out immediately without evidence of "thinking through" the situation.	Leaves seat to sharpen a pencil when teacher is talking; tells teacher her hair is dirty and looks bad; uses socially unacceptable language or gestures.
Expressive language	Difficulty with word recall; poor organization of conversation; speaks off topic; rambles; written work is equally tangential and disorganized.	Uses "thing," "you know" rather than the noun or verb; tells long, unrelated story to the class; telling or writing about how to complete a science experiment is out of order and disorganized.
Receptive language	Poor comprehension of vocabulary; inability to sequence or follow multiple directions.	Even though able to talk all the time, unable to follow through on what he or she is told to do; appears not to hear what teacher says and asks for multiple repeats.
Pragmatic language	Difficulty with taking turns, maintaining, and requesting in conversations; inability to monitor quality of conversation; poor comprehension of humor and puns; use of socially unacceptable words.	Unable to maintain adequate social space with other students; touches the teacher to gain attention; calls out to the teacher numerous times when told to wait; keeps talking when others indicate they are disinterested; does not laugh at other students' jokes; cannot use slang that others would accept; curses at the teacher or at peers.
Executive functioning	Difficulty with many of the processes listed here, plus an inability to recognize strengths and weaknesses.	Does not recognize when homework was completed correctly and may not do the same type of assignment well the next day; cannot outline what behaviors were successful in the classroom; does not describe what problems are experienced when trying to follow directions.

affecting classroom participation. The behaviors are simply examples of what can occur in the classroom but should serve to stimulate discussion about processes that may be affecting the capacity for learning in a specific student and what behaviors might occur in a particular classroom.

When transition from hospital or rehabilitation facility to school is planned, reports are generated that usually describe challenges to the cognitive–communicative processes. Additional information should be provided in the report about what the behaviors that reflect the problem areas might look like in the classroom. Provision of such information would be most beneficial to teachers prior to a school reintegration when preplanning adequate structure and academic outcomes for the student is the most beneficial.

Another challenge when planning proactively for the student is to consider the developmental changes that may affect future growth and learning. Lash[20] stated that, in the case of children and adolescents, the saying "time heals all wounds" should be "time reveals all wounds." DePompei and Blosser[26] also suggested that the child may not grow out of the disability, but rather may grow into it.

As child and adolescent brains mature, the challenges of adapting to a more complex world increase. As the child grows, learning in school becomes more difficult, social and behavioral expectations increase, and adult expectations for community living, work, relationships, and quality of life emerge.[27] Data show that moderate to severe brain injury is usually characterized by increasing functional disability as the child ages and can impact the normal development that is expected. This phenomenon has been well described by clinicians and researchers, and it is variously called the *latent effects* or *neurocognitive stall* associated with pediatric TBI.[28,29] Thus, children and adolescents may not meet developmental milestones as they struggle with new learning and cognitive development. This neurocognitive stall may emerge despite the child seeming to have recovered cognitive abilities commensurate to his or her preinjury level.[28] Hence, as the child/adolescent grows, and new learning and cognitive development does not keep pace, he or she falls further behind peers. Figure 25.3 depicts child growth, brain injury, and neurocognitive stall.

Thus, three developmental perspectives to keep in mind with this population include the following:

1. A previous base of knowledge may allow the student to score within normal limits on standardized tests immediately after the injury. Over time, as new learning should happen, the student is unable to keep up with curricular demands and begins to fail. Often, parents are not aware of this potential problem and schools do not recognize the connection to the TBI.

2. Developmental milestones may not be reached as the student grows. Ability to reason abstractly, use deductive or inductive problem-solving skills, organize homework for multiple teachers or subjects can be affected several years after the injury. This change in learning potential is sometimes not related back to the TBI when it occurs many years after the initial injury.

3. The brain of a student is in a constantly developing and changing mode. Myelination of brain cells continues to impact learning potential for years after the injury. Thus, the student who begins to fail as pragmatic, social skills, and adult personality traits should be emerging is not often identified as continuing to have challenges as a result of a TBI that occurred years earlier and teaching strategies that may help are not considered.

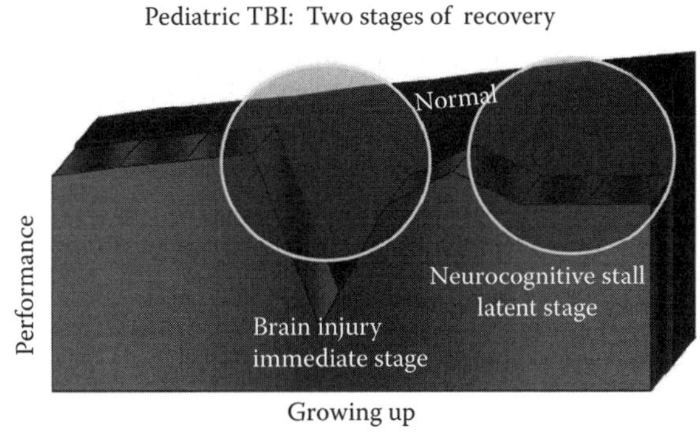

FIGURE 25.3 (See color insert following page 528.)
Depiction of child growth, brain injury, and neurocognitive stall. (Chapman, S., *Brain Injury Professional, 3*(4) 10–73, 2006.)

25.2.1 The Case of John

John was injured in a car crash the summer between kindergarten and first grade. He was unconscious at the scene and was hospitalized for 2 days with a diagnosed TBI and a broken leg. His preschool and kindergarten academic records indicated that he was a normally developing child with prereading and math skills intact. He was able to read introductory first grade materials and was communicating with ease in all academic and social situations. After the crash, he entered first grade, where he continued to demonstrate adequate learning skills in first and second grade. His grades were passing to outstanding in all academic areas. However, he began to stutter at the end of first grade and, by the end of second grade, had been referred to the speech–language pathologist. He began failing most academic requirements for reading and language arts in the third grade and, by fourth grade, was referred to special education for a complete evaluation. School personnel considered him to be learning disabled (LD) and no reference to the TBI was made in any evaluation. There were no assessments of cognitive processing completed.

John is an example of a youngster who performed well after his initial injury on previously learned information but who failed to meet developmental milestones as he grew. Because there was no annual evaluation in place, his learning difficulties were not recognized until they became severe, and interventions that may have facilitated learning were not instituted in a timely fashion. When the problems were recognized, the association with the TBI was lost, and he was diagnosed as LD rather than TBI.

25.3 The Effect of Cognitive–Communicative Challenges on Learning and Behaving in the Classroom

25.3.1 The Interrelationship of Language, Executive Functioning, and Self-Regulation for a Child with Cognitive–Communicative Problems

Singer and Bashir[30] discussed the concept that language, executive functioning, and self-regulation (behavior) are interrelated and emphasized that using metacognition for academic success is critical. They stated that the role of language in both executive functioning and the self-regulatory process is not yet well acknowledged but is essential to both processes. Vygotsky[31] stated that speech plays a central role in the development of self-control, self-direction, problem solving, and task performance. He argued that speech is learned during the course of social interaction, and is the medium for learning and knowing how to regulate personal behavior. Wertsch[32] and Bashir et al.[33] suggested that children learn appropriate language and then use verbal scripts to regulate thinking that guides participation in the learning and communication demands of school. Children use these scripts to respond to the varied discourse styles and instructional demands of teachers and other communication partners. Through the use of scripts, children acquire appropriate behaviors for learning.[34] "In school, language becomes both the object of knowledge and the means through which knowledge is acquired. Thus, within the early school years, and beyond fourth grade in particular, the role of language becomes almost inextricably intertwined with executive functioning and the self-regulatory process."[30, p.267] In this conceptual framework, language skills form a base for development of executive functioning and self-regulation and become an integral part of those functions.

25.3.2 Challenges to Language, Executive Functioning, and Self-Regulation for a Child with Cognitive–Communicative Problems

When a student with TBI is faced with learning and behaving challenges, teachers and therapists should appreciate the part that language plays in the development of executive functioning skills that can lead to increased self-monitoring. The student with cognitive–communicative problems will be at risk in any learning situation and will also have problems with the development of executive functioning and self-regulation skills. Teachers and therapists will often try to modify behaviors in the classroom without first assessing and intervening with language-based learning. Thinking about development and treatment from Singer and Bashir's[30] framework may be beneficial when developing plans for educational intervention.

Cognitive–communicative problems can be directly related to problems with curricular-based knowledge and skills areas. Each grade level has published curricula that guide teachers in knowing what should be achieved during the academic year. The relationship of language demands on the curriculum and the effect on a child with TBI is outlined in Figure 25.4. (The information in this figure is intended to provide an idea of what the curriculum demands could be and is not intended to be all inclusive.) By obtaining the curriculum for a specific grade level and reading through the knowledge and skills expected, a therapist or teacher should be able to anticipate the challenges to the student with TBI and propose teaching modifications that account for the learning challenges of the student.

Language Demands on the Curriculum: Implications for the Student with Traumatic Brain Injury

The student will often face challenges with language skills within the curriculum. Following are examples of the demands and possible interventions.

ENGLISH AND LANGUAGE ARTS

Language Demands on Curriculum	Challenges to Student with TBI	Possible Proactive Solutions
1. Interpret "wh" questions in spoken and written form.	1. Lack of problem solving skills to sort out different meanings of key words to aid in answering "wh" questions.	1. Teach main idea of "wh" questions (who means person, what means fact, etc.).
2. Process grammatical structures, sometimes rapidly.	2. Slowed information processing—unable to sort rapidly; inability to learn new grammatical structures and use functionally.	2. Give information at slower pace; review grammatical structures and help to use functionally in spoken and written output.
3. Understand abstract word meanings (antonyms and synonyms).	3. Difficulty knowing similarities and differences.	3. Teach similarities and differences and how to recognize in spoken and written materials.
4. Employ accurate recall and use of retrieval for word meanings and facts.	4. Short- and long-term memory problems.	4. Encourage vocabulary development within specific curriculum areas by use of memory devices, such as notebooks, associations, and categorization.
Add specific language demands for your client.	**List possible problem areas.**	**Suggest interventions for the therapist and teacher.**

FIGURE 25.4
Language demands on the curriculum. Implications for the student with TBI. (From Blosser, J. and DePompei, R., *Pediatric Traumatic Brain Injury: Proactive Interventions*, 2nd ed., Delmar, New York, 2002, pp. 298–301. With permission.)

SOCIAL STUDIES (HISTORY AND GEOGRAPHY)

Language Demands on Curriculum	Challenges to Student with TBI	Possible Proactive Solutions
1. Employ temporal terms, concepts, and relationships.	1. Difficulty with episodic and temporal events.	1. Use compensatory strategies for episodic memory.
2. Knowledge of past, present, and future.	2. Unsure of relationships that include time plus space.	2. Teach concepts of time and make relationships functional.
3. Use of organizational and sequencing abilities.	3. Poor development of executive functioning.	3. Supply compensatory strategies for sequencing and organization.
4. Ability to take notes from lecture, identify main ideas and supporting information.	4. Inability to locate main ideas and lack of recognition of supporting data.	4. Teach main idea versus supporting data.
5. Ability to recall and retrieve related information.	5. Memory impairments for recall.	5. Develop compensatory strategies for recall and retrieval.
Add specific language demands for your client.	**List possible problem areas.**	**Suggest interventions for the therapist and teacher.**

MATHEMATICS

Language Demands on Curriculum	Challenges to Student with TBI	Possible Proactive Solutions
1. Ability to use syntactic and semantic components of language to solve verbal math problems.	1. Difficulty with semantic aspects of word problems.	1. Aid in finding the main idea of the verbal math problem—what information is needed to solve the problem.
2. Recall and use "math language" when needed—many complex concepts are carried in a few words: "divide," "multiply," "add."	2. Unable to recall the concept associated with a single word, misses the instruction to "add."	2. Teach the meaning of single words that carry considerable— intent aid in recall of the concepts and processes underlying the single word.
3. Employ sequencing skills to complete a process.	3. Sequencing skills are often impaired.	3. Work on meaningful, functional sequencing skills.
4. Use language to understand the word problem and then complete the math to solve the problem.	4. Poor recall, inability to find relevance within the word problem. (Oftentimes, the child with TBI can do the math if he/she can understand the words that formulate the problem.)	4. Develop ability to find the main question within the problem and associate the concepts necessary to solve it.
Add specific language demands for your client.	**List possible problem areas.**	**Suggest interventions for the therapist and teacher.**

SCIENCE

Language Demands on Curriculum	Challenges to Student with TBI	Possible Proactive Solutions
1. Knowledge of concepts such as more than/less than, when/then, before/after.	1. Inability to recognize relationships and concepts that are not concrete in nature.	1. Teach relationships within the word pairs.
2. Recognition of cause and effect.	2. Inability to recognize relevance of cause and effects.	2. Aid in recognizing the relevance of cause and effect.

FIGURE 25.4 (continued)

3. Recall of specific terms and processes.	3. Vocabulary development may be sporadic and inability to recall newly learned words is problematic.	3. Devise memory strategies and compensatory aids for new vocabulary.
4. Demonstration of learned knowledge in projects that often require sequencing of events and steps.	4. Problems sequencing.	4. Employ memory aids for sequencing multiple steps (including written cues).
Add specific language demands for your client.	**List possible problem areas.**	**Suggest interventions for the therapist and teacher.**

Blosser, J. and DePompei, R., *Pediatric Traumatic Brain Injury: Proactive Interventions*, 2nd ed., Delmar, New York, 2002, pp. 298–301.

FIGURE 25.4 (continued)

25.3.3 The Case of John (continued)

John was evaluated and found to have the following curricular-based learning challenges:

Language Arts: Vocabulary development essentially stopped after first grade. He demonstrated word-finding problems, and fluency difficulties were based in his lack of ability to express himself verbally. The following dialog is a language example of John's discussion about his need for a computer.

Therapist: "Is there anything else that would help you?"

John: "Yeah, to have my old own special *thing* (gestures typing) so I, I, I, um, can work all, all of my, my, um, assignments on one *thing* because of what I'm to a sharing a bunch of *things* with a bunch of other students and I cannot do that."

Therapist: "Books? Like your books in class? Is that what you are sharing?"

John: "No, no! My, ah, own own, ah *laptop computer*. See once first I use one *thing*, ev, ever, everybody else wan to use it."

The same word-finding problems were also reflected in spelling and writing attempts. His reading and spelling were found to be at the second grade, third month level. Writing was at kindergarten, ninth month level. He used gestures well and was often assumed to be communicating better than his language capacity indicated he could.

History: John was unable to understand concepts of time and place and could not deal with "when" questions. He could not sequence temporal events and experienced difficulty with most history-based concepts.

Science: John had no concepts for sequencing beyond two steps. He was unable to use deductive reasoning and saw no cause–effect relationships.

Math: John was able to complete most addition, subtraction, multiplication, and division problems. He could not apply the math skills to word problems.

25.4 Treatment of Cognitive–Communicative Strengths and Needs: An Integrative Approach for School

Cognitive–communicative and behavioral deficits following TBI will require special interventions throughout the student's education. Although long-term deficits following TBI are well documented, empirical research on the effectiveness of particular instructional practices for dealing with subsequent learning problems in students with TBI is lacking.[35,36] Given this absence of research, Ylvisaker et al.[37] stated that teachers must examine effective teaching practices and proven instructional interventions for students with other types of learning difficulties. They recommended identifying students by functional need and connecting identified needs with research-based strategies.

25.4.1 Identifying Student Needs

Determining the individual needs of a student will require careful evaluation of the student's functioning. To obtain a comprehensive picture of the student's functioning, assessment information from a variety of sources (e.g., neuropsychology, speech pathology, occupational therapy) should be combined with functional evaluation of the child's skills. Pearson[38] recommended that, in addition to assessment of underlying cognitive processes (how deficits in short-term memory, long-term memory, sequencing, or organization affect performance in the classroom), team members should be readily able to answer questions such as the following:

- At what grade level does the student read? What is the average reading rate for the child's age and how does the child compare with peers?
- Can he do grade level math? Does he use his fingers to calculate?
- Can he follow classroom directions (single step, multistep)?
- Can he correctly sequence steps?
- Can he write? Is he able to keep up taking notes? Is the writing legible?

Evaluation of actual task performance in settings where the student's adaptive skills are called into play is critical, because assessments given under ideal conditions do not reflect the kind of difficulty a student may face in a busy classroom with less guidance and structure. Ongoing functional assessment of the student in the school environment is required to determine the student's current functioning and needs accurately to develop interventions.

This segment discusses two methods for such interventions. First, suggestions for addressing underlying cognitive processes in the classroom are presented. This is followed by a discussion of teaching techniques that may aid the acquisition of academic skills. It is hoped that use of these strategies will establish outcomes for the student that develop independence for learning and generalization of what was learned to new situations.

25.4.2 Strategies for Addressing Underlying Cognitive Processes

Results of the comprehensive evaluation may reveal that the student has a number of specific deficits in underlying cognitive processes. To determine which teaching methods may be most effective in meeting an individual student's particular needs, educators need to examine instructional interventions and teaching practices that have proved effective for addressing similar deficits in students with other types of learning difficulties. For example, organizational impairments following TBI will necessitate proved instructional strategies for organization, such as task analysis (breaking a given task into components or steps) and advanced organizational support (providing an oral or written preview of information to be covered in a lesson). Lack of strategic learning ability will require specific strategy instruction, such as the teaching of word identification strategies, paragraph writing strategies, test-taking strategies, and so forth (see Deshler et al.[39] for a comprehensive review of strategy research and methods). Weak executive function skills will call for instruction in self-regulation procedures (e.g., goal setting, self-monitoring).[40] In addition, a variety of effective teaching practices that have been found to be correlated positively with student achievement (e.g., the provision of structured lessons, guided practice, immediate feedback, clearly stated expectations, frequent review, and small-group instruction) may be particularly beneficial for meeting the needs of students with TBI.[35]

In conjunction with matching specific teaching methods to identified needs, a number of teaching strategies and accommodations should also be considered to address problem areas. These strategies can be used successfully in general education settings or in the context of special education environments. A sampling of common deficits following TBI are identified next, followed by examples from the comprehensive lists of teaching strategies for students with brain injuries by Tyler et al.[36] and Tyler and Mira.[40]

25.4.2.1 Attention/Concentration

To improve attention and concentration, educators should

- Reduce distractions in the student's work area (remove extra pencils, books, and so on)
- Provide preferential seating (an area that has the least amount of distraction and is closest to where instruction is taking place)
- Divide work into small sections and have the student complete one section at a time
- Establish nonverbal cueing system (e.g., eye contact, touch) to remind the student to pay attention

25.4.2.2 Memory

To aid memory, educators should

- Teach the student to use external aids such as notes, timers, calendars, electronic organizers, such as personal data assistants or smartphones, and assignment books as self-reminders to compensate for memory problems
- Frequently repeat and summarize key information
- Use visual imagery, when possible, to supplement oral content
- Teach the student to categorize or "chunk" information
- Relate new information to the student's relevant prior knowledge
- Demonstrate techniques such as mental rehearsal and use of special words or examples as reminders
- Ask the student to rehearse and summarize information verbally

25.4.2.3 Organization

To improve organization, educators should

- Provide the student with written checklists of steps for complex tasks
- Color-code the student's materials for each class (textbook, notebook, supplies)

- Provide an assigned person to review the schedule at the start of the school day and organize materials for each class
- Supply outlines coordinated to class lectures (require the student to take notes within each section)
- Teach the student to use a personal data assistant to organize the day

25.4.2.4 Decreased Speed of Processing

To help the student compensate for decreased speed of processing, the educator should

- Deliver instruction in small increments
- Allow the student to have additional time to process information and complete tasks
- Provide sufficient time for the student to respond to verbal questioning
- Pair verbal instructions with written instructions
- Allow the student to take exams in settings that do not have time restraints

25.4.2.5 Problem Solving

To help the student to develop problem-solving skills, the educator should

- Have the student generate possible solutions to problems as they arise during an activity
- Teach the student the steps involved in problem solving (e.g., identify problem, list relevant information, evaluate possible solutions, create an action plan)

25.4.3 Addressing Academic Deficits

Following a TBI, a student may require specialized assistance or accommodations to continue to participate in the regular curriculum. A number of adaptations that will increase the success of student learning can be provided during the teaching of academic subject matter. Tyler et al.[36] provided the following examples of suggested techniques for addressing underlying deficits while teaching subject matter.

25.4.3.1 Math

Educators should

- Demonstrate mathematical concepts using concrete items. Allow the student to use manipulative times to solve math problems.
- Create functional activities for the student to practice mathematical concepts (e.g., planning a budget, purchasing small items from a school store).
- Practice word problems with pictures or stories that relate personally to the student.
- Allow the student to use a calculator to aid solving multiple-step problems.

25.4.3.2 *Reading*

Educators should

- Review key vocabulary words prior to reading material
- Highlight key words with colored marker
- Provide the student with key questions to answer before reading
- Ask the student to summarize content orally after reading small segments of a large passage

25.4.3.3 *Writing*

Educators should

- Provide for alternative response modes for work (e.g., let the student dictate responses, tape record answers)
- Allow the student to take exams orally
- Provide specialized writing paper (e.g., raised lines)

In some cases following TBI, even with accommodations, a student may no longer be able to acquire information and skills using traditional methodologies and curriculum provided in the general education settings. In such cases, a specialized intensive instructional approach is required. One such specialized approach—Direct Instruction (DI)—was identified by Glang et al.[41] as an evidence-based instructional model that shows particular promise for students with TBI because it combines "systematic analysis and design of content and careful instructional delivery for attacking complex academic content and mastering critical basic academic skills."[p.246]

Using the DI model, carefully designed curriculum materials are delivered in a highly structured, systematic, instructional manner that incorporates several teaching practices that have been consistently linked to pupil achievement outcomes (see Adams and Engleman[42] for a comprehensive description of the model and summary of research). Educators can apply the DI model to existing curriculum, or use one of the numbers of readily available commercially published DI materials for teaching reading, mathematics, and spelling.

There is significant evidence supporting the use of DI with many populations of children, with and without disabilities, and in preliminary studies. DI techniques have been shown to be effective in teaching both academic and behavioral skills to children with brain injuries.[43] Glang et al.[43] stated the DI model is thought to be effective with children with brain injury because it specifically addresses many of the common learning problems typical of these students. For example, DI provides rapid instructional pacing and high levels of student engagement that address attention and concentration difficulties. The model also provides sufficient practice of skills, teaches generalizable strategies, and delivers corrective feedback to address difficulties students with brain injury face in learning new concepts and information.

25.4.4 Assessing Teaching Strategies

Once instructional practices are used, the effectiveness of these practices must be continually evaluated. Also, because of the rapidly changing needs of the student following TBI, ongoing functional assessment of the student in the school environment is required to determine the student's current functioning accurately.

25.4.4.1 The Case of John (continued)

Based on results of the comprehensive evaluation and functional assessments, the Individualized Education Program (IEP) team developed an educational program to meet John's unique learning needs. John received specialized instruction in reading and language arts. John's special education teacher used commercially developed DI reading and spelling materials, which provided the structure, practice, and immediate feedback John needed to succeed. The special education teacher provided support for John in his regular education history, science, and math classes. By assisting John with developing timelines and sequencing information, providing visual–spatial displays, and preteaching content vocabulary, John was able to participate in the general education curriculum. Special accommodations, such as reduced writing requirements, preferential seating, and peer assistance were provided throughout the day. John also received school-based speech–language services for 30 minutes three times per week. During this time, John's word-finding problems were addressed. The decision to stimulate language and not work directly with the fluency problem was based on the thought that, with increased expressive competence, fluency patterns of repetition and word substitution would decrease. Shortly after the IEP was implemented, John began showing progress. John's family and teachers reported that, in addition to making academic gains, John's emotional well-being had also improved since he had begun receiving the help he needed.

25.5 Laws and Regulations That Affect Education, Provision of Services, and Transition for Students with Traumatic Brain Injury

Because of long-term physical, cognitive, language, and psychosocial difficulties, students with TBI may require special education services, special assistance, or accommodations. Students can access such services under the Individuals with Disabilities Education Act (IDEA) or Section 504 of the Rehabilitation Act.

25.5.1 IDEA

IDEA, an outgrowth of the Education for All Handicapped Children Act of 1975 (P.L. 94-142), guarantees a free appropriate public education for children 3 to 21 years old. To receive services under IDEA, a multidisciplinary team must evaluate and determine a student to have a qualifying condition that requires special education services. Since 1990, IDEA has recognized TBI as one of the categories that qualify students for special education services. Once the team has determined a student is eligible for special education, an IEP must be devised and carried out. The IEP is, essentially, a document that describes the action plan for the student's educational program and serves as a contract between parents and the school for the delivery of educational services to the student.

Through IDEA, a full continuum of special education placement options, ranging from homebound services to placement in the general education classroom with special education support, is available. Regardless of setting, the term *special education* means specially designed instruction to meet the unique needs of the student and may include direct skills instruction, the teaching of compensatory strategies, and vocational education, as well as the provision of modifications and accommodations. Related services, such as speech–language therapy, occupational therapy, physical therapy, counseling, adaptive physical education, and behavior management services, are also available through IDEA.

According to Tyler and Savage,[44] because of the underlying medical cause of the disability, the resulting deficits, and the evolving needs of the child, IEPs written for students with TBI require procedures that vary from traditional IEP development. For example, information from a variety of sources and disciplines outside the school system needs to be translated to determine current levels of functioning. Goals need to address cognitive processes rather than strictly academic impairments, and IEP reviews need to be conducted more frequently (e.g., every 2 to 3 months, initially) to address dramatically changing needs. In addition, the student's initial IEP should be a joint venture among the health care facility, the school, and the family.

25.5.2 Section 504

Not all students need, or are eligible for, special education, even though a brain injury may affect learning. With classroom adjustments and curriculum modifications, a student may still be able to participate in the general education program by receiving services under Section 504 of the Rehabilitation Act of 1973. Section 504 is a civil rights act that protects the civil and constitutional rights of persons with disabilities. According to Section 504, schools receiving federal financial assistance may not discriminate against individuals with disabilities. Because some students with disabilities may need adjustments or modifications to benefit from their educational program, classroom teachers and school staff are required to provide them. Unlike IDEA, Section 504 is a regular education management responsibility.

To receive services under Section 504, a person must be considered disabled. According to Section 504, a person may be considered disabled if the individual (1) has a mental or physical impairment that substantially limits one or more major life activities (e.g., walking, breathing, learning, working); (2) has a record of such an impairment; or (3) is regarded as having such an impairment. To determine eligibility for Section 504, a student must be evaluated by a team of individuals who are familiar with the student. The evaluation typically consists only of gathering documented information from a variety of sources and, because most students with TBI have documentation from outside sources, additional evaluation may not be required. The team then reviews the evaluation data to determine the nature of the disability and how it affects the student's education.

To document services, a Section 504 plan describing services or accommodations is developed by the team. The plan lists specific adjustments to the learning environment and modifications to the curriculum. The plan also indicates who is responsible for carrying out and evaluating each adjustment or modification. Based on the student's needs, any number of accommodations can be provided with a 504 plan. They include environmental, curriculum, methodology, organizational, behavioral, and presentation strategies. Tyler and Wilkerson[45] offer information about accommodations that may be provided through a Section 504 plan. Table 25.2[45] provides a sampling of their suggestions for possible accommodations to meet common concerns following brain injury.

Because Section 504 protections extend to a larger population of students than IDEA, Section 504 should be considered as a venue for receiving needed support for students

TABLE 25.2

Section 504 Plan Accommodation

Consider the following accommodations for students qualifying for 504 services:

Memory Deficits

    Written, as well as verbal, direction for tasks

    Frequent review of information

    Monitored planner (check-off system)

Fatigue

    Reduced schedule

    Planned rest break

Fine Motor Difficulties

    Note taker for lectures

    Oral examinations

    Scribe for essays

Processing Delays

    Increased time to complete assignments/tests

    Extended time to provide verbal answers

    Complex directions broken into steps

Attention

    Visual and/or verbal prompts

    Preferential seating (away from distracting areas of the classroom, often in the middle of the classroom beside a well-organized student)

Technology

    Computer/word processor for responding and homework

    Use of communication devices

Source: Tyler, J. and Wilkerson, L., *Section 504 Plan Checklist for a Student with a Brain Injury,* 2nd ed., Lash & Associates Publishing/Training, Wake Forest, NC, 2008.

who do not qualify for services under IDEA. In addition, because IDEA does not apply to students who have graduated from high school or those who have reached age 22, Section 504 serves as the vehicle for obtaining services in postsecondary settings.

25.6 Transitioning Students with Traumatic Brain Injury

Following a TBI, transitioning is often thought of as a one-step activity of moving a child from the hospital to the school. Although the importance of careful planning for school reintegration has been well documented in the literature,[2–4,23–25] there are a number of other important transitions that occur throughout a student's education career. In reality, transitioning occurs repeatedly throughout the lifetime of the student with TBI. Certainly, the student will transition from medical interventions to home, school, and community. Once in school, the child will encounter transitions with the passage from grade level to grade level, the change from elementary to middle school, and middle to high school. Beyond that, the student will transition from high school to postsecondary education, employment, and community living. Specialized planning for all these transition points is required because each can present formidable challenges for students with TBIs resulting from cognitive and behavioral impairments that make it difficult for students to adjust to changes in environments, routines, and expectations.[42]

IDEA requires that, beginning at age 16, a transition plan for movement out of school to postschool activities, employment, independent living, and community participation is included in the student's IEP. Based on students' needs, preferences, and interests, specific outcomes must be identified and supported by transition services, which may include academic support, community-based education focused on employment, functional and independent living skills, personal and social content, and career awareness. Because the same cognitive–communicative challenges exist for all transitions, planning for any transition must be completed with as much proactive planning and anticipation of challenges as the IEP process requires.

The following sections describe the steps for planning transitions. It should be noted that the steps are the same whether the transition is from hospital to school, within school, or from school into community.

25.6.1 Step One: Plan in a Timely Manner

One of the keys to adequate planning is taking sufficient time to devise a well-thought-out plan that accommodates individual strengths and needs. Transition planning should occur well in advance of the time of the actual event. Therefore, hospitals should contact schools well in advance of an anticipated return date (preferably, as soon as the child is hospitalized). School staff should begin planning for in-school transitions months prior to the child's move to a different grade level or school. Transition plans focusing on vocational, postsecondary educational, and community living must be in place beginning at age 16, if determined appropriate by the IEP team.

25.6.2 Step Two: Develop Transition Plans That Are Specific to the Strengths and Needs of the Student

All members of the team should be prepared in advance of the meeting. Some questions that the student and family should think about prior to the meeting include the following:

- What type of education is desired? Regular education, special education services, trade school, 2-year college, 4-year college, none?
- What vocational tracks may be of interest?
- What type of independent living might be desired?
- What leisure activities are of interest?
- What are the student's hopes and dreams for the future?
- What strengths does this student have to achieve any of these desires?
- What challenges to achieving these goals might exist?
- How can a specific plan be devised to address these challenges during in the next few years?
- Who will need to participate to work toward these goals?
- What environmental supports or modifications will be needed to facilitate success?
- What evaluation tools will be used to determine whether there is movement toward achieving these goals?

- Who will participate with the student to determine whether the goals are being met or whether they should be altered?
- How often will a reassessment of this plan be completed?

25.6.3 Step Three: Be Involved in the Meetings

Decisions and plans must be completed at the meeting. Lash et al.[46,47] provide outlines for parents, students, teachers, and advocates that address skills necessary for planning reintegration to school or preparing for work and adulthood. They outline necessary skills of assessment, information gathering, referral, service coordination, advocacy, and evaluation as essential to the planning and implementation process. In addition, there are websites that have been developed to aid individuals and families in advocating for educational and community living needs.[25,27] Refer to these sources for an in-depth discussion of these areas. The discussion should focus on the resources and teaching strategies necessary to aid the student in the classroom and beyond.

25.6.3.1 Resources

- What community resources might be available? For example, Office of Accessibility located on every state college or university campus, Bureau of Vocational Rehabilitation Services (Rehabilitation Services Commission), work–study programs at high school, volunteer opportunities in the community.
- What other agencies might be able to help? Drug and Alcohol Boards, YMCA, Medicare, Departments of Mental Health or Mental Retardation/Developmental Delay, Family Services, Independent Living Centers?
- What opportunities for transportation, housing, and personal assistance might exist through agencies, churches, and social or private organization?

25.6.3.2 Strategies

- What cognitive challenges may need to be accommodated and how will these behaviors appear in the classroom, workplace, or community?
- What accommodations might work (planners, coaches, reminders, adapted equipment, reduced schedules, technology applications for accommodation, note takers, communication devices)?
- Who should be involved in ensuring these accommodations are provided and are ongoing in support of the student?

25.6.4 Step Four: Maintain Contact with the Hospitals, Schools, and Community Resources throughout the Entire Education of the Student

As the student transitions from setting to setting, do not assume the plan or information is being transferred from teacher to teacher, supervisor to supervisor, or school to school. Annual reviews of progress and modifications of plans are essential to continued success.

It is also crucial that the plan be shared with all individuals who work with the student at work, school, or in the community whenever there is a change in personnel or location throughout the year. Be prepared to provide parents with a notebook of personal information related to their child that they can share with a variety of agencies as they advocate during transitions. A checklist for transitioning is depicted in Figure 25.5.

25.6.4.1 *The Case of John (continued)*

When John was 14, the checklist was used to establish a transition plan for him. The planning team consisted of John, his grandmother (legal guardian), the director of special education, two classroom teachers, the work–study coordinator, a speech–language pathologist, a representative of the Rehabilitation Services Commission, and a representative of a local rehabilitation center that held a grant to effect school-to-work transition for youth with disabilities.

The original plan included assessing John for his vocational interests as well as discussion about his challenges in academic and social areas. His strengths included fine motor coordination, outgoing personality, math computation, use of gestures to augment communication attempts, and mechanical aptitude. John was placed in regular classes that emphasized managing skills for daily independent living, home economics, art, and math. He was placed in an LD classroom for assistance with language arts. He began in a vocational school where he learned auto mechanics. He had a job coach with him for all new classes. He attended the local rehabilitation facility 2 days a week where he was taught additional job skills, which included socialization skills training, assistance with strategies for following directions, and self-advocacy training. He called periodic meetings of his IEP and transition teams to discuss progress and additional challenges. Accommodations were made, at his request, for training for job personnel about his poor organization, and he provided an in-service regarding his communication challenges and how he adapted to them. Over the following 3 years, adaptations to his transition plan were completed six times. Training of personnel regarding John's strengths and needs was completed four times as situations in teaching, coaching, and employment changed.

Currently, John is employed half days at a local car dealership, where he is apprenticing as an auto mechanic. He continues his academic work for the other half day where he attends two regular classes and continues with the assistance of the LD teacher. He continues to be challenged academically in language arts. He should graduate this spring at age 19, and the car dealership anticipates hiring him into a full paying position.

25.7 Summary

This chapter has focused on the cognitive–communicative challenge that can emerge after TBI. These challenges often are overlooked in the struggle to provide adequate educational programming. When strategies are used consistently and personnel collaborate to provide ongoing transition and intervention, students can modify behaviors and become contributing adult members of society. These plans can be modified for youth with many levels of severity. Although all will not transition to gainful employment, college, or independent living, it is our belief that all can be accommodated into society for a better quality of life. Hippocrates suggested long ago that we use our skills for those who are mildly injured and also for those who are severely injured—that they all deserve our attention and efforts. We think he is right!

A Transition Planning Guide

1. Identify key players at each agency.	
2. Determine what policies and procedures exist for all agencies involved.	
3 Provide all pertinent information about the student, including tests, cognitive challenges, behaviors that can be anticipated.	
a. Obtain all written records.	
b. Generate a profile of student strengths and challenges.	
c. Identify the challenges that may interfere with the successful performance of the student.	
d. Provide samples of present work levels that represent capabilities and levels of performance.	
4. Relate the challenges and strengths to the new setting.	
a. Discuss accommodations needed.	
b. Offer choices based on the demands of the setting and the needs of the student.	
5. Determine the agency's readiness to accommodate the student.	
a. Provide adequate staff training	
b. Assess environment for necessary changes to accommodate physical, cognitive needs.	
6. Determine what assessments may be needed for placement in the agency.	
7. Outline strategies for supporting performance.	
8. Determine which placement, personnel can best meet student needs.	
9. Observe the environment to determine any supports not in place or additional strategies that can help.	
10. Maintain ongoing communication of all involved parties after that plan is begun.	
11. Modify the plan as often as indicated and PRIOR to a serious problem emerging.	
12. Outline a plan of action if problems emerge so staff can be proactive, rather than reactive.	
13. Outline a functional evaluation plan to determine what is working and what should be changed.	
14. Maintain contact among the key personnel identified in step 1.	
15. Add any other steps pertinent to this student.	

FIGURE 25.5

Transition planning guide.

References

1. Savage, R. and Wolcott, G., *Educational Dimensions of Acquired Brain Injury*, Pro-Ed, Austin, TX, 1994, Ch. 1.
2. Blosser, J. and DePompei, R., *Pediatric Traumatic Brain Injury: Proactive Interventions*, 2nd ed., Delmar, New York, 2002, Ch. 2.
3. Goldberg, A., *Acquired Brain Injury in Childhood and Adolescence*, Charles C. Thomas, Springfield, IL, 1996, Ch. 12.
4. Yeates, K. O. and Tylor, G. H., Behavior problems in school and their educational correlates among children with traumatic brain injury, *Exceptionality*, 14(3), 141–154, 2006.
5. DiScala, C., Onsberg, S., and Savage, R., Children hospitalized for traumatic brain injury: Transition to postacute care, *Journal of Head Trauma Rehabilitation*, 12(2), 1–10, 1997.
6. Bedell, G. M., Haley, S. M., Coster, W. J., and Smith, K. W., Participation readiness at discharge from inpatient rehabilitation in children and adolescents with acquired brain injuries, *Pediatric Rehabilitation*, 5(2), 107–116, 2002.
7. Condalucci, A., *Interdependence: The Route to Community*, CRC Press, Boca Raton, FL, 1991.
8. DiScala, C., *National Pediatric Trauma Registry Biannual Report*, Research and Training Center, Tufts University School of Medicine, Boston, MA, 2001.
9. Bedell, G. M. and Dumas, H. M., Social participation of children and youth with acquired brain injuries discharged from inpatient rehabilitation: A follow-up study, *Brain Injury*, 18(1), 65–82, 2004.
10. DePompei, R., *School Reintegration for Youth with TBI: Issues and Recommendations for Change*, Lecture presented at the Fourth International Brain Injury Association conference, Turin, Italy, 2001, May 8.
11. Condalucci, A., *The Essence of Interdependence*, LA Publishing, Wake Forest, NC, 2008, Ch. 4.
12. Condalucci, A., *Community and Cultural Shifting*, CRC Press, Boca Raton, FL, 2001.
13. Condalucci, A., *Cultural Shifting*, LA Publishing, Wake Forest, NC, 2002.
14. Condalucci, A., *Together Is Better*, LA Publishing, Wake Forest, NC, 2008.
15. Condalucci, A., *Opening the Doors to Community*, LA Publishing, Wake Forest, NC, 2002.
16. DePompei, R. and Blosser, J. L., Managing transitions for education, in M. Rosenthal, E. Griffeth, J. Kreutzer, and B. Pentland (Eds.), *Rehabilitation of the Adult and Child with Traumatic Brain Injury*, 3rd ed., F. A. Davis, Philadelphia, 1999, Ch. 23.
17. Farmer, J. E., Clippard, D. S., Luehr-Wiemann, Y., Wright, E., and Owings, S., Assessing children with traumatic brain injury during rehabilitation: Promoting school and community reentry, *Journal of Learning Disabilities*, 29(5), 532–548, 1996.
18. Fraser, R. T., Career development in school-to-work transition for adolescents with traumatic brain injury, in M. Ylvisaker (Ed.), *Traumatic Brain Injury Rehabilitation: Children and Adolescents*, 2nd ed., Butterworth-Heinemann, Newton, MA, 1998, Ch. 19.
19. Kraemer, B. R. and Blacher, J., An overview of educationally relevant effects, assessment, and school reentry, in A. Glang, G. Singer, and B. Todis (Eds.), *Students with Acquired Brain Injury: The School's Response*, Paul H. Brookes Publishing Company, Baltimore, MD, 1997, Ch. 1.
20. Lash, M., Family centered case management: Preparing parents to become service coordinators for children with ABI, in G. Singer, A. Glang, and J. Williams (Eds.), *Children with Acquired Brain Injury: Educating and Supporting Families*, Paul H. Brookes Publishing, Baltimore, MD, 1996, 79–98.
21. Smith, S. M. and Tyler, J., Successful transition planning and services for students with ABI, in A. Glang, G. Singer, and B. Todis (Eds.), *Students with Acquired Brain Injury: The School's Response*, Paul H. Brookes Publishing Company, Baltimore, MD, 1997, Ch. 6, 185.
22. Arroyos-Jurado, E., Paulsen, J. S., Ehly, S., and Max, J. E., Traumatic brain injury in children and adolescents: Academic and intellectual outcomes following injury, *Exceptionality*, 14(3), 125–140, 2006.

23. Hux, K. and Hacksley, C., Mild traumatic brain injury: Facilitating school success, *Intervention in School and Clinic*, 32(3), 158–165, 1996.
24. Hawley, C. A., Ward, A. B., Magnay, A. R., and Long, J., Outcomes following childhood head injury: A population study, *Journal of Neurology, Neurosurgery, and Psychiatry*, 75(5), 737–742, 2004.
25. Ylvisaker, M., Adelson, D., Braga, L. W., Burnett, S. M., Glang, A., Feeney, T., Moore, W., Rumney, P., and Todis, B., Rehabilitation and ongoing support after pediatric TBI: Twenty years of progress, *Journal of Head Trauma Rehabilitation*, 20(1), 95–109, 2005.
26. DePompei, R. and Blosser, J. L., Traumatic brain injury in young children, in T. L. Layton, E. Crais, and L. Watson (Eds.), *Handbook of Early Language Impairment in Children: Nature*, Thompson Learning-Delmar, Albany, NY, 2000, Ch. 7.
27. Glang, A. and Todis, B., *TBI Transition System* (*T-BITS*): *Systematic Hospital-to-School Transition for Students with Traumatic Brain Injury*, U. S. Department of Education, National Institute of Disability and Rehabilitation Research (NIDRR), October 2006–September 2011, CFDA #84.133A-10, Washington, DC, 2006.
28. Chapman, S. B., Neurocognitive stall: A paradox in long-term recovery from pediatric brain injury, *Brain Injury Professional*, 3(4), 10–13, 2006.
29. Hendryx, P. M. and Verduyn, W. H., Diagnosis and treatment strategies for the latent sequelae of head trauma in children, *Journal of Cognitive Rehabilitation*, 13(3), 9–11, 1995.
30. Singer, B. D. and Bashir, A. S., What are executive functions and self-regulation and what do they have to do with language-learning disorders?, *Language, Speech, and Hearing Services in Schools*, 30(3), 265–273, 1999.
31. Vygotsky, L., *Thought and Language*, MIT Press, Cambridge, MA, 1962, 41.
32. Wertsch, J. V., *Mind as Action*, Oxford Press, New York, 1998, 146.
33. Bashir, A. S., Conte, B. M., and Heerde, S. M., Language and school success: Collaborative challenges and choices, in D. Merritt and B. Calcutta (Eds.), *Language Intervention in the Classroom*, Singular Publishing, San Diego, CA, 1998, Ch. 1.
34. Cazden, C. B., *Classroom Discourse: The Language of Teaching and Learning*, Heinneman-Butterworth, Portsmouth, NH, 1988, 96.
35. Tyler, J. and Grandinette, S., Effective teaching strategies for students with acquired brain injury, *Brain Injury Source*, 38, 2003.
36. Tyler, J., Blosser, J., and DePompei, R., *Teaching Strategies for Students with Brain Injuries*, Lash & Associates Publishing/Training, Wake Forest, NC, 1999.
37. Ylvisaker, M., Todis, B., Glang, A., Urbanczyk, B., Franklin, C., DePompei, R., Feeney, T., Maxwell, N. M., Pearson, S., and Tyler, J. S., Educating students with TBI: Themes and recommendations, *Journal of Head Trauma Rehabilitation*, 16(1), 76–93, 2001.
38. Pearson, S., *How Should We Help? Placement, Instructional Strategies, and Social Issues*, Paper presented at the Brain Injury Association of America 21st annual symposium, Minneapolis, MN, 2001, Jul. 26.
39. Deshler, D. D., Ellis, E. S., and Lenz, B. K., *Teaching Adolescents with Learning Disabilities: Strategies and Methods*, 2nd ed., Love, Denver, CO, 1996.
40. Tyler, J. S. and Mira, M. P., *Traumatic Brain Injury in Children and Adolescents: A Sourcebook for Teachers and Other School Personnel*, 2nd ed., Pro-Ed, Austin, TX, 1999.
41. Glang, A., Ylvisaker, M., Stein, M., Ehlhardt, L., Todis, B., and Tyler, J., Validated instructional practices: Application to students with traumatic brain injury, *Journal of Head Trauma Rehabilitation*, 23(4), 243–251, 2008.
42. Adams, G. L. and Engelmann, S., *Research on Direct Instruction: 25 Years Beyond DISTAR*, Educational Achievement Systems, Seattle, WA, 1996.
43. Glang, A., Singer, G., Cooley, E., and Tish, N., Tailoring direct instruction techniques for use with elementary students with brain injury, *Journal of Head Trauma Rehabilitation*, 7(4), 93–108, 1992.
44. Tyler, T. and Savage, R. C., Students with traumatic brain injury, in F. E. Obiakor, C. A. Utley, and A. F. Rotatori (Eds.), *Advances in Special Education: Psychology of Effective Education for Learners with Exceptionalities*, JAI Press, Stamford, CT, 2003, 299–323.

45. Tyler, J. and Wilkerson, L., *Section 504 Plan Checklist for a Student with a Brain Injury*, 2nd ed., Lash & Associates Publishing/Training, Wake Forest, NC, 2008.
46. Lash, M. and Cluett, R., *A Manual for Managing Special Education for Students with Brain Injury*, Lash & Associates Publishing/Training, Wake Forest, NC, 1998.
47. Lash, M., Kahn, P., and Wolcott, G., *When Your Teenager Is Injured: Preparing for Work and Adulthood*, Research and Training Center, Boston, MA, 1997.

26

The Contribution of the Neuropsychological Evaluation to Traumatic Brain Injury Rehabilitation

Jay M. Uomoto

CONTENTS

26.1 Introduction

One of the earliest accounts of the physical, neurocognitive, and neurobehavioral consequences of acquired brain injury was penned by renowned neurologist Kurt Goldstein[1] in
his book published in 1942, *Aftereffects of Brain Injuries in War*. In this comprehensive volume, Goldstein[1] described characteristic symptoms of patient's with acquired brain injury
based upon his clinical experiences in monitoring and treating numerous patients after
combat, some over the course of 10 years. Goldstein[1] observed precise insights regarding
the scope and genesis of disorders of motor output, sensory input, visuospatial, brainstem,
and frontal lobe functions. His neurologic insights converged with his methods of assessment of cognitive functions and impairments, and described his approach to what would
today be considered elements of the neuropsychological evaluation. These investigations
are carried out for the following reasons:

- To evaluate some of the mental functions usually separated in psychology, such as
  memory and attention.

- To evaluate the patient's general level of performance. Some mental and physical
  performances are investigated over a period of time. The results obtained here are
  also useful for our judgment of the subject's capacity in general.

- To ascertain the circumscribed mental defects, in detail, as a basis for procedure
  in retraining.

- To study the subject's working capacity in special kinds of labor.[p.92]

It is important to observe that much of what Goldstein[1] wished to accomplish with what
he termed *psychologic laboratory examinations* defines the essential goals of the neuropsychological evaluation in the context of traumatic brain injury (TBI) rehabilitation. These
goals are defined as (1) comprehensively delineating the cognitive impairments that have
resulted from TBI: (2) evaluating cognitive assets and deficits to describe thoroughly the
patient's overall functional capacities: (3) utilizing neuropsychological findings in the service of rehabilitative therapies: and (4) integrating neuropsychological insights into the
enterprise of improving quality of life, including return to work, school, and community
reentry.

The use of the term *neuropsychology* is often attributed to Sir William Osler in an address
to the Phipps Psychiatric Clinic at Johns Hopkins Hospital in 1913.[2] During this address,
Osler underscored the importance of paying close attention to the interactions between
brain function and psychiatric disorder in clinical medicine. Although this term largely
lay dormant for decades thereafter, Osler's comment portended what has become characteristic of modern neuropsychology. Here, this same convergence of physical and psychological realms defines the field as the study of brain–behavior relationships.[3] Although
utilized for different purposes in a broad range of neurologic conditions, in TBI rehabilitation, the neuropsychological evaluation can be critical to defining plans of care in
executing effective rehabilitation therapy. Neuropsychological testing procedures have
been used in rehabilitation settings for at least 40 years, primarily for the four purposes
just listed. The practice of neuropsychology in TBI rehabilitation has been enhanced by
advances in advanced neuroimaging techniques, prospective outcome research, advances
in understanding the neurobiology of cognition, and unlocking some of the mysteries
associated with neuroplasticity. The neuropsychological evaluation will likely continue to

augment imaging and other neurobiologic approaches to understanding the consequences of TBI.

26.2 The Context of the Neuropsychology of Traumatic Brain Injury

26.2.1 Pathophysiology and Neuropsychological Functioning in Traumatic Brain Injury

TBI is often the result of acceleration and deceleration forces that are applied to the head and brain. When the skull remains intact, this is referred to as a *closed head injury*. In an *open head injury*, skull integrity is breached where a blunt trauma to the head may result in a depressed skull fracture. Penetrating head wounds resulting from a projectile (e.g., a bullet) entering through the skull would be considered an open head injury. Lucas and Addeo[4] delineate mechanisms of the *primary injury* and *potential secondary effects*. In open head injury, the primary effects include brain tissue damage along the missile track, intracranial bleeding, and meningeal and cerebral lacerations. With closed head injury, brain contusions and hemorrhages can occur, and the common phenomenon of *diffuse axonal injury* (DAI) frequently occurs. Filley[5] states that varying degrees of DAI occur in TBI when shearing forces act on the long fibers of the white matter of the cortex as a result of acceleration (e.g., a stationary head struck by a moving object) and deceleration (e.g., a moving head stopped by a stationary object) actions, common to what occurs in motor vehicle accidents. The gray matter of the cortical mantle moves across the deeper white matter structures of the cortex, producing stretching and shearing forces along the axons, and producing DAI. The extent and severity of DAI is thought to be reflected in gross outcome measurements of the depth and length of coma.

Neuroimaging techniques have advanced to be able to understand the phenomena of DAI. Diffusion tensor imaging (DTI) allows for white matter fiber tracking, especially in combination with functional magnetic resonance imaging (MRI) techniques.[6] Abnormalities in the white matter in such disease processes as multiple sclerosis, stroke, and schizophrenia have been found using this technology. Arfanakis et al.[7] compared DTI against conventional computed tomography (CT) and MRI in those with mild TBI (MTBI) with 24 hours of injury and control participants. None of the head CT scan results in the MTBI group showed abnormalities, whereas both conventional magnetic resonance images and diffusion-weighted images showed abnormal signal intensity that was consistent with edema or petechial hemorrhage. These authors[7] concluded that DTI may, in fact, be a sensitive measure of DAI in MTBI.

White matter changes in those with moderate to severe TBI have been demonstrated using DTI technology. Greenberg et al.[8] followed a group of those with TBI (Glasgow Coma Scale score of 12 points or less, posttraumatic amnesia (PTA) more than 1 hour, and positive acute head CT or MRI findings at 4.5 and 29 months postinjury using DTI. Fractional anisotropy values, a measure of white matter integrity, were compared for the two time points, and these researchers found a decline in white matter fractional anisotropy values, specifically in the frontal and temporal lobes in this moderate to severe group of those with TBI. These findings were seen as consistent with a similar study conducted by Ng et al.[9] using brain MRI technology who also found progression of atrophy at 4.5 months and 2.5 years post-TBI. Such neuroimaging findings suggest that there may be continued white matter progression during the postacute phase in those with MTBI, and it remains unclear whether these changes correlate with neuropsychological findings. Nevertheless, neuropsychological test findings may be a useful tool to understand whether there are declines in neurocognitive functioning in some individuals during the postacute phase. On the other hand, improvement in neuropsychological findings in light of white matter progression might argue for the effects of cognitive–compensatory mechanisms of change that improve the functional status of the person after TBI.

Three areas of the brain appear to be most susceptible to DAI after TBI. According to Filley[5], these are the *brainstem, cerebral hemispheres,* and *corpus callosum.* Executive functioning, working and recent memory deficits, and impairments in complex information processing are commonly found as neuropsychological deficits in TBI. What Luria[10] referred to as *cortical tone* can also be seen, particularly early postinjury. In this instance, the patient demonstrates difficulty regulating and maintaining alertness and focused attention to the task at hand. These common neurobehavioral problems correlate with Filley's[5] three common regions of DAI after TBI. Filley[11] also found that the superimposition of cortical lesions with DAI produced poorer neurobehavioral outcomes in TBI than with DAI alone. Thus, in TBI, the neuropsychological outcomes can be widespread and pervasive, covering a number of neurobehavioral syndromes and an array of cognitive impairments.

Because of the inner skull structures upon which the brain rests, particularly vulnerable are the *orbitofrontal* and *anterior temporal convexity* regions of the cortex. From a purely localized point of view, impairments in these regions explain common neurobehavioral syndromes of disinhibition and decreased regulation of behavior seen in these patients. Aharon-Peretz and Tomer[12] note that brain dysfunction after TBI is always diffuse with frontal dysfunction common secondary to DAI. In TBI—especially because DAI can be prevalent, resulting in dysfunction across many areas of the cortex—there is no specific or common neuropsychological profile, save generalities regarding memory, attention, and executive functioning. Complicating the neuropsychological picture is the fact that there are numerous frontal to subcortical circuits where any lesion along these pathways, although not necessarily localized to the frontal lobe, can result in the same neurobehavioral syndrome. Likewise, as a result of the network of connections between frontal and subcortical structures, the same lesion in two different individuals with TBI may have an entirely different cognitive and neurobehavioral outcome. Luria[10] spoke of the integrated nature of higher cortical functions nearly 30 years ago, even before the advent of functional neuroimaging technology:

> That is why mental functions, as complex functional systems, cannot be localized in narrow zones of the cortex or in isolated cell groups, but must be organized in systems of concertedly working zones, each of which performs its role in complex functional system, and which may be located in completely different, and often far distant, areas of the brain.[p.31]

Although dysfunction along the orbitofrontal–subcortical circuit can produce behavioral disinhibition, impairments in the *dorsolateral-subcortical* circuit underlie executive cognitive processes. Chow and Cummings[13] describe this circuit as controlling processes such as organizational strategies, memory retrieval, ability to shift sets and concepts, and response inhibition. These cognitive processes are commonly assessed by neuropsychological testing procedures. Impairments in the *anterior cingulate–subcortical* circuit results in apathy, initiation deficits, reduced responsivity to tactile sensory input, and paucity of verbal output. Mayberg[14] proposed that dysregulation in the cortical–limbic circuit can account for mood disorders and, particularly, depression. More recently, problems in modulation in the cortical–limbic circuit may even have implications for the types of effective therapy (e.g., cognitive behavior therapy) for those who show evidence of dysregulation in this region of the brain.[15,16] These findings have implications for those with TBI for whom rates of depression and mood disorders are known to be high. Such high rates are likely to have significant correspondence with underlying neurobiologic cortical–limbic circuitry and dysregulation.

26.2.2 Neuropsychological Recovery after Traumatic Brain Injury

Recovery of cognitive functions and reduction of neurobehavioral consequences have been studied throughout the years. One of the earliest and influential of these prospective studies was conducted by Dikmen et al.[17] and Dacey et al.,[18] who studied a cohort of adult TBI patients and a friend control group at 1, 12, and 24 months postinjury. Neuropsychological impairments across many domains of cognitive functions were found at each time interval, the extent of cognitive impairment at each being related to the length of coma. Improvements occurred during the first year, consistent with other studies[19] on cognitive recovery. Dikmen et al. also found further, but more specific, types of cognitive improvement occurring during the second year postinjury; however, the extent of recovery was dependent on severity of injury.[17,18] More recent studies have also examined the rate of neuropsychological recovery within the first year postinjury. Kersel et al.[20] found 31% to 63% of recovery in such functions as simple and complex attention, verbal memory, executive functioning, and perceptual abilities. Novack et al.,[21] prospectively, found improvements in memory, processing speed, language, and constructional abilities at 6 and 12 months postinjury. Gains in community reintegration, but continued deficits in driving abilities, were also found in that study, in which severity of the TBI determined the amount of recovery.

Several prospective studies have been conducted to date, many over the course of many years post-TBI. For example, neuropsychological recovery was followed over a 23-year period by Hessen et al.[22] In their study, 119 participants, 92% of whom had MTBI (45 children, 74 adults), underwent an initial comprehensive neuropsychological test battery that consisted primarily of the Halstead-Reitan Neuropsychological Battery and the Wechsler Memory Scale—Revised. They found that those who sustained an MTBI in which PTA was more than 24 hours or PTA was less than 24 hours but with abnormal electroencephalographic findings within the first 24 hours predicted poor neuropsychological outcomes after 23 years versus using those same predictors in the adult population. They concluded that children with MTBI may be more vulnerable to long-term neuropsychological dysfunction than adults. A recent study by Draper and Ponsford[23] found that, after a 10-year follow-up, cognitive impairments persisted and were associated with initial injury severity. Neuropsychological tests that differentiated those with TBI from control subjects were those that tapped into attention, information processing speed, memory, and executive functioning. Much replication is needed to verify these findings, such that reliable and key predictors of neurocognitive and neurobehavioral outcomes can be identified.

Neuronal injury and glial cellular damage have been shown to account for some of these neuropsychological impairments, both shortly after injury (2 weeks) and more distant to the injury (6 months).[24] DAI has also been related to the rate of recovery of cognitive functions.[25] These studies led to the idea that the majority of neuropsychological recovery occurs within the first 2 years postinjury. This notion has been more recently challenged by Sbordone et al.,[26] who found cognitive, social, physical, and emotional improvements beyond 2 years postinjury. These researchers suggest that recovery continues for at least 10 years postinjury—a finding that is highly discrepant with the earlier prospective studies. It is important to note, however, that the latter research was conducted with a retrospective research design that relies upon judgment of recovery compared with preinjury status up to 10 years in the past. A balance between the earlier prospective work and the retrospective study by Sbordone et al.[26] was struck in a recent longitudinal study of neuropsychological recovery at 1 and 5 years postinjury by Millis et al.[27] Neuropsychological data from the National Institute on Disability and Rehabilitation Research Traumatic Brain Injury Model Systems of Care were analyzed in which recovery of attention, recent memory, oral word fluency, cognitive efficiency, visuoconstructive, sensory–motor, and reasoning abilities was variable across the 5 years. Using a change index score, they found that 22.2% of the sample demonstrated cognitive improvement, whereas 62.6% remained unchanged and 15.2% declined. Clear improvement was shown to occur most on measures of information processing speed, visuoconstruction ability, and verbal recent memory.

Neuropsychological evaluations completed during the early postacute phase of recovery can be predictive of longer term functional outcomes. Green et al.[28] demonstrated that global neuropsychological test aggregate scores (including simple attention, executive function, memory, and speed of processing) were predictive of latter productivity. Productivity in this study was measured as a dichotomous variable that included paid or volunteer employment, and other life activities (e.g., school, parenting roles). Neuropsychological variables likely reflect cognitive capacity, general brain integrity, and specific indices of brain–behavior functioning that impact everyday activities, often referred to as the *ecological validity* or neuropsychological test scores. Key to this relationship between neuropsychological test outcomes and everyday functioning appears to be the correspondence between the cognitive domain of the test and the outcome measure. According to Chaytor and Schmitter-Edgecombe,[29] this correspondence is highly moderated by "the population being tested, the approach utilized . . . the person completing the outcome measure (significant other vs. clinician), illness severity, and time from injury until evaluation."[p.181]

Finally, these longitudinal studies implicate a somewhat sobering clinical picture of successful reintegration into community, vocational, and school activities for the patient who has sustained a TBI. It is often helpful to use the findings of these longitudinal studies in the clinical setting. For example, Boake et al.[30] studied the use of neuropsychological testing data to predict long-term productivity after TBI. Testing completed prior to discharge from the acute inpatient rehabilitation setting was predictive of competitive employment or enrollment in full-time regular education. They found that tests of memory had prognostic value (Wechsler Memory Scale–Revised, Rey Auditory Verbal Learning Test). Furthermore, the Trail Making Test (particularly, Part B) had significant prognostic value regarding long-term productivity. They note this may be the case with Trail Making because of its sensitivity to multiple cognitive domains. Leahy and Lam[31] found that the Stroop Color–Word Test discriminated individuals with TBI who were competitively employed or were enrolled in degree-oriented education. Again, this may be the result of the demands of this test for several cognitive abilities, including complex attention, executive functioning, response inhibition, and speed of processing. These kinds of information can be useful in sequencing rehabilitative therapies throughout the postacute phase of the patient's care to target realistic goals better for the patient in the short and long term. Testing during the inpatient rehabilitation phase may identify TBI patients at high risk for poorer productive outcomes, and the process of planning for subsequent rehabilitation can begin early.

26.2.3 Neuropsychological Testing versus Neuropsychological Assessment

Before discussing the variety of neuropsychological evaluation approaches and test procedures, it is important to differentiate the process of *assessment* as opposed to the technical aspects of *testing*. *Testing* refers to only one aspect of the examination, usually the actual standardized administration and scoring of a battery of neuropsychological tests. Testing can usually be performed by a technician who has been trained in the standardized administration of an array of neuropsychological tests, often referred to as a *psychometrist*, *neuropsychometrist*, or *psychology technician*. Many neuropsychologists elect to administer their own tests during which first-hand observation of the qualitative aspects of the patient's performance may be deemed important. A*ssessment*, in the context of the neuropsychological examination, refers to the comprehensive *process* of evaluating the patient and includes multiple sources of input. These can include review of medical records; patient interview; informant interviews; performance-based measures (neuropsychological tests); paper-and-pencil questionnaires (e.g., personality questionnaires, concussion symptom inventories); direct observation of the patient in the testing setting and in real-world settings; and information gathered upon feedback of testing results. Assessment begins at the very first contact with a referral source or with the patient and is concluded when feedback is provided to all interested parties. Table 26.1 describes the various components involved in the neuropsychological assessment process. Not all components are necessarily included in every neuropsychological examination. The neuropsychologist may use various components depending upon the referral question.

These components comprise an in-depth examination of the patient that covers a broad range of brain–behavior relationships. In the context of brain injury rehabilitation, the neuropsychological assessment provides an active ingredient to planning interventions and defining cognitive rehabilitation strategies that may be executed by the interdisciplinary rehabilitation team. The neuropsychological assessment becomes this active ingredient as a result of the fact that information regarding deficits will, oftentimes, define the obstacles that potentially interfere with the patient's benefit from rehabilitation therapy. For example, if a patient evidences marked recent verbal memory impairment, verbal instruction alone to complete a set of exercises prescribed by the physical therapist may be problematic. Furthermore, the patient may have trouble recalling the proper sequence of steps for completing an exercise or activity of daily living. Knowledge of the type and extent of the verbal recent memory problem will be useful to the therapist to adjust the method of therapy delivery. The therapist may decide to pair verbal instruction with visual demonstration of the exercise set, and provide the patient with pictures of the steps of an exercise routine. Breaking down a complex set of steps into component parts, and training by procedural mastery and repetition of the activity of daily living sequence may be necessary, based on this information about verbal memory impairment. To understand fully a patient's memory capacity, both in terms of assets and deficits, many of these components are necessary for the accurate determination of that patient's memory abilities. Utilizing deficit information (what constitutes the patient's cognitive limitations or vulnerabilities) paired with preserved and asset information (abilities that remain intact and those for which the patient may excel and capitalize upon) provides significant information to rehabilitation therapists in crafting an effective approach to their intervention. It is in the application of the neuropsychological test findings to the care of the TBI patient that the assessment becomes a powerful instrument to improve the functional status of the patient.[32]

TABLE 26.1

Components of the Neuropsychological Evaluation

Step	Component of the Evaluation	Comment
1.	First contact with referral source	Ascertain questions to be answered by the assessment, shaping the referral question to best respond to a consultation request, begin determination of the assessment approach, define other data that may be of assistance for completing the evaluation.
2.	First contact with patient, family, employer, or other party	Understand the patient and family's conceptualization of TBI relative to the need for the assessment; examine discrepancies between patient's insights regarding the TBI versus family/friends' view; align expectations among provider, referral source, and patient/family/employer/other, of what will be accomplished by the examination; obtain information regarding preinjury medical, academic, psychological, and psychosocial status.
3.	Medical record review post-TBI	Examination of early records, including field observations of the patient (e.g., Glasgow Coma Scale scores, emergency medical technician observations, observer observations, if available), emergency room observations of retrograde amnesia, loss of consciousness, posttraumatic amnesia to assist with grading severity of TBI; evidence for early behavioral agitation; tracking the chronology of events postinjury, including medications, treatments, neurosurgical interventions, medical complications and co-occurring conditions, progression of the symptom complex, rehabilitation therapy, patient and family response to the rehabilitation process.
4.	Other record review	Examination of educational records to assist with determination of preinjury cognitive and intellectual functioning level, history of psychiatric impairment, mental health service utilization and substance abuse, determination of premorbid neuropsychological risks or condition, preinjury medical history, and service utilization that may be contributory to the current evaluation.
5.	Preinterview questionnaires	Background information may be ascertained on demographics, logistics, medical history, psychological history, notation and rating scales of past and current symptoms, educational attainment and performance; provides information to structure the clinical interview. Examine for discrepancies between self-report, informant reports, record review; set agenda for seeking potential resolution of consistencies during clinical and informant interviews.
6.	Clinical interview, patient	Review medical and psychosocial history, ascertain current symptom complex from the patient's point of view; assist in determining congruency with early head injury severity indices; determine awareness of neuropsychological and neurobehavioral deficits; assist with ascertaining the patient's experience of quality of life post-TBI; obtain observational mental status functioning; determine contributory conditions to cognitive dysfunction, including depression, anxiety, anger/irritability, fatigue and sleep disturbance, pain symptoms and progression, substance use/abuse, medication (prescribed and over-the-counter medications and supplements) use/abuse/polypharmacy. Determine provisional co-occurring psychiatric diagnoses.
7.	Clinical interview, informants (e.g., family member, friend, teacher, coworker, employer)	Review variable mentioned earlier for the clinical interview with the patient to examine for congruency of that information and to obtain further details; obtain information to judge premorbid compared with post-TBI functioning; assist with the alignment of expectations for treatment and recovery of function in the patient.

TABLE 26.1 (continued)

Components of the Neuropsychological Evaluation

Step	Component of the Evaluation	Comment
8.	Neuropsychological testing	Administration of neuropsychological tests by the neuropsychologist (or other trained and licensed health care professional) or psychometrist (a person trained in the standardized administration of neuropsychological and psychological tests). The length of the examination varies depending upon the referral question; can extend from a brief mental status examination to a full day or two of testing. Interspersed with actual testing are rest breaks and a break for a meal if completed during the day. Development of interpersonal rapport and therapeutic alliance during standardized administration is key to obtaining maximal testing results. Testing may involve administration by both the psychologist and/or psychometrist, and computer-assisted administration of tests. Validity testing (determination of effort and symptom enhancement) may occur near the beginning of the testing session and/or interspersed throughout the testing session. Administration of psychological tests of mood, personality, pain perception, sleep, coping, quality of life, and functional outcome measures (for activities of daily living; instrumental activity of daily living).
9.	Test scoring and interpretation	The neuropsychologist and/or psychometrist scores test protocols; computer scoring programs may be used; generation of test score summary sheets; behavioral observations of test administration is recorded to assist in determining validity of obtained test scores. Depending on the outcome at this stage, further testing may be ordered to clarify or expand certain domains that are assessed.
10.	Report generation	A comprehensive report is generated that incorporates the information acquired; referral questions are answered within the body of the report. A listing of recommendations along with time frames and sequence of importance may be included. Some neuropsychologists may elect to delay the completion of a comprehensive report until after the feedback session to include information obtained during that session. Report length is frequently determined by the referral question and context (e.g., medical center/hospital-based reports may be shorter in length than forensic neuropsychological evaluation reports). Reports may be written for specific audiences, including referring physicians and health care providers, school settings, attorney and forensic settings, case managers, vocational rehabilitation counselors, and so forth.
11.	Feedback session	Feedback regarding the results of the examination is explained to the patient, family members, or others, together or separately. Modification of the report may occur depending upon new questions that may arise; recommendations are made to the patient and family; other providers may be invited to the feedback session, depending upon clinical need and with the permission of the patient; feedback may be provided to case managers, vocational counselors, educational specialists, or other health care providers. Verbal and written feedback to referring sources may accompany the delivery of the report.

26.2.4 Neuropsychological Assessment Orientations

A number of training programs and subsequent models of neuropsychological assessment has emerged since the beginning of clinical neuropsychology. Often related to a particular researcher or research program, an array of orientations or approaches to neuropsychology has emerged.[33] All have been applied in brain injury rehabilitation and have provided an active ingredient to the process of recovery of function in TBI. One large survey of neuropsychological test usage, neuropsychology battery choice, and theoretical orientation found specific clusters of usage.[34] These clusters included fixed battery orientations such as the Halstead-Reitan Neuropsychological Battery and Luria-Nebraska Neuropsychological Battery approaches. The Arthur Benton Laboratory orientation, process, hypothesis testing, and eclectic clusters of test usage was also identified. Currently, there is no consensus on which approach or battery is most appropriate for those with TBI, and the quality of the examination is likely more a function of the training, experience in researching or working with TBI, and experience in applying sets of neuropsychological tests with this population. The major approaches are noted in the following sections with key references that describe the approach in greater detail.

26.2.4.1 Fixed-Battery Approach

The fixed-battery approach refers to the administration of a uniform set of neuropsychological tests across all patients evaluated. This provides for a systematic comparison of patients across the same sets of tests. The fixed-battery approach usually incorporates tests that cover a full range of brain–behavior functions, including sensory–motor, language, attention and concentration, memory, visuoconstructive, visuospatial, information processing speed, and executive functioning domains.

Among the most commonly utilized fixed-battery approaches is the *Halstead-Reitan Neuropsychological Test Battery* (HRNB).[35–38] First developed by Ward Halstead in 1947 and later modified by Ralph Reitan in 1955, the HRNB consists of eight core tests: Category Test, Tactual Performance Test, Speech Sounds Perception, Seashore Rhythm, Finger Oscillation, Trail Making Test, Aphasia Screening Examination, and the Reitan-Klove Sensory Perceptual Examination. It generates the Halstead Impairment Index, which provides a gross indication of impairment severity. A General Neuropsychological Deficit Scale can also be generated from the HRNB that provides indications of level of performance, pathognomonic signs, pattern analysis, and lateralization indicators. Other tests are often used in conjunction with the HRNB, including the Wechsler Adult Intelligence Scale–Revised (WAIS-R) and third edition versions, measures of recent memory, further measures of sensory–motor integrity, and personality functioning (e.g., Minnesota Multiphasic Personality Inventory-2).

Another widely used fixed-battery approach is the *Luria-Nebraska Neuropsychological Battery* (LNNB) developed by Charles Golden et al.[39–42] Utilizing testing procedures of Alexander Luria[43] and systematized by Anne-Lise Christiansen,[44,45] the LNNB was developed to capture some of Luria's original bedside examination methodology, organized into a psychometric format. Although having been highly criticized in the past on the basis of reliability and validity, these criticisms have given way to the cumulative empirical research regarding its enduring psychometric soundness and clinical utility. There are two published versions of the LNNB, Form I and Form II, the latter of which has been thought to be particularly useful with older adults.[46] The LNNB allows for actuarial interpretations, based upon the empirical research on the instrument in different populations, as well as allows for qualitative analysis, particularly on the item analysis level of interpretation. It is a rich clinical instrument that can be useful in the rehabilitation setting because it allows the clinician to apply LNNB findings to an analysis of intact versus impaired functional cognitive systems. The LNNB consists of 11 clinical scales (Motor Functions, Rhythm, Tactile Functions, Visual Functions, Receptive Speech, Expressive Speech, Writing, Reading, Arithmetic, Memory, Intellectual Processes); five summary scales (Pathognomonic, Left Hemisphere, Right Hemisphere, Profile Elevation, Impairment); eight localization scales (Left Frontal, Left Sensory–Motor, Left Parietal–Occipital, Left Temporal, Right Frontal, Right Sensory–Motor, Right Parietal–Occipital, Right Temporal); and 28 factor scales that assist the clinician in illuminating elevations on the clinical scales. Currently, the LNNB-II is only computer scored. The computer scoring options for the LNNB-I can be done by mail-in or fax transmittal. There has not been an update for local computer scoring for the Windows environment, which requires the use of the older DOS operating system. This may be indicative of the decline and demand for usage of this battery. For children, the *LNNB–Children's Version*, *NEPSY-II*, and the *Cognitive Assessment Scales* are available as fixed-battery approaches, and reflect some of the principles that Alexander Luria forwarded.

For older adults, the *Kaplan-Baycrest Neurocognitive Assessment* provides an option of a neuropsychological test battery that is standardized for this population. For those with TBI who present with marked cognitive impairment, the *Severe Impairment Battery* will provide information beyond the standard mental status examination without overtaxing the examinee.

One of the newest neuropsychological test batteries to be published that allows for both a fixed-battery and flexible-battery approach (i.e., the battery can be tailored to the needs of the clinical situation and patient) is the *Neuropsychological Assessment Battery* (NAB).[47] The NAB consists of a screening battery that allows for an overview of specific cognitive domains. Those domains that are impaired on the screening battery can then be followed up by specific modules, eliminating the need to administer the full NAB battery. The full NAB battery could also be administered at the discretion and preference of the clinician as well. A particular benefit of this battery is that embedded in each of the cognitive modules (attention, language, memory, spatial, executive) are "daily living tests" that emphasize ecological validity. For example, in the spatial module, there is a subtest that requires map reading and analysis.

26.2.4.2 Flexible-Battery Approach

In flexible-battery approaches, the neuropsychologist may use a different set of tests, depending upon the referral question and the type of neurologic problem being analyzed. The *hypothesis-testing approach* that has been championed by Muriel Lezak[48] is based on the idea that the presentation of the patient and the referral question generate initial hypotheses regarding the neurocognitive condition of the patient. Tests are selected to test these clinical hypotheses. Confirmation and rejection of specific hypotheses can then lead to further neuropsychological testing to follow up clinical observation of test performance by the patient. Tests such as the WAIS, Rey-Osterrieth Complex Figure Test, Rey Auditory Verbal Learning Test, and the Wisconsin Card Sorting Test are used particularly in TBI because of the nature of commonly found impairments in this population. Although using many standardized tests that those from other orientations administer, the hypothesis-testing approach is characterized by sequential steps in reasoning, and iterative clinical decision making when conducting the neuropsychological evaluation. Lezak[48] describes this process as follows:

> The diagnostic process involves the successive elimination of alternative possibilities, or hypotheses…. The examiner formulates the first set of hypotheses on the basis of the referral question, information obtained from the history or informants, and the initial impression of the patient. Each diagnostic hypothesis is tested by comparing what is

known of the patient's condition (history, appearance, interview behavior, test performance) with what is expected for that particular diagnostic classification. As the examination proceeds, the examiner can progressively refine general hypotheses … into increasingly specific hypotheses.[48, p.101]

26.2.4.3 Process Orientation Approach

Original Lurian methodology called for the qualitative analysis of the patient's performance on tasks that the clinician uses. Anne-Lise Christensen[44] organized a set of Luria's behavioral neurology-oriented procedures into a systematic set of tasks called *Luria's Neuropsychological Investigation*. The approach calls for a set of procedures, including the preliminary conversation (Stage 1), which is the clinical interview. The next step involves the examination of motor, auditory, kinesthetic, and visual analyzers (Stage 2), followed by examination of specific cognitive functions (Stage 3) based upon performance of earlier stages of the examination. During Stage 4 of the examination (syndrome analysis), the clinician identifies the neuropsychological syndrome according to Luria's localization of functional systems in the brain. Luria's Neuropsychological Investigation has been used for the purposes of brain injury rehabilitation and has been used specifically to evaluate those with TBI.[45] Although less frequently referred to as a process instrument and falling under the category of a fixed-battery approach, the LNNB has, from its inception, involved a qualitative and process approach via the item analysis interpretation and syndrome analysis. The rich clinical item content of the LNNB continues to lend itself to qualitative analysis and can, itself, augment a number of approaches to neuropsychological assessment.

Another popular approach to the neuropsychological examination of patients with neurologic disorders has been led by Edith Kaplan,[49] called the *Boston Process Approach*. It often combines the use of fixed neuropsychological tests, but within a framework of examining not only the score outcome, but also the types and processes of the errors involved.[49] Kaplan et al.[50] utilize standardized tests, such as the Wechsler Memory Scale or the WAIS-R, and modify the administration procedures to introduce methods of scoring the protocol to analyze errors and to test the limits of the patient's cognitive capacity. Additional items and multiple-choice formats are added to the instrument to analyze better the performance of the patient. The WAIS-R as Neuropsychological Instrument (WAIS-R-NI) is a good example of this approach[50] in which the patient's constructions of the Block Design test are tracked and certain kinds of errors (e.g., constructing the block patterns outside of the gestalt of the square) may be more indicative of right hemispheric impairment. Another example of the application of the Boston Process Approach is the use of the Rey Complex Figure test. Many neuropsychologists examine the quality of the copy portion of the test (i.e., examination of the reproduction of the patient's drawing of a complex geometric figure) for such pathognomonic signs as rotation, distortion of the figure, poor planning in the visuoconstruction aspects of the design, loss of details, and problems in aligning angles and intersections of the design. Many examiners will assist in their analysis of the reproduced design by handing the examinee a different colored pencil at specific time intervals or after completion of specific elements of the design to recount better the examinee's construction, allowing for a qualitative analysis of the drawing. The Boston Qualitative Scoring System for the Rey-Osterrieth Complex Figure was devised to quantify several elements and error categories of a patient's design reproductions.[51]

26.3 Content of Neuropsychological Assessment

When reviewing several neuropsychological testing procedures, it is important not only to describe the instrument and cognitive domain that it represents, but in the context of TBI rehabilitation, the ecological validity implications are paramount. As mentioned earlier in this chapter, ecological validity refers to a test's ability to predict everyday functioning. Sbordone[52] describes this concept as follows:

> Ecological validity can be defined as the functional and predictive relationship between the patient's performance on a set of neuropsychological tests and the patient's behavior in a variety of real-world settings (e.g., at home, work, school, community). This definition also assumes that demand characteristics within these various settings are idiosyncratic and fluctuate as a result of their specific nature, purpose, and goals.[p.16]

The neuropsychological examination done in the context of TBI rehabilitation is not often used to identify lesions, but rather is used for the purposes of ecological validity. They are useful when attempting to predict the patient's functioning in the environment, and to assist with predicting the patient's behavior in "idiosyncratic" settings that do not remain static. One of the problems with neuropsychological testing, according to Sbordone,[53] is that neuropsychological tests, by themselves, do not predict everyday behaviors or vocational functioning well. It is, therefore, incumbent upon the neuropsychologist to translate assessment findings into meaningful statements about a particular patient, with specific deficits, under specific environmental conditions (e.g., inpatient rehabilitation unit setting, safety issues in being home alone without supervision, a job setting with noise distractions, college chemistry classroom setting). Therefore, ecological implications of particular testing procedures are stated for the testing procedures described in the following sections.

26.3.1 Cognitive Screening and Mental Status Examinations

Instruments that provide global information about general cognitive functioning can be useful in the assessment of patients with TBI to provide a brief look at level of ability. This tends to occur during the early phases of recovery when the patient may not be capable of engaging in a more complex or comprehensive examination. Table 26.2 provides a listing of common cognitive screening measures and their characteristics. These measures provide some coverage of important cognitive domains such as recent memory, attention, visuospatial analysis and visuoconstruction skills, and abstracting and executive functioning skill (e.g., Dementia Rating Scale, Cognistat, Repeatable Battery for the Assessment of Neuropsychological Status [RBANS], Scales of Cognitive Ability for Traumatic Brain Injury). Others provide a global index of cognitive functioning (Mini-Mental State Examination, Clock Drawing Test). Although not used for diagnostic purposes, these tests are helpful when trying to determine whether a more comprehensive battery of neuropsychological tests may be recommended. Many of these tests are performed by those other than neuropsychologists, including speech pathologists, occupational therapists, psychiatrists, physical medicine and rehabilitation physicians, and neurologists.

TABLE 26.2

Tests of Cognitive Screening and Mental Status Examinations

Test	Comment
Cognistat (Neurobehavioral Cognitive Status Examination)	Assesses five major areas: language, constructional ability, memory, calculation skills, and reasoning/judgment.
Dementia Rating Scale-2 (and alternate form)	Provides subscales scores for attention, initiation/perseveration, construction, conceptualization, and memory; yields a total score.
Mini-Mental State Examination (Folstein)	Standard measure of mental state based on the 30-point scale; widely used for gross dementia detection; runs the risk of a high false-negative rate.
Repeatable Battery for the Assessment of Neuropsychological Status	Brief measure of immediate memory, language, visuospatial/constructional, attention, and delayed memory; an alternate form is available for repeat testing.
Screening Test for the Luria-Nebraska Neuropsychological Battery	Very brief measure that determines whether a full LNNB may be helpful; screener includes stimulus materials for adults and children.
Screening module of the Neuropsychological Assessment Battery (NAB)	Contains sections that correspond to the main cognitive modules of the full NAB: attention, language, spatial, memory, and executive functions. Provides recommendations for administering the cognitive module for clinical clarification if not giving the full NAB.
Scales of Cognitive Ability for Traumatic Brain Injury (SCATBI)	Measures cognitive and linguistic abilities and deficits; specifically tailored to those with TBI. The five subtests are perception/discrimination, orientation, organization, recall, and reasoning.
Shipley-2 (formerly the Shipley Institute of Living Scale)	Measures components of cognitive ability: crystallized knowledge (that acquired through experience and education) and fluid reasoning (learned through logic, problem solving, ability to learn new information). Vocabulary test measures crystallized knowledge; fluid reasoning assessed through sequence completion tasks, analysis of block patterns (Kohs cube designs); calculates an impairment index for adults, which is based on the discrepancy between vocabulary and abstracting scores.

26.3.1.1 Ecological Implications

These measures can help the rehabilitation team answer such questions as the following:

- Does the patient have the mental capacity to understand his or her own cognitive condition?
- To what extent is the patient oriented and in need of supervision?
- Can the patient be expected to follow a schedule or keep up with simple instructions?
- What is the gross capacity of the patient to learn routines and carry over instruction from one time or setting to another?
- What is the gross attention ability of the patient?
- Is there evidence for cognitive impairment that requires more in-depth neuropsychological evaluation?
- Is there any relative preservation of cognitive ability that can be capitalized upon for simple tasks?

If the patient fails aspects of these cognitive screening measures, the rehabilitation team may need to provide interventions such as the posting of a calendar in the patient's room for orientation purposes, cue the patient to the tasks at hand and encourage learning by repetition, determine the length of a session based on level of sustained attention, and train the patient to the setting and not assume transfer of learning to a new setting. Some measures, such as the RBANS, allow for repeat administration during which tracking cognitive improvements can occur. This may be particularly important when making discharge plans and organizing postacute services. The usefulness of RBANS is also underscored by its strength in distinguishing cognitive problems in those with TBI compared with noninjured control subjects, where moderate to strong specificity has been found to detect those with TBI.[54]

Cognitive screening measures may also be helpful in tracking the TBI patient's cognition in determining transfers to and from subacute and acute rehabilitation settings. The patient's ability to engage in 3 hours per day of rehabilitative therapy may depend upon the cortical arousal level and integrity of sufficient sustained attention and orientation to benefit from this intensive level of therapy. In special situations, such as the patient with combined spinal cord injury and TBI, making initial judgments about cognition may determine length of stay. In this clinical situation, decreased learning capacity and memory may result in the patient requiring more supervision, cues, and reminders, and repetitive learning of such activities as executing proper transfers, self-catheterization, and repositioning to avoid decubitus ulcers.

26.3.2 General Level of Performance

> Perhaps someone with expert knowledge of the human brain will understand my illness, discover what a brain injury does to a man's mind, memory, and body, appreciate my effort, and help me avoid some of the problems I have in life.[55, p.xxi]
>
> **—From L. Zasetsky in A. R. Luria's** *The Man with a Shattered World*

A. R. Luria's method of behavioral neurology often involved the detailed examination of the patient,[55] as indicated in the previous quote. His observations of the patient laid the foundation to understand brain–behavior relationships and are used as examples of what occurs after TBI. His patient, Lieutenant Zasetsky, suffered a penetrating head injury from a bullet wound during World War II. Well described by Kaczmarek et al.,[56] Zasetsky was shot in March 1943, leaving him with significant deficits of memory, language, writing capacity, and executive functioning. Luria tracked this soldier's recovery and struggles for more than 25 years, chronicling by biography and Zasetsky's own writings the aftereffects of a severe brain injury. Aspects of generalized cognitive impairment and specific realms of cognitive deficits are highlighted by Zasetsky's case history and will be referred to throughout the remainder of this chapter.

Based upon a larger set of neuropsychological test findings, indices of general neuropsychological performance and impairment serve similar functions as cognitive screening measures. They tend to have greater reliability because they are based upon scale scores summed across several domains rather than item-level scores. As mentioned earlier, the Halstead Impairment Index is one of the more commonly cited general performance indices that have been used in outcome research in patients with TBI. The Neuropsychological Deficit Scale, also noted earlier, is a score that is derived from a wider set of HRNB tests. The LNNB can generate its own impairment index, utilizing elevations on specific clinical scales and the pathognomonic scale. One limitation of the use of general impairment scores is that they are unable to describe in detail the specific cognitive problems that can

TABLE 26.3

Measures of General Levels of Performance

Measure	Comment
Halstead Impairment Index	Calculation of the 7 indexed tests of the HRNB; ranges from 0.0 to 1.0, with latter meaning 7 out of 7 of the tests fall in the impaired range.
General Neuropsychological Deficit Scale	Calculated off of 42 variables from the adult HRNB and allied procedures; higher scores indicate more impairment; each of the 42 scores falls in four score ranges (0 = perfectly normal; 1 = normal to mild impairment; 2 = mildly to moderately impaired; 3 = severely impaired performance); total GNDS scores fall into the following ranges: 0–25 (normal), 26–40 (mild impairment), 41–67 (moderate impairment), 68 and higher (severe impairment); total maximum score is 168 on the GNDS.
Luria-Nebraska Neuropsychological Battery—Form 1—Impairment Indices	The LNNB Impairment Index is calculated by examining the difference between the obtained T-score and the Critical Level; similar in conception as the NDS above. In addition, there are other general measures of performance embedded within the LNNB: Pathognomonic, Left Hemisphere, Right Hemisphere, Profile Elevation, Impairment, and the Power/Speed calculation.
Wechsler Adult Intelligence Scale—4th Ed. (WAIS-IV)	FSIQ not generally considered a neuropsychological measure; helpful in estimating long-term cognitive abilities; General Ability Index reflects robust and crystallized abilities for comparison to fluid abilities.
Kaplan Baycrest Neurocognitive Assessment	Evaluates a broad range of functioning, including attention/concentration, immediate memory, delayed memory, verbal fluency, spatial processing, and reasoning/conceptual shifting.
MicroCog: Assessment of Cognitive Functioning	Evaluates attention/mental control, memory, reasoning/calculation, spatial processing, reaction time, information processing accuracy, information processing speed, cognitive functioning and cognitive proficiency; this is a computer-assisted administration system.

explain problems in everyday functioning in the person with TBI. Table 26.3 presents measures of general neuropsychological level of performance.

26.3.2.1 Ecological Implications

An index of general performance is an indication of overall neuropsychological integrity and can be used to judge and predict a patient's ability to function independently in global life functions. A Halstead Impairment Index of 0.9 (i.e., 90% of the indexed tests on the HRNB fell in the brain-impaired range) would alert the rehabilitation team that the patient's cognitive reserve is limited to compensate independently for cognitive deficits in real-world settings. That patient's capacity to generalize learned skills independently to new settings may be limited. This is a result of the fact that an HRNB II of 0.9 indicates a broad range of impaired higher level cognitive functions—cognitive skills that are needed to bear upon complex tasks and behaviors. Likewise, an LNNB Impairment Index that falls in the mild range may be associated with a greater potential for independent living where compensatory strategy training, modifications to the home environment, and training the patient with organizational aids may be feasible and effective. A mild level of general impairment does not necessarily connote mild impairments across all tests in a battery, and could mean normal functioning on some tests combined with severe problems on specific tests. Compensating for the cognitive problem that falls in the severely impaired range (e.g., utilizing a memory aid for scheduling appointments and organizing information that impacts everyday functioning) may require the assistance of a rehabilitation therapist or family member to implement in everyday tasks or contexts. Depending on the time post-TBI, these general indices of impairment may take on different significance. A highly impaired General Neuropsychological Deficit Scale (GNDS) at 1 month postinjury, improving to a mild level of general impairment within 3 months in a person with a moderate to severe TBI bodes well for longer term prognosis. Contrasting this effect with a high GNDS at 5 years postinjury may suggest that further spontaneous recovery, to a larger extent, is highly unlikely given the persistence of significant and global cognitive impairment in that individual. Fluctuations in impairment indices across time may be reflective of situation specific or changes in co-occurring conditions (e.g., marked sleep disorders and coexistence of significant psychiatric or substance use issues).

26.3.3 Sensory–Motor Integrity

> When the doctor learned what my first name was, he'd always address me that way and try to shake hands when he came over. But I couldn't manage to clasp his hand.... Suddenly, I'd remember and try to shake hands again but would only manage to touch his fingers.[55, p.46]

> —L. Zasetsky

Output of motor movement for everyday routine actions (e.g., picking up a jar, using the steering wheel while driving, folding the laundry) may, on the surface, appear to be a reflexive action without involving higher level cognitive actions. Execution of motor programs cannot occur without the recursive feedback of tactile and sensory–perceptual inputs. The regulation of these sensory–motor circuits requires higher level cognition in many cases, especially when learning new motor actions. Luria[57] posited that verbal mediation is a significant driver of human actions, what he described as the regulatory function of speech. Thus, the integration of higher cortical functions with motor movements and the ability to interpret tactile inputs is intricate. The interplay of motor functions and higher order processes occur and are relevant for consideration in brain injury rehabilitation. Table 26.4 describes commonly used tests of motor functions.

26.3.3.1 Ecological Implications

Whether motor input impairment occurs in the peripheral nervous system (e.g., peripheral neuropathy), in the spinal cord (e.g., nerve impingement), at the subcortical level (e.g., cerebellar contusion), or at the cortical level (e.g., subdural hematoma along the motor cortex), impairment in higher level abilities can be affected. Reduced motor input resulting from tactile sensory discrimination problems interferes with judgment of distance in low-light settings, for example. Centrally mediated problems, such as dysmetria, may be compounded by impairments in sensory motor inputs. Training patients to scan and sweep their tactile environment may be less successful when sensory motor input of the fingers or hands is impaired. Reduced tactile discrimination and motor dexterity may prove disruptive to those patients who may work on an assembly line, as an electrician, as a musician that utilizes fine motor movement (e.g., violinists), and other professions that require fine motor dexterity. Organization of the motor act is measured by Item 21 of the LNNB that requires the patient to clench–extend the fingers alternatively between both hands. Cognitive functions that are brought to bear on this item include fine motor speed, alteration and switching of

TABLE 26.4

Tests of Sensory–Motor Functioning

Test	Comment
Motor Scale—LNNB	Multifactorial scale that examines simple motor output abilities to motor programs that require tertiary zone abilities; used clinically and in research contexts as a stand-alone measure.
Tactile Functions Scale—LNNB	Assesses a wide range of tactile input abilities, including tactile-spatial analysis, two-point discrimination.
Reitan-Klove Sensory Perceptual Examination	Given as a part of the HRNB to assess sensory-motor integrity; includes tests of tactile, auditory, and visual modalities.
Finger Oscillation Test	Part of the HRNB; motor speed and lateralization hypotheses can be assessed.
Hand Dynamometer—Grip Strength	Motor output strength and lateralization of deficits can be assessed.
Grooved Pegboard, Purdue Pegboard Test	Motor dexterity and speed is assessed; lateralization can be assessed.
Benton Finger Localization	Localization of fingers—conditions include hands visible and hands hidden from view.
Benton Motor Impersistence	Maintenance of movement and posture is assessed.
Benton Tactile Form Perception	Assesses spatial analysis and tactile recognition; assesses stereognosis.
Tactual Performance Test	Part of the HRNB; though multifaceted in nature, the TPT requires significant tactile-spatial analysis. This test is particularly helpful when testing those with vision impairments where visuoconstruction memory tests cannot be administered. Tactile-spatial problem-solving functions are also assessed by this test.

motor acts (thus requiring organization and rapid sequencing), and the ability to translate visual representation and verbally mediated instructions into accurate motor actions. Impairment on this item has implications for learning by visual demonstration, difficulty keeping and maintaining a sequence, and difficulty in maintaining motor coordination. All of these may be required to keep up with the instructions of the physical therapist to learn the proper way to range the arm, or may implicate problems in coordinating syncopated movements in gait training (i.e., proper equal weight bearing on both feet, swinging the arms alternatively to maintain balance during gait). Changes in tactile–spatial discrimination (Items 70 and 71 of the LNNB measure two-point discrimination distance; aspects of the Reitan-Klove Sensory Perceptual Examination, such as Finger-Tip Number Writing) can impair the patient's ability to use fine motor dexterity for such tasks as accurately executing keyboarding on the computer; or, for a person with low vision, the ability to discriminate Braille symbols; or the mechanic who needs tactile senses to reach and manipulate parts on an engine carburetor that is not visible. Deficits of motor integrity can affect writing output ability, the ability to manipulate and utilize tools, and could affect a person's ability for recreational and leisure pursuits, such as doing needlepoint or playing golf.

One patient with TBI that I evaluated was a liver transplant physician who evidenced problems on the Tactile Functions Scale of the LNNB, with emphasis upon problems in his left (nondominant) hand. The patient described the need to use his left hand to reach underneath the liver while using his right hand to manipulate surgical instruments. The tactile senses of the left hand were required to identify structures of the liver and provide kinesthetic input regarding the position of the liver during transplantation procedures, and thus required judgments that had to be made on a moment-to-moment basis during surgery. With impairments of these functions, the patient could no longer take the lead in doing transplant surgery. This illustrates one example of the critical nature of sensory–motor integrity to higher order abilities in a functional task.

26.3.4 Language Functioning and Pragmatics of Communication

> By this time, I could remember a great many letters by associating them with different words, but when I tried to visualize a particular letter—"k," for example—or hunt up a word for it, I needed quite a bit of time in order to recognize it and point it out to my teacher.[55, p.68]

> —L. Zasetsky

The intricate relationship between higher mental processes and spoken language, according to Vocate,[57] was central to Luria's view of cognition: "He [Luria] argues that 'mind' is impossible without its synergetic relationship with spoken language and that both arise from the physical reality of the human brain and human society."[p.129]

She goes on to summarize Luria's thought by stating that "spoken language is the means by which the individual becomes capable of conscious and voluntary processes"[p.143] and that language "is a component in the complex functional systems of other higher mental processes."[p.146] Indeed, language acquisition is a lynchpin to the acquisition of knowledge and engagement in the sociocultural environment. When there is dysfunction of language ability after TBI, there usually exists significant disruption in the patient's ability to interact with the social environment (e.g., family members, coworkers, friends). Language dysfunction also has implications for other cognitive processes that rely on receptive language functions, such as recent verbal memory ability. In the western world, where there is heavy reliance on language abilities, deficits in language and communication skills can be disabling. Another aspect of language includes the pragmatics of communication. These may include such variables as excessive verbal output, paucity of verbal output, tangential prose, and circuitous narrative verbalizations. Verbal interruptions and decreased ability for conversation turn exchange can also be a part of pragmatic communication. Although the latter pragmatics issue may be best assessed by observation, language-based neuropsychological tests can be useful in providing tasks that elicit problems with communication pragmatics. Table 26.5 describes common neuropsychological tests that evaluate language functioning in the patient with TBI. The larger language batteries (e.g., Multilingual Aphasia Examination, Boston Diagnostic Aphasia Examination, Western Aphasia Battery) are each able to classify aphasia syndromes: global, mixed transcortical, Broca's, transcortical motor, Wernicke's, transcortical sensory, conduction, and anomic aphasias. Key variables that are assessed to ascertain these subtypes include tasks of spontaneous speech, fluency, naming, comprehension (auditory and nonverbal), repetition, reading, and writing. It should be noted that speech therapists are expert in language assessment. There is considerable overlap between measures used by speech therapists and by neuropsychologists.

26.3.4.1 Ecological Implications

Language impairment after TBI can come in many forms, including different forms of aphasia, impairments of oral word fluency, and disorders of pragmatic communication skills. Expressive language disturbances influence everyday activities, such as use of the telephone. If a patient cannot properly communicate safety conditions over the telephone, that patient's safety at home, without continuous supervision, is threatened. Paraphasias can disrupt interpersonal communications and can be experienced as markedly frustrating to the patient. A dynamic can quickly develop with well-meaning family members and

TABLE 26.5

Tests of Language Ability and Dysfunction

Test	Comment
Woodcock Johnson Psycho-Educational Battery, 3rd ed.	A battery of tests of academic achievement that contains subtests that examine written and oral language usage and reading comprehension abilities.
Multilingual Aphasia Examination, 3rd ed.	Focuses on oral expression, spelling, oral verbal comprehension, reading, and the assessment of articulation.
Boston Diagnostic Aphasia Examination, 3rd ed.	Comprehensive set of measures that correspond to a full range of aphasia types.
Token Test	Commonly used to evaluate the ability to follow commands of increasing complexity.
Boston Naming Test	Confrontation naming task that allows for semantic and phonemic cueing; can be used separately from the Boston Diagnostic Aphasia Examination.
Controlled Oral Word Association Test	Measures word fluency; executive processing may influence performance on this test.
Neurosensory Center Comprehensive Examination for Aphasia	Consisting of 24 subtests, it also includes tests that evaluate visual and tactile function. These latter tests are given when a task that requires visual or tactile functions are impaired, thus allowing for discrimination of primary language from competing reasons for the presence of impairment.
Reitan-Indiana Aphasia Screening Examination	Part of the HRNB; tasks are easily passed by normal adults; identifies pathognomonic signs of aphasia; tends to be a gross screening measure of language requiring further detailed examination.
Western Aphasia Battery–Revised	Evaluates reading, writing, calculation ability, and nonverbal skills; yields an aphasia quotient, cortical quotient, auditory comprehension quotient, oral expression quotient, reading quotient, and writing quotient.

friends, who will assist the patient by filling in the correct word or speaking for the person with TBI. Global aphasics experience marked limitations in independent living ability as a result of the limits imposed by both receptive and expressive language abilities. Speech pathologists are adept at identifying, evaluating, and treating an array of aphasic disorders. In the context of rehabilitation, knowing the nature of communication problems that arose from the TBI can assist other therapists in their work with the patient. For example, those with receptive language impairments experience problems with following instructions presented by the therapist. They may require alternate modalities (visual presentation) or multiple modality (presenting information by use of both visual and procedural–kinesthetic input) instruction to accomplish a task. For example, a patient with both expressive and receptive language dysfunction may need to have the therapist demonstrate how to put on an ankle–foot orthosis, but may also need the therapist to direct his or her hands and legs physically to learn the procedure, and minimize the sole use of verbal instruction.

26.3.5 Working Memory and Complex Attention Processing

> I try a little harder to remember and make sense of the person's remarks. And when I talk to my mother or sisters, I have to strain my nerves and memory even more to understand what they're saying to me so that I know what I'm to do or say.[55, p.93]
>
> —L. Zasetsky

Working memory refers to that ability to register and manipulate information. Baddeley[58] referred to this concept as the central executive system. It requires the patient to hold initially encoded information while being able to manipulate that information and store the newly manipulated information for immediate future use. Working memory is invoked when executing mentally, for example, a four-digit subtraction task. Often, visual representation, auditory attention, retrieval of long-term information, and executive abilities can be used in working memory tasks. After information has been initially processed, information can then be encoded into recent memory storage.

Encoding of information requires the person to process that information at a rate commensurate with signal reception. For example, when a person is listening to a lecture in a classroom, the instructor may deliver information in multiple modalities (visual computer-generated slides, talking to those slides, talking somewhat quickly and sometimes tangentially). The delivery of that information may affect the listener who is trying to attend to these multiple modalities, filter out information that is irrelevant to the task at hand, and process these multiple modalities at a rate of multitasking that allows for an adequate level of encoding and storage of that information. Being able to process such information requires all four aspects of cognitive processing as proposed by Luria[10] and further explicated by J. P. Das, known as *PASS Theory*.[59] This theory conceptualizes brain–behavior functioning in terms of four dynamic processes that are brought to bear by a cognitive challenge: planning, arousal–attention, simultaneous, and successive (PASS) processing components. Thus, complex attention processing involves multiple components of cognition that work in concert. The PASS model can be assessed through neo-Lurian–based instruments such as the Cognitive Assessment Scales, Kaufman Short Neuropsychological Assessment Procedure, the Kaufman Adolescent and Adult Intelligence Test, and the LNNB. The model lends itself to much application in neurorehablitation[60] and can describe tasks that occur in everyday functioning.

Another aspect of complex attention processing includes the tradeoff between processing speed and accuracy of processing. Accuracy can include the error rate that occurs during a cognitive task with a specific time limit or task completion constraint. Battistone et al.[61] argue that some individuals with TBI may, in fact, have difficulties in allocating their cognitive resources to a challenging task. Some show problems with processing capacity, others demonstrate volitional actions toward slowed processing. Both processes of processing capacity and invoked cautiousness may play a role in problems with effective encoding of information.

Conceptually, there is a close relationship between working memory and recent memory abilities. Individuals with TBI have difficulty in working memory that some believe is a result of dysfunction of the central executive system, and is related to higher order executive functioning deficits.[62] Some argue that patients with TBI do not, primarily, exhibit problems in working memory but in recent memory processes of encoding, consolidation, retention, and retrieval.[63] Complex attention processing includes the ability to sustain and focus attention on a task. Alternating and divided attention also come under this category of cognition. The research literature clearly shows that attention deficits are common among those with TBI (e.g., Van Zomeren et al.[64]). Impairments in attention appear to occur across the spectrum of TBI, including MTBI, with the latter showing impairments on tests of attention that requires information processing speed.[65] Table 26.6 presents some common measures of working memory and complex attention.

26.3.5.1 Ecological Implications

Working memory and processing speed impairments can be significantly disabling as a result of the need for this aspect of cognition in most human activities. Although those

TABLE 26.6

Working Memory and Complex Attention Processing Measures

Test	Comment
Working Memory Index–WAIS-IV	Comprised of the arithmetic, digit span, and letter–number sequencing subtests.
Processing Speed Index–WAIS-IV	Comprised of the digit symbol-coding and symbol search subtests; requires motor writing output.
Speech–Sounds Perception	From the HRNB; measures sustained auditory attention; ability to perceive verbal information accurately; is sensitive to the presence of brain damage.
Seashore Rhythm Test	From the HRNB; measures focused auditory attention and presence of brain damage.
Rhythm Scale	From the LNNB; assesses sustained and focused attention; examines pitch perception.
Paced Auditory Serial Addition Test	Sustained attention test; significant demands on working memory; information processing speed is also assessed without the need for motor writing output; used frequently in TBI; there are several versions of this test that include different internumber timed intervals.
Ruff 2 and 7 Selective Attention Test	Measures both accuracy and speed of selective attention; normative sample includes those with TBI.
d2 Test of Attention	Speed and accuracy of selective attention is measured; can be used with children and adults.
Brief Test of Attention	Assessment of auditory divided attention; broad normative base.
Visual Search and Attention Test	Visual letter and symbol cancelation task; examines ability to sustain visual attention.
Continuous Performance Test	Examines lapses in attention, vigilance, and impulsive responses.
Auditory Consonant Trigrams Test	Evaluates alternating and divided attention in the auditory modality; executive functioning also influences performance; has been referred to in the literature as the *Brown-Peterson Test*.
Digit Vigilance Test	Produced for visual tracking and target selection of visual stimuli.
Stroop Color–Word Test	Attention, cognitive flexibility, and response inhibition are assessed; commonly used are the Golden and Trenerry versions. A similar version of this test appears in the Delis-Kaplan Executive Function System and is called the *Color–Word Interference Test*. The latter adds a switching component to the task, likely invoking executive abilities.
Test of Everyday Attention	Evaluates divided, alternating, selective, and sustained attention; approach uses everyday materials that may better approximate real-world situations.
Symbol Digit Modalities Test	Visual tracking, motor speed; comparisons between written and oral performances can be provided.
Trail Making Tests, Parts A and B	Part of the HRNB; cognitive flexibility and speed of information processing are assessed; other similar versions include the Comprehensive Trail Making Test and, from the Delis-Kaplan Executive Function System, the Trail Making Test.
Color Trails Test	Similar concepts as Trail Making Test but uses colors instead of letters; can be given without verbal instruction; alternative research forms are available.

without brain injury may function at a preconscious level, for those with brain injury, working memory impairments can be experienced as confusion, derailment, and poor task maintenance. Working memory impairments are evidenced early after TBI, and may significantly contribute to PTA. During acute rehabilitation, clinicians may be required to cue the patient to the task at hand, and may need to direct the patient through the component steps of a task. In the patient with severe TBI, an occupational therapist may need to break down the morning ritual of brushing the teeth and washing the face into much smaller parts. This type of incapacity can be puzzling to family members, who may assume that the patient may have forgotten how to brush the teeth (i.e., long-term memory loss) when, in fact, that patient has difficulty registering information related to the context of teeth brushing and may have difficulty not only with simultaneously processing positioning the tooth brush appropriately while alternating the brushing motion but also in making the decision regarding when to discontinue the task. Difficulties with alternating and divided attention can result in the patient being easily distracted from the task at hand. In an office environment, a secretary with divided attention problems may not be able to focus attention on the telephone while, in the background, coworkers are moving about the room. This is akin to the cocktail party phenomena where most without brain injury may be able to focus on one conversation while ignoring others, then turn the attention to another speaker, again without being distracted by extraneous conversations. The patient with TBI may have difficulties shifting the focus of attention efficiently and will encode incomplete information and may incorporate information from extraneous conversations as a result of difficulties sifting out appropriate auditory stimuli. Referring to the PASS model, these situations may overtax the simultaneous and successive cognitive functions of the person with TBI, with the net result being that of poor encoding of relevant information and, later, poor retrieval of information. In everyday conversations, the rate of verbal delivery of information from a speaker may outdistance the rate of processing available to the person with TBI. Teaching family members and significant others ways of slowing their pace of conversation, and allowing for breaks and repetition when needed, can benefit the listener who may have trouble with simultaneous and successive processing of verbal information. Often, patients will describe being easily overstimulated and overwhelmed when there are too many noise or visual distractions in the immediate environment. Although many will describe this as "multitasking," the same PASS model demands are in play, and as a result of TBI, that individual may not be able to process information because of deficits in each of the four PASS components, leading that person to feel anxious or frustrated in these multitasking situations. Reading tasks can be affected by impairments in visual sustained attention. Tracking words across the page with the aid of a ruler or use of a finger to cue eye movement can help compensate for a patient's difficulties with sustaining attention on the written text. Having patients articulate the words aloud while they read may also assist with self-cueing and focusing attention on a reading task.

26.3.6 Speed of Information Processing

As noted earlier, several neuropsychological tests judge the accuracy and speed of information processing. Individuals without brain injury are usually capable of completing tasks both accurately and within a reasonable period of time. After TBI, one or both aspects of information processing may be impaired. With the publication of the WAIS-III, and the advent of the WAIS-IV comes four indices that are derived by factor analysis of the subtests of the test. The Verbal Comprehension, Perceptual Organization, and Working Memory Indexes require accurate responses, and the patient is penalized less for time of completion. An exception to this is the Block Design test in which the correct response is recorded but more points are awarded with a more rapid correct response. The Processing Speed Index provides a measure of information processing efficiency. Speed of information processing for response inhibition, as measured by the Stroop Color–Word Test, and motor output speed on the Purdue Pegboard has been shown to be associated with general functional outcomes (operationalized by the Glasgow Outcome Scale) in patients with moderate to severe TBI.[66] The analysis of speed versus accuracy is also obtainable on tests such as the Ruff 2 and 7 Selective Attention test, in which selective attention accuracy (errors of omission and commission) and amount of information processed (accurate target detection speed) are measured. The relative mix of accuracy and speed can be calculated from a subset of items from Form I of the LNNB termed the *Power and Speed Indexes*. As with most neuropsychological tests, there are few that purely measure a particular construct. For example, the Stroop Color–Word Test measures information processing speed and response inhibition, as well as shift set maintenance. There is considerable overlap between attention abilities and information processing speed. Table 26.6 also includes measures of information processing speed.

26.3.6.1 Ecological Implications

During the acute inpatient stay, the patient is often engaged in many rehabilitative therapies, each with different tasks and learning goals. The rate of learning these routines and benefiting from treatment may depend on the patient's capacity for information processing speed. It may be important, therefore, to pace the patient through a mobility or ambulation exercise in a way that does not exceed the patient's ability to keep up with instructions. Repetition of instruction and slowing the rate of verbal output on the therapist's part can improve the patient's understanding of the task. During the postacute phase, therapists may elect to improve either accuracy or speed, depending upon the task to be mastered. Those patients in whom behavioral impulsivity and disinhibition may be problematic may benefit from an approach that focuses on pacing the speed of response and inserting verbal self-cueing methods between the instruction and execution of the task. In making job modifications, the patient with brain injury may require that tasks be done on a project-driven basis rather than a time-to-work product basis. It may not be possible for the patient to work full-time and produce the amount of work prior to TBI, but working part-time, on a limited set of projects, may better accommodate speed of information processing deficits. Resolving these processing speed problems may require a clear assessment of the patient's current capacities, and slowing building their efficiency by working on accuracy (reduced rate of errors), then increasing speed while not increasing error rate.

26.3.7 Recent Memory Functioning

> I used to spend all my time lying on my right side or sitting up for a little while trying to recall some of my past. I couldn't remember anything at will, whereas, when I wasn't thinking about anything in particular, some words would occur to me along with the tunes of different songs. I'd hum to myself.[55, p.89]
>
> —L. Zasetsky

Recent memory is a multifaceted concept covering verbal, visual, and tactile spatial domains, as well as episodic (event-related memory) and procedural (recall and reproduction of actions) aspects. Although the scope of this chapter does not allow for a thorough review of memory functioning in TBI, some highlights are in order to describe ecological implications better. For a comprehensive discussion of the neuropsychology of memory, see Squire and Schacter,[67] and Tulving and Craik.[68]

A number of studies have examined memory dysfunction in TBI. A common measure of recent memory is the California Verbal Learning Test, 2nd Edition (CVLT-II), where Wiegner and Donders[69] found attention span, learning efficiency, delayed recall, and inaccurate recall to be components of memory disorder among patients with TBI. Patients with TBI have been found to have a rapid rate of forgetting new information and difficulties with the consolidation of new material.[70] Material-specific memory, or that ability to recall information based on the properties of the stimulus material (verbal, visuospatial), has been found to underlie episodic memory in TBI.[71] Capitalizing upon enhancing stimulus materials may, therefore, assist the learning process in this population.

Recent memory ability and new learning skills are intimately linked, seen both in the neuropsychological evaluation of these skills, but also observed in everyday situations. This is consistent with the literature that states that memory deficits in those with TBI can also be attributable to general cognitive deficits, particularly in those with moderate to severe TBI.[72] Frontal system deficits and the self-regulatory and self-monitoring aspects of the frontal–subcortical system may play a significant role in the registration, encoding, storage, and retrieval of information. Those with self-awareness deficits may not pay attention to information that could be judged to be important to recall at a later time. Those with disinhibition syndromes may not have the sustained attention necessary to register important information, and therefore, storage of such relevant information may be incomplete. Thus, memory functions are highly regionalized from a brain–behavior perspective, and evaluating key components to the process of storage and retrieval is a critical aspect of neuropsychological evaluations in those with TBI. Unlike focal strokes, those with TBI may demonstrate an array of regional brain dysfunction that can affect functional memory ability in a variety of ways. Thus, examination of attention processes, working memory mechanisms, information processing speed efficiency, and executive abilities is crucial to understanding the nature of memory deficits in those with TBI.

Another aspect of memory that is not easily ascertained is prospective memory capacity. Henry et al.[73] refer to this form of memory as "memory for future intentions."[p.457] This form of memory also requires executive abilities including planning, anticipation, and self-monitoring functions. Although many tasks examine recent declarative or episodic memory functions, few are geared to determine prospective intent. Two available tests that measure this aspect of memory include the Cambridge Prospective Memory Test, and the Rivermead Behavioural Memory Test, Third Edition, and these are noted in Table 26.7.

In clinical practice, recent memory tests assess immediate recall of information for which efficient encoding of information is required. Immediate recall paradigms include both verbal (e.g., word-list learning tasks on the CVLT-II) and visual (e.g., Immediate Recall of the Rey Complex Figure Test) components. Delayed recall of initially presented material across 20- to 30-minute time intervals is common among memory tests. The examiner will usually administer other neuropsychological tests/tasks during the time between immediate and delayed recall portions of the test, thus introducing an element of alternating, focused, and divided attention. This can be helpful in evaluating the person with TBI in that delayed recall may be affected by distracting tasks or stimuli, thus interfering with retrieval of previously learned information.

Recognition trials in which the patient must choose among several verbal or visual stimuli to identify what was initially presented assess recall accuracy, and false-positive and

TABLE 26.7

Recent Memory Functioning Tests

Test	Comment
Wechsler Memory Scale (WMS)-IV, Wechsler Memory Scale-IV	Normed with WAIS-III/WAIS-IV; WMS-IV includes expanded normative base for older adults; includes indices for auditory memory, visual memory, visual working memory, immediate memory, delayed memory.
California Verbal Learning Test	Word-list learning test of verbal memory; many indices can be calculated, including the effect of interference, category cues, and recognition on memory performance; norming includes TBI; adult and children's versions are available; short forms and alternate forms also available.
Rey Auditory Verbal Learning Test	Word-list learning test; several different norm tables are available; different word lists are also available.
Buschke Selective Reminding Test	Word-list learning test; widely used in research with TBI; executive functioning ability influences test performance.
Memory Assessment Scales	Measures recent verbal and visual memory across 12 subtests.
Tactual Performance Test	Part of the HRNB; measures incidental tactual memory; requires problem solving, tactile spatial analysis, and speed of information processing.
Cambridge Prospective Memory Test	Evaluates ability to remember future intentions.
Rivermead Behavioural Memory Test–3	Evaluates everyday memory ability; includes elements of prospective memory; expanded normative groups; includes the Novel Task Test, which evaluates a person's ability for new skill learning.
Rey Complex Figure and Recognition Trial	Measures visuospatial memory; provides a recognition trial; can measure visuoconstruction ability and planning ability; qualitative scoring systems are available for other versions of this test.
Extended Complex Figure Test	Similar to the Rey Complex Figure test paradigm; adds recognition and matching tasks to differential visuospatial memory recall and recognition from visuoconstruction difficulties. Includes matching and recognition scores for left and right fields of the complex Figure; includes a short form.
Brief Visuospatial Memory Test	Visuospatial memory is assessed; six alternate forms are available.
Test of Memory and Learning, 2nd ed.	Core indices are verbal memory, nonverbal memory, and composite memory. Note: These three same indices by the test authors appear as a part of the Reynolds Intellectual Assessment Scale. Also contains supplementary indices: verbal delayed recall, learning, attention and concentration, sequential memory, free recall, and associate recall.
Memory Scale–LNNB	Brief scale containing an array of items for immediate visual and verbal recall; word-list learning includes predictive judgments made by the patient in calculating the error score. An item from the LNNB Memory Scale appears as a part of the Screening Test for the LNNB.

false-negative rates. Recall trials often require rote retrieval of information and are generally more difficult for the patient. Recognition trials allow for an assessment of storage capacity (i.e., if the patient accurately recognizes information, it is assumed to be stored). Verbal and visual stimuli may be placed within a context such as a paragraph story that has a beginning, middle, and end; visual stimuli may be recognizable objects or pictures. Other recent memory tests may require the patient to impose an organizing principle (e.g., word-list learning tests such as the Bushcke Selective Reminding Test or the Rey Auditory Verbal Learning Test) to recall stimuli. Still others may cue the patient to categorize earlier presented information (e.g., on the California Verbal Learning Test, the examiner asks the patient for all of the tools and vegetables that are on the list). Table 26.7 presents some common memory tests that are utilized in the context of brain injury rehabilitation.

26.3.7.1 Ecological Implications

Among the various types of cognitive problems presented by the patient with TBI, memory disorders may be more easily treated with the use of compensatory strategies (cf., executive functioning problems). Upon identifying the type of memory problem the patient presents, other functional systems may be used to compensate. A traditional example is the patient with recent verbal memory deficits in delayed recall for which a memory book and training on the routine use of the memory book can capture information that may be lost as a result of recall deficits. Using an organization strategy, assuming relatively intact new learning and executive ability, allows for the patient to utilize the memory aid successfully. A patient with the same verbal memory deficit may be aided by training to visualize information to be recalled, and to learn new information in multiple modalities including visual and tactile, and by verbal repetition.

Rehearsal of important information, paired with cueing techniques (e.g., a watch alarm, using visual reminders such as a green dot placed in strategic places in the house or work setting), may also aid recall accuracy. Consistency of recall of information may require compensatory or environmental manipulations that assist with complex attention problems that may play into recall deficits. Reducing extraneous noise in the environment may allow the patient to encode and store needed information better. Improving lighting conditions during reading activities may also improve encoding of written material, thus improving storage efficiency. One of the difficulties in training the patient in compensatory memory techniques is the problem of "remembering to remember," otherwise known as *metacognition*. Supervisory attention and executive abilities must be intact, to a certain degree, in order for the patient with TBI to utilize memory aides successfully. With the proliferation of personal computers and personal digital assistants, assistive technology may show promise in developing compensatory aides for this population. Unfortunately, those with TBI will often have executive functioning problems. This poses an additional challenge in the brain injury rehabilitation setting in which multiple and integrated compensatory techniques may need to be trained and integrated into the patient's daily routine.

26.3.8 Visuospatial Analysis and Visuoconstruction Ability

Ever since I was wounded, I've had trouble sometimes sitting down in a chair or on a couch. I first look to see where the chair is, but when I try to sit down, I suddenly make a grab for the chair since I'm afraid I'll land on the floor. Sometimes that happens because the chair turns out to be further to one side than I thought.[55, p.47]

—L. Zasetsky

Not only would he "lose" the right side of his body (an injury to the parietal area of the left hemisphere inevitably produces this symptom), sometimes he thought parts of his body had changed—that his head had become inordinately large, his torso extremely small, and his legs displaced. It seemed to him that, in addition to the disintegration of objects he perceived, parts of his body had undergone some form of fragmentation.[55, p.42]

—A. R. Luria

Impairments of visuospatial and visuoconstructive abilities can occur after TBI and may take on many different forms. The patient may evidence problems with visuospatial analysis of graphical percepts. On Block Design of the WAIS-IV, for example, the patient may not be able to construct visual designs using different patterned and colored blocks, and may lose the whole or gestalt of the design. More esoteric problems in TBI may present, for example in Gerstmann's Syndrome,[74] where the combination of agraphia (difficulties in motor writing with spelling and word order altered), acalculia (deficits in execution of arithmetic calculations), finger agnosia (inability to name or move a designated finger after it has been labeled), and right–left confusion (discrimination of instructions that require orientation of the right vs. left side of the body) occurs. Any or all of these components can be evidenced in TBI, likely resulting from the cortical proximity of brain regions that mediate these activities (emphasis on the left parietal region). Impairments of perceptual–motor integration refer to the general inability of the patient to visualize information properly, translate the visual percept into an accurate cognitive representation, and then execute an accurate motor response, such as copying a design that corresponds to the original percept. In constructional dyspraxia, the patient's written reproductions of designs may be distorted and rotated, with evidence of loss of the spatial configuration of the original visual stimuli. Assembly of materials may be impaired as a result of visuoconstruction impairments. Table 26.8 shows some common tests of visuospatial and visuoconstruction skills.

26.3.8.1 Ecological Implications

Mechanical abilities rely heavily on intact visuoconstruction skills. During the early phases of rehabilitation, activities of daily functioning can be affected by impairments of these skills. Dressing activities that require sequencing of steps and accurate right–left

TABLE 26.8

Visuospatial Analysis and Visuoconstruction Ability Tests

Test	Comment
Perceptual Reasoning Scale–WAIS-IV	Composed of core subtests of block design, matrix reasoning, and visual puzzles; supplemental subtests are picture completion and figure weights.
Rey–Osterrieth Complex Figure Test	Design reproductions can indicate impairments of perceptual–motor integration.
Benton Judgment of Line Orientation	Measures visuospatial judgment.
Benton Visual Form Discrimination	Measures visual accuracy and discrimination ability.
Benton Facial Recognition	Ability to match unfamiliar faces is tested; can assess prosopagnosia.
Benton Right–Left Orientation	Measures the ability of the patient to identify body parts accurately on the appropriate side of the body.
Hooper Visual Organization	Allows for the measurement of visuospatial integration without a motor response.
Line Bisection Test	Measures problems with visual neglect, precision of spatial alignment.
Visual Object and Space Perception Battery	Eight subtests measure spatial perception, spatial estimation, and spatial localization.
Visual Functions Scale–LNNB	Items measure visuospatial, visuoconstruction, and visual judgment abilities; executive functioning abilities are required for some of these items.

orientation skills may be impaired. Therapists will often face the patient when demonstrating a technique or skill, and this requires the patient to translate what is seen to actions, requiring accurate right–left orientation. Rather than facing the patient, it may be beneficial to work side-by-side to reduce the need for the patient to translate the visual orientation of the task. Later, during the postacute phase, community mobility, driving ability, and detailed activities, such as filling out a job application or organizing the kitchen, may be affected by visuoconstruction impairments. Pathfinding skills may need to be aided by verbal instruction, enhanced visual cues, and rehearsal of the task to encourage procedural learning. The person with TBI may have trouble navigating, judging distances, and negotiating the living environment, or have trouble with mobility in the community as a result of visuospatial deficits. Reading ability may also be affected where dyslexia (impairments in reading) may have a component of dysgraphia; in combination, they reduce reading efficiency. Large-print materials and cueing techniques may be helpful in these situations. Alternate learning systems, such as books on tape, may be needed as well.

26.3.9 Executive Functioning Capacity

> I can't understand how wood is manufactured, what it is made of. Everything—no matter what I touch—has become mysterious and unknown. I can't put anything together myself, figure anything out, or make anything new. I've become a completely different person, precisely the reverse of what I was before this terrible injury.[55, pp.98–99]
>
> —L. Zasetsky

The term *executive* in executive functioning ability is a term apropos to the construct being measured. It refers to the capacity to encode and utilize information from a variety of sources, process that information quickly and efficiently, and then engage in decision making based on those inputs—much like what a business executive engages in on a daily basis. Executive processes are most often associated with frontal lobe functioning, and a plethora of research has been conducted to examine the executive abilities associated with this brain region (see Miller and Cummings[75] for a comprehensive examination of the human frontal lobes). Luria[10] described executive abilities as residing within the tertiary zone of the brain, and is the unit responsible for the "programming, regulating, and verifying mental activity."[p. 43] What Luria and Tsvetkova[76] also understood was the interconnections of the tertiary zones with other zones in the brain, and delineate a neuropsychology of problem solving not only involving the frontal lobes, but also implicating parietal–occipital and basal–frontal functional systems.

A significant amount of research has been devoted to understanding the nature of executive functioning impairments in TBI and the extent to which such deficits are remediable. Executive functioning deficits, measured by the Wisconsin Card Sorting Test and the Tower of Hanoi/London Test, are related to acute neurophysiologic damage in TBI survivors.[77] A study by Greve et al.[78] demonstrated that patients with TBI can be clustered into four different executive functioning groups: (1) intact performance, (2) impaired response maintenance, (3) problem-solving impairment, and (4) impairments in ability to shift cognitive set. Executive functioning ability may also overlap with neurobehavioral impairments such as emotional dyscontrol and reduced motivation.[79] Changes in executive functioning can be related to recovery in TBI.[80] Busch et al.[81] conducted a factor analytic study of 104 participants with TBI at 1 year postinjury. They identified three factors within the neuropsychological data, the first of which reflected *higher order executive functions* including two subcomponents of self-generative behavior and cognitive flexibility/set shifting. A second factor was represented by *mental control* and *working memory*, whereas a third factor was composed of *memory error measures.* They note that their factor model was characteristic of the 1986 Stuss and Benson model of executive functioning.

According to a well-known model of frontal systems by Stuss and Benson,[82,83] self-awareness is the highest human cognitive capacity that is served by a number of other executive abilities. Figure 26.1 depicts the Stuss–Benson model.

The model is consistent with Lurian theory, with the tertiary zone comprising the first three tiers of the model, and the fourth tier related to Luria's secondary zone. These aspects of executive functioning are well represented in many of the tests used by neuropsychologists (Table 26.9).

26.3.9.1 Ecological Implications

A problem noted by Cripe[84] in connection with testing for executive abilities is the ability to generalize test findings to real-world settings. In the clinical setting, testing occurs in a controlled environment with a minimization of distractions, usually administered by an examiner who can cue and encourage the patient's behavior. This is in contrast to real-world settings that are less structured and require the patient to impose structure and organization to function, require planning and self-initiation on the part of the patient, and in which the environment may be competitive in nature in the absence of a test examiner who can encourage and redirect the behavior of the patient. Neuropsychology laboratory tests may not best represent what the patient can and cannot do in the real-world environment.

Nevertheless, tests of executive functioning can be predictive of outcome. A study by Sherer et al.[85] found that the Trail Making Test (Part B) is particularly effective in predicting productive outcomes in patients with TBI. This is thought to be true because of this test requiring dual-task performance (simultaneous processing) and speed of information processing. Although not specifically cited as tests of executive functioning, tests like the Trail Making Test or Color Trails Test require cognitive flexibility, dual-task performance, alternating attention, working memory, and speed of processing, and all work together in concert. This harkens back to what Luria[10] described as the regulation and verification of higher mental processes. These represent complex and high-level cognitive skills and are

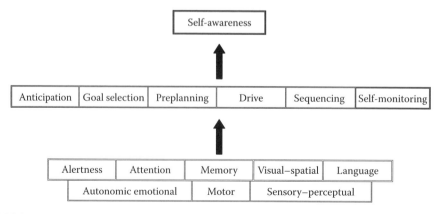

FIGURE 26.1
The Stuss–Benson model of frontal system functioning.

TABLE 26.9

Tests of Executive Functioning

Test	Comment
Delis–Kaplan Executive Function System	Battery of executive functioning tests, many that parallel existing and commonly used executive function tests; advantage of subtests that are standardized to compare scores across executive functioning domains. Consists of the following tests: Trail Making Test, Verbal Fluency Test, Design Fluency Test, Color–Word Interference Test, Sorting Test, 20 Questions Test, Word Context Test, Tower Test, Proverbs Test.
Wisconsin Card Sorting Test	Used widely in clinical and research contexts; shorter 64 trial version available; examines problems with perseveration and ability for novel problem solving.
Category Test, Booklet Category Test, Short Category Test	From the HRNB; short version available; booklet version available but not recommended for use with the standard HRNB battery.
Trail Making Test, Color Trails Test, Comprehensive Trail Making Test	Attention, speed of information processing, and cognitive flexibility are measured.
Stroop Color–Word Test	Response inhibition aspect relates to executive functioning ability.
Cognitive Estimation Test	Examines the ability to make estimated judgments on everyday types of activities and items.
Ruff Figural Fluency Test	Design fluency is assessed; nonverbal equivalent to word fluency test.
Executive Control Battery	Executive dyscontrol; qualitative analysis of performance is assessed.
Intellectual Processes–LNNB	Evaluates higher order cognitive skills, many that require executive abilities.
Frontal Lobe Score–LNNB	Comprised of specific items throughout the LNNB that have been found to be impaired in patients with frontal lobe damage.
Iowa Gambling Task	Evaluates decision-making impairments related to frontal system damage. Emulates a gambling task of card selection and net earnings based on decisions made of card selection. Learning component is also included in the task.
Behavioral Assessment of the Dysexecutive Syndrome	A multiple subtest measure geared toward obtaining ecologically valid data of executive functioning; includes a questionnaire of behavioral symptoms of executive functioning problems that can be filled out by the patient and by a collateral informant.

not easily rehabilitated. A meta-analysis conducted by Kennedy et al.[86] reviewed 15 studies that met inclusion criteria for analysis, and included studies that used metacognition strategy instruction as method of executive function remediation. Their analysis showed promise for this method, as well as for interventions that focus on verbal reasoning skill and multitasking training. Remediation of executive abilities may be difficult because high-level processes are required to benefit from interventions. Providing compensatory strategies for cognitive abilities that serve executive skills, such as assistance for complex attention, recent memory, and visuoconstruction deficits, will likely have an impact on the patient's net executive functioning capacity. Specific strategies for directly managing executive functioning ability often rely upon approaching the patient on many fronts. This includes providing consistent and continuous feedback (e.g., audio and videotaped feedback, immediate feedback on tasks), structuring the patient's problem-solving approaches, and assisting the patient in organizing and simplifying the home or work environment.

There is considerable interplay between executive functioning and a person's ability for coping with everyday stressors and tasks. As studied by Krpan et al.[87] executive functions are related to coping skills for individuals with TBI. Each individual varies to the extent, and in what situations, one may used problem-focused coping (i.e., that involves planning, examination of solutions) or other forms of coping such as emotion-focused coping (handling stressors through regulating emotions). Not surprisingly, the study by Krpan et al.[87] demonstrated that higher executive functioning was associated with use of problem-focused coping, whereas poorer executive functioning related to emotion-focused coping, the latter of which they referred to as *escape avoidant* strategies of coping. For the rehabilitation professional who works with a person with TBI who demonstrates executive dysfunction, interventions that teach problem-solving skills, modeling of planning behaviors, and assist with improving self-monitoring skills will be beneficial. At the same time, it may be important to assist that person to learn and regulate emotions, use self-calming techniques, and other ways to minimize the interference of escape avoidant behaviors. The authors go on to state: "For example, a rehabilitation protocol might involve teaching people to use a conscious process to select adaptive coping strategies, how to effectively use emotion focused coping strategies, and perhaps even how to decode and adaptively respond to emotional or stressful stimuli (i.e., affective regulation)."[87, p.44]

Component analyses of the task at hand (e.g., studying for a college examination) can reveal steps in which executive dysfunction can impair the task at hand (e.g., trouble with organization of study notes). These types of analyses may be used to identify strategies for remediation or compensation, rather than attempting to find a treatment approach for executive abilities in general. Further strategies can be found in Eslinger,[88] Sohlberg and Mateer,[89] and Wilson.[90,91]

26.3.10 Mood Functioning

> It's depressing, having to start all over and make sense out of the world you've lost because of injury and illness, to get these bits and pieces to add up to a coherent whole.[55, p.xxi]

> —L. Zasetsky

Mood impairments and personality functioning are important aspects of functioning in the patient with TBI. Although the assessment of mood states and interpersonal propensities are not considered neuropsychological variables in and of themselves, it is an essential element of the evaluation to understand the whole person. Clearly, mood disorders are common in TBI[92] and may be a function of the neurobiology of neuropsychological disorder.[93] Premorbid cognitive ability appears to be related to experienced distress in individuals after TBI.[94] One of the difficulties faced by clinicians in assessing mood after TBI is the fact that many measures rely on self-report (e.g., MMPI-2, Beck Depression Inventory) and some, like the Symptom Checklist-90-Revised, may not have been standardized on TBI populations,[95] leading to distortion on the profiles produced by these types of measures.[96]

Included within the larger concept of mood are dysphoria, anxiety, irritability, and anger as the primary four aspects of mood. The clinician evaluating mood components will often need to obtain and integrate information from multiple sources to understand best the patient's level and type of mood functioning. Self-report measures and the clinical interview (and careful monitoring of mental status variables during the interview), coupled with informant observations and questionnaires, can be an effective way of ascertaining mood in the person with TBI. Examination of mood fluctuations throughout a given day or week may be helpful to identify any diurnal patterns, situational circumstances, and interpersonal dynamics that may be contributory to mood presentation. Some commonly utilized measures are listed in Table 26.10.

TABLE 26.10

Tests of Mood

Test	Comment
Beck Depression Inventory/Beck Anxiety Inventory	Self-report measures of depression and anxiety (respectively); can sometimes be difficult for a severely cognitively impaired patient to complete.
Geriatric Depression Scale	Self-report measure of depression, normed for older adults; yes/no format.
Center for Epidemiological Studies Depression Scale	Commonly used in research; self-report represents a balance between mood, somatic, and cognitive aspects of depression.
Hamilton Depression Rating Scale	Used frequently in psychiatric research; structured interview results in clinician rating; a self-report version is available.
State–Trait Anxiety Inventory	Self-report measure that examines state anxiety and trait anxiety.
State–Trait Anger Expression Inventory-2	Measures various aspects of anger expression, including state anger and trait anger; an anger expression index is provided as well.
Minnesota Multiphasic Personality Inventory-2 (MMPI-2/MMPI-RF)	Standard personality inventory that has been used extensively in TBI; measures mood states, coping, and interpersonal propensities.
Personality Assessment Inventory	Comprehensive measure of mood, coping, interpersonal propensities, and treatment response indicators.
Millon Behavioral Medicine Diagnostic	Measures interpersonal coping methods in response to medical illness; assesses mood states and treatment responsivity indicators; rooted in Millon Theory.
Neuropsychological Impairment Scale	This questionnaire comes in two report forms: self-report and informant report. Measures aspects of perceived cognitive impairments, but also includes items related to affect that may be playing a role in self-reported cognitive symptoms.
Neuropsychology Behavior and Affect Profile	Evaluates changes in personality and emotion after brain injury.
Neurobehavioral Function Inventory	Patient self-report and informant (family) report forms are available; includes depression, somatic symptoms, memory/attention, communication deficits, aggression, and motor deficit scales.
Neurobehavioral Rating Scale	Measures aspects of mood and behavior that represent consequences of brain injury.

26.3.10.1 Ecological Implications

Mood dysfunction, including depression, anxiety, irritability and anger, can result in excess disability in psychosocial functioning and in cognitive functioning.[97] Treatment of depression can result in improved cognitive functioning, as found by Fann et al.[98] The criteria for major depressive disorder includes concentration deficits, and its alleviation may, in turn, result in some cognitive improvement. In the patient with TBI, other neurobehavioral conditions, such as apathy and reduced affect regulation, may mimic depression, and such symptoms may overlap with depression. In either case, depression can be appropriately assessed when utilizing multiple sources of data including self-report (e.g., Beck Depression Inventory, Geriatric Depression Scale); structured interview formats (e.g., Hamilton Depression Rating Scale); and collateral observations by family, rehabilitation staff, and friends. Coping skills of the patient can moderate some of the effects of mood disorder in patients with TBI; however, the patient's capacity to use psychological coping strategies may be dependent upon the intactness of executive abilities. Reduced self-awareness can act to reduce the frequency with which patients may deem it necessary to change their own behavior and invoke coping strategies (e.g., use of positive self-statements in response to stressful situations). A combination of pharmacotherapy and psychotherapy may therefore prove beneficial to the patient who presents with mood disorder following TBI. Many patients with mood disorder find general mood benefits from physical reactivation through physical therapy and home exercise programs. Reengagement in pleasant activities[99] may also have mood elevating benefit. After TBI, the patient's ability to engage independently in community recreation and leisure pursuits may be limited. Postacute rehabilitation strategies that target recreation and leisure skill improvement will also have the added benefit of improving or maintaining euthymic mood. Other moderating variables that play a role in mood stabilization and cognition include chronic pain, sleep disturbance and fatigue, current medication regimen, and substance use—all of which should be assessed at the time of defining rehabilitation goals.

26.4 Directions for the Future

One of the most frequently cited case studies of TBI is the tragic case of Phineas Gage, the railroad foreman who sustained a devastating penetrating head injury in 1848 when a tamping iron was driven through his left frontal lobe, secondary to a blast. Macmillan[100] documents some of the changes that Gage's physician, John Harlow, observed in his patient shortly after the accident: "Remembers passing and past events correctly, as well before as since the injury. Intellectual manifestations feeble, being exceedingly capricious and childish, but with a will as indomitable as ever; is particularly obstinate; will not yield to restraint when it conflicts with his desires."[100, p.91]

Gage experienced a dramatic change in his life—from being a successful railroad worker to working as a side show for the Barnum and Bailey Circus, displaying the tamping iron and touted as "the only living man with a hole in the top of his head."[100, p.98] Stuss et al.[101] comment on Gage: "Although he miraculously survived and demonstrated good physical recovery and many preserved cognitive abilities, his emotional behavior and personality were so significantly changed that his friends stated that he was a different person: 'No longer Gage.'"[101, p.349]

This story has been repeated numerous times when examining the neuropsychological consequences of TBI. Little has changed regarding common neuropsychological and neurobehavioral outcomes in TBI. Yet we clearly know more about the specific neurobiologic mechanisms of dysfunction and regional brain metabolism that is altered in TBI; refinements in assessment technology have allowed for more precise tracking of effective rehabilitation strategies. From Phineas Gage, we have a clear delineation of the task in front of rehabilitation professionals: to push not only for *care*, but to begin working on *cure*.

The future continues to hold promise for survivors of TBI, especially with regard to research into neuroplasticity. Basic research approaches will likely lead to more transitional research involving the enhancement of recovery[102] and the implementation of neuroprotective measures early post-TBI. Clinical protocols that call for the regular use of neuropharmacologic agents of cognitive enhancers are likely to enhance functional improvement. Further research into the synergistic effect of combined evidence-based cognitive rehabilitation procedures with cognitive enhancers is likely to illumine a biopsychosocial approach to treating TBI.

In a special issue devoted to neuroplasticity in the journal *Brain Injury*, the well-known researcher and neurorehabilitation expert Paul Bach-y-Rita[103] provided a review of the major mechanisms known and thought to be responsible for recovery after brain injury. The influence of nonsynaptic neurotransmission, also known as *volume transmission,* during which neurotransmitters are dispersed through the extracellular fluid to distant receptor sites may be responsible as a mechanism to capitalize upon for functional reorganization of brain functions. Advances in understanding the action of neurotransmitters in vulnerable areas of the brain after TBI (e.g., dorsolateral frontal system) may lead to pharmacologic strategies for neuroprotection and recovery. Understanding the concept of "multiplexing" or the flexibility of function that neural cells and fibers perform may also lead to new techniques of neurorehabilitation. Others have postulated the importance of neuronal stimulation as a means to facilitate neuroplasticity after acquired brain injury.[104]

These new directions in research will certainly expand the role of neuropsychology in the rehabilitation setting, with the neuropsychologist filling roles as an assessor and interventionist. Perhaps the interventionist role may be termed *restorative neuropsychology* as we learn more from the neurosciences regarding the enhancement of recovery in those with TBI.

References

1. Goldstein, K., *Aftereffects of Brain Injuries in War: Their Evaluation and Treatment,* Grune & Stratton, New York, 1942.
2. Bruce, D., On the origin of the term "neuropsychology," *Neuropsychologia,* 23(6), 813–814, 1985.
3. Kolb, B. and Whishaw, I. Q., *Fundamentals of Human Neuropsychology,* 6th ed., W. H. Freeman, New York, 2008.
4. Lucas, J. A. and Addeo, R., Traumatic brain injury and postconcussive syndrome, in P. J. Snyder and P. D. Nussbaum (Eds.), *Clinical Neuropsychology: A Pocket Handbook for Assessment,* 2nd ed., American Psychological Association, Washington, DC, 351–380, 2006.
5. Filley, C. M., *The Behavioral Neurology of White Matter,* Oxford University Press, New York, 2001.
6. Le Bihan, D., Mangin, J.- F., Poupon, C., Clark, C. A., Pappata, S., Molko, N., and Chabriat, H., Diffusion tensor imaging: Concepts and applications, *Journal of Magnetic Resonance Imaging,* 13(4), 534–546, 2001.
7. Arfanakis, K., Haughton, V. M., Carew, J. D., Rogers, B. P., Dempsey, R. J., and Meyerand, M. E., Diffusion tensor MR imaging in diffuse axonal injury, *American Journal of Neuroradiology,* 23(5), 794–802, 2002.
8. Greenberg, G., Mikulis, D. J., Ng, K., DeSouza, D., and Green, R. E., Use of diffusion tensor imaging to examine subacute white matter injury progression in moderate to severe traumatic brain injury, *Archives of Physical Medicine and Rehabilitation,* 89(12 Suppl.), S45–S50, 2008.
9. Ng, K., Mikulis, D. J., Glazer, J., Kabani, N., Till, C., Greenberg, G., Thompson, A., et al., Magnetic resonance imaging evidence of progression of subacute brain atrophy in moderate to severe traumatic brain injury, *Archives of Physical Medicine and Rehabilitation,* 89(12 Suppl.), S35–S44, 2008.
10. Luria, A. R., *The Working Brain: An Introduction to Neuropsychology,* Basic Books, New York, 1973.
11. Filley, C. M., Cranberg, L. D., Alexander, M. P., and Hart, E. J., Neurobehavioral outcome after closed head injury in childhood and adolescence, *Archives of Neurology,* 44(2), 194–198, 1987.
12. Aharon-Peretz, J. and Tomer, R., Traumatic brain injury, in B. L. Miller and J. L. Cummings (Eds.), *The Human Frontal Lobes: Functions and Disorders,* 2nd ed., Guilford Press, New York, 540–551, 2006.

13. Chow, T. W. and Cummings, J. L., Frontal–subcortical circuits, in B. L. Miller and J. L. Cummings (Eds.), *The Human Frontal Lobes: Functions and Disorders*, 2nd ed., Guilford Press, New York, 25–43, 2006.

14. Mayberg, H. S., Limbic–cortical dysregulation: A proposed model of depression, *The Journal of Neuropsychiatry and Clinical Neurosciences*, 9(3), 471–481, 1997.

15. Goldapple, K., Segal, Z., Garson, C., Lau, M., Bieling, P., Kennedy, S., and Mayberg, H., Modulation of cortical–limbic pathways in major depression: Treatment-specific effects of cognitive behavior therapy, *Archives of General Psychiatry*, 61(1), 34–41, 2004.

16. Kennedy, S. H., Konarski, J. Z., Segal, Z. V., Lau, M. A., Bieling, P. J., McIntyre, R. S., and Mayberg, H. S., Differences in brain glucose metabolism between responders to CBT and venlafaxine in a 16-week randomized controlled trial, *The American Journal of Psychiatry*, 164(5), 778–788, 2007.

17. Dikmen, S., Machamer, J., Temkin, N., and McLean, A., Neuropsychological recovery in patients with moderate to severe head injury: 2 Year follow-up, *Journal of Clinical and Experimental Neuropsychology*, 12(4), 507–519, 1990.

18. Dacey, R., Dikmen, S., Temkin, N., McLean, A., Armsden, G., and Winn, H. R., Relative effects of brain and non-brain injuries on neuropsychological and psychosocial outcome, *The Journal of Trauma*, 31(2), 217–222, 1991.

19. Levin, H. S., Gary, Jr., H. E., Eisenberg, H. M., Ruff, R. M., Barth, J. T., Kreutzer, J., High, Jr., W. M., et al., Neurobehavioral outcome 1 year after severe head injury. Experience of the Traumatic Coma Data Bank, *Journal of Neurosurgery*, 73(5), 699–709, 1990.

20. Kersel, D. A., March, N. V., Havill, J. H., and Sleigh, J. W., Neuropsychological functioning during the year following severe traumatic brain injury, *Brain Injury*, 15(4), 283–296, 2001.

21. Novack, T. A., Alderson, A. L., Bush, B. A., Meythaler, J. M., and Canupp, K., Cognitive and functional recovery at 6 and 12 months post-TBI, *Brain Injury*, 14(11), 987–996, 2000.

22. Hessen, E., Nestvold, K., and Anderson, V., Neuropsychological function 23 years after mild traumatic brain injury: A comparison of outcome after paediatric and adult head injuries, *Brain Injury*, 21(9), 963–979, 2007.

23. Draper, K. and Ponsford, J., Cognitive functioning ten years following traumatic brain injury and rehabilitation, *Neuropsychology*, 22(5), 618–625, 2008.

24. Herrmann, N., Curio, N., Jost, S., Grubich, C., Ebert, A., Fork, M., and Synowitz, H., Release of biochemical markers of damage to neuronal and glial brain tissue is associated with short and long term neuropsychological outcome after traumatic brain injury, *Journal of Neurology, Neurosurgery, and Psychiatry*, 70(1), 95–100, 2001.

25. Tofil, S. and Clinchot, D. M., Recovery of automatic and cognitive functions in traumatic brain injury using the functional independence measure, *Brain Injury*, 10(12), 901–910, 1996.

26. Sbordone, R. J., Liter, J. C., and Pettler-Jennings, P., Recovery of function following severe traumatic brain injury: A retrospective 10-year follow-up, *Brain Injury*, 9(3), 285–299, 1995.

27. Millis, S. R., Rosenthal, M., Novack, T. A., Sherer, M., Nick, T. G., Kreutzer, J. S., High, Jr., W. M., and Ricker, J. H., Long-term neuropsychological outcome after traumatic brain injury, *Journal of Head Trauma Rehabilitation*, 16(4), 343–355, 2001.

28. Green, R. E., Colella, B., Hebert, D. A., Bayley, M., Kang, H. S., Till, C., and Monette, G., Prediction of return to productivity after severe traumatic brain injury: Investigations of optimal neuropsychological test and timing of assessment, *Archives of Physical Medicine and Rehabilitation*, 89(12 Suppl.), S51–S60, 2008.

29. Chaytor, N. and Schmitter-Edgecombe, M., The ecological validity of neuropsychological tests: A review of the literature on everyday cognitive skills, *Neuropsychological Review*, 13(4), 181–197, 2003.

30. Boake, C., Millis, S. R., High, Jr., W. M., Delmonico, R. L., Kreutzer, J. S., Rosenthal, M., Sherer, M., and Ivanhoe, C. B., Using early neuropsychological testing to predict long-term productivity outcome from traumatic brain injury, *Archives of Physical Medicine and Rehabilitation*, 82(6), 761–768, 2001.

31. Leahy, B. J. and Lam, C. S., Neuropsychological testing and functional outcome for individuals with traumatic brain injury, *Brain Injury*, 12(12), 1025–1035, 1998.

32. Johnstone, B. and Farmer, J. E., Preparing neuropsychologists for the future: The need for additional training guidelines, *Archives of Clinical Neuropsychology*, 12(6), 523–530, 1997.

33. Uomoto, J. M., Application of the neuropsychological evaluation in vocational planning after brain injury, in R. T. Fraser and D. C. Clemmons (Eds.), *Traumatic Brain Injury Rehabilitation: Practical Vocational, Neuropsychological, and Psychotherapy Interventions*, CRC Press, Boca Raton, FL, 1–69, 2000.

34. Retzlaff, P., Butler, M., and Vanderploeg, R. D., Neuropsychological battery choice and theoretical orientation: A multivariate analysis, *Journal of Clinical Psychology*, 48(5), 666–672, 1992.

35. Halstead, W., *Brain and Intelligence: A Qualitative Study of the Frontal Lobes*, University of Chicago Press, Chicago, IL, 1947.

36. Jarvis, P. E. and Jarvis, J. T., *The Halstead-Reitan Neuropsychological Battery: A Guide to Interpretation and Clinical Applications*, Psychological Assessment Resources, Odessa, FL, 1994.

37. Reitan, R. M. and Wolfson, D., *The Halstead-Reitan Neuropsychological Test Battery: Theory and Clinical Interpretation*, Neuropsychology Press, Tucson, AZ, 1993.

38. Broshek, D. K. and Barth, J. T., The Halstead-Reitan Neuropsychological Test Battery, in G. Groth-Marnat (Ed.), *Neuropsychological Assessment in Clinical Practice: A Guide to Test Interpretation and Integration*, Wiley, New York, 223–262, 2000.

39. Golden, C. J., Purisch, A. D., and Hammeke, T. A., *Luria-Nebraska Neuropsychological Battery: Forms I and II*, Western Psychological Services, Los Angeles, CA, 1995.

40. Golden, C. J., Warren, W. L., and Espe-Pfeiffer, P. (Eds.), *LNNB Handbook: 20th Anniversary, Volume I: A Guide to Clinical Interpretation and Use in Special Settings*, Western Psychological Services, Los Angeles, CA, 1999.

41. Golden, C. J., Warren, W. L., and Espe-Pfeiffer, P. (Eds.), *LNNB Handbook: 20th Anniversary, Volume II: Selected Reprints on the Luria-Nebraska Neuropsychological Battery from the International Journal of Clinical Neuropsychology*, Western Psychological Services, Los Angeles, CA, 1999.

42. Golden, C. J., Freshwater, S. M., and Vayalakkara, J., The Luria Nebraska Neuropsychological Battery, in G. Groth-Marnat (Ed.), *Neuropsychological Assessment in Clinical Practice: A Guide to Test Interpretation and Integration*, Wiley, New York, 263–292, 2000.

43. Luria, A. R., *Higher Cortical Functions in Man*, 2nd ed., Basic Books, New York, 1980.

44. Christensen, A.- L., *Luria's Neuropsychological Investigation: Manual and Test Materials*, Spectrum, New York, 1975.

45. Christensen, A.- L. and Caetano, C., Luria's neuropsychological evaluation in the Nordic countries, *Neuropsychological Review*, 9(2), 71–78, 1999.

46. MacInnes, W. D., Gillen, R. W., Golden, C. J., Graber, B., Cole, J. K., Uhl, H. S., and Greenhouse, A. H., Aging and performance on the Luria-Nebraska Neuropsychological Battery, *The International Journal of Neurosciences*, 19(1–4), 179–189, 1983.

47. White, T. and Stern, R. A., *Neuropsychological Assessment Battery: Psychometric and technical manual*, Psychological Assessment Resources, Lutz, FL, 2003.

48. Lezak, M. D., *Neuropsychological Assessment*, 4th ed., Oxford University Press, New York, 2004.

49. Kaplan, E., A process approach to neuropsychological assessment, in T. Boll and B. K. Bryant (Eds.), *Clinical Neuropsychology and Brain Function: Research, Measurement, and Practice*, American Psychological Association, Washington, DC, 125–167, 1988.

50. Kaplan, E., Fein, D., Morris, R., and Delis, D. C., *WAIS-R as a Neuropsychological Instrument: WAIS-R-NI Manual*, Psychological Corporation, New York, 1991.

51. Stern, R. A., Singer, E. A., Duke, L. M., Singer, N. G., Morey, C. E., Daughtrey, E. W. and Kaplan, E., The Boston qualitative scoring system for the Rey-Osterrieth Complex Figure: Description and interrater reliability, *The Clinical Neuropsychologist*, 8(3), 309–322, 1994.

52. Sbordone, R. J., Ecological validity: Some critical issues for the neuropsychologist, in R. J. Sbordone and C. J. Long (Eds.), *Ecological Validity of Neuropsychological Testing*, CRC Press/St. Lucie Press, Delray Beach, FL, 15–42, 1996.

53. Sbordone, R. J., Limitations of neuropsychological testing to predict the cognitive and behavioral functioning of persons with brain injury in real-world settings, *Neurorehabilitation*, 16(4), 199–201, 2001.

54. McKay, C., Wertheimer, J. C., Fichtenberg, N. L., and Casey, J. E., The Repeatable Battery for the Assessment of Neuropsychological Status (RBANS): Clinical utility in a traumatic brain injury sample, *Clinical Neuropsychologist*, 22(2), 228–241, 2008.

55. Luria, A. R., *The Man with a Shattered World: The History of a Brain Wound*, Harvard University Press, Cambridge, MA, 1972.

56. Kaczmarek, B. L. J., Code, C., and Wallesch, C.-W., The fractionation of mental life: Luria's study of Lieutenant Zasetsky, in C. Code, C.-W. Wallesch, and A. R. Lecours (Eds.), *Classic Cases in Neuropsychology*, Vol. II, Psychology Press, New York, 131–144, 2003.

57. Vocate, D. R., *The Theory of A. R. Luria: Functions of Spoken Language in the Development of Higher Mental Processes*, Lawrence Erlbaum Associates, Hillsdale, NJ, 1987.

58. Baddeley, A., *Working Memory*, Oxford University Press, New York, 1987.

59. Das, J. P., A neo-Lurian approach to assessment and remediation. *Neuropsychological Review*, 9(2), 107–116, 1999.

60. Uomoto, J. M., Older adults and neuropsychological rehabilitation following acquired brain injury, *Neurorehabilitation*, 23(5), 415–424, 2008.

61. Battistone, M., Woltz, D., and Clark, E., Processing speed deficits associated with traumatic brain injury: Processing inefficiency or cautiousness?, *Applied Neuropsychology*, 15(1), 69–78, 2008.

62. McDowell, S., Whyte, J., and D'Esposito, M., Working memory impairments in traumatic brain injury: Evidence from a dual-task paradigm, *Neuropsychologia*, 35(10), 1341–1353, 1997.

63. Curtiss, G., Vanderploeg, R. D., Spencer, J., and Salazar, A. M., Patterns of verbal learning and memory in traumatic brain injury, *Journal of the International Neuropsychological Society*, 7(5), 574–585, 2001.

64. Van Zomeren, A. H., Brouwer, W. H., and Deelman, B. G., Attentional deficits: The riddles of selectivity, speed, and alertness, in N. Brooks (Ed.), *Closed Head Injury: Psychological, Social, and Family Consequences*, Oxford University Press, New York, 74–107, 1984.

65. Cicerone, K. D., Clinical sensitivity of four measures of attention to mild traumatic brain injury, *Clinical Neuropsychologist*, 11(3), 266–272, 1997.

66. Asikainen, I., Nybo, T., Muller, K., Sarna, S., and Kaste, M., Speed performance and long-term functional and vocational outcome in a group of young patients with moderate or severe traumatic brain injury, *European Journal of Neurology*, 6(2), 179–185, 1999.

67. Squire, L. R. and Schacter, D. L. (Eds.), *Neuropsychology of Memory*, 3rd ed., Guilford Publications, New York, 2003.

68. Tulving, E. and Craik, F. I. M. (Eds.), *Oxford Handbook of Memory*, Oxford University Press, New York, 2005.

69. Wiegner, S. and Donders, J., Performance on the California Verbal Learning Test after traumatic brain injury, *Journal of Clinical and Experimental Neuropsychology*, 21(2), 159–170, 1999.

70. Vanderploeg, R. D., Crowell, T. A., and Curtiss, G., Verbal learning and memory deficits in traumatic brain injury: Encoding, consolidation, and retrieval, *Journal of Clinical and Experimental Neuropsychology*, 23(2), 185–195, 2001.

71. Vanderploeg, R. D., Curtiss, G., Schinka, J. A., and Lanham, Jr., R. A., Material-specific memory in traumatic brain injury: Differential effects during acquisition, recall, and retention, *Neuropsychology*, 15(2), 174–184, 2001.

72. Vakil, E., The effect of moderate to severe traumatic brain injury (TBI) on different aspects of memory: A selective review, *Journal of Clinical and Experimental Neuropsychology*, 27(8), 977–1021, 2005.

73. Henry, J. D., Phillips, L. H., Crawford, J. R., Kliegel, M., Theodorou, G., and Summers, F., Traumatic brain injury and prospective memory: Influence of task complexity, *Journal of Clinical and Experimental Neuropsychology*, 29(5), 457–466, 2007.

74. Critchley, M., The enigma of the Gerstmann's syndrome, *Brain*, 89(2), 183–198, 1966.

75. Miller, B. L. and Cummings, J. L. (Eds.), *The Human Frontal Lobes: Functions and Disorders*, 2nd ed., Guilford Publications, New York, 2006.

76. Luria, A. R. and Tsvetkova, L. S., *The Neuropsychological Analysis of Problem-Solving*, Paul M. Deutsch Press, Orlando, FL, 1990.

77. León-Carrión, J., Alarcón, J. C., Revuelta, M., Murillo-Cabezas, F., Dominguez-Roldán, J. M., Dominguez-Morales, M. R., Machuca-Murga, F., and Forastero, P., Executive functioning as outcome in patients after traumatic brain injury, *The International Journal of Neuroscience*, 94(1–2), 75–83, 1998.

78. Greve, K. W., Love, J. M., Sherwin, E., Mathias, C. W., Ramzinski, P., and Levy, J., Wisconsin Card Sorting Test in chronic severe traumatic brain injury: Factor structure and performance subgroups, *Brain Injury*, 16(1), 29–40, 2002.

79. Tate, R. L., Executive dysfunction and characterological changes after traumatic brain injury: Two sides of the same coin?, *Cortex*, 35(1), 39–55, 1999.

80. Ferland, M. B., Ramsay, J., Engeland, C., and O'Hara, P., Comparison of the performance of normal individuals and survivors of traumatic brain injury on repeat administrations of the Wisconsin Card Sorting Test, *Journal of Clinical and Experimental Neuropsychology*, 20(4), 473–482, 1998.

81. Busch, R. M., McBride, A., Curtiss, G., and Vanderploeg, R. D., The components of executive functioning in traumatic brain injury, *Journal of Clinical and Experimental Neuropsychology*, 27(8), 1022–1032, 2005.

82. Stuss, D. T. and Benson, F. D., Neuropsychological studies of the frontal lobes, *Psychological Bulletin*, 95(1), 3–28, 1984.

83. Stuss, D. T. and Benson, F. D., *The Frontal Lobes*, Raven Press, New York, 1986.

84. Cripe, L. I., The ecological validity of executive function testing, in R. J. Sbordone and C. J. Long (Eds.), *Ecological Validity of Neuropsychological Testing*, CRC Press/St. Lucie Press, Delray Beach, FL, 171–202, 1996.

85. Sherer, M., Sander, A. M., Nick, T. G., High, Jr., W. M., Malec, J. F., and Rosenthal, M., Early cognitive status and productivity outcome after traumatic brain injury: Findings from the TBI model systems, *Archives of Physical Medicine and Rehabilitation*, 83(2), 183–192, 2002.

86. Kennedy, M. R., Coelho, C., Turkstra, L., Ylvisaker, M., Moore Sohlberg, M., Yorkston, K., Chiou, H.- H., and Kan, P.- F., Intervention for executive functions after traumatic brain injury: A systematic review, meta-analysis and clinical recommendations, *Neuropsychological Rehabilitation*, 18(3), 257–299, 2008.

87. Krpan, K. M., Levine, B., Stuss, D. T., and Dawson, D. R., Executive function and coping at one-year post traumatic brain injury, *Journal of Clinical and Experimental Neuropsychology*, 29(1), 36–46, 2007.

88. Eslinger, P. J. (Ed.), *Neuropsychological Interventions: Clinical Research and Practice*, Guilford Publications, New York, 2005.

89. Sohlberg, M. M. and Mateer, C. A., *Cognitive Rehabilitation: An Integrative Neuropsychological Approach*, Guilford Publications, New York, 2001.

90. Wilson, B. A., *Case Studies in Neuropsychological Rehabilitation*, Oxford University Press, New York, 1999.

91. Wilson, B. A., Compensating for cognitive deficits following brain injury, *Neuropsychology Review*, 10(4), 233–243, 2000.

92. Perino, C., Rago, R., Cicolini, A., Torta, R., and Monaco, F., Mood and behavioural disorders following traumatic brain injury: Clinical evaluation and pharmacological management, *Brain Injury*, 15(2), 139–148, 2001.

93. Reitan, R. M. and Wolfson, D., Emotional disturbances and their interaction with neuropsychological deficits, *Neuropsychology Review*, 7(1), 3–19, 1997.

94. Skell, R. L., Johnstone, B., Schopp, L., Shaw, J., and Petroski, G. F., Neuropsychological predictors of distress following traumatic brain injury, *Brain Injury*, 14(8), 705–712, 2000.

95. Leathem, J. M. and Babbage, D. R., Affective disorders after traumatic brain injury: Cautions in the use of the Symptom Checklist-90-R, *Journal of Head Trauma Rehabilitation*, 15(6), 1246–1255, 2000.

96. Slaughter, J., Johnstone, G., Petroski, G., and Flax, J., The usefulness of the Brief Symptom Inventory in the neuropsychological evaluation of traumatic brain injury, *Brain Injury*, 13(2), 125–130, 1999.

97. Fann, J. R., Uomoto, J. M., and Katon, W. J., Sertraline in the treatment of major depression following mild traumatic brain injury, *The Journal of Neuropsychiatry and Clinical Neurosciences*, 12(2), 226–232, 2000.

98. Fann, J. R., Uomoto, J. M., and Katon, W. J., Cognitive improvement with treatment of depression following mild traumatic brain injury, *Psychosomatics*, 42(1), 48–54, 2001.

99. Teri, L. and Uomoto, J. M., Reducing excess disability in dementia patients: Training caregivers to manage patient depression, *Clinical Gerontologist*, 10(4), 49–64, 1991.

100. Macmillan, M., *An Odd Kind of Fame: Stories of Phineas Gage*, MIT Press, Cambridge, MA, 2000.

101. Stuss, D. T., Gow, C. A., and Hetherington, C. R., "No longer Gage": Frontal lobe dysfunction and emotional changes, *Journal of Consulting and Clinical Psychology*, 60(3), 349–359, 1992.

102. Stein, D., Brailowsky, S., and Will, B., *Brain Repair*, Oxford University Press, New York, 1995.

103. Bach-y-Rita, P., Theoretical basis for brain plasticity after a TBI. *Brain Injury*, 17(8), 643–651, 2003.

104. Cecatto, R. B. and Chadi, G., The importance of neuronal stimulation in central nervous system plasticity and neurorehabilitation strategies, *Functional Neurology*, 22(3), 137–143, 2007.

27

Evaluation of Traumatic Brain Injury Following Acute Rehabilitation

Mark J. Ashley

CONTENTS

27.1 Introduction

The field of traumatic brain injury (TBI) rehabilitation has changed considerably during the past 30 years. The field was born during the late 1970s from a need realized largely by the private insurance community in the United States. People with TBI were living far longer than ever before and rehabilitation efforts for these individuals were not well developed.

During the early 1980s, a number of hospital- and nonhospital-based rehabilitation programs developed utilizing a variety of program models and concepts. The number of facilities available to people with TBI increased dramatically during the mid 1980s, only to contract again during the early 1990s with the advent of managed care. Early rehabilitation

efforts were largely developed using treatment techniques developed for other populations and applied to the TBI population. The past 30 years have seen a great deal of refinement of interventions and improved predictably of outcome.

The impact of managed care on TBI rehabilitation has been considerable,[1,2] as it has been
in many areas of medicine. Perhaps the largest single impact, however, can be seen in
the amount of treatment provided to people with TBI. The 1980s saw a broadening of
insurance coverage for rehabilitation for people with TBI, but as managed care took hold,
significant decreases in length of stay (LOS) were noted. The average LOS for acute hospitalization decreased from 29 days in 1990 to 19 days in 1999. LOS for acute rehabilitation
hospitalization decreased from 48 days to 28 days from 1990 to 1999, respectively. It is clear
that severity of injury did not change during this time.[3] Kreutzer et al.[2] reported decreases
in lengths of stay averaging 3.65 days or 8% annually for acute and inpatient rehabilitation
treatment of TBI between 1990 and 1996.

It can be argued that alternative treatment settings allowed LOS to be decreased as
noted earlier for these periods, and it is likely that such availability did, in fact, contribute
to shorter LOS. The point, however, is that these individuals were discharged from acute
care settings far earlier than had ever been accomplished before. Consequently, alternative
care settings were increasingly faced with individuals who were admitted with ongoing
medical needs or with, perhaps, as yet unrecognized problems. The trend toward shorter
LOS has sharpened and provides a substantial challenge to the families and professionals involved with this population. The evaluation of a person with TBI becomes far more
complicated than ever before as a result.

TBI, unlike any other diagnosis, can impact an exceptionally broad spectrum of systems.
In addition, recovery from TBI can occur over a protracted course of time,[4-11] with residual
deficits observable for many individuals on a lifetime basis. TBI will impact the injured
person and his or her immediate family for life for persons who sustain moderate to severe
injury.[12-18] Data suggest that even a small percentage of people who sustain mild TBI will
experience symptoms that persist for months or years postinjury.[19,20]

Evaluation of a person with TBI, then, truly requires a great deal of investigation, time,
and thoroughness. Unfortunately, many forces conspire to thwart the completion of such
evaluative efforts. Discharge planners have relatively little notice of impending discharge
requirements. They are plagued with lack of financial coverage for ongoing rehabilitation
or placement in supervised settings for many individuals. Discharge planners understand
that families are ill-equipped to provide all the necessary care for an injured family member, but often have no choice in such placements. Discharge planners may be unaware of
resource availability as a result of the busy nature of their caseload and a resultant inability to research discharge options carefully that may exist locally, regionally, or nationally.

Discharge planners can be proactive when working with a brain injury rehabilitation
unit. Identification of potential discharge options for continued rehabilitation treatment
at the time of admission or very nearly after admission will allow postacute treatment
facilities maximum time to check benefits and negotiate payer acceptance of admission to
a postacute treatment setting. This allows the acute treatment team the broadest array of
discharge options to be developed and with far less time pressure. Early referral does not
have to constitute a commitment to transfer a patient to any particular follow-on setting.
Early referral does not necessarily imply that the patient will require evaluation at that
time—only that benefits can be checked and negotiations started. Postacute rehabilitation
facilities have developed relationships and means of explaining their work to payers and
they are skilled at facilitating access to ongoing treatment. This can ease the burden for the
discharge planner considerably. The discharge planner should maintain a resource center

of discharge options along with materials that describe those options to the rehabilitation team, patient, and family. The discharge planner can also ensure that the medical record is readily accessible to the evaluator, and that the appropriate consents have been completed. The record should contain a recommendation from one or more physicians involved in the patient's care depicting the need for ongoing postacute rehabilitation for the payer's benefit.

The evaluation of a person with TBI is frequently required on short notice and must be conducted in a busy, if not harried, environment in which insufficient time has not allowed for complete collection and collation of necessary information for the evaluator. The evaluation today must be conducted far more quickly, without sacrificing thoroughness or accuracy. More than ever, discharge planners and others need to know the results of the evaluation rapidly, whether an individual is acceptable for admission to the next level of rehabilitation, and whether the individual can be admitted to that next level. The evaluation, then, must be conducted quickly and thoroughly, a report of the findings generated, and all parties informed of the findings and available ongoing treatment options, often in the span of 24 to 48 hours. The evaluator must be supported by a team of professionals who can react quickly to the demands of today's rehabilitation and funding milieu. Of course, some evaluations may be conducted in a home, skilled nursing facility, jail, or psychiatric hospital. In many of these situations, there is far less time pressure to complete the evaluation.

This chapter outlines the comprehensive nature of information that should be collected during an evaluation. It should be recognized that complete collection of the information to follow is unlikely in today's rehabilitation and funding environment; however, information that is not collected should be earmarked for later collection, should the evaluation recommend progression to the next level of rehabilitative intervention or admission to another care setting. It should also be understood that the intention of this chapter is to provide information to the facility-based evaluator who must conduct evaluations at the bedside, in the home, or in another institution. Thus, the evaluation outlined is not designed to be exhaustive, but rather to identify the major issues at hand. Some of these issues may require much more extensive workup than is intended to be represented here.

27.2 Preparation

> So much of our time is preparation, so much is routine,
> and so much retrospect, that the pith of each man's genius
> contracts itself to a very few hours.
>
> **—Ralph Waldo Emerson**

Evaluations proceed best when the evaluator has the opportunity to prepare in advance of the evaluation. Demographic information such as name, age, date of birth, date of injury, social security number, home address, telephone numbers, insurance carrier information, and so on, should be recorded for easy reference during the evaluation. Precious time will not be taken up by these activities in this manner. The evaluator should be very familiar with the complexity of TBI and with the scope of service availability on a local, regional, and national level. All too often, evaluations are conducted to determine whether an individual is appropriate for admission to a specific rehabilitation or assisted living setting. This does not pose a significant problem when the individual is appropriate for admission; however, the evaluator has an ethical responsibility to recognize when an individual may be better served in an alternate environment. To accomplish this, evaluators should be aware of services offered at a variety of settings, other than that in they are employed. Careful consideration must be given to advice offered for the types of treatments or care that should be delivered next for an individual as well as to where those services might be available. Occasionally, evaluations are conducted for the sole purpose of securing an admission to a facility, in which case the evaluator has breached ethical principles.[21]

The evaluator is best served by review of medical records prior to seeing the individual. Collection of medical records can be quite challenging. Medical records are available from treatment centers; however, access to the records can be quite difficult. Medical records departments are charged with maintenance of confidentiality and are frequently overwhelmed in their workload. Although some states have requirements for timed compliance with requests for medical records, obtaining records via mailed or even hand-delivered requests can be exceptionally arduous. Thus, discharge planners or referring physicians or other professionals can facilitate access to records for an evaluator.

Medical records are often more readily available in the files of workers' compensation carriers and, sometimes, accident and health carriers because these companies strive to pay only those bills that are accompanied by medical records. The availability of such records can be useful in cases when the individual being evaluated was injured sometime in the past. It will not always be possible to review the entire medical record prior to completion of the evaluation. The evaluator's role, then, is to note which records have and have not been reviewed and to begin the process of obtaining the balance of the records for immediate review and consideration upon receipt. Incomplete record availability should be noted in the evaluation report, and the report should be amended should newly received information materially change any information or recommendations in the report.

Review of the medical record should begin with records created at the time of injury. The accident scene detail should be reviewed to attempt to determine the nature of the injury, likely levels of force encountered by the body, details pertaining to level of observed consciousness, length of elapsed time to emergency medical treatment, reported patient status, and Glasgow Coma Scale (GCS) score observed at the scene.[22] The GCS is used to both assess the severity of injury and track the course of recovery. Mild brain injury is defined by a GCS score of 13 to 15 points. A rating of 9 to 12 points is classified as a moderate injury and a rating of 3 to 8 points is classified as a severe injury. In instances when the GCS is used to document the course of recovery, notation of medications being administered over the interval should be made because medications can materially impact ratings of depth of coma.[23] Blood alcohol levels can also confound GCS scores and should be noted. Emergency room records may reveal information as indicated earlier and will begin documentation of the observed injuries upon presentation to the emergency department. Increasingly, details such as level of consciousness and trauma scores are being placed and monitored in the charts as emergency departments become more sophisticated in their approach to TBI intervention. These data points are important to collect because they bear upon most outcome predictions available in the literature.

As the medical record progresses, it is tempting to confine one's review to the more easily read typewritten reports. Clearly, these records provide a fairly comprehensive review of a case; however, important details may be found in the handwritten nursing, therapy, and physician notes. As the evaluator reviews the case, questions will arise regarding how and when developments occurred, or conflicting information may be found in different portions of the medical record. The answers to such questions can often be found in such handwritten notes. The record is best understood when reviewed and presented in the evaluation report in chronologic order.

Care should be given to noting admission and discharge dates, especially in the case of multiple-facility involvement. All conditions diagnosed must be included in the report, together with a detailed review of medications, their effects, and reasons for use and discontinuation. The evaluator is well advised to structure the collection of information to increase the likelihood that the most thorough evaluation will be completed. To that end, Appendix 27A provides an evaluative format that is useful in structuring the evaluation and report preparation processes. Information that is not collected is obvious by its absence and, as the evaluator considers finishing the evaluation and whether enough information has been gathered, the form provides a means for such assessment.

The evaluator should approach each evaluation in as uniform a manner as possible. Some of the sections reviewed in this chapter require use of some minimal equipment and familiarity with certain procedures. Standardized reporting of level of disability is strongly suggested by accreditation agencies[24] and should begin at the time of the evaluation. The evaluator will need rating scale forms available, with the heading information already completed. This will speed completion of the rating scales, increasing the likelihood that they are completed. Scales most often used are the GCS, Rancho Los Amigos Scale,[25] the Disability Rating Scale,[26] and the Functional Independence Measurement Scale.[27]

The evaluation is conducted for the purpose of determining the history and current status of the individual with an eye toward determination of the need or propriety of additional treatment or placement. The evaluator should have a thorough working knowledge of various treatment approaches and techniques available to be in the best position to make recommendation about ongoing treatment delivery. Although the focus is largely upon the injured individual, the evaluator has a role to play in education of the individual's family and friends as well as the professionals currently involved with the person. As such, evaluations will require an investment of energy and time unlike that seen in many other diagnostic groups. Evaluations of people with TBI may require well more than 2 to 4 hours, and still remain incomplete. There is a huge amount of information necessary to collect that will shape the rehabilitative effort, and current and future discharge planning. Information collected during the evaluation will set the stage for the more in-depth clinical assessments to be conducted after an individual is admitted to the next level of care being considered. Although it may be tempting to put off collection of some information until after the admission, the propriety of that very admission may be impacted by advanced knowledge of key variables. Prognostication of outcome is often requested at the time of evaluation and the accuracy of such prognostication can only be detrimentally affected by a lack of comprehensive information.

The evaluation should begin with answers to the questions below:

- What is the purpose of the evaluation?
- Who requested the evaluation to be completed?
- What is expected following the evaluation and by whom?
- Who are the various people who are to be involved in the evaluation?
- What specific questions have been posed to be answered by the evaluation?

The evaluation's purpose may be to determine whether an individual is ready for the admission to a next level of care or treatment. It may be conducted for medical–legal purposes. Insight into the purpose of the evaluation is often, although not always, provided by the person who requests the evaluation. The purpose may or may not be well articulated. The evaluation may be conducted at the request of a person behind the scenes, with or without the encouragement of the people currently involved in the individual's care. Some diplomacy may be in order. It is quite important to understand what is expected as an outcome of the evaluation. Because there is so much information that can be collected in an evaluation, the amount of time to complete the evaluation will be dependent upon what those expectations are. Evaluators should be very clear regarding what information they may be expected to provide, what opinions they may be asked to provide, and the information they will have to obtain to answer those questions adequately. The people involved can be quite variable from case to case.

Likewise, roles played by these parties may not be obvious. It should not be assumed that a person's spouse is the primary decision maker, for example. Some spouses defer to parents, siblings, friends, or others. Thus, the evaluator must determine who the key players are and their roles to ensure that communication flows smoothly before, during, and after the evaluation. It is usually advisable to have the major players present and/or available during the evaluation. The evaluator can use their presence as an opportunity to educate them regarding the findings of the evaluation, either as the evaluation unfolds or in summary at the end of the evaluation. Caregivers, understandably, have information as their most intense need and desire.[28,29]

The evaluation can be conducted using a variety of formats in combination with one another. Direct interview and assessment of the injured person may or may not be possible as a means of information collection. It may be necessary to glean information from observation of the injured person as he or she interacts with other allied health professionals or with family and friends. It will be important to be able to interview these parties as well, to obtain information that is unlikely to be well represented in the existing medical record. This includes information concerning preinjury matters such as educational achievement, vocational history, social and family history, and, sometimes, medical history. In the event that information is relied upon from medical records to substantiate a particular matter, care should be taken to note the currency of the report because recovery in TBI sometimes occurs at unpredictable rates.

27.3 Evaluation

27.3.1 Current Medical Status

The person's current medical status is a primary focus of the evaluation, especially in these days of shortened hospital LOS. Current medical status cannot be truly understood, though, without reference to medical history, both prior to and since injury. Every effort should be made to review medical history information thoroughly. Laboratory studies should be reviewed for reported abnormalities, with particular attention paid to neuroendocrine function,[30,31] blood dyscrasia, serum anticonvulsant levels, prothrombin times, infectious disease reports, and alkaline phosphatase levels. Current medical status reporting should include a detailed review of bowel and bladder status and continence. This should include catheter requirements, stool softeners, levels of independence and awareness, and any medical issues noted. Dietary status should review nutritional intake, swallowing status, and level of independence. A good depiction of the history of swallowing evaluations is in order in the event that the person has dysphagia.

A full description of medications, dosages, and indications should be provided. Medication history since injury should be reviewed and reported chronologically, together with indications, effects, and reasons for discontinuance. Seizure history, or its absence, should be noted. All allergies must be clearly documented. The individual's most current height and weight statistics, together with behavioral health concerns, such as alcohol or substance abuse, must be reported.

Dental status should be reviewed, either via the records or via examination.[32] Broken or missing teeth will need to be addressed. The reliance upon dentures, orthotics, or dental appliances should be noted. The oral cavity should be examined for description of the dentition and gums. Some anticonvulsants and other medications can cause gum hyperplasia.[33] Oral hygiene and level of independence and efficiency should be reported. Oral tactile defensiveness may be a clue to painful teeth or gum. Inspection of the buccal cavities for food residue may suggest lingual motility or swallowing problems.

It is important to review the person's sleep, because sleep disorders following TBI appear to occur related to the TBI.[34,35] Check for sleep routine, including bedtime, rising time, nighttime awakening, reasons for awakening, and how the person feels upon awaking in the morning. Note caffeine or other stimulant intake, as well as medications or substances used to induce or maintain sleep. Discussions of sleep can be found in Chapters 11 and 31.

The person's preinjury medical status should be documented. This should include the person's personal history as well as family history that might become contributory to developing health concerns in the future. This should include both physical and emotional health issues. Careful investigation should be conducted into the history of previous trauma to the head or whiplash because this information may be instrumental in understanding the postinjury course of recovery, particularly in the case of mild TBI.[36]

Lastly, medical interventions that may be necessary in the future should be recorded, such as revisions of orthopedic appliances, gastrostomy, tracheostomy sites, cranioplasty, and so on. Such procedures may be best undertaken either prior to or during additional rehabilitation, depending upon the nature of the case. In addition, knowledge that more than one surgical procedure will be necessary in the future may allow for scheduling of both procedures under a single anesthesia.

27.3.2 Audiometry

Audiometric evaluation is not generally performed during the early phases of rehabilitation for TBI. When formal audiometry has been undertaken, the dates of testing and detailed findings should be reported. In instances when formal testing has not been undertaken, observation of the individual's functioning within the environment can provide valuable insight into audiometric function. Historical information is of great importance to be gathered during this process. It is important to know whether there was a blow to the head, the integrity of the tympanic membranes, and whether otorrhea was reported.[37,38] Each of these is important for the possible identification of disarticulation of the ossicular chain within the middle ear.[37,38] Temporal bone fractures may result in cochlear or vestibular damage.[37,38] A blow to the head in the temporal region may impair cranial nerve VII function by damaging the nerve as it exits the skull, possibly impacting either lacrimation alone or lacrimation and salivation.[39,40] In addition, historical information, such as exposure to noise of a chronic nature in the pursuit of recreational or vocational interests, might portend the development of sensory–neural hearing loss. Of course, sensory–neural hearing loss of this type does not arise from the TBI but may complicate communicative and other restorative efforts. Likewise, an individual's chronic exposure to ototoxic medications, such as certain antibiotics and aspirin, might lead to loss of hearing. Reports of tinnitus are common and may be described in varying terms. Terms used by the person to describe tinnitus can be important in understanding its underlying cause. A high-pitched whistling or buzzing sound is most often experienced. The tone is most noticeable in quiet areas and is masked by normal environmental noise levels. Some tinnitus, though, is reported as a roaring and may suggest significant otologic pathology, such as posttraumatic Ménière's. The evaluator must note these issues as well as whether the tinnitus is constant or variable.

Behavioral observation and interview may assist in identification of hearing loss. The evaluator should note whether the individual with lesser communicative abilities attempts to read lips or localize environmental sounds, exhibits an auditory startle reaction, or turns the head to one side during conversation. The individual may report the presence of ringing in the ears, whistling, buzzing, or in some instances, a roaring sensation in the ear. The latter is often accompanied by a sense of oral fullness and fluctuating hearing loss. Further discussion of audiologic and vestibular issues can be found in Chapters 6 and 7.

27.3.3 Cognition

Evaluation of cognition begins with assessment of orientation to person, place, time, and date. These questions are simply asked; however, the evaluator's name should not be used as a reference point. Rather, the name of an individual more familiar to the injured person should be selected.

The presence of attentional deficits can be determined either by observation or by interview with other professionals involved with the individual. An attempt should be made to determine whether the individual's ability to persist with a task (persistence) is better or worse than the individual's ability to persist with mental activities (concentration). It is important to discern a difference, if any, between these two types of attentional tasks.[15,41]

Further investigation into attentional skills can be conducted by evaluation of whether an individual is able to change between activities efficiently and without a loss of information. Some individuals will be unable to change from one activity to another and will exhibit perseverative tendencies. Others may be able to change between activities but do so slowly and lose information in the process. Finally, the evaluator should attempt to determine whether the individual is able to demonstrate vigilance by screening large amounts of information for a target stimulus.

Evaluation of very brief attentional store mechanisms, such as iconic (visual) and echoic (auditory), can be easily undertaken in the scope of a field evaluation. The examiner can prepare cards, as demonstrated in Appendix 27B, for presentation of iconic store stimuli. The presentation of several 3 × 5 cards with three rows of three letters each[42] can be utilized, presenting each card briefly. Examiners should note that the card is presented anywhere from 2 to 5 seconds and, following presentation and removal of the card from sight, examiners indicate which row they would like the person to recall. As the examiner goes through various cards, the row requested should be chosen randomly and the accuracy of response noted. Line recall should be somewhere in the neighborhood of 75% and card recall in the neighborhood of 90%, with a small amount of rehearsal. Echoic store can be evaluated by the presentation of randomly presented numbers, zero to nine. Normal performance is in the neighborhood of six to seven numbers forward recall and four to five numbers backward recall.[43] The task can be further complicated by asking the person to order presented numbers from largest to smallest, thereby assessing both immediate recall and working memory.

Central to the processes of cognition is an individual's ability to identify perceptual attributes of objects and events in their environment.[15] The evaluator should attempt to discern the individual's fluency with this task by presenting up to three objects and asking the individual to provide a description. The examiner can model the description or can enumerate the variables desired, such as color, size, weight, shape, function, detail, texture, and construction. The total time required and the spontaneity of response, after the task is demonstrated, should be noted. The degree to which the evaluator needs to assist the individual in coming up with features should be noted. To undertake this evaluation, the examiner might describe an object to the patient using the eight previously detailed features. A pencil could be 5 inches long, three eighths of an inch in diameter, hexagonal in shape, yellow, pointed, cylindrical, weighing approximately a half ounce, be constructed of wood, have a graphite point or rubber eraser, and be used for writing. The individual is asked to carry out a similar description with up to three objects. This task should be able to be completed in less than 30 seconds per object, and notation of any perseverative response should be made. Of particular interest is whether an individual focuses on the object's function versus a description of how the object is constructed.

Next, the evaluator should determine the degree to which the individual is able to use perceptual features to categorize. This can be done with objects that are common and within the environment. It may be necessary to model the task for the individual. The evaluator should observe whether the individual is able to categorize, and determine which methods and techniques are used for categorization (see Chapter 19). As part of the evaluation of categorization, the examiner should attempt to determine whether the individual can decide which items do not belong in an examiner-defined category. Use of real objects allows the examiner to create a group of objects that share a perceptual feature and to determine whether the individual can decide what attribute is shared by all the objects. For example, grouping of four or five metal objects should elicit a response that all the objects are made of the same material or of metals. Next, the evaluator should determine whether the individual can decide which objects do not belong in a particular category. The evaluator can determine whether the person can extend categorical boundaries by asking questions such as "Can a chair be used as a ladder?," followed up by a request for a description of how this could be undertaken. Individuals who are very concrete and unable to extend categorical boundaries will answer the question in the negative. If an individual answers the question in the affirmative, the evaluator should determine whether the response is a randomly selected one or, in fact, is based upon sound reasoning. The intention is to identify the ability to alter the function of an object to an acharacteristic function based upon a particular feature. In the pencil example, the pencil could be used as a lever or as a weapon. The examiner can show the person an object and ask them to name three other objects not currently in the room that share a named feature with the one being shown, again noting responses, time to complete, and reasonableness of responses. Repetitive responses are not acceptable, and the patient should be encouraged to come up with novel responses.

Proverb interpretation can be undertaken to determine the degree to which an individual is functioning at an abstract reasoning level. In addition, drawing a floor plan of the room in which the individual is sitting, including windows, walls, doors, and placement of furniture, as well as a floor plan of the place where the individual lives, can provide additional insight into visual perceptual skills, as well as abstraction capabilities. In the instance when the proverb is literally interpreted, it becomes apparent that the individual is functioning at a fairly concrete level. Floor plan execution and proverb interpretation can yield information about the individual's ability for planning, sequencing, cognitive distance,[44] visual imagery, and visual praxis.[45]

The ability to sequence can be evaluated by asking the individual to go through a detailed description of how to change a tire, or bake a cake, or some other gender- and experience-appropriate example. In a somewhat similar vein, problem solving can be evaluated by asking the individual what they would do in the event of a given scenario. One such example might be: "What would you do if you came home and found a family member lying on the floor, unconscious, and bleeding heavily from a deep cut on the arm?" Acceptable responses should be noted, as well as the time required to provide those responses. After an acceptable response is obtained, the examiner adds a complication, such as being unable to awaken the person. A logical response might be that they would then call for help. The next complication added would be that the telephone does not work. A logical response to this complication might be to leave the individual and go to a neighbor's for help. Finally, the complication that the neighbors are not home can be provided. Some individuals will become quite frustrated with these task complications, others will provide unique and unrealistic responses to the complications, and still others will be able to provide a reasonable response to the complications. The response pattern should be noted, as well as the time to respond.

Next, it is important to evaluate whether learning is rule governed or nonrule governed.[46] A deck of cards can be utilized to evaluate an individual's abilities in this regard. First, the cards are slowly dealt, face up, into two piles, which are separated on the basis of whether they are black or red. The individual is asked to tell the examiner the rule the examiner is using to place a card in either pile. The individual should be able to identify a rule within 5 to 10 cards per pile. If the individual is able to identify the rule properly, the examiner should continue by simply changing the pile into which the red cards and black cards are delivered (to the converse pile). Again, the individual should be able to tell the examiner that the rule has changed and what the new rule is. This is an evaluation of a "reversal shift" capability. The testing progresses with the examiner changing the rule entirely, placing face cards in one pile and nonface cards in the other. Again, determination of the change in rule and the nature of the rule is the target for this "nonreversal shift" activity. Care should be taken to evaluate the level of capability and/or frustration present during this task, and the task should be discontinued if the individual is unable to complete the task or becomes frustrated with it. Previous administration of the Wisconsin Card Sorting Test may provide the information that can be obtained from this procedure. Whether the individual is a reflective thinker or has an impulsive thought style should be evaluated and noted as cognitive tempo.[15] Speed of processing should likewise be evaluated.

Through much of the evaluation of cognition, the examiner can rely both on formalized evaluative procedures that might have been undertaken by professionals involved in the case and by observation of the individual's behavioral interaction with the environment and individuals in it. In this method, behavior is used as a representation of cognition.[47]

27.3.4 Education

The educational history of the individual should be obtained by interview with family, as well as a review of academic records. Those individuals who are in the process of completing or have completed high school may have academic records available to them personally. In any event, academic records can be requested of grade school and high school institutions and should be reviewed to gain insight into both academic performance and the possibility of previous observations or notations regarding injuries, attentional deficits, learning disabilities, or behavior problems.

All too often, a formal or informal academic skills evaluation is absent from a rehabilitative evaluation. In many instances, these areas are relegated to the speech pathologist or occupational therapist. In some specialized facilities, however, educational specialists are utilized to evaluate and remediate these skill sets.

In a field evaluation, a cursory look at mathematics, reading, writing, money management, and telephone skills is in order. For mathematics, the individual's ability should be evaluated to count with a random number of objects; add and subtract with objects or without; identify sizes; write number symbols up to 100; count by 2s, 5s, and 10s up to 50; add and subtract without renaming up to three columns; add and subtract with renaming up to three columns; multiply one digit by one digit; multiply two digits by one digit; distinguish the value of a decimal fraction compared with a whole number; and find a percentage of a whole number. Reading skills, such as the ability to recognize random letters in the alphabet, read simple sight words, read functional sources (e.g., labels, newspapers, signs), and answer three comprehension questions about material read from a functional source, should be evaluated. Spelling and writing skills can be evaluated by asking individuals to write any given letter of the alphabet; copy a sentence; write two or three sentences about themselves; and spell two of four words at a sixth grade reading level (e.g., direction, activity, vegetable, gentle).

A history should be taken pertaining to money management skills. It should be determined who managed money in the family and the extent to which the injured individual participated in those activities. It should include experience with the management of real money, such as coin identification and making change, as well as whether the individual utilized a checkbook and how he or she managed the checking account. Finally, telephone skills can be evaluated by asking the individual to dial a number, determining whether the appropriate communicative techniques are utilized for the telephone, whether the individual is aware of emergency phone skills, and whether the individual is able to use a telephone directory. Discussion regarding money management skills with the family will allow determination of whether responsibilities have been given over to a family member or caregiver since injury.

The evaluator may wish to bring along grade-level, standardized math and reading exercises, and problems to be used in the evaluation. Care should be taken not to assume capabilities not demonstrated. It is often tempting, based upon an individual's educational or vocational experience or, sometimes, based upon their linguistic skills, to forgo this portion of the evaluation.

27.3.5 Family

It should go without saying that collection of information pertaining to the family will be of great help in determining key players and their roles. It may be that the evaluation setting will not lend itself to a casual collection of this information or complete access to this information in that family members may or may not be present in all settings. In any event, the information should be collected, either by direct interview or telephone interview. The individual's marital status and prior experience with marriage/divorce should be discerned. Previous spouse/partner names and dates of marriages/domestic partnerships should be collected. All children from current and/or former marriages should be identified by name and age. Siblings, also, should be identified by name, age, and location.

It is often helpful to attempt to discern siblings' occupational endeavors. These individuals may be quite insightful during treatment, may have worked in similar or identical fields, may be helpful in identification of vocational aptitudes and skills, and may represent potential vocational placement options following completion of the medical rehabilitation. The parents' names, ages, locations, occupations, and marital status should be obtained as well.

Of greatest interest is the family's education and awareness of the diagnosis, individual deficit areas, and knowledge of the short- and long-term outlook for their family member. Often, families, although they may have been given access to some information, report that they feel quite at a loss to predict a longer term outcome for the injured individual or themselves.[29] Reviewing the evaluation findings with the family, in detail, will both serve as an educational opportunity and an opportunity to determine gaps in their knowledge and to provide education. Many families report a frustration with the lack of information, and a coincidental relief when their questions can be answered by an evaluator, either about past, current, or future events. The evaluator will be interested to know whether the family has had counseling or is currently involved in counseling. In addition, discharge options should be discussed with the family, determining their wish to be involved, their ability to be involved, and the degree of involvement they wish to have.

Conservatorship or guardianship issues can be quite varied from state to state and circumstance to circumstance. That is to say, some individuals may have no guardianship or conservatorship proceedings involved in their case. Others, however, may have a conservatorship over finance, a conservatorship over person, a conservatorship over both, a power-of-attorney arrangement, or some other arrangement. Likewise, some individuals may not have any of these in place and the evaluator may be in a position to advise that these matters be considered with the family's legal counsel. Family members are often poorly informed regarding the role of guardianship or conservatorship proceedings that may have been undertaken or may have been recommended. Consequently, it is always a good policy to obtain copies of any conservatorship or guardianship proceedings so that the evaluator and/or treating facility can be aware of the nature of the proceedings and the impact upon the individual's rights and liberties those proceedings may or may not have.

27.3.6 Occupational/Physical Therapy

Investigation of occupational and physical therapy status should begin with a review of the patient's treatment history and discussion with any currently involved professionals in these disciplines. Current information provided by these professionals can truncate the evaluation time and with no compromise of accuracy. Active and passive range of motion is of interest in the upper and lower extremities, head and neck, and trunk. These can be directly assessed or observed as the individual moves in the environment. Likewise, strength in the upper and lower extremities, as well as head, neck, and trunk, should be determined. The evaluator can note functional capabilities or can proceed through formal strength grading by physical examination. Sensation and proprioception should be evaluated. Comments regarding overall muscle endurance, as well as cardiopulmonary endurance, should be provided. Of interest in sensation testing is appreciation to light touch, to touch discrimination, and to temperature differentiation in all four extremities. Facial sensation is discussed in Section 27.3. 8. Likewise, proprioceptive awareness of the upper and lower extremities should be evaluated. When evaluating stereognosis, the evaluator should be careful that the individual does not see the object being placed in either hand. As the individual names the object, care should again be taken to note whether naming difficulties are present in both hands or only the left hand. A deficit in stereognostic naming in the left hand may point to a callosal lesion.[48] If language impairment is present, the evaluator may ask the individual to identify the object he or she was holding from a group of objects.

The presence or absence of clonus in the upper and lower extremities should be noted. The evaluator is interested in fine motor coordination and dexterity. This can be observed through direct assessment, object manipulation, or finger-to-thumb opposition, progressing through each of the four fingers. Gross motor skills, such as the ability to roll from a supine to prone position and back, assume a quadruped position, assume tall kneeling, assume half kneeling, and stand from a half-kneeling position, will be important to the physical therapist. The individual's ability for transfers should be assessed as indicated from floor to chair or wheelchair, from wheelchair to chair, wheelchair to bed, bed to wheelchair, wheelchair to car, and wheelchair to toilet.

Balance should be evaluated for both sitting and standing, if possible. The evaluator can assess an individual's abilities for challenged and unchallenged sitting and standing balance, one-foot balance, and heel–toe walking. Weight shift during ambulation should be noted, as well as posture, both sitting and standing. Gait should be evaluated for pace; required devices (such as orthotics, canes, walkers); trunk rotation; and reciprocal arm swing, and should include smooth and uneven surfaces. If the individual requires a wheelchair, the type of wheelchair should be noted.

Evaluation of vestibular sensitivity should include review of complaints of headaches, nausea, vomiting, dizziness, lightheadedness, or a feeling of imbalance. Historical information may point to vestibular dysfunction, such as falls that occurred in low-light conditions, loss of balance in the shower, while dressing or playing with the children, reliance upon night-lights, a feeling of imbalance, fear of heights or stairs, or discomfort or motion sickness following car rides or activities that require plane changes. The evaluator may wish to conduct a marching-in-place exercise, with eyes open and eyes closed, or other vestibular tests the evaluator may be comfortable with (see Chapter 6). Walking in a straight line, forward and backward, with eyes open and eyes closed can help to identify vestibular involvement. Deviation will be toward the side of involvement.[49] Of course, care must be taken to provide for proper safety precautions in guarding the person from falls with any balance or coordination testing. These activities should not be undertaken without proper training. Cerebellar testing can be done by heel-to-shin maneuver, finger-to-nose maneuver, and reciprocal alternating movements of the upper extremities.

The ability to complete activities of daily living is of great interest. This should include hygiene, toileting, dressing, grooming, feeding, meal planning, shopping, meal preparation, laundry, and household cleaning. The degree to which the individual participates in these activities, the level of independence exercised, and the degree to which the individual participated in these activities prior to injury will all be important. Part and parcel to the evaluation of activities of daily living skills is a review of the individual's typical daily routine. This should simply include a description of the individual's time to awaken and all activities generally engaged in throughout the day until bedtime. Careful evaluation of the person's ability to initiate tasks as either part of routine or apart from routine should be conducted.[50] Essentially, the evaluator needs to construct a conception of the individual's daily and/or weekly schedule of activities. This should be contrasted to the daily or weekly schedule of activities the individual engaged in prior to injury. Driving habits prior to injury can be discussed as a part of this undertaking and the individual's ability to drive following the injury should be documented. Different states have different requirements regarding reporting to their motor vehicle departments, and the evaluator should be aware of those reporting requirements and/or whether the individual's injury or seizure condition, if present, has been reported. Finally, it may be advisable to tell the patient and family that driving should not be undertaken until the individual is fully and carefully evaluated for visual, vestibular, motor, and cognitive capacity to drive safely.

Evaluation of gustation and olfaction is not often done. The evaluator may wish to carry a standard set of scratch-and-sniff patches to test olfaction. The presence of deficits in olfaction is fairly common following TBI[51] and should be suspected when the individual suffers weight loss, loss of appetite, or diminished meal volume consumption. Likewise, these same behaviors may point to difficulties with dentition and/or swallowing.

27.3.7 Psychosocial

Among the many areas TBI impacts in a person's life, perhaps none can be more profound than the changes in personality that are attributed to TBI by injured individuals, their families, and their friends.[29] A reasonable goal for rehabilitation is to attempt to return the individual to his or her preinjury lifestyle as much as possible. To that end, it becomes quite important to understand the individual's personal history. Information such as where the individual was born and raised, how frequently he or she moved, a military service history, social history, and religious affiliation will provide great insight into preinjury personality.

An evaluation of the individual's ability to describe his or her deficits and limitations should be conducted. The evaluator should attempt to discern how comprehensibly the individual can describe his or her deficits and the degree of assistance needed to do so. Difficulties in acknowledgment or acceptance of disability should be identified, documented, and described. These skills can bear significantly on outcome and need to be recognized and treated early.[52] The individual may have difficulty as a result of cognitive processing problems, denial, rationalization, projection, repression, suppression, displacement, sublimation, or regression. The evaluator should obtain an idea of the individual's self-concept. How does the individual see himself? Does the individual demonstrate a consistency of self from preinjury to current status? Does the individual see himself as others do? Finally, the evaluator should attempt to determine the impact of the injury on self-esteem.

It is important to attempt to determine the degree to which the family is supportive of the individual, is understanding of the individual's deficits and limitations, and is able to participate in a rehabilitative milieu. Problem areas in the family should be identified, in particular because they may impact the rehabilitative undertaking. A similar approach should be taken with friends, attempting to determine the quality and quantity of visitations or interactions.

The preinjury personality may have been more formally assessed somewhere in the individual's treatment. Formalized testing and dates, as well as report summarization, should be included in the evaluation. In addition, the family's characterization of the preinjury personality and the individual's characterization should be reported. Information about membership in organizations, hobbies, recreational interests, preinjury goals, and current goals should be collected. The evaluator will need to request information regarding social and legal history. Results of formal neuropsychological and/or psychological testing should be reported, with the dates of testing, the tests administered, and the findings.

Discussion of sexuality may be conducted either during the psychosocial portion of the evaluation or in the medical portion. The evaluator should attempt to discern the individual's ability to engage in various levels of social interaction and maintenance of social boundaries. Family may be best able to provide a historical reference to the person's expression of sexuality prior to injury. This should be compared with behavior following injury. It is important to attempt to determine whether emotional and sexual intimacy, libido, or ability to perform have been altered or impaired since injury.

TBI often impacts an individual's ability to handle frustration or to engage in socially appropriate behaviors. These deficits may manifest in impulsive anger, verbal aggression, physical aggression, or in behavioral manifestations that are outside of societal norms. The evaluator must note episodes of impulsive anger, frustration, verbal aggression, physical aggression, and any behaviors that have been noted to be problematic. The individual or family should be able to provide insight into coping mechanisms prior to injury and may be able to provide insight into current strategies. It is important to evaluate how the individual shows frustration, whether he or she engages in withdrawal or aggression, and whether there is anxiety, nervousness, psychosomatic complaint, lability, or depression. Information may be available regarding previous psychological or psychiatric treatment. The evaluator should discern whether paranoia, hallucinations, delusions, addictions, depression, regression, or psychosomatic complaints have been noted or observed. The individual's motivational capabilities should be identified, both for those areas in which the individual seems highly motivated or, perhaps, "overly motivated," as well as a lack of motivation or initiation.

27.3.8 Speech–Language Pathology

Deficits of interest in speech/language pathology following TBI are typically in the areas of cognition, motor speech disorders, dysphagia, language disorders, fluency, and voice. As part of the evaluation of motor speech disorders and dysphagia, an oral peripheral examination is undertaken. Observation of the facial symmetry, at rest and during movement, is undertaken to determine whether any asymmetries are present. Facial sensation should be evaluated at all three branches of cranial nerve V[39,40] because this nerve is particularly vulnerable to injury in the temporal region where it exits the skull. The mandibular rest position is noted, as well as the ability to extend and lateralize the mandible and any joint pain. Position of the tongue, at rest and in various maneuvers, is noted, again, with an expectation for no tremor, no fasciculations, and symmetry of movement. An oral peripheral examination form is included in Appendix 27C of this chapter. It is not likely that the evaluator will conduct an otoscopic examination; however, otoscopic examination has probably been performed and the results should be noted. Likewise, swallowing is most generally evaluated at the acute level and the most recent swallowing evaluation, as well as the history of evaluation of dysphagia, should be noted. The evaluator should look for consistency in the management of foods, liquids, secretions, and radiographic evaluation of swallowing. The examiner can undertake a quick apraxia assessment by asking the individual to undertake several activities without demonstrating those activities. These include stick out your tongue, blow, show me your teeth, pucker your lips, bite your lower lip, whistle, lick your lips, clear your throat, cough, smile, and puff your cheeks. Articulatory agility, or the ability to make various speech sounds clearly and quickly, should be noted. Throughout the evaluation, the individual's ability to maintain topic can be determined.[53,54] Any difficulties with fluency (stuttering) should also be noted. Should a fluency disorder be present, the evaluator should determine whether this preexisted the injury. Voice can be characterized as breathy, nasal, hoarse, soft, or loud. Evaluation of intonational changes in conversation should be included because their absence can materially impact communicative intent and success.[55] History of endotracheal intubation should be noted and an attempt should be made to determine pulmonary capacity. A nasal quality in voice may suggest a velopharyngeal paresis.[56]

TBI does not generally result in pure receptive or expressive aphasias as are often demonstrated in cerebral vascular accidents. However, evaluation of expressive and receptive language skills should be undertaken and/or test results reported. Most frequently observed are difficulties with anomia, paraphasias, and neologisms. A *paraphasia* is a whole-word substitution, such as "tar" for "car." *Neologisms* are nonsense words or syllables.[57,58] Finally, the ability to communicate intent should be assessed with a description of the means utilized to communicate.

27.3.9 Vision

A visual evaluation early after TBI is difficult to undertake and is, therefore, often postponed. Clearly, cranial nerve involvement (see Chapter 7) is often included in a neurologic evaluation, and some workup of visual perceptual skills may be available in the occupational therapy history. The evaluator should note whether the individual had prescriptive lenses prior to injury and for what purpose, as well as whether those lenses are currently available and in use. Documentation of complaints of visual acuity should be included and any formal ophthalmologic examination that has been undertaken should be reported, with dates and results. Individuals may report difficulty seeing, blurred vision, double vision, changes in vision with fatigue, difficulty reading, and, in some instances, may report image persistence (being able to see an object after looking away from it) or lack of recognition of familiar objects, places, or persons.[59,60] Some of these reports may not be spontaneous and may require the evaluator's active investigation.

The evaluator can test visual fields to confrontation and can evaluate ocular motility and gaze convergence. Evaluation of visual fields is conducted by covering one eye and moving an object from the ear forward into the lateral field of the uncovered eye. The person is asked to maintain a straight-ahead focus and indicate the earliest point at which the object comes into the peripheral field of vision. The maneuver is repeated from over the head to check superior quadrants, under the chin to evaluate inferior quadrants, and the opposite side of the head to the covered eye to evaluate nasal fields. The entire process is repeated for the other eye. Evaluation of ocular motility is performed by asking the person to track, with eyes only, the movement of an object that is moved in front of the person from left to right to left, up and down, and in a circle. The evaluator is looking for smooth and convergent movements of the eyes, without overshooting or jerky movement, which could imply brainstem involvement of cranial nerves III, IV, VI, or VIII.[61,62] Finally, behavioral observation may help to discern the presence of visual field cuts or neglect, such as when an individual bumps into objects or appears to miss information in the environment predominantly in a particular visual field or quadrant. Here again, it is important to advise the patient and family of any findings in visual fields because these particularly can impact driving and safety.

Information about visual perceptual skills may be available from the occupational therapy department or from ophthalmologic or optometric evaluation. Of interest are depth perception, binocular or stereo vision, visual figure–ground, visual praxis, and visual organization skills. The examiner may wish to carry subtests of standardized visual perceptual tests to investigate visual perceptual skills.

27.3.10 Vocation

The individual's preinjury vocational endeavors should be chronicled in the evaluation. This should consist of a chronologic review of at least the last 10 to 15 years of employment, complete with job position, companies, locations, and salaries. A complete vocational history provides a great deal of information about an individual's work ethic, intellectual capability, social experience, and vocational experience. If large gaps in employment history are noted, reasons for unemployment should be determined. Likewise, if an individual has a history of frequent job changes and positions of short duration, reasons for those job changes should be listed. An individual who frequently changes jobs may have a history of inappropriate social skills as they pertain to job settings, or difficulties with maintaining employment. By the same token, some professions, by their very nature, subject an individual to frequent changes in employer. Consequently, any conclusions drawn regarding an individual's work ethic, personality, or vocational history should be drawn from a comprehensive review of these factors. This section should culminate with the job held at the time of injury or the most recent position and salary. Families or injured individuals, themselves, may be able to provide insight into positions the individual disliked and liked, as well as goals the individual had and/or has. The individual's goals for vocational involvement should be determined, together with the family's goals and expectations. Finally, any vocational evaluation or testing that has been completed should be reported, with dates and results.

27.4 Report Preparation

Appendix 27A in this chapter and, indeed, the very format of this chapter, can be used in report preparation. Findings under each heading can be listed within their own subsection in a report; however, the most important section of the report is likely to be the Impressions and Recommendations section. This section of the report must be clear, concise, and able to answer most questions of most readers. Unfortunately, reports are read by many varied professionals and it is not possible to anticipate all questions, nor is it advisable. Thus, when the report is prepared, it should be prepared with the referral questions in mind, very clearly stated, and answered as clearly as possible in the Impressions and Recommendations section.

A good practice is to utilize standardized scale reporting in an effort to quantify the individual's functioning status in a means that may be immediately understandable across treatment settings. Scales that allow this are the Disability Rating Scale, the Rancho Los Amigos Scale, the GCS, and the Functional Independence Measure. The level of disability should be characterized in terms of the scale or scales utilized. The referral question should be posed and answered, with a listing of factors that will positively influence attainment of any identified goals, and factors that will impede attainment of those same goals. It is often best to list recommendations in a numbered fashion, and it may be helpful to both the preparer of the report and its readers if these recommendations follow the general outline of the report in order. Consequently, following the outline of this chapter, recommendations of a medical nature would be provided first, followed by audiometry, cognition, education, family, occupational and physical therapy, psychosocial, speech–language pathology, vision, vocation, and impressions/recommendations.

The report should include whether the individual is an appropriate candidate for admission to a specific care setting or treatment setting, if this question has been raised. The report should answer whether ongoing rehabilitative services are in order and the expected outcome of those services, if rendered, together with time and cost expectations. Again, this information should be provided only if requested as the primary purpose of the evaluation. Should the individual not be an appropriate candidate for a particular program, it is felt that the evaluator should attempt to provide alternate suggestions for the referral source, injured individual, and/or family. The report should conclude with information about how to contact the evaluator with questions or comments.

27.5 Summary

The evaluation of a person with TBI poses a considerable challenge to the professional. The evaluation is rarely complete enough, and time allotted for evaluation is all too often insufficient. In any evaluation, there will almost universally be more information needed than provided, and the goal to be realized is the successful collection of a maximal amount of information in the time allotted. The evaluator should develop a sense for which information is most important and germane, and a routine within the treatment setting for a collection of information that may not have been available at the time the evaluation was conducted. The evaluation should be viewed as a preliminary venture that sets the stage for a team of professionals to become involved in more in-depth diagnostics and evaluations. Treatment plans that will subsequently be established will be preferentially or detrimentally impacted by the quality of this initial evaluation. It is my contention that allied health professionals in the field of TBI have an ethical responsibility to put forth the effort necessary to conduct a thorough, comprehensive, and accurate evaluation.

References

1. Ashley, M. J., Persel, C. P., and Krych, D. K., Changes in reimbursement climate: Relationship among outcome, cost, and payer type in the postacute rehabilitation environment, *Journal of Head Trauma Rehabilitation*, 8(4), 30–47, 1993.
2. Kreutzer, J. S., Kolakowsky-Hayner, S. A., Ripley, D., Cifu, D. X., Rosenthal, M., Bushnik, T., Zafonte, R., Englander, J., and High, W., Charges and lengths of stay for acute and inpatient rehabilitation treatment of traumatic brain injury 1990–1996, *Brain Injury*, 15(9), 763–774, 2001.
3. U.S. Department of Education, National Institute on Disability and Rehabilitation Research, Traumatic brain injury facts and figures, *The Traumatic Brain Injury Model Systems National Data Center*, 5(1), 2000.
4. Eames, P., Cotterill, G., Kneale, T. A., Storrar, A. L., and Yeomans, P., Outcome of intensive rehabilitation after severe brain injury: A long-term follow-up study, *Brain Injury*, 10(9), 631–650, 1996.
5. Wood, R. L., McCrea, J. D., Wood, L. M., and Merriman, R. N., Clinical and cost-effectiveness of postacute neurobehavioural rehabilitation, *Brain Injury*, 13(2), 69–88, 1999.

6. Gray, D. S. and Burnham, R. S., Preliminary outcome analysis of a long-term rehabilitation program for severe acquired brain injury, *Archives of Physical Medicine and Rehabilitation*, 81(11), 1447–1456, 2000.

7. Bell, K. R. and Tallman, C. A., Community reentry of long-term institutionalized brain-injured persons, *Brain Injury* 9(3), 315–320, 1995.

8. Johnston, M. V. and Lewis, F. D., Outcomes of community reentry programmes for brain injury survivors. Part 1: Independent living and productive activities, *Brain Injury* 5(2), 141–154, 1991.

9. Ashley, M. J. and Persel, C. S., Traumatic brain injury recovery rates in postacute rehabilitation of traumatic brain injury: Spontaneous recovery or treatment? *Journal of Rehabilitation Outcome Measurement*, 3(4), 15–21, 1999.

10. Fryer, L. and Haffey, W., Cognitive rehabilitation and community readaptation: Outcomes from two program models, *Journal of Head Trauma Rehabilitation*, 2(3), 51–63, 1987.

11. Ashley, M. S., Persel, C. S., and Krych, D. K., Long-term outcome follow-up of postacute traumatic brain injury rehabilitation: An assessment of functional and behavioral measures of daily living, *Journal of Rehabilitation Outcome Measurement*, 1(4), 40–47, 1997.

12. Lezak, M. D., Brain damage is a family affair, *Journal of Clinical and Experimental Neuropsychology*, 10(1), 111–123, 1988.

13. Brooks, N., Campsie, L., Symingtom, C., Beattie, A., and McKinlay, W., The five year outcome of severe blunt head injury: A relative's view, *Journal of Neurology, Neurosurgery, and Psychiatry*, 49(7), 764–770, 1986.

14. Marsh, N. V., Kersel, D. A., Havill, J. H., and Sleigh, J. W., Caregiver burden at 1 year following severe traumatic brain injury, *Brain Injury*, 12(12), 1045–1059, 1998.

15. Muma, J. R., *Language Handbook: Concepts, Assessment, Intervention*, Prentice Hall, Englewood Cliffs, NJ, 1978.

16. Perlesz, A., Kinsella, G., and Crowe, S., Psychological distress and family satisfaction following traumatic brain injury: Injured individuals and their primary, secondary and tertiary carers, *Journal of Head Trauma Rehabilitation*, 15(3), 909–929, 2000.

17. Corrigan, J. D., Bogner, J. A., Mysiw, W. J., Clinchot, D., and Fugate, L., Life satisfaction after traumatic brain injury, *Journal of Head Trauma Rehabilitation*, 16(6), 543–555, 2001.

18. Tennant, A., MacDermott, N., and Neary, D., The long-term outcome of head injury: Implications for service planning, *Brain Injury*, 9(6), 595–605, 1995.

19. Auerbach, S. H., The postconcussive syndrome: Formulating the problem, *Hospital Practice* [*Off Ed*], 22(10A), 9–10, 12, 1987.

20. Klonoff, H., Low, M. D., and Clark, C., Head injuries in children: A prospective five year follow-up, *Journal of Neurology, Neurosurgery, and Psychiatry*, 40(12), 1211–1219, 1977.

21. McMahon, B. T. and Shaw, L. R., *Work Worth Doing: Advances in Brain Injury Rehabilitation*, PMD Press, Orlando, FL, 1991.

22. Teasdale, G. and Jennett, B., Assessment of coma and impaired consciousness: A practical scale, *Lancet*, 2(7872), 81–84, 1974.

23. Giacino, J. T., Ashwal, S., Childs, N., Cranford, R., Jennett, B., Katz, D. I., Kelly, J. P., et al., The minimally conscious state: Definition and diagnostic criteria, *Neurology*, 58(3), 349–353, 2002.

24. The Commission on Accreditation of Rehabilitation Facilities, *Medical Rehabilitation Standards Manual*, Commission on Accreditation of Rehabilitation Facilities, Tucson, AZ, 2002.

25. Hagen, C., Malkmus, D., and Durham, P., *Levels of Cognitive Functioning*, Rancho Los Amigos Hospital, Downey, CA, 1972.

26. Rappaport, M., Hall, K. M., Hopkins, K., Belleza, T., and Cope, D. N., Disability rating scale for severe head trauma: Coma to community, *Archives of Physical Medicine and Rehabilitation*, 63(3), 118–123, 1982.

27. Uniform Data System for Medical Rehabilitation, Functional Independence Measure (FIM), State University of New York, Buffalo, NY, 2009.

28. McPherson, K. M., McNaughton, H., and Pentland, B., Information needs of families when one member has a severe brain injury, *International Journal of Rehabilitation Research*, 23(4), 295–301, 2000.

29. McMordie, W. R., Rogers, K. F., and Barker, S. L., Consumer satisfaction with services provided to head-injured patients and their families, *Brain Injury,* 5(1), 43–51, 1991.

30. Kelly, D. F., Gonzalo, I. T., Cohan, P., Berman, N., Swerdloff, R., and Wang, C., Hypopituitarism following traumatic brain injury and aneurysmal subarachnoid hemorrhage: A preliminary report, *Journal of Neurosurgery,* 93(11), 743–752, 2000.

31. Lieberman, S. A., Oberoi, A. L., Gilkison, C. R., Masel, B. E., and Urban, R. J., Prevalence of neuroendocrine dysfunction in patients recovering from traumatic brain injury, *Journal of Endocrinology and Metabolism,* 86(6), 2752–2756, 2001.

32. Zasler, N. D., Devany, C. W., Jarman, A. L., Friedman, R., and Dinius, A., Oral hygiene following traumatic brain injury: A programme to promote dental health, *Brain Injury,* 7(4), 339–345, 1993.

33. Silverstein, L. H., Garnick, J. J., Szikman, M., and Singh, B., Medication-induced gingival enlargement: A clinical review, *General Dentistry,* 45(4), 371–376, 1997.

34. Castriotta, R. J. and Lai, J. M., Sleep disorders associated with traumatic brain injury, *Archives of Physical Medicine and Rehabilitation,* 82(10), 1403–1406, 2001.

35. Masel, B. E., Scheibel, R. S., Kimbark, T., and Kuna, S. T., Excessive daytime sleepiness in adults with brain injuries, *Archives of Physical Medicine and Rehabilitation,* 82(11), 1526–1532, 2001.

36. Carlsson, G. S., Svardsudd, K., and Welin, L., Long-term effects of head injuries sustained during life in three male populations, *Journal of Neurosurgery,* 67(2), 197–205, 1987.

37. Martin, F. N., *Introduction to Audiology,* Prentice Hall, Englewood Cliffs, NJ, 286, 1975.

38. Goodhill, V. and Guggenheim, P., Pathology, diagnosis, and therapy of deafness, in L. E. Travis (Ed.), *Handbook of Speech Pathology and Audiology,* Prentice Hall, Englewood Cliffs, NJ, 279, 1971.

39. Willis, W. D., Jr. and Grossman, R. G., *Medical Neurobiology,* 2nd ed., C. V. Mosby, St. Louis, MO, 1977.

40. Smith, C. H. and Beck, R. W., Facial nerve, in T. D. Duane and E. A. Jaeger (Eds.), *Biomedical Foundations of Ophthalmology,* Vol. 1, J. B. Lippincott, Philadelphia, PA, 1–16, 1983.

41. Muma, J. R., *Language Handbook: Concepts, Assessment, Intervention,* Prentice Hall, Englewood Cliffs, NJ, 1978.

42. Anderson, J. R., *Cognitive Psychology and Its Implications,* W. H. Freeman, San Francisco, CA, 1980.

43. Lezak, M. D., *Neuropsychological Assessment,* Oxford University Press, New York, 1976.

44. Muma, J. R., *Language Handbook: Concepts, Assessment, Intervention,* Prentice-Hall, Englewood Cliffs, NJ, 1978.

45. Fisher, A., Murray, E., and Bundy, A., *Sensory Integration: Theory and Practice,* F. A. Davis, Philadelphia, PA, 1991.

46. Muma, J. R. and Muma, D., *Muma Assessment Program: MAP,* Natural Child Publishing, Lubbock, TX, 1979.

47. Mann, L. and Sabatino, D. A., *Foundations of Cognitive Process in Remedial and Special Education,* Aspen Publishers, Rockville, MD, 1985.

48. Guyton, A. C., *Basic Neuroscience,* 2nd ed., W. B. Saunders, Philadelphia, PA, 1991.

49. Mumenthaler, M., *Neurology,* Thieme Medical Publishers, New York, 1990.

50. Levin, H. S., Grafman, J., and Eisenberg, H., *Neurobehavioral Recovery from Head Injury,* Oxford University Press, New York, 1987.

51. Jennett, B. and Teasdale, G., *Management of Head Injuries,* F. A. Davis, Philadelphia, PA, 273, 1981.

52. Prigatano, G. P., Disturbances of self-awareness and rehabilitation of patients with traumatic brain injury, *Journal of Head Trauma Rehabilitation,* 20(1), 19, 2005.

53. Snow, P., Douglas, J., and Ponsford, J., Conversational discourse abilities following severe traumatic brain injury: A follow-up study, *Brain Injury,* 12(11), 911–935, 1998.

54. Hartley, L. L. and Jensen, P. J., Narrative and procedural discourse after closed head injury, *Brain Injury,* 5(3), 267–285, 1991.

55. Moncur, J. P. and Brackett, I. P., *Modifying Vocal Behavior,* Harper & Row, New York, 1974.

56. Boone, D. R., *The Voice and Voice Therapy*, 2nd ed., Prentice Hall, Englewood Cliffs, NJ, 1977.

57. Clark, H. and Clark, E., *Psychology and Language*, Harcourt, Brace, Jovanovich, New York, 1977.

58. Goodglass, H. and Kaplan, E., *The Assessment of Aphasia and Related Disorders*, Lea & Febiger, Philadelphia, PA, 1972.

59. Bouska, M. J., Kauffman, N. A., and Marcus, S. E., Disorders of the visual perceptual system, in D. A. Umphred (Ed.), *Neurological Rehabilitation*, 2nd ed., C. V. Mosby, St. Louis, MO, 1990.

60. Lepore, F. E., The neuro-ophthalmologic case history: Elucidating the symptoms, in W. Tasman and E. A. Jaeger (Eds.), *Duane's Clinical Ophthalmology*, Vol. 2, J. B. Lippincott, Philadelphia, PA, 1–6, 1995.

61. Farber, S. and Zoltan, B., Visual–vestibular systems interaction: Therapeutic implications, *Journal of Head Trauma Rehabilitation*, 4(2), 9–16, 1989.

62. Goodwin, J. A., Eye signs in neurologic disease, in W. J. Weiner and C. G. Goetz (Eds.), *Neurology for the Non-Neurologist*, 2nd ed., Harper & Row, Philadelphia, PA, 1989.

Appendix 27A: Patient Examination Report

CLIENT:	XXXXXXXXXX
AGE:	XX
DATE OF BIRTH:	XXXXXXXXXX
SOCIAL SECURITY NUMBER:	000-00-0000
DATE OF INJURY:	XXXXXXXXXX
CARRIER CASE MANAGER:	XXXXXXXXXX
CLAIM NO.:	XXXXXXXXXX
REINSURANCE:	XXXXXXXXXX
	XXXXXXXXXX
	XXXXXXXXXX
CONTACT:	XXXXXXXXXX
	XXXXXXXXXX
	(000) 000-0000
DATE OF EVALUATION:	August 18, 1995
DATE OF REPORT:	August 24, 1995

An onsite patient examination was conducted of Mr. Xxxxxx Xxxxxxxxx on August 18, 1995. The examination was conducted at the request and authorization of Mr. Xxxxxx Xxxxxxx, Assistant Vice President, Xxxxxxx Xxxxxxxxxxx Corporation. Present and/ or interviewed during the examination were Mr. Xxxxxx Xxxxxxxxx, Ms. Xxxx Xxxxx, Mr. Xxxxxx Xxxxxxx, and Mrs. Xxxxx Xxxxxxxxx. The examination was conducted by Xxxx X. Xxxxxx, XX, XXX-XXX, XXX, Xxxxxxxxx Xxxxxxx of Xxxxxx xxx Xxxxx Xxxxxx in Xxxxxxx, California. The examination was conducted in Dr. Xxxxx Xxxx'x office.

MEDICAL HISTORY:
AUDIOMETRY:
COGNITION:
EDUCATION:
FAMILY:
OCCUPATIONAL/PHYSICAL THERAPY:

PSYCHOSOCIAL:
SPEECH–LANGUAGE PATHOLOGY:
VISION:
VOCATION:
VOCATIONAL REHABILITATION:
IMPRESSIONS/RECOMMENDATIONS:

> Sincerely,
> NAME OF ORGANIZATION
> Name and Credentials of Examiner
> Title of Examiner

Appendix 27B: Iconic Store Cards

T	Q	M
C	Z	R
K	G	J

N	D	Q
H	K	X
T	Z	P

M

J

D

A

F

R

T

M

E

A

Y

O

W

F

L

E

R

B

A

C

M

D

T

K

Z

O

V

S	J	P
W	O	G
B	X	H

B	T	F
O	M	S
L	E	N

X	T	F
L	A	H
U	V	N

P   F   H

T   R   M

O   Y   L

L   Z   G

U   C   B

N   W   P

D   S   W

L   Q   B

U   G   J

Appendix 27C: Oral Peripheral Evaluation

Client Name   **Date**

Facial Symmetry

Rest:	Normal	Right Droop	Left Droop
Smile:	Normal	Right Weak	Left Weak
Labial Strength:	Normal	Weak	
Pucker:	Normal	Weak	
Facial Sensation:	V 1	V 2	V 3

Mandible

Rest Position:	Normal	Low	
Jaw Extension:	Normal	Right	Left
Jaw Lateralization:	Normal	Right Absent	Left Absent
Resistive Closure:	Normal	Weak Right	Weak Left

Tongue

Rest:	Normal	Right Atrophy	Left Atrophy
Tremor:	Absent	Present	
Protrusions:	Normal	Right Deviation	Left Deviation
Fasciculations:	Absent	Present	
Protrusion Strength:	Normal	Weak	
Elevation:	Normal	Weak	
Lateralization (in cheek):	Normal	Right Weak	Left Weak
Diadochokinetics:	Normal	Depressed	_____
Oral Mucosa:	Normal	Lesion(s): Describe	_____
		Mass: Describe	_____

Velopharyngeal Mechanism

Rest:	Normal	Right Droop	Left Droop
Clefts:	Absent	Present	
Ah:	Normal	Right Droop	Left Droop
Hypernasality:	Yes	No	
Gag:	Absent	Present	

Hearing: _____

Swallowing: Liquids   _____
                  Solids   _____

Vital capacity: (3 trials)
Sustained phonation: ah _____   s _____   z _____

Apraxia Battery

1. Stick out your tongue
2. Blow
3. Show me your teeth
4. Pucker your lips
5. Bite your lower lip
6. Whistle
7. Lick your lips
8. Clear your throat
9. Cough
10. Smile
11. Puff your cheeks

Dentition:	Good Repair		Poor Repair	
Dentures:	Maxillary		Mandibular	
Occlusion:	Normal	I	II	III
Describe	_____			

Corrective Lenses:	Yes	No	

Hearing Aids:	Yes	No	1 or 2
Type	_____		

Dysarthria:	Yes	No	
Severity:	Mild	Moderate	Severe

Apraxia:	Yes	No	
Severity	Mild	Moderate	Severe

Other: _____

_____

_____

Smoking:	Yes	No	How
			Much? _____

Recommendations: _____

_____

_____

_____

Speech/Language Pathologist

Part III

Case Management Themes

28

External Case Management of Brain Injury: An Overview

Jan Wood

CONTENTS

28.1 Introduction

People with traumatic brain injury (TBI) present with some of the most challenging and complex deficits related to injury of any diagnostic group. Injury to the central nervous system impacts the individual so pervasively that most systems are either directly impaired or indirectly impaired because of their interdependence with other impaired systems. As case managers think more pragmatically and less physiologically, they can see a direct translation of physical system impairments and the havoc these impairments wreak on the more functional systems of family, work, and socialization. Of course, all systems relate to one another and, as such, treatment of a specific system will necessarily impact other systems as well. The rehabilitation of a person with TBI requires a wide variety of professional services and tremendous coordination of effort to be appropriately comprehensive.

Since the late 1970s and early 1980s, advances in the field of trauma care and neuro-surgery have allowed victims of TBI to survive the initial insult and live longer than ever before. As a result, the needs of people with TBI are constantly changing, and the demands placed upon family members and caregivers to locate appropriate resources and treatment continue for the remainder of that individual's life. The availability of resources and treatment is ever changing, and thus, there has been a growing demand to have one person coordinate these services within the scope of that individual's funding resources.

Funding sources can be public (i.e., Medicare/Medicaid), private (as in accident and health or workers' compensation insurance), or simply personal funding provided by the individual or family members. In the past, coordination of complicated resources and treatment fell to social workers, nurses, claims adjustors, family members, and caregivers. Today, the case coordinator role is given the title of case manager.[1]

28.2 Case Management: Roles and Responsibilities

Case management is not new to the world of catastrophic disability. Although records of case management services can be found in the early 1900s, it was not until World War II that soldiers with complex injuries survived to live productive lives. Thus developed a need for intervention on behalf of injured individuals for coordination of necessary medical services. The proponent of this innovative concept, seeing case management as a means of controlling costs while providing the most appropriate services allowable under policies, was the insurance industry.

The field continued to grow and case management has increasingly been recognized as an essential part of health care delivery and financing systems. In 1993, through the discussion and study of the National Case Management Task Force, the Case Management Society of America approved a definition of case management. In 2002, the Case Management Society of America developed Standards of Practice and modified the definition. The definition of case management[1] is as follows: "Case Management is a collaborative process of assessment, planning, facilitation, and advocacy for options and services to meet an individual's health needs through communication and available resources to promote quality cost-effective outcomes."[p. 5]

With this definition and the Case Management Society of America role functions of assessment, planning, facilitation, and advocacy in mind, the case manager should positively impact the lives of people with brain injuries, enhancing medical care and the quality of life available to these individuals. Case managers are truly advocates, and if a survivor of brain injury were likened to a wheel, the case manager would be at the hub.

As the hub of this important process, the case manager should have basic knowledge of the following key areas: funding sources, treatment resources, social welfare benefits, vocational rehabilitation services, medicine, and most important, acceptance of disability and social issues. Case managers should operate with a knowing eye, utilizing current knowledge of available medical and therapeutic technologies; be able to provide or obtain authorizations for needed equipment and services to current caregivers; write comprehensive, cohesive reports; and conduct themselves well on the telephone. They need to have an understanding of family dynamics. They need to oversee the dollars and the sense of all that is necessary to relieve the effects of the brain injury.

The case manager should follow a process that includes the following basic elements:

- Identification of high-risk/high-cost cases
- Assessment of the person, the person's needs, and the treatment goals
- Development of a treatment plan, in conjunction with the health care team and attending physician that is responsive to the needs and goals of the person
- Implementation of needed services in a cost-effective and organized manner
- Ongoing evaluation of the treatment plan in relationship to the desired outcome
- Evaluation of case management interventions to promote quality services and evaluation of the effectiveness of case management relative to the desired and/or optimal outcomes

There are two general types of case management services: internal and external. Internal case managers are directly employed by companies that utilize case management services, such as insurance companies, hospitals/facilities, and health maintenance organizations. External case managers are contracted to represent an insurance company, a hospital, or an attorney. Internal and external case managers differ in their individual roles and how they work throughout the case management process. They do hold in common the combined roles of coordinators and educators/facilitators.

Those case managers who are internal case managers follow procedures that are governed by their employer. Case management services are quality controlled and cost driven, and the case managers are interested in achieving positive outcomes and client independence. Many times, they have direct authority to be the decision maker. Other times, they report directly to an in-house supervisor, an adjuster, a claims manager, or a utilization review coordinator.

Within a hospital or facility-based internal case management program, the case manager coordinates all the services that are available through that particular facility, based on the client's needs. In addition, they may become involved in discharge planning. It is possible that an in-house hospital or facility case manager could work directly with an insurance internal or external case manager. This can be an ideal situation in the continuum of care with maximized outcomes.

External case managers are contracted for case management services for a specific disability or to do an evaluation and make recommendations for medical treatment and services. The scope of case management services is dependent upon the agreed contract. If hired by an attorney, the case manager may be asked only to do an evaluation and make recommendations to life care planners regarding lifetime care and the continuation of rehabilitation. In other situations, an insurance company may contract with the case manager to provide the full range of case management coordination and services. In this instance, the case manager does not have the authority to be the decision maker, but reports to someone within the company with their recommendations. The case manager would then receive the authority to provide the recommended services.

Whether a case manager is an internal case manager or an external case manager, the common goal remains to facilitate maximum independence through the provision of rehabilitation treatment, services, and education. In working with a person with a TBI, the case manager identifies needs, facilitates communication, recommends appropriate treatment plans, develops and coordinates services, monitors and assesses ongoing progress, and monitors cost of the case.[2] To achieve these objectives, it is imperative that the case manager has early involvement in the case. Delay in involvement can lead to fragmentation of care and services. Ideally, case managers should be in contact with the trauma facility, the physician, and the injured individual within the first 24 to 48 hours following injury. They should establish early personal contact with the family. This will allow collaboration of claims and rehabilitation personnel and development of an early understanding of the individual with the brain injury, the family, and the interaction between the two.[2]

28.3 The Role of Family

The case manager needs to obtain a preinjury history regarding the primary language, educational achievement, and work history of the injured individual. Consideration should be given to cultural perceptions of disability and rehabilitation because this may have an effect on recovery and family involvement. The existence of substance abuse problems should be determined. The family situation should be assessed to determine whether there are small children, teenagers, elderly adults, or extended family issues to be considered. The case manager should also be aware of any family members that have substance abuse problems. The primary spokesperson for the family must be identified. This may be the spouse, a parent, a sibling, or even a friend. There should be a discussion of benefits that focuses on what services are available to the injured individual and the family in the way of monetary, medical, and rehabilitative support.

The case manager should make the family aware of medical and rehabilitative facilities, their relative assets and liabilities, and that programs are appropriate for their family member. Transfers should be facilitated, as quickly as possible, to an appropriate medical or rehabilitation center.[3] Thus, the education of the family is a primary duty of the case manager. This education should begin early so that the family can gain experience and confidence in making decisions with regard to continued care and treatment options available to their loved one. Another benefit is that families can better assist in observing the quality of care that is being provided.

The case manager needs to be aware that the family is put in a new role that will forever change the dynamics of that family unit. This change requires support and understanding. Family centered care was developed to address the needs and services required by families who have assumed the caregiver role. Also known as *family focused* care, family centered care is based on the assumption that the family, when provided appropriate information, rather than health care professionals, may know what is best for the client.[4,5] One study identified four key themes that family caregivers of TBI survivors view as important, including (1) the search for information, trust, and understanding; (2) the search for support; (3) the need to speak on behalf of the survivor; and (4) navigating the system.[6] Through the use of the Internet, some families are becoming more aware of their options and are better able to make appropriate decisions. It is evident that the client and family cannot be viewed separately, but should be viewed as a whole unit requiring complex and continuous support and services from the health care community.[7]

Discussion should be held with the injured individual, the family, and the carrier regarding all medical and rehabilitation issues. After meeting with the injured individual, the family, the carrier, the physicians, and the treating staff, outcome goals should be established and discharge planning discussed. Ideally, these goals should be agreed upon prior to the commencement of treatment and all parties should be in agreement, including the injured individual, when possible, the carrier, the family, the treating staff and physician, the case manager, and the attorney. At the same time, identification of potential sources of conflict must be made. These may include the influence of secondary gain motivators, such as supplemental income, third-party litigation, immigration status, or issues pertaining to family adjustment.

Careful monitoring of the treatment process should be ongoing to track progress toward, and achievement of, treatment goals. This is time intensive and may require daily contact with the injured individual, the family, and the facility; however, the case manager should never lose sight of the goal of independence and should be aware of the time to reduce involvement and allow independence. Communication is an integral part of this process and, as such, the case manager needs to be able to address the concerns of the individual, the family, the carrier, and the treatment team accurately, diplomatically, and comfortably.

28.4 Funding Sources and Benefits

The case manager must operate within the limitations of the funding sources that are available to the survivor of brain injury.[8] Typically, there are four main funding sources: (1) public funding, (2) accident and health insurance, (3) workers' compensation insurance, and (4) third-party liability.

28.4.1 Public Funding

Public funding may consist of Medicare,[9] Medicaid (which, in California is called MediCal), Department of Vocational Rehabilitation, Veterans' Administration Benefits, State Victims of Violent Crimes funds, school district funds, or governmental health insurance funds, such as those used in the national health care programs of Canada, England, Australia, and many European countries. The case manager needs to be able to identify quickly what can be authorized under these programs because there are varying limitations regarding what equipment, services, and other benefits can be provided.

It is always useful to understand the motivations that drive decisions made by personnel of different funding sources regarding authorization, or withholding of same, for treatment. Generally, sources such as state or federally funded ones are less motivated to provide rehabilitation services. Usually, they are primarily interested in whether a service is allowed under existing guidelines, as well as whether the provider of those services is registered with, or authorized by, the funding organization. Unfortunately, there is often less interest in the person's need for services or in whether prescribed services will enhance quality of life, reduce the cost of care, or provide long-term reduction in cost of care by reducing level of dependence.

On the other hand, some governmental funding sources may be more interested in what services are required and less with what they will cost. This is the case, particularly, for those individuals covered by governmental insurance plans outside the United States. Some governmental plans are beginning to use case management services, however, in an effort to gain a better understanding of resource availability and exercise some control over resource utilization.

The case manager attempting to utilize public funding sources will need to be persistent in pursuit of such funding. It is sometimes useful to encourage families to call upon elected officials to enlist their support in securing funding. Bureaucratic systems require a great deal of time and effort to obtain funding. In some cases, it is helpful to be aware of public law that may mandate provision of services (e.g., Public Laws 94 to 142 pertaining to school district funding) or to be aware of precedent cases that may have been funded for similar services (e.g., Veterans' Administration funding).

28.4.2 Accident and Health Insurance

Most policies have limits regarding the amount of money that can be spent over the lifetime of an individual or have time limitations on certain services such as a 60- or 90-day limitation for rehabilitation. The more severe limitations are typically seen with health maintenance organization plans. There is usually more flexibility available under nonhealth maintenance organization accident and health policies. In any situation, the case manager must determine the most appropriate treatment plan within the scope of the available benefits. It is important that contact be made as quickly as possible, particularly in the situation when there are time limitations involved in benefit availability.[10]

In some instances, it becomes necessary to provide services other than those specifically allowed under the insurance contract to facilitate the best treatment for the person with brain injury. Successful arguments can frequently be made regarding the advisability of extension of contract coverage for services or facilities that are not usually covered. These arguments are often successful when presented in terms of the cost savings to be realized on an immediate basis by utilization of the alternative or noncovered services or facilities. An example of this would be the use of skilled nursing facility benefits to fund participation in a postacute rehabilitation facility.

The case manager should be aware that arrangements such as these are not usually made at the claims level. Many companies utilize internal case managers, nurses, or physicians to assist in such determinations and maintain oversight on catastrophic cases for the carrier. Thus, the external or independent case manager may need to request that the carrier's case manager become involved in any decision regarding provision of extracontractual services. The external case manager then acts as a liaison between the accident and health insurer and the injured to facilitate appropriate services.

Once again, the motivation of the carrier will come into play in the decision-making process for provision of services. Generally speaking, the driving force tends to be one of short-term cost containment. This arises from the fact that, often, the accident and health contract has specific time limitations applicable to benefit provision. This varies, however, with whether the injured individual was the employee covered by the policy or a family member of same.

When the injured person is also the employee, contract coverage may be terminated at 1 year after the last premium is paid by the employer. Of course, the COBRA (Consolidated Omnibus Budget Reconciliation Act) protection may extend the coverage period; however, these monthly premiums are expensive and therefore prohibitive for many persons, especially when household income drops by the amount of the injured person's paycheck. When the individual with brain injury is a family member of the employee, however, contract coverage will continue unless the employee changes employment or the employer changes accident and health companies. In the circumstance of an injured dependent, the carrier may take a somewhat long-term view of the case with short-term cost containment becoming less crucial.

In any event, the case manager should be prepared to discuss how a recommended treatment plan will provide either more service for the same amount of money, thereby requiring less treatment time overall, or how the treatment plan will provide the same treatment for less money. The case manager should not choose or recommend a facility on the basis of cost but, rather, should communicate the benefits of a chosen facility to a potentially reluctant carrier.[11]

28.4.3 Workers' Compensation

Those individuals who have been injured while on the job come under the umbrella of workers' compensation with a limited number of exceptions (Jones Act for seamen and railroad workers). Workers' compensation is a "no fault" system that allows for all medical treatment that is reasonable and necessary to cure and relieve the effect of the injury. In cases when the individual is seriously injured, medical treatment may be required over the remainder of that individual's life.

Since 2005, most states have introduced legislation to reform workers' compensation laws. These bills include the establishment of Medical Fee Schedules, adoption of the Medicare Fee Schedule as the standard, deployment of penalties to reform inappropriate behaviors, adoption of nationally based treatment guidelines, electronic exchange of data from provider to payer, electronic exchange of data from insurer and claim administrator to the state compensation boards, redefinition of accident/injury/illness, establishment of utilization review programs, and the development of workers' compensation provider networks. The networks mirror the health care networks provided to employees by employer-sponsored health care benefits plans with one exception. Worker's compensation networks cannot limit the total amount paid out on any given employee for the life of a claim like health benefits program.[12] The case manager must have knowledge of these issues to select the most appropriate treatment and goals for the industrially injured.[13,14] The case manager should also be attuned to differences in workers' compensation benefits and their administration because these benefits vary from state to state.

As is sometimes seen with accident and health coverage, workers' compensation carriers may utilize an internal case management staff. This staff may be separate from, or part of, the claims staff. In any event, it may be necessary for the external case manager to coordinate with a carrier's internal case management staff.

In the past, the workers' compensation carrier was generally motivated to reduce the long-term costs associated with care for a catastrophically injured worker by provision of the best medical and rehabilitative services early on during the recovery process. With mandated utilization review and nationally recognized treatment guidelines, the carrier has become interested in short-term cost savings, shorter lengths of stays, and the appropriateness of less expensive treatment facilities. The workers' compensation carrier needs to know the broad and long-term perspective on how cost and quality of care interact on both a short- and long-term basis. The case manager must be in a position to demonstrate how this will be accomplished by any medical or rehabilitative venue that is to be proposed using the guidelines and review systems that are available.

28.4.4 Managed Care

Today's managed care programs evolved from the concern of third-party payers and benefit providers about seemingly uncontrollable and spiraling health care costs. In addition to the number of health claims filed, it appeared that the administration of care services lacked any formal mechanism by which costs and expenses could be monitored. Third-party payers responded by developing plans that returned control of heath care administration to the funding source through simple, contractual arrangements with selected care providers within a local community network. The purpose of contracting with selected physicians and facilities was simply to control costs.[15] The basis of managed care is dependent on four principles:

1. Networking of physicians, hospitals, and other providers into organized groups to facilitate cost-effectiveness of health care services.
2. A team of health care professionals and administrators that examines the resource usage pattern in patient care usually conducts utilization reviews.
3. Assignment of a primary care physician who functions as a gatekeeper for service delivery.
4. Payment capitation—predetermined payment rates for service.

Managed care has nearly 100% market penetration in many parts of the United States. Under this model, individuals are quickly moved through the system.[16] Lengths of stays in hospital and rehabilitation facilities are greatly reduced. Managed care plans typically cover only 60 days of rehabilitation and sometimes provide no rehabilitation at all. Managed care plans rarely cover home and community-based health care services, such as nursing and personal assistance services. Managed care plans often have annual or lifetime caps for certain conditions or treatments. Consumers are often denied benefits based on narrow definitions of "medical necessity" because these definitions are based on the health care needs of the "average person." The case manager working in this environment must be aware of what benefits are available and what is necessary to supersede the contracts to obtain services.[15]

28.4.5 Third-Party Liability

Claims that fall within third-party liability are the result of injuries that may have occurred at work or in an automobile accident but have a causation that is from a third party. For example, a worker at a furniture maker, working with a saw that suddenly blows apart, pieces striking the worker in the head, may initially appear to be solely a worker's compensation claim but, upon investigation, faulty equipment from the saw manufacturer is the true cause. Litigation is pursued by both the worker's compensation carrier for reimbursement of benefits that have been paid and by the injured worker for damages and future benefits that occurred as the result of the faulty saw. Falling within this group of claims are injuries that are the result of medical malpractice, product liability, employers' liability, individual negligence, and subrogation.

Case management for litigation cases can be quite different from other types of case management. The litigious process often requires that positions concerning both immediate and long-term care need to be taken. Because the litigation process can be simplistically viewed as one of negotiation, the parties to this process may adopt views and positions that are seemingly extreme. The parties move through a process that will culminate in a settlement or judgment with which all parties must live.

The parties to the defense often have a goal of minimizing the financial impact of any case. Some approach the process by expert evaluation and testimony. Others combine evaluation and testimony with attempts to direct the care and rehabilitation of the injured individual. The case manager may be in a position to provide expert testimony and/or case management services pertaining to required treatment or care.

The parties for the plaintiff often have the goal of securing required treatment for the individual. They also attempt to address long-term needs of the individual to ensure that these needs may be used to secure appropriate care and/or treatment for the individual. They may also be asked to participate in expert testimony or life care planning.

Because litigation cases may not always have intact funding sources for securing care and treatment, the case manager may need to solicit services for the injured individual on a lien basis. Care should be taken to disclose the nature of the case to the provider carefully, allowing the potential provider of service to discuss the legal issues with the individual's attorney. The merits of the actual legal case may impact the willingness of the treating facility to accept the case on a lien basis. The case manager should be aware that, in cases when less than ideal judgments or settlements are reached, the case manager and/ or providers may be approached, after the fact, to discount bills substantially. Thus, these cases carry some financial risks not typical to other types of funding.

The case manager must be vigilant regarding the fact that some cases may have third-party litigation pending even though the primary payer source is workers' compensation or accident and health insurance. The presence of pending third-party litigation has been observed, in some cases, to impact negatively the overall direction of ongoing rehabilitation efforts.

In cases when there is no other funding source available, the case manager may be able to utilize public funding sources, either singly or in combination, to secure care and/or treatment for the injured individual. These sources may also file a lien for payment for the services that they provide. Care should be taken to advise all parties that the care and/ or treatment is being provided on the basis of what can be paid for, as opposed to what is ideal for the individual, to avoid undesirable liability issues later on.

28.5 Life Care Planning

Life care planning is an effective method for the prediction of future care costs and was introduced in 1985 as a guideline for determining damages in civil litigation cases. Life care planning has continued to grow, change, and modify the scope of practice associated with brain injury case management.

A life care plan is defined as follows: "A dynamic document based upon published standards of practice, comprehensive assessment, data analysis, and research that provides an organized, concise plan for current and future needs with associated costs for individuals who have experienced catastrophic injury or have chronic health care needs."[17, p.iii]

In the field of case management, the life care plan is produced by a life care planner. The planner should be certified and should have an understanding of brain injury. The life care planner must obtain and review a complete copy of the medical records, including nurse's notes, physician orders, emergency records, admission and discharge reports, and laboratory and radiographic reports. An initial interview should take place with the appropriate people, including the injured person, family members, and caregivers. Topics to be discussed should include the living situation, medications, supplies, and equipment used. A review of all daily activities should be included. It is also necessary to consult with the treatment team and the treating physician to obtain information regarding future medical care and treatment. The life care plan should include frequency of the service or treatment, cost, duration of the treatment, source of information, and, perhaps, vendors for the services. Research should be done with regard to life expectancy to determine the need for future changes in living arrangement resulting from aging with a brain injury.

Life care plans serve several purposes: (1) to assist the attorney in determining the value of the brain injury case for settlement purposes, (2) to assist the insurance carrier to determine and set the financial reserves on the brain injury case, and (3) to assist the treating physician to set long-range goals and living arrangements.

Certified life care planners have standards of practice and ethical values that they follow.

> These values include:
>
> - All individuals with catastrophic disabilities have worth and dignity.
> - Life care plans are designed to facilitate and maximize functional capacity and independence for persons with catastrophic disabilities.
> - The systematic process of life care planning and related catastrophic case management is conducted in an objective and fair manner within the context of family, community, and employment systems.
> - Comprehensive and integrated services are the focus of life care planning and based on individual involvement, personal assets, and a sense of equal justice from all involved parties."[18, p.16]

Each life care plan requires creativity, compassion, and the realization that lives have changed forever. The life care plan may be the best and only opportunity to put some of the broken pieces back together and offer hope for the future.[17]

Many life care plans are used to determine the settlement value of a claim. Because of the changing needs of a brain-injured individual, especially those with moderate to severe injury, a structure settlement would be the most appropriate form of settlement. A structure settlement is a settlement used to purchase an annuity from a life insurance company. It is recommended that the life insurance company have a rating from AM Best, which rates the company's financial stability. The better the rating, the better the financial stability. It provides monthly funds to take care of the medical needs of the injured individual. It may also provide funds for monthly finances. All funding is based upon a thorough analysis of the future needs of the individual, usually based on a life care plan and any long-term financial benefits the individual may be entitled to receive, such as permanent disability in workers' compensation. Consideration must also be made regarding any Medicare benefits or Social Security disability benefits the individual may be receiving. Should this situation occur, Medicare requires a set-aside be arranged for monies that would cover medical care that Medicare might pay for in the future. Within the structure settlement, a set-aside account is funded. After the initial setup monies, annual funds are deposited into an account with the sole purpose of paying for medical expenses, including doctor visits, hospitalization, physical therapy, and prescription drugs.

28.6 Cost Analysis

Ideally, the case manager should be informed of a new case within the first 24 to 48 hours. The case manager will be better able to take charge of the case and direct the injured individual to the appropriate programs. It may be necessary to educate the claims departments on the various programs that will be needed to ensure maximum independence for the TBI survivor. This can be accomplished by presenting a cost–benefit analysis, along with recommendations on the appropriate course of care. The analysis is one means to ensure the optimal delivery of care to a person with a brain injury by suggesting alternatives in treatment plans. The case manager reviews the cost savings of providing long-term care with minimal rehabilitation versus a more aggressive rehabilitation program, and the costs that are required to provide this program. The case manager should review the analysis with one eye on functional outcome. Should the selection of a program that may cost more produce a better outcome, the cost savings are realized later when the patient has stabilized. The cost of long-term placement may seem more economic within the first few years of the case; however, a cost–benefit analysis will be able to show that more aggressive rehabilitation will save money in the long term. Cheaper is not always better.

28.7 Continuum of Care

With the development of brain injury programs, the traditional modes of fragmented medical and rehabilitation treatment are no longer appropriate to meet the complex needs of this population.[18] The ideal system flows from onset of the injury/disease and is designed to achieve the maximum recovery and lowest long-term costs. This may include early acute management, treatment in an acute rehabilitation center, and treatment in a postacute rehabilitation center. These may be followed by outpatient or home and community rehabilitation programming, and may continue with long-term care, thereby illustrating the continued need for case management services. As people with a brain injury enter this system, their needs tend to evolve with each step in the recovery process. Education of both the injured individual and the family should be ongoing throughout the continuum of care.

The continuum of care begins in the field with emergency care, followed by admission to the emergency room or trauma center. After possible surgical intervention, the individual may be transferred to the intensive care unit or general medical unit, remaining in an acute hospital setting. Depending upon the severity of the injury, the individual may be transferred to an acute rehabilitation center or begin to receive structured rehabilitative therapies while in the intensive care unit or acute setting. Should the individual remain in a comatose or persistent vegetative state, a coma stimulation program may be initiated in an attempt to improve arousal and level of awareness.

Postacute rehabilitation services, covering both transitional living facilities and community reentry programs, were developed during the late 1970s in direct response to the less than desirable discharge options available at that time following acute rehabilitation. In the majority, these are community-based residential programs, and they serve to facilitate reentry or reintegration into society at the highest functional level possible for a given individual. As such, they are often an appropriate interim step between the acute rehabilitation hospital and return to home. When necessary, the individual may continue on to a day treatment or outpatient program, where ongoing rehabilitation and vocational issues can be further addressed. Behavioral rehabilitation programs exist for those individuals who exhibit severe neurobehavioral problems during recovery that are difficult to control.[19]

When home is not a suitable discharge option, a supervised or supportive living program may be considered as a logical next step. These are usually group living situations, which often use resources within the community for day activities. In addition, specialized long-term care facilities exist for those individuals who require skilled nursing or constant monitoring or who, for other reasons, including neurobehavioral problems, are not able to return to the home and community from which they came.

28.8 Facility Assessment

The case manager must certainly have up-to-date information regarding resources that can be utilized for a given individual's continuum of care. This places a great deal of responsibility on the case manager to develop a thorough understanding of available resources. The question that must be carefully and critically posed, then, concerns what to look for in a brain injury rehabilitation program.[3,8,9,16]

The following outlines a number of areas that the case manager should be aware of when assessing a facility (see the Appendix for the checklist form):

   I. Facility experience
     A. Has the facility been open longer than 2 years?
     B. Does the program specialize in brain injury?
     C. Does the program handle behavioral clients?
     D. Does the program specialize in community reentry?
     E. Does the program specialize in cognitive retraining?
     F. Does the program specialize in vocational rehabilitation?
     G. Does the program specialize in return to work?
     H. Does the program have a supportive living program?
  II. Personnel qualifications
     A. Does the program employ all professional staff?
     B. Does the program employ or contract with
        1. A physical therapy staff?
        2. An occupational therapy staff?
        3. A speech–language pathology staff?
        4. An educational staff?
        5. A neuropsychology staff?
        6. A clinical psychology staff?
        7. A nursing staff?
        8. A recreational therapy staff?
        9. A social services staff?
        10. A community staff?
     C. Do these staff members have professional licenses?
     D. Are these licenses available for review?
     E. Is each professional assigned to one facility 100% of the time?

    F. Do licensed professionals provide more than half the treatment for their discipline?

    G. Are assistants used to provide treatment?

    H. Does the assistant provide more than half the treatment?

    I. Is the assistant certified?

    J. Does the program have a medical director?

    K. Does the program regularly obtain medical consultations for patient health issues?

    L. Does the program regularly obtain medical consultation for patient program issues?

    M. Does the program have a core of senior staff with more than 2 years of experience?

    N. Has the core of senior staff been employed by this program longer than 2 years?

III. Peer review

    A. Is the opinion of the professional community outside the program favorable?

    B. Does the program seek input for programming purposes from the case manager?

    C. Does the program consider the case manager part of the treatment team?

    D. Is the staff able to answer questions concisely, in layperson terms?

    E. Do the answers make sense?

    F. Is senior and treating staff available for consultations or to answer questions?

    G. After discharge, does the program continue to follow the client?

IV. Services provided

    A. Is the program residential?

    B. Is therapy performed in the residential setting?

    C. Is therapy performed in a separate setting from the living environment?

    D. Is therapy conducted in a community setting?

    E. Is more than half of therapy conducted on a one-on-one therapist-to-client basis?

    F. Are the programs custom tailored to meet the individual's needs?

    G. Is the program able to prepare the client for the intended discharge setting?

V. Patient evaluation criteria

    A. Was the preadmission evaluation performed by other than marketing staff?

    B. Did the evaluation include a thorough review of medical records?

    C. Were goals stated in the evaluation?

    D. Did the evaluation include an estimate of discharge living status?

    E. Did the evaluation provide a length of time the program will take to accomplish the goals stated in the evaluation?

    F. Did the evaluation include a detailed projection of treatment costs?

    G. Did the evaluation provide you with more information than you had before the evaluation?

VI. Communication and documentation

    A. Does the program provide detailed weekly reports?

    B. Are the reports clear, concise, and easy to read?

    C. Are goals reevaluated on a monthly basis?

    D. Are goals set appropriately?

    E. Do treaters educate the injured individual?

    F. Do treaters educate the family?

VII. Price structure

    A. Is fee-for-service billing available?

    B. Is the program billing easily audited?

    C. Are complete reports provided in the billing?

    D. Does the program participate in discounting practices?

    E. Does the program charge for evaluation services?

    F. If the program charges a *per diem* rate, is the number of hours of therapy and treatment defined?

    G. Does the program bill according a fee schedule?

28.9 Working with the Person with TBI

Many case managers work not only with catastrophic cases but also with other disabilities that would not be considered catastrophic injuries. TBI, spinal cord injury, and burn injury differ from any other diagnosis in that the involvement of a case manager has the potential for lasting the longest period of time.

The majority of TBI individuals will have long-lasting demonstrable deficits. The process of recovery and rehabilitation is a long-term one. The need for environmental structure and environmental modification cannot be overstated with this population. Of course, the rehabilitation process seeks to reduce the dependence upon environmental modification and structure. However, it is fair to say that various levels of severity of injury, together with varying personalities, will culminate in equally variable needs for environmental modification and structure.

Perhaps one of the most striking differences in case management of the TBI individual has to do with the pervasiveness of deficits. There seems to be no other disability in which functional realms are so diversely impacted. TBI can affect all aspects of living, including cognitive, emotional, psychological, physical, communicative, social, educational, recreational, perceptual, visual, intellectual, vocational, and, most important, changes in family structure.

It is important to realize that, as the case manager interacts with the individual and his or her family, the very nature of observed changes in personality for the injured individual and for roles and responsibilities within the family mandates an interaction with the individual and his or her family on a highly personal and private level. It is far too easy to misinterpret these changes and to be caught up in them. It is also easy to personalize behaviors of either the injured individual or his or her family. It is of paramount importance that the case manager be able to be of support to the injured individual and family yet, at the same time, maintain a professional distance that will allow maintenance of objectivity in the long term.

The psychological and emotional impact of case management of the those with TBI on the case manager can be considerable. As such, the case manager must frequently evaluate the level of personal involvement contrasted to personal detachment to maintain professional objectivity efficaciously.

The case manager should ensure that treaters have a full understanding of preinjury dynamics involved in personality, family, social, academic, vocational, and medical matters. There is perhaps no stronger influence on outcome than preinjury characteristics in these areas. There is, frequently, assumption made about skill sets in one or more of these areas by allied health professionals. Likewise, there is, often, projection of personal morals, values, and cultural norms by allied health professionals to their patients. The case manager should be ever vigilant for these occurrences and should attempt to ensure that the medical and rehabilitative care is directed by the morals, values, and cultural norms of the injured individual and his family. Counseling can be invaluable in the pursuit of a good balance therein.

The case manager needs to be aware of the role of iatrogenesis in the management of the TBI individual. Iatrogenesis refers to treatment-induced conditions and can arise not only from surgical intervention but from pharmacologic intervention as well. The case manager should scrutinize all pharmacologic and surgical interventions and consider them together with other life events that may be occurring concomitantly in the injured individual's life. It is not uncommon to find that iatrogenic conditions (e.g., medication side effects) are treated inappropriately. Medication side effects may very well be treated by additional medications rather than by titration of medication dosage.

The case manager should realize that there is perhaps no other disability category in which intensity of treatment and dollars expended, especially early on, equate with dollar savings and better outcomes in the long term.[19,20] The case manager should understand that, in the vast majority of cases, the TBI individual is quite capable of learning. As a consequence, therapy should be conducted in a fashion that facilitates learning and has, as its basis, the idea that the brain-injured individual can, in fact, learn.

28.10 Summary

The case manager carries on a delicate balance of meeting the needs of the TBI person and meeting the needs of all other parties involved. It is not uncommon for financial or legal parties, in particular as referral sources, to wield significant pressures for the case manager to utilize specific approaches to the rehabilitation process. The case manager must carefully evaluate the influence of all motivators on decisions of a case. The primary rule of thumb to be followed is that, if the injured individual will gain substantial benefit from a particular treatment, all other parties will benefit. The temptation may be present to lean in the direction of a plaintiff or defense attorney, for example, or in the direction of a parent or spouse. However, the case manager must be able to maintain a neutral high ground that focuses on the needs of the injured individual first, considering the needs and desires of others secondarily.

The goal of the case manager in a brain injury case is to impact the individual's life positively to minimize long-term changes in living and occupational status, and to improve independence and minimize disability level. All goals should support each other and must be congruent with each other. The case manager is the individual's advocate, who speaks for that individual across teams and disciplines to keep the decision makers focused. As the rehabilitation process proceeds, case managers should broaden their role and help injured individuals and their family advocate for themselves.[21]

The case manager is an integral part of the rehabilitation process and, as such, has a responsibility to enhance the overall process. Good, thorough rehabilitation is a winning scenario for society, the funding sources, the family, the case manager, and, most important, the person with TBI.

References

1. Case Management Society of America, *Standards of Practice for Case Management*, rev., CMSA, Little Rock, Arkansas, 2002.
2. Gambosh, M. F., Who's in charge?, *Continuing Care*, 28, 1991.
3. Durgin, C. J., Rath, B., and Dales, E., The cost of caring: Balancing the human and economic factors when justifying costs of brain injury rehabilitation, *Continuing Care*, 10(10), 21–23, 29–30, 1991.
4. Titler, M. G., Bombei, C., and Schutte, D. L., Developing family focused care, *Critical Care Nursing Clinics of North America*, 7(2), 375–386, 1995.
5. Rutledge, D. N., Donaldson, N. E., and Pravikoff, D. S., Caring for families of patients in acute or chronic health care settings, part 1, *Online Journal of Clinical Innovations*, 3(2), 1–26, 2000.
6. Smith, J. E. and Smith, D. L., No map, no guide: Family caregivers' perspectives on their journeys through the system, *Care Management Journals*, 2(1), 27–33, 2000.
7. Goodman, D. L., Durham, R., and Easterling, P., Continuum of care approach to severe traumatic brain injury, *Journal of Care Management*, 8(3), 31–36, 2002.
8. Batavia, A. I., Book reviews: The payment of medical rehabilitation services: Current mechanisms and potential models, *Journal of Rehabilitation Administration*, 14, 90, 1990.
9. France, R. G. and Goodrich, D. F., The Medicare prospective payment system: Implications for rehabilitation managers, *Journal of Rehabilitation Administration*, 12, 33, 1988.
10. Kowlsen, T., The balancing act, *Continuing Care*, 18, 1991.
11. McNeill, B. E., A case manager's guide to provider evaluation, *Case Management Advisor*, 1990.
12. Brown, T., Legislative trends in workers' compensation, *Case in Point*, 78, 69–71, 2008–2009.
13. McIntyre, K. J., Marriott medical management: Nurses help cut work comp medical bills, *The Case Manager*, 32, 1991.
14. Goka, R. S., Case management: A rehabilitation physician's perspective, *Journal of Insurance Medicine*, 23(4), 252–255, 1991.
15. May, V. R., Turner, T., Taylor, D., and Rubin, S., The life care planning process and certification: Current trends in health care management, part 1, *Journal of Care Management*, 6(1), 38–46, 2000.
16. Demoratz, M., Community reintegration following a brain injury, *Care Management*, 7(5), 35–37, 2001.
17. Weed, R. O., *Life Care Planning and Case Management Handbook*, CRC Press, Boca Raton, FL, 1998.
18. May, V. R., Turner, T., Taylor, D., and Rubin, S., The life care planning process and certification: Current trends in health care management, part 2, *Journal of Care Management*, 6(2), 9–20, 2000.

19. Ashley, M. J., Krych, D. K., and Lehr, R. P., Cost/benefit analysis for postacute rehabilitation of the traumatically brain-injured patient, *Journal of Insurance Medicine*, 22(2), 156–161, 1990.
20. Ashley, M. J., Persel, C. S., and Krych, D. K., Changes in reimbursement climate: Relationship among outcome, cost, and payer type in the postacute rehabilitation environment, *Journal of Head Trauma Rehabilitation*, 8(4), 30–47, 1993.
21. Moss, E. and Maxfield, D., Crucial conversations for health care: Speak up and help others do the same, part III, *Professional Case Management*, 12(3), 178–180, 2007.

Appendix

Facility Experience	Yes	No	Comments
Has the facility been open longer than 2 years?			
Does the program specialize in brain injury?			
Does the program handle behavioral clients?			
Does the program specialize in community reentry?			
Does the program specialize in cognitive retraining?			
Does the program specialize in vocational rehabilitation?			
Does the program specialize in return to work?			
Personnel Qualifications	**Yes**	**No**	**Comments**
Does the program employ all professional staff?			
Does the program employ or contract with			
— a physical therapy staff?			
— an occupational therapy staff?			
— a speech–language pathology staff?			
— an educational staff?			
— a neuropsychology staff?			
— a clinical psychology staff?			
— a nursing staff?			
— a recreational therapy staff?			
— a social services staff?			
— a community staff?			
Do the previously mentioned staff have professional licenses?			
Are these licenses available for review?			
Is each professional assigned to one facility 100% of the time?			
Do the licensed professionals provide more than half the treatment for their discipline?			
Are assistants used to provide treatment?			
Does the assistant provide more than half the treatment?			
Is the assistant certified?			
Does the program have a medical director?			
Does the program regularly obtain medical consultations for patient health issues?			

	Yes	No	Comments
Does the program regularly obtain medical consultation for patient program issues?			
Does the program have a core of senior staff with more than 2 years of experience?			
Has the core of senior staff been employed by this program longer than 2 years?			
Peer Review	**Yes**	**No**	**Comments**
Is the opinion of the professional community outside the program favorable?			
Does the program seek input for programming purposes from the case manager?			
Does the program consider the case manager part of the treatment team?			
Is the staff able to answer questions concisely, in layperson terms?			
Do the answers make sense?			
Is senior and treating staff available for consultations or to answer questions?			
After discharge, does the program continue to follow the client?			
Services Provided	**Yes**	**No**	**Comments**
Is the program residential?			
Is therapy performed in the residential setting?			
Is therapy performed in a separate setting from the living environment?			
Is therapy conducted in a community setting?			
Is more than half of therapy conducted on a one-on-one, therapist-to-client basis?			
Are the programs custom tailored to meet the individual's needs?			
Is the program able to prepare the client for the intended discharge setting?			
Patient Evaluation Criteria	**Yes**	**No**	**Comments**
Was the preadmission evaluation performed by other than marketing staff?			
Did the evaluation include a thorough review of medical records?			
Were goals stated in the evaluation?			
Did the evaluation include an estimate of discharge living status?			
Did the evaluation provide a length of time the program will take to accomplish the goals stated in the evaluation?			
Did the evaluation include a detailed projection of treatment costs?			
Did the evaluation provide you with more information than you had before the evaluation?			
Communication and Documentation	**Yes**	**No**	**Comments**
Does the program provide detailed weekly reports?			
Are the reports clear, concise, and easy to read?			

Are goals reevaluated on a monthly basis?			
Are goals set appropriately?			
Do treaters educate the injured individual?			
Do treaters educate the family?			
Price Structure	**Yes**	**No**	**Comments**
Is fee-for-service billing available?			
Is the program billing easily audited?			
Are complete reports provided in the billing?			
Does the program participate in discounting practices?			
Does the program charge for evaluation services?			
If the program charges a *per diem* rate, is the number of hours of therapy and treatment defined?			

29

Litigation and Settlement Options for the Brain-Injured Survivor

William L. E. Dussault

CONTENTS

29.1 Introduction

Individuals who have experienced traumatic brain injuries are often involved in litigation to obtain financial recoveries for the injuries they have experienced. Personal injury attorneys who work in this area typically do a wonderful job in the traditional aspects of litigation and settlement of the legal case. However, they are often completely unfamiliar with the long-term consequences of obtaining funds on behalf of the disabled client without proper planning for the long-term use and management of the funds. The same lack of awareness of the impact that resources generated from a personal injury claim held by a disabled person will have on that individual's public benefit eligibility will also make a well-intended gift or contribution from a third party have disastrous consequences for the disabled individual.

In the United States, a social service delivery system has been created over the last 35 years to assist individuals who experience disabilities. The system elements include, but are not limited to, publicly funded case management, housing of many different varieties and levels of supervision, monthly income, medical and therapy support, special education, vocational services, and social services. These services have many things in common; they are hard to obtain, require diligent advocacy, and are often inadequate in scope and nature. But they also share the feature of providing a basic level of support for the disabled individual that, if properly coordinated and managed with the individual's private resources, can significantly extend the availability of the private resources and improve the quality of life for the injured survivor.

The purpose of this chapter is to provide a basic overview of these benefit programs (collateral source benefits) and to advise how private resources from litigation or other sources may be managed in such a way as to maintain public benefit eligibility while still allowing private use of resources to supplement the public benefits.

29.2 Public Collateral Source Benefit Analysis

There are a number of federally funded public programs available for persons who have experienced catastrophic injuries and consequent disabilities. The services and funding offered through these programs can enhance their lives, and, in many instances, increase their independence. The plaintiff's personal injury attorney needs to be aware of the various benefit programs for several reasons. First, there is an argument that, as the client's "attorney of record," the attorney has an obligation, under the Rules of Professional Conduct, to assist the client with all of the client's legal needs. This certainly includes the right to various benefits that arise resulting from the client's disability (see RPC 1.2(c) re. *Scope of Representation, ABA Model Rules of Professional Conduct,* 3rd ed., Center for Professional Responsibility, American Bar Association (1996)). Second, the attorney acts in the capacity of a fiduciary, especially for a client the attorney knows, or in the exercise of reasonable professional judgment, ought to know, has limited capacity to act on his or her own behalf. The attorney cannot ignore the information regarding the client's injuries that has been collected to support the client's claim for damages. The standard of care owed to the disabled client from the attorney as a fiduciary is, arguably, much higher and should include the duty to advise of programs that are or should be available to the client. Third, through accessing various public benefit services on behalf of the client, the attorney can assist the client to obtain financial, medical, rehabilitative, and supportive services during the pendency and subsequent to the completion of the litigation process. This will assist both the client and the attorney in managing the stresses of an otherwise very difficult time. Finally, by gaining access to and working with public benefit programs, the attorney can create valuable allies in developing evidence of the client's long-term injuries and damages. As tort reform proposals continue to mutate, new rules on the admissibility of evidence on collateral source benefits are being generated and implemented on a state-by-state basis around the country. For example, in the states of Florida and Arizona, it may now be possible for defendants in a medical malpractice action to present testimony of collateral source benefits that may be used to offset the plaintiff's life care plan (see Florida Statute Ann. § 768.76 (West Supp. 1998)). Absent evidence of continued eligibility for these benefits after settlement of the litigation, the introduction of benefit evidence may result in a recovery that limits or eliminates the very benefits that were used to reduce the recovery.

Private programs for those with disabilities can be extraordinarily expensive. Individuals with disabilities have a constellation of publically funded benefit programs available to them if they meet various eligibility criteria. The extensive social service delivery system that has been created in the public sector is haphazard and uncoordinated within and among the local, state, and federal levels. Single point-of-entry systems where consumers of public disability services can obtain information or access to all of the services available do not exist. Confusion between the various service delivery agencies is the norm. Lack of information between agencies at the various government levels is typical.

The majority of funding available for publicly supported benefit programs is generated through, or in conjunction with, funding available under the Social Security Act, Chapter 42 of the U.S. Code. Most people are not aware of the number of different programs established by Congress under the aegis of this Act. All planning for individuals with disabilities must first consider the need for continued eligibility for local, state, and federal benefit programs funded through the Social Security Act (SSA). *Knowledge of the four basic, disability-related SSA benefit programs is critical.*

29.2.1 Programs That Provide Income

29.2.1.1 Social Security Retirement Benefits (SSDI): Title II, 42 U.S.C.§ 402–431

This is the principal disability and retirement income program for American workers, funded by FICA tax contributions. Disabled workers or individuals of retirement age will receive benefits. To be eligible for disability benefits under Title II (known as SSA or Social Security Disability Insurance [SSDI]) a worker must meet two tests. First, the worker must have worked and contributed sufficient funds into the Social Security system, and second, the worker must meet a disability standard.

An individual may become eligible for these benefits if they have worked a sufficient number of qualifying quarters of employment. For the typical worker, this will require that the individual has worked in 20 of the most recent 40 calendar quarters prior to an injury. A minimum amount of FICA payments will have to have been made for the worker in those 20 calendar quarters of employment. Unmarried, dependent children and grandchildren of a deceased worker or worker 65 years of age who are younger than 18 or older than 18 and disabled prior to age 22, qualify for benefits on their deceased/retired parent's or grandparent's account.

The disability definition requires that the individual be medically disabled with sufficient severity that the individual is precluded from performing "substantial, gainful activity" (competitive employment with earnings of $980.00 per month or more as of 2009, indexed annually). Title II benefits are not "means" tested; the disabled individual's assets and unearned income are irrelevant. Payment of the monthly benefit is typically made by direct deposit to the disabled person's bank account or to a "representative payee" appointed to receive and manage the payment for the disabled person by the Social Security Administration. A worker will become eligible for Title II benefits 5 months after the date the disability occurs.

29.2.1.2 *Supplemental Security Income (SSI): Title XVI*

This program provides a guaranteed minimum income to the elderly, blind, and disabled who have not made adequate contributions to their personal Social Security accounts and who do not qualify for payments under another's Social Security account to qualify for a specific minimum amount of SSDI. Currently, SSI provides a federal cash supplement of approximately $674 per month as of January 2009, indexed annually. Some states also provide supplemental payments that increase the total monthly amount received.

Eligibility for SSI is based on the same disability requirements as in SSDI noted earlier *and* upon financial need. There is no requirement for past employment or payment of FICA taxes by benefit applicants. SSI payments are not available to "inmates of a public institution," such as jails or prisons and residents of Medicaid- (known as "MediCal" in California) funded state residential or nursing care facilities. Eligibility is "means" tested (i.e., the applicant must have assets "available" to him or her of less than $2000.00, exclusive of certain "exempt" resources such as the ownership of a home, a vehicle, a burial plan and/or funeral plot worth not more than $1500.00, personal furnishings, tools of a trade, and a "plan of self-support"). A "plan of self-support" is a written plan outlining how a disabled person intends to become self-supporting. The plan must be approved by the local Social Security office and, with that approval, can generally be funded with up to $6000.00 per year. Income tests are also applied.

SSI eligibility is determined through local Social Security Administration offices. Case workers utilize the Programs Operations Manual System (POMS) as a guideline for determining eligibility. Access to the relevant POMS can be found at http://policy.ssa.gov/poms.nsf/aboutpoms.

29.2.2 Programs That Provide Medical Assistance

29.2.2.1 *Medicare: Title XVIII*

This program provides hospital (Part A), supplemental medical insurance benefits (Part B), and prescription medication coverage (Part D) for eligible participants. Congress is currently exploring possible revisions to these coverages. To receive Medicare, an applicant must be eligible for Social Security Title II benefits (SSDI). If the applicant is filing against his own account but is still younger than retirement age, as would be the case with an injured worker, or if the applicant is someone other than the individual against whose Social Security account the benefits are based (i.e., disabled dependent children or adults receiving benefits on a deceased parent's account), a 2-year waiting period is required from the applicant's date of eligibility for SSDI benefits before Medicare coverage is effective.

For individuals who have sustained a catastrophic injury, the typical waiting period is 29 months, comprised of the 5-month waiting period for SSDI and the 24-month waiting period from that initial eligibility date for Medicare. For an injured worker who receives medical insurance through work, COBRA health care continuation coverage is available for the full 29 months, but only if an election to continue coverage is made at the date of termination of employment.

The Medicare program provides only listed hospital and doctor's services, as well as some coverage for prescriptive medications. Payment is made through a local contracting agency acting on behalf of the Social Security Administration. Payment is not means tested, but coverage is limited. Some pharmaceuticals, durable medical equipment, custodial care, and residential care are not covered and there are significant copayments and deductibles for covered services and medications.

The Medicare prescription drug benefit (Part D) began in January 2006. Although many people are finding a cost benefit in the new plan, it remains controversial. The choices that must be made by the eligible beneficiaries are complex and require some intense scrutiny of complicated paperwork. Some beneficiaries are finding that costs of prescriptions under Part D are higher than they were on their prior prescription coverage plans. A basic knowledge of Part D can be obtained at www.medicare.gov following the link titled "prescription drug plan." There will still be significant deductibles and copayments even after the full benefit becomes effective. In addition, the private companies offering the coverage under Part D are not required to have all drugs available. The participant must check each company's formulary or list of available drugs to be sure the drugs they need are covered under the plan that is selected. There is substantial controversy over the cost of this plan and it may yet be reviewed and revised.

Figure 29.1 provides a convenient summarization of the income and medical coverage entitlement programs available to persons with traumatic brain injury.

29.2.2.2 Medicaid: Title XIX

29.2.2.2.1 General

Medicaid is a federally funded, state-administered, program with individual states being given a great deal of flexibility in use of funds. This program generally provides a wider variety of services than the Medicare program. Eligibility for this program is based on SSI (Title XVI) criteria for both disability and need. If an applicant meets eligibility requirements, there is no waiting period for benefit eligibility.

The Medicaid program currently provides a significant portion of state-sponsored medical care: acute care, immediate postacute care, and long-term residential care and some in-home support programs for individuals with disabilities that arise as a result of catastrophic injuries. Congress is currently considering revisions of the Medicaid Title of the SSA to emphasize usage of Medicaid dollars for community programs to encourage independence for individuals with disabilities. Medicaid funding for community-oriented programs is provided through a variety of state specific "waiver" programs. Each state applies to the Centers for Medicare and Medicaid Services (CMS) to request that the requirement that federal money be used in institutional residential programs be "waived" for a specific community-oriented population or purpose. The waivers are subject to annual review by CMS and are dependent on federal funding. Each state has at least one waiver program. Traumatic brain injury or home and community-based service waivers are among the most common.

INCOME

TITLE II – SOCIAL SECURITY ACT 42 U.S.C. § 402 DISABILITY, RETIREMENT, AND SURVIVOR'S BENEFITS (SSDI)	TITLE XVI – SOCIAL SECURITY ACT 42 U.S.C. § 1380 SUPPLEMENTAL SECURITY INCOME (SSI)

(1) Direct monthly cash benefit paid to eligible person or representative
 	
(2) Eligibility is dependent upon:
  (a) Disability, and
  (b) Contribution to Social Security system
 	
(3) <u>Not</u> means-tested
 	
Establishes eligibility for:
	(1) Direct monthly cash benefit paid to eligible person or representative
	
	(2) Eligibility is dependent upon:
	  (a) Disability, and
	  (b) Means-tested –
	    (i) Assets and resources
	    (ii) Income test
	
	(3) Contribution to Social Security system is <u>not</u> required for eligibility
	
	Establishes eligibility for:

  MEDICAL & CARE COVERAGE

TITLE XVIII – SOCIAL SECURITY ACT 42 U.S.C. § 1395 – MEDICARE	TITLE IXX – SOCIAL SECURITY ACT 42 U.S.C. § 1396 – MEDICAID

(1) Managed through local private contractors
 	
(2) Medical insurance program, eligibility for which is dependent upon eligibility under Title II – <u>not</u> means tested
 	
(3) Three types of benefits:
  (a) Part A – Hospital Benefits
  (b) Part B – Physician and out-patient services benefits
  (c) Part D – Medications
 	
(4) Program requires payment of deductibles, co-payments, premiums, and many goods and services are not covered
	(1) Managed through state agency under state and federal rules – complex
	
	(2) Is means-tested – generally related to SSI eligibility, but may be extended above SSI means-tested clients for certain benefit categories
	
	(3) Numerous services and items covered, including:
	  (a) Physicians, hospital, many therapies, prescriptions medications, and some medical devices
	  (b) Community and In-home care
	  (c) Long-term care (institutional care)
	  (d) May even pay Medicare premiums

FIGURE 29.1
Summarization of the income and medical coverage entitlement programs.

Under some of the Medicaid waiver programs, some or all of the income, assets, and resources tests for the actual recipient or related family members may be disregarded in determining eligibility for specific collateral source benefits. The following is an example of a "waiver" program that is available in many states:

In-home medical assistance for severely disabled children with substantial medical needs, often including aides/attendants, with the waiver applying to the home care costs, so that those children will not have to be institutionalized at greater cost.

The type of program just described is intended to help families to keep their severely disabled children at home and out of institutions. A family with a middle-class income generally cannot afford the noninsured costs to do this without some form of assistance. It is important to recognize that waiver programs vary from state to state, and a family's reliance upon a waiver program could eliminate or restrict interstate residence changes as a result of financial impossibility.

Medicaid is generally considered to be the most important of the federal benefit sources for individuals with disability. For that reason, more detailed information concerning Medicaid is set forth in the next section.

29.2.2.2.2 Details

Because of the interplay between federal funding and state administration, there are multiple levels of statuary, regulatory, and guideline authority for implementing the Medicaid program. Medicaid is codified at Title XIX of the Social Security Act, 42 U.S.C. § 1392 *et seq.*

(a) State Medicaid programs are governed by two general sets of requirements:

   (i) Those states that follow the SSI statute and regulations found at Title XVI of the Social Security Act, 42 U.S.C. § 1382.

   (ii) Those states that follow the more restrictive requirements that were in place at the time the Medicaid statute was established. The more restrictive states that are not limited to the SSI Rules are known as the Section 209(b) states. There are 14 209(b) states: Connecticut, Hawaii, Illinois, Indiana, Minnesota, Missouri, Nebraska, New Hampshire, North Carolina, North Dakota, Ohio, Oklahoma, Utah, and Virginia (*see* 42 U.S.C. § 1396a(f)).

(b) The primary means of determining eligibility for Medicaid are categorical.

   (i) Specific groups or categories of people are eligible if they fall within the group criteria. The major eligible categories include those persons who meet the Temporary Assistance to Needy Families (TANF) requirements and those individuals in need who meet the eligibility requirements for SSI for the elderly, blind, and disabled (the medically indigent).

   (ii) States have the option of qualifying individuals for Medicaid long-term care support as "medically needy" at income levels that are above the SSI eligibility criteria.

   (iii) Funding for Medicaid programs is provided jointly by federal and state resources. Federal statutes, regulations, and policies provide general guidelines for the program, whereas states are authorized, within certain limits of flexibility, to establish requirements on eligibility for state-operated, but partially federally funded, programs. The federal regulations are at 42 CFR 430 *et seq.* (For the Code of Federal Regulations, see http://www.access.gpo.gov/nara/cfr/cfr-table-search.html.) The CMS (formerly the Health Care Financing Administration [HCFA]) promulgates program instructions and guidelines to the states in a transmittal collectively entitled the "State Medicaid Manual," which can also be found in the Commerce Clearing House Service Medicaid and Medicare Guide. (For the "State Medicaid Manual," see http://cms.hhs.gov/manuals/45_smm/pub45toc.asp.)

   (iv) For institutionalized persons, states are generally prohibited from using eligibility criteria more restrictive than those used by the SSI Program (42 U.S.C. § 1396 A(a)(10)(C)). (For the U.S. Code, see http://www.cms.hhs.gov/Manuals/PBM/itemdetail.asp?filterType=none&filterByDID=-99&sortByDID=1&sortOrder=ascending&itemID=CMS021927) Guidance on various Medicaid issues can be found in the federal SSI statute at 42 U.S.C. § 1381–1383, the federal SSI Regulations 20 CFR 416 *et seq.*, and in the federal SSI SI-POMS.

(v)   Although the SSI income and resource limits (noted briefly previously) have been generally used as the basis for Medicaid eligibility for single individuals, amendments to the Medicaid eligibility rules enacted since 1988–1989 have resulted in significant changes applicable to married couples. In addition, resource and income limitations vary depending on whether a state is an SSI/categorical state or a 209(b) state. It is not within the scope allotted to this chapter to attempt to present the income and resource limitations on a state-specific basis. Each attorney or family will have to take the responsibility to review the state income and resource limitations for single and married persons who may be in need of Medicaid eligibility within the particular state of residence.

Prior to October, 1989, each state was given broad latitude in establishing the resource eligibility requirements for Medicaid-funded, long-term care. The result was very substantial intrastate variability in eligibility for Medicaid funded benefits.

(c)   Effective in October 1989, the Medicare Catastrophic Coverage Act (MCCA) of 1988 at Title III, Section 3, made important changes in the Medicaid program for long-term care residential options (acute care hospitals and nursing homes). The relevant provisions of the Act and the technical amendments made to it by the Family Support Act of 1988 are codified at 42 U.S.C. § 1396p(c) (Transfers of Assets) and 42 U.S.C. § 1396r-5 (Other Provisions). More changes were made in the Revenue Reconciliation Act of 1989. That 1989 federal amendment set forth minimum federal eligibility standard parameters that were required to be met by each state.

(i)   The eligibility criteria for single (unmarried) individuals for Medicaid assistance remained pursuant to the SSI/209(b) categorical models that were then being used by each state. The SSI eligibility criterion required that, to be eligible on a means-tested basis, the individual had to have total resources actually available to the individual of less than $2000.

(ii)   For SSI purposes, a resource is cash or other liquid assets and any other real or personal property that an individual (or spouse, if any) owns and could convert to cash to obtain food and shelter. If the individual had the right, authority, or power to liquidate the property, it was considered a resource.

(iii) In determining resources that count against the applicant's eligibility, certain exclusions were established, which included the following:

(1) An individuals' home, regardless of value (modified as of 2005; described later), so long as the home is the principal place of residence of the applicant. The home exclusion also applied to any contiguous land and related buildings.

(2) Household goods and personal effects of reasonable value (generally considered up to $2000). Most states do not do an exhaustive review of personal property in determining eligibility.

(3) A vehicle of value up to $4500 unless used for medically necessary or employment-related transportation, in which case no value limit applies (i.e., lift-equipped van) (value limitation removed in 2005).

(4) Burial plots or funeral plans of value up to $1500 each.

(5) Life insurance with face value of up to $1500. If face value exceeded $1500, cash surrender value counted against the $2000 resource limitation. Term-life insurance would not count as a resource.

(6) Certain federal reparations and settlement funds.

(iv) Eligibility standards for married couples were significantly modified by the MCCA of 1989.

(1) States were allowed to elect an exempt resource allocation to be set aside for the nondisabled spouse who would continue to live in the community when the disabled spouse went to a hospital or facility for long-term care. States could choose from a low of $12,000 to a high of $60,000 as the exempt resource amount. The exempt resource amount was indexed and increases on an annual basis since 1989. The maximum exemption, as of the year 2009, is approximately $109,560.00 for the nondisabled spouse.

(2) The couple's home, regardless of value, was determined to be exempt, provided that the home was transferred in ownership interest from the disabled and institutionalized spouse to the community spouse within 1 year of the institutionalized spouse's date of entry into a care placement under the Medicaid Financing Program.

(3) Both spouses were allowed to have all of the remaining exempt resources as indicated in subparagraph (c)(iii), (1) through (6), above.

(4) The MCCA provisions established time penalties if resources were transferred to anyone other than an applicant's spouse without full value being received in return (an uncompensated transfer). Those penalties were found at 42 U.S.C. § 1396 p(c). The amendments established a 30-month look-back period. If uncompensated transfers were made within the 30-month period, a penalty disqualification time was established in which an applicant could not receive Medicaid. The maximum length of the penalty period was 30 months. This penalty period has since been amended (described later).

(5) The MCCA established provisions regarding the treatment of grantor trusts created for the purpose of qualifying disabled individuals for Medicaid benefits. Those restrictions were initially found at 42 U.S.C. § 1396 a(k). Trusts established for the purpose of qualifying individuals for Medicaid were termed *Medicaid Qualifying Trusts* (MQTs). An MQT was defined as a trust or similar legal device established other than by will by an individual or an individual's spouse under which the individual may be the beneficiary of all or part of the payments from the trust and the distribution of such payments is determined by one or more trustees who are permitted to exercise any discretion with respect to distributions to the applicant. If discretion was available, the Social Security Administration was entitled to presume that payments would be made under the discretionary provisions, regardless of whether the trustee agreed to make the payments. The anomaly here is that an MQT, in fact, disqualified the beneficiary for Medicaid.

Both the provisions concerning transfer of assets and the provisions regarding the treatment of trusts were significantly amended by the 1993 Omnibus Budget Reconciliation Act (OBRA) Amendments to the

Medicaid statute. The 1993 OBRA Provisions are codified in pertinent part at 42 U.S.C. § 1396 p(a) through (e). Estate recovery requirements, transfer of asset rules, treatment of trusts, and definitions for transfer and trust provisions were all impacted by the recent amendments.

(d) Particular attention should be paid to subparagraph (c) of the 1993 amendments regarding the transfer-of-asset rules. There are no penalties for the transfer of ownership of assets between spouses. For example, assume that one spouse became seriously injured and expensive acute and postacute long-term care had to be provided. The couple had modest means, such as a house, car, and several thousand dollars in the bank. Perhaps the couple also had a modest retirement or IRA account of less than the community spouse exempt resource allowance in their state. The disabled spouse (or an appropriately authorized legal representative) could transfer ownership of all the assets owned by the disabled party or the couple to the nondisabled spouse. The disabled spouse would then qualify for Medicaid funding to pay for the needed extended care.

For transfers of assets to individuals other than a spouse, a transfer penalty period or look-back period would be imposed. The look-back period is computed under a complicated formula that resulted in disqualification for benefits for a period of up to 36 months for transfers of assets to a third party when the asset transfer was made without the donor receiving full-value compensation in return. The 36-month period is not capped. If an application for benefit eligibility was made within a 36-month look-back period, it is possible that a penalty period of longer than 36 months could be imposed. Assume an injured client had bank accounts and stocks worth $40,000.00. The client's family approached the attorney to determine if the funds could be preserved during the pendency of the development of the personal injury claim for which counsel had been employed. There are a series of strategies that were available to allow preservation of some or even all of the funds they include. Rather simple transfers to third parties could then be made in a manner that would preserve at least 50% percent of the funds. More complex transactions could have been structured to preserve all of the funds and pay them out for the client's use over an extended period of time.

(i) A penalty period of up to 60 months was called for when a transfer of assets belonging to the disabled grantor or his or her spouse was made to a trust for the benefit of the disabled grantor or spouse.

(ii) The trust provisions contained significant limitations on the use of trusts in Medicaid planning. Planning with trust options are discussed later.

(e) On December 14, 1999, the Foster Care Independence Act of 1999 (P.L. 106-169) was signed into law to be effective January 1, 2000. Provisions of this law brought the SSI eligibility criteria into congruence with the Medicaid Trust requirements. From January 1, 2000, forward, SSI and Medicaid used the same eligibility provisions as far as what constituted exempt resources held in trusts. Section 205 of this law provides, generally, that trusts established with the assets of an individual (or spouse) *will be* considered a resource for SSI eligibility purposes. It also addresses when earnings or additions to trusts will be considered income. For our purposes, the key issue in this legislation is the provision of an exception to the statutory rules for counting assets in trusts that parallel the provisions in Medicaid from sections 1917(d)(4)(A) of the SSA (42 U.S.C. § 1396p(d)(4)(A). For purposes of SSI eligibility, the exceptions are known as Medicaid trust exceptions. Although these exceptions are also SSI exceptions, the Social Security Administration also refers to them as Medicaid trust exceptions to distinguish them from other exceptions to counting trusts provided in the SSI law (e.g., undue hardship) and because the term has become a term of common usage. New POMS clarifying the relationship between the SSI and Medicaid Trust rules were issued on January 13, 2009, at POMS 01120.200-204.

(f) The Medicaid amendments included in the Deficit Reduction Act of 2005 reflect the most significant changes to the eligibility requirements for the program since OBRA '93. Although the language of the amendments indicates they are to become effective as of February 8, 2006, there has been a delay in many states in implementing the changes included in the 2005 amendment. In some states, it took as long as twelve to eighteen months to effect the new amendments on a state level. Check your state to determine the effective date of the changes in that state.

The amendments build on and extend some of the provisions of OBRA '93 in an attempt to reduce the planning tactics available to qualify middle and upper income individuals and families for Medicaid-funded benefits and services. Among the more significant changes, the look-back period of 36 months mentioned earlier has been extended to 60 months whether the transfer of assets is to a trust or an individual. Perhaps most important, the date on which the look-back period commences has been changed from the date of the actual transfer to the date when the individual requires the care for which funding is sought. Under the prior statute, if Mrs. Jones made a transfer (by gift) of $300,000 to her children on June 1, 2005, a 36-month look-back or penalty period would begin on that date. Under the new statute, up to a 60-month penalty period would be imposed but would not start to run until the individual requested Medicaid-funded services.

Annuities were often recommended as a way to "hide" resources in an exempt status and delay payment through postdeath or balloon payments that were not actuarially sound given the annuitant's actual life expectancy. New requirements for annuities have now been established. In order for the resources placed into the annuity to be considered exempt, the annuity must be irrevocable and nonassignable. It must be actuarially sound using the Social Security Administration tables and it must be in actual payment status with equal payments to be made over the term of the annuity. If a payment is to be made upon the death of the annuitant, the state Medicaid agency must be the first remainder beneficiary up to the full amount of the death payment or the amount of Medicaid assistance paid, whichever is less. The only exceptions to the beneficiary designation provisions occur where a surviving spouse or disabled or minor child survives the annuitant. The statute and regulations are unclear if structured settlement annuities are included in these new restrictions.

Where a beneficiary previously was allowed to maintain a home of any value as an exempt resource, the value of the home has now been limited to $500,000 ($750,000 as a state option). If a Medicaid applicant lives in a continuing care facility, a refundable entrance fee is considered an available resource for purposes of eligibility to the extent the individual is able to use the funds. This may require the rewriting of entrance fee contracts for these facilities either to grant a right of use of the funds for cost of care or to give the state a recovery right on a fee that is refundable only on the residents death.

As indicated here, SSI and SSDI benefits provide income via monthly payments of cash to the individual. Medicare and Medicaid provide health care coverage. Through state-specific Medicaid waiver programs, housing and attendant care is also often covered. Because of the substantial amount of funding available to state and local government service delivery agencies through the Medicaid budget, states tend to adopt the Medicaid financial eligibility criteria for entrance into many of their purely state-funded programs. Group living arrangements, including independent assisted living, foster care, adult family homes, group homes, institutional placements, and intermediate and skilled nursing placements, are often funded, in whole or in part, through this system. Day activity programs ranging from adult day care, work training, sheltered workshop, and competitive vocational placement programs may also depend on Medicaid or SSI eligibility. Case management services and social and recreational programs are also tied to this broad-based, disability-related, social service delivery system.

The loss of SSI and Medicaid eligibility will often preclude the ability of an individual with disability to access most, if not all, of the other programs available in the system. Unfortunately, the availability of private funding, such as through a personal injury settlement or judgment, will not guarantee that the individual can buy access to the same system that is available if the individual meets the SSI and Medicaid eligibility criteria. The government has a limited number of placements available within the publicly supported system. Government contracts routinely restrict access to those placements by significantly reducing public payments available to service delivery providers who accept private payment for services. The disabled individual is caught in a "Catch 22." Even if they have funds available, the use of the available funds is foreclosed by the government agencies' insistence that the private service providers reserve their service slots to agency clients. The privately funded disabled individual is often restricted to very few, very expensive, service providers who accept only private paying clients.

To gain the benefit offered by these various programs, one must obviously meet the eligibility criteria. However, it must be acknowledged that the standard of living available to an individual who has nothing but the services provided under the numerous public benefit programs will not be acceptable to most of the clients who will have access to other funds or services. Coordination of the two sources of funding (public and private) is absolutely necessary to provide a reasonably comfortable lifestyle for the disabled person, regardless of age.

In addition to the programs enunciated under the SSA, there are a wide variety of other programs that are established at the federal level that provide services to individuals who experience disabilities as a result of catastrophic accidents. Included among the more common programs are the Individuals with Disabilities Education Act (IDEA) 20 U.S.C. §1400 *et. Seq* (see http://idea.ed.gov), the Developmental Disabilities Act, the Rehabilitation Act, HUD Section 8 rent subsidy provisions, food stamps, loan programs, and so forth.

Beyond federal, means-tested programs, each state offers an assortment of partially or fully state-funded programs and assistance to persons with disabilities, which vary significantly from state to state, but which are usually means tested. For all state programs that are funded with some federal dollars, the states must agree to apply eligibility criteria that are no more restrictive than federal eligibility criteria. States are permitted to enact legislation and pass regulations regarding these programs as long as they do not contradict federal rules, statutes, and regulations on eligibility. Some common state programs include in-home aide or attendant services, vocational training and placement programs, advocacy, and case management programs.

When a settlement or judgment is achieved for an individual who is disabled as a result of a traumatic brain injury, it may be easy to assume that the individual's needs will be met with the proceeds. However, settlements and judgments are seldom adequate to meet lifelong needs for these individuals after deduction for attorneys' fees and costs, and outstanding expenses of the individual that often have accumulated to significant amounts. Federal statute requires that any assistance the individual has received through the Medicaid program be reimbursed. These factors, together with the exponential increases in medical costs we have seen in recent years, make it unlikely that the individual will net enough money from the litigation to provide for a lifetime of care. The ideal is to coordinate use of the settlement or judgment proceeds with benefits under collateral source benefit programs.

If the disabled individual receives title to the settlement or judgment proceeds, the result will certainly be ineligibility for Medicaid, SSI, and other "needs" based programs. To maximize the possibility that the disabled person will receive lifelong benefit from the settlement or judgment proceeds, it is vital to retain or establish eligibility for those programs.

In the 1993 OBRA, Congress enacted the first legislation that specifically authorized the use of court-ordered trusts for receipt of assets of disabled persons in conjunction with eligibility for Medicaid assistance. The relevant portion of the Act is codified at 42 U.S.C. § 1396p(d)(4)(A), and is included in the Appendix at the end of this chapter. As a result of this legislation, it is now possible to avoid negative impact on the disabled person's eligibility for Medicaid and many other federally funded disability-related benefit programs by directing settlement and judgment proceeds into properly crafted, court-ordered, special needs trusts.

29.3 Proper Selection of Management Devices

29.3.1 Guardianship/Conservatorship

These are the traditional vehicles for managing income, assets, and resources of persons who experience disability. Unfortunately, assets held in a guardianship or conservatorship belong to the disabled person who is subject to the court's intervention (sometimes called a *ward*) and preclude eligibility for needs-tested benefit programs if they exceed the prescribed limits. If the client is able to work and earn an amount that precludes benefit eligibility, and is expected to be able to continue working to retirement age despite the disability, placing settlement or judgment proceeds into a guardianship or conservatorship may not result in harm to the client. Even so, the expense and time required to maintain a guardianship or conservatorship are considerations that may make this option unattractive for managing settlement or judgment proceeds. The need to seek court approval for changes in investments, which greatly reduces the guardian/conservator's ability to respond to market changes, is also of concern.

Although guardianship or conservatorship may not be the optimum method for managing settlement or judgment proceeds, it can provide important protections for a disabled person who has cognitive deficits. A guardian or conservator of the estate could be appointed for a disabled adult to protect him or her from entering into exploitive contracts or from being exposed to other financial abuses. Appointment of a guardian of the person may be important to ensure adequate medical attention, for authority to give informed medical consents, and for making residential and other personal arrangements for the disabled person.

29.3.2 Spendthrift/Support Trusts

This type of trust arrangement may be adequate for a disabled individual who does not have ongoing medical needs, who is able to reside at least semi-independently, and who is able to earn a wage that is adequate, or almost adequate, to allow self-support, especially if employment benefits include medical insurance. An asset protection trust can be crafted to protect against exploitation and against creditors. However, the drawback to a "support" trust is that, if the disabled individual is unable to sustain long-term employment or sustains a subsequent injury, the trust will effectively bar eligibility for SSI and Medicaid.

29.3.3 Special Needs/Supplemental Trusts

This is the type of trust that complies with the requirements of 42 U.S.C. § 1396p(d)(4)(A) of the 1993 OBRA and prevents the assets directed to the trust from being considered available to the disabled beneficiary. Properly drafted and implemented, the resources held in the trust are considered exempt from consideration in determining benefit eligibility. This type of trust will not, by itself, ensure eligibility for SSI and Medicaid collateral source benefits. The disabled beneficiary must still meet all the disability criteria, and all the income, assets, and resources to which the applicant holds title must fall within financial eligibility criteria. If the other eligibility criteria are not met at the time such a trust is established, the special needs supplemental trust still provides all of the protections of a spendthrift support trust, while protecting the beneficiary's possible future need and eligibility for collateral source benefits.

29.3.4 Structured Settlement Annuities

Structured settlement annuities are frequently suggested and may play some role as part of a settlement achieved for a disabled person. Great care needs to be exercised here because this option has come under serious criticism in the economic climate since 2008. It must be remembered that such an annuity is a potentially lifelong investment of the disabled beneficiary's funds with little or no option for revision after purchase. Flexibility in the use of the funds and in responding to changing investment climates is not possible with a structured settlement annuity. There is no inherent protection against inflation offered, and the purchasing power of the annuity payments will decrease over time. The financial security of the issuing insurance carrier is of great concern as this chapter is being written. The financial ratings systems in place to guide insurance product purchasers have come under great criticism and are difficult to rely on at this point, so these annuities must be very carefully considered in advance.

The Internal Revenue Code sections 104 and 130, which authorize the use of a structured settlement annuity to provide tax-free income to the beneficiary, specifically provide that they are nonassignable and should not be sold or borrowed against. A secondary "gray market" has developed for the purchase of the annuities, but substantial discounts off the current value are required. It is important that sufficient settlement proceeds be left liquid over and above any selected annuity to meet unexpected needs that may, and often do, arise. A good rule of thumb for the few cases that might warrant the use of this product is that no more than one third of the net settlement available to the client be used to fund any such structure. Any structure included as part of a settlement for the disabled client should be designed to meet that client's specific anticipated needs. For example, if the client has home medical equipment that needs to be replaced every 5 years, that known need should be a factor. If the client is expected to require major surgery that may not be covered by medical insurance (or Medicaid, if eligibility is anticipated), that known need should also be a factor in designing the pay-out stream of the annuity. If the client requires a wheelchair lift-equipped van for transportation and it is expected that the vehicle will need to be replaced every 5 years, that known need should be a factor.

To obtain the income tax advantage that ostensibly results from a structured annuity settlement, the structure must typically be purchased by a defendant. For catastrophic cases, the purported tax advantage of the structured settlement annuity is usually nullified. The injured client will have medical deductions on his personal tax 1040 form that will minimize or eliminate most, if not all, income tax on the income generated on investment of the settlement funds. Maximization of income through careful investment becomes a paramount goal superseding any limited advantage generated by the tax-free income generated through the annuity. The actual rate of return generated on such an annuity is fixed as of the date of purchase. When interest rates are generally low, it must be remembered that, in this type of annuity, they will not adjust as the investment climate shifts. On the other hand, if there are concerns about undue influence for inappropriate or unnecessary expenditures because of family or other situations of the disabled person, a structured settlement annuity held in a trust may provide enhanced conservation and protection to the beneficiary. A structured settlement annuity can be made payable directly to a court-ordered trust that is established for the benefit of a disabled person.

29.4 Selection and Format of Fiduciary/Investment Manager

29.4.1 Types of Trustees

The trustee is responsible for management and investment of the trust assets and, depending upon the format of the trust agreement, is sometimes responsible for determining trust disbursements. There are several types of entities that often serve as trustees to manage special needs and other kinds of trusts. Each type of entity offers advantages and disadvantages, and a variety of factors must be considered in selecting the entity best suited to a given trust arrangement. The three most commonly used entities are institutional trustees, private trustees, and broker advisor/trustee affiliations.

29.4.1.1 Institutional Trustees

This term refers to banks and trust companies, which are traditionally the most commonly designated professional trustees. Fees among bank and trust company trustees are frequently on the higher end of the spectrum, but can often be negotiated. It is often the case that the fees for investment management services performed by bank trustees are not fully disclosed when the bank is promoting its services. Be sure to ask if separate investment fees result when the bank uses its own investment funds or those of an affiliated company. A primary advantage in using a bank or trust company as a trustee generally ensures competent, experienced management that is familiar with the relevant state and federal legislation and regulations controlling trust activities.

However, unless the specific institution has experience with special needs trust management, bank and trust company management goals may conflict with the beneficiary's needs. These institutions are most accustomed to administering trusts that contain clear and unambiguous disbursement instructions. In special needs trusts, all disbursements are discretionary. The traditional bank trust management focus is to increase and enhance the trust corpus, only making disbursements that are required. No disbursements are *required* in a special needs trust. As a result, before designating a bank or trust company as trustee, it is vital to ascertain that institution's familiarity with special needs trusts and its understanding of its role under them. If the trust is placed with a bank or other professional trustee, it is very important that the trust document clearly outline the duties and obligations of the trustee, especially as they relate to expenditures that will preserve benefit eligibility, yet still meet the disabled beneficiary's needs. General provisions granting the trustee immunity for improper distributions should be avoided.

29.4.1.2 Private Trustees

This term includes private individuals who may simply be related to or friendly with the beneficiary, and professional persons with a background that will assist them in trust management. A significant advantage to naming a private trustee is increased responsiveness to the beneficiary's evolving situation and needs. Conversely, it is also a risk that the private trustee could become unduly influenced by the beneficiary or the beneficiary's family. A private trustee is likely to serve at a comparatively low fee, but is likely to require substantial legal and accounting assistance, at trust expense. A private trustee would generally be required by the court to be bonded or insured, the cost of which would also be at trust expense. Unless the private trustee has investment expertise, investment returns are likely to be lower than would be seen in management by an institutional trustee. In addition, unless the private trustee has a great deal of experience with public benefit coordination or employs a benefit compliance manager, he or she is not likely to be familiar with the special restrictions that apply to a special needs trust.

29.4.1.3 Broker Advisor/Trustee Affiliations

Use of a specifically designated broker in conjunction with a professional trustee to manage trusts is a recent development that has evolved to meet the unique demands of special needs trusts. In this arrangement, a professional trustee (either an institutional or private trustee) is named to "hold" and manage trust assets, whereas a broker or brokerage is designated to manage trust investments. Brokers are usually better informed about various markets and investment opportunities and quicker to act on that information than are banks and trust companies. Investment performance is often better than that of a bank or trust company when this arrangement is used. The broker/brokerage is prohibited by Securities and Exchange Commission regulations from acting as a fiduciary, hence the two-part trustee arrangement. A drawback to this arrangement is that some duplication of fees generally occurs. Careful negotiations prior to appointment of the broker and professional trustee can minimize that drawback. Similarly, the broker and the trust company will need assistance to comply fully with ensuring that distributions from the trust do not compromise benefit eligibility.

29.4.2 Trust Disbursement Committees/Co-trustees

A trust disbursement committee or co-trustee is often designated in court-ordered special needs trusts to serve in conjunction with a financial trustee. The committees actually serve as a co-trustee with full fiduciary responsibility and liability for the decisions they are called upon to make. By majority vote, these co-trustees decide on trust expenditures that are intended to benefit the disabled beneficiary. They are usually comprised of three voting positions, one of which can be held by an immediate family member or shared by the parents of the disabled beneficiary. Most courts will not approve a disbursement co-trustee that is controlled by the beneficiary's family, to minimize opportunities for conflict of interest and self-dealing. Appropriate persons to fill two of the three voting positions might include nurses, physicians, counselors, therapists, vocational or rehabilitation advisors, teachers, close family friends, and members of the clergy. It is important that the entities filling the nonfamily co-trustee positions be able to act independently and not be under undue influence of any of the other parties.

The use of this type of co-trustee committee usually increases not only the responsiveness, but also the appropriateness, of disbursements made for the disabled beneficiary over those that might be authorized by a trustee alone. The co-trustees usually assign different duties among themselves, with each voting position having or acquiring expertise in specific and relevant areas, such as familiarity with local service providers. The co-trustee committee often evolves into a highly effective case management team that is able to advocate for the beneficiary with third parties, such as government agencies, and maximize the combined benefits of government and private programs and insurance in conjunction with carefully selected trust disbursements. In addition, these "teams" often develop long-term personal relationships with, and personal investment in, the beneficiary.

Family members usually serve on these committees without fee, particularly if those family members received loss of consortium or other direct compensation for the beneficiary's injuries. They are compensated for expenses. In situations when family committee members are asked to perform a great deal of legwork, such as seeking out residential arrangements, interviewing aides, and so forth, fees for time spent in those specific projects may be appropriate. Other committee members are usually compensated for their time and expenses. Although this may, at first glance, appear to be costly, it is often less expensive than paying more traditional professional trustee's hourly fees for services rendered in investigating and determining trust expenditures.

29.4.3 Collateral Source Benefit Compliance Managers

These are individuals or organizations with expertise concerning government and private benefit programs that provide services to persons who experience disabilities. Those services can be vital in a special needs trust arrangement if eligibility for Medicaid, SSI, and a host of other programs is to be established or preserved. The statutes and regulations concerning these programs undergo frequent change and reinterpretation. There are state-by-state variations on waiver and certain other programs. For example, giving a beneficiary a monthly cash allowance can have a disastrous effect on his or her continuing benefit eligibility. A collateral source benefit compliance manager can assist a trustee or trust disbursement committee in selecting disbursements that allow maximum benefit and flexibility for the beneficiary while avoiding serious consequences to continuing eligibility for needs-based benefit programs.

29.4.4 Primary and Secondary Guardianship/Conservatorship Selection

Although the proper drafting and implementation of a special needs trust to manage settlement and judgment proceeds can minimize negative impact on the beneficiary's program eligibility, there remain a significant number of services that a trust, quite simply, has no authority to provide. Any income or assets to which the beneficiary holds title (such as monthly SSI benefit payments or ownership of a home) are outside the control of the trust. In addition, unless the beneficiary has a valid durable power of attorney, only the beneficiary can make informed medical decisions for him- or herself. If the beneficiary has marginal cognitive capacity, he or she may go without treatment simply because there is no one authorized to grant consent.

Guardianship and conservatorship statutes allow appointment of persons or entities that can provide those services. Although relevant statutes vary from state to state, a guardian of the person generally can be granted court authority over almost all personal decisions the disabled person could make if he or she were able. In some jurisdictions, a guardian's "substitute" consent to elective surgery requires advance court approval. In almost all jurisdictions, nonemergency sterilization procedures may only be authorized by a guardian with advance court approval. For day-to-day personal needs, such as selecting a personal physician or dentist and minor procedures (stitches, root canals), a guardian has general authority to grant consent. Regarding asset management, a guardian of the estate or conservator can receive and manage the disabled person's income, manage personal assets, and negotiate fees and contracts with service providers (outside of the trust). It is important in situations when the guardian of the person and the guardian or conservator of the estate are different entities that they be able to work together for the good of the disabled person.

29.5 Due Diligence

When representing an incapacitated client, the attorney is exposed to greater moral and ethical considerations than when representing a nondisabled client. If the client is so disabled as to benefit from a special needs trust arrangement and the attorney is presenting such an arrangement for consideration by the court, the attorney must exercise due diligence in assisting in locating, evaluating, and selecting the trust management team. Even if the recommendation for a special needs trust and management team is made by a guardian ad litem or next friend, the trust instrument and proposed team is usually selected by counsel and the disabled client's family and thereafter presented for the court, guardian ad litem, or next friend's consideration. Key considerations include those described in the following sections.

29.5.1 Disclosed and Undisclosed Fees

Trustee's fee schedules are generally premised on the assumption they would have full responsibility for all trust activities. Special needs trusts often have disbursement activity directed by a co-trustee or trust disbursement committee that is separate and apart from the professional or financial trustee. As a result, reductions from standard fees should be negotiated with trustees for special needs trusts whenever possible. In addition to the fees taken under the standard fee schedules, most trustees provide supplemental services that are billed on an hourly or per type of asset basis. Supplemental services might include preparation of tax returns, accounting services, real estate management, and investment services. It is important to obtain a full disclosure of specific services that are covered by the a proposed trustee's fee schedule, what services are not included, what expenses are included and what are not, and what hourly fee rates are charged for the staff members that will work on the trust account. What initially appears to be a bargain fee schedule rate may result in very high fees if many basic services are billed separately from the schedule.

When a broker/trustee arrangement is utilized, counsel should negotiate with both the broker and trustee to ensure that double charging for investment services is minimized. Brokers are sometimes willing to discount their fees, whereas trustees may be more difficult to convince to reduce their fees proportionate to the time they would have spent making investment decisions. It is their position that they continue to bear liability for trust investments so must be compensated for the risk. Although this may be true, most broker/trustee arrangements are between sister organizations and, if that is indeed the case, counsel should argue that the risk is between the organizations and should not result in fee doubling to the trust.

29.5.2 Insurance/Bonding

In evaluating prospective trustees, counsel should determine whether the prospective trustee carries blanket bonding or fiduciary insurance. Obtaining approval of a trustee that subsequently fails in its fiduciary duty to an incapacitated client's trust can place counsel in a position of liability. Some courts will require that the trustee be bonded or insured, at least regarding the trust. If the trustee does not carry appropriate insurance, the cost of purchasing that coverage regarding the trust is a factor that must be considered as a cost of using that trustee. Watch for state court rules or statutes that govern the type of protective devices (bonds, blocked accounts, insurance, and so forth) that should or must be in place to protect the trust beneficiary from violations by a trustee.

If any significant portion of the settlement will be structured, it is wise for counsel at least to inquire about obtaining an underlying guarantee on the structure. Many of the carriers that currently issue structured settlement annuities are in difficult financial positions and have sought or are reputed to be seeking federal "bail-out" funding. Prior company failures, such as the Executive Life Insurance Company failure, left some annuitants receiving pennies on the dollar for their anticipated income. Due diligence on the issuing company requires more than just the assurances of the issuing or selling brokers.

29.5.3 Experience with Type of Settlement Device

When comparing prospective trustees, it is often worth considering payment of higher fees for a trustee that has significant experience with and understanding of special needs trusts. Inexperienced trustees can generate a great deal of excess fees in the process of familiarizing their staff with interpretation of the terms and conditions of a special needs trust. Costly errors, such as allowing inappropriate expenditures that result in loss of benefit eligibility, are more likely to occur with an inexperienced trustee. Remember, most co-trustees who are selected to serve as a member of trust disbursement committees are initially inexperienced regarding special needs trust expenditures themselves. An experienced trustee can provide guidance if inappropriate expenditures are authorized, often avoiding negative consequences. If a sole trustee is selected to manage a special needs trust, experience becomes even more important. Beneficiaries of special needs trusts are often unable to determine their own needs or the impact that disbursements will have on any benefits they may receive, so cannot be relied upon to seek appropriate disbursements from the trustee. A sole trustee of a special needs trust must be proactive in remaining aware of the beneficiary's ongoing situation and needs, and must also develop information on and contacts with resources for meeting those needs. We have seen inexperienced trustees happily invest and manage special needs trusts for years, increasing the corpus, without making any disbursements for the beneficiary because none had been requested.

29.6 Estate Planning Considerations

There are a number of estate planning issues that must be considered aside from establishing an appropriate method for receipt and management of settlement or judgment proceeds for the person who has experienced a traumatic brain injury. Areas that should be reviewed are the estate plan for the disabled individual and estate plans for his or her family members.

29.6.1 Estate Planning for the Brain Injury Survivor

29.6.1.1 Will/Power of Appointment

Whenever possible, the survivor of a traumatic brain injury should have a will. The injured person should be carefully evaluated by medical and legal professionals to determine whether he or she has testamentary capacity. If there is sufficient capacity, a will should be drafted by appropriate counsel reflecting the injured person's wishes. It would be wise to accumulate and retain evidence of testamentary capacity and perhaps even to videotape the will's execution. That will would control all assets to which the injured person holds title.

In addition, the will may control disposition of assets remaining in a court-ordered special needs trust established for the injured person after satisfaction of the statutory Medicaid lien. Many of these trusts contain provisions directing distribution upon the beneficiary's death to his or her heirs at law or pursuant to the beneficiary's will, if any. The attorney drafting the trust will need to determine the laws that apply to this type of trust in the state in which it is to be implemented to be sure that the beneficiary does not retain any rights under the common law to revoke the trust. Designating a specific remainder beneficiary in the trust must be considered not only as part of the beneficiary's estate plan, but also as a means of eliminating the beneficiary's right to terminate the trust. If the assets remaining in the trust at the beneficiary's death can pass pursuant to a will, it is important for the injured person to understand the extent of assets his or her will can control before he or she decides on a distribution scheme.

In some instances, a court-ordered trust or local statutes may allow the beneficiary to designate remainder trust beneficiaries through a power of appointment. It is unclear whether the standard of capacity for execution of a power of appointment rises to the level of testamentary capacity. If testamentary capacity is in doubt but marginally possible, it may be wise to obtain a separate power of appointment reflecting the injured person's distribution instructions. It would be important to accumulate and retain evidence of capacity, again even to the extent of videotaping the document execution.

If the injured person does not have capacity to execute a will, assets to which he or she holds title will pass at his or her death in accordance with the laws of intestate succession applicable to his or her state of residence.

29.6.1.2 Power of Attorney

A power of attorney is a formally written document granted by one individual (the principal) to a second individual who is designated as an attorney in fact (AIF). Each state has statutes governing the creation and use of powers of attorney. First and foremost, it is necessary to determine that the injured person has legal capacity to execute a power of attorney.

Generally, it is possible, and sometimes advisable, to name more than one individual and/or entity as the AIF, but it is always prudent to designate a substitute in the event the primary AIF is unable to serve. A properly drafted power of attorney should specify the authority that is to be shared or transferred from the principal to the AIF. In some states, it may be possible to combine a delegation of authority over financial matters with delegation of authority over personal and health care matters. A general power of attorney typically grants authority from the principal to the AIF upon execution of the document. A durable power of attorney (sometimes called a *springing power of attorney*) becomes effective upon the disability of the principal. In a combined general and durable power of attorney, the authority of the AIF commences upon execution and continues through disability until either written revocation by the principal or the principal's death.

Powers of attorney should be specifically drafted to meet the client's express wishes. In a durable power of attorney, the client should select the criteria to be used in determining when the disability comes into existence. The client should be counseled on the nature and extent of authority that is or will be transferred to the AIF. Gifting, estate planning, the creation or revocation of trusts, management of specific assets, real property transactions, and tax issues must be expressly addressed. Health care directives should be incorporated into the power of attorney and reference to the Health Insurance Portability and Accountability Act of 1996 must be expressly included to allow access to information and health care records.

Again, it is critical to remember that the principal must be capable of understanding the nature of the document and the extent of authority being transferred at the time the document is executed in order for the power of attorney to be valid. The client should also be counseled that the power is primarily an assistive device and offers only minimal protection. The existence of even a durable power does not deprive the principal of the right to make decisions on his or her own, up to and including the decision to revoke the power. This may be true even after the criteria for disability established in the document have been met.

29.6.2 Estate Planning for the Brain Injury Survivor's Family Members

29.6.2.1 Wills

The use of a carefully drafted will is essential in preparing estate plans for people who have a family member who experiences disabilities. One must attempt to maintain the disabled family member's eligibility for the basic government services, both to maximize the resources available to meet that disabled person's needs and to ensure access to the public service delivery system. This must be done with a recognition that those basic government services are not going to be adequate to meet all of the disabled person's needs.

In almost all cases, spouses, parents, grandparents, and other relatives should consider making arrangements to the effect that the disabled person does not own or receive legal title to their money, real estate, or other assets, whether transferred by will, inheritance, or gift. This may be good advice even if the disabled person is "legally competent" and only experiences physical or sensory disability. The disabled individual should not be designated as a direct beneficiary of any life insurance or retirement programs.

A basic will is the cornerstone of the estate plan. Each family member should consult an attorney with training in estate planning who is also aware of the need to provide special planning for the family member who experiences a disability. A special needs trust will be utilized as the basic planning mechanism. This type of special needs trust should not contain the state lien reimbursement language that must appear in the litigation settlement trust. Funds that are generated from the family or other third parties should not be commingled with the funds from the settlement and should not be placed into the litigation special needs trust. Family estate planning requires consideration of personal, financial, federal estate tax planning, and state inheritance tax issues relevant to the state in which the family resides. Planning for disability is less state specific, because the most important benefit programs for individuals with disabilities are federal in origin. The majority of disability related programs are based upon federal statutes, as noted earlier.

As part of the basic estate plan, the disabled family member should be specifically acknowledged in the will and excluded from any direct inheritance. The exclusion should be explicit. A will could state "I expressly leave nothing to my child, JOHN DOE, except my love and affection, knowing he will be adequately provided for otherwise." Any bequest intended for the disabled family member, whether that family member is a spouse, child, grandparent, or other relative, should be directed to a special needs trust for that person's benefit. That trust can either be included in the will as a "testamentary trust," or created prior to death as a "living trust," which is discussed more fully in the next section. If a living trust is established, the will should then include "pour-over" provisions directing the funds intended for the disabled person's benefit to the *trustee* of the living trust. The pour-over language must specifically identify the living trust—for example, "The Smith Living Trust for the Benefit of Johnnie Smith Under Agreement Dated January 10, 2009."

29.6.2.2 Living Trusts

Living irrevocable trusts are another planning option. This is most useful when money or other assets are or will be set aside during the lifetime of the grantor (maker of the gift). A living trust is created in a separate document and not included within a will. To be valid, some asset must be placed into the name of the trust at, or shortly after, the date of creation. The beneficiary of a living trust who is disabled cannot be given any right to compel payments from the trust or terminate the trust in whole or in part in his or her own favor. When a living trust is used as a vehicle for tax planned gifts, a limited right of withdrawal, or "Crummey" power, is usually included. Care must be taken in this regard because access to the gifts available through a Crummey power will disqualify the trust beneficiary from needs-tested benefit programs for at least the period during which the power remains open. For Medicaid, the disqualification period could be for several months after the right of withdrawal expires. The grantor must weigh the grantor's possible gift and estate tax benefit against the cost of the beneficiary's loss of eligibility for needs-tested government benefit programs.

An increasingly popular option is the "Irrevocable Life Insurance Trust," or living trust funded with life insurance. The use of insurance within a special needs trust (SNT) is totally appropriate and recognized as a proper financial planning tool in this field. It is especially important when the special needs beneficiary is likely to outlive his or her parents. In today's era of modern medicine, we are seeing large numbers of even severely disabled or injured persons outlive their adjusted life expectancies, sometimes many years beyond what was anticipated. Funding a trust with life insurance generally provides excellent return on the investment, with funds becoming available when they are most needed—after the loss of the care and supervision of a parent.

Term insurance is an effective and inexpensive funding device for younger families to place into a trust. Premium cost can be reasonable for a significant amount of coverage. Whole life policies may also be used at a somewhat higher premium cost, but with the added advantage of the accumulation of cash value in the policy. This builds an immediate principle in the trust.

If the cost of premiums is an issue, a "second-to-die" policy instead of term life is attractive. The "second-to-die" policies are guaranteed to pay upon the second insured party's death. There is no risk that the trust will not receive the policy proceeds as long as the beneficiary outlives both parents. This is very appealing because it guarantees future funding at low cost.

The purchase of any insurance should take place within the trust to avoid negative estate tax consequences to the insured. Use of a Crummey power may be desirable because the amount of the premium that may be gifted to the trust each year to fund the insurance premiums will not usually be large enough to impact the beneficiary's eligibility for needs-tested benefit programs. If a trust beneficiary who is granted a Crummey withdrawal power to a current trust deposit meant for payment of insurance premiums is already receiving SSI or Medicaid, access to the right of withdrawal will negatively impact ongoing benefits.

If a life insurance trust is not desired, life insurance proceeds can also be directed to testamentary trusts (trusts in wills). If this option is used, the proceeds should be directed to the trustee of the "testamentary trust established in my Last Will and Testament dated _____ or as hereafter amended, for the benefit of my disabled child/spouse/grandchild, _____, to be held, managed, and distributed pursuant to the terms and conditions of that testamentary trust." Life insurance proceeds should *not* be directed to the disabled individual.

29.6.2.3 Special Needs Trust Provisions

Whether a testamentary or living SNT model is chosen, there are certain critical provisions that must be included within the trust language. The trust must be a discretionary supplemental spendthrift trust. It must be designed to protect the trust assets and income from the claims of creditors, including the state. The assets in the trust will actually be owned by the trust, and not by the disabled beneficiary. Hence, if the trust is properly drafted, the trust assets cannot be considered to preclude the beneficiary's financial eligibility for local, state, and federal government benefit and service programs. The trust should also provide a structure for the management of the assets on behalf of an individual with disabilities who may lack the capacity to appreciate fully the complexities of investment and management of substantial sums of money.

It is not the main purpose of an SNT to pay for the basic food, shelter, and medical needs of the disabled person. The government benefit programs are intended to cover those needs. The stated purpose of the trust might read as follows:

> *Purpose:* The express purpose of this trust is to provide for JOHN DOE extra and supplemental care, maintenance, support, and education in addition to and over and above the benefits JOHN DOE otherwise receives as a result of his handicap or disability from any local, state, or federal government, or from any other private agencies, any of which provide services or benefits to handicapped persons. It is the express purpose of the trustor to use the trust estate only to supplement other benefits received by the beneficiary. To this end, the trustee may provide such resources and experiences as will contribute to and make the beneficiary's life as pleasant, comfortable, and happy as feasible. Nothing herein shall preclude the trustee from purchasing those services and items that promote the beneficiary's happiness, welfare, and development, including, but not limited to, vacation and recreation trips away from places of residence, expenses for traveling companions if requested or necessary, entertainment expenses, supplemental medical and dental expenses, social services expenses, and transportation costs. This trust is to be considered as a discretionary, and not a basic support, trust. The trust estate shall not be used to provide basic food and shelter nor be available to the beneficiary for conversion for such items, unless all local, state, and federal benefits to which the beneficiary is entitled as a result of disability have first been applied for those purposes or the trustee has determined that full or partial benefit eligibility is not in the beneficiaries best interest. This trust is to be irrevocable except as provided in Article _____, entitled "Term," set forth below.

The trustee must be given complete discretion to determine when, and under what circumstances, payments should be made on behalf of the disabled individual. The key to financial eligibility for the government benefits will be the "availability" of the resources to the disabled person. If the disabled individual has the ability to demand distribution of the resources, as would be the case in a basic support trust or a trust that requires annual distribution of income and principal, then the resources contained in the trust or to be distributed in that year will count against the child for financial eligibility for benefits. The primary question appears to be whether the disabled child can receive state assistance without the state having any enforceable rights to contributions from the trust. An example of a paragraph establishing full discretion is as follows:

> *Discretion:* The trustee shall have absolute and unfettered discretion to determine when and if the beneficiary needs regular or extra supportive services and provisions as referred to in the paragraphs above. The trustee may make or withhold payment at any time and in any amount as the trustee deems appropriate in the exercise of his or her discretion. The exercise by the trustee of his or her discretion shall be conclusive and binding on all persons.

Payments from the trust should be made directly to the individuals or companies who provide goods or services to the disabled beneficiary. If the trust, or any other third party for that matter, makes payments of cash to the disabled individual or pays for basic food or shelter for the disabled individual, the cash or value of the item provided must be reported to the benefit agencies. That amount will be deducted from the individual's level of benefits. Sample payment language might read as follows:

> *Payments:* All payments from this trust that do go to the benefit of the beneficiary are to be direct payments to the person or persons who supply either goods or services to the beneficiary at the request of the trustee. However, the trustee may exercise discretion in allowing the beneficiary such periodic allowances for personal spending money as the trustee shall deem appropriate.

One of the advantages of establishing a trust for an individual with disabilities is that the person who creates the trust can determine to whom any assets remaining in the trust will pass after the disabled person's death. It is important to designate a beneficiary who will be entitled to take the remaining balance in the trust at the disabled person's death. That secondary, or residual, beneficiary then has a legal interest in the trust, providing additional protection from state claims for repayment that could be made against the disabled beneficiary's interest.

A spendthrift provision is the traditional way to provide protection in a trust against claims by the creditors of the beneficiary—in this case, the disabled individual. Such a provision acknowledges that the disabled beneficiary has no legal interest in the trust until disbursements are actually made on his or her behalf. Statute and common law on spendthrift provisions may vary widely from state to state. Therefore, state specific legal review is necessary. Sample spendthrift language reads as follows:

> *Spendthrift:* The beneficiary shall have no interest in either the principal or income of this trust. The assets of this trust shall in no way be assignable or alienable by or through any process whatsoever. The assets of the trust shall not be subject to garnishment, attachment, levy, or any other legal process of any court from any creditor of any beneficiary, nor shall the assets be an asset in any future bankruptcy of any beneficiary. Furthermore, because this trust is to be conserved and maintained for the special needs of the impaired beneficiary throughout his lifetime, no part of the corpus thereof, neither principal nor undistributed income, shall be construed as part of the beneficiary's "estate" or be subject to the claims of voluntary or involuntary creditors for the provision of goods, care, and services, including residential care, by any public entity, office, department or agency of the State of _____ or any other state, county, municipal, federal or other governmental entity, department or agency, except specifically provided for otherwise in this instrument.

Under most court decisions interpreting such trusts, the intent of the trustor is one of the key deciding factors in implementing the trust. The trustee should have the ability to determine when, if, and how payments are to be made on behalf of the disabled beneficiary. It may even be well to go so far as to allow the trustee to deny payment for such basic and elemental needs as food, housing, and clothing. A clear statement of the trustor's intent to supplement, and not supplant, other sources of income to the beneficiary, including local, state, and federal benefit programs, is vital. The drafter could even include a provision that requires the principal of the trust to be distributed to a third party in the event that the trust assets are used to disqualify the trust beneficiary from government program eligibility. A sample statement of intent follows:

> *Trustor's Intent:* It is the intention of the trustor in executing this trust to provide benefits for the beneficiary without interfering with or reducing the benefits to which he or she is entitled under the social services agencies of the State of _____, its successor agencies, and/or any other state or federal agency or department, and to maximize the benefits to the beneficiary. Accordingly, regardless of any provisions in this instrument to the contrary, if in the trustee's opinion, a distribution called for herein would not

achieve its full economic benefit as intended because of physical, emotional, legal, or other disabilities or reasons, the trustee may withhold such distribution or benefits or a portion thereof until such time as the trustee feels that the fully intended benefit would be accomplished by the distribution.

Because trust distributions may subject the beneficiary to federal and other tax liability, a provision allowing the trust to make distributions to cover that liability should be included.

Taxes: The trustee shall pay any income tax liability of JOHN DOE that results from income received by the trust but properly reported on JOHN DOE's income tax return, such amount to be specified in writing and delivered by JOHN DOE's tax accountant or tax preparer to the trustee. The trustee shall rely conclusively on this amount. The funds used to pay any such tax liability shall be paid directly to the appropriate tax authority and shall not be available to JOHN DOE. Any such funds are not a resource of JOHN DOE and should not be treated as a distribution of income for purposes of Medicaid or SSI qualification.

In some situations, disabled family members may lose eligibility for collateral source benefits as a result of improvement in their health, employment that provides income over the federal poverty standard, or other reasons. In these cases, the disabled person may be left with insufficient assets and resources to pay rent or buy food. Thus, incorporating language that recognizes this type of problem and provides a safety net for the disabled family member is important.

POMS: Disbursements from the principal or income of the trust estate in accordance with the purpose provision above shall be made subject to the provisions of the Social Security Act, Regulations and Programs Operations Manual System (POMS) in such a manner that distributions shall not be considered as income to the beneficiary under the definition of that term as provided therein, during any period of time when, in the judgment of the trustee, the beneficiary is, or should be, receiving means-tested local, state, or federal disability-related benefits that are funded in whole or in part with funds originating under the Social Security Act (42 U.S.C., as now or hereafter amended) or related funding sources, or to which the beneficiary is, or should be, categorically eligible as a result of the beneficiary's receipt of Supplemental Security Income. During any period of time when JOHN DOE is, or should be, receiving such benefits and as long as distributions from this trust do not exceed the level of income that would allow preservation of eligibility for such benefits under the Act, Regulations, and POMS, any such distributions shall be considered allowable by the trustee under the terms of this trust agreement. Should JOHN DOE not be eligible for such benefits or should the trustee determine that it is not in his best interest to seek or maintain such eligibility, this restriction on distributions shall not apply, provided that all distributions from this trust shall be for the sole benefit and in the best interest of JOHN DOE.

The suggestions made in this chapter should not be used without the assistance of an attorney who is intimately familiar with all the eligibility criteria applicable to all the local, state, and federal benefit programs available to individuals with disabilities. This is a new and very helpful area of practice for individuals with disabilities and their families. It allows us to provide extended services to maximize the benefits available to disabled consumers while still providing for an enhanced quality of life through the coordination of public benefits and private resources.

Appendix: 42 U.S.C. § 1396p(d)(4)(A) 01/02/01

(4)   This subsection shall not apply to any of the following trusts:

(A)   A trust containing the assets of an individual under age 65 who is disabled (as defined in section 1382c(a)(3) of this title) and which is established for the benefit of such individual by a parent, grandparent, legal guardian of the individual, or a court if the State will receive all amounts remaining in the trust upon the death of such individual up to an amount equal to the total medical assistance paid on behalf of the individual under a State plan under this subchapter.

(B)   A trust established in a State for the benefit of an individual if—

   (i)   the trust is composed only of pension, Social Security, and other income to the individual (and accumulated income in the trust);

   (ii)   the State will receive all amounts remaining in the trust upon the death of such individual up to an amount equal to the total medical assistance paid on behalf of the individual under a State plan under this subchapter; and

   (iii)   the State makes medical assistance available to individuals described in section 1396a(a)(10)(A)(ii)(V) of this title but does not make such assistance available to individuals for nursing facility services under section 1396a(a)(10)(C) of this title.

(C)   A trust containing the assets of an individual who is disabled (as defined in section 1382c(a)(3) of this title) that meets the following conditions:

   (i)   The trust is established and managed by a non-profit association.

   (ii)   A separate account is maintained for each beneficiary of the trust, but, for purposes of investment and management of funds, the trust pools these accounts.

   (iii)   Accounts in the trust are established solely for the benefit of individuals who are disabled (as defined in section 1382c(a)(3) of this title) by the parent, grandparent, or legal guardian of such individuals, by such individuals, or by a court.

   (iv)   To the extent that amounts remaining in the beneficiary's account upon the death of the beneficiary are not retained by the trust, the trust pays to the State from such remaining amounts in the account an amount equal to the total amount of medical assistance paid on behalf of the beneficiary under the State plan under this subchapter.

30

Ethical Challenges in Funding Treatment and Care in Traumatic Brain Injury: An Argument for National Health Insurance

Thomas R. Kerkhoff, Stephanie L. Hanson, and Zoë N. Swaine

CONTENTS

30.1 Introduction

Increasing health care costs in the United States during the past 35 years have proved difficult to control for both governmental and private health insurance entities. For approximately 47 million Americans (15% of the population), access to affordable health care is not available. In addition, during the past 40 years, health care spending has outstripped revenue by 2.5% annually, with increasing numbers of patient safety and quality problems.[1,2] This harsh reality is amplified when attempting to provide treatment and care for those individuals who are catastrophically injured, requiring expensive trauma and acute care services, rehabilitation, and lifelong support services, as exemplified by traumatic brain injury (TBI). The current sources of U.S. health care funding include (1) federal government programs that are, to a limited extent, universal in access, but population and mission specific (Public Health, Medicare, Medicaid, Military Health System, and Veterans' Administration Health System); (2) private health insurance policies available through employers or social organizations (e.g., American Association of Retired Persons) and for direct purchase that embrace contract law as the mechanism for determining allocation/rationing of health services for premiums paid; and (3) indigent care offered, most often, through specific health care providers (HCPs), with financial losses offset, to a limited extent, by state budget contributions earmarked for indigent care.

In 1999, Banja[3] wrote about the ethical implications of adverse reimbursement practices regarding brain injury rehabilitation. He cited several barriers to third-party reimbursement and patient advocacy: erosion of employer-based insurance, controversies over medical necessity determinations, and conflicts of interest among providers within the role of patient advocate and the Employee Retirement Income Security Act (ERISA) preemption. He posed remedies to these barriers, including universal access through compulsory participation (citing inevitable evolution toward such a system in industrialized countries), procedural language to allow for appeals of medical necessity denials based on unreasonable risk of harm, and emphasis upon fiduciary responsibility, including increased rehabilitation outcome research to counter contentions that much of rehabilitation treatment is "experimental" or "unproved." Kerkhoff et al.[4] echoed a portion of a proposal put forth earlier by Stern et al.[5] for consideration of national health system reform supporting universal health care access modeled after public utilities in the United States to address ethical and health policy concerns regarding the health care system.

A decade has passed since these works were published. Casual observation of the current health care system in the United States finds the same barriers in place and no sweeping reform in the health care delivery system in the interim. However, Wilensky[2] asserted that the United States has been a country of incremental change during the past several decades, given the absence of a clear legislative majority in Congress. Comprehensive reform is not predicted to occur until the Medicare and Medicaid funding mechanisms run into crisis (estimated to occur between 2012 and 2016), especially given existing political divisiveness surrounding potential solutions (e.g., restructuring coverage, taxation) to address escalating costs and lack of universal coverage.

More important, since the early 1990s, public opinion about the health care system has reflected inconsistent attitudes. Wilensky[2] cites public opinion polls reflecting important disconnects in attitudes about health care. She reported that the majority of people (57%) believe that the nation has a health care crisis, but nevertheless report being satisfied (64%–80%) with their own health care. Reform is characterized in public opinion by improved care for the nation, while the individual sacrifices quality of care. Finally, most individuals say that employers should be required to provide health insurance coverage (54%), but *not* at the expense of job cuts (63%).

It is in this environment of fundamental uncertainty about the goals and structure of the U.S. health care system that we present this chapter for consideration. To provide structure to this chapter, we will utilize the ethical decision-making model developed by Hanson et al.[6] to illustrate ethical issues embedded within the fiscal management of the health care system, especially as it impacts rehabilitation of individuals with TBI (Table 30.1). First, the critical incident—an event or circumstance that spurs ethical debate—will be formulated. Next, ethical principles and concepts relevant to the critical incident will be presented. Historical context and key stakeholders will be put forth. Then, related organizational and legal concepts will be explored. Following the development of background information, alternative resolutions will be proposed, with a desired outcome selected between the competing resolutions. Finally, critical commentary will conclude the chapter.

30.2 Critical Incident

Individuals who are involved in incidents that cause TBIs are typically triaged at the scene via the emergency medical service and transported to trauma centers or hospital emergency departments that provide lifesaving emergency care. This early response system is guaranteed under the Emergency Medical Treatment and Active Labor Act.[7] Survivors proceed within the acute medical care process toward stabilization in intensive care units. Survivors with health insurance, or those who reside in health care facilities that offer indigent care, may have access to inpatient comprehensive or nursing home-based subacute rehabilitation for limited stays depending upon patient need. When that segment of the recovery process is completed, follow-up services may be available through community-based care systems (e.g., home health care, outpatient rehabilitation treatment, residential and transitional living facilities). Finally, depending upon the state of residence, state-subsidized and private organization-sponsored case management, vocational rehabilitation, and support/advocacy services may be available.

TABLE 30.1

Ethics Case Analysis Model

Stage	Description
I. Critical Incident	Trigger event identified via formal review mechanisms (e.g., continuous quality improvement) and/or individual professional judgment; should warrant an ethics consult
II. Ethical Principles, Standards, or Concepts	Need to be identified and specified in pursuit of an ethics case analysis or formal consult
III. Historical Context and Key Stakeholders	Investigation of contextual factors and individual players that impacted the critical incident; include time frame, individuals/organizations; subsets of contextual factors include (1) *biological* (e.g., disease, injury, lab data); (2) *psychological* (emotional state, trait); (3) *social* (peer or external influences); (4) environmental (*products and technology* [e.g., food, drugs, transportation systems], *natural* [e.g., population, climate, air quality], and *services, systems,* and *policies* [e.g., health care system, educational system, hospital system, costs]).
IV. Organizational and Legal Concepts	Further defining medicolegal and organizational regulations, policies, or rules/laws that influence the situation; does not replace legal consultation
V. Resolution	Secure the commitment of stakeholders to negotiate collaboratively and propose alternative solutions; develop a consensus action plan, balancing benefits and costs; specify the desired outcome
VI. Disposition	Evaluate the actual versus desired outcome; if necessary, modify the resolution to approximate the desired outcome; apply relevant post hoc clinical/legal case precedents, practice standards, and research literature to assist in resolving any substantial differences between the desired and actual outcomes

Source: Hanson, S. L., Kerkhoff, T. R., and Bush, S. S., *Health Care Ethics for Psychologists: A Casebook*, American Psychological Association Press, Washington, DC, 2005.

Although service delivery components exist in each phase of the progression through treatment and long-term support, variability in access to and availability of services within and across states is substantial.[8,9] Concrete funding limitations emerge early during the care process because of financial pressures to discharge survivors quickly. Based upon the Centers for Medicare and Medicaid Services (CMS) guidelines,[9,10] dollar reimbursement amounts are allocated to specific diagnoses and linked to specified lengths of stay in acute care, which influence health care decision makers such as providers and administrators. Increasing numbers of survivors without sufficient health insurance or other sources of funding fall out of the care system at each juncture or transition point along the way. In addition, the experience of clinicians, such as speech–language pathologists, suggests that inadequate coverage limits "their ability to provide care consistent with recognized standards."[11, p. 3] The realistic need for episodic lifelong intervention services for individuals with TBI poses an extreme challenge to the already stressed health care funding and service delivery systems. Thus, the vaunted continuum of care in TBI is, in fact, an aspirational goal yet to be achieved, rather than a matter of standardized care.

The broad view of the current problem is best understood in the context of the lack of federally mandated universal access to health care and the variability of health care service delivery environments within and across states. This fact necessarily leads to segmentation of the population into special interest groups, of which survivors of TBI and their family members are but one example. Thus, effective campaigns to change the current health care system to meet the needs of such special interest groups apply differential pressures within the national health care system vis-à-vis the general population, creating resource imbalances within a system of limited funding and service resources. By ignoring a view to the consequences for the larger health care system, it is frankly easier, from both a political and financial perspective, to make smaller scale incremental changes to subcomponents of the health care system. However, the upshot of such a social dynamic is a lack of coordinated reform (e.g., planning, finances, service development and delivery, research) within the larger health care system—a situation that perpetuates the health care crisis.

30.3 Ethical Principles and Concepts

30.3.1 Autonomy: An Individual's Right to Self-Determination

Respect for autonomy is strongly upheld by federal and state legislation.[12] Imposition of financially based access criteria regarding basic required health care services poses an unacceptable health care exclusion (limitation in options, choice) for those who are economically disadvantaged. This untenable ethical reality is validated in the face of no specified right to health care contained in the U.S. Constitution. Freedom of choice should be free from manipulation or coercion based in large measure on financially motivated contractual relationships, as is the case with private health insurance. Although attention to controlling health care costs is certainly an important and ethically valid concept within the business of health care, treatment decisions heavily influenced by profit motive are substantially at risk for ignoring the public good and the rights of the individual in self-determination.[13]

30.3.2 Beneficence: Provision of Beneficial Health Care Services

Facilitating good in the context of health care delivery includes providing adequate primary, secondary, and tertiary care to those with legitimate health care needs. Both Banja[3] and Beauchamp and Childress[12] have argued that HCPs have an ethical obligation to help those in need by virtue of the technical skill they possess to address that need. Availability of and access to beneficial and proven health care services are the foundation upon which the call for standardized health benefit language/plans is based.[2,5] This provision presupposes that sufficient rehabilitation research data exist regarding clinical outcomes of specific prevention and intervention procedures.[3,14–16]

30.3.3 Nonmaleficence: Do Not Harm; Prevent Harm

Limiting or excluding individuals with legitimate health care needs from access to needed services contravenes the ethical principle of nonmaleficence. Potential for harm resulting from inaction ignores the concept of due care or what the individual is entitled to by virtue of need. Resorting to the concept of "medical necessity" (contractually based insurance coverage) as a limiting or exclusionary factor in provision of funds for valid health-related needs focuses too narrowly upon biology and "ignores interventions geared toward the person being functional, self-directive, autonomous, and independent."[3, p.753] In addition, financial incentives linked to abbreviating the scope of care or using less expensive alternatives that "jeopardize patients' care"[3, p.749] are equally untenable, posing a conflict of interest upon the care provider as both a patient advocate and professional under contract to an insurance company. On the other hand, providing needless and costly care drains resources from an already strained health care system, a limited public resource, perpetuating problems with inconsistent coverage and inadequate care.

30.3.4 Justice: Fair and Equitable Access to and Allocation of Needed Health Care Services

Access to needed health care should be unimpeded by the happenstance of injury or socioeconomic position (e.g., natural and social lotteries).[12] Economic discrimination regarding access has been an unfortunate characteristic of the U.S. health care system from its inception. However, the fee-for-service model historically did allow for deferred payment or even bartering to offset costs of care, as the individual and HCP usually had a personal working relationship. The ever-increasing economic gulf between upper and lower classes has simply exaggerated the issue of unfair access. Banja[3] argues for a national patients' bill of rights, consolidation of political and social will to change the current managed care system, and consumer advocacy (including court challenges) to create momentum for a more equitable health care system. As Ruger[17] has suggested, an equitable health care system is one in which protection is provided to those who are disadvantaged (e.g., poor, ill). He argues that good health expands individual productivity, thereby contributing to the economy. On the other hand, the aggregated cost of being uninsured creates an economic drain.

The equitable distribution of resources is a shared responsibility among different layers of the health care system (e.g., consumer, provider, fiscal agent). On the politicoeconomic side of the argument, universal coverage means mandates and entitlements, which necessitates subsidizing the uninsured and costs real money, while risking displacement of the current insurance system.[2]

30.3.5 Intersecting Ethical Concepts and Conflicts of Interest: Opposing Social Forces Impacting Health Care Provider Clinical Decision Making

HCPs who rely on federal and private insurance reimbursement for health care service delivery costs are often faced with the responsibility of balancing clinical decision making with the financial implications of those decisions. When the act of balancing costs with service delivery is performed with a goal of meeting standards of care (beneficence, nonmaleficence) and being fiscally responsible regarding utilization of limited health care financial resources (justice), this process enhances provision of efficient and effective services. However, when the provider is offered financial incentives (direct or indirect) to deny or limit services, or to offer less expensive alternatives that might compromise quality of care in service of economic self-interest (personal or organizational), conflicts of interest arise.[3,14] Likewise, when health care funding entities prioritize resource allocation decisions from a financial perspective to maximize profit for investors, a legitimate function of business operations, the individual in need of health care services may experience increased risk of harm and restricted choice. Weber[13] emphasizes the importance of considering the rights of the individual as the first ethical priority when making business decisions in health care.

It is of crucial importance that the patient–HCP relationship be founded on the premise of the ethical obligations to act in good faith, keep promises and vows, fulfill agreements, and maintain adaptive fiduciary relationships.[3] As such, the HCP must attempt to avoid constraints upon performing proper care. The act of a payer (managed care organization [MCO]) not authorizing or denying care (as medically unnecessary), requiring lower cost/lower quality alternative care, prohibiting the offer of a second opinion or other reasonable alternative treatments, and post hoc reimbursement denials for medically necessary treatments already provided compromises fiduciary responsibility. In addition, when the payment authorization or nonauthorization message is communicated by the payer to the provider for relay to the patient, the patient–HCP relationship can be negatively impacted because of diffusion of responsibility. The rationale sometimes used by payers that the service is not being denied, only payment, is simply an obfuscation. These two components of health care are inextricably interdependent.

30.4 Historical Context and Key Stakeholders

When evaluating ethical challenges created for the TBI population by organizational structures and fiscal operations within the U.S. health care system, it is important to consider individuals with TBI in the broader context of catastrophic injuries for which lifetime insurance caps can prove woefully inadequate and can be further nested within the even larger system in which a significant pool of individuals lack access to adequate health care. It is only within this panoramic view of the current health care system that we can properly assess the scope of the problem of health care funding limitations.

Mappes and DeGrazia[18] have highlighted commonly accepted goals of health care within industrialized nations, including universal access, cost controls, comprehensive benefits, freedom of choice and freedom from hassle for patients, and quality of care. They also cite statistical information that puts these goals into perspective within the United States. In 1986, 37 million citizens lacked health insurance. By 2004, the number rose to between 44 and 45 million people and is currently estimated to be between 47 and 48 million individuals (one sixth of the U.S. population).[18]

Poorly controlled health care costs are another aspect of the problem. In 1986, 11% of the gross domestic product (GDP) was devoted to health care. In 1994, health care costs rose to 14% of the GDP. In the mid to late 1990s, the percentage leveled off in response to initial managed care controls, but began to rise steeply at double-digit rates between 2000 and 2004. In 2003, it represented 15.2% of the GDP. The current per capita health expenditure in the United States is $5,711,[19] more than any other industrialized country. Mappes and DeGrazia[18] reported that even good private health care insurance plans have limited mental health and no dental care. Many have limited coverage for rehabilitation, and long-term and chronic care, commonly "forcing" members (via denial of authorization or reimbursement to health care facilities) to leave hospitals before they feel well. This is coupled with challenges regarding restrictive billing codes for services, such as the limited application of medical codes for rehabilitation psychology services, resulting in reduced reimbursement. Disparate state Medicaid programs lead to piecemeal legislation in efforts to reform state programs as problems arise. With the exception of prescription assistance, the United States lags behind countries such as Canada, Germany, Britain, Italy, France, and Sweden for comprehensiveness.

Freedom of choice is limited under managed care, and multiple layers of administrative costs have characteristically made the current system more costly and less efficient than promised. Universal care systems abroad, with significantly less administrative complexity, offer more choice in HCPs and hospitals, along with reduced hassle during provision of service with quality of care reported to be comparable with that received by well-insured Americans.[19] Finally, the U.S. health care system has defined quality of care in terms of expensive technology, rather than providing quality basic care to those in need.

Let us now briefly consider TBI in its own right. Reynolds et al.[20] reveal that TBI is the leading cause of death and disability in persons younger than 45, and that injury rates are highest among families with the lowest income levels. Public health policy regarding TBI varies greatly among states and has been limited in relation to patient need. For example, eligibility delays for Medicaid funding (state-administered programs) requires facilities and HCPs to admit patients with a promise of funding, but no guarantee. This process relies upon health care facilities honoring duty to care and timeliness of admission for rehabilitation treatment, which in turn promotes better outcomes[21] and takes advantage of the opportunity to influence plasticity in neuronal recovery.[22] However, this harsh financial reality has resulted in increasing service denials because funding has not materialized in a number of cases, and facilities cannot continue to operate without predictable sources of revenue. How did our health care system arrive at this point in time? In the next section, we briefly explore the evolution of our health care delivery system.

30.4.1 Medicare, Medicaid, and Rehabilitation

Braddom[14] presents a concise developmental summary of the Medicare program from its inception in 1965 to the present. Currently, more than one in every seven Americans is insured by Medicare, and it is predicted this will increase to one in five Americans by 2030.[23] To manage costs created by ever-expanding enrollment, during the mid 1980s, Medicare shifted from a cost-based system to a predetermined payment system based on diagnosis. It has continued to use prospective payment, managed health plans, reimbursement caps, and restriction of services (e.g., home health) in an attempt to contain costs.[23,24] A turning point for individuals with disabilities occurred in 1972, when Medicare began to fund health care services for those with disabling conditions lasting more than 24 months. However, those same individuals lost private insurance after qualifying for Social Security Disability Income (SSDI). From the rehabilitation facility perspective, the Medicare policy makers also attempted to manage the service delivery sector and contain costs by offering financial incentives.

The rehabilitation continuum is composed of several postacute care pathways: inpatient rehabilitation facilities, subacute nursing facilities, long-term care hospitals, outpatient services, and home health care in-home rehabilitation treatment.[21] Although the fiscal control methodology has changed during the past 25 years (e.g., 75% rule, Prospective Payment Systems [PPS][25]), the CMS has attempted to alter the proportional impact of these rehabilitation sectors by varying financial reimbursement formulas.[10] This market influence is accomplished via fiscal intermediaries (i.e., private contractors) who administer the funding process per geographic region. It is notable that funding criteria vary by region, despite uniform regulations published by CMS.[26] In recent years, policy shifts regarding rehabilitation have resulted in measurable changes in the rehabilitation service delivery system. Varied research studies investigating effects of policy changes after the fact have documented a leveling off of the number of inpatient rehabilitation facilities, dramatic reductions in transitional and residential living programs, and shortening treatment duration in home health care rehabilitation services in favor of subacute rehabilitation programs. Hoffman et al.[27] proposed that the PPS may not be appropriate for inpatient rehabilitation facilities managing individuals with TBI as opposed to other rehabilitation diagnoses. The authors linked this to the number of outliers that fall outside PPS guidelines. Chan[21] reported that 13% of the entire Medicare budget in 2005 was accounted for by postacute care. Because Medicare pays for approximately 70% of postacute care, its policy-making actions in the area are the bellwether for the nation. DeJong et al.[28] found that PPS implementation caused a shift in services toward those individuals with stroke who sustained moderate impairment and away from those who sustained severe impairment. Frymark and Mullen[29] discovered that inpatient rehabilitation facilities responded to the PPS by decreasing lengths of stay for patients with cognitive impairment, discharging patients home at lower functional levels, despite increasing intensity of cognitive rehabilitation treatment during the shortened stays. They concluded that the natural healing course could not be financially manipulated by market forces. The findings of Frymark and Mullen[29] are consistent with those of Kreutzer et al.,[30] who studied acute care and rehabilitation lengths of stays for four model system TBI programs over a 7-year period. They found that inpatient rehabilitation stays for persons with TBI dropped 8% annually, from a mean of 47.7 days in 1990 to 29.5 days in 1996, whereas charges simultaneously increased by 7% annually. This compares with rising costs of 3.1% for general goods and services, and 5.8% for medical care during that same time period. Kaplan's[9] study reported a reduction in inpatient rehabilitation and long-term care beds nationally in response to the PPS. Hoffman[31] revealed that the PPS decreased inpatient rehabilitation referrals, while increasing referrals to skilled nursing facilities. McCue and Thompson[32] found that the PPS effectively decreased acute hospital lengths of stay, not resulting in increased mortality, but in higher likelihood of discharge to home while still medically unstable, or discharge to another facility rather than home. Mellick et al.,[33] for example, found that individuals with TBI funded by government payers were overrepresented in long-term care. Clearly, market forces were shaping decisions regarding care needs for patients who might otherwise have received inpatient rehabilitation care.

Chan[21] describes the current Medicare payment system as "balkanized" in its differential treatment of multiple and insular segments.

> We lack the confidence in our payment systems because we do not really know where to place our incentives. We do not have enough information on efficacy, much less on effectiveness, to identify the treatments that we should be encouraging and for which type of patients. Thus, we must find ways to break down the barriers between provider types to enhance research in this area.[p.1523]

Chan[21] argues that the essential goal is for empirical research focused upon optimal treatments, settings, timing, and intensity to influence policy development, rather than purely economic factors. By extension, without a coherent national health policy, such integrative research cannot easily be sponsored or conducted.

Clohan et al.[34] put forth several recommendations to address the need for understanding the effects of policy changes upon the complex Medicare system. First, develop new measures and improve existing measures of patient characteristics, treatment contents, and long-term outcomes. The focus must be on differences among individual patients and the effect of those differences on long-term outcomes in postacute care. Second, integrate the postacute system of care so that outcome measures are uniform. The present silo system reinforces cost shifting and disincentives to provide the most cost-effective sequence of postacute care services. Timing of data collection needs to account for variation among recovery trajectories. Third, create partnerships among payers, providers, and research to access the universe of available relevant data. Fourth, provide universal access to effective services and reduce access to ineffective ones. Defining effective services, however, necessarily begins a dialogue regarding rationing. Other research suggests that it might be possible to incorporate enrollee preferences within the context of cost containment strategies that could potentially contribute to program expansion based on tradeoffs accepted.[35]

Reynolds et al.[20] made recommendations to address coordination of funding streams at the state level (Medicaid) regarding individuals with TBI, including implementing a TBI registry linked to service coordination available to all persons, regardless of funding source. They noted a fragmentation of responsibility within and across states, as vested interests carved out political territory. They also recommended that states (1) reexamine their home and community-based service (HCBS) Medicaid waivers to determine whether they can meet the needs of persons who are newly injured and (2) establish a mechanism to serve as payer of last resort to cover all necessary rehabilitation for newly injured persons with TBI. Finally, rehabilitation services should be of high quality and should be delivered in a cost-effective manner.

30.4.2 Managed Care

Perhaps a more accurate label for this health care business process is *managed care funding.* Pozgar[7] states that most MCOs have evolved into administrative units, disbursing funds to contracted health care service delivery organizations to offset the costs incurred by delivering services. These funds are collected by health care insurance organizations (MCOs) via contract subscriptions (i.e., plans) paid by employers and individuals. The cost of varied plans is calculated upon types of health care services covered. The expectation on the part of subscribers is that the funds contributed to the MCO will be used to share the cost of health care service delivery incurred by the individual, who also pays a portion of the health care service cost via copays. In return, the MCO attempts to ensure quality of service delivery by creating selective credentials-based criteria for enrolling providers and exercising exclusionary power regarding acceptable types of services covered. The insurance business mechanism underlying this financial arrangement rests upon the assumptions that (1) the pool of monies collected by the MCO will be greater than the outlay of funds to pay for health care services and (2) a desirable proportion of subscribers are healthy and in little need of health care services beyond preventive care. The monies remaining after health care costs are paid out in the form of reimbursement, plus any administrative fees collected from subscribers and service delivery contractors, are retained by the MCO as revenue. Furthermore, the MCOs use allocation strategies that set health care reimbursement outlay to keep profit margins of HCPs lean. These contractual details are negotiated with providers during the periodic contract renewal process. Simply stated, this is the process of applying competitive market pressure upon health care delivery organizations to reduce their costs. Financial incentives are used to facilitate efficient operating processes to reap a more beneficial rate of reimbursement. As note earlier, the CMS uses similar service delivery system controls in its efforts to keep ever-rising health care costs under better control.

Braddom[14] offers a historical perspective. He states that the U.S. federal government twice rejected the notion of national health insurance. The first instance occurred in 1916, when the American Medical Association recommended such a program to Congress. It would have required raising taxes, triggered union objections, and smacked of socialism. Then, after World War II, President Harry Truman proposed emulating the national health care system then emerging in Britain. Congress again responded that such a program would be too expensive and socialistic, concluding that the federal government would not be an effective administrator of such a program. As a consequence, the fee-for-service health service delivery model arose, with out-of-pocket payment and emerging private health insurance companies filling the funding gap, assisted by the tax exempt status of employer premium contributions, a benefit that continues today. Similarly, employers, eager to attract new workers as the economy rebounded from the war years, offered health insurance benefits to prospective employees. Although this system developed quickly, over the next 20 years, the costs related to providing health services rose at an alarming rate. It is important to remember that the era beginning in the early 1970s—health-related technology development—burgeoned, creating the compelling social perception that acquiring high technology was fundamental to providing high-quality health care. Curiously, this developing component of the health care system brought with it even higher costs, and reduced access to its benefits for those without funding resources. Concerned with this potentially threatening economic trend, Congress (firmly believing that the private business sector and competitive market forces would provide answers to this economic challenge) began actively to support the new concept of managed health care in the form of Health Maintenance Organizations (HMO), such as the HMO Act of 1973.

Pozgar[7,] defines managed care as "the process of structuring or restructuring the health care system in terms of financing, purchasing, delivering, measuring, and documenting a broad range of health care services and products."[p. 446] As can be seen in this description, managed care is rooted in the business profit motive as a given driver of the system. An unfortunate consequence of adopting a commercial service industry-derived model and applying its tenets to health care is that market forces result in cyclic expansion and contraction related to profit and cost containment: the business "life span" cycle. Thus, startup, growth in services and facilities, maturity of those services, and predictable decline as the competitive market forces introduce "new and improved" services and products introduce unintended disorganization into the provision of health care. In addition, publicly held health care networks are built on business models that attempt to respond to pressures to meet predicted quarterly earnings that may or may not materialize and are not necessarily motivated by health-related indices. This can be seen in competition for market share among the bewildering numbers of variations of MCOs as they vie for healthy subscribers who switch from one plan to another as incentives change.[7]

This consumer behavior pattern emulates that seen with the highly competitive cell phone industry and its constantly changing technology and service arrangements, which result in consumers frequently jumping among plans, products, and services. Changing among health insurance plans on a frequent basis serves only the goals of financial drivers of the system, not the actual provision of care. The upshot of this approach is that the system can never quite establish an equilibrium that allows the continuum of care (the dynamic process that attempts to coordinate transitions between health care system components) to work consistently and effectively. The funding system is volatile, whereas the health service delivery segment must remain stable, consistent, and adherent to standards of care that are founded on the ethical concepts of due care, unencumbered choice, informed consent, beneficial treatment, avoidance of harm, compassion, veracity, and so forth.[12] Some costs are arguably unjustly spent in the interest of profit margins (e.g., nonessential advertising with claims that are made independent of HCP input).[36] It is not surprising that administrative costs of managed care insurance plans constitute $.30 of the U.S. health care dollar.[2]

Understanding funding for TBI treatment and care must necessarily incorporate consideration of contextual influences on service needs and, thus, financial burden. Biologic aspects of TBI include the nature of the injury—damage to the brain and central nervous system on a continuum of severity from mild to profound. Anatomic factors like location and extent of lesions, the nature of the injury (blunt shearing trauma, penetrating trauma, accompanying circulatory compromise) will also impact recovery. The functional changes encountered with such injuries are myriad, as the essential cognitive/intellectual, emotional, and behavioral processing centers are impaired. Such injuries require emergency treatment—often lifesaving, medical stabilization (treatment of intercurrent conditions related to the mechanism of injury), rehabilitation interventions, and long-term care and support, especially if the injuries are moderate to severe. It is quite obvious that the survivors of such injuries pose a challenge to the health care system in terms of expensive, intensive emergency and acute medical intervention, and lifelong funding and support/care services. There are also a sizeable number of individuals who have survived non-TBIs. Causes of such injuries include infection, neurotoxic agents, varied encephalopathies, and varied neurologic diseases (e.g., multiple sclerosis), the evaluation, treatment, and care needs of which are equally pressing and complex. Survivors with diseases that cause decline in function over time result in an increasing burden upon care partners and the health care funding system. The fragmentation among advocacy efforts tends to impede coordination of resources to serve populations with similar needs.

Psychological stressors related to such dramatic changes in the life of the survivor and family/social support systems have been catalogued in extensive research during the past several decades.[37–39] The incidence of depression and substance abuse in people with TBI compared with the uninjured population is somewhat higher, especially during the first 2 years after injury.[40,41] The emotional distress related to the initial injuries can be addressed during the acute care and rehabilitation phases of recovery. Long-term emotional support must be available in the survivor's community, with episodic need for intervention as life challenges arise. These services can be conceived as falling on a continuum from individual assessment and treatment through residential neurobehavioral programs and vocational rehabilitation. In addition, support services for family care partners providing daily assistance to survivors can ameliorate stress and risk of emotional burnout[42] (also, see parallels in Iezzoni and Ngo[43]). It has also been shown that a well-functioning postacute care and support system can serve as a diversion mechanism from lapses in judgment that can bring individuals with TBI to the unwanted attention of the justice system.[44]

Social aspects of the health care funding problems facing survivors of TBI and their families can be construed as being local, regional, and national in scope. Local social influences are exemplified by changes in social support networks after injury, and the presence or absence of social support agencies in local communities. Disparities between urban and rural health care delivery systems are well documented.[20] The communication-based technology supporting "telerehabilitation" may serve to bridge the gap between urban and rural service delivery systems.[45] However, this technology remains in its early stages of development, and Medicaid funding is sporadic at best. Regional influences are noted in the variability in state laws and regulations governing health care, especially populations with special needs, like survivors of TBI. Because the Medicaid system is managed by the states rather than the federal government, those survivors who have Medicaid support are subject to varying types of resources and intensity of service.[20,46]

At the national level, there has been a social ambivalence regarding health care funding. National opinion polls have consistently identified the need for health care system reform, while simultaneously documenting reluctance to consider such reform if increased employment or taxation burdens would be required to effect change.[2,3] Since the early 1990s, one of the few significant and broad legislative successes was the 1997 passage of the State Children's Health Insurance Program (SCHIP), which provides health care coverage to children from low-income families (up to 200% of poverty and, thus, above the Medicaid limits; see www.cms.hhs.gov/NationalSCHIPPolicy for a program overview). The program, under the CMS, is financed jointly by the federal and state governments but managed by the states, such that eligibility and benefits vary depending upon state of residence. However, all state programs provide a core set of services that, for most states, includes rehabilitation-related services such as occupational, physical, and speech therapy, and substance abuse and mental health services.[47] Enrollment in SCHIP increased from 660,351 in 1998 to 6.6 million children in 2006. Similar attempts to provide broad-based coverage for the millions of uninsured adults, however, have been fraught with problems. Ambivalence, coupled with political agendas focused upon reelection, states' rights, and avoidance of taxation issues, has resulted in the continuing lack of a cohesive national health care policy, as well as delaying needed reforms to Social Security and Medicare and Medicaid programs.

Environmental influences also vary by situation. The circumstances surrounding a traumatic injury can facilitate or hinder service delivery upon entry into the continuum of care. Such influences can include time to first intervention, distance from the scene to emergency hospital treatment, distribution of postemergency facilities (e.g., inpatient rehabilitation unit), and social agency support across the course of recovery (contrasting urban and rural communities). Variation in environmental factors needs to be factored into any reform of the larger health care system, as the care delivery interface is located within the communities of the individuals in need of health care.

30.4.3 Key Stakeholders

Key stakeholders are those involved in or influencing funding decisions. In this section, we discuss common stakeholders affecting delivery of care to individuals with TBI.

30.4.3.1 *TBI Survivor and Family*

Survivors of TBI number 1.4 million annually in the United States. From 1995 to 2001, the average annual number of hospitalizations for persons with TBI was 235,000 and the number of emergency room visits was 1.1 million.[41] It is estimated that 5.3 million survivors of TBI who are hospitalized require lifelong assistance with activities of daily living.[48] The extraordinarily expensive treatment and lifelong nature of care and support place emotional and financial burdens upon the whole family system. Addressing access to adequate funding mechanisms relieves survivors and families of unneeded concern regarding financial hardship when facing the prolonged and uncertain recovery course is challenging enough. Care partner advocacy should rightly focus upon obtaining optimal treatment and care.

30.4.3.2 Health Service Delivery Systems and Health Care Providers

Providing appropriate high-quality services, regardless of ability to pay, needs to remain the primary focus of this stakeholder group. Although responsible and effective financial resource management is a necessary component of service provision, having to consider treatment denials or curtailing service quantity or intensity resulting from inadequate funding should not be a priority focus of service providers at the treatment interface. Such budgetary considerations need to be addressed at the level of organizational policy making. Care provided to the indigent population should be formalized within the state welfare and Medicaid systems. Formal recognition of this invaluable service would offer a guarantee of state financial support for humanitarian efforts, reducing risk for the health care organization.

Health care organizations are bound by organizational and clinical practice regulations and standards. These accreditation processes offer some measure of social legitimacy to quality of care provided by those organizations receiving such recognition. Service delivery organizations are primarily dependent upon external funding mechanisms to remain financially viable. Ethical, professional, and governmental standards prohibit forgoing provision of required services or compromising care quality for an individual in need in the absence of ability to pay. Individual HCPs are bound by discipline-specific ethics codes and professional practice standards. Such quality control mechanisms typically encourage provision of *pro bono* services when financial barriers to treatment arise.

30.4.3.3 Managed Care Organizations

These organizations, in their many operational variants, apply service sector business practices to funding health care via contractual relationships with organizations and individual practitioners. Decision-making models developed for noncritical commercial services and products that focus on employee productivity, marketing, sales, and resource allocation (in this instance, health care funding dollars) are utilized for the purposes of generating revenue and profit for investors. Delivery of health care services is typically accomplished via MCO employees (as in HMOs) or contracted providers (organizations and clinicians), with the MCO acting solely in an administrative role. Weber[13] specified ethical obligations upon organizations providing any component of health-related service. Ethical priorities include honoring basic individual rights, individual self-interest, interests of the organization, and public/community good. Generating profit is a valid aspect of health care business enterprises, but it cannot be produced at the expense of benefit to those persons served and to the community in which the organization resides.

Two ethically worrisome challenges arise when the health care funding administrator is separated from the subscriber. First is the practice of making "medical necessity" determinations regarding contractual limitations at a distance from the patient primarily via clinical record review and occasional discussions with treating HCPs. Geographic and social distance from the recipient of care promotes dilution of responsibility for the insurance company's decision makers. Service providers become subject to point-of-contact financial discussion—both positive and negative. Responsibility for communicating this information to the patient/insurance plan subscriber often falls on the provider of the health service for whom the patient seemingly has easier access. Although providers are ethically obligated to discuss charges anticipated in the context of the patient's informed consent, only when providers encourage patients to contact their insurance provider directly regarding funding decisions and reimbursement is responsibility shifted back to the decision-making agent.

Second, the rationale for minimizing the detrimental effect of nonauthorization or denial of services to a patient is often that lack of funding does not preclude provision of services. This response can be construed as an attempt to shift responsibility and risk of treatment limitations of the contractual relationship between the insurance plan and the patient/ subscriber to the provider/patient relationship. The patient will characteristically look to the provider to rectify the wrong perceived in funding denial by providing needed treatment irrespective of funding limitations.

30.4.3.4 Private Sector Advocacy Organizations

These organizations may function in a diagnosis-specific role (e.g., Brain Injury Association, national and state chapters), or in broader health care advocacy roles (charitable foundations). The responsibility to coordinate advocacy efforts remains limited as long as there is an absence of national health policy to provide a set of unifying priorities.

30.4.3.5 State Government

During the course of administering Medicaid programs and waivers (e.g., HCBS), funding streams are often directed to meet the state-specific needs of its citizens. Variability across states is evident when national surveys are conducted to study such programs.[20] The challenge remains in coordinating service delivery across state boundaries in such a manner that state rights are not significantly compromised. This is most parsimoniously interpreted as still having degrees of freedom to meet health care needs unique to specific states.

30.4.3.6 Federal Government

The opportunity facing the federal government is best understood in the context of unifying disparate existing health care components into a coherent system of health care funding and service delivery. This would require investigation of best health care practices among the Active Military Health System, the Veterans' Administration, Public Health, and Medicare and Medicaid programs. In addition, adoption of proven infrastructure and funding mechanisms would be necessary to distribute equitably and make accessible needed health care services across the nation.

30.5 Organization and Legal Concepts

The legal case examples sampled for this chapter (Table 30.2) represent legal challenges to existing laws and regulations. Although such case decisions often serve as precedents for other courts across the country, the process of effecting change by accretion is both time-consuming and labor intensive. Dramatic and imminent change in the national health care system is unlikely to occur via this incremental corrective vehicle. Rather, an

TABLE 30.2

Relevant Legal Precedents

Case Precedent	Source	Description
Karsten v Kaiser Foundation Health Plan	536 U.S. 355 (2002)	Malpractice against HMO, asking paid medical bills be considered damages.
Katskee v Blue Cross Blue Shield of Nebraska	515 N.W. 2d 645 (Nebraska, 1994)	Insurance coverage metric as disease related to functions of the body over solely biologic entities.
Olmstead v LC	527 US 581 (1999)	U.S. Supreme Court decision mandates offering community-based services to individuals with severe disabilities who would otherwise require institutionalization.
Pegram v Herdrich	Pegram 120 s.Ct. at 2149–2151	No HMO could survive without some incentive connecting physician reward with treatment rationing; under ERISA, treatment decisions do not have to be made solely in the interest of the participants and beneficiaries.
Shea v Esensten	107 F.3d 625 (8th Cir. 1997)	Knowledge of financial incentives that affect a physician's decisions to refer patients to specialists is material information requiring disclosure.
Wickline v State of California	192 Cal.App.3d 1630; cert. granted, 231 Cal. Rptr. 560 (1986); review dismissed, case remanded, 239 Cal. Rptr. 805 (1987)	Physicians who comply without protest to limitations imposed by a third-party payer might bear legal responsibility for the outcome—related to do no harm

effective use of legal challenges is optimized in fine-tuning relevant legislation as problems with implementation or application arise. For example, although the Supreme Court openly affirmed in *Pegram v Hardrich* that our country has long supported financial incentives for providers as part of HMO operations, it also indicated that ERISA does not apply to such relationships. The court opened the door at the state level for legal challenges to such financial arrangements. Some states have imposed financial incentive restrictions as a consequence.[49] Humbach,[50] in an effort to call attention to perceived wrong-doing in the health insurance industry, proposed and specified a prosecution strategy to invoke criminal statute. Keying off the worrisome findings of Ware et al.[51] summarizing the Medical Outcomes Study regarding HMOs, the authors explain that the problem with civil penalties upon MCOs is that the burden of a fine can be passed along to the subscribers in the form of higher premiums as a cost of doing business. Criminal penalties cannot be shifted. The central concept revolves around the following two questions: Were the policy makers aware of risk to the patient and was the patient's life shortened or health impaired as a result of such policy decisions? Humbach[50] further targets the executives of health insurance companies for "administrative errancy," viewing criminal law as a tool of social policy and deterrent impact. Although this approach to increasing social awareness concerning problems with health care funding is unlikely to garner substantial support, it demonstrates that other means exist to encourage or complement development of national health policy.

Federal and state health-related legislation has, for the past several decades, been focused upon provision of needed regulation, funding streams, and mandated services for specific populations (Table 30.3). Even the original Medicare legislation in 1965 focused initially upon providing health care for retirees. Only in 1973 was that legislation broadened

TABLE 30.3

Relevant Legislation

Legislation	Source	Description
Americans with Disabilities Act (ADA)	Public Law 101-336, 1991	Prohibits discrimination against people with disabilities: (1) employment practices, (2) provision of state and local government services, (3) public accommodations and commercial facilities, (4) telecommunications, (5) miscellaneous (e.g., historic buildings, congressional hearings).
Emergency Medical Treatment and Active Labor Act (EMTALA)	Pozgar (2004, 252), secondary source: 42 U.S.C.A. 1395dd (3)(A) (C)(1), 1992	Hospitals required to provide either stabilizing treatment or an appropriate transfer for patients with emergency medical conditions.
Employee Retirement Income Security Act of 1974 (ERISA)	Pozgar (2004, 469)	Designed to ensure that employee welfare benefit plans conform to a uniform body of benefit law; preempts state law affecting employee benefit plans; does not regulate plan contents.
Ethics in Patient Referral Act (Stark Act)	Part of Omnibus Budget Reconciliations Act of 1989; Pozgar (2004, 469)	Prohibits physicians (HCPs) who have ownership interest or compensation arrangements with a clinical laboratory from referring patients to that lab; requires all Medicare providers to report names and provider personal identification numbers of all physicians (HCPs) or immediate relatives with ownership interests in the provider entity.
Health Care Quality Improvement Act of 1986 (HCQIA)	Pozgar (2004, 469)	Provide those persons giving information to professional review bodies and those assisting in review activities immunity from damages that may arise from adverse decisions that affect a physician's (HCP's) medical staff privileges; does not extend to civil rights litigation or suits filed by United States or state attorneys general.
Health Insurance Portability and Accountability Act of 1996 (HIPAA)	http://cms.hhs.gov/hipaa/, Pozgar (2004, 26)	Establishes national standards for electronic health care transactions and national identifiers for HCPs, health plans, and employers; addresses privacy of health data.
Medicare Waiver for Employment Services, 1981	Amended Social Security Act, section 2176 of Public Law 97-35—Omnibus Budget Reconciliation Act, Home and Community Based Services (HCBS)	Finances noninstitutional, long-term services in the community as long as costs are no higher than that of institutional care.
Safe Harbor Regulations	56 Fed. Reg. 35 952; codified at 42 C.F.R. 1006 951-953; Pozgar (2004, 480)	Describes how HCPs should structure financial arrangements to be exempt from prosecution by the Department of Justice and Federal Trade Commission.
Tax Equity and Fiscal Responsibility Act of 1982 (TEFRA)	Braddom (2005)	Specified the upper limit that Medicare could be billed by an inpatient rehabilitation facility (IRF) for an inpatient admission; individual facility cost reimbursement limits based on charges in 1982.
State Children's Health Insurance Program Act of 1997 (SCHIP)	Social Security Act Section 2108(a)	Program provides federal matching funds to help states expand health care coverage to children from low-income families. States must assess progress made in reducing the number of uninsured children.

(continued)

TABLE 30.3 (continued)

Relevant Legislation

Legislation	Source	Description
Title XIII of the Public Health Service Act—HMO Act of 1973	42 U.S.C. 300 1995	Intended to grow HMOs as cost-effective private sector health service delivery systems; amendments: 1976, eased restrictions on open enrollment, community rating, medical staffing; 1978, financial disclosures; 1981, solvency protection; 1986, certain HMO grant and loan programs abolished.
Traumatic Brain Injury Act (TBI Act); amended 2000, reauthorized 2008	Public Law 104-166, Washington, DC: U.S. Government Printing Office, 1996; Public Law 106-310, as amended 2000; S. 793 signed into law April 28, 2008	Grants to states to improve access to services for individuals and families with traumatic brain injury; and enhanced research (via National Institutes of Health), prevention and surveillance (via Center for Disease Control and Prevention) efforts.
Workforce Investment Act (WIA)	Public Law 105-220, August 7, 1998	Goals: increase occupational skills, employment retention and earnings of participants with disabilities in three funding streams: adults, dislocated workers, youth.
Work Incentive Improvement Act—Ticket to Work	Public Law 106-113, November 17, 1999	Created a payment system that allows an approved community rehabilitation provider to receive outcome-based payments for employment services to SSDI and Social Security Income consumers.

Sources: Pozgar, G. *Legal Aspects of Health Care Administration,* 9th Edition, Jones & Bartlett Publishers, Boston, MA, 2004; Braddom R., *Archives of Physical Medicine and Rehabilitation,* 86(7), 1287–1292, 2005.

to encompass individuals with disabilities. The next broad view legislation was the Americans with Disabilities Act in 1991. Despite its widespread effect upon the nation, it was focused upon eliminating discriminatory practices and barriers in the workplace and public venues. More recently, the TBI Act of 1996 provided legislative encouragement for developing community services, access to research, prevention, and surveillance. These legislative priorities address the mission of the Public Health Service and avoid the most difficult and expensive components of the continuum of care, emergency and acute intervention, and end-of-life care. In order for the tort system to function efficiently and effectively in the process of fine-tuning legislation, sweeping health system reform legislation must first be enacted.

30.6 Resolution

30.6.1 Alternative A: Maintain the Current Health Care System

Keeping in mind that approximately 47 million American citizens currently lack effective access to health care services, let us summarize the current multicomponent health care system. The federal government administers (providing funds, treatment/care delivery, and other services) in the following venues: (1) Military Health System, serving active duty military personnel and their families; (2) Veterans' Administration Health System, serving military service veterans and family members with service-connected health problems; (3) Medicare and Medicaid, serving eligible (tax contributions to the system and financial means testing) seniors, the poor, and individuals with disabilities; (4) Public Health, providing prevention and basic health services to selected populations, and epidemiologic research support; and (5) health-related research support through grant-funding agencies (e.g., National Institutes of Health, National Institute of Disability and Rehabilitation Research [NIDRR]). Ancillary to these direct health care support components is Social Security (SSDI, Social Security Income), which also offers economic support to eligible seniors and individuals with disabilities.

State governments administer Medicaid programs for those qualified, providing contracted basic health services. In addition, states administer vocational rehabilitation programs serving individuals with disabilities. Many of these programs have attempted to privatize in recent years, with variable success.[52,53] State governments provide funding for indigent care and in support of children's health services for the economically disadvantaged. Variability among state-supported health programs is widely acknowledged. We are most familiar with programs offered in Florida. A notable example of creative state government-supported health care is exemplified by the Brain and Spinal Cord Injury Program (administered within the Department of Health and funded via a trust fund based upon a percentage of driving under the influence and red light-running traffic fines). Stewart and Zafonte[46] provide a thorough description of this program. It has been heralded as a disability case management model worthy of emulation, as has occurred in both Texas and Georgia.[8,20] Finally, state government can facilitate the private sector's involvement in providing health-related programs for its citizen via grants to support residential and transitional living programs, as well as supported employment programs. Some of these programs also receive private funding from insurance and structured legal settlements. Traditionally, states have funded adaptive community-based residential living, treatment, and vocational support models serving individuals with developmental delays for decades, a program model that could be adapted to serve survivors of TBI.

As noted earlier, the private-sector managed care industry has evolved, to a major degree, into funding administrative entities. These companies operate within the structure of contract law, providing criteria-based health service funding for a variety of selected health services. The funding is designed to promote health, weighted toward prevention and hospital-based services, and to attempt to curb rising health care costs via financial incentives for cost containment.

Managed care efforts, after the first few years of trimming unnecessary health delivery costs, have not been successful in curbing the dramatic rise of health care costs.[21] In addition, as noted previously, quality of health care in the U.S. system has been called into question.[18] Employers have balked at their rising portion of employee health insurance premiums, opting to either curtail benefits (especially costly rehabilitation, mental health, and dental) or to stop offering health insurance as a benefit.[14] HCPs have been forced to staff large departments to process insurance claims, each with complex and variable reimbursement procedures.

Indigent care is typically provided by large medical centers with stated missions that include providing treatment irrespective of ability to pay. Individuals with economic disadvantages are often provided equal-quality service geared primarily toward emergency and acute inpatient treatment. Beyond that, depending upon the complexity of the medical system, individuals can receive rehabilitation services. Typically, rehabilitation services are provided with a specified dollar amount that can be applied to the *per diem* rehabilitation facility rate, therapy services, and required adaptive equipment.

Currently, undocumented aliens presenting in emergency departments for treatment typically receive needed emergency care. However, the ability to provide secondary and tertiary care (including rehabilitation services) to this population is highly variable across health care systems and remains a sensitive political issue that has yet to be resolved.

Let us now consider the ethical principles and concepts explained earlier in relation to the current health care system.

30.6.1.1 Respect for Autonomy

Freedom to choose HCPs is highly variable among the variety of health insurance plans (governmental and private). Absent a mandatory national health insurance system in which all HCPs are enrolled, true freedom of choice is necessarily limited. Similarly, disclosure of covered health services, an essential component of informed consent, has traditionally been inconsistent. Until legally challenged, gag rules were supported in the interest of MCO profit, preventing true informed consent by patients. However, consent processes are necessary to defend resource allocation rules ethically. A detailed discussion of informed consent in the context of managed care is provided by Emanuel.[36] He notes that consumer market choice reflects consent only if a reasonable range of choices is available. He concludes that establishing consent would require sustained commitment on the part of MCOs, especially given the lack of knowledge regarding best practices for acquiring consent at an organizational level. With this commitment, several benefits might be realized, such as support for service limits.

30.6.1.2 Beneficence

The health care system and funding mechanisms that drive them are focused upon benefiting individuals in need of health care. The methods of providing that benefit are highly variable, with frequently encountered barriers to accessing needed resources being economic and contractual limitations of health insurance plans.

30.6.1.3 Nonmaleficence

Preventing harm (especially medical errors) is an active goal within the U.S. health care system.[1] However, there appears to be a conceptual disconnect between provision of health services and funding those same services, even though they are necessarily interrelated and interdependent. Individuals avoid seeking necessary services because of limited coverage and perceptual concerns driving exclusionary criteria (e.g., mental health coverage). In addition, financial incentives or caps discouraging high cost but important comprehensive procedures (e.g., neuropsychological testing) can result in misdiagnosis and/or mistreatment. When elective services are considered, the funding process enjoys ethical distance from the freely chosen and optional health care service.

30.6.1.4 Justice

Within the current health care system, costs are rising, reflected in the rising percent of the GDP spent on health care. Cost containment methods have relied heavily on employer-based insurance plans plus government-sponsored programs and have been variable. The current health care system is inequitable and overly restrictive in its funding procedures.

It is lacking in unfettered universal access to basic health care services, favoring those who are economically advantaged and can purchase services out of pocket from HCPs with open panels. Thus, problems in both access and just allocation exist.

30.6.1.5 Duty to Care

HCPs, within their areas of competence, must be able to provide needed health care to anyone presenting in need of service. Financial restrictions upon providing basic health care services are ethically untenable. The ability to provide needed health care is presumed in the obligation to receive what is owed (return to health) based on the principle of due care.

30.6.1.6 Conflict of Interest

With the successful legal challenge to the concept of "gag clauses" contained in employment contracts between HCPs and MCOs, financial constraints can no longer be the reason that information (availability of alternatives, second opinions) is kept from patients.[7] However, financially based restrictions upon validly requested basic service delivery (affecting length of stay, type, duration, and intensity of services) continue to place HCPs and health care organizations alike in an untenable ethical situation. MCOs have used expensive equipment (e.g., argumentative communication devices) to reduce costs, such as limiting sophisticated testing and referrals to specialists who provide more costly care. On the other hand, financial incentives linked to improved health do not necessarily create a conflict of interest.

30.6.1.7 Benefits

- Status quo avoids difficult choices involving competing political forces and funding realities.
- The private health insurance business sector continues to derive profit from health funding administration.
- Taxation remains unchanged with respect to health care.
- Consumers familiar with current systems are not imposed upon toward alternative structures they must navigate anew.

30.6.1.8 Costs

- A sizeable minority of citizens has limited or no access to basic health services.
- Increasing health care costs are negatively impacting the economy. The looming budget crisis within the Medicare and Medicaid systems, as well as Social Security, will impact within the next 8 years.
- The quality of health care in the United States continues to lag behind that of other industrialized countries (near the bottom of the 13 most advanced industrialized countries), based on what Kawachi[54] surmises as economic inequality. MCOs have not ensured improved health care for the cost efficiencies gained. It has also been argued that private insurance is more costly to administer than public insurance.[2,24]

- Employers, especially small businesses, faced with paying increasing health insurance premiums for employees are likely to continue to curtail or eliminate health care benefits, especially when adverse selection is at play (i.e., plans selected for healthier beneficiaries; conversely, enrollees gravitate toward plans that provide for specific personal health needs).

30.6.2 Alternative B: Two-Tiered Health Care System—Universal Basic Health Care (NHI), Plus Elective Services Available for Private Pay

Beauchamp and Childress[12] have proposed a two-tiered system of health care that includes providing universal access to a decent minimum of health care (government funded) while preserving the opportunity to purchase additional services beyond the minimum for those with the ability to pay (out-of-pocket private insurance). A national health insurance program would provide universal access to preventive and treatment services, including mental health and rehabilitation, addressing the current ethical and economic concerns of the current system. Given performance and cost data from existing health care systems within the federal government's purview (Military Health System, Veterans' Administration Health System, Medicare and Medicaid), and information from other countries' national health system,[18] the processes of health service delivery, cost containment, and policy governing the operation of such a system are available to implement a national health insurance program.

For individuals with disabilities, routine prevention, treatment, and care services would be provided under the National Health Insurance (NHI) system. Current Medicaid waiver programs like HCBS would be preserved and subsumed under the NHI system. Information gleaned from postacute treatment and care for individuals with TBI could be utilized to design a uniform and comprehensive cost-effective system of long-term care and support infrastructure (transitional living, residential treatment for neurobehavioral problems, vocational development programs, care partner assistance, and case management).[46]

This complex undertaking would require increased taxes or other creative funding sources. DeGrazia,[24] who favors a single-payer system for health care, critiques several proposals for acquiring universal coverage while addressing costs (e.g., tax credits; incremental expansion of Medicare, Medicaid, and SCHIP; employer mandates) put forth by the 2008 U.S. presidential candidates. Federally mandated participation in such an NHI plan would be understood, as well as development of rules and regulation governing operation, along with a continuing oversight mechanism to ensure both quality care and cost controls. Selection of preventive, diagnostic, treatment, and care services to be included in the category of basic health care would require careful consideration.

Caution would need to be exercised to ensure that health care resulting from catastrophic events that produce lifelong health care needs be included, along with more routine medical procedures. Balancing costs of short duration expensive interventions (surgeries, emergency treatment, technology-intensive specialty diagnostics or treatment) with long-term care and support for chronic conditions will be a challenge in crafting an effective comprehensive health system. An example of an approach to address this balance is provided by Israel, which uses a system in which new technologies are routinely evaluated based on guiding criteria (e.g., number of individuals who would benefit, potential to prevent death or morbidity, financial burden) and then rated as having a specific priority level for consideration for addition to the core set of services.[19]

Let us again consider implications of a proposed (two-tiered) reform to the health care system in terms of ethical principles and concepts.

30.6.2.1 Respect for Autonomy

Choice of provider would be facilitated, given mandatory participation in the NHI by all HCPs. In addition, choice for elective services beyond basic health care would be available to those individuals with the ability to pay.

30.6.2.2 Beneficence

The system's balance would be swung back toward the welfare of the individual, without at-the-bedside limitations imposed upon individuals by financial constraints. In meeting their ethical obligations regarding duty to care, the HCPs would be free to focus solely upon provision of appropriate quality health care services to those in need, constrained only by standards of practice and discipline-specific codes of ethics.

30.6.2.3 Nonmaleficence

Potential harm caused by denial or delay of health care would be reduced by universal access to a single-payer national health insurance program because questions regarding whether one qualifies for basic services would no longer be relevant. Consistent with due care, the individual citizen would be provided needed basic health services without economic discrimination.

30.6.2.4 Justice

Provision of the opportunity for access to both basic and elective health care services allows for equitable distribution of health care resources within the sociocultural context of the United States, while maintaining centralized control over costs. For example, administrative efficiencies and cost savings would be realized through removal of or streamlined processes for marketing, billing, eligibility screenings, and fee structures. Ensuring fair procedures regarding both policy making (with input from providers and consumers alike during system development) and health care decision making for the individual reinforce the notion of equity in meeting the health care needs of the populace.

30.6.2.5 Conflict of Interest

The separation of the processes of cost containment and provision of health care obviates this ethical confound.

30.6.2.6 Benefits

- Reforming the U.S. health care system offers the chance to redress inequities in provision of needed care and increase quality of care.
- The health insurance industry would continue to profit from the elective procedure component of the two-tiered system.
- Proper disclosure of expenditures incurred by a national health insurance program would offer the taxpayer the opportunity to evaluate its effectiveness and offer modifications through the legislative process.

- Health care cost containment would become a reality without the vagaries of open market economic forces. Firm budgetary data would allow knowledgeable consideration of the consequences of NHI upon Medicare and Medicaid programs, along with Social Security.

- The layered approach remains consistent with fundamental American values regarding market influence on elective care.

- A transparent appeals process for service denial could exist as an opportunity to educate the public and review current practices.

- Consumers should experience greater autonomy in provider selection.

30.6.2.7 *Costs*

- An initial period of disruption would accompany sweeping change in the health care system on a national scale. However, as has been noted within the managed care era of U.S. health care, such dramatic changes are relatively quickly accommodated and ways to maximize care efficiency explored within the newly established operational parameters.

- Employers would be relieved of the burden of providing health insurance premium offsets to employees. Some may elect to provide cost-reduced elective health insurance benefits under a group risk pool rationale for those employees seeking to avail themselves of elective health care services as an incentive for employment.

- Increased taxes would likely be inevitable, but this fact must be reconciled with the elimination of private health insurance premiums, out-of-pocket copays, and possible reduction in taxes related to Medicare and Medicaid programs (assuming restructure).

- Lack of incentives may discourage providers from participating or providing high-quality care. Although this is a risk, we believe it is offset by simplification of processes that are currently overly bureaucratic and cumbersome (e.g., billing). Providers may find they gain time that can be redirected toward increased patient care.

30.7 Disposition

It is clearly recognized that the political challenges will be many and that intermediate steps and compromise may be necessary (see Menzel[55] for example) to move significantly toward universal coverage and/or a single payer for that coverage in the United States. However, a budgetary crisis in the Medicare and Medicaid systems is looming and may force such change under duress if planned action is not taken.[2] With the advent of the Obama administration, the nation has yet another clear opportunity to engage in the complex process of planning and implementing health care reform to address the inequities in care delivery and costs experienced across the current health care system.

30.8 Additional Commentary

Although no system of health care reform satisfies all ethical concerns and challenges currently created by the U.S. health care system, providing a basic minimum of care to all citizens is a necessary, but not sufficient, component of change. It is acknowledged that this model inherently favors increased numbers of individuals covered over more comprehensive care offered to fewer individuals. Although support for this model for some is based on the belief that every American is entitled to receive care in a just society, for others it is also based on the belief that not doing so is ultimately more costly. Consider, for example, that lack of health insurance leads to delayed diagnosis, life-threatening complications, and 18,000 premature deaths in the United States each year.[56] Therefore, the long-term costs of not providing minimum care strain the system in a manner that universal care would constructively impact. In addition, creating a system perceived to embody easier access would help shift system entry for underserved patients away from costly emergency care and toward lower cost preventative care.

   National health care reform does not imply complete separation of fiscal responsibility from individual health care practice, however. This exclusive separation would be ethically untenable. Specifically, it would be unjust to drain resources by recommending a higher cost procedure for which empirical data exist to support equal or better outcomes for a lower cost procedure. It is important to recognize, however, that the focus of this decision for the HCP is rightfully on health outcome; thus, beneficence drives the decision with the secondary consideration being the principle of justice, whereby cost containment creates a pool of dollars for future distribution of resources toward additional available health services. Similarly, elective care available in the two-tiered system cannot operate unconstrained regardless of the patient's autonomous choice or treatment availability. One only has to consider the challenges created by end-of-life care to acknowledge the complexities of balancing ethical contingencies in treatment decisions. Checks and balances must always exist to maximize fulfillment of ethical obligations across potentially competing principles.

   As noted earlier, health care models cannot require HCPs in the field to make decisions driven by cost containment. Decisions must be based on beliefs in beneficent care and effective outcome. Therefore, disturbing questions, such as should a patient forfeit his or her right to care if knowingly engaging in behavior documented to result in costly treatment (e.g., unsafe sexual behavior, smoking, noncompliance with medication regimens resulting in serious complications) become moot. Health care providers must be able to evaluate and treat based on presenting diagnosis and not past behavior; otherwise, the ethical foundation upon which most health care disciplines is built crumbles. National health care reform argues against such restrictions but favors an informed process to determine minimum care.

   Perhaps the most fundamental challenge of establishing universal care, then, is to define the core upon which this model rests: What type of care and how much of that care is every citizen entitled to? How does one weigh qualitative factors, such as patient suffering? Should some care that is known to reduce morbidity and mortality (e.g., prenatal screening) be mandated, such as childhood immunizations currently are, versus simply made available? Our country has strong legal underpinnings favoring respect for autonomy so such a heavy-handed approach is unlikely and would place providers at odds with patients exercising their right of free choice, compromising the patient–provider relationship. However, this dilemma nevertheless raises the issue of what is informed choice in a national health care system?

Sabik and Lie[19] compared priority setting in eight countries and found two major approaches to establishing basic care. Norway, the Netherlands, Sweden, and Denmark began with commissions determining abstract principles governing decision priorities, and Israel, New Zealand, the United Kingdom, and Oregon in the United States established governing commissions that recommended the specific services to be covered. In general, Sabik and Lie[19] found that the priority-setting principles had little effect on health policy. On the other hand, the policies of the commissions that had decision-making authority for services covered (i.e., the countries/state taking the second approach) were implemented, although not without limitations, revisions, and challenges (see, for example, comments provided by Wailoo et al.[57] on the system used in the United Kingdom). Sabik and Lie[19] further concluded that priority setting should be led by health care experts and that we will be challenged to create an appropriate balance between these panels and some degree of public involvement in decision making. The difficulty in translating community values into health care policy is echoed by Ubel.[58] Sabik and Lie[19] suggest a core component of public involvement should be that citizens are provided the rationale for decisions made. As Emanuel[36] has discussed, this involvement could also take multiple other forms, ranging from citizens being informed about minimum care recommendations with the opportunity to provide feedback on relative value to citizen representatives on the commissions setting the rules for inclusion or exclusion. Thus, consideration of participant values establishes an organizational level of respect for autonomy. However, although various participation methods have been used for more than a decade, they have lacked empirical scrutiny.[59,p. 95] Ubel[58] suggests that multiple methods for measuring community values should be used and offers discussion that combines these methods with ethical analysis. He suggests that, through the use of multiple measurement strategies, any existing consensual community preferences can be identified. However, prior to incorporating these values into health care policy, they must be vetted empirically to prevent discriminatory practices against vulnerable populations, such as individuals with TBI. Other research suggests that, with appropriate information, the public is willing to participate in exercises involving the allocation of limited resources and may also be willing to abide by group decisions regarding service priorities.[35,60]

30.9 Summary

Universal health care does not eliminate the need for rationing because there will always be a limited health care budget. Conversely, however, ethical concerns do not inherently arise from the limited pool of dollars available. Ethical concerns arise when the rules surrounding resource accessibility and/or allocation appear unjust, nontransparent, or ambiguous, for which the current U.S. health care system has been soundly criticized. Minimum care begins to address the inequities within the current U.S. health care system reflected in the 47 million uninsured Americans. To implement the system successfully, decisions regarding minimum care must be socially (publicly) endorsed, which require rules that are perceived to be unambiguous and equitable. The question of justice comes into clear focus based on whether and how resources are accessed and distributed. Although we can never totally separate financial incentive from health care decisions, creating a system that prevents providers from withholding services or not disclosing service limitations in the interest of profit is more consistent with beneficent care, patient autonomy, and a just system. It is acknowledged, however, that national health care reform cannot simply be mandated and expected to be fully actualized without addressing fundamental values and historical barriers, such as representation of minority providers and lack of consideration of cultural factors that significantly influence access to care even when care is available. For example, minorities have been found to be underrepresented in inpatient rehabilitation care.[33] Active community representation after the priority-setting schema is established may prove critical in legitimizing a system to which disenfranchised citizens will respond by changing their health care behavior. However, translating community values into health care policy is complicated at best. Significant research is needed to understand the role of the public in influencing broad health policy and ultimate social acceptance of, and thus, informed consent to, any major reform effort intended to balance beneficent care with justice. In addition, educating the public regarding the service needs of individuals with TBI is an ongoing challenge. Consider, for example, the findings of Mellick et al.,[33] who analyzed postacute hospital pathways for persons with TBI enrolled in a statewide Traumatic Brain Injury Registry and Follow-up System. Almost 65% of individuals were discharged home from acute hospitalization *without follow-up services* (i.e., no inpatient rehabilitation, outpatient care, or long-term care), *including 54.3% of persons with moderate TBI and 23.5% of persons with severe TBI.* As Norma B. Anderson, then president of ASHA, has stated, "insurance companies, the health care system, and the public all need to become far more informed and accepting about TBI so that it becomes much better known and understood, and treatment for optimal recovery becomes widely available."[11, p.3]

There is no question that even after a universal system of care is established, the need for strong advocacy for individuals with TBI remains. Advocating for inclusion of services based on the development of new technologies or stronger empirical support for specific assessment and intervention strategies will be critical to advancing TBI care. Any health care reform process will have to address the fundamental design problem of current health care systems with foci that has been on acute care without adequately addressing the lifelong service needs of people with disabilities and other chronic health issues.[61] Both individuals and organizations, such as local Brain Injury Association (BIA) chapters and discipline-specific associations, will play key roles in influencing evolving policy regarding standard care for persons with TBI. In addition, similar to existing systems, individual providers and organizations will likely still need to assist persons with TBI and their families in appealing denial decisions and seek to reconcile inconsistent implementation of regulations across states. This is especially true during times of transition, an example of which is the multiyear transition being undertaken by the CMS, which has been moving away from separate regional carriers for Part A and Part B and is, instead, implementing the 15 Medicare Administrative Contractors handling all Part A and B claims processing based on geographic region. This change is the result of the Medicare Modernization Act, and as noted earlier, is an attempt to reduce costs by streamlining claims processing. This type of transformation is just one example illustrating that changes in implementation over time are a forgone conclusion of any health care reform process, and organizations that have traditionally held strong advocacy positions for persons with TBI will continue to be critical to influence the direction of health care coverage and access.

Advocacy also remains the lynchpin of successful legislative efforts to ensure appropriate focus on TBI policy that either directly or indirectly impacts health care reform. For example, S. 793, the TBI Act of 2008, was signed into law on April 28, 2008, authorizing appropriations and modifying state grants via the Department of Health and Human Services for tracking TBI occurrence and supporting TBI rehabilitation. Ultimately, these types of successes are the result of the tireless efforts of many at multiple levels of our social structure who are interested in ensuring that beneficent care for persons with TBI remains possible, regardless of the health care system used. Given the current presidential candidates' positions on health care reform, we will likely continue to see employer-based programs coupled with expansion of existing public programs, at least in the near term.[24] Advocacy will be needed as much, if not more, to ensure that the disenfranchisement of a significant number of U.S. citizens, including persons with TBI, does not occur in any system whose intent is ultimately to improve health care for all of its citizens.

References

1. Kohn, L. T., Corrigan, J. M., and Donaldson, M. S., *To Err Is Human: Building a Safer Health System*, National Academies Press, Washington, DC, 1999.
2. Wilensky, G., *The Politics of Health Care Reform*, presented at the University of Florida, College of Public Health and Health Professions, 50th Anniversary Lecture Series, Gainesville, FL, 2008, Apr. 11.
3. Banja, J., Patient advocacy at risk: Ethical, legal and political dimensions of adverse reimbursement practices in brain injury rehabilitation in the U.S., *Brain Injury*, 13(10), 745–758, 1999.
4. Kerkhoff, T., Hanson, S., Guenther, R., and Ashkanazi, G., The foundations and application of ethical principles in rehabilitation psychology, *Rehabilitation Psychology*, 42(1), 17–30, 1997.
5. Stern, L., Rossiter, L., and Wilensky, G., Ethics, health care, and the Enthoven proposal, *Health Affairs*, 1(3), 48–63, 1982.
6. Hanson, S. L., Kerkhoff, T. R., and Bush, S. S., *Health Care Ethics for Psychologists: A Casebook*, American Psychological Association Press, Washington, DC, 2005.
7. Pozgar, G., *Legal Aspects of Health Care Administration*, 10th ed., Jones and Bartlett, Sudbury, MA, 2007.
8. Kitchener, M., Ng, T., Grossman, B., and Harrington, C., Medicaid waiver programs for traumatic brain and spinal cord injury, *Journal of Health and Social Policy*, 20(3), 51–66, 2005.
9. Kaplan, S., Growth and payment adequacy of Medicare postacute care rehabilitation, *Archives of Physical Medicine and Rehabilitation*, 88(11), 1494–1499, 2007.
10. Centers for Medicare and Medicaid Services, *Inpatient Rehabilitation Facility PPS and the 75% Rule*, U.S. Department of Health and Human Services, Washington, DC, 2007.
11. American Speech–Language–Hearing Association, ASHA Poll: Inadequate insurance coverage hinders the public's recovery from traumatic brain injury, June 19, 2007, http://www.asha.org/about/news/tbievent/tbipressrelease.htm (accessed December 11, 2007).
12. Beauchamp, T. L. and Childress, J. S., *Biomedical Ethics*, 5th ed., Wiley, New York, 2001.
13. Weber, L., *Business Ethics in Healthcare: Beyond Compliance*, Indiana University Press, Bloomington, IN, 2001.
14. Braddom R., Medicare funding for inpatient rehabilitation: How did we get to this point and what do we do now?, *Archives of Physical Medicine and Rehabilitation*, 86(7), 1287–1292, 2005.
15. Cicerone, K. D., Dahlberg, C., Kalmar, K., Langenbahn, D. M., Malec, J. F., Berqquist, T. F., Felicetti, T., et al., Evidence-based cognitive rehabilitation: Recommendations for clinical practice, *Archives of Physical Medicine and Rehabilitation*, 81(12), 1596–1615, 2000.

16. Cicerone, K. D., Dahlberg, C., Malec, J. F., Langenbahn, D. M., Felicetti, T., Kneipp, S., Ellmo, W., et al., Evidence-based cognitive rehabilitation: Updated review of the literature from 1998 through 2002, *Archives of Physical Medicine and Rehabilitation*, 86(8), 1681–1692, 2005.

17. Ruger, J. P., The moral foundations of health insurance, *QJM: An International Journal of Medicine*, 100(1), 53–57, 2007.

18. Mappes, T. and DeGrazia, D., *Biomedical Ethics*, 6th ed., McGraw Hill, New York, 2005.

19. Sabik, L. M. and Lie, R. K., Priority setting in health care: Lessons from the experiences of eight countries, *International Journal for Equity in Health*, 7(4), 2008. http://www.equityhealthj.com/content/pdf/1475-9276-7-4.pdf.2008.

20. Reynolds, W. E., Page, S. J., and Johnston, M. V., Coordinated and adequately funded state streams for rehabilitation of newly injured persons with TBI, *Journal of Head Trauma Rehabilitation*, 16(1), 34–46, 2001.

21. Chan L., The state-of-the-science: Challenges in designing postacute care payment policy, *Archives of Physical Medicine and Rehabilitation*, 88(11), 1522–1525, 2007.

22. Lehr, Jr., R. P., Therapy, neuroplasticity, and rehabilitation, in M. J. Ashley (Ed.), *Traumatic Brain Injury: Rehabilitative Treatment and Case Management*, 2nd ed., CRC Press, Boca Raton, FL, 2004, 303–316.

23. Moon, M., Medicare, *New England Journal of Medicine*, 344(12), 928–931, 2001.

24. DeGrazia, D., Single payer meets managed competition: The case for public funding and private delivery, *Hastings Center Report*, 38(1), 23–33, 2008.

25. Stineman, M. G., Prospective payment, prospective challenge, *Archives of Physical Medicine and Rehabilitation*, 83(12), 1802–1805, 2002.

26. Callahan, C., Billing reimbursement: 2008 Update, Paper presented at the APA, Division 22, RP 2008 Rehabilitation Psychology Conference, Tucson, AZ, 2008, April 4, http://www.cms.hhs.gov/InpatientRehabFacPPS/Downloads/IRF_PPS_75_percent_rule_060807.pdf (accessed January 17, 2008).

27. Hoffman, J. M., Doctor, J. N., Chan, L., Whyte, J., Jha, A., and Dikmen, S., Potential impact of the new Medicare Prospective Payment System on reimbursement for traumatic brain injury inpatient rehabilitation, *Archives of Physical Medicine and Rehabilitation*, 84(8), 1165–1172, 2003.

28. DeJong, G., Horn, S. D., Smout, R. J., and Ryser, D. K., The early impact of the inpatient rehabilitation facility prospective payment system on stroke rehabilitation case mix, practice patterns, and outcomes, *Archives of Physical Medicine and Rehabilitation*, 86(12, Suppl. 2), S93–S100, 2005.

29. Frymark, T. B. and Mullen, R. C., Influence of the prospective payment system on speech–language pathology services, *American Journal of Physical Medicine and Rehabilitation*, 84(1), 12–21, 2005.

30. Kreutzer, J. S., Kolakowsky-Hayner, S. A., Ripley, D., Cifu, D. X., Rosenthal, M., Bushnik, T., Zafonte, R., Englander, J., and High, W., Changes and lengths of stay for acute and inpatient rehabilitation treatment of traumatic brain injury 1990–1996, *Brain Injury*, 15(9), 763–774, 2001.

31. Hoffman, J., Change in inpatient rehabilitation admissions for individuals with TBI after implementation of the Medicare IRF-PPS, Presented at State of the Science Symposium on Post-Acute Rehabilitation: Setting a research agenda and developing an evidence base for practice and public policy, Crystal City, VA, 2007.

32. McCue, M. J. and Thompson, J. M., Early effects of the prospective payment system on inpatient rehabilitation hospital performance, *Archives of Physical Medicine and Rehabilitation*, 87(2), 198–202, 2006.

33. Mellick, D., Gerhart, K. A., and Whiteneck, G. G., Understanding outcomes based on the postacute hospitalization pathways followed by persons with traumatic brain injury, *Brain Injury*, 17(1), 55–71, 2003.

34. Clohan D. B., Durkin E. M., Hammel J., Murray, P., Whyte, J., Dijkers, M., Gans, B. M. N., Graves, D. E., Heinemann, A. W., and Worsowicz, G., Postacute rehabilitation research and policy recommendations, *Archives of Physical Medicine and Rehabilitation*, 88(11), 1535–1541, 2007.

35. Danis, M., Biddle, A. K., and Goold, S. D., Enrollees choose priorities for Medicare, *The Gerontologist*, 44(1), 58–67, 2004.
36. Emanuel, E. J., Justice and managed care: Four principles for the just allocation of health care resources, *Hastings Center Report*, 30(3), 8–16, 2000.
37. Prigatano, G. P. and Gupta, S., Friends after traumatic brain injury in children, *Journal of Head Trauma Rehabilitation*, 21(6), 505–513, 2006.
38. Prigatano, G. and Fordyce, D., *Neuropsychological Rehabilitation after Brain Injury*, Johns Hopkins University Press, Baltimore, MD, 1986.
39. Winstanley, J., Simpson, G., Tate, R., and Myles, B., Early indicators and contributors to psychological distress in relatives during rehabilitation following severe traumatic brain injury: Findings from the Brain Injury Outcomes Study, *Journal of Head Trauma Rehabilitation*, 21(6), 453–466, 2006.
40. Corrigan J. D., Substance abuse as a mediating factor in outcome from traumatic brain injury, *Archives of Physical Medicine and Rehabilitation*, 76(4), 302–309, 1995.
41. Langlois, J. A., Rutland-Brown, W., and Wald, M. M., The epidemiology and impact of traumatic brain injury: A brief overview, *Journal of Head Trauma Rehabilitation*, 21(5), 375–378, 2006.
42. Toseland, R., *Caregiver Education and Support Programs: Best Practices Models*, Monograph, Family Caregiver Alliance, San Francisco, CA, 2004.
43. Iezzoni, L. I. and Ngo, L., Health, disability, and life insurance experiences of working-age persons with multiple sclerosis, *Multiple Sclerosis*, 13(4), 534–546, 2007.
44. Brain Injury Association of Massachusetts, Prevention Programs—Gateway Diversion Program, http://www.biama.org/whatdoes/gateway.html (accessed April 28, 2008).
45. Palsbo, S. E., Medicaid payment for telerehabilitation, *Archives of Physical Medicine and Rehabilitation*, 85(7), 1188–1191, 2004.
46. Stuart, M. and Zafonte, R., Fighting the silent epidemic: The Florida Brain and Spinal Cord Injury Program, *Journal of Head Trauma Rehabilitation*, 19(4), 329–340, 2004.
47. Rosenbach, M., Ellwood, M., Irvin, C., Young, C., Conroy, W., Quinn, B., and Kell, M., Implementation of the State Children's Health Insurance Program: Synthesis of State Evaluations, 2003, http://www.cms.hhs.gov/NationalSCHIPPolicy/07_EvaluationsAndReports.asp#TopOfPage (accessed SCHIP FY 2001 Report to Congress June 10, 2008).
48. Brain Injury Association of America, Facts about traumatic brain injury, http://biausa.org/elements/aboutbi/factsheets/factsaboutbi_2008.pdf (accessed April 28, 2008).
49. Bloche, M. G. and Jacobson, P. D., The Supreme Court and bedside rationing, *Journal of the American Medical Association*, 284(21), 2776–2779, 2000.
50. Humbach, J. A., Criminal prosecution for HMO treatment denial, *Special Law Digest: Health Care Law*, 282, 9–49, 2002.
51. Ware, J. E., Bayliss, M. S., Rogers, W. H., Kosinski, M., and Tarlov, A. R., Differences in 4-year health outcomes for elderly and poor, chronically ill patients treated in HMO and fee-for-service systems: Results from the Medical Outcome Study, *Journal of the American Medical Association*, 276(13), 1039–1047, 1996.
52. Goodall, P. and Ghiloni, C. T., The changing face of publicly funded employment services, *Journal of Head Trauma Rehabilitation*, 16(1), 94–106, 2001.
53. Vaughn, S. L. and King, A., A survey of state programs to finance rehabilitation and community services for individuals with brain injury, *Journal of Head Trauma Rehabilitation*, 16(1), 20–33, 2001.
54. Kawachi, I., Why the United States is not number one in health, in J. Morone and L. Jacobs (Eds.), *Healthy, Wealthy, and Fair: Health Care and the Good Society*, Oxford University Press, New York, 2005. Excerpted from B. Steinbock, J. Arras, and A. London (Eds.), *Ethical Issues in Modern Medicine: Contemporary Readings in Bioethics*, McGraw Hill, New York, 2009, 222–230.
55. Menzel, P. T., A path to universal access, *Hastings Center Report*, 38(1), 34–36, 2008.
56. Institute of Medicine, *Insuring America's Health: Principles and Recommendations*, National Academies Press, Washington, DC, 2004.

57. Wailoo, A., Roberts, J., Brazier, J., and McCabe, C., Efficiency, equity, and NICE clinical guidelines, *British Medical Journal*, 328(7439), 536–537, 2004.

58. Ubel, P. A., The challenge of measuring community values in ways appropriate for setting health care priorities, *Kennedy Institute of Ethics Journal*, 9(3), 263–284, 1999.

59. Abelson, J., Eyles, J., McLeod, C. B., Collins, P., McMullan, C., and Forest, P. G., Does deliberation make a difference? Results from a citizens panel study of health goals priority setting, *Health Policy*, 66(1), 95–106, 2003.

60. Danis, M., Biddle, A. K., and Dorr Goold, S., Insurance benefit preferences of the low- income uninsured, *Journal of General Internal Medicine*, 17(2), 125–133, 2002.

61. Emanuel, E. J., The problem with single-payer plans, *Hastings Center Report*, 38(1), 38–41, 2008.

31

Discharge Planning in Traumatic Brain Injury Rehabilitation

Mark J. Ashley and Susan M. Ashley

CONTENTS

31.1 Introduction

Traumatic brain injury (TBI) has the potential to visit upon an individual tremendous change and, in some cases, devastation to life as it might have been known to the person prior to injury. Although professionals struggle to find better ways to mitigate the effects of brain injury, treatment must ultimately come to an end. When it does, the fruits of the discharge planning process become more or less apparent. Discharge planners faces tremendous challenges at all levels of care, not the least of which is developing a firm understanding of the broad impact of brain injury upon the person.

To be most effective in discharge planning, it is important to understand the impact of TBI on the individual, family, and society. Jennings[1] eloquently summarizes the writings of March et al.[2] as follows:

TBI is a complex nexus of symbols, norms, relationships, both interpersonal and intrap-ersonal perceptions and negotiated identities, and caregiving activities. TBI brings forth a new character on the social stage. There enters a person with a different set of memories, feelings, capacities, abilities, and needs placed in a family ecosystem where he is at once an intimate and a stranger. His very presence violates boundaries of many different kinds and provides nearly everyone involved with a serious chal-lenge to their repertory of ordinary social skills and responses. Role reversal and role distance become endemic, everyday issues. Women must relearn how to be wives or mothers, and men, husbands or fathers. Children, now sadly perhaps the wiser or more quick-witted, must reconstruct a relationship with a parent. The entire kinship system shakes.[1, p. 34]

Jennings goes on to say:

Then, because TBI plays such havoc with what Thomas Hobbes called the "small mor-als" of everyday life (the etiquette of cursing, table manners, personal grooming, and the like), the large morals—the human rights and rules of nondiscrimination, dignity, respect, and social justice—that really matter to our humanity become even more cru-cial than they ordinarily are. TBI tests not so much things like patience (although it does do that), but more significantly and tellingly, it tests respect, justice, and love.[1]

Jennings suggests:

The primary duty of the family with respect to the person with TBI is not so much protection from bodily harm, nor the promotion of best interests, at least as that term is commonly understood. Instead, familial and caregiving duties should revolve around practices needed to sustain the person's human flourishing or quality of life as a person. Providing comfort and safety, mere guardianship, is not enough.[1]

There are a number of practical challenges to discharge planning that bear some com-ment. First, length of stay (LOS) in medical treatment and rehabilitation has been impacted by huge decrements. Since 1990, the overall LOS for acute hospitalization and for hospital-based rehabilitation has decreased markedly for persons with TBI.[3,4] Overall, hospitaliza-tion rates for TBI decreased by 50% from 1993 to 1996. Kreutzer et al.[4] reported acute care LOS averaged between 22 to 29 days between 1990 and 1994, and decreased to less than 20 days in 1995, and an average of 16 days in 1996. Average LOS for acute rehabilitation hos-pitalization decreased from 47.74 days in 1990 to 29.49 days in 1996. They attributed these changes to concurrently occurring changes in overall delivery of medical services resulting from the impact of managed care. It seems reasonable, nonetheless, to conclude that earlier discharges from shorter LOS are likely to complicate the discharge planner's job. In 2009, LOS for hospital-based treatment of brain injury less than 14 days is not uncommon.

At the same time that societal trends toward lesser treatment increase, discharge plan-ners are left with fewer discharge options and an ever present need for pragmatism in securing a suitable discharge scenario for a given patient. The process of discharge plan-ning varies with the setting in which it is undertaken, the amount of information that is available to the discharge planner, and resources that may be available for ongoing care for the individual. And, as if the process was not complicated enough, the discharge planner is dealing with a disease that is likely the most complicated in its impact and ramifications for the individual, the family, and society.

It is therefore difficult to approach the subject of discharge planning with a single view because of the different levels of treatment from which discharge planning must occur—that is, acute hospitalization, hospital-based rehabilitation, or various postacute rehabilitation settings. Rotondi et al.[5] identified a trend of inconsistent findings in the professional literature regarding the needs of caregivers and persons with injury that resulted in confusion or disparate reporting of needs. They undertook a longitudinal data collection process using semistructured interviewing of individuals with injury and their caregivers across four postinjury phases: (1) acute care, (2) inpatient rehabilitation, (3) return home (a transitional period typically lasted about 3 or 4 months after discharge from inpatient care), and (4) a postreturn home phase that could be described as "life in the community." Of greatest interest are the findings relative to phases 3 and 4 pertaining to the longer term discharge picture. First, there are differences in the reported needs between individuals with injury and their caregivers. This is consistent with other literature in this area and points to the need to consider both individuals with injury and caregivers in treatment formulation. Six themes were identified as important across all phases: (1) understanding injuries, treatments, and consequences; 2) emotional and mental health of persons with TBI; (3) financial assistance; (4) guidance; (5) family emotional and mental health; and (6) finding and evaluating providers. In the longest term phases, additional themes of importance included the following: (1) reassessment of the person with TBI, (2) community integration, (3) support group, (4) support from family and friends, (5) care coordination, (6) respite services, and (7) life planning. These findings point to the needs individuals with injury and their caregivers have for differing types of information, services, and support over time.

Families are not always ready to take in information when professionals are ready to provide it. Professionals may provide information and terminology that is too complex to be understood or may provide that information at a time when the family or the individual with injury are unable to understand it. The findings of Rotondi et al.[5] strongly support the need for the development of an easily accessible system of information that is designed to meet the diverse needs of the entire population of individuals living with brain injury and their caregivers, as they progress along the continuum from injury to long-term living. In addition, treaters engaged in the earliest phases are well advised to understand the kind of information that is relevant to the person with injury and their caregivers at points in time in which these early treaters are involved. Knowledge of the long-term information, service, and support needs can be utilized by early treaters to begin to prepare individuals with injury and their caregivers for the longer term. It is unlikely, however, that treaters during the early phases will successfully provide a complete preparation for the long term. For those individuals and/or families who tend toward a desire to terminate treatment quickly during the early phases, thinking that return home will mean a return to normal functioning, this information may be useful in encouraging them to complete treatment as recommended and prepare them better for the longer term. Finally, these findings are particularly pertinent when one considers that the predominant service delivery model is one that is "front-end loaded" with medical and rehabilitative services. The latter two phases are far less impacted by availability of medical and rehabilitative services, resulting in the need for individuals with injury and their caregivers to "go it alone."

Discharge planners frequently must focus on the immediate discharge environment following a treatment setting. Although this is quite important, such an approach does not tend to prepare the person or the caregivers for the longer term. As the field of TBI rehabilitation has matured during the past 25 years, it has become increasingly possible to consider other aspects of outcome. Outcome has traditionally encompassed self-care skills, independent living skills, and return to work. Although the importance of vocational skills cannot be overstated, there is no dependable nor reliable means of securing well-designed vocational rehabilitation services for persons who have sustained TBI.[6,7] So issues such as caregiver preparation and burden, the impact of catastrophic disability upon family systems and family members, and factors such as life satisfaction and health-related quality of life have emerged as viable concerns in discharge planning as they bear upon the viability and durability of many discharge placements.

The medical model tends to focus upon medical issues, with less attention paid to issues of life satisfaction.[8] Regardless of the level of disability following injury and the cessation of treatment, life satisfaction for the injured person and the caregivers should be a major consideration of any assessment of outcome. Ultimately, of course, the degree to which sequelae of TBI are resolved during rehabilitation will bear substantially on level of life satisfaction achieved by the injured person.

Because relatively little attention is afforded to the arena of life satisfaction in discharge planning, many of the issues in this chapter will bear directly or indirectly on this topic. People survive TBI. The question ought to be how well they and their caregivers survive the immense trauma inflicted by the injury itself and the absolute upheaval of life that often follows. To that end, discharge planners should work to identify not only the next immediate care or treatment setting, but also they should also work with their treatment team and community resources to pull together educational materials and resources that will address the issues described in this chapter. The intent should be to attend to both the immediate and long-term needs of persons with TBI and their caregivers.

Most discharges from treatment occur as events planned and agreed upon among all parties. A special circumstance is encountered, however, when an individual with TBI makes a choice to stop treatment in a manner that is often referred to as *against medical advice*. In these instances, many ethical questions arise that must be addressed by the treatment team, the discharge planner, and caregivers.[9] The treatment team and caregivers may face the decision of recommending competency hearings to attempt to continue to provide recommended treatment. Simply put, a person's refusal to follow treatment advice willingly cannot become a reason to proceed to discharge. Banja et al.[9] submit that clinicians have an ethical responsibility to attempt to convince people of the need for continued treatment in language they can comprehend, and may also have a responsibility to recommend competency proceedings. Should competency proceedings be undertaken, it is incumbent upon the treatment team to provide clear, objective, and convincing evidence that relates to people's ability to care for themselves, obtain and maintain employment, know what to do in an emergency, and be aware of and practice safe sexual precautions. Banja et al.[9] point out that many people with TBI can present relatively well to an adjudicator who is unfamiliar with brain injury. Thus, the treatment team must be prepared with hard facts and objective data.

Discharge disposition may also be heavily influenced by the type of funding available to the injured person. Chan et al.[10] reviewed 1271 cases of moderate to severe TBI and the frequency with which individuals were placed in skilled nursing facilities (SNFs) or rehabilitation facilities. Those not included in the study were people with Medicare or self-insurance coverage, people who were discharged to home or transferred to another facility, people who left against medical advice, and people who were incarcerated. It was clear that people with Medicaid coverage were more likely to have been injured by assault and had longer LOS. People with Medicaid coverage were much more likely to be discharged to an SNF than to a rehabilitation setting. People with fee-for-service insurance coverage had shorter acute LOS and were most likely to be transferred to rehabilitation settings. People with health maintenance organization coverage had a higher percentage of referral to SNFs, although the difference did not reach statistical significance. The implications for recovery of function are not entirely clear for those people less likely to be transferred to a rehabilitation setting, although research with a stroke population showed a clear advantage in outcome for those people who received rehabilitative treatment.[11]

Discharge disposition may also be impacted by whether a physical medicine and rehabilitation specialist has been involved in the case, either for treatment or consultation. Wrigley et al.[12] reviewed the discharge disposition for 756 people with TBI and found a significant difference in disposition related to the presence or absence of the specialist. The study also showed direct and indirect injury severity indicators, marital status, and age-impacted likelihood of referral to rehabilitation settings. The impact of age was such that older people were more likely to be referred.

The purpose of this chapter is twofold: to offer a broadened view of discharge planning that extends years beyond injury and to provide insights into the nature of the long-term problems encountered, with methods of addressing these problems. Much of the discussion in this chapter involves postdischarge caregivers, their needs, concerns, and education. The ethical implications of relegating the care of a person with TBI to what is, usually, a lay population without adequate financial, clinical, educational, or other resources is not a focus of this chapter. In fact, it is highly doubtful that one could reasonably conclude that sufficient resources are allocated to people with TBI and their caregivers in general. This chapter approaches the issues from the perspective of what can be done within current limitations of the managed care environment.

31.2 Early Problem Identification During Follow-Up

The sequelae of TBI can be many and varied, with relatively little congruency between any two injured persons. In fact, it is only with the perspective gained by rehabilitative experience with large numbers of persons who have survived TBI that one gains a view of the wide variety of these sequelae, successful and unsuccessful approaches to them, and some commonalities that can be found in subgroups of the whole population. It is this experience that illustrates the importance of regularly scheduled follow-up contact with persons and their caregivers to identify problems before they become complicated or develop into insurmountable obstacles requiring major changes in the person's life. Such follow-up should be conducted in the days and weeks immediately after discharge and in the months and years that follow.

Job coaching, as an example, has come to be widely recognized as a successful means of accomplishing return to work.[13–15] The job coach functions to train the individual, ensure that the assigned work is completed, identify barriers to success, and find requisite solutions for those identified barriers. The concept of early problem identification is equally valid when applied to the broader picture of the person's family, social, academic, and/or vocational experience after discharge. Properly educated caregivers can sometimes be quite successful in setting up more effective discharge scenarios and maintaining them; however, they must be able and willing to participate in the early identification of problem areas and have access to resources for ideas on management of those problems. Ideally, the discharge planner has been able to provide good educational preparation of relevant potential barriers that specific caregivers might encounter for their family member, as well as act as an ongoing resource for the person and caregiver. In fact, the entire rehabilitation team can often be helpful in answering questions caregivers may encounter postdischarge. The discharge planner can act as an interface to the team or facilitate more direct contact. Measures such as educational lectures, resource centers, websites, educational materials, continued consultation for ideas, and problem solving following discharge can all contribute to the ongoing education of persons and their caregivers.

As problems develop postdischarge—and they do—they often proceed to develop greater complications than necessary only because their significance is either not recognized early on, their cause or end point may not be recognized, or a reasonable solution to the problem cannot be identified by the people involved. Discharge planning should include the preparation of a Caregiver Manual (Appendix 31A) that seeks to address known areas of concern for an injured person, as well as the more likely long-term complications that may be encountered, and methods for either avoiding those complications or methods to address them when they occur. Likewise, consultation should be conducted with postdischarge treaters to ensure that these individuals are properly briefed on the specifics of the case, that adequate records have been transmitted, and that an invitation for ongoing consultation by the discharging team has been offered. This accomplishes both a continuity of care and treatment approach and provides the postdischarge treaters with some depth of experience that they, as individual treaters outside a comprehensive rehabilitation milieu, may be lacking.

31.3 Avoiding Reinjury

The literature is fairly clear about the additive nature of injury to the brain seen with repetitive traumas.[16] Likewise, the literature is clear regarding the susceptibility of persons to reinjury following a first or second TBI.[17] As a hallmark of success of rehabilitation and in a desire to increase overall life satisfaction, normalization of routine and activities is generally viewed rather positively. Return to some aspects of life, however, may be contraindicated following TBI.

In general, the person's desired social, vocational, and recreational pursuits must be considered with regard to balancing the level of risk for reinjury with the need to be productive and meaningfully engaged in life. There is no clear-cut, easy approach to admonition regarding such matters. For example, it may or may not be advisable to limit an individual's use of a bicycle. Although it is clear that such use should always be done with a helmet, some persons will have visual field, vestibular, or other physical deficits that make reinjury far more likely. Others may find that bicycle use is a sole method for transportation to engage in other life activities. In many cases, the best that can be accomplished is a careful review of the intended vocational and recreational activities for the potential of reinjury. Subsequent identification of high-risk activities should be made for the person, the family, and the employer with a discussion of the risks and benefits of engaging in each activity. Sexual activity, dating, job safety, and return to risky recreational pursuits (e.g., motocross, skiing, or snowboarding) are only some examples of issues that will arise and need to be considered long term. Recommendations for activity restrictions may be permanent or temporary depending on the circumstance.

These discussions need to begin early during the rehabilitation process as they often represent major shifts in activities from which life satisfaction derives. People often have some difficulty adjusting to the idea that their lives will be affected over the long term.[18–20] It is often beneficial if they can be helped to view these changes as educated choices they are making to alter their lifestyles as a reasonable response to a major event in their lives, as opposed to changes that are *imposed* by well-meaning health care providers and/or family members, or by the injury itself. In some cases, persons with acquired brain injury have significant difficulty in understanding the nature of changes in their abilities.[21,22] They may persist with expectations that can no longer be justified based upon their actual capabilities. Early identification of such discrepancies must be undertaken during the rehabilitative process, aggressively addressed during treatment, and reflected in the discharge planning.[23]

31.4 Activities and Activity Levels

Human beings are prepared from a very early age to become productive in later life. That productivity is expressed, ever increasingly, through vocational endeavors, although this is often preceded by educational preparation of one sort or another. Productivity in later life is a major source of interpersonal interaction and socialization. Those activities and facets of life that contribute to life satisfaction are largely contained within, or derived from, the pursuit of avocational and vocational interests and the subsequent social interplay that occurs.

Perhaps the harshest reality following TBI for those persons unfortunate enough to be left with significant residual deficits is the lack of access to those events and affairs in life that represent the pinnacle achievements of our adulthood and all that we are prepared to participate in lifelong. Loss of the ability to work can have demoralizing effects.[24] Social isolation and the resulting depression that often accompanies it arises largely from an inability to access avocational or vocational activities meaningfully and independently following TBI.[8,25] In fact, in the United States, there is not a real societal push to provide for return to such activities. Funding for rehabilitation into these activities is not sufficient nor appropriate,[26] with the possible exception of the workers' compensation system in some states. Even workers' compensation systems may frequently fail to undertake vocational rehabilitation adequately with this population.

The discharge planner must encourage the treatment team, injured person, caregivers, and funding source to recognize the rich therapeutic and life satisfaction benefits associated with immediate and long-term actualization of active and meaningful engagement in living. The patient must be prepared to complete as many activities of daily living (ADLs) as possible and as independently as possible before discharge. The discharge environment should encourage the injured person's participation in ADL completion and foster continued growth in areas of difficulty on a day-to-day basis. All too often, however, persons are not left to dress themselves or feed themselves because to complete these activities to the level of independence that they may be capable of requires too much time. Caregivers may be pressed for time or patience and choose to complete the task for the injured person. Some caregivers watch the injured person struggle to complete a given series of tasks and conclude that the frustration is so great as to be emotionally painful for the person or themselves. Sometimes these caregivers can "love too much," attempting to reduce frustration by eliminating the task altogether or completing it for the person. The problem is that people respond to the level of environmental expectation. Caregivers who complete basic activities for the individual inadvertently strip the person of a righteous sense of individuality and independence while unwittingly perpetuating, perhaps, an unnecessary level of dependence. The key is to educate caregivers and injured persons alike to identify reasonable levels of environmental support and expectation to create an environment that is hospitable, yet one that fosters continued improvement.

Discharge planning should include a detailed and comprehensive resource analysis of available venues for meaningful engagement in the real world (see Appendix 31A). Although this may be premature at a given level of treatment, engaging in this pursuit with an injured person and/or the caregivers can provide them with insight into the long-term nature of the problems before them and teach them to undertake the resource analysis on an ongoing basis. The resource analysis should include options for volunteer activity, return to school, or return to work, as well as information about more immediate care and treatment needs, such as pharmacy location, current and future professional contact information, durable medical equipment suppliers, and support groups. The process should review the proper timing of return to school or work to avoid premature return to either of these activities. The emotional trauma of failure in either of these environments can be considerable, and great care should be undertaken to effect a properly timed return to these activities. It is often helpful to identify family and friends' vocational and avocational interests as potential sources of assistance early during the vocational rehabilitation process.

Likewise, the discharge planner must provide the injured person and caregivers with information regarding how best to bring about a return to school or work. Unfortunately, most state-funded vocational rehabilitation programs are woefully inadequate for this population.[7] This information should include education about the laws that may govern the return and proper preparation for the return, both of the injured person and the people in the return environment. The discharge planner should prepare a list of resources that are available to help in returning to school or work. These may include specific persons within, or who can consult with, a school district, departments for students with special needs at a community college or university setting, or state-sponsored vocational rehabilitation service information. Chapter 25 of this text provides an excellent discussion of issues relative to returning to school. Some cities have active support groups that assist persons in resource identification, return to work, adjustment to disability, day care, and assisted living.

Return to work is usually best when it is accomplished on a protracted and gradual basis. The employer of injury should be reserved as a final placement. It is usually best to preserve this placement, reserving it for the last vocational placement. Because vocational rehabilitation following brain injury is actually more akin to vocational therapy, return to work may require involvement in several less demanding positions that are intentionally limited in their scope, and have specific purposes of reestablishing basic worker characteristics and gradually increasing the level of task complexity and responsibility to be carried by the injured worker. It is incumbent upon the discharge planner to prepare the injured person and caregivers properly with information that allows them to undertake this process with or without professional assistance. Equally important is the caregivers' preparation to recognize a return to work that is premature or poorly timed. A more detailed discussion of return to work can be found in Chapter 23 of this text.

31.5 Family Systems

The statistics regarding survival of family systems following return of a person with TBI to the home are disturbing. Families report increased depression, decreased ability to express feelings, decreased time and energy for social or recreational activity, and a tendency toward exercising increased control following severe TBI.[27] Lezak[28] has suggested that the emotional disturbances and disorders of executive function in the family member with TBI contribute distinctively to family burden. Education, counseling, and emotional support are recommended for families. Lezak's observations were substantiated by a study that systematically examined family system outcome following brain injury.[29] Distressed family functioning across all domains was identified by family members. The return of a person with TBI to the home is first met with great pleasure. Lezak[30] identified six stages of families' reactions after the stresses of having the injured family member at home are experienced. Pleasure is replaced by bewilderment and anxiety as the families' energy dwindles. Optimism diminishes and guilt, depression, despair, and mourning follow the bewilderment. Families undergo a reorganization and, finally, an emotional disengagement.[30] Separation, divorce, behavioral problem development in children, or departure from the home by nearly adult children or siblings are all expected consequences. Emotional responses vary somewhat by position in the family. Mothers, fathers, and siblings appear to react differently to the stresses of TBI within the family.[31-35] First, parents report increased global marital distress, reduced expression of affection, and a feeling of less spousal understanding in families in which children between 15 and 24 years of age have TBI.[33] Mothers report greater dissatisfaction with spousal support than fathers.[33,35] Mothers are more likely to be under a physician's care than fathers, are more likely to be using psychotropic medications, and tend to express negative emotion more than their husbands.[33] Rosenberg[34] studied spousal reaction following mild head injury. Half of the wives reported a high degree of negative impact in their relationships resulting from changes following TBI. Lyth-Frantz[35] compared marital relationship impact between couples with a child with TBI and couples with a child without disabling conditions. The effect of TBI was to decrease marital satisfaction, decrease satisfaction with parent–child relationships, produce greater family enmeshment, create a perception that the family's fate was a function of circumstances beyond the family's control, and decrease interest and involvement in intellectual, cultural, and physically oriented recreation. Next, siblings report that family stress is the greatest problem encountered following TBI in another sibling[32] and they show significant signs of emotional distress.[31] Coping strategies used by siblings are suppression of frustrations,[32] wishful thinking, avoidance, and self-blame.[31] The emotional trauma inflicted upon a family is tremendous and predisposes most families to disruption of the family system, sometimes with devastating consequences like marital separation or divorce, development of behavioral problems in noninjured siblings, and challenges to the parent–child bonds between parents and noninjured siblings Wongvatunyu and Porter[36] used a phenomenologic method to describe changes in family systems from interviews with seven mothers of TBI survivors in summarizing those changes 6 months or more after injury. The individuals with injury ranged from 20 to 36 years of age at the time of interview and ranged from 6 months to 20 years postinjury. Care requirements ranged from independence with ADLs to complete dependence. Communication problems ranged from none to unable to communicate verbally, and cognitive and behavioral difficulties ranged from memory difficulties to impaired speed of processing for motivation and anger problems.

Five basic themes were identified from this research: (1) getting attention from each other for different reasons now, (2) getting along with each other since the injury, (3) facing new financial hurdles, (4) going separate ways down this new path, and (5) splitting family members apart against their will. This unique line of investigation allows tremendous insight into real-world difficulties faced by families over the long term. Some mothers reported family members simply did not understand what had happened to the injured person, whereas one mother viewed her family as being afraid and uncertain of what to say or how to act. One mother indicated her husband and family members were scared of direct involvement with her injured son, acting as though they might hurt him when they handle him. Mothers noted that some family members could not accept the changes they saw in the injured family member. Some felt more attention was paid to the individual's limitations than was warranted. Some mothers reported that other family members thought the mothers were too attentive to the injured young adults—"mothering her a little too much."

Under the theme of "getting along with each other since the injury," there were reports that some family members were getting along like normal, some got along better than prior to injury, and some were struggling to get along since the injury.

Financial difficulties included secondary costs associated with the injury. In one instance, the injured individual was married and had four young children, all of whom were facing financial problems as a result of a lack of regular income. The grandparents, now caretakers of the adult son with brain injury, participated in the financial caregiving of the son's family. One mother quit her job to care for her son and divorced after the injury. The son's father would occasionally help out financially, but eventually his support waned. Those mothers who mentioned financial changes viewed them as fundamental and long-lasting.

Two mothers moved out of the family home with the injured young adult child to another community that was close to a rehabilitation facility. The mothers believe that such separations were very difficult for the families, with one mother stating, "It's changed all their lives. It's torn the family up." Another mother stated, "It's just nothing there anymore. No family life or anything."

Married mothers reported slightly more help than single mothers from family members. There were some reports of positive changes within the family after injury, noting that some relationships have improved or were closer than before.

Uysal et al.[37] reviewed parenting skills of individuals with TBI and their spouses, the effects of parental TBI on children, and the effects of parental TBI on levels of depression for all family members in a review of 16 families in which one parent had a TBI. One premise for this investigation is that people of child-rearing age are represented in the frequency of TBI, increasing the likelihood that children in these families will be affected by the TBI sequelae. Difficulties such as attention to detail, the ability to divide attention, memory difficulties in particular for events and conversations, time management difficulties, and organizational deficits would seemingly impact parenting. In addition, affective and behavioral symptoms such as irritability, aggression, mood swings, anxiety, social withdrawal, and depression could potentially impact family interactions. Lastly, inability to function vocationally would bring about not only financial challenges, but also difficulties in the modeling of a work ethic.

In that study, parents with TBI reported less encouragement of cognitive competence, less achievement, and less conformity in their children compared with parents without TBI. Children's ratings showed only a difference in the parent behavior ratings along the dimensions of "lacks control." Overall, the differences appeared to involve less goal setting, less encouragement of skill development, less emphasis on obedience to rules and orderliness, less promotional work values, less nurturing, and lower levels of active involvement with children. Parents with TBI and their children had a greater tendency toward depression.

Members of a family can generally be expected to survive the immediate and long-term consequences experienced when a family member is injured. However, the quality of that survival should be actively discussed and planned. Families function in complicated patterns of individual and group behaviors and settle into a manner of living that becomes more or less the norm for that group. As catastrophic injury and disability enter the picture, the customary rhythm of a family is severely disrupted.[27,28] Family resources of time, attention, financial resources, and energy tend to become focused on the injured family member, sometimes to the near exclusion of all other needs. This phenomenon has been partially described as a *command performance* wherein a family member meets unbelievable physical and emotional demands on a protracted daily basis, seemingly without regard for his or her own needs, health, and welfare. Although such a "crisis" mode of operation can be useful for short periods of time, a diagnosis of TBI usually heralds the family embarkation upon a prolonged change in their way of living.

During the early stages of rehabilitation, families are sometimes reluctant to believe outcome prognostications that may be provided, viewing them as inaccurate and pessimistic. Many families report having been told that their family member may die, and if they do not die, that they may be severely disabled. These comments are often interpreted as being told their family member was going to die or that they would be severely disabled for the rest of their lives. The result is a loss of credibility suffered by treaters down the line, through no one's fault but circumstance alone. Such misperceptions may be avoided by active pursuit of a planned educational format by the treatment team that covers a number of topics regarding the nature of injuries sustained, their treatment, and both near- and long-term issues for caregivers.

During these early stages of rehabilitation, families respond best to access to information about their specific family member's condition and possible future care requirements. McMordie et al.[38] found a high sense of hopelessness communicated by professionals to families and injured people, as reported in postdischarge surveys. Provision of a range of possible outcomes is easier to accept for many families and probably most accurate. This approach engenders a desire for more information about which outcome might be best achieved and how. McMordie et al.[38] also found the greatest consumer dissatisfaction with information provision—specifically, information about available resources, long-term outcome, and personality change following TBI. Resource centers that provide families and injured persons with detailed information that is easy to understand and readily available can be most helpful. McPherson et al.[39] support these assertions in their finding that families interviewed just 6 weeks after discharge from acute rehabilitation indicated their primary need was more information, although these needs were not spontaneously presented. Instead, their need for information required prompting to be made known.

Likewise, counseling from either experienced staff or other family members can be helpful in preparing families for the challenges that lie ahead. An analogy to racing can be useful, comparing the coming weeks, months, and years to a marathon, rather than a sprint of a few days or weeks. Of course, treaters are often reluctant to engage in such discussions for fear of unnecessarily removing the element of hope from the picture for patients and/or their families. Great sensitivity is required in the pursuit of information provision, education, and preparation while continuing to encourage realistic levels of hope.

Families are rarely ready to hear the need to care for themselves, feeling as though such a response would be unwise, risky, selfish, or all of these. They are, likewise, not prepared to hear that their family member is either perilously close to death, as in the early stages of moderate to severe injuries, and that, should they survive, they should begin to plan for such huge changes in their lives. Given the very short time frames associated with acute hospitalization, the discharge planner may be reluctant to contribute to the stresses of an already overwhelmed family. This dilemma contributes to the lack of preparedness most families report.

Families must be encouraged both to plan and return actively to normalized patterns of family living. The initial disruption of such patterns can develop into a new norm for families if allowed to continue unchallenged. Families may need assistance in learning to discuss their concerns and fears. Although this may be expected of younger family members, facilitated discussions with adult family members and friends can be exceedingly helpful for those participating directly and in modeling how to conduct such discussions with children, siblings, extended family, and friends in the future. In fact, families should be directed to talk openly about their concerns and fears, especially facilitating these discussions between couples, parents and children, and family members and friends. This should include factual information about injuries sustained, treatments provided, future treatment needs, and preparation for future stages in recovery and return home. Families need to be educated about the various treatment facilities that may be available locally, regionally, and nationally. They should be made aware of the various levels of care frequently encountered, including acute care, acute rehabilitation, subacute care, residential and outpatient postacute services, home and community treatment, and assisted living services. They should be provided with all the treatment options and an explanation regarding which will be available to them based upon financial constraints individual to their situation. Although some of these services may not be appropriate or even available, the discussion will help the family to understand, from a slightly different perspective, the challenges they will be facing. This information can be provided in the form of informational pamphlets, counseling sessions, or other educational formats.

Families may need assistance in identification of assumptions within the family that may bias services that an injured person receives. Topics such as cost, geography, expertise of treaters, and objective comparison of various treatment options can be helpful. Treaters must recognize the need to investigate treatment options available locally, regionally, and nationally and balance this with the somewhat parochial tendencies professionals gravitate toward with reference to beliefs regarding their own competencies and those available at other treatment settings. Many professionals believe they are able to provide for their patient's needs adequately, but this belief may inadvertently portend a blinding to other more specialized or expert services available. This is particularly poignant for treaters at the acute and postacute rehabilitative treatment level. Because LOS has decreased for acute hospitalization and acute rehabilitation services,[3,4] professionals must familiarize themselves with the multitude of postacute treatment options available today and actively advocate for their patient's access to these highly specialized models of treatment.

Parents of injured children naturally rally around the injured child, all too often subjugating the needs of siblings and themselves. This approach may be acceptable on a very short-term basis; however, it should not be encouraged on a protracted basis. An aunt, uncle, family friend, or grandparent usually cannot supplant a parent for children. Parents should be encouraged and assisted in frank, age-appropriate discussions with siblings about the injury and the future. Of course, care must be taken to consider the emotional health and readiness of each child on a case-by-case basis, but generally speaking, children deal best with factual information. In addition, the family will be challenged as never before to deal with high levels and ranges of emotion and may be unprepared to recognize key differences in coping strategies exercised by different people in the family circle. Failure of family members to recognize and deal appropriately with such differences in coping strategies can lead to tremendous misunderstandings and misgivings. As has been evidenced in numerous families, such misperceptions have actually contributed to deterioration and, sometimes, dissolution of family structures.

Gan et al.[40] undertook research to identify predictors of family system functioning after acquired brain injury. Greater distress and family functioning was noted by individuals with acquired brain injury, mothers, spouses and siblings. Fathers and offspring did not report greater distress in family functioning. Problem solving was observed to be an area of difficulty, along with rule changes in the family.

An overall increase in responsibilities has been previously reported, along with challenges of adjusting work responsibilities to manage time and availability for care for the individual injury.[32,41] Hall et al.[41] found gender to be associated with family functioning—in particular, for families of females with acquired brain injury. They speculate that impulsivity, a lack of inhibition, egocentricity, and a change in the nurturing nature of the individual might constitute "out of role" behavioral change. Finally, their study indicated the importance of utilizing a family systems approach in dealing with the immediate and longitudinal consequences of brain injury within families.

Families will need information on the importance of establishing and using a structured routine after the injured person returns home. Ironically, structure leads to freedom. The injured person will need as much external assistance as possible in organizing the environment and events. Predictable routines will aid in organization of the return home for all parties and will enhance the redevelopment of self-care skills, in particular. Some families function well with such direction because they functioned in a structured fashion prior to injury. Other families, however, may not have functioned in such a way and may need a fair amount of help in learning to do so. Families need to understand the importance of a regular schedule for waking/sleeping, medications, meals, hydration, exercise, and completion of ADLs. An approach that is haphazard not only causes confusion, but also brings risk associated with missed medications, meals, fluids, or rest. Likewise, because rehabilitation is maximized repetition, complete participation in ADLs to the fullest extent possible by the injured person will bring about the fastest return of these skills.

Lastly, caregivers should be advised regarding the provision of feedback and consequences for inappropriate behaviors they may encounter. Sometimes, families are at a loss regarding whether feedback should be provided for asocial behaviors. Although feedback can be overdone, generally, it is best for the family to be taught to deliver appropriate feedback and consequences for asocial behaviors. They should be taught how to deliver consequences immediately after the behaviors occur. If a behavior analyst or psychologist is available, such programming should begin in the treatment setting, with instruction given to caregivers on continuation of the programming following discharge. A more detailed discussion of behavioral interventions is included in Chapter 20 of this volume.

31.6 Caregiver Concerns

Responsibility for caring for the individual, long after formal rehabilitation has ended usually falls to the family. The role of caregiving is demanding and typically lasts for the lifetime of the individual. Families are often ill-prepared to take on caregiving responsibilities.[42] Issues reported by family members include family strain, depression, burden, anxiety, psychological distress, social isolation, loss of income, and role strain.[41,43–51]

Reduced and restricted LOSs have resulted in placement of persons with TBI in the home setting far earlier than is, perhaps, best for the individual, in some cases. The burden placed upon caregivers cannot be overstated. Caregivers are faced with a myriad of potential medical complications that may not have been adequately identified during hospitalization or may not have manifested during that time. Most homes are not built with the anticipation of dealing with the needs of a person with physical handicaps, and in a similar vein, most families are not equipped to deal with the pervasive demands created by a person with medical, physical, cognitive, communicative, and/or behavioral problems.

Studies indicate that depression, anxiety, anger, fatigue, mood disturbance, and family dissatisfaction are frequently encountered by the injured person and by caregivers alike.[50] These complaints are reported by many levels of involvement by caregivers, extending well beyond the primary caregiver to secondary and tertiary caregivers. The primary caregiver is most often a woman, usually a wife or mother.[1,50] In a population studied in which the mean age of the person with TBI was 28 years, 64% of caregivers were the parent of the injured person and 25% were the spouse.[1] The mean age of the caregiver was 44 years, suggesting a fairly long future of management of such responsibilities. Seventy percent of the caregivers lived in the same residence as the injured person.

Measures of life satisfaction demonstrate a progression as chronicity increases. During the first year after injury, employment was associated with life satisfaction whereas age, marital status, social integration, and depressed mood were not. However, during year 2 postinjury, employment, social integration, and depressed mood were associated with life satisfaction.[8] This progression may be the result of the recognition of the permanence of sequelae of the brain injury as time progresses. Given the findings on the relationship between quality of life and employment, it appears that persons with TBI who are able to become gainfully employed or productive on a day-to-day basis experience greater life satisfaction.[8,25]

Kreutzer et al.[52] reviewed employment stability patterns during the first 4 years after TBI and found that minority participants were more than twice as likely to experience unstable employment patterns. A contribution to postinjury differences in outcome has been suggested to be related to preinjury differences between racial groups in the United States that include lower educational levels, lower income, less employment stability, and poor insurance coverage for minority populations. Minority group members are more likely to have violence as an etiology injury.[53,54] One study indicated that more than one third of African-American subjects have violence as an etiology for injury compared with less than 3% of white subjects.[55] Examination of racial differences in caregiving patterns, caregiver emotional function, and sources of emotional support following TBI showed that proportionately fewer African-American caregivers were spouses compared with white caregivers. Caregivers as "other relatives or friends" were two times more prevalent in African-American caregiving. The largest nonspouse, nonparent caregiver group was siblings in the African-American study sample, followed by other relatives, grown children, and boyfriends/girlfriends. Less than 5% of caregivers fell into any of these categories for white caregivers. The majority of caregivers lived with patients in both groups. The study demonstrated adverse effects of emotional distress and satisfaction with life as level of disability increased, and there were no differences between racial groups along these parameters. More whites than African-Americans received psychological treatment or counseling.[56,57]

Caregivers should be prepared for their responsibilities both to endure over a long period of time and for their burden of care to increase over time, especially as severity of injury increases.[43,58] Brooks et al.[43] found that the 10 most frequently encountered problems reported by relatives remained either stable or increased, in the majority, from 1 year postinjury to 5 years postinjury (Table 31.1). In fact, the largest increase in frequency of reporting was in the area of disturbed behavior at 5 years. Threats or gestures of violence increased from 15% at year 1 to 54% at year 5. Twenty percent (20%) of relatives reported their family member to have been physically violent, involving actual assault at year 5, an increase from 10% at 1 year postinjury.

Caregivers may need to take on the role of nurse, therapist, educator, counselor, vocational rehabilitation counselor, social worker, case manager, and life care planner in addition to their other responsibilities. Holland and Shigaki[59] point out that education of a caregiver early during the acute treatment phase may be limited in its efficiency because of the disruption of the continuum of recovery that can be encountered as a result of a lack of rehabilitation programming continuity from acute rehabilitation through community reentry. They suggest a three-phase approach to provision of educational materials to caregivers, according to the phase of recovery of their family member. Holland and Shigaki[59] suggest that a resource listing of published educational material and local care resources be provided, over time, to caregivers, and they provide a listing of such bibliographic resources for the reader. DePompei and Williams[60] outline a family-centered counseling approach that is useful during rehabilitation. Acorn[61] developed a guide for community-based family education and support groups to provide education regarding TBI and its sequelae, enable families to identify community resources, and build support networks among families with TBI.

TABLE 31.1

The Ten Problems Most Frequently Reported by Relatives at 5 Years ($N = 42$)

	Percent Relatives Reporting	
Problem	**1 Year**	**5 Years**
Personality change	60	74
Slowness	65	67
Poor memory	67	67
Irritability	67	64
Bad temper	64	64
Tiredness	69	62
Depression	51	57
Rapid mood change	57	57
Tension and anxiety	57	57
Threats of violence	15	54

Source: Brooks, N., Campsie, L., Symington, C., Beattie, A., and McKinlay, W., *Journal of Neurology, Neurosurgery, and Psychiatry,* 49(7), 764–770, 1986. With permission.

31.7 Seizure Hygiene

The overall incidence of posttraumatic epilepsy (PTE) is estimated at about 5% for all persons with nonmissile head injury.[62] The incidence of PTE following moderate head injury is 1.6% and, following severe head injury, is 11.6%.[63] Overall incidence for PTE has been noted to be as high as 25% and up to 35% for persons comatose for 3 weeks or more.[64] In the 1980s, seizure prophylaxis was somewhat common in the United States, whereas in Europe, the more prevalent approach was that of the "free first fit." Anticonvulsant coverage was provided in the United States to attempt to prevent the first seizure, whereas in Europe, such coverage was provided after evidence of a first seizure. A study by Temkin et al.[65] demonstrated no real long-term benefit associated with prophylaxis coverage, and as a result, this practice in the United States has slowly decreased. In fact, a more considered approach to prophylaxis is generally followed, taking into account the nature of the injury and the likelihood of PTE associated with that type of injury.

PTE can first occur many years postinjury.[66,67] It is important to advise persons with TBI and their families about their relative risk for the development of seizures and factors that are within their control that may impact the nature of a given seizure disorder. Families should be educated regarding what constitutes seizure activity. Grand mal seizures are easily recognized, whereas partial motor seizures may be less recognizable. Clearly, complex partial seizures are least recognizable, although they constitute a surprisingly high percentage of seizure prevalence following acquired brain injury.[68] Complex partial seizure disorders are difficult to diagnose and may be misinterpreted as psychiatric conditions by caregivers and professionals alike.

Medication compliance represents a primary area of concern. The person must understand the medication regimen that has been prescribed. This includes the importance of compliance with the timing of medication administration and understanding whether and when a missed dosage can be made up. For example, missed dosages of dilantin or phenobarbital, although best taken at prescribed times, can be taken at any time during the same 24-hour period that the missing dosage is prescribed. Tegretol, on the other hand, cannot be handled in a like manner. Education must be provided regarding the specific characteristics and options of a given anticonvulsant coverage.

Likewise, it is important for persons and their families to understand whether an anticonvulsant can be abruptly stopped. The cessation of medication may be because of a prescription lapse, unavailability of the medication resulting from travel, forgetfulness, financial concerns, incarceration, or a directive from an uninformed health care provider, family member, or friend, or the injured person simply stops the medication. Some anticonvulsants and antispasmodics require a tapering, so that seizures are not actually precipitated.

It is also wise to educate regarding sleep, rest, and stress. Many persons with seizure disorders experience increases in the frequency of seizure activity with increased fatigue and stress. Education regarding monitoring of drug levels during periods of diarrhea or constipation can be important for the person with a relatively fragile seizure disorder because drug absorption can be impacted by such conditions.

Information regarding maintenance of adequate hydration should be provided. People who live in arid climates, who may travel extended distances by airplane, or engage in outdoor activities such as hiking, backpacking, or river trips should be advised to monitor decaffeinated and nonalcoholic fluid intake carefully, both by noting the quantity per day and the frequency and nature of urination. Education regarding the diuretic effect of alcohol and caffeine should be provided.

Lastly, some anticonvulsants may interact with other drugs, either increasing or decreasing the other drug's effectiveness, or increasing or decreasing the serum levels of the anticonvulsant coverage.[69] Specific information about these drug interactions must be provided to the person and his or her family so they may monitor future prescription use for potential interactions. Although this is a role that is best filled by the health care provider and/or a pharmacy, these individuals may be unable to fill this role because of a lack of information or lack of access to the person's complete medical history.

31.8 Depression

Depression has become identified as a significant long-term complication by numerous authors.[50,70–72] Studies that look out 3 to 7 years postinjury point to depression as a major complaint by both injured persons and their caregivers.[70–72] The advent of the selective serotonin reuptake inhibitor class of antidepressants has been an important development in the treatment of persons with TBI.[73] This particular class of drugs appears to be tolerated well, in general, and has a low complication rate.

Persistent depression with older adults has been investigated. A systematic review of depression in the elderly after TBI was reported by Menzel.[74] She reported the prevalence of depression ranged from 1.8% to 8.9% in community-residing elders. This increased 25% for those residing in nursing homes and long-term care settings. Menzel[74] reported the prevalence of depression in the overall TBI population ranged from 15.3% to 42%. Levin et al.[75] reviewed 41 individuals with TBI ranging from mild to moderate severity and averaging 67.9 years of age. The individuals were assessed at an average of 33.9 days postinjury and reassessed at an average of 218 days and then again at 411 days postinjury. Depression was evaluated using the Geriatric Depression Scale. Overall, there was no significant difference in depression levels reported based on severity of injury. At the initial assessment, 24% had mild to moderate levels of depression, 7% had severe levels of depression, and 68% had no evidence of depression. At the second assessment interval, 30 of the original 41 individuals were reassessed and, of eight individuals with clinically significant levels of depression at the first evaluation, 50% continued to show evidence of depression. Clinically significant levels of depression were found in 18% of the remaining individuals who did not initially endorsed depression. At the time of the third assessment, 25 individuals remained and, of them, 12% continued to have clinically significant levels of depression.

Rapoport et al.[76] assessed the impact of major depression and psychosocial functioning, psychological distress, and postconcussion symptoms outcomes following mild to moderate TBI in 477 individuals. Respondents averaged 67.12 years of age. The prevalence of major depression at 2 months postinjury was 15.6%. Although 18.2% of individuals had a history of depression prior to injury, none of them had major depression at baseline postinjury. Of those who were depressed at baseline, half (55.6%) of those who were followed at 1 year still met the criteria for major depression, even though 80% were being treated with antidepressants.

The etiology of depression appears to be twofold: biochemical and situational. Social isolation is considerable and arises from diminished real-world interaction. This diminution can be traced, in part, to a lack of avocational or vocational involvement, together with frequently impaired interpersonal skills.[77,78] Both contribute to substantial social isolation. Most persons with TBI are quite able to recognize the differences in their lives comparing pre- and postinjury status. In the absence of meaningful involvement in the regular work-a-day world, feelings of isolation, frustration, and depression are commonly reported. Discharge planners should educate injured persons and their caregivers to participate in fitness and aerobic exercise routines that have been medically approved to assist with fatigue and depression. It is wise to educate regarding the symptoms of depression. This should include agitated depression, panic attacks, and anxiety.

The discharge planner can address this issue by education and encouragement to establish meaningful involvement to the person's capability postdischarge. Likewise, the discharge planner can make the injured person and the caregivers aware of counseling services; church or community support groups that may operate recreational, avocational, or vocational activities; and the value of use of antidepressant medications in consultation with their physician. There must be a careful tie-in to development and maintenance of appropriate activity levels and meaningful involvement in both the home and community.

Many people with TBI report frustration at the loss of choices and control in their lives postinjury. Aware caregivers can provide an increasing array of choice and control in daily decision making, gradually turning more and more control over to the injured person as he or she is able to accept it. Because this is an ongoing and continually changing process, caregivers need to understand the need to be vigilant and reexamine choice/control issues on a regular basis. Families sometimes attempt to exert maximal control after a family member is catastrophically injured,[27] perhaps in an attempt to limit their exposure to future disastrous events. Some gain control over other aspects of life previously managed by the injured person (e.g., finances) and are reluctant to give up or share that control. Still others sense a need to exert control to prevent a person with impaired judgment from becoming financially, legally, emotionally, sexually, or socially encumbered beyond his or her capability. The need to protect stands in opposition, in some cases, to the pursuit of life satisfaction and participation in age-appropriate activities. The interaction of risk with freedom of choice and balancing rights to self-determination, life satisfaction, and safety should be actively discussed on an ongoing basis.

These matters can become quite complicated and most families are best assisted by professional counseling. Discharge planners are well advised to make contact with mental health professionals in an injured person's home area that are experienced with TBI and can offer occasional assistance and counseling on an as-needed basis.

31.9 Sleep

Sleep disturbance is a relatively common complication following TBI. Sleep disturbance can be manifest in three primary problems: (1) sleep apnea/hypopnea, (2) periodic limb movement disorder (PLMD), and (3) hypersomnolence (excessive daytime sleepiness). Interruption of sleep is a fairly common complaint following TBI and may be related to routine, diet, psychological issues, or sleep hygiene. Education should be provided regarding each of these impacts to the injured person and his or her caregivers because they may be most easily addressed. More complicated issues, such as sleep apnea/hypopnea, PLMD, and hypersomnolence, may require medical intervention. It is beyond the scope of this chapter to review sleep disorders thoroughly. Rather, the intent is to review some of the more common issues that may be encountered following TBI.

In the general population, the prevalence of sleep apnea/hypopnea is estimated to be between 2% and 4%.[79] PLMD is estimated to occur in 5% of the population[58,80] and hypersomnolence occurs in 0.3% to 13% of the general population, depending upon definitions used.[81,82] By contrast, sleep apnea/hypopnea has been evidenced in 11.3% of persons with TBI, PLMD in 25.4%, and hypersomnia in 29.6%[83] in a study of 71 consecutively enrolled persons admitted to a postacute residential rehabilitation program. An interesting finding in that study was that persons with hypersomnolence were often unable to perceive their hypersomnolence and the researchers suggested routine sleep laboratory evaluation. Castriotta and Lai[84] studied 10 persons with TBI who reported hypersomnolence. These individuals averaged 110 months postinjury. Treatable sleep disturbances consisting of obstructive sleep apnea, upper airway resistance syndrome, central sleep apnea, and/or narcolepsy were found in all 10 subjects. Three individuals had a preinjury history of hypersomnia and, of these three, two actually sustained TBI from motor vehicle collisions while driving, with the suspicion that they may have fallen asleep at the wheel.

Finally, in a study of 184 persons who complained of excessive daytime sleepiness after head or neck injury, multiple sleep latency testing showed mean sleep onset time of less than 5 minutes in 28% of the subjects and less than 10 minutes in 82%.[85] Awareness of hypersomnolence did not correlate with the objective findings. Sleep-disordered breathing occurred in 32% of the persons studied.

Sleep has been associated with cognitive function, behavioral functioning, and psychological health.[83,86–88] Likewise, sleep apnea has been associated with motor vehicle collisions[89,90] and unintentional injuries.[91] These data reflect potential contributory factors to an initial TBI, as well as to likelihood of reinjury, either resulting from trauma or chronic hypoxemic events.

The discharge planner should provide education regarding signs and symptoms associated with sleep disturbances, as well as information regarding diagnosis and treatment in cases when these issues have not been thoroughly investigated prior to discharge.

31.10 Long-Term Psychological Issues

There are numerous issues with regard to psychological well-being that persist beyond the initial brain injury. Bergland and Thomas[92] used a case study approach to describe changes in functioning for 425 adolescents who sustained TBI. Seventy-five percent of the individuals' parents reported a change in the persona of the individual was recognized by that individual. Parents decided exaggerated emotions and behavioral excess or deficit contributed most to the impression of the different personality. Worry, anxiety, fear, frustration, anger, and withdrawal were frequent emotional reactions of individuals when confronted with the reality of their injury in everyday environments. A loss of ability and self-esteem were reported with these changes in awareness. Parents reported increased time and effort for all activities was required and that this added to the strain and difficulty of managing life postinjury. The impact on social relationships was such that, although friends were supportive of the individual during hospitalization, relationships tapered off after the permanence of deficits became apparent. This was hurtful and disappointing to most of the adolescents, and the parental response was one of intense pain at the sight of their child's suffering, with parental attempts to buffer the loss and hurt for their child. Most reported difficulty in establishing and maintaining new friendships, as well as confusion and hurt over lost friendships.

Parents discussed the disappointment, loss, and grief associated with the perceived loss of their child's future. Conflicts that affected family roles, marriage, and sibling relations were reported. For those who returned to school, many reported an unrealistic workload at school and a lack of understanding and insufficient assistance within the school setting and with managing classroom responsibilities and work load. A few quit school because of academic or injury-related difficulties. Most returning students and families reported the return-to-school experience to be difficult, disappointing, and frustrating.

Hibbard et al.[93] utilized the Structured Clinical Interview for Diagnostic and Statistical Manual of Mental Disorders–IV (DSM-IV) personality disorders to survey for 12 axis II personality disorders in 100 individuals with TBI between the ages of 18 and 65. The individuals averaged 40 years of age and 7.6 years postinjury. The highest prevalence of axis II disorders were antisocial personality disorder, obsessive–compulsive personality disorder, paranoid personality disorder, and narcissistic personality disorder. Personality changes endorsed by more than 30% of the sample postinjury reflected loss of self-confidence, attempts to cope with cognitive and interpersonal failures, and negative affect problems. Hibbard et al.[93] felt the findings argued against a specific TBI personality syndrome and supported, instead, the diversity of personality disorders reflective of the persistent challenges and compensatory coping strategies developed.

Hibbard et al.[94] reported the incidence of mood, anxiety, and substance use disorders in individuals with TBI following review of 100 adults between the ages of 18 and 65 years who averaged 8 years postinjury at the time of the study. Data were collected by interview and the authors attempted to identify diagnoses of major depression, dysthymia, bipolar disorder, anxiety diagnoses of panic disorder and phobia, and substance use disorders. A significant percentage of individuals presented with substance use disorders prior to TBI. The most frequent axis I diagnoses were major depression and specific anxiety disorders: posttraumatic stress disorder, obsessive–compulsive disorder, and panic disorder. They found 44% of individuals presented with two or more axis I diagnoses postinjury. Individuals with a history of pre-TBI axis I disorders were more likely to develop post-TBI major depression and substance use disorders. Rates of disorder resolution were similar for individuals regardless of preinjury psychiatric histories. Anxiety disorders were least likely to remit.

Draper et al.[95] investigated the relationship between demographic variables, injury severity, cognitive functioning, emotional state, aggression, alcohol use, and fatigue at 10 years postinjury following TBI in 53 individuals ranging in severity of injury from mild to very severe. Generally speaking, the incidence of clinically significant anxiety increased in a stepwise fashion with severity of injury, with the exception of distinguishing between severe and very severe injuries for which clinically significant anxiety was 33% and 22%, respectively. Interestingly, the presence of clinically significant depression decreased as severity of injury increased, ranging from 67% in mild injuries to 35% in very severe injuries. Individuals with more severe anxiety and depression had poorer psychosocial functioning. Fatigue and aggression were also found to be important issues at 10 years postinjury. Aggression was a significant problem for 12% of individuals studied, and fatigue was found to be a strong contributing variable. High levels of alcohol use were also associated with more severe aggression, with 32% of participants using alcohol at "potentially harmful levels."

Hawley and Joseph[96] surveyed 165 individuals with TBI to investigate long-term positive psychological growth. Follow-up was conducted a mean of 11.5 years postinjury. Evidence showed that individuals are capable of positive growth following brain injury. There was no difference noted between those with mild versus severe injury. The degree to which an individual experienced positive growth was negatively correlated with anxiety and depression present at follow-up, suggesting a positive outlook was associated with low anxiety and depression. Higher levels of growth appeared to be associated with better psychological adjustment.

Hoofien et al.[97] reviewed psychiatric symptomatology, cognitive abilities, and psychosocial functioning in 76 individuals with severe TBI, averaging 14.1 years postinjury, comparing findings of individuals with injury with those of their families.

Figure 31.1 illustrates elevations in psychiatric symptomatology related to hostility, depression, anxiety, psychoticism, obsessive–compulsive, somatization, and phobic-ideation reflecting overall psychiatric distress for individuals with injury. Figure 31.2 illustrates psychiatric distress reflected by families of individuals with brain injury. Family members showed elevations in anxiety, hostility, somatization, depression, and phobic ideation. Correlations were observed between psychiatric symptoms and behavior patterns. High levels of distress correlated with greater exhibition of behavioral disturbance and difficulty in acceptance of disability. Significant negative correlations were observed between level of functioning and acceptance of disability, indicating that the lower the acceptance of disability, the higher the psychological symptomatology. Persistent deficits in intelligence, memory, learning, manual speed, and dexterity were noted.

Of 76 individuals with severe TBI (mainly, coma duration of 14 days) in the study, 28 were reported as competitively employed. Eighteen were considered engaged in noncompetitive employment settings. Only 10 individuals reported salary as their main source of income, with 45 individuals reporting their main source of income to be compensatory allowances,

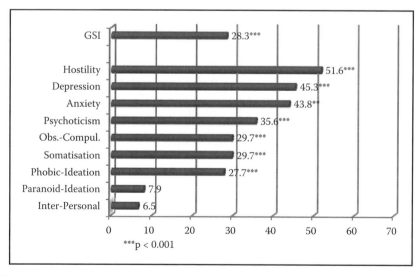

FIGURE 31.1
Percentage of patients with significantly elevated Symptom Checklist-90-R (SCL-90-R) and Global Severity Index (GSI) scores. ***p < .001. (From Hoofien, D., Gilboa, A., Vakils, E., and Donovick, P. J., *Brain Injury*, 15(3), 189–209, 2001. With permission.)

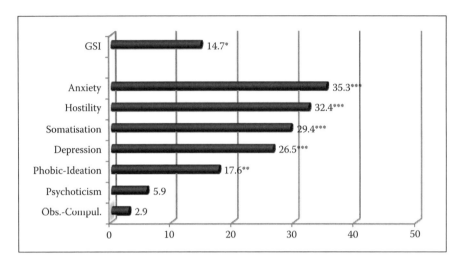

FIGURE 31.2
Percentage of family members with significantly elevated SCL-90-R and GSI scores. *p < .05, **p < .01, ***p < 0.001. Note: Paranoid ideation and interpersonal sensitivity were endorsed below the 95 percentile. (From Hoofien, D., Gilboa, A., Vakils, E., and Donovick, P. J., *Brain Injury*, 15(3), 189–209, 2001. With permission.)

three relying mainly on family support, and 18 identifying various combinations of the two as their main source of income.

With reference to family functioning, significantly fewer individuals were married, and the prevalence of divorce was higher when compared with the cultural norm. Social functioning was evaluated by reports of numbers of friends and type of social engagement. Participants reported an average of 2.7 friends, whereas 19 individuals reported they had no friends at all outside the family. Five indicated they had no social support at all.

In a small preliminary study, McGrath and Linley[98] found some evidence for progression in what they referred to as *posttraumatic growth following acquired brain injury*. In comparing matched samples in which one group averaged 7 months postinjury and the other group averaged 10 years postinjury, it was possible to discern some progression in posttraumatic growth over time. Items that were most strongly endorsed for both groups included the following: (1) appreciation of life, (2) relating to others, (3) personal strength, (4) new possibilities, and (5) spiritual change. The 10-year postinjury group had higher endorsement of a change in understanding of spiritual matters whereas this area was not endorsed in the 7-month postinjury group. McGrath and Linley[98] suggested that positive change may take many months to develop and that "a degree of unpleasant engagement with the reality of the long-term situation may be necessary."[p.772]

Finally, Powell et al.[99] investigated the time course and characterized positive psychological changes after TBI, comparing two groups of individuals with brain injury in a long-term follow-up study. The first group was comprised of 23 individuals who averaged 1.7 years postinjury and the second group was comprised of 25 individuals who averaged 11.6 years postinjury. The authors looked for correlation between posttraumatic growth and other factors, such as life satisfaction, anxiety, depression, and severity of injury. They investigated individuals' subjective perceptions of their experiences, the significance of the event for them, positive and negative lifestyle and personal changes that had been made, perceptions of good and bad advice for coping, and the factors that aided with adjustment. Not surprisingly, life satisfaction was found to be negatively correlated with anxiety and depression, and positively correlated with the degree to which individuals endorsed perceptions that their lives had been ruined.

Figure 31.3 illustrates factors that have been identified as helpful in adjustment to life after injury and suggests that social support from family and friends, and personal skills were most helpful. Figure 31.4 illustrates perceived positive changes in self and lifestyle with the two most frequently endorsed findings being that the individual appreciated people in life more and had positive changes in lifestyle. Figure 31.5 illustrates advice that was found to be helpful, with the two most frequently reported being "It takes time; you will improve; time is a healer" and "Don't give up; have a positive attitude." Advice that was considered to be the worst is illustrated in Figure 31.6, with the two most frequently reported as "Act as if nothing happened" and pessimistic comments offering no hope.

31.11 Crisis Management

Few families can be expected to be prepared to manage the various types of crises that arise for persons with TBI and their caregivers. Davis et al.[100] conducted research using a triangulated research strategy involving both qualitative and quantitative methods to understand better the experience of crisis following brain injury. Triangulation involved information derived from individuals with brain injury, their families, and professionals involved in their care in community-based settings.

When crisis is usually thought of as a temporary state of upset and disorganization, the results of these authors' work suggested that the experience of crisis after brain injury is somewhat different. Although crisis is usually thought of as time limited, crisis following brain injury was more regularly characterized as "never ending." Participants described crisis as a lifelong condition during which coping was dependent upon an individual's ability to redefine one's identity. There was indication that crisis varied in intensity from time to time, but it was never really absent. Davis et al.[100] described crisis as receding somewhat, leaving the individual and family with a "precarious homeostasis" during periods of crisis recession.

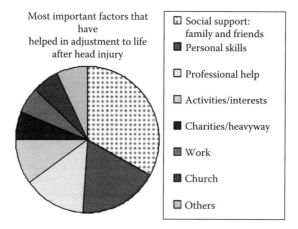

FIGURE 31.3
Whole-sample response to the question: What are the most important factors that have helped in adjustment to life after head injury? (From Powell, T., Ekin-Wood, A., and Collin, C., *Brain Injury*, 21(1), 31–38, 2007. With permission.)

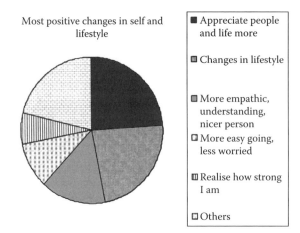

FIGURE 31.4
Whole-sample response to the question: What are the most positive changes in yourself and your lifestyle following your head injury? (From Powell, T., Ekin-Wood, A., and Collin, C., *Brain Injury*, 21(1), 31–38, 2007. With permission.)

Simply put, crises emerge when the nature and number of demands exceed the existing capacities of an individual or a system.[101] After brain injury, both the nature and number of demands change drastically. Individuals and families are placed in a confusing series of circumstances, the likes of which they have most likely not experienced in life before. Circumstance, terminology, and potential interventions are all new, and the personal circumstances of the individual with injury change substantially as a result of the brain injury itself. Both subtle and dramatic changes can be found in a wide variety of areas of function and capability, some of which may be apparent to the individual or family whereas some remain to be discovered over time. Some of these changes actually impact the individual's ability to cope, such as difficulties with memory, judgment, impulsivity, or anger control. Support in crises is important and comes from social structures that involve family, friends, and educational and/or work settings. Ironically, in many instances, the availability of these very systems changes as a result of the injury. The result is that a crisis,

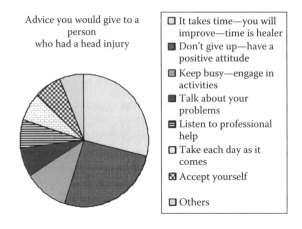

FIGURE 31.5
Whole-sample response to the question: What is the best advice you would give to a person that had just had a head injury? (From Powell, T., Ekin-Wood, A., and Collin, C., *Brain Injury*, 21(1), 31–38, 2007. With permission.)

The two worst pieces of advice you could give
to somebody after a head injury

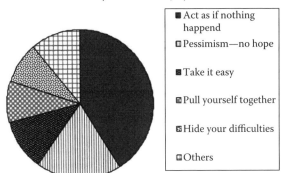

- Act as if nothing happend
- Pessimism—no hope
- Take it easy
- Pull yourself together
- Hide your difficulties
- Others

FIGURE 31.6
Whole-sample response to the question: What is the worst advice you could give to somebody after a head injury? (From Powell, T., Ekin-Wood, A., and Collin, C., *Brain Injury*, 21(1), 31–38, 2007. With permission.)

once initiated, is compounded by limitations in coping mechanisms as well as availability of support structures contributing to a slowed or lesser resolution of crisis.

Crises can include financial, social, medical, and legal matters. In general, it can be very useful to attempt to prepare injured persons and their caregivers by collecting information they may need in the event of certain situations arising. The injured person should be provided a succinct medical history that can be conveyed to emergency personnel as needed. Likewise, this information should be provided to health care providers who will continue to care for the injured person upon returning home. A list of past treaters and their contact information can be quite helpful.

The discharge planner should see that discussions have been held with the injured person and the caregivers regarding treatment authorization requirements, advanced directives, and durable power of attorney for health care arrangements. Obtaining durable power of attorney agreements can be expensive and, as a result, may not be undertaken. Likewise, guardianship or conservatorship proceedings can be expensive and less likely to be undertaken. Information should be provided to caregivers concerning experienced legal resources within their vicinity, and the advantages and disadvantages associated with advanced directives, durable power of attorney for health care arrangements, and competency proceedings.

31.12 Home Adaptations

It is most likely that an individual's home will require some sort of modification to assist in the management of the injured person. Fortunately, there are a number of inexpensive and reliable electronic means to address some difficulties encountered following TBI.

Impairments of smell and taste represent a common area of concern. Smoke, natural gas, and carbon monoxide detectors are available at fairly low cost, although, as battery operated devices, they pose a challenge for the memory impaired in terms of proper maintenance. Caregivers need instruction in establishing a food-labeling procedure for storage of food because spoiled food cannot be detected with impaired smell, taste, or, in some cases, vision or judgment. Clearly labeled food that indicates a "do-not-use-after" date can be helpful.

Visual and balance impairments may necessitate the introduction of additional lighting to bedroom, hallway, closet, bathroom, basement, and garage areas. Many persons after TBI have balance that relies heavily upon visual input because vestibular and proprioceptive inputs are diminished.[102] Consequently, low-light conditions increase the likelihood of a loss of balance and/or fall, increasing the risk of reinjury.

Accessibility must be considered for the physically challenged individual. This includes access and egress from the living environment, and moving around within the environment safely. Access and egress should be considered from the perspective of ramping, as well as time required to egress from various areas of the home. Locks on doors may need to be modified to allow the person with dexterity problems easy operation in the event of an emergency. Thumb bolt, push button, or automatic locks may be helpful. Locks that are code operated may help with problems associated with dexterity or lost keys. It is necessary to consider doorway widths, bathroom fixture access, hot water temperature control, transfer bars or equipment, height and elevation angle of the bed, and placement, height, and sturdiness of furniture. Kitchen safety can be addressed by consideration of electrical disabling of large appliances at the circuit breaker box and placement of a lock on the access door to the circuit breaker box. Stovetops, ideally, should have the controls at the front of the cooking surface. It may be necessary to place nonbreakable dishes in lower cupboards for easier access, as well as frequently used foodstuffs.

Persons with oral dysarthria, balance impairments, seizure disorders, or other serious health conditions should be advised to obtain a MedicAlert bracelet that will allow public safety officials a means of independent verification of a condition. This can be crucial in obtaining needed medical attention and also in avoiding inappropriate incarceration under the mistaken impression of public intoxication.

Consideration should be given to the utilization of portable telephone equipment in the home, with backup fixed equipment. The portable phone should have an extended-life battery capability and a loud, continuously sounding page/find feature because memory difficulties may make finding the portable phone difficult. Placement of multiple phones should be considered for the physically challenged person. Phones are available with very large buttons for easy dialing for the visually or physically challenged person. Likewise, phones that allow for light indicators for incoming calls and volume adjustment can be useful for the hearing impaired. Lastly, an easily operated answering machine can be helpful in managing communications, along with preprogrammed cell phones.

Systems are available that allow for telephonic alerts to be delivered in the event of an emergency. The system operates when a remote medallion worn by the user is activated. This can be useful for people with balance problems, seizure disorders, and so forth. The system contacts either a service or a user-defined contact to relay the emergency message.

Bathrooms should be equipped with grab bars around the shower/tub and toilet areas. Hand-held shower wands can be helpful for the physically challenged person. Bath benches that are nonslip and nonslip floor coverings for the shower/tub area and adjacent flooring should be considered. It may be necessary to remove glass shower door fixtures, both for access and safety in the event of a loss of balance. Bowed shower rods and curtains can provide extra space in the shower. Ground fault interrupt electrical receptacles should be installed in the vicinity of water, such as in bathrooms and kitchens.

Remote electrical control devices can be helpful in managing the environment. These include remotes for common equipment like televisions and radio/stereo units, but can also be purchased to control lighting and other electrical appliances. Such units are referred to as *BSR* or *X-10 units* and function by transmission of a signal through existing electrical wiring to specially installed light switches or electrical outlets.

In general, home evaluations are conducted by occupational and/or physical therapy staff members. These individuals are quite skilled in conducting these evaluations. It can be useful to have a community resource catalog available to caregivers that lists vendors of equipment and services.

Some individuals own weapons and keep them in their living environments. The existence of weapons in the home should be explored, and recommendations made for their management. Safety becomes an issue not only for the physically or judgment-impaired person, but also for the depressed person.

The Internet continues to evolve and offer increased access to services. Shopping for many items can be safely conducted via the Internet, and social contact can likewise be enhanced. Some communities have grocery and pharmacy ordering and delivery available via Internet services. Of course, the Internet is also a place of vulnerability for social and financial matters. E-mail contact with an established list of friends and professionals can be quite useful. Chat rooms can be risky and difficult to use. Resources such as useful websites or services, identified in advance for the injured person and the caregiver, can be provided. Families may want to consider the use of certain potential filters for the protection of the individual.

31.13 Financial Planning

Families need help in preparing for the loss of income usually associated with TBI. Osberg et al.[103] reviewed missed work days and financial consequences for parents of TBI children. Table 31.2 shows the percentage of families reporting various problems at 1-month and 6-month postdischarge intervals sorted by severity of injury. A high percentage of parents reported a loss of work time and injury-caused financial problems.

In a long-term outcome survey conducted of more than 300 families averaging 7 years postinjury, the mean reduction in monthly earnings for the injured person was more than $1000 per month in 1997 dollars.[70] On a family basis, mean monthly income reduction 7 years postinjury was more than $400, suggesting that other family members had either obtained employment or sought higher wages, perhaps in response to the loss of an income. It should be noted that virtually all persons in this study had insurance of one sort or another that provided funding for their rehabilitation. This is important in that some of these individuals were covered by either liability or workers' compensation coverage, both of which are likely to provide some income on a long-term basis. This is obviously not the case for persons without such coverage. The income loss may be markedly higher for people without these types of coverage.

Families should be encouraged to review their budgets and spending plans immediately. Larger purchases should be reconsidered or postponed. Refinancing, consolidation, or restructuring of family debt may become important. Again, most families are overwhelmed with the changes in their day-to-day reality and will not have considered these long-term issues. The discharge planner may be able to provide a resource list of lenders willing to assist with debt restructuring, refinancing, consumer education, and so on. In some instances, families may have other income resources they can call upon to assist with short-term financial needs as they adjust to a lower income as a family unit. These can be

TABLE 31.2

Percentage of Families Agreeing or Strongly Agreeing by Injury Severity Score

	Injury Severity		
	Mild (n = 36)	**Moderate (n = 30)**	**Severe (n = 14)**
One Month Postdischarge			
Financial Problems			
The injury is causing financial problems[c]	17	27	79
Additional income is needed[b]	11	17	50
Work Problems			
Time is lost from work	36	47	57
I am cutting down the hours I work[a]	17	30	57
I stopped working because of child's injury[a]	3	17	29
Six Months Postdischarge			
Financial Problems			
The injury is causing financial problems[b]	14	20	57
Additional income is needed[b]	6	10	43
Work Problems			
Time is lost from work[b]	22	27	71
I am cutting down the hours I work[c]	0	7	57
I stopped working because of child's injury[b]	0	10	29

[a]$p < .05$, [b]$p < .01$, [c]$p < .001$.

Note: An example of how to read this table is as follows. Among the 36 children with mild injuries, 17% of families reported the injury is causing financial problems versus 27% among the 30 families of children with moderate injuries, and 79% of the 14 families of children with severe injuries. Table footnote c indicates that the percentage differences across the three severity groups are significant at the .001 level.

Source: Osberg, J. S., Brooke, M. M., Baryza, M. J., Rowe, K., Lash, M., and Kahn, P., *Brain Injury*, 11(1), 11–24, 1997. With permission.

found in retirement funds, whole-life insurance policies, and supplemental disability policies. Families may need to consider the sale of certain assets both to generate income and to reduce indebtedness.

End-of-life issues are difficult for many families to discuss and plan for, either with or without TBI. Yet, the financial consequences of death can be considerable. Estate planning can identify useful tools to assist a family to plan for the death of caregivers. Simple review of a family's likely net worth will determine whether formal tools such as trusts might be helpful in reducing tax consequences, asset protection, and preservation of maximal funding for the injured family member. Life insurance policies, both individual and second-to-die policies, may be warranted to help in providing some funding for care. It can be helpful for parents to discuss their intentions for the use of proceeds from their estate upon their death with noninjured siblings, especially if a decision is made to reserve those proceeds primarily or entirely for the injured family member. As families age, different estate planning approaches may be appropriate. For example, a family with several young children may be inclined to plan estate distributions for the benefit of all the children. However, as children become adults who are providing for themselves, the family may change its direction of estate proceeds to benefit those who are unable to provide for themselves.

Lastly, the discharge planner should provide information and/or application forms necessary for Social Security Income, Social Security Disability Income, and/or Financial Aid to Dependent Children. More information on financial planning can be found in Chapter 29 of this volume.

31.14 Additional Rehabilitation Timing

Some persons with TBI recover over a period of time that is fairly concise and confined in duration. Others, however, seem to experience recovery in a less time-contiguous fashion. Still others may experience a fairly good period of recovery and success following discharge, only to experience postdischarge complications that cause the individual to regress to a lesser level of functioning. A return to rehabilitation services can sometimes be useful in furthering the recovery of an individual or in reestablishing a previously attained level of function. Many studies report functionally significant improvements and reduced disability levels achieved during later application of rehabilitation services after chronic placement in institutional or home settings.[104–117] These studies conclude that, in individuals with moderate to severe brain injury, substantial functional and neurobehavioral impairment can be reasonably expected to achieve statistically significant functional improvements following application of "late" rehabilitation. The literature, however, does not provide a thorough review of the characteristics of those persons who respond well to late rehabilitation, at least not enough to provide a clear delineation of that group from one that will not benefit.

The propriety of additional rehabilitation depends upon the reasons for a lack of progress in earlier rehabilitation attempts or the reasons for deterioration from previously achieved levels of functioning. Brain injury is not a degenerative diagnosis. Regression or deterioration observed following brain injury can be traced to either a medical, psychological/emotional, or environmental etiology. The key is to identify accurately which of these may be active as reasons for a decline in function and determine whether they can be reversed or changed. One example might be the identification of iatrogenic complications associated with inappropriate pharmacologic intervention. Another might be a change in a family system in which an undue amount of overdependence was fostered for many years, only to require further intervention when the responsible family member or caregiver was no longer available or able to provide care. This might occur in the sudden death of a parent or a decline in health of a caregiver resulting from advancing age. Again, regularly scheduled follow-up contact may allow identification of such situations and allow the discharge planner to advocate proactively for additional rehabilitative services.

31.15 Summary

The world of health care has changed tremendously during the past two decades and, alarmingly, more so during the past few years. Shorter LOSs and decreasing financial resources have increased the level of acuity with which people are discharged from treatment settings, and the level of disability with which people are returned to home environments. Ongoing care and treatment is relegated, many times, to the injured person and his or her caregivers. The burden for discharge planning cannot fall to a single individual on a treatment team, but rather must be dealt with by the entire team and, institutionally, by the resources developed and made available by the treating facility. Whether viewed as a part of patient care, advocacy, or community service, the creation of resource and information centers provides a vital service to persons with TBI and their families. Caregivers must be encouraged to maintain contact with previous care providers and to manage and participate actively in follow-up activities.

The responsibilities carried by discharge planners are immense and the information suggested herein materially adds to an already overwhelming workload. A checklist is provided in Appendix 31B to assist the discharge planner in both approaching and organizing a discharge for a person with TBI and as an outline for services that the discharge planner might encourage to be developed, institutionally, to support excellence in discharge planning.

References

1. Jennings, B., The ordeal of reminding: Traumatic brain injury and the goals of care, *The Hastings Center Report*, 36(2), 29–37, 2006.
2. Marsh, N. V., Kersel, D. A., Havill, J. H., and Sleigh, J. W., Caregiver burden at 1 year following severe traumatic brain injury, *Brain Injury*, 12(12), 1045–1059, 1998.
3. The Traumatic Brain Injury Model Systems National Data Center, Traumatic Brain Injury Facts and Figures, The Traumatic Brain Injury Model Systems National Data Center, Englewood, CO, 1997.
4. Kreutzer, J. S., Kolakowsky-Hayner, S. A., Ripley, D., Cifu, D. X., Rosenthal, M., Bushnik, T., Zafonte, R., Englander, J., and High, W., Charges and lengths of stay for acute and inpatient rehabilitation treatment of traumatic brain injury 1990 to 1996, *Brain Injury*, 15(9), 763–774, 2001.
5. Rotondi, A. J., Sinkule, J., Balzer, K., Harris, J., and Moldovan, R., A qualitative needs assessment of persons who have experienced traumatic brain injury and their primary family caregivers, *Journal of Head Trauma Rehabilitation*, 22(1), 14–25, 2007.
6. Burns, P. G., Kay, T., and Pieper, B., *A Survey of the Vocational Service System as It Relates to Head Injury Survivors and Their Vocational Needs*, Grant no. 0001229, New York State Head Injury Association, 1986.
7. Goodall, P., Lawyer, H. L., and Wehman, P., Vocational rehabilitation and traumatic brain injury: A legislative and public policy perspective, *Journal of Head Trauma Rehabilitation*, 9(2), 61–81, 1994.
8. Corrigan, J. D., Bogner, J. A., Mysiw, W. J., Clinchot, D., and Fugate, L., Life satisfaction after traumatic brain injury, *Journal of Head Trauma Rehabilitation*, 16(6), 543–555, 2001.
9. Banja, J. D., Adler, R. K., and Stringer, A. Y., Ethical dimensions of caring for defiant patients: A case study, *Journal of Head Trauma Rehabilitation*, 11(6), 93–97, 1996.
10. Chan, L., Doctor, J., Temkin, N., MacLehose, R. F., Esselman, P., Bell, K., and Dikmen, S., Discharge disposition from acute care after traumatic brain injury: The effect of insurance type, *Archives of Physical Medicine and Rehabilitation*, 82(9), 1151–1154, 2001.
11. Retchin, S. M., Brown, R. S., Yeh, S. C., Chu, D., and Moreno, L., Outcome of stroke patients in Medicare fee for service and managed care, *Journal of the American Medical Association*, 278(2), 119–124, 1997.
12. Wrigley, J. M., Yoels, W. C., Webb, C. R., and Fine, P. R., Social and physical factors in the referral of people with traumatic brain injuries to rehabilitation, *Archives of Physical Medicine and Rehabilitation*, 75(2), 149–155, 1994.
13. Brantner, C. L., Job coaching for persons with traumatic brain injuries employed in professional and technical occupations, *Journal of Applied Rehabilitation Counseling*, 23(3), 3–14, 1992.
14. Wehman, P. H., Kreutzer, J. S., West, M. D., Sherron, P. D., Zasler, N. D., Groah, C. H., Stonnington, H. H., Burns, C. T., and Sale, P. R., Return to work for persons with traumatic brain injury: A supported employment approach, *Archives of Physical Medicine and Rehabilitation*, 71(13), 1047–1052, 1990.
15. Hajfey, W. J. and Abrams, D. L., Employment outcomes for participants in a brain injury work reentry program: Preliminary findings, *Journal of Head Trauma Rehabilitation*, 6(3), 24–34, 1991.

16. Carlsson, G. S., Syardsudd, K., and Welin, L., Long-term effects of head injuries sustained during life in three male populations, *Journal of Neurosurgery*, 67(2), 197–205, 1987.

17. Annegers, J. F., Grabow, J. D., Kurland, L. T., and Laws, Jr., E. R., The incidence, causes, and secular trends of head trauma in Olmstead County, Minnesota, 1935–1974, *Neurology*, 30(9), 912–919, 1980.

18. Felmingham, K. L., Baguely, I. J., and Crooks, J., A comparison of acute and postdischarge predictors of employment 2 years after traumatic brain injury, *Archives of Physical Medicine and Rehabilitation*, 82(4), 435–439, 2001.

19. Ezrachi, O., Ben-Yishay, Y., Kay, T., Diller, L., and Rattok, J., Predicting employment in traumatic brain injury following neuropsychological rehabilitation, *Journal of Head Trauma Rehabilitation*, 6(3), 71–84, 1991.

20. Zuger, R. R., Vocational rehabilitation counseling of traumatic brain injury: Factors contributing to stress, *Journal of Rehabilitation*, 59(2), 28–30, 1993.

21. Ben-Yishay, Y. and Diller, L., Cognitive remediation in traumatic brain injury: Update and issues, *Archives of Physical Medicine and Rehabilitation*, 74(2), 204–213, 1993.

22. Giacino, J. T. and Cicerone, K. D., Varieties of deficit unawareness after brain injury, *Journal of Head Trauma Rehabilitation*, 13(5), 1–15, 1998.

23. Prigatano, G. P., Fordyce, D. J., Zeiner, H. K., Roueche, R., Peppig, M., and Wood, B. C., Neuropsychological rehabilitation after closed head injury in young adults, *Journal of Neurology, Neurosurgery, and Psychiatry*, 47(5), 505–513, 1984.

24. Miller, L., Back to the future: Legal, vocational, and quality-of-life issues in the long-term adjustment of the brain-injured patient, *Journal of Cognitive Rehabilitation*, 10(5), 14–20, 1993.

25. Tennant, A., MacDermott, N., and Neary, D., The long-term outcome of head injury: Implications for service planning, *Brain Injury*, 9(6), 595–605, 1995.

26. Sim, J., Improving return-to-work strategies in the United States disability programs, with analysis of program practices in Germany and Sweden, *Social Security Bulletin*, 59(3), 41–50, 1999.

27. Boyle, G. J. and Haines, S., Severe traumatic brain injury: Some effects on family caregivers, *Psychological Reports*, 90(2), 415–425, 2002.

28. Lezak, M. D., Brain damage is a family affair, *Journal of Clinical and Experimental Neuropsychology*, 10(1), 111–123, 1988.

29. Gan, C. and Schuller, R., Family system outcome following acquired brain injury: Clinical and research perspectives, *Brain Injury*, 16(4), 311–322, 2002.

30. Lezak, M. D., Psychological implications of traumatic brain damage for the patient's family, *Rehabilitation Psychology*, 31(4), 241–250, 1986.

31. Orsillo, S. M., McCaffrey, R. J., and Fisher, J. M., Siblings of head-injured individuals: A population at risk, *Journal of Head Trauma Rehabilitation*, 8(1), 102–115, 1993.

32. Willer, B., Allen, K., Durnan, M., et al., Problems and coping strategies of mothers, siblings, and young adult males with traumatic brain injury, *Canadian Journal of Rehabilitation*, 3(3), 167–173, 1990.

33. Thompson, A. M., Parental marital functioning following TBI in an adolescent/young adult child, PhD dissertation, Michigan State University, Michigan. Retrieved December 22, 2009, from Dissertations & Theses: A&I (Publication No. AAT 9706570), 1996.

34. Rosenberg, L. E., The effects of traumatic brain injury on spouses, PhD dissertation, The University of Wisconsin, Madison, Wisconsin. Retrieved December 22, 2009, from Dissertations & Theses: A&I (Publication No. AAT 9736066), 1997.

35. Lyth-Frantz, L., Traumatic brain injury of a child: Effects on the marital relationship and parenting. PhD dissertation, State University of New York at Buffalo, New York. Retrieved December 22, 2009, from Dissertations & Theses: A&I (Publication No. AAT 9822169), 1998.

36. Wongvatunyu, S. and Porter, E. J., Changes in family life perceived by mothers of young adult TBI survivors, *Journal of Family Nursing*, 14(3), 314–332, 2008.

37. Uysal, S., Hibbard, M. R., Robillard, D., Pappadopulos, E., and Jaffe, M., The effect of parental traumatic brain injury on parenting and child behavior, *Journal of Head Trauma Rehabilitation*, 13(6), 57–71, 1998.

38. McMordie, W. R., Rogers, K. F., and Barker, S. L., Consumer satisfaction with services provided to head-injured patients and their families, *Brain Injury*, 5(1), 43–51, 1991.

39. McPherson, K. M., McNaughton, H., and Pentland, B., Information needs of families when one member has a severe brain injury, *International Journal of Rehabilitation Research*, 23(4), 295–301, 2000.

40. Gan, C. and Schuller, R., Family system outcome following acquired brain injury: Clinical and research perspectives, *Brain Injury*, 16(4), 311–322, 2002.

41. Hall, K. M., Karzmark, P., Stevens, M., Englander, J., O'Hare, P., and Wright, J., Family stressors in traumatic brain injury: A two-year follow-up, *Archives of Physical Medicine and Rehabilitation*, 75(8), 876–884, 1994.

42. Man, D. W., Family caregivers' reactions and coping for persons with brain injury, *Brain Injury*, 16(12), 1025–1037, 2002.

43. Brooks, N., Campsie, L., Symington, C., Beattie, A., and McKinlay, W., The 5 year outcome of severe blunt head injury: A relative's view, *Journal of Neurology, Neurosurgery, and Psychiatry*, 49(7), 764–770, 1986.

44. Brooks, N., Campsie, L., Symington, C., Beattie, A., and McKinlay, W., The effects of severe head injury on patient and relative within seven years of injury, *Journal of Head Trauma Rehabilitation*, 2(3), 1–13, 1987.

45. Ergh, T. C., Rapport, L. J., Coleman, R. D., and Hanks, R. A., Predictors of caregiver and family functioning following traumatic brain injury: Social support moderates caregiver distress, *Journal of Head Trauma Rehabilitation*, 17(2), 155–174, 2002.

46. Gillen, R., Tennen, H., Affleck, G., and Steinpreis, R., Distress, depressive symptoms, and depressive disorder among caregivers of patients with brain injury, *Journal of Head Trauma Rehabilitation*, 13(3), 31–43, 1998.

47. Kreutzer, J. S., Gervasio, A. H., and Camplair, P. S., Primary caregivers' psychological status and family functioning after traumatic brain injury, *Brain Injury*, 8(3), 197–210, 1994.

48. Livingston, M. G., Brooks, D. N., and Bond, M. R., Patient outcome in the year following severe head injury and relatives' psychiatric and social functioning, *Journal of Neurology, Neurosurgery, and Psychiatry*, 48(9), 876–881, 1985.

49. Minnes, P., Graffi, S., Nolte, M. L., Carlson, P., and Harrick, L., Coping and stress in Canadian family caregivers of persons with traumatic brain injuries, *Brain Injury*, 14(8), 737–748, 2000.

50. Perlesz, A., Kinsella, G., and Crowe, S., Psychological distress and family satisfaction following traumatic brain injury: Injured individuals and their primary, secondary, and tertiary carers, *Journal of Head Trauma Rehabilitation*, 15(3), 909–929, 2000.

51. Wade, S. L., Taylor, H. G., Drotar, D., Stancin, T., Yeates, K. O., and Minich, N. M., A prospective study of long-term caregiver and family adaptation following brain injury in children, *Journal of Head Trauma Rehabilitation*, 17(2), 96–111, 2002.

52. Kreutzer, J. S., Marwitz, J. H., Walker, W., Sander, A., Sherer, M., Bogner, J. et al., Moderating factors in return to work and job stability after traumatic brain injury, *Journal of Head Trauma Rehabilitation*, 18(2), 128, 2003.

53. Burnett, D. M., Kolakowsky-Hayner, S. A., Slater, D., Stringer, A., Bushnik, T., Zafonte, R., et al., Ethnographic analysis of traumatic brain injury patients in the national Model Systems database, *Archives of Physical Medicine and Rehabilitation*, 84(2), 263–267, 2003.

54. Hart, T., Bogner, J., Whyte, J., and Polansky, M., Attribution of blame in accidental and violence-related traumatic brain injury, *Rehabilitation Psychology*, 48(2), 86–92, 2003.

55. Hart, T., O'Neil-Pirozzi, T. M., Williams, K. D., Rapport, L. J., Hammond, F., and Kreutzer, J., Racial differences in caregiving patterns, caregiver emotional function, and sources of emotional support following traumatic brain injury, *Journal of Head Trauma Rehabilitation*, 22(2), 122–131, 2007.

56. Corrigan, J. D., Bogner, J. A., Mysiw, W. J., Clinchot, D., and Fugate, L., Life satisfaction after traumatic brain injury, *Journal of Head Trauma Rehabilitation*, 16(6), 543–555, 2001.

57. Tennant, A., Macdermott, N., and Neary, D., The long-term outcome of head injury: Implications for service planning, *Brain Injury*, 9(6), 595–605, 1995.

58. Bixler, E. O., Kales, A., Vela-Bueno, A., Jacoby, J. A., Scarone, S., and Soldatos, C. R., Nocturnal myoclonus and nocturnal myoclonic activity in a normal population, *Research Communications in Chemical Pathology and Pharmacology*, 36(1), 129–140, 1982.

59. Holland, D. and Shigaki, C. L., Educating families and caretakers of traumatically brain injured patients in the new health care environment: A three phase model and bibliography, *Brain Injury*, 12(12), 993–1009, 1998.

60. DePompei, R. and Williams, J., Working with families after TBI: A family centered approach, *Topics in Language Disorders*, 15(1), 68–81, 1995.

61. Acorn, S., An education/support program for families of survivors of head injury, *Canadian Journal of Rehabilitation*, 7(2), 149–151, 1993.

62. Jennett, B., *Epilepsy After Non-Missile Head Injuries*, 2nd ed., Heinemann, London, 1975.

63. Annegers, J. F., Grabow, J. D., Groover, R. V., Laws, E. R., Elveback, L. R., and Kurland, L. T., Seizures after head trauma: A population study, *Neurology*, 30(7 Pt. 1), 683–689, 1980.

64. Guidice, M. A. and Berchou, R. C., Posttraumatic epilepsy following head injury, *Brain Injury*, 1(1), 61–64, 1987.

65. Temkin, N. R., Dikmen, S. S., Wilensky, A. J., Keihm, J., Chabal, S., and Winn, H. R., A randomized, double-blind study of phenytoin for the prevention of posttraumatic seizures, *New England Journal of Medicine*, 323(8), 497–502, 1990.

66. Yablon S. A., Posttraumatic seizures, *Archives of Physical Medicine and Rehabilitation*, 74(9), 983–1001, 1993.

67. Dalmady-Israel, C. and Zasler, N. D., Posttraumatic seizures: A critical review, *Brain Injury*, 7(3), 263–273, 1993.

68. Jennett, B. and Teasdale, G., *Management of Head Injuries*, F. A. Davis, Philadelphia, 1981.

69. Ramsay R. E. and Pryor F., Epilepsy in the elderly, *Neurology*, 55(5 Suppl. 1), S9–S14, 2000, Discussion, S54–S58.

70. Ashley, M. J., Persel, C. S., and Krych, D. K., Long-term outcome follow-up of postacute traumatic brain injury rehabilitation: An assessment of functional and behavioral measures of daily living, *Journal of Rehabilitation Outcomes Measurement*, 1(4), 40–47, 1997.

71. Rosenthal, M., Christensen, B. K., and Ross, T. P., Depression following traumatic brain injury, *Archives of Physical Medicine and Rehabilitation*, 79(1), 90–104, 1998.

72. Satz, P., Forney, D. L., Zaucha, K., Asarnow, R. R., Light, R., McCleary, C., Levin, H., et al., Depression, cognition, and functional correlates of recovery outcome after traumatic brain injury, *Brain Injury*, 12(7), 537–553, 1998.

73. Zafonte. R. D., Cullen, N., and Lexell, J., Serotonin agents in the treatment of acquired brain injury, *Journal of Head Trauma Rehabilitation*, 17(4), 322–334, 2002.

74. Menzel, J. C., Depression in the elderly after traumatic brain injury: A systematic review, *Brain Injury*, 22(5), 375–380, 2008.

75. Levin, H. S., Goldstein, F. C., and MacKenzie, E. J., Depression as a secondary condition following mild and moderate traumatic brain injury, *Seminars in Clinical Neuropsychiatry*, 2(3), 207–215, 1997.

76. Rapoport, J. J., Kiss, A., and Feinstein, A., The impact of major depression on outcome following mild-to-moderate traumatic brain injury in older adults, *Journal of Affective Disorders*, 92(2–3), 273–276, 2006.

77. Sale, P., West., M. D., Sherron, P. D., and Wehman, P. H., Exploratory analysis of job separation from supported employment for persons with traumatic brain injury, *Journal of Head Trauma Rehabilitation*, 6(3), 1–11, 1991.

78. Rao, V. and Lyketsos, C. G., Psychiatric aspects of traumatic brain injury, *Psychiatric Clinics of North America*, 25(1), 43–69, 2002.

79. Young, T., Palta, M., Dempsey, J., Skatrud, J., Weber, S., and Badr, S., The occurrence of sleep-disordered breathing among middle-aged adults, *New England Journal of Medicine*, 328(17), 1230–1235, 1993.

80. Ancoli-Israel, S., Kripke, D. F., Klauber, M. R., Mason, W. J., Fell, R., and Kaplan, O., Periodic limb movements in sleep in community-dwelling elderly, *Sleep*, 14(6), 496–500, 1991.

81. Benbadis, S. R., Perry, M. C., Sundstad, L. S., and Wolgamuth, B. R., Prevalence of daytime sleepiness in a population of drivers, *Neurology*, 52(1), 209–210, 1999.

82. D'Alessandro, R., Rinaldi, R., Cristina, E., Gamberini, G., and Lugaresi, E., Prevalence of excessive daytime sleepiness, an open epidemiological problem [letter], *Sleep*, 18(5), 389–391, 1995.

83. Masel, B. E., Scheibel, R. S., Kimbark, T., and Kuna, S. T., Excessive daytime sleepiness in adults with brain injuries, *Archives of Physical Medicine and Rehabilitation*, 82(11), 1526–1532, 2001.

84. Castriotta, R. J. and Lai, J. M., Sleep disorders associated with traumatic brain injury, *Archives of Physical Medicine and Rehabilitation*, 82(10), 1403–1406, 2001.

85. Guilleminault, C., Yuen, K. M., Gulevich, M. G., Karadeniz, D., Leger, D., and Philip, P., Hypersomnia after head–neck trauma: A medicolegal dilemma, *Neurology*, 54(3), 653–659, 2000.

86. Findley, L. J., Barth, J. T., Powers, D. C., Wilhoit, S. C., Boyd, D. G., and Suratt, P. M., Cognitive impairment in patients with obstructive sleep apnea and associated hypoxemia, *Chest*, 90(5), 686–690, 1986.

87. Greenberg, G. D., Watson, R. K., and Deptula, D., Neuropsychological dysfunction in sleep apnea, *Sleep*, 10(3), 254–262, 1987.

88. Montplasir, J., Bédard, M. A., Richer, F., and Rouleau, I., Neurobehavioral manifestations in obstructive sleep apnea syndrome before and after treatment with continuous positive airway pressure, *Sleep*, 15(Suppl. 6), S17–19, 1992.

89. Young, T., Bluestein, J., Finn, L., and Palta, M., Sleep-disordered breathing and motor-vehicle accidents in a population-based sample of employed adults, *Sleep*, 20(8), 608–613, 1997.

90. Teran-Santos, J., Jimenez-Gomez, A., and Cordero-Guevara, J., The association between sleep apnea and the risk of traffic accidents, Cooperative Group Burgos-Santander, *New England Journal of Medicine*, 340(11), 847–851, 1999.

91. Horstmann, S., Hess, C. W., Bassetti, C., Gugger, M., and Mathis, J., Sleepiness-related accidents in sleep apnea patients, *Sleep*, 23(3), 383–389, 2000.

92. Bergland, M. and Thomas, K., Psychological issues following severe head injury in adolescence: Individual and family perceptions, *Rehabilitation Counseling Bulletin*, 35(1), 5–22, 1991.

93. Hibbard, M. R., Bogdany, J., Uysal, S., Kepler, K., Silver, J. M., Gordon, W. A., et al., Axis II psychopathology in individuals with traumatic brain injury, *Brain Injury*, 14(1), 45–61, 2000.

94. Hibbard, M. R., Uysal, S., Kepler, K., Bogdany, J., and Silver, J., Axis I psychopathology in individuals with traumatic brain injury, *Journal of Head Trauma Rehabilitation*, 13(4), 24–39, 1998.

95. Draper, K., Ponsford, J., and Schönberger, M., Psychosocial and emotional outcomes 10 years following traumatic brain injury, *Journal of Head Trauma Rehabilitation*, 22(5), 278–287, 2007.

96. Hawley, C. A. and Joseph, S., Predictors of positive growth after traumatic brain injury: A longitudinal study, *Brain Injury*, 22(5), 427–435, 2008.

97. Hoofien, D., Gilboa, A., Vakil, D., and Donovick, P. J., Traumatic brain injury (TBI) 10–20 years later: A comprehensive outcome study of psychiatric symptomatology, cognitive abilities, and psychosocial functioning, *Brain Injury*, 15(3), 189–209, 2001.

98. McGrath, J. C. and Linley, P. A., Post-traumatic growth in acquired brain injury: A preliminary small scale study, *Brain Injury*, 20(7), 767–773, 2006.

99. Powell, T., Ekin-Wood, A., and Collin, C., Post-traumatic growth after head injury: A long-term follow-up, *Brain Injury*, 21(1), 31–38, 2007.

100. Davis, J. R., Gemeinhardt, M., Gan, C., Anstey, K., and Gargaro, J., Crisis and its assessment after brain injury, *Brain Injury*, 17(5), 359, 2003.

101. Callahan, J., Crisis in theory and crisis intervention in emergencies, in P. M. Kleespies (Ed.), *Emergencies in Mental Health Practice: Evaluation and Management*, 22–40, Guilford Press, New York, 1998.

102. Jury, M. A. and Flynn, M. C., Auditory and vestibular sequelae to traumatic brain injury: A pilot study, *New Zealand Medical Journal*, 114(1134), 286–288, 2001.

103. Osberg, J. S., Brooke, M. M., Baryza, M. J., Rowe, K., Lash, M., and Kahn, P., Impact of childhood brain injury on work and family finances, *Brain Injury,* 11(1), 11–24, 1997.
104. Cope, D. N., Cole, J. R., Hall, K. M., and Barkan, H., Brain injury: Analysis of outcome in a post-acute rehabilitation system. Part 1: General analysis, *Brain Injury,* 5(2), 111–125, 1995.
105. Johnston, M. V. and Lewis, F. D., Outcomes of community re-entry programmes for brain injury survivors. Part 1: Independent living and productive activities, *Brain Injury,* 5(2), 141–154, 1991.
106. Ashley, M. J. and Persel, C. S., Traumatic brain injury recovery rates in postacute rehabilitation of traumatic brain injury: Spontaneous recovery or treatment?, *Journal of Outcomes Measurement,* 3(4), 15–21, 1999.
107. Fryer, L. and Haffey, W., Cognitive rehabilitation and community readaptation: Outcomes from two program models, *Journal of Head Trauma Rehabilitation,* 2(3), 51–63, 1987.
108. Eames, P., Cotterill, G., Kneale, T. A., Storrar, A. L., and Yeomans, P., Outcome of intensive rehabilitation after severe brain injury: A long-term follow-up study, *Brain Injury,* 10(9), 631–650, 1996.
109. Wood, R. L., McCrea, J. D., Wood, L. M., and Merriman, R. N., Clinical and cost effectiveness of post-acute neurobehavioural rehabilitation, *Brain Injury,* 13(2), 69–88, 1999.
110. Gray, D. S. and Burnham, R. S., Preliminary outcome analysis of a long-term rehabilitation program for severe acquired brain injury, *Archives of Physical Medicine and Rehabilitation,* 81(11), 1447–1456, 2000.
111. Ashley, M. J., Schultz, J. D., Bryan, V. L., Krych, D. K., and Hays, D. R., Justification of postacute traumatic brain injury rehabilitation using net present value techniques: A case study, *Journal of Rehabilitation Outcomes Measurement,* 1(5), 33–41, 1997.
112. Ashley, M. J. and Krych, D. K., Cost/benefit analysis for post-acute rehabilitation of the traumatically brain injured patient, *Journal of Insurance Medicine,* 22(2), 156–161, 1990.
113. High, W. M., Roebuck-Spencer, T., Sander, A. M., Stuchen, M. A., and Shere, M., Early versus late admission to postacute rehabilitation: Impact of functional outcome after traumatic brain injury, *Archives of Physical Medicine and Rehabilitation,* 87(3), 334–342, 2006.
114. Prvu-Bettger, J. A. and Stineman, M. G., Effectiveness of multidisciplinary rehabilitation services in postacute care: State-of-the-science: A review, *Archives of Physical Medicine and Rehabilitation,* 88(11), 1526–1534, 2007.
115. Turner Stokes, L., Cost-efficiency of longer stay rehabilitation programmes: Can they provide value for money?, *Brain Injury,* 21(10), 1015–1021, 2007.
116. Turner Stokes, L., Paul, S., and Williams, H., Efficiency of specialist rehabilitation in reducing dependency and costs of continuing care for adults with complex acquired brain injuries, *Journal of Neurology, Neurosurgery, and Psychiatry,* 77(5), 634–639, 2006.
117. Worthington, A. D., Matthews, S., Melia, Y., and Oddy, M., Cost–benefits associated with social outcome from neurobehavioural rehabilitation, *Brain Injury,* 20(9), 947–957, 2006.

Appendix 31A: Family Manual Outline

NAME:

DATE OF BIRTH:

DATE OF INJURY:

INJURY: (In layman's terms)

LOCATION OF INJURY:

GENERAL APPROACH:
(Discuss [1] what has been used in therapy for activity of daily living completion, [2] what to expect that the client needs for assistance, [3] specific areas of deficit and how they affect performance, [4] behaviors exhibited, and [5] what tasks are priority and *have* to be completed and which tasks should be encouraged.)

BEHAVIOR:
(Make note of all behaviors, including but not limited to physical aggression, angry language, exiting, stealing, self-abuse, nonparticipation, sexually aberrant behavior, and property abuse. This section should also include how to provide reinforcement and what approach to use to gain participation and compliance.)

AMBULATION STATUS:
(Include level of independence with ambulation, what type of assistive device is needed and the type of supervision required.)

SPEECH:

VISION:

ADAPTIVE EQUIPMENT:

ACTIVITIES OF DAILY LIVING:

A.   Hygiene and Grooming: (Include information on showering ability, oral care, combing hair, applying makeup, and so forth, with how much assistance needed.)

B.   Dressing: (Include how much assistance is needed and any adaptive equipment.)

C.   Toileting: (Note level of independence, including limitations.)

D.   Medication: (Note who should be responsible, times, any special instructions.)

E.   Meal Preparation: (Include level of assistance needed for all meals.)

F.   Eating: (Include level of help needed, type of diet, any special dietary needs or restrictions.)

G.   Bedtime/Wake-Up/Alarm Clock: (Structure should be maintained as much as possible to maintain abilities. Include techniques used to gain compliance.)

H.   Laundry: (How often and what assistance is needed.)

I.   Dishes: (Note assistance level needed.)

J.   Mail Retrieval (if appropriate):

K.   Time Management: (Note level of ability.)

L.   Travel: (Include how the client will be transported, with level of assistance needed.)

M.   Grocery Shopping: (List help needed for shopping list, money, food storage, and so on.)

N.   Money Management: (Note level of involvement and who is responsible.)

OUTINGS/LEISURE ACTIVITIES:
(Include type of activities the client can and likes to participate in. Set expectations for the outing if maladaptive behavior exists.)

DAILY ROUTINE:
(Outline a typical day for weekdays and weekends, including any help needed such as a checklist.)

VOCATIONAL/AVOCATIONAL INVOLVEMENT:
(Include responsible parties, level of participation, supervision needed, and so forth.)

NURSING/MEDICAL ISSUES:
(Include current medications, any specific care issues or restrictions, allergies, and so forth.)

THERAPEUTIC HOME PROGRAMS:
(List activities from the therapists that the client can do at home. Outline the goal and procedure for the activity using pictures, videos, and so on.)

Appendix 31B: Discharge Planning Checklist

NAME: _____

DATE OF ESTIMATED DISCHARGE: _____

GUARDIAN/CONSERVATOR: _____

DISCHARGE ADDRESS: _____

I. LIVING ACCOMMODATIONS

  A. Apt. _____ Home _____ Rented _____

     Owned _____Group home/assisted living _____

     Other _____

  B. Cleaning needs:

     1. Self or family _____

     2. Outside agency _____

  C. Home modification needs/considerations:

     Home assessment needed: Yes _____No _____

      1. Lighting needs: _____

      2. Door locks: _____

      3. Bathroom fixtures: _____

      4. Hot-water temperature control: _____

      5. Doorway widths: _____

      6. Ramps: _____

      7. Transfer bars: _____

      8. Stovetop controls: _____

      9. Ground fault interrupt electrical receptors:_____

    10. Remote electrical controls: _____

    11. Shower:

       a. Roll-in shower

       b. Hand-held wand

       c. Grab bars

       d. Bath bench

       e. Shower chair

    12. Alarms:

       a. Smoke alarm

       b. Carbon monoxide detector

       c. Natural gas detector

       d. Home security system

    13. Room accessibility:

       a. Furniture placement

       b. Nonskid rugs

       c. Carpet pile

    14. Other: _____

              _____

              _____

              _____

D. Equipment needs:

1. Resource catalog/vendors
2. Answering machine/emergency response system
3. Specialized vehicle

   Type:

   a. Automobile

   b. Van

   c. Electric scooter

   Maintenance: _____

4. Wheelchair

   Type: _____

   Maintenance: _____

   Special Modifications: _____

   Own or rent: _____

5. Walker

   Type: _____

   Maintenance: _____

   Own or rent: _____

6. Cane

   Type: _____

7. Other: _____

   _____

   a. ADL equipment

      1. Grooming/hygiene: _____

      2. Dressing/cooking: _____

      3. Recreational: _____

      4. Ergonomics: _____

   b. Orthotics

      1. Splints: _____

      2. Ankle/foot orthosis: _____

      3. Slings: _____

      4. Other: _____

E. Supplies: (Identify supplies that will be needed on an ongoing basis.)

1. Incontinence supplies: _____

2. Feeding supplies: _____

3. Eye glasses: _____

4. Medical identification bracelet: _____

5. Other: _____

II. SUPERVISION/CAREGIVER NEEDS

    A. Hours Required

<table>
<tr><td></td><td>Weekday</td><td>Weekend</td></tr>
<tr><td>1. AM</td><td>_____</td><td>_____</td></tr>
<tr><td>2. PM</td><td>_____</td><td>_____</td></tr>
<tr><td>3. Overnight</td><td>_____</td><td>_____</td></tr>
</table>

    B. Type

        1. Family _____

        2. Agency _____

        3. Nursing _____

    C. Respite alternatives: _____

    D. Responsible party postdischarge: _____

    E. Recommended daily structure: _____

    F. Caregiver manual that is client specific with anticipated complications: (See outline in Appendix A.)

III. COMMUNITY RESOURCE ANALYSIS

    A. School options

    B. Work options

        1. Volunteer

        2. Day treatment

        3. Sheltered employment

        4. Competitive employment

        5. Department of Rehabilitation

    C. Transportation

    D. Shopping

    E. Hospitals/urgent care/emergency services

    F. Banks

    G. Religious information

IV MEDICAL

    A. Medical history: (Include medical precautions and concerns as well as past treaters with contact information.)

_____

_____

_____

_____

_____

_____

_____

_____

_____

_____

B. Physicians:

   1. Primary physician: _____

   _____

   _____

   2. Physiatrist: _____

   _____

   _____

   3. Neurologist:_____

   _____

   _____

   4. Psychologist:_____

   _____

   _____

   5. Orthopedist:_____

   _____

   _____

   6. Ophthalmologist: _____

   _____

   _____

   7. Dentist: _____

   _____

   _____

8. Other: _____

_____

_____

C. Therapy: (days/hours)

PT _____OT _____ SP _____Counseling _____

Job Coach _____

Location: _____

D. Medications:

Name	Pharmacy	Physician

Known allergies: _____

Seizure history: Yes/No _____Date of last seizure: _____

Prescription obtained: Yes/No _____

E. Dietary recommendations: _____

_____

_____

F. Swallowing precautions: _____

G. Restrictions:

1. Driving: _____

2. Bicycling: _____

3. Heights: _____

    4. Lifting: _____

    5. Power equipment use: _____

    6. Standing/sitting: _____

    7. Chemical/hazardous materials: _____

    8. Working overhead: _____

    9. Sports participation: _____

  10. Other: _____

         _____

         _____

V. BEHAVIOR

A. Type:

Physical _____

_____

Cognitive _____

_____

B. Plan and expectations: _____

_____

_____

C. Crisis plan: _____

_____

_____

VI. CLIENT/FAMILY EDUCATION: (Provide information in the following areas.)

A. Seizures

B. Drug interactions

C. Long-term effects of TBI

    1. Second impact syndrome

    2. Depression

    3. Alcohol/drug

    4. Sleep hygiene

    5. Hydration

    6. Bowel/bladder

    D. Community support systems

    E. Treatment authorizations

       1. Advance directives

       2. Durable power of attorney for heath care

    F. Therapeutic home programs

    G. Guardianship/conservatorship, if needed

    H. Public assistance, if needed

    I. Behavior interaction/approach

VII. FINANCIAL PLANNING

    A. Family budget review

       1. Restructure debt

       2. Use retirement, life insurance for short-term needs

    B. Public assistance

       1. SSI

       2. SSDI

       3. Medicaid/Medicare

       4. State-specific benefits (e.g., victims of violent crimes, regional center, low-income housing, disabled phone and electric rates, Easter Seals, Crippled Children's Society (CCS), service organizations)

VIII. ADDITIONAL RECOMMENDATIONS

_____

_____

_____

Completed by: _____ Date: _____

Client signature/reviewed with: _____

Print name: _____ Date: _____

Index

NOTE: Page numbers followed by f indicate figures; t indicates tables.